Consultative Hemostasis and Thrombosis

Consultative Hemostasis and Thrombosis

Craig S. Kitchens, M.D.
Professor of Medicine
University of Florida
Chief, Medical Services
Malcom Randall Veterans Administration Medical Center
Gainesville, Florida

Barbara M. Alving, M.D.
Deputy Director
National Heart, Lung, and Blood Institute
National Institutes of Health
Bethesda, Maryland

Craig M. Kessler, M.D.
Professor of Medicine and Pathology
Georgetown University School of Medicine
Chief, Division of Hematology and Oncology
Washington, D.C.

W.B. SAUNDERS COMPANY
An Imprint of Elsevier Science
Philadelphia • London • New York • St. Louis • Sydney • Toronto

W.B. SAUNDERS COMPANY
An Imprint of Elsevier Science

The Curtis Center
Independence Square West
Philadelphia, Pennsylvania 19106

CONSULTATIVE HEMOSTASIS AND THROMBOSIS   ISBN 0-7216-8264-2

Copyright © 2002, Elsevier Science (USA). All rights reserved

No part of this publication may be reproduced or transmitted in any form or by any means, electronic or mechanical, including photocopy, recording, or any information storage and retrieval system, without permission in writing from the publisher.

Printed in the United States of America

Last digit is the print number: 9 8 7 6 5 4 3 2 1

Dedication

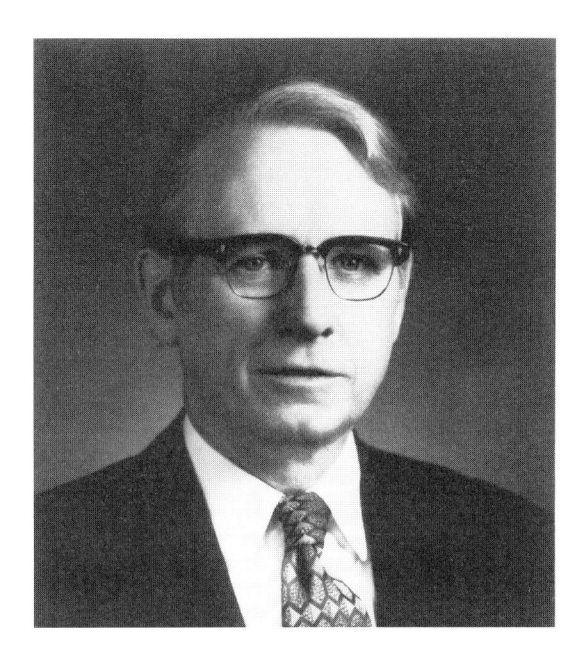

With pride and humility, the editors dedicate this text to our mentor, C. Lockard Conley, M.D. We three editors were fellows together in his Division of Hematology at Johns Hopkins in the early 1970s.

Dr. Conley, a native of Baltimore, received his medical degree from Columbia University College of Physicians and Surgeons in 1940. After an internship and residency at Presbyterian Hospital in New York, he joined the Army Air Corps, where he studied aviation physiology, concentrating on the effects of high altitude hypoxia. In 1946, he joined the Department of Medicine at Johns Hopkins University, serving as the chief of the Division of Hematology until his retirement in 1986. During those four decades his division helped shape the future of hematology, in part by training hematology fellows who, through their research, academic, and clinical positions, have impacted at national and international levels.

During his four decades of leadership, modern hematology took root, developed, and expanded. The Hematology Division at Johns Hopkins University was at the forefront of many activities. Dr. Conley, working with colleagues and fellows, made early and important observations on disseminated intravascular coagulation (particularly as a consequence of hemolytic transfusion reactions), provided the initial descriptions of the contact coagulation system which led to the discovery of factor XII, recognized what we now call the lupus anticoagulant, and investigated the role of platelets in the early acceleration phase of coagulation. In addition, Dr. Conley and colleagues made seminal observations regarding thalassemia and other hemoglobinopathies, providing the original description of homozygous hemoglobin C disease and recognizing the implications of hereditary persistence of hemoglobin F. These latter observations arguably were instrumental in the research path taken by Dr. (Sir David) Weatherall, another "Conley fellow" and author of the Foreword of this text.

Dr. Conley is known as a master clinician, research hematologist, and mentor. His greatest satisfaction, however, was not in his personal accomplishments, which he modestly downplayed, but rather in the success of his fellows. It was almost impossible to convince Dr. Conley to include his name on a manuscript. In fact, none of the editors has actually coauthored a paper with Dr. Conley, although we all tried on multiple occasions. He led young investigators and clinicians in the most natural of ways without intimidation or domination, inspiring them to do their best largely because of the excitement and joy of new discoveries. A physician of the highest integrity and intellectual rigor, he insisted on equally high standards for his fellows. All fellows were required to present clinical or laboratory observations in a clear, well-reasoned fashion and to understand what was known about the area of research or clinical interest and what was yet to be known. He was the patient's chief advocate and also a master detective and investigator of disease processes; he consistently sought to reconcile clinical findings with current knowledge of pathophysiology. These aspects of Dr. Conley's character resulted in the unraveling of numerous hematologic mysteries.

Dr. Conley's intelligence, inquisitiveness, and kindness, as well as self-effacement and humility complement his natural leadership skills; these attributes have been recognized and deeply appreciated by his colleagues and by his patients. He has received a Mastership as well as a Distinguished Teacher Award from the American College of Physicians, and he ascended through the leadership ranks of the American Society of Hematology, serving as its president 1975–76. His advice and consultation have been sought by innumerable institutions, foundations, and other groups.

The editors are gratefully indebted to Dr. Conley, not only for having trained us to be hematologists, but also to respect the investigative aspects as well as the art and practice of medicine.

Craig S. Kitchens, M.D.
Barbara M. Alving, M.D.
Craig M. Kessler, M.D.

Contributors

Amal M. Abu-Ghosh, M.B.B.S.
Research Assistant
Department of Pediatrics
Division of Hematology/Oncology
Georgetown University Medical Center
Washington, D.C.
  General Aspects of Thrombocytopenia, Platelet Transfusions, and Thrombopoietic Growth Factors

Victoria Afshani, M.D.
Clinical Associate
University of Pennsylvania Health System
Philadelphia, Pennsylvania
  Management of Bleeding Disorders in Pregnancy

Barbara M. Alving, M.D.
Deputy Director
National Heart, Lung, and Blood Institute
National Institutes of Health
Bethesda, Maryland
  The Antiphospholipid Syndrome: Clinical Presentation, Diagnosis, and Patient Management

Anne Angiolillo, M.D.
Assistant Professor of Pediatrics
George Washington University School of Medicine and Health Sciences
Attending Physician
Department of Hematology/Oncology
Children's National Medical Center
Washington, D.C.
  General Aspects of Thrombocytopenia, Platelet Transfusions, and Thrombopoietic Growth Factors

Jack E. Ansell, M.D.
Professor of Medicine
Boston University School of Medicine
Vice Chairman for Clinical Affairs
Department of Medicine
Boston University Medical Center
Boston, Massachusetts
  Outpatient Anticoagulant Therapy

Kenneth A. Bauer, M.D.
Associate Professor of Medicine
Harvard Medical School
Chief, Hematology Section
VA Boston Healthcare System
Director, Thrombosis Clinical Research
Beth Israel Deaconess Medical Center
Boston, Massachusetts
  Thrombophilia

Richard C. Becker, M.D.
Professor of Medicine
University of Massachusetts Medical School
Director, Cardiovascular Thrombosis Research Center
Director, Anticoagulation Services
University of Massachusetts Memorial Medical Center
Worcester, Massachusetts
  Hemostatic Aspects of Cardiovascular Medicine

Scott D. Berkowitz, M.D.
Adjunct Associate Professor of Medicine
Duke University Medical Center
Durham, North Carolina
Medical Director, Clinical Research Thrombosis and Hemostasis Team
AstraZeneca Pharmaceuticals
Wayne, Pennsylvania
  Hemostatic Aspects of Cardiovascular Medicine
  Antithrombotic and Thrombolytic Agents

Rhonda L. Bohn, M.P.H., Sc.D.
Instructor in Medicine
Brigham and Women's Hospital
Harvard Medical School
Boston, Massachusetts
  Nonhemophilic Inhibitors of Coagulation

Charles D. Bolan, LTC, USA, MC
Associate Professor of Clinical Medicine
Uniformed Services University of the Health Sciences (USUHS)
Visiting Scientist
Department of Transfusion Medicine
Warren G. Magnuson Clinical Center
National Institutes of Health
Bethesda, Maryland
Transfusion Medicine and Pharmacologic Aspects of Hemostasis

Mitchell S. Cairo, M.D.
Professor of Pediatrics
Columbia University
Director, Pediatric Cancer Research
Director, Pediatric Blood and Marrow Transplantation
Children's Hospital of New York
Columbia University
New York, New York
General Aspects of Thrombocytopenia, Platelet Transfusions, and Thrombopoietic Growth Factors

Alice J. Cohen, M.D.
Assistant Clinical Professor of Medicine
Columbia University
College of Physicians and Surgeons
New York, New York
Director, Hematology and Oncology
Newark Beth Israel Medical Center
Newark, New Jersey
Hemophilia A and B

Mary Cushman, M.D., M.Sc.
Associate Professor of Medicine and Pathology
University of Vermont
Attending Physician
Fletcher Allen Health Care
Burlington, Vermont
Novel Risk Factors for Arterial Thrombosis

Katan C. Davae, M.D.
Department of Cardiovascular and Interventional Radiology
Harvard University
Brigham and Women's Hospital
Boston, Massachusetts
Inferior Vena Caval Interventions in Thromboembolic Disease—The Viewpoint of Vascular Radiology

Virginia Davenport, R.N.
Clinical Research Nurse
Columbia University
New York, New York
General Aspects of Thrombocytopenia, Platelet Transfusions, and Thrombopoietic Growth Factors

Thomas G. DeLoughery, M.D.
Associate Professor
Oregon Health and Sciences University
Portland, Oregon
Hemorrhagic and Thrombotic Disorders in the Intensive Care Setting

Professor Amiram Eldor*
Tel-Aviv University Ramat-Aviv, Israel School of Medicine
Director, Institute of Hematology
Tel-Aviv Sourasky Medical Center
Ichilov Hospital
Tel Aviv, Israel
Management of Thrombophilia and Antiphospholipid Syndrome During Pregnancy

Miguel A. Escobar, M.D.
Instructor in Medicine
University of North Carolina at Chapel Hill
Division of Hematology and Oncology and the Center for Thrombosis and Hemostasis
Chapel Hill, North Carolina
Less Common Congenital Disorders of Hemostasis

Bruce L. Evatt, M.D.
Clinical Professor of Medicine
Emory University School of Medicine
Chief, Hematologic Diseases Branch
Centers for Disease Control
Atlanta, Georgia
Hemostatic Aspects of Patients with Human Immunodeficiency Virus/Acquired Immunodeficiency Syndrome

Bruce M. Ewenstein, M.D., Ph.D.
Assistant Professor of Medicine
Harvard Medical School
Director, Boston Hemophilia Center
Brigham and Women's Hospital and Children's Hospital
Boston, Massachusetts
Nonhemophilic Inhibitors of Coagulation

Charles W. Francis, M.D.
Professor of Medicine and of Pathology and Laboratory Medicine
University of Rochester School of Medicine and Dentistry
Rochester, New York
Antithrombotic and Thrombolytic Agents

James N. George, M.D.
Professor of Medicine
University of Oklahoma Health Sciences Center
Oklahoma City, Oklahoma
Immune Thrombocytopenic Purpura

*Deceased

David L. Gillespie, M.D.
Chief, Division of Vascular Surgery
Uniformed Services University
Bethesda, Maryland
Assistant Chief, Vascular Surgery
Walter Reed Army Medical Center
Washington, D.C.
Prevention, Diagnosis, and Treatment of the Postphlebitic Syndrome

David Green, M.D., Ph.D.
Professor of Medicine
Northwestern University Medical School
Attending Physician
Northwestern Memorial Hospital
Chicago, Illinois
Prevention and Treatment of Venous Thromboembolism in Neurologic and Neurosurgical Patients

William D. Haire, M.D.
Professor
Department of Internal Medicine
Section of Oncology and Hematology
University of Nebraska Medical Center
Omaha, Nebraska
Deep Venous Thrombosis and Pulmonary Embolus

John A. Heit, M.D.
Associate Professor of Medicine
Mayo Medical School
Consultant, Division of Cardiovascular Diseases
Mayo Clinic
Rochester, Minnesota
Neuraxial Anesthesia and the Anticoagulated Patient: Balancing the Risks and Benefits

W. Craig Hooper, Ph.D.
Section Chief
Molecular and Hemostasis Laboratory
Hematologic Diseases Branch
Centers for Disease Control and Prevention
Atlanta, Georgia
Hemostatic Aspects of Patients with Human Immunodeficiency Virus/Acquired Immunodeficiency Syndrome

Terese T. Horlocker, M.D.
Professor of Anesthesiology
Mayo Clinic
Chair, Section of Orthopedic Anesthesia
Rochester, Minnesota
Neuraxial Anesthesia and the Anticoagulated Patient: Balancing the Risks and Benefits

McDonald K. Horne III, M.D.
Senior Clinical Investigator
Department of Laboratory Medicine
Warren G. Magnuson Clinical Center
National Institutes of Health
Bethesda, Maryland
Hemostatic Testing and Laboratory Interpretation

Mark R. Jackson, M.D.
Associate Professor of Surgery
University of Texas Southwestern Medical Center
Dallas, Texas
Topical Hemostatic Agents for Localized Bleeding

Craig M. Kessler, M.D.
Professor of Medicine and Pathology
Georgetown University School of Medicine
Chief, Division of Hematology and Oncology
Washington, D.C.
A Systematic Approach to the Bleeding Patient
Hemophilia A and B
Thrombocytosis

Craig S. Kitchens, M.D.
Professor of Medicine
University of Florida
Chief, Medical Services
Malcom Randall Veterans Administration Medical Center
Gainesville, Florida
The Consultative Process
Purpura and Related Hematovascular Lesions
Disseminated Intravascular Coagulation
Venous Thromboses at Unusual Sites
Surgery and Hemostasis

Harvey G. Klein, M.D.
Professor, Medicine and Pathology
Johns Hopkins School of Medicine
Chief, Department of Transfusion Medicine
Warren G. Magnuson Clinical Center
National Institutes of Health
Bethesda, Maryland
Transfusion Medicine and Pharmacologic Aspects of Hemostasis

Kiarash Kojouri, M.D.
Internal Medicine Resident
University of Oklahoma Health Sciences Center
Oklahoma City, Oklahoma
Immune Thrombocytopenic Purpura

Barbara A. Konkle, M.D.
Associate Professor of Medicine and Pathology and Laboratory Medicine
University of Pennsylvania
Director, Penn Comprehensive Hemophilia and Thrombosis Program
Philadelphia, Pennsylvania
Thrombotic Risk of Oral Contraceptives, Postmenopausal Hormone Replacement, and Selective Estrogen Receptor Modulators

Mark N. Levine, M.D., M.Sc.
Professor of Clinical Epidemiology and Biostatistics
Professor of Medicine
Buffett Taylor Chair of Breast Cancer Research
McMaster University
Medical Oncologist
Cancer Care Ontario Hamilton Regional Cancer Center
Hamilton, Ontario, Canada
Hemostatic and Thrombotic Disorders of Malignancy

Minetta C. Liu, M.D.
Assistant Professor of Medicine
Department of Medicine
Division of Hematology/Oncology
Department of Oncology
Georgetown University Hospital
Washington, D.C.
A Systematic Approach to the Bleeding Patient

B. Gail Macik, M.D.
Associate Professor of Medicine and Pathology
University of Virginia Health System
Division of Hematology/Oncology
Charlottesville, Virginia
Near-Site Testing in Hemostatic Disorders

Michael F. Meyerovitz, M.D.
Associate Professor of Radiology
Harvard Medical School
Cardiovascular and Interventional Radiology
Brigham and Women's Hospital
Boston, Massachusetts
St. Vincent Hospital
Worcester, Massachusetts
Inferior Vena Caval Interventions in Thromboembolic Disease—The Viewpoint of Vascular Radiology

Prabhas Mittal, M.D.
Clinical Fellow
Department of Blood and Marrow Transplantation
University of Texas M.D. Anderson Cancer Center
Houston, Texas
Thrombocytosis

Joel L. Moake, M.D.
Professor of Medicine
Baylor College of Medicine
Associate Director, Biomedical Engineering Laboratory
Rice University
Houston, Texas
Thrombotic Thrombocytopenic Purpura

Sean D. O'Donnell, M.D.
Assistant Professor of Surgery
Uniformed Services University of the Health Sciences
F. Edward Herbert School of Medicine
Bethesda, Maryland
Chief and Program Director
Vascular Surgery
Walter Reed Army Medical Center
Washington, D.C.
Prevention, Diagnosis, and Treatment of the Postphlebitic Syndrome

Kathleen G. Putnam, S.M.
Research Assistant
Divisions of Pharmacoepidemiology and Pharmacoeconomics
Brigham and Women's Hospital
Boston, Massachusetts
Nonhemophilic Inhbitors of Coagulation

Margaret V. Ragni, M.D., M.P.H.
Professor of Medicine
Division of Hematology/Oncology
Director, Hemophilia Center of Western Pennsylvania
University of Pittsburgh Medical Center School of Medicine
Pittsburgh, Pennsylvania
Liver Disease, Organ Transplantation, and Hemostasis

A. Koneti Rao, M.D.
Professor of Medicine, Thrombosis Research and Pathology
Associate Dean for MD-PhD program
Temple University School of Medicine
Philadelphia, Pennsylvania
Disorders of Platelet Function

Margaret E. Rick, M.D.
Professor of Medicine
Uniformed Services University of the Health Sciences
Assistant Chief, Hematology Service
Warren G. Magnuson Clinical Center
National Institutes of Health
Bethesda, Maryland
von Willebrand Disease

Frederick R. Rickles, M.D.
Professor of Medicine and Pediatrics
George Washington University School of Medicine and Health Sciences
Associate Vice President for Health Research, Compliance and Technology Transfer
George Washington University
Attending Physician
George Washington University Hospital and the Children's National Medical Center
Washington, D.C.
Hemostatic and Thrombotic Disorders of Malignancy

Paul M. Ridker, M.D., M.P.H.
Associate Professor of Medicine
Harvard Medical School

Director, Center for Cardiovascular Disease
  Prevention
Brigham and Women's Hospital
Boston, Massachusetts
  Novel Risk Factors for Arterial Thrombosis

Harold R. Roberts, M.D.
Professor of Medicine
University of North Carolina at Chapel Hill
Attending Physician
University of North Carolina Hospitals
Chapel Hill, North Carolina
  Less Common Congenital Disorders of Hemostasis

Patricio Rosa, M.D.
Assistant Professor of Surgery
Uniformed Services University of Health Science
Bethesda, Maryland
Chief, Vascular Surgery Service
Tripler Army Medical Center
Staff Surgeon
Kaiser-Permanent Mdana Lua Medical Center
Honolulu, Hawaii
  *Prevention, Diagnosis, and Treatment of the
    Postphlebitic Syndrome*

Stephanie Seremetis, M.D.
Medical Director
Biopharmaceutical Division
Novo Nordisk BioPharmaceuticals
Princeton, New Jersey
  Management of Bleeding Disorders in Pregnancy

Steven Stein, M.D.
Assistant Professor of Medicine
University of Pennsylvania
Assistant Professor
Hospital of University of Pennsylvania
Philadelphia, Pennsylvania
  *Thrombotic Risk of Oral Contraceptives,
    Postmenopausal Hormone Replacement, and Selective
    Estrogen Receptor Modulators*

Michael Streiff, M.D.
Assistant Professor of Medicine
Johns Hopkins Medical Institutions
Baltimore, Maryland
  *Inferior Vena Caval Filters: A Hematologist's
    Perspective*

Theodore E. Warkentin, M.D.
Professor, Department of Pathology and Molecular
  Medicine
Department of Medicine
McMaster University
Associate Head
Transfusion Medicine, and Hematologist, Service of
  Clinical Hematology
Hamilton Regional Laboratory Medicine Program
Hamilton, Ontario, Canada
  Heparin-Induced Thrombocytopenia

Jeffrey Zwicker, M.D.
Clinical Fellow in Medicine
Harvard Medical School
Boston, Massachusetts
  Thrombophilia

NOTICE

Medicine is an ever-changing field. Standard safety precautions must be followed, but as new research and clinical experience broaden our knowledge, changes in treatment and drug therapy may become necessary or appropriate. Readers are advised to check the most current product information provided by the manufacturer of each drug to be administered to verify the recommended dose, the method and duration of administration, and contraindications. It is the responsibility of the treating physician, relying on experience and knowledge of the patient, to determine dosages and the best treatment for each individual patient. Neither the Publisher nor the editor assume any liability for any injury and/or damage to persons or property arising from this publication.

The Publisher

Preface

The editors are pleased to present *Consultative Hemostasis and Thrombosis* as a new, midsized textbook that is user friendly and acutely focused on information for the busy consultant requiring in-depth information. All of the 50 physicians whom we invited to contribute to this project responded enthusiastically, providing further support for the role of this book in filling a unique and useful niche. The orientation of this book is toward evaluation and management of patients with hemostatic or thrombotic disorders. The reader is referred to other sources for greater in-depth information pertaining to the basic sciences providing the foundation of clinical practice. The first three sections (General Information, Hemorrhagic Processes, and Thrombotic Processes) discuss the basic hemostatic and thrombotic disorders. The following three sections (Pharmacologic Agents, Women's Issues, and Special Considerations) focus on the rapidly evolving interdisciplinary aspects of hemostasis and thrombosis, which involve hematologists, cardiologists, invasive radiologists, transfusion medicine specialists, obstetricians, intensivists, hepatologists, and anesthesiologists. The ever-widening array of drugs and therapeutics is thoroughly reviewed. It is our hope and belief that the reader will find the text up-to-date, authoritative, useful, and readable.

The editors were saddened to learn that Professor Amiram Eldor of Tel-Aviv, Israel, the author of Chapter 29, Management of Thrombophilia and Antiphospholipid Syndrome During Pregnancy, was killed in an airline crash on November 24, 2001 while returning from a scientific meeting in Europe. Dr. Eldor was an outstanding physician and scholar; his chapter will serve as a strong testament to his empathy, knowledge and dedication to the pregnant patient suffering from thrombotic disorders.

Craig S. Kitchens, M.D.
Barbara M. Alving, M.D.
Craig M. Kessler, M.D.

Foreword

One of the paradoxes of a career in academic medicine is that the older you get the more often you are asked to comment on subjects that are completely outside your field of competence. On this occasion, however, despite knowing next to nothing about the subject, I have at least some excuse for responding to the kind request of the editors of this new work to write a short foreword, partly because the problems of thrombosis and hemostasis touch on almost every branch of medical practice, but mainly because this book is dedicated to Dr. C. Lockard Conley, a one-time mentor and long-time friend.

I had the great pleasure of working with Lock Conley at Johns Hopkins Hospital as a Fellow in Hematology for several years in the early 1960s. Of all the remarkable physicians with whom I have had the privilege of associating over the years I can think of no one who had more influence on the way I came to think about patient care and medical research. First and foremost he was (and still is) a superb clinician who, although he had wide knowledge and expertise right across the field of hematology, was also a very able general internist. His analysis of patients, and the breadth of his approach to their problems, was an ideal model for those who worked in his department, whether they were medical students, house staff, or trainees in hematology. On rounds he had a remarkable facility to get to the core of a clinical problem, backed by an encyclopedic knowledge of the medical literature. I am often reminded of sessions with Lock when I listen to those who have recently rediscovered evidence-based medicine. Quoting everything of any value that had been written on a particular topic, he would pounce in a flash on any loose or misinformed thinking. He combined this ability with an Oslerian faculty for learning by clinical experience, of which he had a wealth; marrow reporting sessions with him using a double-headed microscope were some of the most stimulating teaching experiences that I have ever had.

Lock Conley was not prescriptive about much of the research that went on in his department. Rather, he produced a good working environment and often allowed his young trainees to follow their own inclinations. He was always willing to discuss and criticise what we were doing and was a great value when we were writing up results for publication. He would never allow any ambiguity or loose prose and insisted on numerous drafts, all of which he vetted. But unless he had been heavily involved in the design or execution of the work he would never allow his name to appear on a paper. He was, first and foremost, a clinical research worker who took problems from the ward or clinic and, in doing so, made major contributions in the fields of coagulation and the abnormal hemoglobins. Although he did not personally become involved in the later cellular or molecular aspects of hematology he generously encouraged me to use his department as a base for collaborative studies with the Biophysics Department at Hopkins, which allowed me to move into this field just as it was developing, a typical example of his farsighted approach to everything he did.

Lock Conley had an enormous influence on all the young people who spent time in his department. He taught and expected the very highest standards of clinical practice, and nurtured a highly critical approach to evaluation of the medical literature and to personal research. But above all, his total integrity set standards against which his young colleagues could measure themselves throughout their careers. At first meeting he was rather formidable, but as one got to know him it became clear that he was a man of tremendous warmth and humanity who was extremely loyal to all those that had worked for him, many of whom, like myself, became close friends, both with him and his delightful wife Edith.

It seems particularly fitting therefore that the three former students of Lock who have edited this excellent book have dedicated it to him. The fields of thrombosis and hemostasis, which he did so much to develop, have undergone a remarkable transition over recent years, particularly following the applications of molecular and cell biology to the study of diseases which result from defects in the extremely complex biological system that maintains the fine balance between hemostasis and pathological thrombosis. Although this book covers some of the "new science" of this field, its main focus is on its clinical applications. Hence it will be of broad interest, not only to hematologists but to physicians in every field of medicine. It is a particularly apt recognition of a hematologist who was, above all, a first class generalist who practised holistic medicine in the best sense of the term. I wish this excellent book every success.

Sir David Weatherall, FRS
Regius Professor of Medicine
Oxford, England

Contents

Color Plates follow page 154

PART I
GENERAL INFORMATION 1

Chapter 1
The Consultative Process 3
Craig S. Kitchens, M.D.

Introduction 3
Extent of the Consultation 4
Reason for Consultation 5
Consultant's Point of View 7
Duties of the Referring Physician and the Consultant 8
Timing 8
How to Do the Consultation 9
Recommendations 9
Concerns 10
Outcomes 10
When Should a Consultant Request Consultation? 13

Chapter 2
Hemostatic Testing and
Laboratory Interpretation 15
McDonald K. Horne III, M.D.

Physiologic Hemostasis 15
Laboratory Evaluation of the Procoagulant System 16
Assays of the Natural Anticoagulant Proteins 20
Laboratory Evaluation of Platelet Function 20
Assays of the Fibrinolytic System 24

Chapter 3
A Systematic Approach to the
Bleeding Patient 27
Minetta C. Liu, M.D. and Craig M. Kessler, M.D.

The Clinical Evaluation 27
The Basic Laboratory Evaluation 31
Management of Acute Hemorrhagic Episodes 37

PART II
HEMORRHAGIC PROCESSES 41

Chapter 4
Hemophilia A and B 43
Alice J. Cohen, M.D. and Craig M. Kessler, M.D.

Introduction/Epidemiology/Genetics 43
Prenatal Diagnosis/Carrier Testing 44
Postnatal Diagnosis 44
Clinical Features of the Hemophilias 45
Laboratory Characteristics 47
Therapeutic Modalities for the Hemophilias 48
DDAVP 51
Ancillary Treatments 51
Prophylaxis/Indwelling Venous Access Device 51
Treatment Complications 52
Infectious Complications of Replacement Therapy in Hemophilia: HIV, Hepatitis, and Parvovirus B19 53
Gene Therapy 54

Chapter 5
Less Common Congenital Disorders
of Hemostasis 57
Harold R. Roberts, M.D. and Miguel A. Escobar, M.D.

Disorders of Fibrinogen 57
Prothrombin Deficiency (Hypoprothrombinemia and Dysprothrombinemia) 61
Factor V Deficiency 63
Factor VII Deficiency 64
Factor X Deficiency 65
Factor XI Deficiency 66
Deficiency of the Contact Factors 67
Familial Combined Factor Deficiencies 69
α_2-Plasmin Inhibitor Deficiency 70
α_1-Antitrypsin Pittsburgh 70
Protein Z Deficiency 70
Consultation Considerations 70
Medico-Legal Issues 71
Cost-Containment Issues 71

xvii

Chapter 6
Nonhemophilic Inhibitors of Coagulation 75
Bruce M. Ewenstein, M.D., Ph.D., Kathleen G. Putnam, S.M., and Rhonda L. Bohn, M.P.H., Sc.D.

Laboratory Diagnosis 75
Acquired Inhibitors of Factor VIII 77
Inhibitors of the Vitamin K-Dependent Proteins 83
Inhibitors of Factor XI 84
Inhibitors of Factor V 84
Inhibitors of Fibrinogen and Factor XIII 85
Inhibitors of von Willebrand Factor 85

Chapter 7
von Willebrand Disease 91
Margaret E. Rick, M.D.

Historical Overview 91
Physiology and Structure-Function Relationships 91
Clinical Presentation 93
Diagnosis 94
Classification 95
Acquired von Willebrand Disease 97
Treatment 97

Chapter 8
General Aspects of Thrombocytopenia, Platelet Transfusions, and Thrombopoietic Growth Factors 103
Anne Angiolillo, M.D., Amal M. Abu-Ghosh, M.D., Virginia Davenport, R.N., and Mitchell S. Cairo, M.D.

Historical Perspective 103
Physiologic Thrombopoiesis 103
Pathophysiology and Classification 104
Thrombocytopenia and Platelet Transfusion Therapy 105
Platelet Collections and Transfusions 107
Risks of Platelet Transfusion Therapy 107
Thrombopoietic Growth Factors 109

Chapter 9
Immune Thrombocytopenic Purpura 117
James N. George, M.D. and Kiarash Kojouri, M.D.

Historical Aspects of Understanding the Pathogenesis of ITP 117
Evaluation of a Patient Presenting with Isolated Thrombocytopenia 119
Differential Diagnosis of ITP 121
Management 123
Management of ITP in Pregnant Women and Their Newborn Infants 127

Chapter 10
Disorders of Platelet Function 133
A. Koneti Rao, M.D.

Overview of Physiology 133
Disorders of Platelet Function 133
Consultation Considerations 145

Chapter 11
Purpura and Related Hematovascular Lesions 149
Craig S. Kitchens, M.D.

Historical Perspective 149
Microvascular Structure-Function Interrelations 150
Pathophysiologic Categories of Purpura 152
Consultation Considerations 161
Laboratory Evaluation 162
Cost Containment 162
Treatment Issues 162
Medical-Legal Considerations 162

Chapter 12
Disseminated Intravascular Coagulation 165
Craig S. Kitchens, M.D.

Historical Overview 165
Physiology and Pathophysiology 166
Causes of DIC 167
Initiation of DIC 167
Comments About Two Representative Causes of DIC 169
Differential Diagnosis of DIC 171
Consequences of DIC 173
Treatment of DIC 174
Consultation Considerations 176
Cost-Containment Issues 176
Medical-Legal Considerations 176

PART III
THROMBOTIC PROCESSES 179

Chapter 13
Thrombophilia 181
Jeffrey Zwicker, M.D. and Kenneth A. Bauer, M.D.

Background, Prevalence, and Diagnosis 181
Clinical Implications of Inherited Thrombophilia 187
Approach to Thrombosis 189
Treatment of Thrombotic Events 192

Chapter 14
Deep Venous Thrombosis and Pulmonary Embolus 197
William D. Haire, M.D.

Introduction: The Concept of Venous Thromboembolism (VTE) 197
Etiology and Pathogenesis 197
Prevention 199
Diagnosis 204
Treatment 210
Conclusion 218

Chapter 15
Venous Thromboses at Unusual Sites 225
Craig S. Kitchens, M.D.

Historical Aspects 225
Importance to the Patient and Clinician 226

Mesenteric Vein Thrombosis 226
Splenic Vein Thrombosis 228
Portal Vein Thrombosis 229
Renal Vein Thrombosis 229
Cerebral Venous Thrombosis 231
Hepatic Venous Thrombosis 232
Retinal Vein Thrombosis 234
Axillary and Subclavian Vein Thrombosis 235
Cutaneous Microvascular Thrombosis
   (Purpura Fulminans) 236
Other Sites of Thrombosis 236
Consultation Considerations 238
Laboratory Evaluation 238
Cost Containment 238

Chapter 16
Prevention, Diagnosis, and Treatment of the Postphlebitic Syndrome 243
Patricio Rosa, M.D., David L. Gillespie, M.D., and Sean D. O'Donnell, M.D.

Introduction/Epidemiology 243
Pathophysiology 244
Symptoms 246
Differential Diagnosis 246
Risk Factors 247
Diagnosis 247
Prevention 249
Treatment 250
Consultation Considerations 252
Conclusion 252

Chapter 17
Thrombocytosis 255
Prabhas Mittal, M.D. and Craig M. Kessler, M.D.

Introduction and Epidemiology 255
Pathogenesis of Essential Thrombocythemia 255
Clinical Features and Thrombohemorrhagic
   Complications 257
Prognostic Indicators for Thromboses and Hemorrhage 257
Diagnosis of Essential Thrombocytosis 258
Laboratory Findings of Essential Thrombocythemia 259
Differential Diagnosis 259
Treatment of Essential Thrombocythemia 259

Chapter 18
The Antiphospholipid Syndrome: Clinical Presentation, Diagnosis, and Patient Management 269
Barbara M. Alving, M.D.

Introduction and Historical Comments 269
Antiphospholipid Syndrome: Overview of Clinical
   Manifestations 269
Neurologic Manifestations of the Antiphospholipid
   Syndrome 270
Fetal Loss and the Antiphospholipid Syndrome 271
Thrombocytopenia and the Antiphospholipid Syndrome 271
APA and Cardiac Valve Dysfunction 271
Association of LA with Prothrombin Deficiency 272
LA As a Laboratory Abnormality 272

Immunology and Pathophysiology of APA 273
ELISA for APA (Cardiolipin Assay) 273
Testing for LA 273
Treatment of Patients Who Have the Antiphospholipid
   Syndrome or Laboratory Manifestation of APA
   (LA or ACA) 274
Cost Containment and Medicolegal Aspects of Testing for LA
   and the Antiphospholipid Syndrome 275
Conclusion 276

Chapter 19
Hemostatic Aspects of Cardiovascular Medicine 279
Richard C. Becker, M.D. and Scott D. Berkowitz, M.D.

Historical Perspectives in Cardiovascular Medicine 279
Coronary Atherogenesis 281
Coronary Thrombogenesis 282
Vascular Thrombosis 282
Defining Steps in Arterial Thrombus Formation 283
Current Management of Acute Coronary Syndromes:
   Pharmacologic Therapies 284
Cardioembolism 299
Determining Thromboembolic Risk 301
Mural Thrombosis and Embolic Events 303
Atheromas of the Ascending Aorta 303
Cardiovascular Hemostasis 303

Chapter 20
Novel Risk Factors for Arterial Thrombosis 311
Mary Cushman, M.D., M.Sc. and Paul M. Ridker, M.D., M.P.H.

Subclinical Artherosclerosis 313
Lipid Metabolism Measures 313
Fibrinogen 314
C-Reactive Protein (hs-CRP) and Other Markers of
   Inflammation 315
Impaired Fibrinolysis 317
Hemostatic Activation Markers 317
Total Plasma Homocysteine 317
The Hematologist's Perspective 319
Future Directions in Coronary Risk Prediction 319

Chapter 21
Hemostatic and Thrombotic Disorders of Malignancy 325
Frederick R. Rickles, M.D. and Mark N. Levine, M.D.

Historical Overview 325
Pathogenesis 326
Hemostatic Disorders 328
Thrombotic Disorders 329
Case Scenarios 336

Chapter 22
Thrombotic Thrombocytopenic Purpura 343
Joel L. Moake, M.D.

Historical Review 343
Clinical Manifestations of TTP 344

xx Contents

Laboratory Findings 344
Types of TTP 344
Pathophysiology 345
Causes of TTP 347
Differential Diagnosis of TTP 348
Distinction Between TTP and HUS 348
Treatment of TTP 349
Possible Future Approaches to Therapy 350
Cost Containment 351
Medical-Legal Issues 351
Consultative Considerations 352

Chapter 23
Heparin-Induced Thrombocytopenia 355
Theodore E. Warkentin, M.D.

Historical Overview 355
Terminology 355
Pathogenesis 356
Frequency 356
Clinical Features 357
Differential Diagnosis 362
Laboratory Testing 362
Treatment of HIT-Associated Thrombosis 365
Caveats in Management of HIT 368
Treatment of Isolated Heparin-Induced
 Thrombocytopenia 369
Re-exposure to Heparin of a Patient with Previous HIT 369
Specialized Clinical Situations 369

PART IV
PHARMACOLOGIC AGENTS..........373

Chapter 24
Antithrombotic and
Thrombolytic Agents 375
Charles W. Francis, M.D. and Scott D. Berkowitz, M.D.

Oral Anticoagulants 375
Heparin 378
Low-Molecular-Weight Heparin 380
Danaparoid Sodium 382
Hirudin 383
Argatroban 384
Bivalirudin 384
Fibrinolytic Therapy 385

Chapter 25
Transfusion Medicine and Pharmacologic
Aspects of Hemostasis 395
*Charles D. Bolan, LTC, USA, MC, and
Harvey G. Klein, M.D.*

Synopsis 395
Introduction and Historical Overview 395
Traditional Blood Products 396
Pharmaceutical Agents 400
Other Agents 411

Chapter 26
Topical Hemostatic Agents for
Localized Bleeding 419
Mark R. Jackson, M.D.

Intraoperative and Postoperative Bleeding 419
Available Topical Agents 419
Combinations of Thrombin and Fibrinogen 421

PART V
WOMEN'S ISSUES 425

Chapter 27
Thrombotic Risk of Oral Contraceptives,
Postmenopausal Hormone Replacement,
and Selective Estrogen Receptor
Modulators (SERMs) 427
Steven Stein, M.D. and Barbara A. Konkle, M.D.

Basic Science 427
Oral Contraceptive Use and Thrombosis 427
Hormone Replacement Therapy and Thrombosis 430
Selective Estrogen Receptor Modulators
 and Thrombosis 432

Chapter 28
Management of Bleeding Disorders
in Pregnancy 437
Stephanie Seremetis, M.D. and Victoria Afshani, M.D.

Inherited Disorders of Bleeding in Pregnancy 437
Thrombocytopenia 443
Immune Thrombocytopenic Purpura 443
Alloimmune Thrombocytopenia 445
The HELLP Syndrome 446

Chapter 29
Management of Thrombophilia and
Antiphospholipid Syndrome
During Pregnancy 449
Prof. Amiram Eldor

Venous Thromboembolism in Pregnancy 449
Hereditary Thrombophilias and Venous Thrombosis During
 Pregnancy 450
The Management of Thrombophilia During Pregnancy 451
The Antiphospholipid Syndrome 454
Postpartum Ovarian Vein Thrombosis 455
Arterial Thrombosis During Pregnancy 456
Thrombophilia and Obstetric Complications 456
Antithrombotic Agents for Preventing Obstetric
 Complications 457

PART VI
SPECIAL CONSIDERATIONS..........461

Chapter 30
Surgery and Hemostasis 463
Craig S. Kitchens, M.D.

Surgery for Patients with Congenital Hemostatic Defects 463
Effect of Surgery on Hemostasis 465
Preoperative Hemostatic Testing 468
Invasive Procedures in Patients with Abnormal Coagulation Tests 470
Invasive Procedures for Patients on Anticoagulant Therapy 473
Consultation on Patients with Intraoperative or Postoperative Hemorrhage 474

Chapter 31
Liver Disease, Organ Transplantation, and Hemostasis 481
Margaret V. Ragni, M.D., M.P.H.

Historical Overview 481
Pathophysiology of Coagulopathy Associated with Liver Disease 482
Clinical Diagnosis 484
Laboratory Diagnosis of Coagulopathy Associated with Liver Disease 485
Liver Transplantation 487
Treatment of Transplantation Coagulopathy 488
Treatment of Liver Disease Coagulopathy 488
Future Advances 489

Chapter 32
Hemorrhagic and Thrombotic Disorders in the Intensive Care Setting 493
Thomas G. DeLoughery, M.D.

Bleeding Problems 493
Initial Evaluation 493
Immediate Therapy: Transfusion Therapy 495
Coagulation Defects 497
Thrombocytopenia and Platelet Dysfunction 501
Venous Thromboembolism 505
Catheter Thrombosis 507

Chapter 33
Hemostatic Aspects of Patients with Human Immunodeficiency Virus/Acquired Immunodeficiency Syndrome 515
Bruce L. Evatt, M.D. and W. Craig Hooper, Ph.D.

HIV/AIDS-Associated Thrombocytopenia 515
Bleeding Complications in HIV-Infected Hemophilia Patients Treated with Protease Inhibitors 516
Thrombosis 517
HIV-Associated Thrombotic Microangiopathy: Thrombotic Thrombocytopenic Purpura and Hemolytic-Uremic Syndrome 518

Chapter 34
Outpatient Anticoagulant Therapy 523
Jack E. Ansell, M.D.

Mechanism of Action 523
Pharmacokinetics 523
Warfarin and Drug Interactions 524
Therapeutic Range and Monitoring of Oral Anticoagulants 524
Practical Aspects of Oral Anticoagulation Management 525
Managing the Risks of Oral Anticoagulant Therapy 528
Patient Self-Testing and Patient Self-Management 529

Chapter 35
Near-Site Testing in Hemostatic Disorders 535
B. Gail Macik, M.D.

Overview of Hemostatic Near-Site Testing 536
Overview of Platelet Function Analyzers 536
Overview of Clot-Detection Analyzers 539
Global Assessment of Clot Formation 545

Chapter 36
Prevention and Treatment of Venous Thromboembolism in Neurologic and Neurosurgical Patients 549
David Green, M.D., Ph.D.

Stroke 549
Spinal Cord Injury 550
Neurosurgery 553

Chapter 37
Inferior Vena Caval Interventions in Thromboembolic Disease—The Viewpoint of Vascular Radiology 557
Katan C. Davae, M.D. and Michael F. Meyerovitz, M.D.

History of IVC Interruption in Prevention of Pulmonary Embolism 558
Anatomy and Anomalies of the Inferior Vena Cava 558
Indications and Contraindications to IVC Filter Placement 559
Appropriate Filter Selection 560
IVC Filters Currently Approved for Use in the United States 561
Patient Preparation and IVC Filter Placement 563
Complications of IVC Filter Placement 564
Special Filter Circumstances 564
Future Outlook 565

Chapter 38
Inferior Vena Caval Filters: A Hematologist's Perspective 569
Michael Streiff, M.D.

The Safety and Efficacy of IVC Filters in VTE 569
A Randomized Trial of IVC Filters in the Prevention of Pulmonary Emboli 573

Anticoagulation After IVC Filter Placement: Is it
  Necessary? 573
Anticoagulation Versus IVC Filters for VTE 574
Suprarenal IVC Filters 574
Superior Vena Caval Filters 576
Expanded Indications: IVC Filters in Hip and Knee
  Arthroplasty 576
IVC Filters for Prevention of VTE in Trauma Patients 576
IVC Filters for VTE in Cancer Patients 580
Free-Floating Thrombus: An Indication for IVC Filter
  Placement? 582
IVC Filters for VTE in Other Patient Populations 583
Temporary/Retrievable IVC Filters 583
Indications for IVC Filter Placement 583
Conclusion 584

Chapter 39
Neuraxial Anesthesia and the Anticoagulated Patient: Balancing the Risks and Benefits 589

Terese T. Horlocker, M.D. and John A. Heit, M.D.

Historical Overview 589
Physiologic Responses to Surgery 590
Benefits of Neuraxial Anesthesia and Analgesia 590
Risk Factors for Spinal Hematoma 591
Consultation Considerations 594
Signs and Symptoms of Spinal Hematoma After Neuraxial
  Anesthesia 597

Index 599

PART I

GENERAL INFORMATION

CHAPTER 1

The Consultative Process

Craig S. Kitchens, M.D.

Life is short, and the art long, the occasion fleeting, experience fallacious, and judgement difficult.

Hippocrates[1]

As long as medicine is an art, its chief and characteristic instrument must be the human faculty. We come therefore to the very practical question of what aspects of human faculty it is necessary for the good doctor to cultivate. The first to be named must always be the power of attention, of giving one's whole mind to the patient without the interposition of oneself. It sounds simple but only the very greatest doctors ever fully attain it. It is an active process and not either mere resigned listening or even politely waiting until you can interrupt. Disease often tells its secret in the casual parentheses.

Wilfred Trotter[2]

INTRODUCTION

As a specialist, the hematologist is frequently asked to consult on a patient in order to clarify or solidify the diagnosis, prognosis, or treatment plan of another physician. Consultation is done in either the inpatient or the outpatient setting and can in turn be requested on a stat, urgent, subacute, or leisurely basis. By inference, the referring physician remains the physician in control of the patient's care but the consultant's expertise, experience, judgment, wisdom, and even approval are sought in order to assist the referring physician's concept of the case in its entirety. In this era of cost-containment and managed care, expert evaluation is cost-effective because it may curtail the diagnostic process, limit unnecessary or even ill-directed testing, and shorten overall hospital time as well as minimize patient suffering. A well-directed consultation is the best bargain for all stakeholders.

The diagnostic procedure is a fascinating exercise. It involves the most acute use of our senses and the accurate recording of our observations. It requires a logical synthesis of the central nervous system of the responsible doctor, of information from the patient and his family, from other doctors who have cared for the patient in the past, from colleagues in various specialties who are helping with the immediate problem, and from the laboratory. Prognosis and correct therapy depend upon the correct use of the diagnostic process.

Eugene A. Stead, Jr.[3]

---

[1] Hippocrates (460–370 BC). Hippocrates is considered to be the founder of European medicine. He lived in Greece during the Classic Period and was a contemporary of Socrates, Plato, Herodotus, and others. He is credited with three advances in medicine, namely, the separation of medicine as an art and science from magic, the development of the written detailed study of disease, and the promulgation of the highest of moral standards that characterize the profession. Descriptive bedside medicine was his forte. His writings showed him to be humble, containing frequent admissions of errors in his thinking in order that others might not stumble in the same manner. This timeless aphorism contains all the essential elements of clinical practice in a concise statement.

[2] Wilfred Batten Trotter (1872–1939). Wilfred Trotter was an English sociologist and neurosurgeon who was very interested in the sociologic aspects of medicine. He is credited with originating the term *herd instinct*. He was also a surgeon to King George V. This quote is taken from the chapter entitled "The Art of Being a Physician" by Lloyd H. Smith, Jr., in the 19th edition of the *Cecil Textbook of Medicine* (W. B. Saunders, Philadelphia, 1992).

[3] Eugene A. Stead, Jr. (1908–). Dr. Stead is a primary pillar of American internal medicine. He was born and educated in Atlanta and then went to Boston, where he was strongly influenced by Soma Weiss. He was a pioneer in clinical investigation of the human circulatory system. At 34 years old he returned to Emory as the Chairman of Medicine in 1943 but then was recruited to the new Duke Medical School in Durham, North Carolina, in 1947, where he was Chairman for 20 years, founding and elevating that department of medicine to one of the greatest in the nation. He has trained innumerable professors and chairs of medicine. Dr. Stead is a master of clinical thought, piercing observations, and a keen wit bettered by none. The two quotes are from E.A. Stead, Jr., *What this Patient Needs is a Doctor*, edited by Wagner, Cebe, and Rozer (Carolina Academic Press, Durham, North Carolina, 1978).

Table 1-1 • THE CONSULTATIVE PROCESS

Extent of the consultation
   Confirmatory consultation
   Brief consultation
   Comprehensive consultation
   Urgent consultation on a catastrophically ill patient
   "Undiagnosing" consultation
   The curbside consultation

Reason for consultation
   Helping another physician
   Second opinion requested by the primary physician
   Second opinion requested by the patient
   Second opinion requested by a third-party payor
   Other third parties
   The disgruntled patient or family
   Inappropriate consultations

Consultant's point of view
Duties of the referring physician and consultant
Timing
How to do the consultation
Recommendations
Concerns
Outcomes
   Total agreement
   Supporting consultation
   Finding another physician for the patient
   Consultant assumes primary care of the patient
   Serious troubles
   Redirecting thrust of a workup
   Major disagreements between physicians
   Duration of consultation
   When a diagnosis is not forthcoming

When should a consultant request consultation?

There are many facets of the consultative process, ranging from the extent and reason for the consultation to the nature of recommendations and outcomes expected. These are listed in Table 1–1.

EXTENT OF THE CONSULTATION

It is essential that both the referring physician and the consultant have in mind the extent of consultation requested, which will in turn govern the aim and comprehensiveness of the consultation.

Confirmatory Consultation

In this situation the referring physician is quite comfortable with the diagnosis, prognosis and treatment. He or she generally wishes the consultant to focus on efforts already made and to corroborate those findings. This type is frequent in the second opinion consultation or one in which the referring physician needs encouragement as well as perhaps some advice garnered from the consultant's experience. These consultations are therefore focused, often brief, yet may involve reviewing substantial previously collected data. In general, the consultant does not need to request extra tests.

A subtype of the confirmatory consultation exists when the referring physician does not think the services of the consultant are indicated but, because of uncertainty or pressure from family members, wishes the consultant to document such in the chart. The most frequent reason for not using specific services is severe illness in the patient, which would make the consultant's services worthless, futile, or even contraindicated by unnecessarily extending the dying process. Examples in hematology might include evaluation for mild thrombocytopenia in an intensive care unit (ICU) patient with multiorgan dysfunction syndrome or whether a "hypercoagulable workup" is indicated in an elderly patient dying of carcinomatosis yet manifesting new deep venous thrombosis. The referring physician should indicate to the consultant that services may not be indicated. The consultant should not be reluctant to see such patients.

Brief Consultation

In this consultation, the questions are more broad based and commonly involve long-term questions in an appropriately diagnosed and managed patient such as length of therapy with glucocorticosteroids in a patient with immune thrombocytopenia purpura before one proceeds to splenectomy or the duration of anticoagulant therapy in a patient with hypercoagulability who has developed a major thrombosis. The consultant's long-term experience with many similar patients and knowledge of the literature is often more important than his or her diagnostic or therapeutic acumen.

Comprehensive Consultation

In this situation the referring practitioner may not be a subspecialist but an internist or occasionally another physician who needs comprehensive assistance regarding the diagnosis, prognosis, and therapy. This consultation often is generated by surgeons or obstetricians/gynecologists attending a patient with thrombosis who needs thorough evaluation for hypercoagulability. In these situations the consultant more often than not is the manager of laboratory testing and can do so in a cost-effective manner based on his or her expertise. Key decisions are often made by the consultant with the approval of the referring physician. Occasionally the referring physician will ask the consultant to manage entirely hematologic aspects of the patient's care, which can be easily done conjointly with the referring physician. A common example is consulting with an obstetrician attending a woman with antiphospholipid syndrome. Together they can discuss preconception issues, anticoagulant therapy throughout gestation, and anticoagulant management during and after delivery of the child with the patient and her family.

Urgent Consultation on a Catastrophically Ill Patient

These patients are often hospitalized in an ICU, and may be seen by multiple experts attempting to assist the attending physician in a diagnosis. These consultations require subspecialty expertise and also a solid knowledge of general internal medicine. Anyone may make the single unifying diagnosis that underpins all manifestations in such extremely ill patients. The consultant hematologist may be the first to recognize that thrombocytopenia in a febrile, confused, azotemic patient supports an overall diagnosis of Rocky Mountain spotted fever, thus corroborating all findings made by all previous consultants.

"Undiagnosing" Consultation

Sometimes patients may be incorrectly diagnosed and thus inappropriately sent to the hematologist. In these situations one must be rather careful to exclude explicitly the diagnosis that the referring physician made. It is both professional and cost-effective to rule out the diagnosis that was being entertained. One must carefully garner laboratory data that justifies the negation of the working diagnosis as well as corroborating evidence, such as historical and physical examination findings, that may be incompatible with that diagnosis. It is easier to diagnose a patient incorrectly than to undo a diagnosis. One could argue that higher standards are required for undiagnosing an illness than diagnosing that illness. An example is a physician who seeks your endorsement of his or her diagnosis of protein C deficiency only to learn the protein C level was low because of concurrent warfarin therapy. The incorrect diagnosis not only is wrong but has financial, familial, and insurability ramifications. A forthright consultation will steer the referring physician away from the incorrect diagnosis so that the diagnostic process may be redirected.

The Curbside Consultation

Although many condemn "curbside consultations," they are a fact of professional life. These consults occur serendipitously in the doctors' lounge, in the hallway, or occasionally by phone. They are unofficial and both the "consultant" and the requesting physician must realize any suggestions arising from this act are not based on a real doctor–patient relationship as there is no traditional history, physical examination, and counseling of the patient; therefore a doctor (consultant)–patient relationship is not established. Rather, the requesting physician is inquiring in an unofficial broad manner about generalities that may well apply for a group of patients (e.g., those with mild thrombocytopenia undergoing colonoscopy) yet might not apply to a specific patient (e.g., as above but in a Jehovah's Witness). Giving of one's professional advice, even without compensation, is part of professionalism. Practitioners should not abuse this precept either by repeatedly taking advantage of this courtesy or using the general unofficial advice in a specific official capacity.

A name provides an illusion of clarity where there was mystery and gives illness a tangibility which makes it seem more likely to be overcome. This applies not only to the patient but also to the doctor.

Richard Asher[4]

While a doctor's knowledge may be extraordinarily precise for predicting what would happen to a thousand patients with a given condition, as the denominator becomes smaller, accuracy in prediction attenuates exponentially. It nearly disappears when the sample size recedes to unity, namely, when the doctor is called to prophesy outcome for a single individual. It is difficult to apply statistics to an individual patient. The unique challenge in doctoring is to determine where, if anywhere, a particular patient fits on the Gaussian distribution curve derived from a larger population. The decisive factor is the physician's breadth of clinical experience.

Bernard Lown[5]

REASON FOR CONSULTATION

At first glance it seems intuitive that the reason to consult is to help another physician's management of a patient. Whereas this view is fundamental, it is not all inclusive. Several reasons exist for the consultation and cover the entire spectrum of the consultant–patient interaction.

Helping Another Physician

This is still the most common reason for the consult to be requested. In these situations, the primary physician

---

[4] Richard Asher (1911–1969). Dr. Asher was a keen English clinician and consummate wordsmith. His writings and lecture style clearly showed that he liked what he did, especially excelling at the interface of internal medicine and psychiatry. He coined the term *Munchausen syndrome* as well as *myxedema madness*. His writings and lectures demonstrate that he made cogent observations from the simplest of medical situations and wrote about them in an economical style. This quote comes from a collection of his best essays on how doctors should use words, *Talking Sense* (University Park Press, Baltimore, 1972).

[5] Bernard Lown (1921–). Dr. Lown graduated from Johns Hopkins Medical School in 1942 and spent his clinical years in Boston. He was a cardiologist of the old school, giving most of his credit as a clinician to Dr. Samuel Levine. Dr. Lown taught a whole generation of clinical cardiologists not only cardiology but the art of being a physician, with particular reference to listening to the patient and making a strong, empathetic connection. Dr. Lown's contributions are numerous and include seminal observations on digitalis intoxication, use of lidocaine in arrhythmias, the establishment of DC cardioversion, and the establishment of what would become the modern coronary care unit. He won the Nobel Peace Prize in 1985 for his work in prevention of nuclear war. These quotations are taken from his 1996 book *The Lost Art of Healing* (Houghton, Mifflin, Boston, 1996), which is highly recommended to any physician cherishing aspects we may well be losing as the burden of the technological approach to medicine increases.

requests assistance in the patient's diagnosis, prognosis, or treatment while he or she maintains overall care of the patient.

Second Opinion Requested by the Primary Physician

In this situation the primary physician has made a diagnosis and plan but because of either his or her unfamiliarity with the process or because of the seriousness of the illness, he or she requests a second corroborating opinion. In nearly all cases the patient's care remains with the referring physician.

Second Opinion Requested by the Patient

In this situation the patient either has pressed for a second opinion or may have secured the consultation without informing the primary physician. This circumstance should be elucidated soon in the consultative process and is probably best done so by asking to whom your report should be sent. The patient and family may vary in reasons for pursuing a second opinion but more often than not is the result of a benign motivation. They generally wish the report to go back to the referring physician. That should be done with an opening sentence in the consultation letter stating that the patient sought the second opinion and that your information is being transmitted to the primary physician.

Second Opinion Sought by a Third-Party Payor

Increasingly third-party payors request second opinions, especially if a new diagnosis or planned procedure has significant financial implications. These are worthwhile financially both to the payor but especially to the patient because the correct diagnosis and treatment is always best for the patient. These second opinions should be honored and are part of good modern medicine.

Other Third Parties

Occasionally in disputes regarding quality of care, causation, injury, prognostication, and workers' compensation, an independent medical evaluation (IME) is requested. This is one of the few situations in which a consulting physician is to remain an emotionally neutral party objectively trying to find facts to assist the mediation process while serving as an advocate for neither side. It is of great importance to the consultant to project this neutrality to the patient, his or her family, and both parties of a dispute and to document initially in the report that he or she is not and will not be a provider of care and thus there is no traditional doctor–patient relationship established. Therefore, treatment (unless absolutely emergently so) is not instituted but rather is described in the report, which should be an objective statement of one's findings. Some consultants do not do IME or workers' compensation consults and this should be clearly stated to those who are requesting such consultation.

A physician shall, in the provision of appropriate patient care, except in emergencies, be free to choose whom to serve, with whom to associate, and the environment in which to provide medical service.

AMA Code of Medical Ethics[6]

The Disgruntled Patient or Family

Occasionally a patient has lost all confidence in a practitioner for either real or perceived cause. These patients and especially their families may rail against a physician for either missing or delaying a diagnosis, for treating too rapidly or too slowly, or for a less than perfect outcome. It is generally best to allow some degree of emotional venting by such parties during the consultation visit but soon it should be established that even if the patient is not to return to that initial practitioner, the patient's well-being remains dependent on records, reports, and tests from the other physician. At this time the consultant should discuss with the patient the importance of the background work collected by the primary physician as it serves as the foundation for the consultation. All previous information is useful. Information from the first physician should be requested by the consulting physician (not by the patient) in a nonthreatening but honest manner, preferably face-to-face or by telephone rather than the mail as such direct discourse between the two physicians greatly facilitates the initial practitioner's efforts to elaborate his or her side of the story, to diminish concerns that the patient and consultant may be conspiring against the primary physician, and finally, in fact, to expedite patient care. The new consultant may assume primary care of the patient, find another qualified practitioner appropriate for the patient, or facilitate continued care of the patient by the original physician, especially if there have been only minor misunderstandings between these two parties.

In explaining to patients the failure of other physicians to have reached the correct diagnosis in the past, it should be pointed out that one cannot judge the past by the present. It often takes time for changes to occur to the point where a correct diagnosis is possible.

Philip A. Tumulty[7]

---

[6] American Medical Association Code of Medical Ethics, 1997. This compilation of medical ethics with its supporting case law, opinions, and foundations is extremely concise and well written. Unfortunately, it is not referred to enough by physicians as a foundation for a most important part of modern medical practice.

[7] Philip A. Tumulty (1912–1989). Dr. Tumulty was the master consult physician at Johns Hopkins Hospital and a professor of medicine for many decades. The three editors were fortunate to have worked with Dr. Tumulty as house officers. Dr. Tumulty was the quintessential diagnostician and curator of the art of medicine exemplifying the highest attributes of an internist. His quotes in this chapter are taken from his book, *The Effective Clinician* (W.B. Saunders, Philadelphia, 1973).

Acknowledged mistakes provide potent learning experiences. Admitting them helps ensure that they will not be repeated. The humbling avowal of error prevents doctors from confusing their mission with a divine one. We possess no omniscient powers, only intuition, experience, and a patina of knowledge. These are most effective when one is constantly probing to advance the interest of an ailing human being.

Bernard Lown[5]

Inappropriate Consultations

Occasionally consultations are requested that may be inappropriate. Although a consultant should always be at the service of a physician calling for a consultation, he or she must be on guard against any consultation that reflects adversely on the patient, cost-containment, or the profession. Physicians must minimize inappropriate consultations and identify abuses.

One such inappropriate consultation involves what the author refers to as "institutional elitism." This may occur when a patient is admitted to a hospital for legitimate reasons for an acute hematologic problem. Unless proven otherwise, it should be assumed that chronic problems that are managed by other physicians are adequately treated. Thus, new consultations for these problems need not be generated. An example may be a case of a bipolar patient with acute idiopathic thrombocytopenia (ITP). If one assumes that the patient's chronic bipolar disorder has been appropriately treated for many years by a physician who is regarded as being an expert and with whom the patient and family are perfectly happy, it is inappropriate to ask one's own institutional psychiatrist to see the patient unless one can weave some situation in which the bipolarism or its treatment may have something to do with the acute ITP. Assuming in this illustrative case that the bipolar disorder has nothing to do with ITP, it is best to continue the patient's pharmacologic management and then send a copy of discharge summary to the psychiatrist for his or her office file.

A second, more pervasive form of inappropriate consultation is often referred to as "churning." In this situation, a patient is admitted and each and every system or organ that is abnormal is immediately and with little forethought consulted on by experts. Basic internal medicine expertise should eliminate the notion that every murmur requires an immediate visit from a cardiologist, every wheeze requires a pulmonologist, or every arthritic joint requires a rheumatologist. This thesis is especially true with the very brief length of hospitalizations we currently endure. A consultation should be carefully chosen and the question regarding the management should be focused toward any problem that is relevant to the current clinical setting.

A British study showed that 75 percent of the information leading to a correct diagnosis comes from a detailed history, 10 percent from the physical examination, 5 percent from simple routine tests, 5 percent from all the costly invasive tests; in 5 percent, no answer is forthcoming. Some of the most challenging medical problems I have encountered could be solved only through information provided by the patient. The time invested in obtaining a meticulous history is never ill spent. Careful history-taking actually saves time. The history provides the road map; without it the journey is merely a shopping around at numerous garages for technological fixes.

Bernard Lown[5]

CONSULTANT'S POINT OF VIEW

As a general rule, the consultant should approach the case from the point of view of one having one degree of training more specialized than the referring practitioner. If the referring physician is another hematologist/oncologist, one can more likely than not appropriately review the case from the point of view of a subspecialist (e.g., coagulationist) for that hematology/oncology referring physician. The consultation will thus be quite focused. When another internist refers the patient to the subspecialist, one should regard the patient from the position of a hematologist/oncologist and therefore approach the patient in a more general manner. Therefore, other hematologic matters such as anemia, elevated white count, or splenomegaly can be and should be addressed if they are found by the consultant. When consultation is originated by a noninternist such as a surgeon, obstetrician/gynecologist, or psychiatrist, one must approach the patient from the point of view of a general internist. In these situations one might also want to address elevated blood glucose, hypertension, or a dermatologic process not previously appreciated by the referring doctor. While it is not necessary to address each of these problems oneself, the fact that one has found them when they had not been previously appreciated warrants consideration. One may evaluate these personally or one may wish to refer these patients to a diabetologist, hypertension specialist, or dermatologist, respectively. However, the fact remains that the consultant as an internist has found these items which are of medical importance and clearly part of the overall consultation process. Increasingly patients are being referred to subspecialists by nonphysicians such as dentists, physician assistants, advanced registered nurse practitioners, or even third-party payors. In these situations the consultant must look at the patient as a physician as well as a specialist unless this has clearly been done by someone else. In these situations, the consultant must often ascertain that a patient has had appropriate preventive care (e.g., Pap smears and mammograms) or at least make sure that those very important points have been addressed as well as the question that is being directly asked by the referring healthcare provider.

I do not know a better training for a writer than to spend some years in the medical profession. I suppose that you can learn a good deal about human nature in a solicitor's office; but there on the whole you have to deal with men in full control of themselves. They lie perhaps as much as they lie to the doctor, but they lie more consistently, and it may be that for the solicitor it is not so necessary to know the truth. The interests he deals with, besides, are usually material. He sees human nature from a specialized standpoint. But the doctor, especially the hospital doctor, sees it bare. Reticences can generally be undermined; very often there are none. Fear for the most part will shatter every defence; even vanity is unnerved by it. Most people have a furious itch to talk about themselves and are restrained only by the disinclination of others to listen. Reserve is an artificial quality that is developed in most of us but is the result of innumerable rebuffs. The doctor is discreet. It is his business to listen and no details are too intimate for his ears.

W. Somerset Maugham[8]

DUTIES OF THE REFERRING PHYSICIAN AND THE CONSULTANT

The consultant should focus as directly, efficiently, and cost-effectively as possible on the precise question that the referring physician has formulated. This, of course, depends on the accuracy of the referring physician's question as well as the possibility that the referring physician may have missed some important points. In all cases, the consultant should provide that level of consultation that is best for the patient.

Increasingly the consultant may use a physician extender such as a physician assistant or advanced registered nurse practitioner. Such professionals are usually highly knowledgeable in their area and clearly enhance the efficiency of the busy consultant. It must remain, however, absolutely clear to the referring physician and the patient that the extender is working with the consultant and not independently. If the extender dictates the report, it is wise and reassuring to have joint signatures on the correspondence.

Too little has been made of the duties of the referring practitioner. In this era of brief visits in which time is at a premium, the referring physician cannot simply ask a consult to go in depth into a patient's multiyear history of present illness with multiple hospitalizations, innumerable radiographs, biopsies, and sheaves of laboratory data just to "figure it all out" in a 45-minute consultation. Rather, the referring physician must prepare a brief (one-page) summary of what has happened and construct a chief question that is to be asked of the consultant. If radiographs, biopsies, or other special tests are of importance and pertinent, they must come with the patient, preferably being hand-delivered by the patient directly to the consultant. Mailing important matrial that will be delivered a week after the consultation is perfunctory and disrespectful. On the other hand, if these previous records are not important, they are better not brought as they otherwise will clutter the diagnostic process and further encroach on effective consultation time.

'If I failed to send a letter along with a new referral, which I more often did than not, this man would call me before he saw the patient and bluntly ask, "Dr. Sams, what do you want me to do for this patient?" The first time this happened I was taken aback, for specialists are not usually that open or that direct, and I am afraid I stammered a little with confusion and surprise. Then I learned just as bluntly to reply, 'Prove to me he does not have a brain tumor,' or, 'Tell me she is having migraines,', or, 'I am worried about multiple sclerosis and need you to confirm or deny it,', or even, 'She is a crock and forgive me for dumping on you.'

Ferrol Sams[9]

TIMING

The timing of the consultation plays an important part in determining the tempo and depth of the consultant's evaluation of a patient. For instance, for a coagulation evaluation it is important to know whether the patient is being considered for impending surgery. In this situation one usually is more exhaustive in the consultation because the hemostatic challenge of surgery is imminent. On the other hand, one may be asked to see a patient with postoperative hemorrhage in whom another operation is not being planned in the foreseeable future. It is characteristically difficult to make sense out of postoperative intrahemorrhagic coagulation tests as most diagnostic hemostatic testing is designed to ferret out problems in stable situations. Hemostatic studies from a patient who has been stressed by operation and hemorrhage, and is in the midst of receiving a variety of therapeutic agents and blood products, are difficult to interpret. Another situation involves patients who seek hemostatic evaluation as part of a kindred analysis when another family member, often a first-degree relative, has been found to have a genetic disease such as the factor V Leiden mutation.

---

[8] W. Somerset Maugham (1874–1965). Dr. Maugham was trained at St. Thomas' Hospital in London and used his medical background in his more famous career as a novelist and short-story writer as well as playwright. He wrote more than 60 books. Of special interest to physicians is *Of Human Bondage*. This quote comes from his autobiography, *The Summing Up* (Bantam, Doubleday Dell Publishing Group, New York).

[9] Ferrol Sams (1922–). This American physician was educated at Emory University School of Medicine and still practices in southern Georgia. He is a master storyteller and has written several novels, including *Run with the Horsemen* and *Whisper of the River*. The quotation used comes from *The Widow's Mite* (Peachtree Publishers, Atlanta, 1987).

*Accurate diagnosis and knowledge of the prognosis, both with and without various modes of therapy, should guide the physician in answering three major questions of therapy: **Whether** to treat, **When** to treat, and with **Which** modality.*
Maxwell M. Wintrobe[10]

HOW TO DO THE CONSULTATION

A consultation is fundamentally similar to an admission evaluation of a patient but can be and usually is more focused, since the consultant is answering specific questions posed by the referring physician. Nonetheless, a careful history and physical examination are still in order and should be in depth, particularly regarding the area of expertise of the consultant. If the question posed is clearly focused and the encounter is a simple confirmatory and/or second opinion consultation, the consultation can be brief and therefore very circumscribed with respect to laboratory tests. Stumbling blocks, particularly in the area of coagulation and thrombosis, regard not only *what* labs are reviewed but also *when* the laboratory results were drawn. Every hematologist has had the problem of finding low and then normal protein C and protein S activity levels randomly spread throughout a patient's chart without knowing whether the patient was receiving warfarin therapy at the time of testing. Similarly, a prolonged activated partial thromboplastin time may be the result of a traumatic venipuncture, contaminating heparin, or a true underlying process such as disseminated intravascular coagulation. One cannot simply look at raw laboratory data without knowing what the clinical circumstances were at that time in order to interpret those data. The obverse of this is that when the consultant performs laboratory tests, he or she is expected to state explicitly in the chart the ongoing events at the time those laboratory specimens were collected. It is important to know whether warfarin therapy or heparin therapy was concurrent, whether liver disease was manifest, or if there was a recent massive thrombosis. Otherwise one is unable to convert data into information useful to the patient and the physician.

RECOMMENDATIONS

A consultant's recommendations should be clearly stated and easily found. In urgent cases or especially if information is pivotal in patient management, the referring physician should be called as soon as feasible to discuss the events of the consultation. This rapid communication is then followed up with a more formal consultation note.

In preparing the final report, the consultant should state in the first sentence or two the reason for the consultation. An example may be "Thank you very much for sending this 37-year-old white man with clearcut ITP in consultation for my opinion regarding length of prednisone treatment prior to possible splenectomy." This first sentence thus makes clear at least what your expectations were of the consultation and, if such prove to be wrong, then the consultation can be refocused. For inpatient consultation, particularly when the patient is not on an internal medicine service, one's diagnoses and recommendations are probably best tabulated in a numerical fashion, as the entire history and physical examination and recounting of laboratory data more likely than not will not be read by the busy referring doctor.

Genetic counseling may also be an aspect of the consultation. As examples, when patients are found to have heritable diseases, such as hemophilia or thrombophilia, it is wise to tell both the family and the referring physician that at least first-degree relatives might be screened for the presence or absence of the genetic disease. It is useful for first-degree relatives to know whether they do or do not have the defect, regardless of prior symptomatology or lack thereof, as future therapeutic plans are impacted by either positive or negative diagnosis of such illnesses.

One should be perfectly clear on to whom to send the consultation report. In inpatient work, the report is usually left on the chart for all appropriate persons to see.

In outpatient consultations, the initial copy is sent to that practitioner who referred the patient. Frequently patients wish to have copies of the consultation and this should be honored in almost all respects. In rare situations in which the consultant feels uncomfortable, he or she should inform the patient that it is his or her obligation to send the consultation report back to the referring physician and let the referring physician and patient discuss those matters between themselves. Keep in mind, however, that any report is rightfully discoverable, so if a patient wishes to have a report, such inevitably will be accomplished.

More often than not patients will have seen other physicians who may have a stake in the patient's overall care and so it is pertinent to ask the patient whether he or she wishes to have a copy of the report sent to other health care practitioners who have cared for the patient or may in the near future.

In the special circumstances of IME and workers' compensation cases, the report is sent to the party who requested and paid for the consultation. Here it is not advisable to send copies to other practitioners without the explicit permission of the patient or the parties requesting the IME or workers' compensation evaluation.

---

[10] Maxwell M. Wintrobe (1901–1986). Dr. Wintrobe is considered the father of American hematology. Born and trained in Canada, he joined the faculty at Johns Hopkins in 1929 and then in 1943 became a founding giant at the new medical school in Salt Lake City, where he helped build that service into one of preeminence. A host of American hematologists can trace their academic lineage directly or indirectly through several steps to Dr. Wintrobe. His quotation is taken from the introduction to his textbook, *Clinical Hematology*, first published in 1942. It has been wisely retained by the present editors of the 10th edition (Williams & Wilkins, Baltimore, 1998).

Time after time I have gone out into my office in the evening feeling as if I couldn't keep my eyes open a moment longer. I would start out on my morning calls after only a few hours' sleep, sit in front of some house waiting to get the courage to climb the steps and push the front door bell. But once I saw the patient all that would disappear. In a flash the details of the case would begin to formulate themselves into a recognizable outline, the diagnosis would unravel itself, or would refuse to make itself plain, and the hunt was on.

William Carlos Williams[11]

CONCERNS

Sometimes circumstances develop during the consultation that place the consultant in an unenviable position. One's maturity and professionalism will serve to direct the correct course of action even if initially it seems totally impossible. The fundamental commandment should be to do that which is best for the patient rather than one's own emotional comfort. These dilemmas usually involve the relationship between the referring physician and the patient.

A patient or his or her family may be disgruntled with the original physician. Diagnoses are missed by all practitioners and therapy provided can be incorrect. Bad outcomes should be clearly separated from deviation in standard of care. Tact with honesty and forthrightness should be employed. Often diagnoses that are perfectly clear in retrospect are in fact initiated and validated by prior efforts made on behalf of the patient. Treatments can be controversial and even bizarre treatments have their vocal advocates. One should never openly fault another practitioner without knowing all the facts involved. It is best to limit oneself to what is known and carefully document such in the record as the stated facts may change if and when more data are collected. It is usually wise to refer such cases to a third practitioner or assume the care yourself rather than force the patient and physician back together if care does appear in fact to be suboptimal. One should find a way to discuss this matter with the other physician as such will eventually be revealed in some manner regardless. Early communication will allow the other practitioner to voice facts of which the consultant may not be aware. As mentioned previously, it is often possible to reconcile the patient and the referring physician's problems. Early communication also allows the initial physician, if he or she indeed has practiced below the standard of care, to make amends with the patient or, if appropriate, for the physician to contact his or her risk management personnel sooner rather than later.

Some practitioners may initially be curt, hurried, or disrespectful, or do not offer enough of their time to their patients, but nonetheless, are practicing within the medical-legal standard of care. If reparations cannot be made, the patient is best served by finding an equally intelligent but more humanistic physician.

Some patients are habitually malcontent; this can be determined by both discussion with the practitioner and discovery that the patient is persistently unable to establish and maintain profitable relationships with any healthcare provider. This category may include patients with personality disorders, drug-seekers, and persons with self-induced or factitious illnesses. These are most difficult as their problems are far deeper than just those that apply to one's subspecialty.

What the scalpel is to the surgeon, words are to the clinician. When he uses them effectively, his patients do well. If not, the results may be disastrous.

Philip A. Tumulty[7]

OUTCOMES

Total Agreement

In this situation the consultant totally agrees with the evaluation of the referring physician and consultation serves primarily to add a layer of understanding and confidence to the patient and his or her family. Whereas almost always one can make some minor suggestions, the thrust of the consultation is clearly to agree with and support the diagnosis, prognosis, and treatment plan of the referring physician. In almost all cases the referring physician will continue with the assumption of care of the patient.

Supporting Consultation

Occasionally a physician will refer a noncompliant or doubtful patient to a consultant in order to have the latter reinforce a point with which the referring physician is having difficulty because of poor patient acceptance or compliance. Common examples of this type of consultation include the acceptance of certain diagnoses and especially cessation of smoking. Surprisingly, some patients refuse to accept the determination that they are normal despite all the supporting evidence. They continue to hang on to mildly abnormal laboratory data or minor findings such as normal bruising as evidence for some underlying pathologic process. It is frequent and wise for the referring physician to informally communicate this approach with the consulting physician prior to the consultation. When it is clear that the referring physician will continue to assume care of the patient, the consultation is an opportune time for the consulting physician to strongly reinforce the stance of the referring physician assuming that it is correct. Inappropriate behavior on the part of the patient can be addressed. This may occasionally generate some degree of resentment on the part of the patient, who may report such resentment to the referring physician or even distort details of the consultation. The strong advocacy role played by the consultant physician rightfully justifies the benevolent attempt of the consultant to positively modify the patient's understanding or behavior. One

---

[11] William Carlos Williams (1883–1963). This American physician translated his hard work as a practitioner into everyday-life scenarios that characterized his enormous production of poetry and short stories. The quotation comes from a short story called "The Practice" from the *Autobiography of William Carlos Williams* (New Directions Publishing Company, 1951).

should promptly telephonically alert the referring physician of these events so that the referring physician will be forewarned regarding possible negative opinions of the consulting physician voiced by the patient.

Finding Another Physician for the Patient

It may become clear to the consultant that the referring physician has not made the correct diagnosis, prognostication, or treatment and that perhaps another primary physician should assume care of the patient. The consultant must be prepared to relate this opinion to the referring physician, especially if the patient or his or her family is obviously upset with the referring physician. The consultant, as a neutral third party, can sometimes improve patient care, but it is always still advisable as well as truthful to acknowledge to all parties the foundation work prepared and gathered by the original physician.

Consultant Assumes Primary Care of the Patient

Very rarely the consultant will assume primary care of the patient; this is not an advisable practice to take because if this does occur the relationship between the referring physician and consultant may be eroded. Transference of care is clearly understood whenever a patient moves from an area where he or she was previously attended by the referring physician to the consultant's geographic area. One may occasionally have a patient and his or her family so positively impressed by the attention and clinical sophistication of the consultant that they ask the consultant to assume their care. Flattering that it may be, it is advisable not to do this unless there is absolute agreement from all parties, to include third-party payors. It is not intrinsically unethical but generally should be held at an absolute minimum.

It is not unethical to enter into a patient–physician relationship with a patient who has been receiving care from another physician. By accepting second-opinion patients for treatment, physicians affirm the right of patients to have a free choice in the selection of their physicians.

AMA Code of Ethics[6]

Serious Troubles

Rarely a patient's case has been so mismanaged that there is clear and immediate danger for the patient. If this does occur, the consultant is helping the patient and also potentially the referring physician by extracting the patient from continued mismanagement. If the patient's care is severely compromised and immediate care is necessary, prompt hospitalization at the consultant's facility is a way to address the problem and defuse potential ill will with the referring physician. In this manner, diagnostic and therapeutic procedures can be initiated promptly and the consultant allowed time as well as data to justify this aggressive maneuver to the referring physician. Whether the patient should be returned to the referring physician may be a matter of the preference of both the patient and the referring physician as well as their abilities to continue the correct treatment.

The best way to get a difficult job done is face-to-face or ear-to-ear. Sending notes is never satisfactory.

Eugene A. Stead, Jr.[3]

Redirecting the Thrust of a Workup

The consultant has the benefit of having more time, laboratory data, and response to therapy than the original physician. Occasionally the consultant may suddenly visualize the correct diagnosis, which, while explaining all the findings in the case, is far different from that of the referring physician. At this juncture the diagnostic and therapeutic thrust must be changed from one direction to another. A representative example would be a patient who is being evaluated for anemia and is referred for a bone marrow examination because a myriad of tests have been negative. If during the history the consultant recognizes that fatigue, chills, fevers, weight loss, and night sweats have been overlooked and the consultant is the first to detect a new cardiac murmur, it is clear that the evaluation should be focused more toward infectious endocarditis than anemia of unknown etiology. Rarely do any parties become upset with this new direction, especially when such proves to be correct. Credit again must be given to the foundation of material gathered by the original physicians.

Major Disagreements Between Physicians

This is a most unfortunate situation and, as rarely as it is encountered, usually occurs in the inpatient rather than the outpatient setting. Not all the recommendations that a consultant makes need be carried out by any referring physician and such is certainly the prerogative of the attending physician. No code holds that the attending physician must execute each and every recommendation made by the consulting physician. On some occasions, however, the feelings are so strong and so clear in the mind of the consultant that for the primary physician to continue to ignore the recommendations may well fall below the standard of care in the consultant's opinion. In this situation, frank face-to-face discussion with the attending physician is mandatory. This is particularly true in teaching institutions, where there are several buffers of communication between the consultant faculty member and the attending of record. If these matters cannot be resolved, it may be wisest to sign off a case in writing in the chart. Admittedly this should be a very rare event but it does occur perhaps a few times in a decade among consultants in a very busy consultation service. The note need not be long nor give reasons but simply state that one as the consultant is signing off this case but availability can be reestablished by reconsultation. The consultant might name other consultants who may be contacted on this case.

From the day you begin practice never under any circumstances listen to a tale told to the detriment of a brother practitioner. And when any dispute or trouble does arise, go frankly, ere sunset, and talk the matter over, in which way you may gain a brother and a friend.

William Osler[12]

Duration of Consultation

There is often question about how long one should be involved as a consultant in the outpatient setting as well as the inpatient setting. This question may be more pertinent on an inpatient basis. Some focused questions are effectively answered by an equally focused single note. In other situations, those questions are quickly and efficiently answered with one or two brief follow-up visits to ascertain results of certain requested laboratory data or the response to therapy after which the consultation can be terminated. It is advisable to sign off in writing in the medical record so that it is clear to all parties that one has ceased closely following the patient yet is still available if another question emerges or if things do not go as well as planned.

Some consultations involve "clearing a patient for surgery." All parties should understand that the term "cleared for surgery" implies clearance *at that time.* Therefore, any events that happen later cannot have been considered; a patient is not cleared for surgery in perpetuity. This often must be expressly written in the outpatient consultation as facts can change between the consultation and the actual surgery. For instance, a patient with chronic thrombocytopenia who has a platelet count of 60,000/μL may be cleared for nearly any surgery now but that clearance does not forever hold true. If the patient returns in a year for another operation and the platelet count is now 20,000/μL, the situation has clearly changed. It is wise to signify the limits of the clearance in the body of the consultation. Clearance is not to be confused with a guarantee of success but implies that the risk:benefit ratio is made as favorable as possible for the patient and that parties acknowledge the risk and agree that the perceived benefit is worth that risk.

In general the consultant should follow the case for as long as the expertise is needed. If one is consulted for preparing an individual with hemophilia for surgery, it would be wise for the consultant to see the patient several visits postoperatively as bleeding can either be immediate, intermediate, or sometimes delayed.

When a Diagnosis Is Not Forthcoming

Not all diagnoses can be established. The wise consultant should never feel pressed to force a diagnosis, since an incorrect diagnosis is worse than no diagnosis. In making an incorrect diagnosis, one shuts the window of opportunity to pursue the correct diagnosis. It is wisest to realize and state that one affirmatively knows he or she does not know the answer rather than to force a diagnosis. It often is the responsibility of the consultant to energize the referring physician to continue observation in a conservative course. Failure to do so frequently results in erratic testing and troublesome indecisive therapeutics. If a therapeutic course is taken, it must be maintained sufficiently long enough to have time to either succeed or fail on its own merits while one constantly reevaluates for signs of success or failure as well as entertains another diagnosis. Often the remaining and most important procedure in such cases is observation. With observation, some diagnoses become clear while other cases spontaneously improve.

The essential and wise thing to do is not to force a diagnosis when the answer is not evident, but rather to follow a conservative program of support and periodic reexamination, retaining an open mind as to the basis of the patient's complaints.

Philip A. Tumulty[7]

Once a particular therapeutic program has been launched, give the patient's response to it time to mature and produce clear-cut answers before it is stopped or altered.

Philip A. Tumulty[7]

You can observe a lot just by looking.

Yogi Berra[13]

---

[12] William Osler (1849–1919). Dr. Osler received his M.D. degree from McGill University and was the founding physician of the new Johns Hopkins University. While helping to establish the preeminence of Hopkins, he wrote his *Principles and Practice of Medicine* and subsequently became the Regis Professor of Medicine at Oxford University, the chair presently held by Dr. Weatherall, who was kind enough to write the preface of this text. Dr. Osler wrote prolifically on medical and nonmedical subjects. The quotation used is one of his *Aphorisms.*

[13] Yogi Berra (1925–). Yogi Berra was born in St. Louis, Missouri, and became one of the greatest catchers in baseball history. He is quite well known for his malapropisms, usually now referred to as "Yogi-isms." These have been richly collected in *The Wit and Wisdom of Yogi Berra* by Phil Pepe (Meckler Boos, Westport, Conn., 1988), from which this Yogi-ism was taken.

WHEN SHOULD A CONSULTANT REQUEST CONSULTATION?

Sometimes consultations can be extremely difficult and a well-trained, experienced consultant may find that he or she needs a special laboratory test or special consultation with other experienced experts. These facts are clearly understandable and often for geographic reasons such discussions are made telephonically. It is appropriate to enter such secondary consultation in the body of the report but one should recall that the secondary consultant has not had benefit of seeing the patient first-hand and therefore is relying on the primary consultant's presentation, perception, and understanding of the case. Should blood or biopsy material be referred to yet another consultant, it is best to have the understanding and permission of the patient for reasons of confidentiality as well as the potential for fees generated for services.

There is always a strong impulse to do something to help a sick person, but no action is better than the wrong action.
Philip A. Tumulty[7]

Everyone is ignorant, only on different subjects.
Will Rogers[14]

In order to enhance this chapter, the editor has borrowed the thoughts and words of several highly regarded medical teachers and medical philosophers as well as three physician-writers of renown and two American icons of wit.

[14] Will Rogers (1879–1935). Will Rogers was one of our great American humorists. He was also a showman of great repute. His wit was usually sharp and at times critical. His favorite target was politics and any type of pretention. The quote is from *Will Rogers: Wise and Witty Sayings of a Great American Humorist* (Hallmark, Claremore, Oklahoma, 1969).

CHAPTER 2

Hemostatic Testing and Laboratory Interpretation

McDonald K. Horne III, M.D.

Laboratory testing is an integral part of evaluating a patient for a hemorrhagic diathesis. Although the clinical history is critical in assessing the risk of bleeding, understanding the pathophysiology of the problem, and therefore how to treat it, usually relies heavily on the laboratory results. It is important, therefore, to appreciate both the purpose and the shortcomings of the standard laboratory tests of the hemostatic system.

PHYSIOLOGIC HEMOSTASIS

Physiologic hemostasis begins with vasoconstriction and the accumulation of platelets at the site of injury. Although circulating platelets are normally quiescent, everything changes when they encounter a breach in the vasculature. They tumble along the exposed surface, intermittently detained by interactions between their surface glycoprotein Ibα and von Willebrand factor (vWF) in the subendothelial matrix, and finally adhere to collagen via two receptors, one that binds collagen tightly (integrin $\alpha_2\beta_1$) in a position to interact with a second low-affinity receptor (glycoprotein VI) that transmits a stimulus to the cell.[1-6] This stimulus initiates a series of reactions that converts the platelet membrane glycoprotein complex IIb/IIIa into a binding site for fibrinogen and stimulates the cells to secrete ADP and thromboxane A_2, which activate ("recruit") other platelets in the vicinity. Fibrinogen is a large, bivalent protein that cross-links neighboring platelets into aggregates to begin building a hemostatic plug.

Breaching a blood vessel also exposes membrane-bound tissue factor (TF) in the extravascular tissue to traces of activated factor VII (factor VIIa) that are always present in the plasma.[7] By binding to TF, factor VIIa becomes a potent activator of factor X and initiates the path to the earliest production of thrombin (Fig. 2–1).[8] Although this "tissue factor pathway" is quickly shut down by a specific inhibitor (tissue factor pathway inhibitor, TFPI), coagulation accelerates to a rapid pace because nascent thrombin activates factors V, VIII, and XI to produce additional thrombin. Interaction among the procoagulant proteins is facilitated by platelet activation, which transforms the platelet surface into a platform for the assembly of coagulant complexes.[9] When thrombin cleaves two small peptides from fibrinogen, fibrin monomers are formed and begin to polymerize. Fibrin polymers become cross-linked by activated factor XIII, and soon a macroscopic gel of blood cells in fibrin mesh is organized to stanch the bleeding. Hemostasis has been achieved.

Coagulation is kept localized at the vessel wound by inhibitors that inactivate procoagulant factors leaving the immediate vicinity. Deficiences in these inhibitors may allow the clot to propagate beyond the site to form an obstructing thrombus. Procoagulant proteases (e.g., thrombin and factor Xa) are inhibited by antithrombin in the plasma and by highly active antithrombin that is bound to heparan sulfate on endothelial surfaces. Procoagulant cofactors (i.e., factors Va and VIIIa) are inactivated by activated protein C and its cofactor protein S.

As fibrin polymerizes it binds plasminogen and tissue plasminogen activator (tPA) into the clot and thereby inaugurates the processes that will slowly degrade the hemostatic plug as wound healing proceeds and vessel integrity is restored. This process is tightly regulated by inhibitors of tPA (plasminogen activator inhibitor-1; PAI-1) and plasmin (α_2-antiplasmin; α_2-AP).[10] Deficiencies of these inhibitors predispose to premature clot lysis and recurrent hemorrhage through an incompletely healed vessel wound.

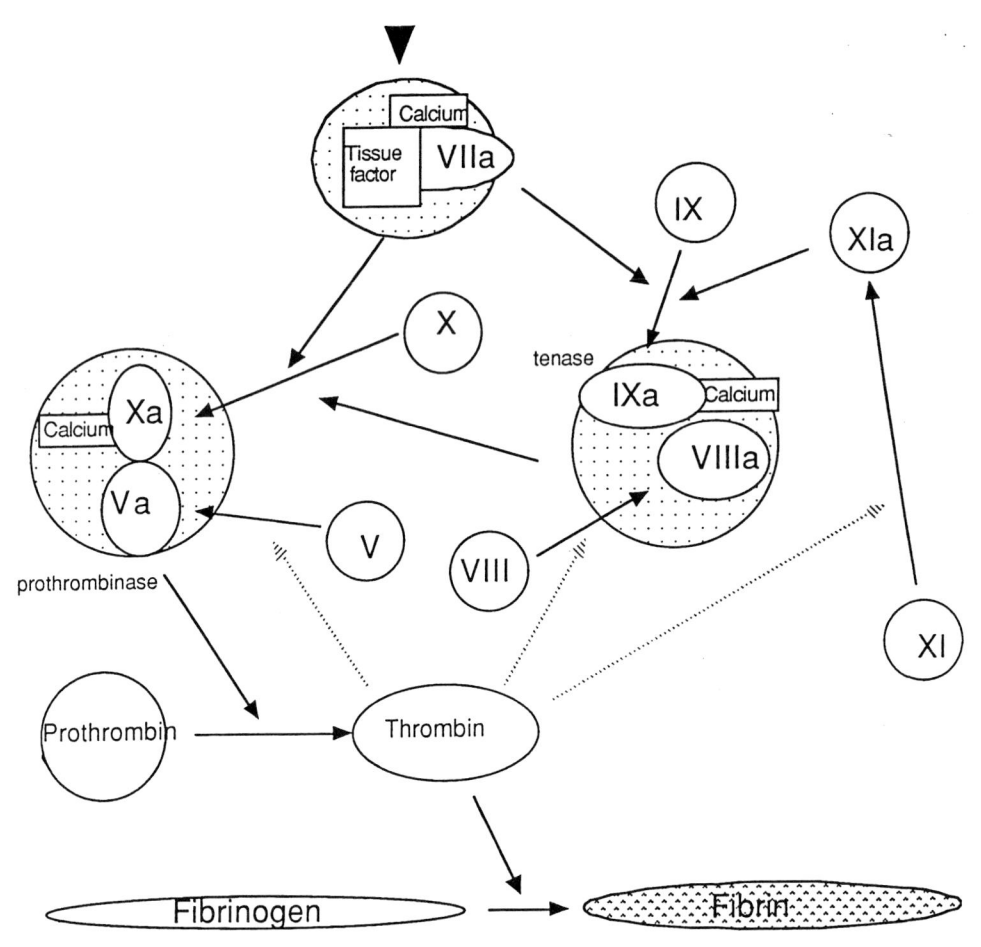

Figure 2–1 Schematic representation of coagulation. The natural process begins with formation of the factor VIIa-tissue factor complex (*top arrowhead*) and ends with the formation of fibrin. Phospholipid surfaces are represented by stippled circles. The complex of lipid, calcium, and factors Xa and Va is referred to as *prothrombinase*, while that including factors IXa and VIIIa is *tenase*. The stippled arrows show the feedback pathways of thrombin to activate factors V, VIII, and XI.

LABORATORY EVALUATION OF THE PROCOAGULANT SYSTEM

There is no truly adequate global laboratory test of hemostasis.[11] Even the seemingly simple in vitro clotting time of whole blood (e.g., the Lee-White clotting time, dating to 1913) is riddled with artifacts. Far more complex assays include thromboelastography, which has recently gained popularity as a guide to intraoperative transfusion support, and electronic measurements of hemostasis at simulated vessel wounds.[12–14] However, broad applications of these techniques have not been adequately evaluated. Laboratory assessment of hemostasis, therefore, is largely based upon assays of isolated portions of this highly complex system. Although far from perfect, these tests can nevertheless elucidate most bleeding disorders.

Prothrombin Time

Although originally intended to measure prothrombin (factor II) concentration, it was later realized that the prothrombin time (PT) measures much more (Fig. 2–2).[11] It is performed by adding tissue factor (in the form of a phospholipid complex, or "thromboplastin," originally derived from brain tissue but more recently prepared as a recombinant protein) and calcium to hypocalcemic (i.e., anticoagulated with citrate) plasma. Tissue factor reacts with factor VIIa to activate the "extrinsic" pathway of coagulation—"extrinsic" because it is stimulated by a substance normally extrinsic to the vasculature, namely, tissue factor. In addition to factor VII, the PT reflects the activities of factor V, factor X, and factor II (prothrombin) assembled with phospholipid and calcium to form the "prothrombinase" complex, which yields thrombin that then produces polymerizing fibrin to form a clot (Figs. 2–1 and 2–2).

Therefore, the PT is sensitive to the activities of factors II, V, VII, X, and fibrinogen, but to different degrees and with different clinical implications (Table 2–1). It is also important to realize that the relationship between PT and the degree of factor deficiency is not linear: the PT prolongs exponentially at lower factor concentrations.

A derivative of the PT is the International Normalized Ratio (INR), which was developed to monitor anticoagulation with warfarin.[15] The difficulty with using the PT

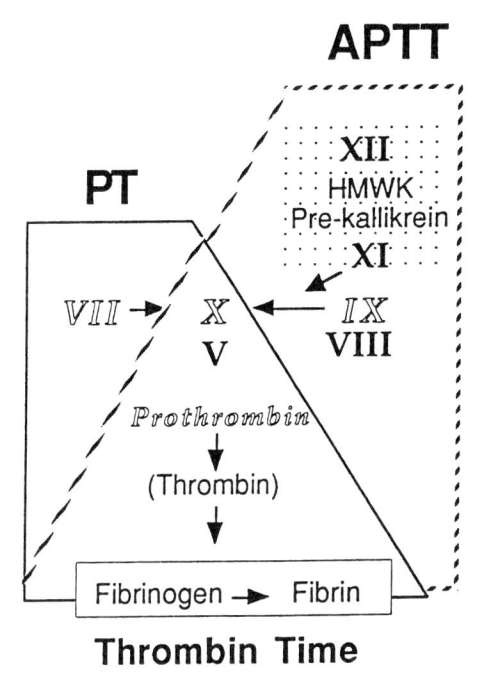

Figure 2–2 Reactions reflected by the prothrombin time (PT), aPTT, and thrombin time. The stippled section encompasses the portion of the intrinsic system that depends upon activation by negatively charge surfaces. Vitamin K-dependent factors (prothrombin, factors VII, IX, and X) are shown in darkened letters.

for this purpose is that the sensitivity of the PT to the degree of anticoagulation created by warfarin is dependent upon the particular reagents and instrument used to measure the PT, and these vary among different laboratories. To compensate for this variability each laboratory must adjust its PT according to the following formula:

$$INR = (Patient\ PT/control\ PT)^{ISI}$$

Table 2–1 • SENSITIVITY OF PT AND aPTT TO PROCOAGULANTS

Procoagulant	Hemostasis[a]	Approximate Level for Normal PT[b]	aPTT[b]
Fibrinogen (Factor I)	50–100 mg/dL	100 mg/dL	60 mg/dL
Prothrombin (Factor II)	20–30%	50%	15%
Factor V	>20%	50%	40%
Factor VII	>10%	50%	NA
Factor VIII	>40%	NA	35%
Factor IX	>30%	Na	20%
Factor X	>20%	60%	25%
Factor XI	>50% (variable)	NA	30%
Factor XII	0	NA	20%

[a] Data from Roberts HR, Bingham MD: Other coagulation factor deficiencies. In Loscalzo J, Schafer AI (eds): Thrombosis and Hemorrhage. Baltimore, Williams & Wilkins, 1998, pp 773–802.
[b] Data from the Hematology Service, Clinical Pathology Department, Warren G. Magnusson Clinical Center, derived using the STA (Diagnostica Stago, Asnieres, France) and provided by Ms. Khanh Nghiem and Dr. Margaret Rick.

in which the "control" is the mid-point of the laboratory's normal range and the ISI (International Sensitivity Index) is a value determined for each batch of each commercial thromboplastin. Thromboplastins that are less sensitive to the effect of warfarin have greater ISIs. The INR should not be used to assess liver function since the test is calibrated specifically for plasma from patients taking warfarin. Its sensitivity to factor deficiencies related to liver disease cannot be predicted.[16]

Although the PT is not used to monitor other anticoagulants, it is prolonged by relatively high concentrations of heparin and by therapeutic concentrations of the newer anticoagulants lepirudin and argatroban.

Activated Partial Thromboplastin Time (aPTT)

This standard assay is performed by adding phospholipid (lacking tissue factor, hence a "partial" thromboplastin) and particulate matter (to activate the "contact" pathway of coagulation, hence the "activated" PTT) to citrated plasma along with calcium. The aPTT is affected by all of the coagulation factors in the "intrinsic" and "common" pathways, although its sensitivity to the individual factors varies somewhat (Fig. 2–2, Table 2–1). While the aPTT is an extremely useful screening test, it does not simulate physiologic coagulant mechanisms even as well as the PT. A severe deficiency of factor XII, for example, markedly prolongs the aPTT but does not cause a bleeding tendency. This apparent discrepancy is due to the fact that in the absence of tissue factor in vitro coagulation is initiated by factor XII that has been activated by "contact" with a negatively charged surface (e.g., glass). The lack of bleeding associated with a deficiency of factor XII, as well as other proteins activated by surface contact (high-molecular-weight kininogen and prekallikrein), confirms that this mechanism is not important for physiologic hemostasis[17,18] (see Chapter 5).

The aPTT is also prolonged by inhibitors of in vitro coagulation, some of which cause excessive bleeding and others of which do not. Clinically important examples include pathologic antibodies to factors VIII, IX, and V. Heparin is another; its presence can be readily identified by normalization of the aPTT after protamine has been added to the plasma. On the benign side are lupus anticoagulants, which prolong the aPTT but are not anticoagulants in vivo.

Inhibitors can be detected by a "mixing study," in which the patient's plasma is mixed (usually 1:1) with pooled normal plasma and is then retested with the aPTT. Because an inhibitor in the patient's plasma will inhibit the mixture as well, the aPTT of the mixture will also be prolonged, though usually not as much as the aPTT of the patient's plasma alone. In contrast, if the patient has coagulation factor deficiencies, the normal plasma will correct these sufficiently to normalize the aPTT of the mixture. A problem with this method, however, is that the definition of a "correction" after mixing is not standard: must the aPTT be within the normal range or must it only be within a few seconds of normal?

The effect of a weak inhibitor may disappear after mixing with normal plasma.

An important caveat is that, unlike other antifactor antibodies, antibodies that inhibit FVIII typically require a period of incubation in order to become apparent. Therefore, in addition to repeating the aPTT immediately after mixing the patient's plasma with normal plasma, a portion of the mixture should be allowed to incubate at 37°C for an hour and then retested with the aPTT.

The aPTT is commonly considered (naively) to be a direct and precise measurement of the antithrombotic activity of heparin, and the clinical goal is to achieve a certain "therapeutic" level, which is usually approximately 1.5 to 2.5 times a "control" value. However, there are several important details underlying this practice that should be appreciated by clinicians who prescribe heparin.[19] Although it is counterintuitive, the prolongation of an in vitro clotting time does not necessarily correlate well with the in vivo activity that arrests thrombosis (as illustrated by factor XII deficiency). In fact, the "therapeutic" or "antithrombotic" dose of heparin was determined by clinical trials that ultimately related clinical outcome to plasma heparin concentration (i.e., units/mL), which was measured by an assay specific for heparin (protamine titration).[20] Therefore, in order to use the aPTT to monitor heparin dosage, each laboratory must determine the range of its aPTT that represents a "therapeutic" heparin concentration.[19,20] By the protamine titration method this range is 0.2 to 0.4 IU/mL and by assay of antifactor Xa activity (amidolytic) it is 0.3 to 0.6 IU/mL. These concentrations might or might not correspond to the commonly referenced goal of 1.5 to 2.5 times a control value. The aPTT is, therefore, a surrogate that is useful for monitoring heparin but has its limitations.

Another important detail is the definition of "control" value. There is sometimes confusion about whether this represents the patient's preheparin aPTT or something else. By the standard definition, however, the "control" aPTT is the mean of the laboratory's normal range for aPTT.[20]

There are also in vivo factors that make the aPTT a less than perfect assay for heparin. Some patients exhibit "heparin resistance," by which is meant that they need an inordinate dose of heparin (e.g., >35,000 units/day) to achieve a therapeutic aPTT.[21] While some of these cases are the result of high levels of heparin binding proteins in the plasma (e.g., platelet factor 4), others are due to elevations of factor VIII, an acute phase reactant that tends to shorten the aPTT but does not reduce the in vivo effectiveness of heparin. In the latter instance, raising the dose of heparin may lead to excessive plasma heparin levels and increase the risk of hemorrhage. The cause of heparin resistance can be clarified by a direct measurement of heparin concentration by one of the methods mentioned above.[19]

Use of the PT and aPTT in Making Clinical Decisions

Although the PT and aPTT are designed to detect as many clinically significant coagulation abnormalities as possible, there are some hemorrhagic diatheses that are missed by these screening tests, and conversely the PT and/or aPTT can be abnormal when no hemorrhagic diathesis exists (Table 2–2). The hemorrhagic risk associated with a prolongation of the PT or aPTT depends upon the underlying factor deficiency(ies), which must be documented with specific assays.[22] The risk obviously also depends on the nature of the hemostatic challenge—e.g., a skin biopsy vs. a tonsillectomy. When single factors are decreased, the risk of bleeding can be predicted from the study of individuals with inherited coagulation factor deficiencies[23] (see Chapter 5). However, when the screening tests are abnormal because of reductions in multiple factors, which is typically the case in acquired coagulopathies, the bleeding risk is not as well established.[24] Nevertheless, clinical observations suggest that if PT and aPTT are less than 1.5 times the mid-normal range, the risk of excessive hemorrhage is minimal.[25–31] Patients taking warfarin, for example, who have an INR of 1.5 can safely have major surgery, and liver biopsies can be performed without completely correcting the PT[22,32] (see Chapter 30). However, the risk of bleeding will be increased by other factors, such as platelet dysfunction (from the use of nonsteroidal anti-inflammatory drugs or the presence of renal insufficiency), ongoing fibrinolysis (as with disseminated intravascular coagulation), or anatomic lesions (such as a gastrointestinal tumor). Therefore, the importance of moderate prolongations of the PT and aPTT must be judged in light of all available clinical information.

Occasionally the PT or aPTT will be shorter than normal, and the question is whether this signifies hypercoagulability. In fact, short aPTTs are not rare in hospitalized patients and are associated with a worse prognosis, including thrombosis, and short PT and aPTTs can both be associated with disseminated intravascular coagulation.[33,34] However, there is no evidence that anticoagulation should be initiated simply because a short clotting time is discovered. A common cause for a short aPTT is elevation of levels of factor VIII, which is also

---

Table 2–2 • USES AND LIMITATIONS OF THE PT AND aPTT IN CLINICAL DECISION-MAKING

Hemorrhagic diatheses with normal PT and/or aPTT
Mild von Willebrand disease or hemophilia
Platelet dysfunction
α_2-Antiplasmin deficiency
Dysfibrinogenemia
Monoclonal gammopathy
Factor XIII deficiency
Vascular or connective tissue abnormalities (see Chapter 11)

Conditions with abnormal screening tests but no hemorrhagic diathesis
Factor XII deficiency
Prekallikrein deficiency
High-molecular-weight kininogen deficiency
Mild to moderate factor VII deficiency
Lupus anticoagulants
Excess citrate anticoagulant (e.g., with hematocrit >60%)

an acute phase reactant.[35] Epidemiologic studies have shown that patients who have had deep venous thrombosis tend to have higher levels of factor VIII than control groups, but an *episodic* elevation of factor VIII is not known to be an independent risk factor for thrombosis.[36] A short PT may be related to an in vitro problem, such as partial activation of factor VII due to an inadequately siliconized tube, or to a traumatic venipuncture, which causes limited activation of coagulation.[37,38] Although higher concentrations of factor VII, prothrombin, and fibrinogen have all been associated with a thrombotic tendency in epidemiologic studies, the implicated levels of these factors are still within the normal range and do not produce a short PT or aPTT.[39,40]

Thrombin Clotting Time

The thrombin clotting time is the simplest clotting assay. It measures only the rate of conversion of fibrinogen to polymerized fibrin in response to added thrombin. As such, it is only sensitive to the concentration and function of fibrinogen and to inhibitors of the conversion reaction. Therefore, it may be prolonged by hypofibrinogenemia, dysfibrinogenemia, heparin (extremely sensitive), fibrin(ogen) degradation products, and high concentrations of immunoglobulin (e.g., in Waldenstrom macroglobulinemia). In addition, patients who have been exposed to topical bovine thrombin may have antibodies that inhibit the clotting time if bovine thrombin is used in the assay.[41]

Fibrinogen Concentration

Fibrinogen is routinely quantitated by an assay that is a variation of the thrombin clotting time. The effect of potential inhibitors, particularly heparin, is minimized by diluting the plasma and using a relatively high concentration of thrombin. This functional assay, however, will not distinguish between hypofibrinogenemia and dysfibrinogenemia. This requires a measurement of fibrinogen mass by either immunologic or chemical methods, both of which are more laborious than the functional test.

Tests for Lupus Anticoagulants

Lupus anticoagulants (LAs) are antibodies to complexes of phospholipid proteins, most commonly β_2-glycoprotein I, that interfere with the in vitro formation of prothrombinase. They cause prolongation of coagulation assays dependent upon phospholipid, such as the aPTT. As discussed above, LA activity persists in a 1:1 mixture of patient plasma and pooled normal plasma. However, if the mixture includes thawed plasma that contained even a few platelets when it was frozen, enough platelet fragments (phospholipid) may be present to adsorb the antibody, resulting in a normal aPTT for the mixture.

Identification of an LA requires demonstrating that the inhibitory activity of the antibody is affected by the amount of phospholipid present in the test mixture. When the phospholipid concentration in a clotting assay is relatively low, the apparent activity of the LA is enhanced. When the phospholipid concentration is relatively high, the activity of the LA is less apparent or even disappears. However, because LAs vary in their reactivity with different lipids, several different assays may be necessary to be certain that an LA is not missed.[42]

The tissue thromboplastin inhibition test accentuates the activity of an LA by using a relatively low concentration of thromboplastin in a prothrombin time assay.[43] However, this test will also be positive when other anticoagulants, such as heparin or specific factor inhibitors, are present or if coagulation factor deficiencies are present. In contrast, in the platelet neutralization test, platelet lysate (a source of phospholipid) is added to the test plasma to determine whether this will shorten the aPTT of the plasma.[43] If it does, the characteristic interaction between an LA and lipid has been demonstrated. A variation of this assay is based upon adding hexagonal phase phospholipid, which is arranged in tubules with the hydrophobic head groups facing inward, in contrast to the more familiar lipid bilayers.[44] The hexagonal configuration is particularly effective in countering LA activity. The commercial assay using hexagonal phase phospholipid is made even more specific by supplementing the patient's plama with normal plasma to replace any factor deficiencies that might confuse the result.

Another commonly used test for LAs is based upon the dilute Russell's viper venom time (dRVVT).[45] Russell's viper venom activates factor X to initiate coagulation, which then depends upon calcium and phospholipid added to the plasma. An advantage of the dRVVT is that it is not affected by deficiencies or inhibitors of factors VII, VIII, IX, XI, and XII (Fig. 2–2). If the dRVVT of the patient's plasma is prolonged, the test must be repeated with a larger amount of lipid (of plant or animal origin), which will shorten the clotting time close to that of normal plasma if an LA is present.[42, 45]

Specific Factor Assays

Routine assays of specific coagulation factors depend upon the availability of plasma samples completely lacking a single factor. These are usually obtained through commercial sources from individuals with inherited factor deficiencies. In the assay the missing factor is supplied by the plasma of the patient under study or by pooled normal plasma (by definition containing 100% of all factors). Therefore, samples of deficient plasma are mixed with varying amounts (dilutions) of patient or normal plasma, and clotting times (PT or aPTT) are measured for each. Patient and normal results are compared. For example, if the clotting time of the patient plasma mixture is the same as the clotting time of a mixture containing a quarter as much normal plasma, the patient's factor level is 25%. By generating a standard curve based upon pooled normal plasma, a factor concentration can be extrapolated for any patient result.

Sometimes the presence of a coagulation inhibitor, such as an LA, can be suspected from the results of a factor assay if serial dilutions of each patient plasma are tested. Diluting the plasma also dilutes any inhibitor, allowing the underlying activity of the coagulation factor to emerge. Therefore, if the calculated factor concentration increases with increasing dilutions of patient plasma, the likely cause is dilution of an inhibitor.

The standard assay for factor XIII is a screening test that is performed quite differently from other factor assays. The patient's plasma is first clotted in the presence of calcium to activate factor XIII. The clot is then placed in a solution of 5 M urea or 1% monochloroacetic acid and observed. Dissolution of the clot in less than 24 hours indicates poor cross-linking of the polymerized fibrin and therefore a probable deficiency of factor XIII, which must be confirmed with a more specific assay.

Factor VIII Inhibitor Assay

The most commonly used test for a factor VIII inhibitor (polyclonal IgG) is the Bethesda assay.[46] A variation of this assay can be used for factor IX inhibitors as well. Various amounts of patient plasma (prepared by serial dilution with buffer) are incubated with pooled normal plasma (a source of factor VIII) for 2 hours at 37°C. During this time the patient's inhibitor reduces the activity of the factor VIII in the normal plasma. Then aPTTs are performed on the plasma mixtures to determine the residual factor VIII activity. The inhibitor, quantitated in Bethesda units, is expressed as the reciprocal of the dilution of patient plasma that reduces the factor VIII of the normal plasma by 50%. For example, if a mixture of one part patient plasma and three parts normal plasma (i.e., a 1:4 dilution of patient plasma) lost half of its factor VIII activity (compared to a control incubated with buffer instead of patient plasma) after 2 hours of incubation, the titer of the patient's factor VIII inhibitor would be 4 Bethesda units. In practice the results from several dilutions of the patient plasma are necessary to extrapolate the dilution that reduces the factor VIII by exactly 50%.

Evaluation of von Willebrand Factor

Von Willebrand factor (vWF) function is routinely measured as "ristocetin cofactor" activity. Ristocetin is an antibiotic that allows vWF to bind to and agglutinate either fresh or fixed platelets. In this assay dilutions of a patient's plasma are mixed with platelets and ristocetin and the lag time to agglutination is measured. The same procedure is also performed with pooled normal plasma, which contains 100% vWF. By comparing the lag times of the patient's diluted plasma with those for normal plasma, the concentration of vWF in the patient sample can be estimated. VWF antigen can also be measured, and its pattern of multimers is analyzed by electrophoresis in agarose gels. The details of these specialized tests are discussed more fully in Chapter 7.

ASSAYS OF THE NATURAL ANTICOAGULANT PROTEINS

The natural anticoagulant proteins, antithrombin and proteins C and S, are most easily measured with functional assays using automated technology. The common functional antithrombin assays measure the inhibition of a known quantity of thrombin added to heparinized plasma and therefore reflect antithrombin's heparin cofactor activity, which is reduced when antithrombin is either quantitatively (type 1 deficiency) or qualitatively (types 2 and 3 deficiencies) abnormal. The most common inherited abnormalities of antithrombin, however, are defects in the heparin-binding domain of antithrombin (type 3 deficiency), which at least in the heterozygous state are rarely associated with thrombosis. Therefore, to assess the thrombotic risk associated with a deficiency of heparin cofactor activity, additional testing is necessary to determine whether antithrombin protein is low (an immunologic assay) or whether the thrombin binding ability of the molecule is impaired (an assay of antithrombin activity in the absence of heparin).[47]

To quantitate protein C functionally the protein must first be activated in patient plasma with thrombin and thrombomodulin or with a snake venom extract. What is actually measured is the ability of the activated protein C to prolong the aPTT (i.e., inactivate factors Va and VIIIa) of normal plasma that has been depleted of protein C.[48]

Quantitation of protein S function is based upon its activity as a cofactor for activated protein C. Activated protein C and factor Va (a substrate for activated protein C) are added to patient plasma, and clotting is initiated by adding calcium. The clotting time depends upon the amount of protein S supplied by the patient's plasma.[49] Immunologic assays of protein S must consider the fact that approximately 60% of the protein is normally inactivated by binding to the complement regulatory protein C4b-binding protein. The unbound (active) and bound forms can be separated by precipitating the latter with polyethylene glycol.[50]

LABORATORY EVALUATION OF PLATELET FUNCTION

Platelet Concentration

Platelet concentration is measured electronically by instruments that detect the cells by their effect on electrical impedance or light scatter. The optical method is more specific since it identifies platelets by their cytoplasmic granularity, whereas impedance technology measures all particles of a given size and therefore may include red cell fragments and exclude very large platelets. Both methods, however, will register a low platelet count if the cells are clumped together. This phenomenon causes "pseudothrombocytopenia," which results from in vitro platelet agglutination occurring in EDTA, the standard anticoagulant for blood counts.[51] Although automated instruments may detect the possibility that this has occurred, clumping must be confirmed by reviewing a peripheral blood smear. The newest automated technology is based upon identifying platelets with fluorescent monoclonal antibodies to the platelet glycoprotein IIIa. This may allow easy detection of platelet clumping.

Template Bleeding Time

Intuitively the template bleeding time would seem to be the most reliable assessment of an individual's hemostatic capacity. Unfortunately it is not.[52] The test was designed to measure primary hemostasis, which depends upon platelet number and function and upon the constriction of the microvasculature. However, the bleeding time does not reliably predict the extent of surgical bleeding and should not be used in presurgical screening.[52,53] On the other hand, it can be useful in suggesting platelet pathology or von Willebrand disease in patients who have already demonstrated a tendency to bleed easily.[54] Note that in this instance it is the history that predicts surgical bleeding, not the bleeding time.

The test is performed by making a shallow incision on the volar surface of an arm maintained at a constant venous pressure of 40 mm Hg with a sphygmomanometer. The size of the cut is controlled with a template of various designs. Every 30 seconds blood oozing from the wound is gently removed by blotting with filter paper until the bleeding stops (typically 3 to 10 minutes). In addition to the factors mentioned above, the bleeding time is affected by the size and number of cut blood vessels, which depend upon the microanatomy of the dermis and subcutaneous tissue and therefore upon age, sex, and body habitus. Therefore, many determinants dispose the bleeding time to poor reproducibility and wide variability among individuals with intact hemostatic mechanisms.

Platelet Function Studies

The traditional laboratory analysis of platelet function is based upon platelet aggregation in response to certain agonists. Although the patterns of aggregation are assumed to reflect platelet physiology, interpretation of the results is complicated by the nonphysiologic in vitro environment of the tested sample, which is hypocalcemic (i.e., anticoagulated with citrate), alkalotic (i.e., equilibrated with room air), platelet-rich plasma (not whole blood) that is rapidly swirling (i.e., not in laminar flow) in a glass cuvette (i.e., not a vascular lumen).[55] A more recent version of this technique uses whole blood and is presumably more physiologic since it allows for possible effects of red and white cells on platelet function.[56] The latest methods measure how quickly platelets plug small holes coated with platelet agonists such as collagen and ADP.[14,57] These systems use whole blood at high shear rates in an effort to simulate physiologic conditions even more closely. Although these newer techniques are promising, their superiority to the traditional platelet aggregation tests is not yet established. Therefore, the following discussion will concentrate on the more commonly used platelet aggregation studies.

Platelet aggregation is usually monitored by light transmission (but electrical impedance methods are also available) through stirred platelet-rich plasma.[58-61] The aggregation responses of a patient's platelets must be compared to those of normal platelets. A problem, however, is that the response of normal individuals is variable. The individual chosen to be the test's "control" typically has vigorous responses to all agonists and therefore this is an appropriate test of the reagents but does not accurately reflect the "normal range." The normal range for a response must be determined in each laboratory by testing many individuals who deny any evidence of abnormal bleeding (despite significant challenges) and who are not taking any medication known to affect platelet function.

Since the platelet responses being tested require metabolic energy, the blood must be freshly collected. The platelet suspension is prepared by gentle centrifugation, adjusted to a standardized platelet count, and placed in the light path of an aggregometer. An agonist is then added, usually ADP, epinephrine, collagen, thrombin, or arachidonic acid. Initially the suspension transmits relatively little light. As the cells are stimulated, their shape changes from discoid to spherical, and the turbidity of the suspension increases slightly (Fig. 2-3). Then the cells begin to form aggregates, which deflect less light, and the suspension becomes clearer. Eventually the aggregates become large enough to be seen by the unaided eye.

Platelet secretion of ATP (from their dense granules) can be simultaneously monitored as luminescence during the course of aggregation if luciferin and luciferase are initially added to the cell suspension in a lumiaggregometer.[60,62] The temporal relationship between platelet aggregation and ATP secretion depends upon the agonist (Figs. 2-3 and 2-4). Thrombin and arachidonic acid cause ATP release that coincides with cell aggregation, whereas ADP and epinephrine stimulate an initial ("primary") wave of aggregation that precedes ATP secretion and is followed by a larger ("secondary") wave that coincides with ATP release (Fig. 2-3).[63-65] With the latter agonists the two waves are often difficult to distinguish, but simultaneous monitoring of ATP secretion identifies the appearance of the second one (Fig. 2-3).

The response to collagen depends upon the dose used. At lower concentrations (e.g., 1 to 2 μg/mL) only a fraction of the platelets are activated by binding to collagen fibrils. The collagen-bound cells release thromboxane A_2, which stimulates and aggregates platelets nearby. With higher doses of collagen there is a greater opportunity for more platelets to be directly activated by collagen and less dependence upon thromboxane A_2 synthesis.[54]

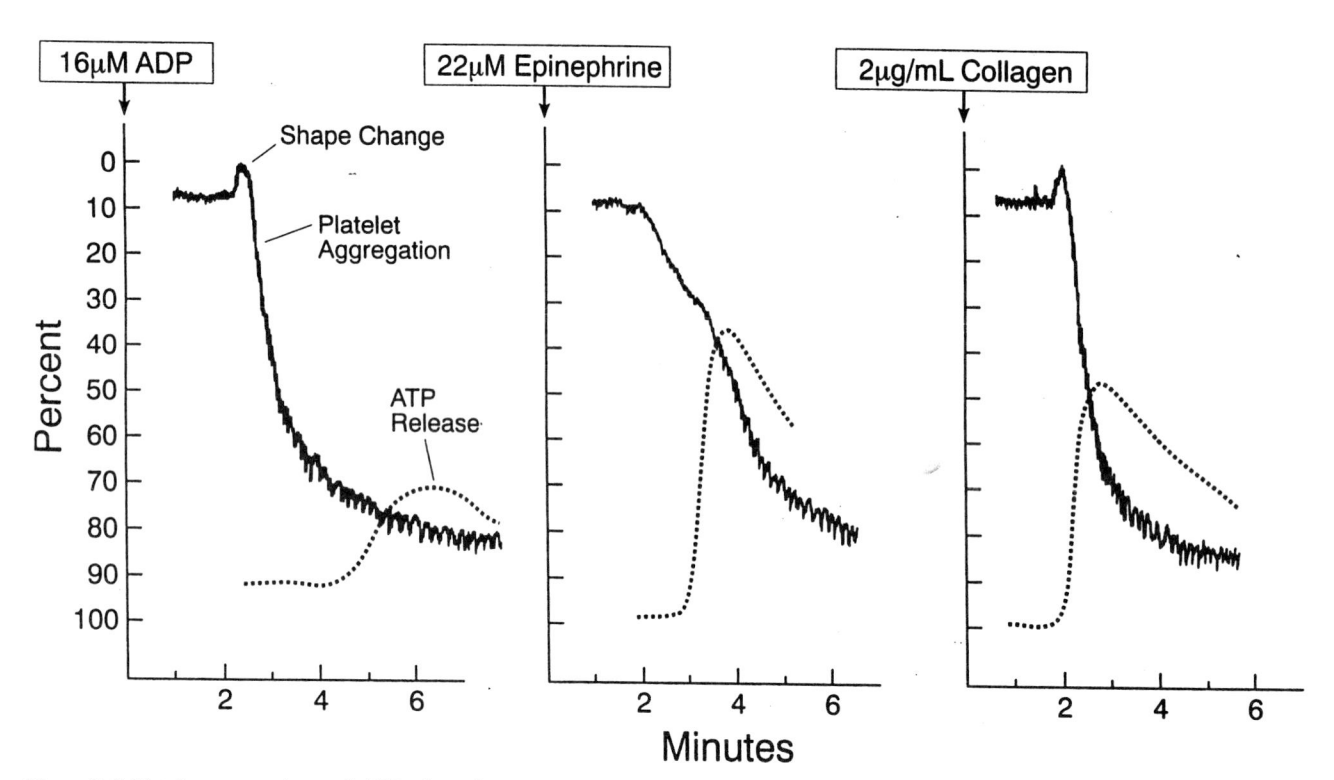

Figure 2–3 Platelet aggregation and ATP release in response to ADP, epinephrine, and collagen. The primary and secondary waves of ADP-induced aggregation (*left panel*) are merged, but the secondary wave can be recognized by the ATP release. Two waves are distinguishable with epinephrine (*middle panel*); ATP release coincides with the second wave. With collagen (*right panel*) there is only one wave of aggregation, and this appears simultaneously with ATP release. Shape change is induced by ADP and collagen but not by epinephrine.

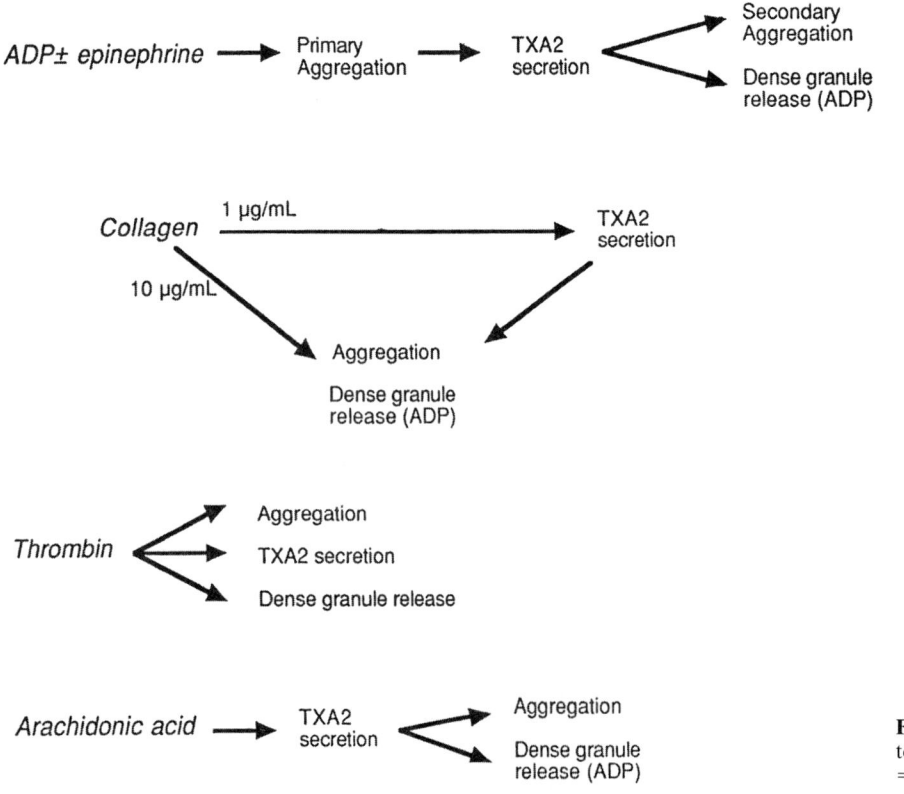

Figure 2–4 Platelet reaction in response to commonly employed agonists. (TXA2 = thromboxane A_2)

Platelets from normal individuals vary considerably in their in vitro response to ADP and epinephrine.[66,67] Members of some families have no response to epinephrine at all yet have no bleeding tendency.[68] Stimulation with ADP is more reliable and offers the possibility of examining the entire repertoire of platelet responses one phase at a time. In an aggregometer ADP generates a shape change (small, transient increase in turbidity) followed by one wave of aggregation (decreasing turbidity) and then another superimposed one that coincides with platelet secretion (Fig. 2–3). The response to epinephrine is similar except that there is no shape change. The collagen response is preceded by a lag phase, during which collagen is polymerizing. Collagen causes shape change followed by a single wave of aggregation simultaneous with secretion of the dense granular contents (e.g., ADP, ATP). The importance of the response to arachidonic acid is that it tests the integrity of the metabolic pathway leading to thromboxane A_2. This pathway is inhibited by aspirin and other nonsteroidal anti-inflammatory drugs. Therefore, aspirin will eliminate not only the response to arachidonic acid but also the thromboxane A_2-dependent secondary waves stimulated by ADP and epinephrine and the thromboxane A_2-dependent portion of the single wave stimulated by low doses of collagen (Fig. 2–4).

Different pathologic defects are characterized by different patterns of aggregation (Table 2–3).[69,70] Rare patients may have significantly reduced or abnormal receptors for collagen or epinephrine, and accordingly their platelets respond poorly to these agonists but normally to other stimulants.[71,72] Patients with Glanzmann's thrombasthenia have absent or abnormal binding sites for fibrinogen, which is essential for cross-linking platelets into aggregates, and therefore none of the agonists make their platelets aggregate. The most common platelet function abnormalities, however, are defects in the ability of the cells to secrete their dense granules, either because the granules are absent or because defects in the thromboxane A_2 pathway (e.g., inhibition of cyclo-oxygenase by aspirin) block the secretory mechanisms[45,73] (see Chapter 10).

Serum Thrombopoietin

Measurement of serum thrombopoietin has become increasingly available to evaluate thrombocytopenia and thrombocytosis. Thrombopoietin appears to be produced constitutively and to be largely bound to megakaryocytes. During amegakaryocytic thrombocytopenia the total mass of platelets and megakaryocytes, and therefore thrombopoietin binding sites, is low, and the concentration of unbound (i.e., serum) thrombopoietin is elevated.[74–76] In contrast, when thrombocytopenia is caused by peripheral destruction of platelets (e.g., in idiopathic thrombocytopenic purpura), thrombopoietin is adsorbed to the expanded megakaryocyte mass, and serum thrombopoietin is low. This relationship, however, does not extend to thrombocytosis, in which thrombopoein levels are frequently high, regardless of whether the thrombocytosis is primary or reactive.[77] Therefore, thrombopoietin levels are more helpful in evaluating thrombocytopenia than thrombocytosis. Because thrombopoietin is synthesized in the liver, liver disease may result in a lower serum level and confuse its interpretation.[76]

Platelet Evaluation by Flow Cytometry

Although flow cytometric evaluation of platelets is not widely available, its potential clinical applications are significant.[78,79] By using a fluorescent dye that binds to RNA, young platelets can be identified. Analogous to the red cell reticulocyte count, the concentration of "reticulated" platelets reflects the level of thrombopoiesis and can be used in evaluating the etiology of thrombocytopenia and to detect early marrow recovery after ablative regimens.[80,81] Although electronically measured mean platelet volume gives similar information, it is subject to in vitro changes and is therefore less reliable.[82] Using fluorescent monoclonal antibodies, rare platelet membrane disorders can be diagnosed and antiplatelet antibodies can be detected.[67,68] Other proteins are present only on the surface of stimulated platelets, and their detection with fluorescent monoclonal antibodies is a

Table 2–3 • PATTERNS OF AGGREGATION IN DIFFERENT PATHOLOGIC DEFECTS

	Aggregation Response					
	ADP	Epinephrine	Collagen (2 µg/mL)	Thrombin	Arachidonic Acid	ATP Release
Agonist receptor defect						
Epinephrine	N	A	N	N	N	N
Collagen	N	N	A	N	N	N
Secretion disorders						
Deficient dense granules	D	D	D	N	D	A
Abnormal secretory mechanism	D	D	A	N	A	A
Deficient fibrinogen receptor (Glanzmann)	A	A	A	A	A	N

N, normal; D, decreased; A, absent.

method for studying in vivo platelet activation. Storage pool deficiency can be documented with mepacrine, a fluorescent material that selectively accumulates in platelet dense granules.[83]

Plasma Glycocalicin

Glycocalicin is a carbohydrate-rich fragment of the platelet membrane glycoprotein Ib and can be detected in plasma by enzyme-linked immunosorbent assay (ELISA).[84–86] Its plasma concentration increases with increased platelet turnover. Although not yet widely available, glycocalicin measurements can be used to evaluate the mechanism of thrombocytopenia.

ASSAYS OF THE FIBRINOLYTIC SYSTEM

Laboratory evaluation of the fibrinolytic system is problematic. There is no screening test comparable to a PT or aPTT for the coagulation system. Attempts to develop global assays have not been satisfactory. A traditional one has been the euglobulin clot lysis time, which measures plasminogen activation but ignores inhibitors of fibrinolysis that are critical in vivo. What is available are assays of individual reactants and products in the fibrinolytic scheme. The most commonly used test is a measure of fibrin degradation products.

Fibrin(ogen) Degradation Products

Fibrin(ogen) degradation products (FDP) are routinely measured with FDP-specific antibodies bound to latex beads. In the presence of FDP the beads agglutinate to form macroscopic aggregates. Although ELISAs are more quantitative, they are also far more laborious and do not yield significantly greater information for clinical purposes. The antibodies used in the assays are of critical importance. The older assays for FDP employ polyclonal antibodies that detect not only all degradation products but undegraded fibrinogen as well. They can only be used to test serum, since any trace of residual fibrinogen will give a false positive result.

Newer assays use monoclonal antibodies that only detect epitopes on the degradation products and therefore can be used to test either serum or plasma.[87] These assays measure either a degradation product shared by both fibrin (FbDP) and fibrinogen (FgDP) or a product of fibrinogen only or fibrin only. The most commonly used assay measures D-dimer, which is a product of cross-linked fibrin.[88] If separate assays for FbDP and FgDP are used, fibrinogenolysis can be distinguished from fibrinolysis. In practice, however, the value of making this distinction is rarely significant. High levels of rheumatoid factor may give false positive results in any of these tests.

D-dimer assays can also used in evaluating patients for deep venous thrombosis. While their sensitivity is high, however, their specificity is low. Therefore, a negative result rules out thrombosis, but a positive result does not necessarily confirm the diagnosis.[89] Only recently has a rapid assay (i.e., performed in less than an hour) with high sensitivity (approximately 100%) become available, making the use of D-dimer quantitation truly useful in evaluating outpatients and avoiding more expensive and/or invasive procedures.[89,90]

Measurement of Reactants in Fibrinolysis

A variety of functional and immunologic assays are available to quantitate plasminogen, α_2-antiplasmin (α_2-AP), tissue plasminogen activator (tPA), and plasminogen activator inhibitor-1 (PAI-1) in plasma. Perhaps the most useful is the functional assay of α_2-AP, which can be deficient on an inherited or acquired basis and a cause of bleeding. Plasminogen analysis is only important in the search for rare causes of thrombophilia (hypofibrinolysis) or to determine whether plasminogen deficiency underlies a patient's apparent resistance the thrombolytic therapy. PAI-1 and tPA assays should only be used as research tools since their role in clinical diagnosis and treatment decisions is currently unclear.[91]

■ REFERENCES

Chapter 2 References

1. Shattil SJ, Kashiwagi H, Pampori N. Integrin signaling: the platelet paradigm. Blood 1998;91:2645–2657.
2. Kulkarni S, Dopheide SM, Yap CL, et al. A revised model of platelet aggregation. J Clin Invest 2000;105:783–791.
3. Watson SP, Gibbins J. Collagen receptor signalling in platelets: extending the role of the ITAM. Immunol Today 1998;19:260–264.
4. Gibbins JM, Okuma M, Farndale R, et al. Glycoprotein VI is the collagen receptor in platelets which underlies tyrosine phosphorylation of the Fc receptor γ-chain. FEBS Lett 1997;413:255–259.
5. Brass LF, Manning DR, Cichowski K, et al. Signaling through G proteins in platelets: to the integrins and beyond. Thromb Haemost 1997;78:581–589.
6. Luscher EF, Weber S. The formation of the haemostatic plug—a special case of platelet aggregation. Thromb Haemost 1993;70:234–237.
7. Morrissey JH, Macik BG, Neuenschwander PG, et al. Quantitation of activated factor VII levels in plasma using a tissue factor mutant selectively deficient in promoting factor VII activation. Blood 1993;81:734–744.
8. Butenas S, van't Veer C, Mann KG. "Normal" thrombin generation. Blood 1999;94:2169–2178.
9. Mann KG. The assembly of blood clotting complexes on membranes. TIBS 1987;12:229–233.
10. Chandler WL. The human fibrinolytic system. Crit Rev Oncol/Hematol 1996;24:27–45.
11. Owen CA. Historical account of tests of hemostasis. Am J Clin Pathol 1990; 93 (suppl 1):S3–S8.
12. Mallett SV, Cox DJA. Thromboelastography. Br J Anaesth 1992;69:307–313.
13. Shore-Lesserson L, Manspeizer HE, DePerio M, et al. Thromboelastography-guided transfusion algorithm reduces transfusions in complex cardiac surgery. Anesth Analg 1999;88:312–319.

14. Li CKN, Hoffmann TJ, Hsieh P-Y, et al. The Xylum Clot Signature Analyzer™: a dynamic flow system that simulates vascular injury. Thromb Res 1998;92:S67–S77.
15. Fairweather RB, Ansell J, van den Besselaar AMHP, et al. College of American Pathologists conference XXXI on laboratory monitoring of anticoagulant therapy. Arch Pathol Lab Med 1998;122:768–781.
16. Kovacs MJ, Wong A, MacKinnon K, et al. Assessment of the validity of the INR system for patients with liver impairment. Thromb Haemost 1994;71:727–730.
17. Colman RW. Biologic activities of the contact factors in vivo. Thromb Haemost 1999;82:1568–1577.
18. Abildgaard CF, Harrison J. Fletcher factor deficiency: family study and detection. Blood 1974;43:641–644.
19. Brill-Edwards P, Ginsberg JS, Johnston M, et al. Establishing a therapeutic range for heparin. Ann Intern Med 1993;119:104–109.
20. Hyers TM, Agnelli G, Hull RD, et al. Antithrombotic therapy for venous thromboembolic disease. Chest 1998;114:561S–578S.
21. Levine MN, Hirsh J, Gent M, et al. A randomized trial comparing activated thromboplastin time with heparin assay in patients with acute venous thromboembolism requiring large daily doses of heparin. Arch Intern Med 1994;154:49–56.
22. Kitchens CS: Prolonged activated partial thromboplastin time of unknown etiology: a prospective study of 100 consecutive cases referred for consultation. Am J Hematol 1988;27:38–45.
23. Roberts HR, Bingham MD. Other coagulation factor deficiencies. In Loscalzo J, Schafer AI (eds): Thrombosis and Hemorrhage (2nd ed), Baltimore, Williams & Wilkins, 1998, pp 773–802.
24. Burns ER, Goldberg SN, Wenz B. Paradoxic effect of multiple mild coagulation factor deficiencies on the prothrombin time and activated partial thromboplastin time. Am J Clin Pathol 1993;100:94–98.
25. Rustad H, Myhre E. Surgery during anticoagulant treatment. Acta Med Scand 1963;173:115–119.
26. Ciavarella D, Reed RL, Counts RB, et al. Clotting factor levels and the risk of diffuse microvascular bleeding in the massively transfused patient. Br J Haematol 1987; 67:365–368.
27. McVay PA, Toy PTCY. Lack of increased bleeding after liver biopsy in patients with mild hemostatic abnormalities. Am J Clin Pathol 1990; 94:747–753.
28. McVay PA, Toy PTCY. Lack of increased bleeding after paracentesis and thoracentesis in patients with mild coagulation abnormalities. Transfusion 1991;31:164–171.
29. Kearon C, Hirsh J. Management of anticoagulation before and after elective surgery. N Engl J Med 1997;336;1506–1511.
30. Devani P, Lavery KM, Howell CJT. Dental extractions in patients on warfarin: is alteration of anticoagulant regime necessary? Br J Oral Maxil Surg 1998;36:107–111.
31. Wahl MJ. Dental surgery in anticoagulated patients. Arch Intern Med 1998;158:1610–1616.
32. Gazzard BG, Henderson JM, Williams R. The use of fresh frozen plasma or a concentrate of factor IX as replacement therapy before liver biopsy. Gut 1975;16:621–625.
33. Reddy NM, Hall SW, MacKintosh FR. Partial thromboplastin time. Prediction of adverse events and poor prognosis by low abnormal values. Arch Intern Med 1999;159:2706–2710.
34. Bick RL. Disseminated intravascular coagulation: pathophysiologic mechanisms and manifestations. Semin Thromb Hemost 1998;24:3–18.
35. Edson JR, Krivit W, White JG. Kaolin partial thromboplastin time: high levels of procoagulants producing short clotting times or masking deficiencies of other procoagulants or low concentrations of anticoagulants. J Lab Clin Med 1967;70:463–470.
36. Koster T, Blann AD, Briet E, et al. Role of clotting factor VIII in effect of von Willebrand factor on occurrence of deep-vein thrombosis. Lancet 1995;345:152–155.
37. Palmer RN, Gralnick HR. Cold-induced contact surface activation of the prothrombin time in whole blood. Blood 1982; 59:38–42.
38. Miller GJ, Bauer KA, Barzegar S, et al. The effects of quality and timing of venepuncture on markers of blood coagulation in healthy middle-aged men. Thromb Haemost 1995;73:82–86.
39. Meade TW, Ruddock V, Stirling Y, et al. Fibrinolytic activity, clotting factors, and long-term incidence of ischaemic heart disease in the Northwick Park Heart Study. Lancet 1993;342:1076–1079.
40. Simioni P, Tormene D, Manfrin D, et al. Prothrombin antigen levels in symptomatic and asymptomatic carriers of the 20210A prothrombin variant. Br J Haematol 1998;103:1045–1050.
41. Ortel TL, Charles LA, Keller FG, et al. Topical thrombin and acquired coagulation factor inhibitors: clinical spectrum and laboratory diagnosis. Am J Hematol 1994;45:128–135.
42. Brandt JT, Barna LK, Triplett DA. Laboratory identification of lupus anticoagulants: results of the second international workshop for identification of lupus anticoagulants. Thromb Haemost 1995;74:1597–1603.
43. Triplett DA, Brandt JT, Kaczor D, et al. Laboratory diagnosis of lupus inhibitors: a comparison of the tissue thromboplastin inhibition procedure with a new platelet neutralization procedure. Am J Clin Pathol 1983;79:678–682.
44. Rauch J, Tannenbaum M, Janoff AS. Distinguishing plasma lupus anticoagulants from anti-factor antibodies using hexagonal (II) phase phospholipids. Thromb Haemost 1989;62:892–896.
45. Triplett DA. Use of the dilute Russell viper venom time (dRVVT): its importance and pitfalls. J Autoimmun 2000;15:173–178.
46. Kessler CM. An introduction to factor VIII inhibitors: the detection and quantitation. Am J Med 1991;91(suppl 5A): 1S–5S.
47. Blajchman MA, Austin RC, Fernandez-Rachubinski F, et al. Molecular basis of inherited human antithrombin deficiency. Blood 1992; 80:2159–2171.
48. Martinoli J-L, Stocker K. Fast functional protein C assay using Protac, a novel protein C activator. Thromb Res 1986;43:253–264.
49. Wolf M, Boyer-Neumann C, Martinoli J-L, et al. A new functional assay for human protein S activity using activated factor V as substrate. Thromb Haemost 1989;62:1144–1145.
50. Edson JR, Vogt JM, Huesman DA. Laboratory diagnosis of inherited protein S deficiency. Am J Clin Pathol 1990;94:176–186.
51. Bizzaro N. EDTA-dependent pseudothrombocytopenia: a clinical and epidemiological study of 112 cases, with 10-year follow-up. Am J Hematol 1995;50:103–109.
52. Rogers RPC, Levin J. A critical reappraisal of the bleeding time. Semin Thromb Hemost 1990;16:1–20.
53. Peterson P, Hayes TE, Arkin CF, et al. The preoperative bleeding time test lacks clinical benefit. Arch Surg 1998;133:134–139.
54. Nieuwenhuis HK, Akkerman J-W N, Sixma JJ. Patients with a prolonged bleeding time and normal aggregation tests may have storage pool deficiency: studies on one hundred six patients. Blood 1987;70:620–623.
55. Han P, Ardlie NG. The influence of pH, temperature, and calcium on platelet aggregation: maintenance of environmental pH and platelet function for *in vitro* studies in plasma stored at 37°C. Br J Haematol 1974;26:373–389.
56. Abbate R, Favilla S, Boddi M, et al. Factors influencing platelet aggregation in whole blood. Am J Clin Pathol 1986;86:91–96.
57. Mammem EF, Comp PC, Gosselin R, et al. PFA-100™ System: a new method for assessment of platelet dysfunction. Semin Thromb Hemost 1998;24:195–202.
58. Yardumian DA, Mackie IJ, Machin SJ. Laboratory investigation of platelet function: a review of methodology. J Clin Pathol 1986;39:701–712.
59. Remaley AT, Kennedy JM, Laposata M. Evaluation of the clinical utility of platelet aggregation studies. Am J Hematol 1989;31:188–193.
60. Holmsen H. Significance of testing platelet function in vitro. Eur J Clin Invest 1994;24(suppl 1):3–8.

61. Storey RF, Heptinstall S. Laboratory investigation of platelet function. Clin Lab Haem 1999;21:317–329.
62. Gould SJ, Subramani S. Firefly luciferase as a tool in molecular and cell biology. Anal Biochem 1988;175:5–13.
63. Charo IF, Feinman RD, Detwiler TC. Interrelations of platelet aggregation and secretion. J Clin Invest 1977;60:866–873.
64. Charo IF, Feinman RD, Detwiler TC. Prostaglandin endoperoxides and thromboxane A_2 can induce platelet aggregation in the absence of secretion. Nature 1977;269:66–69.
65. Kinlough-Rathbone RL, Reimers HJ, Mustard JF, et al. Sodium arachidonate can induce platelet shape change and aggregation which are independent of the release reaction. Science 1976;192:1011–1012.
66. Rossi EC, Louis G. A time-dependent increase in the responsiveness of platelet-rich plasma to epinephrine. J Lab Clin Invest 1975;85:300–306.
67. Johnson M, Ramey E, Ramwell PW. Sex and age differences in human platelet aggregation. Nature 1975;253:355–357.
68. Scrutton MC, Clare KA, Hutton RA, et al. Depressed responsiveness to adrenaline in platelets from apparently normal human donors: a familial trait. Br J Haematol 1981;49:303–314.
69. Day HJ, Rao AK. Evaluation of platelet function. Semin Hematol 1986;23:89–101.
70. Zucker MB. Platelet aggregation measured by the photometric method. Meth Enzymol 1989;69:117–133.
71. Arai M, Yamamoto N, Moroi M, et al. Platelets with 10% of the normal amount of glycoprotein VI have an impaired response to collagen that results in a mild bleeding tendency. Br J Haematol 1995;89:124–130.
72. Rao AK, Willis J, Kowalska MA, et al. Differential requirements for platelet aggregation and inhibition of adenylate cyclase by epinephrine. Studies of a familial platelet $alpha_2$-adrenergic receptor defect. Blood 1988;71:494–501.
73. Lages B, Weiss HJ. Heterogeneous defects of platelet secretion and responses to weak agonists in patients with bleeding disorders. Br J Haematol 1988;68:53–62.
74. Emmons RVB, Reid DM, Cohen RL, et al. Human thrombopoietin levels are high when thrombopoietin is due to megakaryocyte deficiency and low when due to increased platelet destruction. Blood 1996;87:4068–4071.
75. Porcelijn L, Folman CC, Bossers B, et al. The diagnostic value of thrombopoietin level measurements in thrombocytopenia. Thromb Haemost 1998;79:1101–1105.
76. Koike Y, Yoneyama A, Shirai J, et al. Evaluation of thrombopoiesis in thrombocytopenic disorders by simultaneous measurement of reticulated platelets of whole blood and serum thrombopoietin concentrations. Thromb Haemost 1998;79:1106–1110.
77. Cerutti A, Custodi P, Duranti M, et al. Thrombopoietin levels in patients with primary and reactive thrombocytosis. Br J Haematol 1997;99:281–284.
78. Michelson AD. Flow cytometry: a clinical test of platelet function. Blood 1996;87:4925–4936.
79. Schmitz G, Rothe G, Ruf A, et al. European working group on clinical cell analysis: consensus protocol for the flow cytometric characterization of platelet function. Thromb Haemost 1998;79:885–896.
80. Ault KA, Rinder HM, Mitchell J, et al. The significance of platelets with increased RNA content (reticulated platelets). Am J Clin Pathol 1992;98:637–646.
81. Harrison P, Robinson MSC, Mackie IJ, et al. Reticulated platelets. Platelets 1997;8:379–383.
82. Jackson SR, Carter JM. Platelet volume: laboratory measurement and clinical application. Blood Rev 1993;7:104–113.
83. Gordon N, Thom J, Cole C, et al. Rapid detection of hereditary and acquired platelet storage pool deficiency by flow cytometry. Br J Haematol 1995;89:117–123.
84. Steinberg MH, Kelton JG, Coller BS. Plasma glycocalicin, an aid in the classification of thrombocytopenic disorders. N Engl J Med 1987;317:1037–1042.
85. Steffan A, Pradella P, Cordiano I, et al. Glycocalicin in the diagnosis and management of immune thrombocytopenia. Eur J Haematol 1998;61:77–83.
86. Fabris F, Cordiano I, Steffan A, et al. Indirect study of thrombopoiesis (TPO, reticulated platelets, glycocalicin) in patients with hereditary macrothrombocytopenia. Eur J Haematol 2000;64:151–156.
87. Amiral J, Grosley M, Mimilla F, et al. Monoclonal antibodies to different neo-epitopes on fibrinogen and fibrin degradation products. Blood Coag Fibrinol 1990;1:447–452.
88. Gaffney PJ. D-dimer. History of the discovery, characterization and utility of this and other fibrin fragments. Fibrinolysis 1993;7(suppl 2):2–8.
89. Freyburger, G, Trillaud, H, Labrouche, S, et al. D-dimer strategy in thrombosis exclusion. Thromb Haemost 1998;79:32–37.
90. Perrier, A, Desmarais, S, Miron M-J, et al. Non-invasive diagnosis of venous thromboembolism in outpatients. Lancet 1999;353:190–195.
91. Chandler WL, Trimble SL, Loo S-C, et al. Effect of PAI-1 levels on the molar concentrations of active tissue plasminogen activator (t-PA) and t-PA/PAI-1 complex in plasma. Blood 1990;76:930–937.

CHAPTER 3

A Systematic Approach to the Bleeding Patient

Minetta C. Liu, M.D.
Craig M. Kessler, M.D.

The evaluation of patients with hemorrhagic complications is a multistep process that involves a complete history, a detailed physical examination, and a directed laboratory evaluation. The relative emphasis placed on each of these components varies according to each unique clinical situation, but all factors must be considered. Important points of differentiation include localized defects vs. systemic defects, acquired defects vs. inherited defects, and disorders of primary hemostasis (i.e., those related to platelet abnormalities) vs. disorders of secondary hemostasis (i.e., those related to coagulation factor, fibrinogen, or connective tissue abnormalities).

This chapter offers a systematic approach to the patient with either a clinically significant risk of bleeding or an immediate history of spontaneous, excessive hemorrhage. It is important to understand that some clinical situations will not allow for the full comprehensive evaluation and may therefore require a more streamlined approach. An intubated patient who has developed brisk bleeding in the immediate postoperative period, for example, will not be able to provide any information about his personal or family history; a determination of this patient's most likely cause for bleeding will therefore rest on the pertinent physical and laboratory findings. Of primary importance for all consulting hematologists is a realization that the management of coagulation abnormalities—which are often epiphenomena or complications of other medical illnesses—is often empirical and cannot always be approached by a standard algorithm.

THE CLINICAL EVALUATION

Each component of the clinical assessment provides critical information that either supports or excludes the possibility that a true hemorrhagic disorder actually exists. The information garnered from the history and physical examination ultimately guides the direction and extent of the laboratory evaluation and also helps in determining how future bleeding complications can be managed and/or prevented. This multifactorial approach is necessary because the likelihood of false-positive and false-negative diagnoses is high when the decision rests on one component alone. Consider, for example, the process required in order to obtain an accurate medical history. A patient's perception of his or her own bleeding tendency is often either exaggerated or understated: in one study, 65% of women and 35% of men without a laboratory-confirmed bleeding disorder answered the questions as if they did have a bleeding diathesis, while 38% of the women and 54% of the men who had documented von Willebrand disease (vWD) or a documented qualitative platelet disorder answered the questions as if they were completely unaware of their bleeding diathesis.[1]

Obtaining a Detailed History

Several authors have formulated basic comprehensive questionnaires in an effort to simplify and standardize the evaluation of individuals with easy bruising or bleeding.[1–3] The format of these questionnaires generally involves the use of binary (i.e., yes or no) questions that elicit immediate, unambiguous responses from patients; quantitative and qualitative qualifiers are used where appropriate. Examples of questions effectively applied to the present history could include the following:

Have you ever experienced a serious hemorrhagic complication during or after a surgical procedure? The initial assessment of postoperative bleeding complications should differentiate between incomplete surgical ligation or cauterization of blood vessels and the presence of an underlying defect in hemostasis. Clinical suspicion for a bleeding diathesis should be substantiated with objective evidence from the case in question: a description of all wounds and venipuncture sites, an evaluation of all laboratory abnormalities (e.g., worsening anemia, thrombocytopenia, or alterations in the prothrombin time or activated partial thromboplastin time), calculations of the estimated blood loss and subsequent transfusion requirements, knowledge of the means required to stop the bleeding, and documentation of a prolonged hospital stay. In addition, the timing of the hemorrhagic complication in relation to the procedure (i.e., immediate vs. delayed) can provide important clues as well. Intraoperative and immediate postoperative bleeding at the surgical site are often due to defects in primary hemostasis—that is, abnormalities of platelet number, adhesion, and/or aggregation (Table 3–1). In contrast, delayed postoperative bleeding at the surgical site is typically due to coagulation factor deficiencies, qualitative or quantitative disorders of fibrinogen, or vascular abnormalities related to defects in collagen structure (Table 3–2); notably, factor XIII deficiency, fibrinogen deficiency, and several of the collagen disorders are often marked by poor wound healing and subsequent wound dehiscence as well. Furthermore, excessive bleeding from the umbilical cord stump at birth and/or bleeding from the circumcision site are strongly indicative of a severe inherited disorder, whereas bleeding related to abdominal or cardiothoracic surgery in a previously "normal" adult is not. Nevertheless, a number

Table 3–1 • DISORDERS OF PRIMARY HEMOSTASIS

Hereditary Disease States
von Willebrand disease
Glanzmann's thrombasthenia
Bernard-Soulier syndrome
Platelet storage pool disease
Gray platelet syndrome
Wiskott-Aldrich syndrome
May-Hegglin anomaly

Iatrogenic Disease States
Post-transfusion purpura
Drug-induced immunologic thrombocytopenia (e.g., quinine, heparin, sulfonamide antibiotics)
Drug-induced qualitative platelet disorders (e.g., aspirin, NSAIDs, ticlopidine, abciximab, mithramycin)

Acquired Disease States
Autoimmune thrombocytopenic purpura
Disseminated intravascular coagulation
Systemic amyloidosis
Hypersplenism
Aplastic anemia
Uremia
Mechanical platelet destruction from turbulent circulation (e.g., cardiac bypass, severe aortic stenosis)

Primary hemostasis involves formation of the platelet plug. The above is a representative list of potential causes of abnormalities in platelet number, adhesion, or aggregation.

Table 3–2 • DISORDERS OF SECONDARY HEMOSTASIS

Coagulation Factor Abnormalities
Hemophilia A (factor VIII deficiency)
Hemophilia B (factor IX deficiency)
Deficiencies in factor II, V, VII, or X
Acquired inhibitors to specific coagulation factors (e.g., factor VIII or factor V inhibitors)
Factor XIII deficiency

Contact Factor Abnormalities
Factor XI deficiency

Fibrinogen Abnormalities
Afibrinogenemia
Hypofibrinogenemia
Inherited dysfibrinogenemias
Hyperfibrinolysis

Connective Tissue Disorders
Ehlers-Danlos Syndrome
Osler-Weber-Rendu syndrome (hereditary hemorrhagic telangiectasia)
Scurvy (vitamin C deficiency)

Secondary hemostasis involves humoral coagulation subsequent to formation of the platelet plug. The above is a representative list of potential causes of abnormalities in coagulation factors, contact factors, fibrinogen, or the connective tissues.

of cases of factor XI deficiency, mild vWD, and mild Ehlers-Danlos syndrome have escaped diagnosis until later in life when the defect in hemostasis is manifested as mucosal surface bleeding during or after routine surgery.

Have you ever experienced excessive vaginal bleeding immediately after childbirth or perineal bleeding from an episiotomy? Multiparous women should be questioned about each pregnancy in detail with regard to both complications and outcomes. Obstetric histories are particularly important because multiple spontaneous miscarriages and infertility can be associated with both congenital maternal coagulopathies (e.g., factor XIII deficiency and the dysfibrinogenemias) and some acquired syndromes (e.g., anticardiolipin/antiphospholipid syndrome). Interestingly, women who either have mild or moderate vWD or who are carriers of hemophilia A typically do not experience easy bruising or bleeding manifestations during pregnancy, during the delivery, or when they are taking such estrogen-containing compounds as oral contraceptives or hormone replacement therapy. This is most likely related to the increased synthesis of von Willebrand factor (vWF) and factor VIII as acute phase reactant proteins in response to high-estrogen states; the activity levels of these factors begin to fall immediately postpartum and do not reach baseline for weeks (or even longer in women who are nursing). In addition, acquired autoantibodies directed against factor VIII may occur within the first year postpartum after an otherwise normal delivery; this acquired, postpartum hemophilia is marked by pronounced bleeding and bruising as well as by spontaneous remissions and rare recurrences with subsequent pregnancies.[4]

Have you experienced persistent menorrhagia in the absence of fibroids or other uterine abnormalities? Menstrual histories often provide useful clues for an underlying hemostatic defect, particularly in those women with persistent menorrhagia and/or a microcytic anemia despite adequate iron supplementation. A history of severe iron deficiency in a young woman, the use of packed red blood cell transfusions for an anemia of unknown etiology, the need for a dilation and curettage procedure for persistent uterine bleeding, or the need for a hysterectomy to treat menorrhagia should increase the suspicion for an underlying defect in hemostasis. In fact, recent surveys suggest that a significant number of hysterectomies for menorrhagia are performed in women with vWD.[5] Unfortunately, each woman's definition of menorrhagia can be somewhat vague. Numerous bleeding scales have been devised to circumvent this variability, but they are very cumbersome to use. They all attempt to quantitate menstrual blood loss according to the duration of heavy flow (i.e., longer than 3 days), the duration of each menstrual cycle (i.e., longer than 7 days total), and the number of pads or tampons used. The accuracy of this latter factor, however, can also vary as it depends on the individual patient's hygienic habits and fastidiousness. Finally, the need for oral contraceptives to control excessive menstrual bleeding should be noted, since this may also serve as an indicator of the degree of menorrhagia and may also confound the ability to diagnose (vWD) secondary to the acute phase reactivity of the factor VIII and vWF.

Do you experience brisk or prolonged bleeding after minor cuts or exaggerated bruising after minor trauma? Excessive and persistent bleeding or oozing from a relatively minor superficial injury and the appearance of ecchymoses or purpura (especially true hematomas) following minimal trauma may be indicative of an underlying congenital or acquired hemostatic defect. For example, profuse bleeding and the need for prolonged periods of direct pressure for a small paper cut or razor nick are unusual; this crude bleeding time could be a manifestation of qualitative or quantitative platelet defects or of vWD. The loss of deciduous teeth and extractions of molar teeth are also inadvertent but accurate tests of hemostasis; again, immediate bleeding after the initial event is more consistent with a vascular or platelet abnormality, while delayed bleeding and/or rebleeding is more consistent with a coagulation factor deficiency. Finally, poor or delayed wound healing is uncharacteristic of platelet disorders but may be associated with factor XIII deficiency, hereditary dysfibrinogenemia, and Ehlers-Danlos syndrome.

Have you ever developed a hemarthrosis, retroperitoneal hematoma, or soft tissue hematoma in the absence of major trauma? These clinical events are typical manifestations of defects in secondary hemostasis—that is, problems of humoral coagulation subsequent to platelet adhesion and formation of the platelet plug. The hemophilias are good examples of this type of delayed but severe bleeding, which can persist until the involved compartment has achieved self-tamponade. Of note, individuals who develop acquired neutralizing autoantibodies against specific coagulation factors are clinically similar but not identical to those with classic hemophilia; although both patient populations usually present with extensive spontaneous bleeds in critical areas, spontaneous hemarthrosis is remarkably rare in those with acquired coagulation factor autoantibodies but very common in those with classic hemophilia.

Have you ever experienced spontaneous bleeding? A spontaneous hemorrhage is one that occurs in the absence of any identifiable trauma other than the stress of weight bearing. Bleeding that spontaneously originates from the mucous membranes—e.g., epistaxis, melena, or menorrhagia—is more commonly associated with severe thrombocytopenia (defined as a platelet count of $< 10,000/\mu L$), qualitative platelet dysfunction, or severe vWD. Spontaneous hemarthroses and intramuscular bleeds, on the other hand, are more characteristic of certain severe coagulation factor deficiencies. If bleeding is multifocal, an underlying acquired bleeding diathesis, such as disseminated intravascular coagulation, should be suspected. As in all other bleeding situations, an objective clinical and laboratory assessment is critical in order to determine the need for and type of medical intervention. In addition, hematemesis, hematochezia, melena, hemoptysis, and hematuria can occur spontaneously in confirmed hemorrhagic disorders, but a thorough investigation should be pursued in an effort to identify a critical anatomic lesion as the source of bleeding.

Has any member(s) of your family experienced severe bleeding complications, perhaps requiring transfusions of packed red blood cells? The most common congenital hemorrhagic diatheses and qualitative thrombocytopathies follow distinct patterns of inheritance (Table 3–3). One must keep in mind, however, that a negative family history does not necessarily preclude the presence of a familial disorder; patients may not be aware of their family members' medical histories, the genetic defect may be characterized by variable penetrance, the coagulation disorder may lead to a mild bleeding diathesis

---

Table 3–3 • CONGENITAL COAGULOPATHIES AND QUALITATIVE THROMBOCYTOPATHIES

Sex-Linked Recessive Disorders
Hemophilia A (factor VIII deficiency)
Hemophilia B (factor IX deficiency)
Wiskott-Aldrich syndrome

Autosomal Dominant Disorders
von Willebrand Disease
Osler-Weber-Rendu syndrome (hereditary hemorrhagic telangiectasia)
Dysfibrinogenemias

Autosomal Recessive Disorders
Deficiencies in factor II, V, VII, XI, X, or XIII
α_2-Antiplasmin deficiency
Bernard-Soulier syndrome
Glanzmann's thrombasthenia
Gray platelet syndrome
Afibrinogenemia
Hypofibrinogenemia
Type 3 von Willebrand disease

that is not always manifested clinically, or the mutation may have occurred spontaneously. Nonetheless, a careful review of the patient's pedigree may reveal the underlying inheritance pattern to be one of the following: (1) sex-linked recessive, including hemophilia A, hemophilia B, and Wiskott-Aldrich syndrome; (2) autosomal dominant, including vWD, Osler-Weber-Rendu syndrome (hereditary hemorrhagic telangiectasia), and hereditary dysfibrinogenemia; or (3) autosomal recessive, including factor II deficiency, factor VII deficiency, and Bernard-Soulier syndrome.

Do you have any known medical problems? A number of medical conditions are associated with the development of acquired defects in coagulation and/or hemostasis. One of the most well-documented associations is that between the lupus-type anticoagulants and systemic lupus erythematosus, other autoimmune disorders, medications (including phenothiazines and tricyclic antidepressants), acute infections, and some lymphoproliferative disorders. Although the lupus-type anticoagulants do prolong in vitro coagulation assays, the major risk is for thrombosis as opposed to bleeding. Hemorrhagic manifestations can occur, however, in those patients with the lupus anticoagulant who concurrently develop autoantibodies to prothrombin (resulting in a true decrease in the circulating half-life of factor II) or to platelet membrane glycoproteins (resulting in either thrombocytopenia or platelet dysfunction).

Other medical conditions associated with a potential for bleeding complications warrant mention as well. For example, catastrophic and life-threatening hemorrhagic events can occur in cases of acute promyelocytic leukemia as a result of the secondary disseminated intravascular coagulation (DIC) that is induced by the release of tissue factor from the malignant promyelocytes. Uremia secondary to renal failure, on the other hand, is associated with qualitative as opposed to quantitative platelet defects. This is in contrast to severe, end-stage hepatic dysfunction, which can lead to defects in both primary and secondary hemostasis: thrombocytopenia secondary to portal hypertension and hypersplenism; deficient synthesis and postribosomal modification of the vitamin K-dependent clotting factors; low-grade DIC secondary to the decreased clearance of activated procoagulant proteins and the decreased synthesis and clearance of such fibrinolytic modulatory proteins as α_2-antiplasmin, the primary inhibitor of plasmin; and the acquired dysfibrinogenemia of liver disease, in which increased susceptibility to fibrinolytic enzyme degradation may play a key role.[6] In addition, systemic amyloidosis is associated with the development of factor X deficiency as a result of the specific adsorption of the factor X protein by amyloid fibrils[7]; amyloid-induced gastrointestinal malabsorption syndromes may exacerbate this coagulation defect because of vitamin K deficiency. Finally, associations between Gaucher disease and factor IX deficiency and between hypothyroidism, right-to-left cardiac shunts, and Wilms' tumors and vWD have been reported, each with a different underlying etiology.

Do you take any prescription medications, over-the-counter medications, or homeopathic remedies on a regular basis? The use of warfarin or any of the heparin or heparinoid products poses obvious bleeding risks. Antiplatelet agents such as aspirin, cilostazol, clopidogrel, dipyridamole, ticlopidine, the traditional nonsteroidal anti-inflammatory drugs (NSAIDs), and the monoclonal antibody inhibitors directed against the platelet glycoprotein IIa/IIIb complex are of concern as well. Various "alternative medicines"—including the Chinese black tree fungus and large quantities of garlic, vitamin E, vitamin C, and ginger—have also been associated with abnormalities of platelet function as manifested by a prolonged bleeding time and an increased risk for clinically significant bleeding.[8] Physicians and patients alike should also be aware that certain antibiotics are notorious for their ability to affect the synthesis of the vitamin K-dependent clotting factors; cephazolin, levofloxacin, and trimethoprim/sulfamethoxazole are just a few examples. In addition, the penicillins, sulfonamides, and tricyclic antidepressants are among the medications associated with the development of factor VIII autoantibody inhibitors and the lupus-type anticoagulants. Finally, the use of iron supplements should be noted, as this may be related to a previous diagnosis of iron-deficiency anemia secondary to severe or chronic blood loss.

Have you noticed any unusual rashes or easy bruisability? Petechiae, purpura, ecchymoses, and telangiectasias are often indicative of an underlying coagulopathy or vasculitis. Individual descriptions of rashes are variable, and the definition of "easy bruisability" is entirely subjective; both should therefore be qualified with and substantiated by objective physical findings (refer to Chapter 11 for additional information). Suspicious lesions include those that develop spontaneously or with minimal trauma and those that are located over the torso rather than on the extensor surfaces of the extremities. If a patient develops a painful eschar while on warfarin, the possibility of warfarin-induced skin necrosis, a prothrombotic disorder associated with warfarin-induced deficiencies of protein C or protein S, should be considered. Of note, heparin-induced thrombocytopenia with resultant thrombosis may also be associated with severe skin manifestations, although these are typically more variable in nature.

Objective Findings on the Physical Examination

The physical examination of individuals with suspected coagulation disorders should concentrate on detecting gross evidence of bleeding and bruising. This evidence could be petechiae, purpura, ecchymoses, sites of previous or active hemorrhage, or evidence of hemarthroses or hematomas. Table 3–4 summarizes the major clinical manifestations and correlative laboratory data for some of the more common acquired causes of bleeding, particularly in patients without a previous history of hemorrhagic complications. In addition, characteristic cutaneous findings may provide clues to an underlying defect in hemostasis. Examples of this include the following: the joint laxity, skin hyperelasticity, and "tissue paper-thin" scars typical of patients with Ehlers-Danlos syn-

Table 3-4 • ACQUIRED CAUSES OF BLEEDING IN AMBULATORY PATIENTS

Diagnosis	Manifestation	Confirmation
Thrombocytopenia	Petechial bleeding	Platelet count <20,000/μL
Scurvy	Subcutaneous bleeding, especially in confluent sheets	Normal platelet count, dietary history
Acquired hemophilia	Soft tissue hemorrhage	Low factor VIII activity with factor VIII antibody; rarely antibodies to factor V, XI, or XIII
Antibodies against factor II and/or V following use of "fibrin glue"	Soft tissue hemorrhage	History of recent use of "fibrin glue" using bovine products; low levels of factor II and V with antibodies
Amyloidosis	Soft tissue hemorrhage	Variable factor levels; fat pad biopsy for amyloid
Vitamin K deficiency	Soft tissue hemorrhage, hematuria	Dietary history, long PT, PTT; normal TT; low factor II, VII, IX, X levels
Warfarin ingestion[a,b]	Soft tissue hemorrhage, hematuria	Drug history; low factor II, VII, IX, X levels; long PT, PTT; normal TT
Heparin administration[a,c]	Soft tissue hemorrhage	Long PT, PTT; very long TT, heparin level
Factitious purpura	Bizarre pattern of lesions	Normal studies; psychological studies

[a] Inadvertent or surreptitious.
[b] Also caused by "superwarfarin" rodentocide exposure.
[c] Rare cases of heparin production in systemic mastocytosis.

drome; the follicular keratoses, perifollicular purpura with associated "corkscrew hairs," and diffuse petechiae characteristic of patients with vitamin C deficiency and scurvy; the subcutaneous extravasation of blood, "loose-fitting skin," and loss of the subcutaneous fat pad seen in patients with senile purpura; the skin fragility and purplish striae (usually located on the flexor and extensor surfaces of the upper and lower extremities and on the torso) typical of patients with Cushing syndrome; and the macroglossia and nonthrombocytopenic purpura often seen in patients with systemic amyloidosis (see Chapter 11).

Petechiae measure less than 3 mm in diameter, while purpura and ecchymoses both measure greater than 3 mm in diameter. These cutaneous lesions result from the rupture of venules, capillaries, or arterioles in the skin and may be related to a qualitative or quantitative platelet abnormality or vasculitis. Nonetheless, some bruising can occur in the absence of an increased risk of hemorrhage: purpura simplex, a common and predominantly female phenomenon marked by excessive bruising in relation to menses; senile purpura, marked by the development of irregular, reddish-purple ecchymoses on the extensor surface of the upper extremities as a result of the decreased elasticity of blood vessels and subcutaneous fat with age; and psychogenic purpura, marked by bruises that repeatedly occur in areas accessible to the patient, persist for months with a denial of repeated trauma, and resolve only after casting of the affected limb.

Telangiectasias, on the other hand, are blanching lesions frequently detected under the tongue and on the face, oral and nasal mucosa, vermilion border of the lips, chest wall, shoulders, legs, and nail beds. These lesions can occur in association with the normal aging process, with estrogen surges secondary to pregnancy or the use of oral contraceptives or estrogen replacement therapy, with underlying liver disease, and with some of the collagen vascular diseases (e.g., the CREST syndrome, which is characterized by $c$alcinosis, Raynaud's phenomenon, $e$sophageal disease, $s$clerodactyly, and $t$elangiectasias). Mucosal and visceral telangiectasias, on the other hand, are the hallmarks of Osler-Weber-Rendu syndrome (hereditary hemorrhagic telangiectasia) and serve as potential sources of bleeding, arteriovenous malformation, or aneurysms.

THE BASIC LABORATORY EVALUATION

While the findings derived from a comprehensive and careful clinical assessment may increase clinical suspicion for a particular hemorrhagic disorder, laboratory confirmation is required in order to define the specific defect and develop a logical treatment strategy. Basic, readily available, and easily performed screening tests can be used to distinguish between the broad categories of primary hemostatic defects (i.e., platelet disorders) and the humoral coagulation disorders (Table 3-5). Subsequently, more specialized and esoteric assays can be selected to establish the definitive diagnosis (Table

Table 3-5 • BASIC SCREENING TESTS FOR PATIENTS WITH HEMORRHAGIC COMPLICATIONS

Automated complete blood cell count (with platelet count and mean platelet volume)
Peripheral blood smear review
Bleeding time
Prothrombin time (PT)
Activated partial thromboplastin time (aPTT)
Plasma clot solubility assay
Fibrin clot retraction assay

32 PART I   General Information

Table 3-6 • SPECIFIC LABORATORY ASSAYS FOR PATIENTS WITH HEMORRHAGIC COMPLICATIONS

For Suspected Platelet Disorders
Platelet aggregation studies
Bone marrow aspirate and biopsy
Platelet-associated immunoglobulin levels
Electron microscopy for platelet morphology

For Suspected Coagulation Factor Abnormalities
Mixing studies
Fibrinogen levels, D-dimer levels
Specific clotting factor levels
Bethesda assay (for coagulation factor inhibitors)
Thrombin time
Reptilase time
Euglobulin clot lysis assay
Molecular and immunologic fibrinogen assays

Basic Laboratory Tests to Distinguish Between Platelet and Coagulation Defects

A platelet abnormality should be suspected in patients with a history of intraoperative or immediate postoperative hemorrhagic complications, frequent mucosal bleeds in the absence of known trauma, and/or a persistent petechial rash. Quantitative platelet abnormalities are immediately apparent once an *automated blood cell count* is performed and the patient's *peripheral blood smear* is reviewed. Thrombocytopenia, defined as a platelet count of less than 150,000/µL, should be confirmed by direct observation to exclude the laboratory phenomenon of pseudothrombocytopenia,[9-12] in which platelet clumping occurs in vitro in a temperature- and time-dependent manner in the presence of EDTA; the mean platelet volume (MPV) is therefore increased as the clumps of platelets are "sized" as single platelets as they pass through the aperture of automated cell counters. Repeat platelet counts in freshly collected, citrate-anticoagulated whole blood should provide substantially higher, more accurate values because the platelet agglutination in pseudothrombocytopenia typically results from the chelation of calcium ions by the standard EDTA anticoagulant. Phase or manual platelet counts should also reveal more accurate platelet counts

3-6). The panel of tests typically required includes some combination of the following: a complete blood cell count, examination of the peripheral blood smear, a bleeding time, the prothrombin time (PT), the activated partial thromboplastin time (aPTT), the thrombin time, and the fibrinogen concentration. Examples of laboratory profiles for some of the more frequently encountered hemorrhagic disorders are provided in Table 3-7.

Table 3-7 • LABORATORY PROFILES FOR SELECTED DISORDERS ASSOCIATED WITH A DEFECT IN HEMOSTASIS[a]

	Platelet Count	Platelet Size or Morphology	Bleeding Time	PT/INR	aPTT	Plasma Clot Solubility Assay	Standard Platelet Aggregation Studies	Mixing Studies	Fibrinogen Levels	Thrombin Time	Euglobulin Clot Lysis Assay
Disseminated intravascular coagulation	↓	NL	(↑)	(↑)	(↑)	acc	N/I	(+)	(↓)	(↑)	(acc)
Idiopathic thrombocytopenic purpura	↓	abnl	(↑)	NL	NL	NL	N/I	N/I	NL	NL	NL
von Willebrand disease, type 2B	V	abnl	↑	NL	(↑)	NL	abnl*	+	NL	NL	N/I
von Willebrand disease, other	NL	NL	(↑)	NL	(↑)	NL	abnl*	+	NL	NL	N/I
Glanzmann's thrombasthenia	NL	NL	↑	NL	NL	NL	abnl	N/I	NL	NL	N/I
Wiskott-Aldrich syndrome	↓	abnl	(↑)	NL	NL	NL	(abnl)	N/I	NL	NL	N/I
Bernard-Soulier syndrome	↓	abnl	↑	NL	NL	NL	abnl*	N/I	NL	NL	N/I
Gray platelet syndrome	↓	abnl	↑	NL	NL	NL	V	N/I	NL	NL	N/I
Afibrinogenemia/hypofibrinogenemia	NL	NL	(↑)	↑	↑	NL	(abnl)	(+)	↓	↑	(acc)
Congenital dysfibrinogenemias	NL	NL	NL	(↑)	(↑)	NL	(NL)	−	(↓)	↑	acc
Ehlers-Danlos syndrome	NL	NL	(↑)	NL	NL	NL	(abnl)	N/I	NL	NL	NL

[a] Refer to Table 1 of Chapter 5 for a summary of the clotting factor deficiencies.

↑, increased; ↓, decreased; NL, normal laboratory values; abnl, abnormal laboratory test results in favor of the abnormality; *, deficient platelet aggregation by ristocetin only, with normal aggregation to ADP, epinephrine, and collagen; V, results are variable; (), usually but not always; N/I, not indicated; acc, accelerated; +, corrects upon mixing; −, does not correct upon mixing.

since the actual platelet count can be ascertained visually whether or not clumping is present. Finally, platelet size and morphology may help to differentiate between peripheral platelet destruction (which is marked by a higher MPV and an increase in platelet size) and decreased bone marrow production.[13] A morphologic evaluation of the peripheral smear may also distinguish between various congenital etiologies of thrombocytopenia: the gray, vacuolated platelets seen in α-granule deficiency; the basophilic cytoplasmic inclusion bodies (Döhle bodies) found in the granulocytes of patients with the May-Hegglin anomaly; and the microplatelets characteristic of Wiskott-Aldrich syndrome are only a few examples.

If a patient's clinical picture is consistent with a defect in primary hemostasis and the platelet count is within normal limits, a qualitative platelet abnormality should be excluded. The *bleeding time* is a useful screening test in this regard because it allows for a gross indication of overall platelet function and of the activity of those plasma proteins involved in the interaction between platelets and the endothelium (e.g., vWF). The bleeding time is usually normal with platelet counts over 100,000/μL, and it is usually prolonged proportionally as platelet counts decrease from 100,000/μL to 10,000/μL.[14] In idiopathic thrombocytopenic purpura (ITP), however, the bleeding time may be normal despite a quantitative deficiency; this may reflect the fact that the younger, more rapidly generated platelets are larger and "more active" in their capacity to adhere to areas of damaged endothelium and to aggregate with each other to form a platelet plug.

The Duke bleeding time, which involves a prick or incision of the earlobe, was described in 1910 and represents the first recognized method of determining the bleeding time.[15] Over the years, modifications of this test have been proposed in an attempt to improve its sensitivity and reproducibility.[16] The Ivy and Simplate II techniques are the most commonly employed to date. Essentially, a blood pressure cuff is inflated on the upper arm to maintain a consistent pressure of 40 mm Hg. A standardized puncture wound (for the Ivy technique) or vertical incision (for the Simplate II technique) is then made on the ventral aspect of the forearm with a mechanical stylet or spring-loaded razor blade, respectively. Freely dripping blood from the immediate periphery of the wound or incision is blotted every 30 seconds with filter paper, and the time required for the formation of a platelet plug and the cessation of bleeding is recorded as the bleeding time.[17] The "normal" bleeding time varies between 2 to 9 minutes, depending on the exact technique used. In addition, the validity of this test relies on several operator-dependent factors, including the depth of the puncture wound, the length of the incision, the ability to maintain a constant venous pressure, and the method of blotting; there is no question that the bleeding time is reliable only if the test is done carefully by an experienced individual who pays close attention to the proper technique. Standardized, automated techniques have also been designed that examine platelet adhesion to collagen-coated capillary tubes as a means of monitoring and quantitating the degree of in vitro platelet aggregation in response to various agonists[18]; these assays are becoming more widely available, but their exact role in the assessment of bleeding complications remains to be determined (see Chapter 35).

The *prothrombin time* (PT) is an ex vivo coagulation assay performed by adding a commercial source of tissue factor and calcium to the patient's citrate-anticoagulated plasma. The resultant clotting time is traditionally described as a global reflection of the activities of the coagulation factors involved in the common and extrinsic pathways of coagulation—factor V, factor X, prothrombin, fibrinogen, and factor VII. The tissue factor/thromboplastin preparations typically used to activate the clotting process are currently available as standardized reference reagents derived from rabbit brain extracts. Recombinant human tissue factor preparations are also becoming increasingly available, and the PT measured with this source of tissue factor is probably the most reliable in terms of assessing true coagulation factor levels in variants of factor VII deficiency.[19] Other sources of tissue factor do exist, but they are typically used in more specialized circumstances; ox brain sources of tissue factor/thromboplastin, for example, are particularly useful in the detection of the rare congenital coagulopathy, variant factor VII Padua.[20]

Because the numerous tissue factor/thromboplastin reagents possess different procoagulant properties, PT results can vary widely from one laboratory to another—even for the same plasma specimen. The automated machines used for the assay also contribute to this variability. The *International Normalized Ratio* (INR) was developed in order to minimize these differences such that the dose of warfarin can be reliably adjusted regardless of where the PT assay is performed. Each thromboplastin reagent has a unique International Sensitivity Index (ISI), which is derived by comparing its prothrombotic potential against a standard with an ISI of 1.0. The variability seen with the PT results is minimized by calculating the INR as a ratio of the patient's PT to the mean normal PT obtained from pooled normal plasma, which is then raised to the ISI as an exponential power: INR = (patient's PT/mean normal PT)^{ISI}. Although the INR is employed in the safety monitoring and efficacy evaluation of anticoagulation with warfarin, it has not been a useful predictor of potential bleeding complications in patients with either liver disease or congenital coagulopathies in the common or extrinsic pathways.

The *activated partial thromboplastin time* (aPTT), on the other hand, reflects the activities of the coagulation factors involved in the common and intrinsic pathways of coagulation—factor V, factor X, prothrombin, fibrinogen, factor VIII, factor IX, factor XI, factor XII, prekallikrein, and high-molecular-weight kininogen. It is measured by adding a source of phospholipids, a phospholipid surface activator, and calcium to citrate-anticoagulated plasma; the commercially available contact factor activators used in initiating the aPTT reaction typically consist of a phospholipid source (e.g., variable ratios of phosphatidyl serine and phosphatidyl inositol) and one of several surface activating agents (e.g., kaolin, silica, or ellagic acid). Clotting factor activity levels must be decreased to at least 40% of normal in order to affect the aPTT. In addition, a deficiency of prekallikrein, which is one of the components of the contact phase of coagulation, results in a prolonged aPTT that can be corrected with the extended incubation of the patient's plasma with an exogenous source of phospholipid and contact activator at 37°C prior to recalcification. Of note, deficiencies of factor XII, prekallikrein, and/or high-molecular-weight kininogen are not associated with a bleeding diathesis despite the fact that they are associated with prolongation of the aPTT.

Finally, the possibility of factor XIII deficiency or α_2-antiplasmin deficiency should be excluded when all of the basic screening tests are unremarkable and the clinical suspicion for a bleeding diathesis still remains. Factor XIII is a fibrin stabilizing factor that functions in the covalent cross-linking of fibrin strands in the presence of calcium and thrombin. α_2-Antiplasmin, on the other hand, functions in controlling lysis of the fibrin plug through the regulation of plasmin activity. As such, neither qualitative nor quantitative defects in factor XIII or α_2-antiplasmin can be detected by the standard assays used to evaluate clot formation—including the PT/aPTT. The *plasma clot solubility assay* serves as a crude assay for factor XIII deficiency. Under normal conditions, the addition of 1% monochloracetic acid or 5 M urea will not result in dissolution of the clot; if the factor XIII activity level is less than 1%, however, the fibrin clot will rapidly dissolve. α_2-Antiplasmin deficiency may also result in increased urea clot solubility, but α_2-antiplasmin activity levels and antigen levels can and should be directly assessed in order to confirm the diagnosis.

Specialized Tests for Platelet Disorders and Abnormalities in Platelet Binding Proteins

Once a low platelet count is confirmed by direct observation of the peripheral blood smear, further investigations are necessary in order to determine the cause of thrombocytopenia: (1) decreased production due to primary bone marrow dysfunction; (2) secondary thrombocytopenia due to increased peripheral destruction as in ITP, DIC, and thrombotic thrombocytopenic purpura (TTP); or (3) secondary thrombocytopenia due to platelet sequestration by hypersplenism. Although the history and physical examination can be very helpful, an evaluation of the *bone marrow aspirate and biopsy* allows for a direct assessment of the presence or absence of megakaryocytes—often the most useful first step in the diagnostic process. If there is a concomitant macrocytic anemia, red blood cell folate levels and serum B_{12} levels should be checked in order to exclude the possibility of megaloblastic anemia. A sucrose hemolysis test and a Ham's test should also be considered in order to screen for paroxysmal nocturnal hemoglobinuria (PNH) if there is evidence of intravascular hemolysis (e.g., clinical icterus, a low serum haptoglobin, reticulocytosis, hemoglobinuria, or the detection of urinary hemosiderin) with or without evidence of systemic hypercoagulability; the diagnosis of PNH can then be confirmed by flow cytometry of the peripheral blood to assess for such specific erythrocyte membrane protein deficiencies as CD59 (MIRL, or the *m*embrane *i*nhibitor of *r*eactive *l*ysis) and CD55 (DAF, or the *d*ecay *a*ccelerating *f*actor). Finally, all patients with unusual bleeding or bruising and a concomitant malignancy, autoimmune collagen vascular disease, acute infection, liver disease, a recent history of massive trauma, or shock should be assessed for DIC by means of laboratory tests that include a fibrinogen level, quantitation of the fibrin degradation products (or the more useful D-dimer assay), the thrombin time, and the PT/aPTT.

More precise, rapidly performed, noninvasive laboratory approaches that can distinguish between thrombocytopenia secondary to peripheral platelet destruction and primary thrombocytopenia due to a hypoproliferative bone marrow are currently under investigation, but none are in widespread clinical use at this time. Various techniques for the measurement of *platelet-associated immunoglobulin levels* have not been very helpful in the diagnosis of ITP because of technical difficulties and the lack of specificity.[21,22] The measurement of *plasma glycocalicin levels,* on the other hand, has proven to be more promising in its ability to correlate low platelet counts with states of increased peripheral platelet destruction.[23,24] Glycocalicin, the carbohydrate-rich portion of platelet membrane glycoprotein Ib, is proteolytically cleaved from circulating platelets and released into the plasma such that its level increases proportionally with increasing platelet turnover. Although this assay remains investigational, it has been useful in identifying cases of thrombocytopenia secondary to such entities as DIC, ITP, and TTP.

Abnormalities of platelet function as opposed to platelet number, on the other hand, are suspected when the bleeding time is prolonged (refer to Chapter 10 for additional information); these abnormalities can involve either the platelets themselves or the plasma proteins involved in the interaction between platelets and the endothelium. The ingestion of those medications known to have antiplatelet properties—including aspirin, NSAIDs, and some homeopathic remedies—represents the most common acquired cause of an increased bleeding time. Acquired platelet defects are also seen in association with multiple myeloma, myeloproliferative disorders, and uremia, and these diagnoses should be considered given the proper clinical circumstances. Inherited qualitative platelet defects, on the other hand, are typically diagnosed during infancy or childhood and include abnormalities and/or deficiencies in platelet membrane glycoproteins (e.g., glycoprotein Ib/IX in Bernard-Soulier syndrome and glycoprotein IIb/IIIa in Glanzmann's thrombasthenia) as well as deficiencies in platelet secretory granules (e.g., the α-granules in "gray platelet syndrome" and the dense bodies in storage pool disease). Finally, the possibility of vWD must always be considered in patients with a prolonged bleeding time and a suspicious family history, as this entity can occur in up to 1% of the general population (refer to Chapter 7 for additional information). One must appreciate, however, that bleeding times may fluctuate in individuals with mild vWD such that a single normal bleeding time does not exclude the diagnosis; it is therefore recommended that three serial bleeding times be performed at 7- to 10-day intervals when vWD is suspected. Interestingly, recent clinical evidence indicates that complete normalization of the bleeding time is not required for individuals with vWD to achieve normal hemostasis with replacement therapy during routine surgery.[25, 26]

Platelet aggregation studies are readily accessible in most experienced, comprehensive coagulation laboratories and often serve as the primary means of differentiating between these various syndromes. This assay is performed by isolating platelet-rich plasma from the patient's citrate-anticoagulated whole blood at low-speed centrifugation. Standard concentrations of various agonists are added under standardized conditions of temperature and constant agitation. The stimulation of platelet aggregation in vitro is detected by the platelet aggregometer as changes in light transmission through a cuvette containing the treated platelet-rich plasma; by convention, platelet-rich plasma has 0% light transmission, and platelet-free plasma has 100% light transmission when compared to normal controls. The agonists typically used in platelet aggregation studies include adenosine diphosphate, epinephrine, and collagen, although other agents may yield characteristic patterns as well. For example, platelet aggregation studies with arachidonic acid as the agonist can be used to exclude the surreptitious ingestion of aspirin or NSAIDs as the underlying etiology of abnormal, suboptimal platelet aggregation responses to the standard agonists.

The absence of passive platelet agglutination, as opposed to platelet aggregation, in response to the addition of specific concentrations of ristocetin can be helpful, particularly in terms of differentiating between the following syndromes: the classical type 1 and type 2A variants of vWD, which usually display normal or moderately decreased responses to standard concentrations of the agonist; the type 2B variant of vWD, which is characterized by hypersensitive platelets that agglutinate in response to low concentrations of the agonist; the type 3 variant of vWD, which usually has little or no response to standard concentrations of the agonist; and Bernard-Soulier syndrome, which also demonstrates suboptimal platelet agglutination after the addition of standard concentrations of the agonist.

Normal responses in standard platelet aggregation assays will exclude most qualitative platelet defects as the primary cause of easy bruisability or abnormal bleeding, but mild vWD can remain a possibility. As with other useful laboratory studies, variations of the standard platelet aggregation assay have been devised in an effort to increase sensitivity and/or specificity. Platelet aggregation studies can be performed in the absence of an in vitro agonist, for example, to determine if there is any evidence of spontaneous platelet hyperaggregability. Other attempts to increase the sensitivity of platelet aggregation studies include the following: (1) "loading" the dense granules of platelets in platelet-rich plasma with radiolabeled ^{14}C-serotonin and monitoring its release upon platelet activation by various agents; and (2) chemiluminescent-based platelet activation assays that monitor the release of ATP from platelet dense granules. Although these techniques are not yet considered standard practice, they can be useful adjuncts to the platelet factor 4 assay in the detection of heparin-induced thrombocytopenia.[27]

Specialized Tests for Coagulation Factor Abnormalities

An abnormally prolonged PT or aPTT should be confirmed by *mixing studies,* in which the PT and/or aPTT of a 1:1 mixture of patient plasma and normal plasma is measured after 0, 60, and 120 minutes of incubation at 37°C. Complete and persistent correction of the PT and/or aPTT is indicative of a coagulation factor deficiency, considering the observation that all factor levels must be at least 40% of normal in order to attain normal coagulation times. A prolonged assay(s) that either does not correct or only temporarily corrects (i.e., one that is normal at time 0 but prolonged at time 120 minutes), on the other hand, is more consistent with either a lupus-type anticoagulant or a circulating inhibitor that neutralizes the activity of a specific coagulation protein. It should be noted that low titer and low avidity inhibitors result in modest elevations of the PT and/or aPTT and may therefore require more dilute mixtures of patient plasma with normal plasma.

Coagulation factor deficiencies can be divided conceptually into intrinsic, extrinsic, or common pathway defects according to whether the PT and/or aPTT are affected; this is despite the known biologic overlap between the different pathways (e.g., the factor VII/tissue factor complex in the extrinsic pathway can activate factor IX in the intrinsic pathway, and factor XIIa in the intrinsic pathway can activate factor VII in the extrinsic pathway). Isolated prolongation of the PT is suggestive of factor VII deficiency, while isolated prolongation of the aPTT is more consistent with a deficiency of either factor VIII, factor IX, factor XI, factor XII, high-molecular-weight kininogen, or prekallikrein. Finally, prolongation of both the PT and the aPTT can be associated with any one of the following scenarios: multiple factor deficiencies affecting the intrinsic, extrinsic, and/or common pathways of coagulation; isolated factor V deficiency; isolated factor X deficiency; isolated prothrombin (factor II) deficiency; and hypofibrinogenemia (defined as a fibrinogen level of less than 80 mg/dL). A *fibrinogen level* is often the first step toward differentiating between these conditions, as an acquired or congenital fibrinogen deficiency may be the sole explanation for these abnormal coagulation parameters. If, on the other hand, the fibrinogen level is 100 mg/dL or higher and the prolonged PT and aPTT both correct in a mixing study, the presence of one or more clotting factor deficiencies should be suspected. *Specific factor assays* should follow in an effort to pinpoint the defect, and details from the clinical history, family history, and the physical examination may help to streamline this investigation.

If the mixing studies do not correct, the presence of a circulating inhibitor is likely. Inhibitors are neutralizing antibodies directed nonspecifically or specifically against clotting factor proteins. Nonspecific inhibitors are best exemplified by anticardiolipin and antiphospholipid autoantibodies—the so-called lupus anticoagulants that are directed against such phospholipid binding proteins as prothrombin and β_2-glycoprotein I.

Specific inhibitors are either alloantibodies that develop in individuals with severe coagulation factor deficiencies after multiple exposures to specific factor replacement products (e.g., the factor VIII inhibitors encountered in patients with hemophilia A after repeated exposure to factor VIII concentrates) or autoantibodies that develop spontaneously as an autoimmune phenomenon in individuals with previously normal coagulation. The most common specific inhibitors are those against the factor VIII coagulant protein; these inhibitors are usually polyclonal IgG1 or IgG4 antibodies that do not fix complement and interact with factor VIII in a time- and temperature-dependent manner.

Specific clotting factor inhibitors may be quantified using the *Bethesda assay,* which is described below using factor VIII antibodies as an example. Patient plasma (which contains the suspected inhibitor) and control plasma (which does not contain any factor inhibitors) are each incubated with a source of normal factor VIII activity for 2 hours at 37°C; this source could be normal pooled human plasma, recombinant factor VIII concentrate, or porcine factor VIII concentrate. The residual factor VIII activity of each mixture is then measured and converted into the Bethesda inhibitor titer (Bethesda Units per milliliter), which represents the reciprocal of the patient plasma dilution that neutralizes 50% of the added factor VIII.[28] If, for example, a 1/100 dilution of patient plasma produces 50% factor VIII activity when mixed with normal pooled plasma, the inhibitor titer equals 100 Bethesda Units (BU). Of note, the *Oxford assay* has been used to quantify factor inhibitor activity in Europe and is similar to the Bethesda assay except for its 4-hour incubation period; one Oxford Unit is equivalent to 0.8 BU.[29]

An abnormal PT and/or aPTT without confirmatory laboratory evidence of either a coagulation factor deficiency or the presence of a factor inhibitor should prompt further assessment by means of the *thrombin time*. The thrombin time measures the conversion of fibrinogen to fibrin in the final stages of the coagulation pathway by determining the clotting time of undiluted plasma in the presence of excess exogenous thrombin. Of note, concomitant prolongation of the PT, aPTT, and thrombin time strongly suggests the presence of a quantitative or qualitative fibrinogen defect because all of these assays depend on the formation of a fibrin clot as their endpoint. In general, the potential causes of a prolonged thrombin time include elevated fibrinogen-fibrin degradation products or D-dimers, significantly elevated immunoglobulins, and the presence of acquired antibodies against thrombin. Most commonly, however, the thrombin time is prolonged by the presence of heparin or a heparin-like anticoagulant (e.g., hirudin) in the assay mixture. The heparin could either be an exogenous contaminant derived from an intravenous or intra-arterial access line or a constituent of the plasma sample from an anticoagulated patient. Heparin functions as a circulating inhibitor of coagulation, and its effects can be eliminated in coagulation assays with the addition of protamine sulfate or an ion exchange resin; unfortunately, there is no such neutralizing agent for hirudin. In contrast, the *reptilase time* is not affected by the presence of heparin or heparin-like anticoagulants despite the fact that it, like the thrombin time, measures the conversion of fibrinogen to fibrin. Rather, it may be prolonged in association with increased levels of fibrin or fibrinogen degradation products, the dysfibrinogenemias, and high circulating concentrations of abnormal immunoglobulins (e.g., with the monoclonal gammopathies), each of which inhibits the reptilase-induced cleavage of fibrinopeptide A from the fibrinogen α-chains.

The *euglobulin clot lysis assay* is also useful in the evaluation of qualitative abnormalities of fibrinogen. It is based on the ability of plasmin to degrade cross-linked fibrin clots and thus provides a global assessment of the fibrinolytic system. Essentially, plasma is precipitated at a low pH in order to obtain the euglobulin fraction, which predominantly consists of fibrinogen, plasminogen, plasmin, plasminogen activators, and factor XIII. Once the precipitate is redissolved, fibrin clot formation can be initiated with the addition of exogenous thrombin. Under normal conditions, the clot should remain intact for at least 2 hours. If the clot lyses within the first 30 to 60 minutes, however, the possibility of one of the following diagnoses should be entertained: hyperfibrinolysis, dysfibrinogenemia, or factor XIII deficiency.

Finally, the dysfibrinogenemias should be suspected when there is a discrepancy of more than 25% to 30% between the lower fibrinogen concentration when measured as functional protein and the higher fibrinogen concentration when measured as immunologically detectable protein. The definitive diagnosis is based on the identification of a specific structural or molecular defect: (1) confirmation of the abnormal fibrinogen structure using SDS polyacrylimide gel electrophoresis; (2) the evaluation of abnormal fibrinopeptide cleavage and release, as well as of abnormal fibrin polymerization; and (3) a detailed analysis of the mutation site in both the fibrinogen DNA and the fibrinogen gene product. Importantly, structure-function relationships in the congenital dysfibrinogenemias remain unclear and without an established means by which to predict whether or not the abnormal fibrinogen protein will be associated with hypercoagulability or with a bleeding diathesis, poor wound healing, and/or recurrent spontaneous miscarriages.

MANAGEMENT OF ACUTE HEMORRHAGIC EPISODES

It is not always possible to adhere to an algorithmic approach to the bleeding patient. This is especially true in cases of unexpected intraoperative or postoperative bleeding in which immediate intervention is required. Time may not allow for the completion of basic laboratory screening tests prior to the initiation of therapy, so the clinician is often forced to treat the patient empirically. The first priority is to exclude the possibility of incomplete surgical ligation or incomplete cauterization of blood vessels, and this can be done fairly quickly through a careful review of the immediate clinical history and a directed physical examination. Although the results of these coagulation assays are not likely to be available until after the acute situation is resolved, they should be collected prior to any intervention that could affect the results and delay confirmation of the ultimate diagnosis.

One crude but helpful bedside test is the *fibrin clot retraction assay*. This assay is performed by collecting an aliquot of the patient's blood into a plain glass tube that does not contain any anticoagulant (e.g., a serum red-top tube or capillary tube). The blood is carefully observed over time for clot formation at room temperature. A normal response is characterized by clot retraction from one wall of the glass tube, whereas altered clot structure secondary to interference with fibrin formation or with platelet aggregation is marked by gelatinous clot formation without evidence of clot retraction.[30, 31] The fibrin clot retraction assay is therefore a "quick and dirty" test for hyperfibrinolysis, hypofibrinogenemia, dysfibrinogenemia, the presence of fibrin degradation products, thrombocytopenia, and qualitative platelet disorders. It can also be affected by an elevated hematocrit, and the results of this assay should be interpreted accordingly. Interestingly, normal clot retraction may occur despite the absence of factor XIII.[32]

Empirical therapy in these acute bleeding situations typically begins with the administration of standard blood products—platelets, fresh frozen plasma, and cryoprecipitate. Single-donor or pooled random-donor *platelets* should be transfused regardless of the preoperative laboratory values, as the infusion of normal unaffected platelets will transiently compensate for any undiagnosed platelet dysfunction that may be contributing to the bleeding diathesis. This type of scenario has been associated with surgical procedures involving cardiopulmonary bypass, in which both thrombocytopenia and platelet dysfunction can occur immediately after surgery and can last for several days into the postoperative period.

Fresh frozen plasma contains physiologic levels of both the labile and stable components of the coagulation system and is indicated for the replacement of deficient coagulation factors. It may also be administered in cases of massive blood loss requiring the transfusion of more than one blood volume over 24 hours; this is because of a dilutional or "washout" phenomenon of coagulation factors and because of factor consumption from bleeding. In general, three to five units of fresh frozen plasma are needed in order to adequately replace the coagulation factors in an average sized adult (10 to 20 mL/kg body weight). Other plasma replacement products exist and may be considered for their enhanced safety profile despite the greater cost in comparison to single-donor units of fresh frozen plasma. *Solvent detergent-treated pooled frozen plasma*, for example, has an improved viral safety profile because the lipid-enveloped pathogenic blood-borne viruses—including human immunodeficiency virus, hepatitis B, and hepatitis C—are virtually eliminated in the preparative process. In the near future, *psoralen-treated pooled plasma* could provide an additional option for safe replacement therapy because of the intended removal of all nucleic acid-containing organisms. If specific deficiencies of factor VIII or IX are known to exist preoperatively, however, the corresponding *recombinant factor concentrate* should be administered in order to eliminate the potential infectious complications associated with the transfusion of blood products. In addition, recombinant factor VIIa concentrate has recently been used as replacement therapy for individuals with severe factor VIII deficiency and as a pancoagulant in bleeding patients with acquired coagulation factor inhibitors and qualitative or quantitative platelet disorders.[33-36]

Cryoprecipitate, on the other hand, is primarily used to correct quantitative or qualitative fibrinogen abnormalities. It is prepared by thawing fresh frozen plasma at 4°C and removing the supernatant. The remaining precipitate is rich in factor VIII, vWF multimers of various sizes, fibrinogen, fibronectin, and factor XIII. As a rough rule of thumb, one unit of cryoprecipitate per 7 kg of body weight is necessary to increase the plasma fibrinogen level by 75 mg/dL. Formerly, cryoprecipitate was also administered as a source of vWF protein in individuals with vWD; because of its inferior viral safety profile, however, it should be used only when intermediate-purity, viral attenuated factor VIII concentrates are not available.

If the transfusion of platelets, fresh frozen plasma, and/or cryoprecipitate is not able to reverse or prevent active bleeding, the administration of DDAVP, ε-aminocaproic acid, tranexamic acid, or topical fibrin sealants should be considered. DDAVP (1-deamino-8-D-arginine vasopression; desmopressin; Stimate) is a useful therapy for the qualitative platelet defect associated with either uremia or the ingestion of aspirin, for mild or moderately severe hemophilia A, and for vWD (especially type 1). The agent is infused at a dose of 0.3 μg/kg body weight intravenously over 15 to 30 minutes in 50 mL normal saline with a maximum total dose of 20 mg. Although its exact mechanism of action is unknown, DDAVP ultimately produces transient increases in the levels of vWF antigen, factor VIII activity, ristocetin cofactor activity, tissue plasminogen activator, and plasminogen activator inhibitor-type 1. It also increases the circulating concentration of the highest molecular weight von Willebrand factor protein multimers. Because of its antidiuretic effects, DDAVP is associated with a definite risk of water retention, which can lead to a dilutional hyponatremia and seizures—particularly in infants and the elderly; free water intake should therefore be minimized to avoid this risk. Angina pectoris and thrombotic stroke have also been reported as potential complications in older, susceptible patients. The peak drug effect occurs within 30 minutes of administration and usually lasts for at least several hours. Of note, intranasal preparations of DDAVP do exist, but their use is usually reserved for situations of chronic administration and/or prophylaxis for simple surgical procedures in patients with mild hemophilia A or vWD.

ε-aminocaproic acid (EACA; Amicar) and tranexamic acid (Cyclokapron) are antifibrinolytic agents often used in the treatment of acute, severe mucosal hemorrhages secondary to systemic hyperfibrinolysis. They are particularly useful adjunctive therapies in the management of mucosal bleeding, as they modulate the effects of the tissue plasminogen activator that is released when DDAVP is administered. These antifibrinolytic agents are generally well tolerated, although nausea, vomiting, diarrhea, dizziness, malaise, fever, rash, and transient hypotension or cardiac arrhythmias, may occur. EACA may also rarely cause rhabdomyolysis and should therefore be used with extreme caution. Importantly, neither drug should be administered to individuals who also have evidence of hypercoagulability. Finally, fibrin sealants are commercially available as topical procoagulants for active bleeding on surfaces; they are derived from plasma, are virally inactivated, and can be applied easily in the operative setting to sites of active bleeding and anastamosis (refer to Chapter 26 for additional information).[37,38]

■ REFERENCES

Chapter 3 References

1. Wahlberg T, Blomback M, Hall P, Axelsson G. Applications of indicators, predictors and diagnostic indices in coagulation disorders. I. Evaluation of a self-administered questionnaire with binary questions. Methods Inf Med 1980;19:194–200.
2. Coller B, Schneiderman PI. Clinical evaluation of hemorrhagic disorders: bleeding history and differential diagnosis of purpura. In Hoffman R, Benz EJ, Shattil SJ, et al. (eds): Hematology: Basic Principles and Practice, 2nd ed. New York, Churchill Livingstone, 1995.
3. Miller C, Graham JB, Goldin LR, Elston RC. Genetics of classic von Willebrand's disease. II. Optimal assignment of the heterozygous genotype (diagnosis) by discriminant analysis. Blood 1979; 54:137–145.
4. Michiels JJ. Acquired hemophilia A in women postpartum: clinical manifestations, diagnosis, and treatment. Clin Appl Thromb-Hemost 2000;6:82–86.
5. Kadir R, Economides DL, Sabin CA, et al. Assessment of menstrual blood loss and gynaecological problems in patients with inherited bleeding disorders. Haemophilia 1999;5:40–48.
6. Violi F, Basili S, Ferro D, et al. Association between high values of D-dimer and tissue-plasminogen activator activity and first gastrointestinal bleeding in cirrhotic patients. CALC Group, Thromb Haemost 1996;76:177–183.
7. Furie B, Voo L, McAdam K, Furie BC. Mechanism of factor X deficiency in systemic amyloidosis. N Engl J Med 1981; 304:827–830.
8. George JN, Shattil SJ. The clinical importance of acquired abnormalities of platelet function. N Engl J Med 1991;324:27–39.
9. Payne B, Pierre RV. Pseudothrombocytopenia: a laboratory artifact with potentially serious consequences. Mayo Clin Proc 1984;59:123–125.
10. Pegels J, Bruynes ECE, Engelfriet CP, et al. Pseudothrombocytopenia: an immunologic study on platelet antibodies dependent on ethylene diamine tetra-acetate. Blood 1982;59:157–161.
11. Fiorin F, Steffan A, Pradella P, et al. IgG platelet antibodies in EDTA-dependent pseudothrombocytopenia bind to platelet membrane glycoprotein IIb. Am J Clin Pathol 1998;110: 178–183.
12. Bizzaro N. EDTA-dependent pseudothrombocytopenia: a clinical and epidemiological study of 112 cases, with 10-year follow-up. Am J Hematol 1995;50:103–109.
13. Niethammer A, Forman EN. Use of the platelet histogram maximum in evaluating thrombocytopenia. Am J Hematol 1999; 60:19–23.
14. Harker L, Slichter SJ. The bleeding time as a screening test for evaluation of platelet function. N Engl J Med 1972;287:155–159.
15. Duke WW. The relation of blood platelets to hemorrhagic disease: description of a method for determining the bleeding time and coagulation time and report of three cases of hemorrhagic disease relieved by transfusion. JAMA 1910;55:1185–1192.
16. Bowie E, Owen CA Jr. Standardization of the bleeding time. Scand J Haemat Suppl 1980;37:87–94.
17. Koster T, Caekebeke-Peerlinck KMJ, Briet E. A randomized and blinded comparison of the sensitivity and the reproducibility of the Ivy and Simplate II bleeding time techniques. Am J Clin Pathol 1989;92:315–320.
18. Mammem EF, Comp PC, Gosselin R, et al. PFA-100 system: a new method for assessment of platelet dysfunction. Semin Thromb Hemost 1998;24:195–202.
19. Roberts HR, Bingham MD. Other coagulation factor deficiencies. In Loscalzo J, Schafer AI (eds): Thrombosis and Hemorrhage, 2nd ed. Philadelphia, Williams Wilkins, 1998.
20. Girolami A, Cattarozzi G, Dal Bo Zanon R, Toffanin F. Factor VII Padua 2: another factor VII abnormality with defective ox brain thromboplastin activity and a complex hereditary pattern. Blood 1979;54:46–53.
21. Warner M, Kelton JG. Laboratory investigation of immune thrombocytopenia. J Clin Pathol 1997;50:5–12.
22. Warner MN, Moore JC, Warkentin TE, et al. A prospective study of protein-specific assays used to investigate idiopathic thrombocytopenic purpura. Br J Haematol 1999;104:442–447.
23. Steffan A, Pradella P, Cordiano I, et al. Glycocalicin in the diagnosis and management of immune thrombocytopenia. Eur J Haematol 1998;61:77–83.
24. Kunishima S, Kobayashi S, Naoe T. Increased but highly dispersed levels of plasma glycocalicin in patients with disseminated intravascular coagulation. Eur J Haematol 1996;56:173–177.
25. Hanna WT, Bona RD, Zimmerman CE, et al. The use of intermediate and high purity factor VIII products in the treatment of von Willebrand disease. Thromb Haemost 1994;71:173–179.
26. Foster PA. A perspective on the use of FVIII concentrates and cryoprecipitate prophylactically in surgery or therapeutically in severe bleeds in patients with von Willebrand disease unresponsive to DDAVP: results of an international survey. On behalf of the Subcommittee on von Willebrand Factor of the Scientific

and Standardization Committee of the ISTH. Thromb Haemost 1995;74:1370–1378.

27. Walenga J, Jeske WP, Fasanella AR, et al. Laboratory tests for the diagnosis of heparin-induced thrombocytopenia. Semin Thromb Hemost 1999; 25(suppl 1):43–49.

28. Hultin M. Factor VIII inhibitor assays. In Beutler E, Lichtman MA, Coller BS, Kipps TJ (eds): Williams' Hematology, 5th ed. New York, McGraw-Hill, 1995.

29. Rizza CR, Biggs R. The treatment of patients who have factor VIII antibodies. Br J Haematol 1973;24:65–82.

30. Poppa C, Enache F. Plasma clot retraction assay with standard platelet count. Med Interne 1978;16:183–187.

31. Morgenstern E, Korell U, Richter J. Platelet and fibrin strands during clot retraction. Thromb Res 1984;33:617–623.

32. Rao KM, Newcomb TF. Clot retraction in a factor XIII free system. Scand J Haemost 1980;24:142–148.

33. Hedner U, Glazer S, Pingel K, et al. Successful use of recombinant factor VIIa in a patient with severe hemophilia A during synovectomy. Lancet 1988;ii:1193.

34. Lusher JM. Recombinant factor VIIa (Novoseven) in the treatment of internal bleeding in patients with factor VIII and IX inhibitors. Haemostasis 1996;26(suppl 1):124–130.

35. Kristensen J, Killander A, Hippe E, et al. Clinical experience with recombinant factor VIIa in patients with thrombocytopenia. Haemostasis 1996;26(suppl 1):159–164.

36. Peters M, Heijboer H. Treatment of a patient with Bernard Soulier syndrome and recurrent nosebleeds with recombinant factor VIIa. Thromb Haemost 1998;80:352.

37. Dunn CJ, Goa KL. Fibrin sealant: a review of its use in surgery and endoscopy. Drugs 1999;58:863–886.

38. Jackson MR, Alving BM. Fibrin sealant in preclinical and clinical studies. Curr Opin Hematol 1999;6:415–419.

PART II

Hemorrhagic Processes

CHAPTER 4

Hemophilia A and B

Alice J. Cohen, M.D.
Craig M. Kessler, M.D.

INTRODUCTION/EPIDEMIOLOGY/GENETICS

The hemophilias are the best known of the hereditary bleeding disorders. Hemophilia A arises secondary to congenital deficiency of coagulation factor VIII, while those with hemophilia B lack coagulation factor IX. Both are transmitted genetically as X-linked recessive disorders, almost exclusively affecting males whose daughters and mothers are obligate carriers of the gene defect. Hemophilia A occurs in 1 of every 5000 live male births and accounts for approximately 80% to 85% of hemophilia cases. Hemophilia B is far less common, occurring in 1 of every 30,000 live male births. The incidence of these hemophilias is equal across all ethnic and racial groups.

The factor VIII gene comprises 186,000 base pairs and is considerably larger than the factor IX gene, which consists of 34,000 base pairs. These genes are located on particularly fragile portions of the X chromosome. By virtue of its size alone, the factor VIII gene is more susceptible to mutations; this may be an explanation for the greater prevalence of hemophilia A versus hemophilia B (4:1). The incidence of the hemophilias has not changed over the years despite the availability of genetic counseling and prenatal testing of at-risk mothers. Approximately 30% of the hemophilias present as spontaneous mutations, with no prior family histories of coagulation disorders.

Symptomatic hemophilia rarely affects females but can by virtue of any of the following genetic mechanisms: (1) high degree of lyonization of factor VIII or IX alleles in carriers; (2) hemizygosity of the X chromosome in females with Turner syndrome (XO karyotype); or (3) homozygosity in female progeny of hemophilia carriers and affected hemophilic males.[1] Females who are phenotypically hemophilic should undergo a diagnostic evaluation to exclude von Willebrand disease variant types 2N or 3, or testicular feminization syndrome.

The most common mutation of the factor VIII gene, responsible for at least 45% of cases of severe hemophilia A, involves the inversion of intron 22. This results from the translocation and exchange of DNA between either of two "nonfunctional" factor VIII-related genes within intron 22 and areas of homologous DNA within the functional factor VIII gene.[2] The recombination produces disjointed and inverted DNA sequences, preventing the transcription of a normal full-length factor VIII molecule. The coded protein typically possesses no functional or immunologic factor VIII activity in severe hemophilia A.

Less commonly, severe hemophilia A may be due to large gene deletions involving multiple or single domains, small point mutations resulting in the formation of stop codon sequences, or insertions and/or deletions in the gene. Moderate and mild severity hemophilia A are mainly the result of missense mutations; many different point mutations and deletions have been identified in patients with mild or moderate hemophilia A.[3] The incidence of alloantibody inhibitors in individuals with hemophilia A is highest in those with stop mutations in lights-chain domains. This is significant since alloantibodies (and autoantibody inhibitors) are directed against epitopes on the $A_2 > C_2 > A_3$ domains of the factor VIII coagulant protein. The A_2 and A_3 domains normally interact with factor IXa; A_2 interacts with factor Xa; C_2 interacts with phospholipid and von Willebrand factor protein. These inhibitors will block these interactions and interfere with formation of the tenase complex of coagulation.

Numerous point mutations and deletions have been identified in individuals with hemophilia B. These frequently result in the production of a defective, nonfunctioning, but immunologically detectable factor IX protein ("cross-reacting material" or CRM+) in the plasma. Individuals with large gene deletions and nonsense mutations are usually CRM− and are most susceptible to the development of factor IX alloantibodies.[4]

PRENATAL DIAGNOSIS/CARRIER TESTING

The evaluation of carrier status is a critical aspect in the routine medical care of female carriers of the hemophilias and in the management of their future pregnancies. Genetic counseling and testing of obligate carriers and at-risk family members of the propositus with hemophilia may be useful in family and peripartum planning. The most common methods for identification of carrier status include direct gene mutation analysis and linkage analysis using DNA polymorphisms. For patients with severe hemophilia A, the first-line testing is the identification of the intron 22 inversion. In individuals in whom the inversion is not detected or in whom there are no family members available for testing, the more cumbersome and labor-intensive method of linkage analysis can be performed using restriction fragment length polymorphisms (RFLP) to look for DNA polymorphisms.[5] Prior to offering any of testing, patients should be referred to a genetic counsellor who will provide counselling and recommend the appropriate diagnostic testing. Gene mutations of the factor IX gene are more easily detected because it is one third the size of the factor VIII gene. More than 300 mutations of the factor IX gene have been identified, most common are single point mutations.[6]

Techniques for detecting hemophilia in the fetus include chorionic villous sampling at 12 weeks of gestation[7] or amniocentesis at 16 weeks. The risk of miscarriage from these procedures ranges between 0.5% and 1.0%. If DNA testing is unavailable, fetal blood sample using fetoscopy can be performed at 20 weeks to measure factor VIII activity, but is associated with a significant 1% to 6% risk of fetal demise.[8] This technique is not useful for measurement of factor IX levels because they are routinely reduced in newborns along with the other vitamin K-dependent clotting factor proteins. The risks of prenatal testing need to be balanced against the need for knowing the diagnosis prior to delivery or if termination is being considered.

POSTNATAL DIAGNOSIS

The postnatal recognition and diagnosis of hemophilia A or B are facilitated if other family members are known to have hemophilia. The degree of severity of the hemophilia is usually similar in all affected family members. The exception is the so-called Heckathorn disease,[9] in which there is considerable variability of factor VIII levels in family members affected with hemophilia A. Frequently, family members and the details of their medical histories are unavailable at the time of patient presentation. Moreover, approximately 30% of all hemophilia is due to spontaneous mutations in families without prior history of coagulation abnormalities. For instance, Queen Victoria of England appears to have spontaneously mutated her factor VIII gene and then spread it throughout European royalty. Measurement of factor VIII or IX activity in the affected individual is necessary to establish the diagnosis. For hemophilia A, factor VIII coagulant activity can be determined either by a direct functional plasma clot-based assay or by a chromogenic substrate-based assay. Factor IX activity levels also are measured utilizing a plasma clot-based assay. Hemophilia A must be differentiated from von Willebrand disease by the measurement of von Willebrand factor (vWF) antigen and ristocetin cofactor activity, and by examination of the multimeric composition of the vWF protein with SDS gel chromatography, if clinically indicated. Von Willebrand disease variant types 2N and 3 may be phenotypically similar to severe hemophilia A, although the autosomally transmitted inheritance pattern of von Willebrand disease should help to distinguish it from the sex-linked recessive genetic pattern of hemophilia A (see Chapter 7).

When hemophilia is suspected in a fetus of a known carrier, the measurement of the factor VIII or IX activity (or both) should be performed on a cord blood sample. This avoids the need for venipuncture, which can produce clinically important bruising and/or hemorrhage in the severely affected neonate. The diagnosis of hemophilia B in the neonate may be confounded by the fact that factor IX levels (as well as the other vitamin K-dependent proteins) are significantly reduced at birth and may remain so for up to 6 months. Normal plasma activity levels of coagulation factor VIII and IX in patients older than infants range between 0.5 and 1.5 U/mL (50% and 150%). The severity of hemophilia is defined by the measured level of clotting factor activity: severe hemophilia is defined as factor VIII or IX activity below 1% (<0.01 U/mL) and occurs in approximately 50% of affected individuals. Moderate hemophilia occurs in about 10% of affected patients, who have factor VIII or IX levels between 1% and 5% (0.01 and 0.05 U/mL). Mild hemophilia, affecting 30% to 40% of affected patients, have factor VIII or IX activity levels above 5% (above 0.05 U/mL).

Between 2% and 8% of hemophilic infants will develop intracranial hemorrhage and scalp hematoma in the perinatal period.[10] These complications are associated with prolonged and difficult labors, the use of vacuum extraction and forceps to facilitate delivery, the presence of cephalopelvic disproportion, and precipitous delivery.[11] Caesarian section might reduce these bleeding risks, and, recently, the intrauterine transfusion of clotting factor concentrate immediately before delivery has been attempted to prevent such problems. Nevertheless, the most common initial bleeding events in hemophilic children occur in association with circumcision and cord necrosis. Ecchymoses may develop in the first few months of life, but spontaneous hemarthroses, the hallmark of the hemophilias, usually do not occur until approximately 1 year of age with the onset of walking. The development of hematomas at the site of intramuscular injections of routine vaccinations or medications (including the postnatal administration of vitamin K) should increase the suspicion that an abnormality exists. This type of bleeding can be avoided by giving these injections either subcutaneously or after pretreatment with clotting factor concentrates. Oral bleeding due to loss of deciduous teeth, tongue biting, and frenulum injury is common in the young child and may require clotting factor replacement.

Patients with moderately severe hemophilia usually do not experience spontaneous hemorrhagic episodes but minor trauma or surgery can precipitate bleeding unless clotting factor replacement or DDAVP is provided prophylactically. Mild hemophilia may be diagnosed during routine preoperative screening of the coagulation mechanism, which reveals a prolonged activated partial thromboplastin time.[12] These patients can present with bleeding after significant trauma or surgery, but rarely have hemarthroses. Some patients may never have a bleeding event.

CLINICAL FEATURES OF THE HEMOPHILIAS

Intra-articular Bleeding: Hemarthroses and Hemophilic Arthropathy

The most common sites of spontaneous bleeding in individuals with severe hemophilia A and B involve the joints and muscles. The knees (greater than 50% of all events), elbows, ankles, shoulders, and wrists are affected in decreasing incidence.[13] It is the recurrent nature of the bleeds into these joints that results in the degeneration of the cartilage and progressive destruction of the joint space. The pathophysiology of hemophilic arthropathy can be divided into three phases. Following hemorrhage into the joint, iron is deposited into the synovium and chondrocytes of the articular cartilage (the first phase). Subsequently, focal areas of villous hypertrophy develop on the synovial surface, which, because of their friability, will continue to rebleed with normal joint stresses even as routine as weight bearing. This ultimately establishes the "target joint" situation, characterized by recurrent, painful, and destructive bleeds into the same joint.

Associated with the iron deposition is the release of inflammatory cytokines, which recruit macrophages and fibroblasts into the joint space and establish a favorable environment for progression of joint disease. This second phase of hemophilic arthropathy involves the development of chronic synovitis, pain, fibrosis, and progressive joint stiffness with decreased range of motion. Within the joint space can be found hydrolytic and proteolytic enzymes, such as acid phophatase and cathepsin D.[14] In the final stage of hemophilic arthropathy (phase three), the progressive and erosive destruction of the cartilage, narrowing of the joint space, subchondral cyst formation, and eventual collapse and sclerosis of the joint become apparent. Conventional roentgenographs traditionally have been utilized to monitor the progression of hemophilic arthropathy; however, until there are bone changes, the films will appear normal and may underestimate the extent of the joint disease. Magnetic resonance imaging (MRI) is emerging as a useful and sensitive tool for detecting early synovial damage and intra-articular bleeding.

The predominant clinical manifestations of recurrent joint hemorrhage are pain and swelling. Well before the onset of pain, patients describe prickly sensations and burning within the joint as the first signs of bleeding. If the bleeding is allowed to continue, the pain and swelling lead to fixation of the joint in a flexed position until the swelling subsides. The early recognition and treatment of acute bleeding episodes are essential to prevent excessive hemorrhage into the joint space and minimize subsequent joint destruction. The goal of "on-demand" therapy, which is the administration of replacement clotting factor concentrate to treat the acute bleed, is to increase the factor VIII or IX activity levels to 30% to 50% of normal. Occasionally, repeat infusions of factor concentrate are necessary to terminate bleeding and reduce pain, especially for target joints. If significant pain and swelling are protracted, a short course of corticosteroids (prednisone 1 mg/kg/day) may be utilized. This has been more beneficial in children than in adults and should be avoided in patients with human immunodeficiency virus (HIV) infection. Rarely, joint aspirations are performed for routine hemarthroses. They are reserved for patients with intractable pain despite factor replacement therapy or patients with fever and in whom septic arthritis is suspected. Prior to joint aspiration, adequate factor replacement therapy should be administered. Aspiration should be avoided in patients with alloantibody inhibitors because of the increased risks of bleeding complications from the procedure.

Narcotic analgesics frequently are a necessary therapeutic adjunct for pain control and the application of ice packs and avoidance of weight bearing by using crutches will reduce the inflammation and pain attendant with the hemarthrosis. Initiating physical therapy as soon as pain control is achieved will reduce the development of muscle atrophy around the affected joint and prevent permanent flexion contractures. Plaster casting of target joints should not be done.

A secondary prophylaxis regimen of replacement therapy can be of immense benefit to patients with target joints. This consists of administering the appropriate clotting factor concentrate two or three times weekly, respectively, to maintain trough factor activity levels of 1% to 3%. When maintained for at least 3 months this approach should effectively interrupt the cycle of recurrent bleeding.[15] In patients who have developed chronic synovitis that is refractory to medical management, surgical debridement and synovectomy should be considered to reduce the bleeding and pain; however, joint destruction may progress albeit at a much slower pace. This procedure is of most benefit in patients with minimal hemarthropathy.

Radioactive and chemical nonsurgical synovectomies have been utilized on a limited basis, predominantly in Canada and Europe, to break the vicious cycle of hemarthrosis–chronic synovitis–hemarthrosis. These techniques currently are under investigation in the United States. Most radionuclide synovectomies in hemophiliacs have been performed with the β emittor isotopes yttrium-90 (^{90}Y) and phosphorus 32 (^{32}P), which are less likely to be mutagenic and less likely to produce localized inflammatory reactions of the synovium compared to γ emitters.[16] There is a greater than 50% reduction in frequency of bleeding events and pain following radionuclide synovectomy and the range of motion of the joints is stabilized or improved in more than 50% of patients. Unfortunately, with long-term follow-up, the range of motion tends to deteriorate despite this treatment. Chemical synovectomies with osmic acid or rifampacin also reduce the frequency of hemarthroses but both produce acute and painful inflammatory reactions and the overall results are inferior to the radionuclides. The best method to prevent progressive joint destruction is to prevent intra-articular bleeding. The use of primary prophylaxis regimens (twice or thrice weekly treatment with clotting factor replacement therapy, beginning in infancy after the first bleed and continuing indefinitely thereafter) is being studied as a means of achieving this goal.

Intramuscular Hemorrhage

Intramuscular hemorrhages, which are the second most common sites of bleeding in individuals with hemophilia, account for 30% of bleeding events. The location of the intramuscular hemorrhage determines the morbidity of the event. Hemorrhages into large muscles, though extensive, generally resolve without complications, as they are not confined. Bleeding into a closed fascial compartment can lead to significant compression of vital structures with resulting ischemia, gangrene, flexion contractures, and neuropathy (compartment syndrome). Intramuscular hematomas present with localized tenderness and pain and can be associated with low-grade fevers, elevations of serum lactate dehydrogenase (LDH), and large ecchmoses. Bleeding into the psoas muscles and retroperitoneal space can produce sudden onset of inguinal pain and decreased range of motion of the ipsilateral hip, which assumes a markedly flexed position, usually with lateral rotation. Hemorrhage can be life threatening if a large volume of blood is lost. In addition, femoral nerve compression can occur with permanent disability if a compartment syndrome develops. The diagnosis can be made by pelvic ultrasonography or computed tomography (CT).[17] Bleeding into this area needs to be controlled rapidly by raising and maintaining the clotting factor activity to 80% to 100% of normal for at least 48 to 72 hours. Surgery is strictly to be avoided in this situation.

Hematuria

Spontaneous gross hematuria occurs frequently in patients with hemophilia and is usually painless unless intraureteral clots develop. Hematuria can be precipitated by the use of nonsteroidal anti-inflammatory drugs, trauma, or exertion. Pelvic clots, obstructive hydronephrosis, compromised collecting systems, and retroperitoneal fibrosis can be demonstrated on intravenous pyelograms. The cause of spontaneous hematuria in individuals with hemophilia is unknown, but may be due to direct tubular damage by circulating immune complexes formed after clotting factor replacement therapy.[15] Immune complexes may also mediate the development of anaphylaxis and nephrotic syndrome, which can occur with factor IX replacement therapy, particularly when utilized for immune tolerance, in patients with alloantibodies to factor IX.[19] Individuals with large gene deletions of factor IX appear to be at highest risk, and this syndrome has been reported with all commercially available factor IX products.[20] Avoidance of any or all sources of coagulation factor IX for replacement therapy is necessary and recombinant factor VIIa concentrate becomes the treatment of choice for acute bleeding events in these individuals.

Other causes of hematuria that should be considered include infection, neoplasm, and renal or ureteral stones. Nephrolithiasis has been seen most commonly in HIV-infected hemophiliacs taking the HIV protease inhibitor indinavir (Crixivan), which produces crystalluria and calculi consisting of the intact drug.

The general approach to the management of hematuria depends upon the cause; however, the mainstay of treatment initially is hydration. If the hematuria persists beyond several days, clotting factor replacement therapy to raise factor activity levels to 50% of normal should be administered although bleeding might well continue. Antifibrinolytic agents generally should be avoided because of the risk of intraureteral clot formation, which can lead to obstruction of the collecting system and eventual renal failure.

Intracranial Hemorrhage

The most common cause of death from bleeding in patients with the hemophilias is intracranial/intracerebral hemorrhage. Intracranial hemorrhage can occur with minimal trauma, particularly in children, or spontaneously in the absence of identifiable trauma; intracranial hemorrhage is spontaneous 50% of the time in affected adults. HIV-infected hemophiliacs receiving antiretroviral protease inhibitors may have an increased risk of developing spontaneous intracranial (and intramuscular) hemorrhages.[21] Fifty percent of patients with intracranial hemorrhage have neurologic sequelae, and 30% of events result in death. Presenting clinical symptoms usually include headaches, which can be associated with nausea and vomiting and occasional seizures. Whenever an intracranial hemorrhage is documented, suspected, or even remotely possible after head trauma, it is imperative that factor VIII or IX concentrate (appropriate to the type of hemophilia) be administered immediately to achieve 100% of normal factor activity. This treatment must precede any diagnostic testing. The head CT scan may not show evidence of bleeding immediately after the event. In patients who require a lumbar puncture, factor VIII and IX replacement therapy should be given 15 to 30 minutes prior to the procedure to increase the factor activity to 100% of normal. If the patient has not had a recent recovery study to demonstrate the response to factor infusion, a clotting factor level should be performed after the factor has been infused and prior to the procedure. Because of the serious implications if an intracranial bleed is ignored, even patients with mild hemophilia and factor VIII or IX activity levels below 50% of normal should receive clotting factor replacement therapy for severe head trauma.

Gastrointestinal and Oropharyngeal Bleeding

Gastrointestinal bleeding occurs in approximately 10% to 15% of adult hemophiliacs. Anatomic lesions are more common than spontaneous hemorrhage. Peptic ulcer disease, gastritis, and varices should be excluded as sources of bleeding. In those individuals with chronic hepatitis C and cirrhosis, varices as a result of portal hypertension are the leading cause of acute bleeds. Gastrointestinal hemorrhage should be treated with clotting factor replacement to at least 50% of normal activity.

The oropharynx is a highly vascular area and excessive bleeding may occur from small lacerations, a bitten tongue, and even the appearance of a new tooth. Of particular concern are retropharyngeal bleeds that can lead to upper-airway obstruction.[22] This type of hemorrhage is a hematologic emergency and requires clotting factor replacement to levels of 80% to 100% of normal. Bleeding associated with simple dental extractions after local injections of anesthesia can be managed with oral administration of antifibrinolytic agents and topical application of fibrin sealants. If nerve block injections are used for anesthesia of more complex oral surgery, clotting factor concentrate should be administered prior to the procedure to prevent untoward hemorrhage along fascial planes in the neck, which could result in airway compromise. Major oral surgery requires clotting factor replacement to levels of between 25% and 50% of normal along with antifibrinolytic agents administered post surgery for 3 to 10 days. Other comments regarding surgical procedures in hemophiliacs are discussed in Chapter 30.

Pseudotumor Formation in Hemophilia

In 1% to 2% of severe hemophiliacs, hematomas produced by repetitive bleeding episodes continue to enlarge and may encapsulate. They have the appearance of expanding masses on roentgenography and may invade contiguous structures, including bone, muscle, or soft tissue organs. The pseudotumors themselves are composed of old clot and necrotic tissue and arise because of inadequate treatment of bleeding events. Symptoms associated with expanding pseudotumors are related to the size of the encapsulated mass and the degree of compromise of the integrity of the structures they are invading. Noninvasive techniques, such as MRI, ultrasonography, and CT, should be used to diagnose pseudotumors; needle biopsy may produce serious bleeding complications. Operative biopsies and subsequent surgical removal are associated with up to 20% mortality despite adequate coverage with clotting factor concentrates.[23] Improved surgical results may be obtained if the pseudotumor is evacuated and the cavity packed with fibrin sealant.[23] Adequate and immediate clotting factor replacement therapy of acute bleeds should minimize the risk of developing pseudotumors.

LABORATORY CHARACTERISTICS

The diagnosis of hemophilia A and B should be suspected in male patients with unusually easy bruisability and abnormal bleeding, accompanied with an isolated prolongation of the activated partial thromboplastin time (aPTT). Individuals with any of the hemophilias have normal prothrombin times, platelet counts, and platelet function studies. Usually the bleeding times are normal. Mixing studies performed with equal parts of patient plasma and normal pooled plasma incubated at 37°C should show complete and prompt correction of the prolonged aPTT. The correction of the aPTT in the mixture at both 0 and 120 minutes of incubation essentially excludes the presence of an alloantibody inhibitor directed against a specific clotting factor or the presence of a lupus-like anticoagulant directed against phospholipid in the aPTT assay system.

Correction of the aPTT at 2 hours eliminates the likelihood that any weak neutralizing inhibitors are present. Factor VIII allo- and autoantibody inhibitors interact with the factor VIII coagulant protein in a time- and temperature-dependent manner. If a lupus-like anticoagulant is suspected, a diluted phospholipid based assay, such as the dilute Russell viper venom time, the tissue thromboplastin inhibition time, or the platelet neutralization procedure, which utilizes platelets as a source of phospholipid, should be performed to confirm its presence (see Chapter 18). If a clotting factor deficiency is suspected from the mixing study, assays should be performed to determine the activity levels of specific clotting factor proteins in the intrinsic pathway of coagulation, including factors XII, XI, IX, and VIII. Such assays also define the severity of the specific clotting factor deficiency.

In general, specific clotting factor assays are performed utilizing an aPTT-based one-stage clotting time. This assay assumes that the level of factor VIII is rate limiting with all other components of the assay being present at saturating levels. The one-stage aPTT assay is most physiologic of the factor VIII assays.[24] More recently, chromogenic assays have been introduced. The factor VIII:C chromogenic assay is based on the quantity of factor Xa generated in the presence of factor VIII:C, factor IXa, thrombin, calcium, and phospholipid. Chromogenic assays generally yield higher levels of factor VIII activities (1.5 to 2 times) than the standard aPTT based factor VIII:C assay in individuals who have received the B-domain deleted form of recombinant factor VIII concentrate.[25] These differences have not been explained and require further study. Currently, chromogenic assays are utilized routinely by laboratories in Europe, while aPTT-based assays have been the norm in the United States. The options for monitoring B-domain deleted recombinant factor VIII concentrate are to utilize the chromogenic assay or to utilize the one-stage aPTT with the World Health Organization standard. The issues still surrounding the choice of assay include the cost (chromogenic assays costing twice that of aPTT assays), quality control issues (no peer-group controls for the chromogenic factor VIII assay to date in the United States), the monitoring of the B-domain deleted factor VIII concentrate (aPTT assays giving levels at 50% of the chromogenic assays), and the standardization of inhibitor quantitation using the chromogenic assay.

In individuals with low levels of factor VIII activity, especially females, von Willebrand disease type 2 Normandy must be considered. These individuals are phenotypic hemophiliacs with normally functioning vWF protein in ristocetin-based assays but factor VIII binding assays are abnormal due to a genetic point mutation at the binding site for factor VIII on the vWF protein. This results in a significantly decreased plasma circulation time and decreased plasma concentration for factor VIII. Additionally, the inheritance pattern is autosomal rather than X linked. The availability of testing for suspected of having von Willebrand disease type 2 Normandy is limited, and therefore patients should be referred to a hemophilia treatment center for evaluation.

Up to 50% of individuals with severe hemophilia A and 3% to 4% of individuals with hemophilia B will develop alloantibody inhibitors. These neutralizing alloantibodies should be suspected in hemophiliacs in whom the recovery (the % incremental response to clotting factor concentrate 15 to 30 minutes after administration) of clotting factor activity levels is less than 60% of the expected increase above baseline levels. The inhibitor can be quantitated utilizing the Bethesda assay,[26] in which the residual clotting factor activity in a mixture of patient plasma and pooled normal plasma (PNP) is determined with a one stage clotting time. One Bethesda unit (BU) is defined as the amount of antibody in a patient's plasma that causes a 50% decrease in factor VIII activity in PNP after incubation at 37°C for 2 hours. Although this assay originally was developed for use in patients with hemophilia A, the same procedure is useful also for quantitating inhibitors in patients with hemophilia B and individuals with autoantibodies directed against clotting factors.

Autoantibody inhibitors directed specifically against factor VIII (acquired hemophilia) and less commonly against factor IX can occur in individuals with previously normal coagulation. In acquired hemophilia, quantitation using the Bethesda assay may not accurately reflect the bleeding tendency because these autoantibodies follow "type II" pharmacokinetics with a nonlinear neutralization pattern and incomplete inactivation of factor VIII activity even at the highest concentrations.[27]

Low titer inhibitors (low responders) are defined as less than 5 BU, a level which does not rise after reexposure to the clotting factor protein contained in replacement therapies (anamnestic response). High titer inhibitors are defined as greater than 10 BU with significant anamnesis soon after reexposure to clotting factor concentrate (high responders). Individuals with antibody titers between 5 and 10 BU could be either high or low responders, depending on the presence or absence of anamnesis. A modification of the Bethesda assay, the Nijmegen assay, was developed to improve the specificity and reliability in detecting low titer inhibitors in the range of 0 to 0.8 BU. Both the test and control mixtures are buffered with an imidazole buffer to stabilize the pH at 7.4, and the original buffer in the control mixture is replaced with immunodepleted factor VIII deficient plasma to attain comparable protein concentrations in both mixtures.[28] This assay is generally reserved for clinical research studies in which it is important to detect the presence of low titer inhibitors.

THERAPEUTIC MODALITIES FOR THE HEMOPHILIAS

Hemophilia Treatment Centers

Hemophilia treatment centers (HTCs) provide comprehensive medical and psychosocial services to patients and their families with inherited bleeding disorders. Utilizing a multidisciplinary team of nurses, physicians, psychosocial professionals, and laboratory technologists, state-of-the-art care is provided for patients with hemophilia and its complications. A survival advantage for patients with hemophilia has been demonstrated for those patients followed and treated at an HTC.[29] Additionally, HTCs provide cost effective care, can offer Public Health Service (PHS) pricing for clotting factor concentrates, and provide training for home infusion of clotting factor allowing the patient to treat a bleed as soon as it is recognized. In the United States and Canada, HTCs are supported by funding from the federal governments.

Clotting Factor Replacement Therapy with Coagulation Factor Concentrates

Replacement of factor VIII or IX to hemostatically adequate plasma levels for prevention or treatment of acute bleeding is the basis of the management of hemophilia. Treatment should be administered at early onset of symptoms to limit the amount of bleeding and to prevent damage to the surrounding tissues. Replacement therapy should also be administered emergently before surgery to prevent intraoperative bleeding complications or prophylactically to prevent hemophilic arthropathy.

Both factor VIII and factor IX replacement products may be either plasma derived or genetically engineered with recombinant technology utilizing mammalian cell lines transfected with normal human genes that code for clotting factor proteins (Tables 4–1 and 4–2). Factor replacement products are often classified based on their final purity, defined as specific activity (International Units of clotting factor activity/mg of protein). Intermediate purity products have relatively low specific activities (less than 50 U/mg) because they are contaminated with additional plasma proteins including fibrinogen,

Table 4–1 • FACTOR VIII CONCENTRATES LICENSED IN THE UNITED STATES

Type/Product Name	Manufacturer	Method of Viral Inactivation	Specific Activity (IU/mg Protein, Discounting Albumin)
Ultrapure Recombinant			
Recombinate	Baxter Hyland	Immunoaffinity chromatography	>3000
Kogenate FS	Bayer	Immunoaffinity chromatography solvent detergent (TNBP/polysorbate 80)	>3000 (albumin-free formulations)
Hexilate FS	Aventis-Behring		>3000
Re Facto	Genetics Institute (American Home Products)	Immunoaffinity chromatography solvent detergent TNBP/Triton X1000	11,200–15,500 (albumin-free formulation)
Ultrapure Plasma-Derived			
Monoclate P	Aventis-Behring	Immunoaffinity chromatography and pasteurization (60°C, 10 hours)	>3000
Hemofil M	Baxter Hyland Immuno (BHI)	Immunoaffinity chromatography solvent detergent (TNBP/Triton X-100) and terminal heating (25°C, >10 hours)	>3000
Monarc M	Baxter (utilizing volunteer donor plasma collected by American Red Cross)		>3000
Intermediate-Purity and High-Purity Plasma Derived			
Alphanate SD	Alpha Therapeutics	Affinity chromatography solvent detergent TNBP and polysorbate 80 and pasteurization 80°C, 72 hours	8–30
Humate P	Aventis Behring	Pasteurization (60°C, 10 hours)	1–2
Koate DVI	Bayer	Solvent detergent (TNBP and polysorbate 80) and pasteurization 80°C, 72 hours	9–22

Table 4–2 • FACTOR IX CONCENTRATES AVAILABLE IN THE UNITED STATES

Type/Product Name	Manufacturer	Virucidal Technique	Specific Activity (IU/mg Protein, Discounting Albumin)
Ultrapure Recombinant Factor IX			
Benefix	Genetics Institute	Affinity chromatography and ultrafiltration	>200 (albumin free)
Very Highly Purified Plasma-Derived Factor IX			
Alphanine SD	Alpha Therapeutics	Dual affinity chromatography solvent detergent (TNBP and polysorbate 80) nanofiltration	229 ± 23(22)
Mononine	Aventis Behring	Immunoaffinity chromatography sodium thiocyanate ultrafiltration	>160
Low-Purity Plasma-Derived Factor IX Complex Concentrates			
Bebulin VH	Baxter Hyland Immuno (Vienna)	Vapor heat (60°C, 10 hours, 1190 mbar pressure plus 1 hour 80°C, 1375 mbar	2
Konyne 80	Bayer	Dry heat (80°C, 72 hours)	1.25
Profilnine D	Alpha Therapeutics	Solvent detergent TNBP and polysorbate 80	4.5
Proplex T	Baxter Hyland Immuno	Dry heat (60°C, 144 hours)	3.9

fibronectin, and other noncoagulant proteins. High-purity (more than 50 U/mg) and ultra-high-purity (more than 3000 U/mg for factor VIII concentrates; more than 160 U/mg for factor IX concentrates) products contain little or no contaminating plasma proteins other than albumin as a stabilizer. More recently, albumin-free formulations of recombinant "full-length" and B-domain-deleted factor VIII concentrates have become available. Monoclonal antibody-purified, plasma-derived factor IX concentrate and recombinant factor IX concentrate are free of any albumin.

All coagulation factor concentrates, plasma-derived and recombinant, have been subjected to some method of viral inactivation, attenuation, or elimination. These techniques include high dry heating, pasteurization, or solvent detergent extraction utilized singly or in combination. Viral safety may be further enhanced by adding immunoaffinity chromatography (monoclonal antibody purification) and gel filtration chromatography steps to segregate the desired therapeutic clotting factor protein from contaminating proteins and viruses. Viral attenuated plasma-derived factor concentrates have been eradicated of lipid-enveloped viruses such as HIV and hepatitis B and C and there have been no documented transmissions of these diseases since 1985 for factor VIII concentrates and 1990 for factor IX concentrates. Non-lipid enveloped viruses such as hepatitis A and parvovirus B19 are not susceptible to these techniques and sporadic outbreaks have been reported.[30,31]

All patients who are to receive clotting factor concentrates should be vaccinated against hepatitis A and B in infancy. Recombinant factor concentrates by definition will not transmit any of the hepatitides, HIV, or parvovirus B19; however, if they contain human albumin as a stabilizer, there has been theoretical concern that they could transmit the prion(s) associated with Creutzfeldt-Jakob disease (CJD) or new-variant CJD. Up until this time, longitudinal epidemiologic surveillance and autopsy studies analyzing postmortem brain tissue from individuals with hemophilia and other transfusion-dependent populations have not yielded any evidence for transmission of CJD to humans exposed repeatedly to blood products.

All of the commercially available factor VIII replacement concentrates appear to be equally efficacious with equivalent postadministration recovery levels observed for the plasma-derived and recombinant full-length factor VIII preparations. Of note, infusions of the genetically engineered B-domain-deleted factor VIII concentrate, Refacto (Genetics Institute), do not achieve expected factor VIII increments/recoveries when monitored with the one-stage clotting time. When a chromogenic based assay is utilized, factor VIII level increments are as expected.[32] The discrepancies between the one-stage clotting assay and the chromogenic assay with the recombinant B-domain-deleted factor VIII concentrate probably reflect differences in phospholipid content between both assay systems; however, they also bring into question which of the assay systems provides the most accurate indicator of factor VIII optimal dosing in vivo.

The dosing of clotting factor replacement therapy in hemophilia is based on the patient's plasma volume, the distribution of the clotting protein between the intravascular and extravascular compartments, the circulating half-life of the clotting factor in the plasma, and the level of clotting factor activity required to achieve adequate hemostasis or prophylaxis. Dosage is calculated by assuming that 1 U/kg body weight of factor VIII replacement will raise the plasma activity of factor VIII by approximately 0.02 U/mL (2%), and 1 U/kg of factor IX concentrate, which has a larger volume of distribution, will increase plasma factor IX levels by 0.01U/mL (1%). Administration of the recombinant factor IX concentrate may yield recoveries that are 80% of expected at 15 to 30 minutes, requiring a correction factor of 1.2 when calculating the dose to be infused. Not all individuals with hemophilia B demonstrate this variation in recovery, necessitating baseline recovery studies before instituting treatment with the product.

The circulating half-life for factor VIII is 8 to 12 hours, and for factor IX is around 18 hours. Optimal hemostatic plasma levels of factors VIII and IX depend upon the clinical situation. "On-demand" regimens administer factor concentrate at the time of the hemorrhagic event; levels of 30% to 50% of normal clotting factor activity are required to control minor to moderate-severity bleeding, to prevent recurrent hemorrhage, and to support tissue healing. Levels of 50% to 100% clotting factor activity should be achieved and maintained for a minimum of 7 to 10 days to treat or prevent life- and limb-threatening hemorrhage or for major surgical procedures. Routinely, clotting factor replacement therapy is delivered by bolus infusion immediately after reconstitution.

The use of continuous infusion regimens for clotting factor replacement has become more common, especially in the postoperative setting. Continuous infusion maintains a stable and continuous therapeutic level of factor activity without a "peaks and troughs" effect. This translates into decreased total amount of factor infused (and therefore decreased cost of care) and easy laboratory monitoring with random blood samples.[33] None of the clotting factor concentrates have been licensed for use as a continuous infusion. Many of the HTCs have developed their own protocols for preparation, infusion, and standards of safety with little risk of infection. These protocols are developed in cooperation with research pharmacists. How much added albumin is necessary to maintain the stability of the product is not defined. Currently, infusion pumps have not been licensed for use with clotting factor concentrates.

The choice of which clotting factor concentrate to administer to individuals with hemophilia A or B should be individualized; participation of the patient/family in the decision is essential. Consideration should be given to cost, age of the patient, presence of an alloantibody inhibitor, and HIV and hepatitis C virus (HCV) status. In addition, some hemophilia treaters believe that the ultra-high purity factor VIII concentrates, both plasma derived and recombinant, may have a greater tendency to induce alloantibody development.[34,35] Because of this belief, they will not use these products in previously untreated patients. The literature suggests, however, that the increased incidence of alloantibodies with these factor VIII concentrates actually may be related to increased surveillance testing for alloantibodies using very sensitive assays. Intermediate-purity factor VIII concentrates have been shown to inhibit normal lymphocyte immune responses in vitro, probably because of extraneous proteins or the presence of TGF-β in the preparations. Absolute CD4 lymphocyte counts have been shown to decrease more quickly in HIV-seropositive patients with intermediate purity factor VIII concentrates than with ultra-high-purity products[36]; however, this has not been shown to impact on survival in hemophiliacs with acquired immunodeficiency syndrome (AIDS) or with progression of asymptomatic to symptomatic HIV disease. Similar immune effects have been reported with factor IX concentrates.

The choice of which factor IX concentrate to administer should take into account the thrombogenicity potential of the intermediate-purity products, which contain some activated factors II, VII, and X, in addition to IX. Prolonged and repeated use of these intermediate products has been associated with development of disseminated intravascular coagulopathy, stroke, and myocardial infarction, and this risk is increased further in patients with hepatic insufficiency. This may be related to the cumulative and sustained procoagulant effects of the activated clotting factors Xa and IIa, which have considerably longer circulating half-lives than factor IX. Little or no thrombogenicity has been observed with the ultra-high-purity factor IX plasma derived or recombinant concentrates; therefore, these products are more appropriate for immune tolerance induction regimens, primary prophylaxis, and surgery. Despite the risk of thrombogenicity, when used appropriately, intermediate-purity factor IX concentrates are safe and effective.

DDAVP

DDAVP (1-deamino-8-D-arginine-vasopressin) plays an important role in the management of patients with mild hemophilia A. The intravenous infusion of DDAVP at the dose of 0.3 μg/kg of body weight in 50 mL of normal saline over 15 to 30 minutes or intranasal spray of 150 μg/nostril produces a rise in circulating factor VIII:C and vWF protein levels by 2- or 3-fold over the patient's native level by causing a release of factor VIII/vWF from storage sites. The peak effect of the intravenous form is seen in 30 to 60 minutes,[37] while the intranasal form peaks in 60 to 90 minutes[38] after administration. Thus, DDAVP can be given in advance of dental work and minor surgical procedures, or at the time of acute spontaneous or traumatic bleeding events to avoid the need for factor VIII replacement products. DDAVP can be administered every 12 to 24 hours; however, tachyphylaxis often develops because of the depletion of factor VIII/vWF from the storage sites. Common side effects associated with DDAVP use include flushing, hypertension, and retention of free water. This last effect can induce severe hyponatremia, especially in infants and the elderly, and precipitate the onset of seizures. Therefore, free-water fluid intake should be restricted and serum sodium levels monitored in these individuals. Of concern in the elderly population is the occurrence of angina pectoris, stroke, and coronary artery thrombosis; DDAVP should be utilized cautiously in this population. DDAVP releases tissue plasminogen activator from endothelial cells and may stimulate local fibrinolysis, particularly on mucosal surfaces. Therefore, for bleeding in the gastrointestinal or genitourinary tract or in the oropharyngeal area, antifibrinolytic agents (see below) should be administered concurrently with DDAVP.

ANCILLARY TREATMENTS

Antifibrinolytic Agents

Antifibrinolytic agents are a useful but underutilized ancillary therapy in the management of patients with hemophilia A and B. By inhibiting the fibrinolysis of the thrombus by plasmin, antifibrinolytics can maintain the integrity of the clot and prevent hemorrhage. They are particularly useful in the management of mucous membrane bleeding from the oropharynx, nose, and genitourinary tract because the secretions from these sites naturally contain fibrinolytic enzymes. ε-aminocaproic acid (EACA)(Amicar) and tranexamic acid (Cyklokapron) can be administered intravenously, orally, or topically in patients with hemophilia. These medications can be utilized alone or in conjunction with DDAVP for the prevention or control of bleeding. The optimum dose and duration is not well defined but Amicar is usually dosed at 50mg/kg every 6 hours for 3 to 10 days and Cyklokapron is given at a dose of 1.5 g every 6 hours for 3 to 6 days.

Fibrin Glues or Sealants

Fibrin glues, also known as fibrin sealants or fibrin tissue adhesives, are composed of thrombin, fibrinogen, and sometimes factor XIII and antifibrinolytic agents (see Chapter 26). The major benefits have been obtained when the fibrin sealants are combined with continuous or bolus infusions of factor concentrate. A "swish and swallow" regimen with tranexamic acid solution daily for 2 weeks can be used after applying fibrin sealant topically to sites of oral surgery.[39] Fibrin tissue adhesives have been utilized very successfully with a reduction in bleeding in hemophilia patients undergoing orthopedic surgery.[40] The fibrin sealants available in the United States have been virally inactivated.

PROPHYLAXIS/INDWELLING VENOUS ACCESS DEVICE

With the increased safety of coagulation factor replacement products, primary prophylaxis regimens with factor VIII and IX concentrates have become very popular. The goal of primary prophylaxis in the severe hemophilias is to prevent hemarthroses and the subsequent development of hemophilic arthropathy. Primary prophylaxis is initiated prior to or after the first hemarthrosis, usually around the age of 14 to 18 months, at the time that the child begins to walk. Enough clotting replacement therapy is administered to maintain coagulation factor trough levels of 1% to 3% activity, which reduces the incidence of spontaneous hemarthroses. In severe hemophilia A this is usually achieved by infusing factor VIII concentrate on Monday and Wednesday at a dose of 25 to 40 U/kg and on Friday at a dose of 40 U/kg. For severe hemophilia B, dosing with factor IX concentrate at 25 to 40 U/kg occurs twice weekly, usually on Monday and Thursday. Primary prophylaxis has been shown: (1) to decrease the total number and frequency of all bleeding episodes; (2) to decrease the frequency of repetitive joint bleeds; (3) to decrease the rate of deterioration of the joint as observed on X-ray; (4) to decrease the number of days lost from school; and (5) to decrease the number of days spent in the hospital for severe bleeds.

In order to administer clotting factor two or three times per week, it may be necessary to implant an indwelling venous access device when peripheral access is unavailable. This is especially true for small children. Venous access devices consist of Port-a-Caths, which do not require daily care by the family, or Hickman or Broviac catheters. These indwelling venous access devices, however, are the cause of most of the complications associated with prophylaxis. Systemic infections complicate 10% to 50% of chronic venous access devices used in hemophiliacs. Catheter-related thromboses in the upper extremities occur up to 50% of the time. To reduce the risk of thrombosis, it is standard procedure to flush the catheters after use with 20 cc of normal saline and 300 to 500 units of unfractionated heparin (3- to 5-cc volume).

The short-term costs of clotting factor replacement in primary prophylaxis are greater than on-demand therapy; however, the long-term cost savings may be greater with primary prophylaxis if patients' joints are preserved, if their lives are more productive financially and personally, and if expensive surgical interventions can be avoided. Longitudinal randomized controlled studies currently are being conducted to confirm these premises. Secondary prophylaxis can be utilized in patients with target joints who are having recurrent events. Coagulation factor concentrate is administered similarly to primary prophylaxis but over a limited period of 3 to 6 months.

Dental Care

Routine dental treatment can be a major source of morbidity in individuals with hemophilia. The best dental care is aimed at the prevention of dental caries, gingivitis, and periodontal disease. Caries are prevented by periodic fluoride applications. Sealants can be applied to the biting surfaces of molar teeth to reduce the incidence of caries. Gingival disease can be reduced by controlling the development of dental plaque by effective tooth brushing and the use of antibacterial mouth rinses such as chlorohexidine. Early dental care of children with hemophilia provided by a dental team who coordinate their efforts with the hemophilia treatment center is essential. If severe hemophiliacs require extractions or oral or periodontal surgery, clotting factor replacement therapy may be necessary. For mild hemophilia, DDAVP administration immediately prior to the procedure is sufficient. Antifibrinolytic agents should be utilized as adjunctive therapy. The dose and duration of ε-aminocaproic acid (Amicar) therapy is variable but ranges from as low as 500 mg as a total dose for minor work to as high as 50 mg/kg every 6 hours for 3 to 10 days for extensive procedures.

TREATMENT COMPLICATIONS

Inhibitors

The major complication of treatment with coagulation factor concentrates in the hemophilias is the development of alloantibodies directed against factor VIII or IX. The development of these alloantibodies in patients with severe hemophilia A occurs more frequently with the use of ultra-high-purity factor concentrates (plasma derived and recombinant) than with intermediate purity factor concentrates, occurring in 15% to 35% of patients and in 1% to 4% of patients with severe hemophilia B.[41] Approximately 50% of factor VIII or IX inhibitors are low titer and transient. High-titer, high-responding inhibitors are the major clinical concern. Alloantibody inhibitors occur after at least one infusion of factor concentrate and at a median of 9 to 12 exposure days. They do not occur naturally prior to infusion. Most alloantibody inhibitors occur before the age of 20, are usually IgG subclass 4 or 1 immunoglobulins, and follow type 1 pharmacokinetics, characterized by specific and total neutralization of factor VIII or IX procoagulant activity. Risk factors for the development of these inhibitors include severity of hemophilia (patients with severe disease are affected much more than those with moderate or mild disease probably because they are also more heavily treated), age (younger rather than older), race (blacks and Hispanics more commonly affected than Caucasians for factor VIII alloantibodies; Scandinavians more common than other ethnicities for factor IX alloantibodies), family incidence of inhibitors (increased incidence among brother pairs and maternal relatives), and the extent and type of genetic mutation underlying the hemophilia (intron 22 inversion for factor VIII inhibitor; large gene deletions for factor IX inhibitors).

The development of an alloantibody inhibitor should be suspected when active bleeding does not subside despite the administration of clotting factor concentrate in doses deemed sufficient to raise factor VIII or IX activities to adequate hemostatic levels. Once suspected, the alloantibody inhibitor can be detected and measured in the laboratory using the Bethesda assay. By definition, the recovery study, performed by infusing clotting factor concentrate to achieve a level of 100% of normal activity, will yield less than 60% of expected values at 15 to 30 minutes. Ideally, this maneuver should be performed after a "washout period" of 72 to 96 hours without factor administration. The immediate management of inhibitors consists of treating the acute bleeding event; the long-range management involves the reduction/eradication of the inhibitor. Sources of the specific clotting factor should be withheld indefinitely unless immune tolerance induction is to be attempted. This withholding will allow the inhibitor titer to drop spontaneously over time. Acute bleeding events associated with low titer factor inhibitors (less than 5 BU) can be managed by overwhelming the inhibitor with large doses of human clotting factor concentrate (200 U/kg). For high-titer inhibitors, alternative clotting factor concentrates need to be utilized since human factor concentrates cannot overwhelm the inhibitor (Table 4–3). Porcine factor VIII concentrate (Hyate C, Speywood) is particularly useful in allo- or auto-factor VIII antibody situations since there is low cross-reactivity between anti-human factor VIII antibodies and the porcine-derived factor VIII coagulant protein. Porcine factor VIII concentrate is the only inhibitor treatment available that allows for the measurement of factor VIII activity levels after infusion. There has been no documented transmission of blood-borne infectious agents, including parvovirus. Disadvantages of this product include anamnestic antibody generation against human or porcine factor VIII, episodic thrombocytopenia, and rare anaphylaxis.

Infusions of so-called bypassing agents offer another useful treatment modality for bleeding associated with allo- and auto-factor VIII antibodies. These products include factor IX complex concentrates (formerly known as prothrombin complex concentrates, or PCCs) of the unactivated and activated varieties and recombinant factor VIIa concentrate. The PCCs have an increased risk of thromboembolic events and repeat dosing is based on clinical response following infusion. Usual doses range from 50 to 100 U/kg as intravenous boluses every 8 to 12 hours, as needed. Recombinant factor VIIa concentrate (NovoSeven, Novo Nordisk) has a low but finite risk of thromboembolic events, particularly in older individuals, and requires IV bolus infusions to be repeated every 2 to 3 hours at a dose of 90 µg/kg until bleeding is controlled.[42] No useful laboratory measurement is available; factor VII levels are very high and prothrombin times are substantially reduced; neither is predictive for adequate hemostasis. The management of acute bleeding events in hemophilia B complicated with high-titer inhibitors also involves the use of PCCs or recombinant VIIa concentrate.

Immune tolerance induction (ITI) regimens have been devised to reduce the level of alloantibodies against factors VIII and IX. ITI is a prolonged desensitization process in which the immune system production of inhibitory antibody is suppressed permanently after prolonged daily infusions of clotting factor concentrate. During this induction period, anamnestic antibody responses can occur and necessitate the use of one of the bypassing agents to treat acute bleeding events. Successful ITI can be achieved in approximately 50% of high-titer inhibitors, but ITI has been most successful in low titer inhibitors, which have been present for less than a year.[43] More than 60% of individuals achieve inhibitors levels below 1 BU within 6 months of initiating ITI; 80% by 1 year have levels below 1 BU. By 30 months, 90% have been successfully tolerized according to clotting factor kinetics and recovery data. A variety of protocols for ITI have been developed, including high-dose regimens that infuse up 200 U of clotting factor concentrate/kg/day and low-dose regimens of 50 U clotting factor/kg administered daily. Once the inhibitor resolves, patients are then placed on prophylaxis regimens indefinitely with bolus infusions of factor VIII concentrate thrice weekly or factor IX concentrate twice weekly. Some ITI regimens have included initial immunosuppressive therapy with cyclophosphamide or glucocorticosteroids along with infusions of intravenous immune globulin. Because ITI success is better with low-titer inhibitors, occasionally, plasmapheresis is used to acutely decrease a high-titer inhibitor to low titers. This improves the success of clotting factor infusions to reverse bleeding and facilitates the initiation of ITI.

INFECTIOUS COMPLICATIONS OF REPLACEMENT THERAPY IN HEMOPHILIA: HIV, HEPATITIS, AND PARVOVIRUS B19

AIDS was first identified in individuals with hemophilia in 1981, and by 1984 over 90% of patients with severe hemophilia A and 50% with severe hemophilia B were

Table 4–3 • INHIBITOR THERAPY

Type/Product Name	Manufacturer	Method of Viral Attenuation
Hyate: C (porcine factor VIII)	Speywood	None
Autoplex T	Baxter Hyland Immuno (Distributed by Nabi)	Dry heat (60°C, 144 hours)
FEIBA VH	Baxter Hyland Immuno (Vienna)	Vapor heat (60°C, 10 hours, 1190 mbar plus 80°C, 1 hour, 1375 mbar
NovoSeven (recombinant factor VIIa)	Novo Nordisk	Affinity chromatography

HIV seropositive. The HIV virus was contracted from repeated infusions of plasma-derived coagulation factor replacement products in this population of obligate recipients. In 1984, high dry heating and pasteurization techniques for viral attenuation were introduced into the manufacturing process of factor VIII concentrates. Shortly thereafter, solvent detergent treatment regimens were developed. All of these processes were added to the manufacturing of factor IX concentrates in the late 1980s. Combined with strict donor viral screening protocols and intensive donor self-exclusion programs, these viral attenuation processes have prevented any documented HIV or HCV seroconversions with the use of plasma-derived clotting factor concentrates in the United States since the late 1980s. Recombinant factor concentrates would not be expected to transmit these blood-borne pathogenic viruses. Unfortunately, these viral attenuation processes are effective only against lipid enveloped viruses such as HIV, HCV, and hepatitis B virus (HBV), but not against parvovirus B19, hepatitis A virus (HAV), or Creutzfeld-Jakob prions.

Patients with HIV and hemophilia have benefited from the introduction of anti-HIV protease inhibitor medications. An increase in bleeding severity and frequency with unusual sites of bleeding has been a hallmark complication in some hemophiliacs treated with these medications. The cause remains unclear but may involve the development of qualitative platelet defects (see Chapter 33).[44]

Prior to availability of the specific hepatitis B vaccine, hepatitis B was found in as many as 70% to 90% of severe hemophiliacs. HCV seroprevalence is greater than 90% in hemophiliacs treated with plasma-derived factor concentrates prior to 1985. Coinfection of HCV and HIV has high morbidity, increasing the risk of cirrhosis, hepatocellular carcinoma, and liver failure. Currently, treatment with interferon-alpha and ribavirin provides the greatest response rate and longest duration of HCV suppression.[45] The best and most durable responses to this therapeutic regimen are observed in those with the lowest HCV RNA viral titers and with HCV genotypes other than type 1. Unfortunately, hemophiliacs most commonly have been infected with HCV genotypes 1 and 3. All hemophiliacs should be vaccinated against HBV starting at birth or the time of diagnosis, and against HAV at 2 years of age or older if found to be seronegative.

The seroprevalence of parvovirus B19 in hemophiliac is 80%, significantly higher than the normal population matched for age and socioeconomic status. This non-lipid-enveloped virus, like hepatitis A, is not eradicated from plasma derived clotting factor concentrates by currently utilized viral attenuation techniques. Acute parvovirus B19 infection usually is asymptomatic when acquired through blood products; however, rarely, it may induce aplastic anemia or pure red cell aplasia, particularly in the presence of HIV. The vertical transmission of parvovirus in pregnant women may cause hydrops fetalis.

Creutzfeldt-Jakob Disease (CJD) is a rare, incurable fatal degenerative disease of the central nervous system, which has been described as a spongiform encephalopathy. The cause of CJD has been most recently linked to a disease-causing prion protein.[46] CJD is transmitted usually through direct inoculation, most commonly associated with implants of dura mater from infected individuals, administration of growth hormone derived from pituitary glands from infected cadavers, and after transplantation of organs from infected donors. A new variant form of CJD has been described in cattle ("mad cow disease" [bovine spongiform encephalopathy, or BSE]) and has been transmitted to humans via ingestion of contaminated beef. There has never been a reported case of human transmission of CJD from blood transfusions or a blood-derived product; however, prions have been identified in the buffy coat leukocytes of CJD-affected humans and can be transmitted experimentally to rodents after inoculating those cells into the animals' brains. Because of an incubation time as long as 35 years, a definitive conclusion about transmissability potential from human-to-human through blood transfusions cannot be determined readily. To reduce the theoretical risk of CJD transmission to hemophiliacs by pooled plasma-derived clotting factor concentrates, donor pools have been reduced in number; the use of recombinant replacement products has been encouraged and albumin-free formulations of these products have been developed; and screening of blood donors for CJD risks has been implemented. There have been no prospective studies performed to determine the incidence of parvovirus B19 transmission from plasma-derived products. This is not an issue for recombinant products. There have been no documented HIV transmissions from plasma-derived factor VIII concentrates since 1985 nor from factor IX concentrates since 1987, when viral attenuation processes were added to the products. Although sporadic cases of HCV have been reported, this also occurs in the normal population. There have been no epidemics of HCV infection from the virally attenuated factor concentrates.

GENE THERAPY

The use of gene therapy in the treatment of hemophilia A and B has progressed rapidly in recent years. The increase of plasma factor levels to above 1% can make a dramatic difference in the clinical outcomes and quality of life for individuals with hemophilia. Coagulation factors VIII and IX can be synthesized efficiently in a variety of somatic cell types. Thus, the hemophilias are very amenable to gene therapy. A number of viral vectors have been utilized to transfer human factor VIII or IX genes into target cells. These have included retroviral vectors, adenoviral vectors, adeno-associated viral vectors, and lentiviral vectors. Other methodologies currently under investigation for gene transfer in the hemophilias include chimeraplasty, which utilizes RNA/DNA oligonucleotides to activate endogenous repair systems and correct point mutations[47]; the use of host fibroblasts transfected nonvirally with normal human factor VIII or IX genes by electroporation; naked DNA transfer; and various types of plasmid-DNA transfer techniques. Potential complications of gene therapy include the development of inhibitory antibodies,[48] the risk of integrating the transgene into essential genes in the host, and the risk of inadvertent integration of the transgene into the germline with transmission to later generations. Currently, the clinical use of gene therapy in the treatment of the hemophilias remains in early and limited phase I trials. None of these complications has been observed thus far. Seven individuals have received intramuscular injections of an adeno-associated viral vector at three different dose levels for the treatment of their hemophilia B.[49] No inhibitors have been detected. The first reported phase I trial of human gene therapy in hemophilia A has utilized a nonviral ex-vivo somatic cell gene transfer system. Host fibroblasts obtained from a simple skin biopsy are cultured and transfected by electroporation with a B-domain-deleted human factor VIII gene. The transfected fibroblasts isolated from the culture are subsequently implanted into the host's omental fat pad via laparoscopy.[50] To date six individuals with severe hemophilia A have undergone this procedure and no inhibitors have been detected. Three patients have demonstrated sustained increases above baseline of their factor VIII activity levels, ranging between 1% and 4%, and have experienced an associated decrease in their bleeding tendency and factor VIII replacement requirements. Although these and future gene therapy clinical trials in hemophilia A and B may hold the promise of curing these disorders, the simple palliation of disease severity (e.g., rendering a severe hemophiliac into a moderate or mild case) is more realistic and will significantly reduce the morbidity, the mortality, and the cost of treating the disease. There will remain a need for safe, effective, and reasonably priced clotting factor concentrates, even after gene therapy, to provide prophylaxis in the perioperative period, to treat acute traumatic and surgical bleeds, and to initiate ITI if these individuals develop alloantibody inhibitors.

■ REFERENCES

Chapter 4 References

1. Lusher JM, McMillan CW. Severe factor VIII and factor IX deficiency in females. Am J Med 1978;65:637–648.
2. Anatonarakis SE, Rossiter JP, Young M, et al. Factor VIII gene inversions in severe hemophilia A: Results of an international consortium study. Blood 1995;86:2206–2212.
3. Tuddenheam EGD, Schwabb R, Seehafer J, et al. Haemophilia A: database of nucleotide substitutions, deletions, insertions and rearrangements of the factor VIII gene, second edition. Nucleic Acid Res 1994;22:3511–3533.
4. White GC, Beebe A, Nielsen B. Recombinant factor IX. Thromb Haemost 1997;77:261–265.
5. Goodeve AC. Advances in carrier detection in haemophilia. Haemophilia 1998;4:358–364.
6. Giannelli F, Green PM, Sommer SS, et al. Haemophilia B: database of point mutations and short additions and deletions, 7th edition. Nucleic Acid Res 1997;25:133–135.
7. Brocker-Vriends AHJT, Briet E, Kanahi HHH, et al. First trimester prenatal diagnosis of hemophilia A: Two years experience. Prenat Diagn 1988;8:411–421.
8. Gustavvi B, Cordesius E, Lofber L, et al. Fetoscopy. Acta Obstet Gynecol Scand 1979;58:409–410.
9. Ratnoff OD, Lewis JH. Heckathorn's disease: variable functional deficiency of antihemophilic factor (Factor VIII). Blood 1975;46:161–173.
10. Ljung R, Lindgren AC, Petrini P, et al. Normal vaginal delivery is to be recommended for haemophilia carrier gravidae. Acta Paediatr 1994;83:609–611.
11. Towner D, Castro MA, Eby-Wilkens E, et al. Effect of mode of delivery of nulliparous women on neonatal intracranial injury. N Engl J Med 1999;341:1709–1714.
12. Kitchens CS. Occult hemophilia. Johns Hopkins Med J 1980;146:255–259.
13. Arnold, WD, Hilgartner MW. Hemophilic arthropathy: current concepts of pathogenesis and management. J Bone Joint Surg (Am) 1977;59:287–305.
14. Hilgartner MW. Hemophilic arthropathy. Adv Pediatr 1975;21:139–165.
15. Manco-Johnson MJ, Nuss R, Geraghty S, et al. Results of secondary prophylaxis in children with severe hemophilia. Am J Hematol 1994;47:113–117.
16. Siegel HJ, Luck JV, Siegel ME, et al. Hemarthrosis and synovitis associated with hemophilia: clinical use of P-32 chromic phosphate synoviorthesis for treatment. Radiology 1994;190:257–261.
17. Jones JJ, Kitchens CS. Spontaneous intra-abdominal hemorrhage in hemophilia. Arch Intern Med 1984;144:297–300.
18. Rizza CR. Hemophilia and related inherited coagulation defects. In Bloom AL, Forbes CD, Thomas DP, et al. (Eds). Haemostasis and Thrombosis. Churchill Livingstone, London, 1994, p. 827.
19. Ewenstein BM, Takemoto C, Warrier I, et al. Nephrotic syndrome as a complication of immune tolerance in hemophilia B. Blood 1997;89:1115–1116.
20. Warrier I, Koerper MA, DiMichele D, et al. Factor IX inhibitors and anaphylaxis in hemophilia B. J Pediatr Hematol Oncol 1997;19:23–27.
21. Wilde JT. Protease inhibitor therapy. Haemophilia 2000;6:487–490.
22. Kitchens CS. Retropharyngeal hematoma in a hemophiliac. South Med J 1977;70:1421–1422.
23. Rodriguez Merchan EC. The haemophilic pseudotumor. Int Orthop 1995;19:255–260.
24. Lundblad RL, Kingdon HS, Mann KG, et al. Issues with the assay of factor VIII activity in plasma and factor VIII concentrates. Thromb Haemost 2000;84:942–948.
25. Lusher JM, Hillman-Weisman C, Horst D. In vivo recovery with products of very high purity-assay discrepancies. Haemophilia 1998;4:641–645.
26. Kasper CK, Aledort LM, Counts RB, et al. A more uniform measurement of factor VIII inhibitors. Thromb Diath Haemorrhag 1975;34:869–872.
27. Biggs R, Austen DE, Denson KW, et al. The mode of action of antibodies which destroy factor VIII. II. Antibodies which give complex concentration graphs. Br J Haematol 1972;23:137–155.
28. Verbruggen B, Novakova I, Wessels H, et al. The Nijmegen modification of the Bethesda assay for factor VIII:C inhibitors: improved specificity and reliability. Thromb Haemost 1995;73:247–251.
29. Souci JM, Nuss R, Evatt B, et al. Mortality among males with hemophilia: relations with source of medical care. Blood 2000;96:437–442.
30. Mannucci PM, Gdovin S, Gringeri A, et al. Transmission of hepatitis A to patients with hemophilia by factor VIII concentrates treated with organic solvent and detergent to inactivate viruses. Ann Intern Med 1994;120:1–11.
31. Lefrere JJ, Mariotti M, Thauvin M. B19 parvovirus DNA in solvent/detergent-treated anti-haemophilia concentrates. Lancet 1994;343:211–212.
32. Fijnvandraat K, Berntorp E, ten Cate JW, et al. Recombinant, B-domain deleted factor VIII (r-VIII SQ): pharmacokinetics and

initial safety aspects in hemophilia A patients. Thromb Haemost 1997;77:298–302.
33. Martinowitz U, Schulman S, Gitel H, et al. Adjusted dose continuous infusion of factor VIII in patients with haemophilia A. Br J Haematol 1992;82:729–734.
34. Lusher JM, Arkin S, Abildgaard CF, et al. Recombinant factor VIII for the treatment of previously untreated patients with hemophilia. N Engl J Med 1993;328:453–459.
35. Bray GL, Gomperts ED, Courter S, et al. and the Recombinant Study Group. A multicenter study of recombinant factor VIII (Recombinate): safety, efficacy and inhibitor risk in previously untreated patients with hemophilia A. Blood 1994;83:2428–2435.
36. Seremetis S, Aledort LM, Bergman G, et al. Three year randomized study of high purity or intermediate purity factor VIII concentrates in symptom-free HIV seropositive hemophiliacs: effects on immune status. Lancet 1993;342:700–703.
37. Fuente B, Kasper CK, Rickles FR, et al. Response of patients with mild and moderate hemophilia A and von Willebrand disease to treatment with desmopressin. Ann Intern Med 1985;103:6–15.
38. Lethagen S, Harris AS, Nilsson IM. Intranasal desmopressin (DDAVP) by spray in mild hemophilia A and von Willebrand's disease type I. Blut 1989;60:187–191.
39. Rakocz M, Mazar A, Varon D, et al. Dental extractions in patients with bleeding disorders, the use of fibrin glue. Oral Surg Oral Med Oral Pathol 1993;5:280–282.
40. Martinowitz U, Schulman S, Horoszowski H, et al. Role of fibrin sealant in surgical procedures on patients with hemostatic disorders. Clin Orthop Rel Res 1996;398:65–75.
41. Ljung RC. Gene mutations and inhibitor formation in patients with hemophilia B. Acta Haematol 1995;94(Suppl 1):49–52.
42. Key NS, Aledort LM, Beardsley D, et al. Home treatment of mild to moderate bleeding episodes using recombinant factor VIIa (NovoSeven) in haemophiliacs with inhibitors. Thromb Haemost 1998;80:912–918.
43. Ewing NP, Sanders NL, Dietrich SL, et al. Induction of immune tolerance of factor VIII in hemophiliacs with inhibitors. JAMA 1988;259:65–68.
44. Wilde JT. Protease inhibitor therapy and bleeding. Haemophilia 2000;6:487–490.
45. McHutchison JG, Gordon SC, Schiff Er, et al. Interferon Alfa 2b alone or in combination with ribavirin as initial treatment for chronic hepatitis C. N Engl J Med 1998;339:1485–1492.
46. Pablos-Mendez A, Netto E, Defendini R. Infectious prions or cytotoxic metabolites? Lancet 1993;341:159–161.
47. Kotani H, Germann MW, Andrus A, et al. RNA facilitates RecA-mediated DNA pairing and strand transfer between molecules bearing limited regions of homology. Mol Gen Genet 1996;250:626–634.
48. Armstrong E, Fields PA, Arruda VR, et al. Immune responses in hemophilia B mice expressing a species-specific transgene. Mol Ther 2000;1:225–235.
49. Manno CS, Glader B, Ragni MV. A phase I trial of AAV-mediated muscle directed gene transfer for hemophilia B. Blood 2000;96:3459(abstr).
50. Roth DA, Tawa NE, O'Brien J, et al. Non-viral gene transfer of blood coagulation factor VIII in patients with severe hemophilia A. Blood 2000;96:2532(abstr).

# Less Common Congenital Disorders of Hemostasis

Harold R. Roberts, M.D.
Miguel A. Escobar, M.D.

In this chapter the less common congenital disorders of hemostasis will be discussed. These include disorders of fibrinogen; prothrombin; and factors V, VII, X, and XI. In addition, the nonbleeding disorders associated with deficiencies of factor XII, prekallikrein, and high-molecular-weight kininogen will be discussed since these disorders are characterized by prolonged partial thromboplastin times and can be confused with the procoagulant defects that are associated with bleeding. Furthermore, the rare bleeding syndromes of factor XIII deficiency, α_2-plasmin inhibitor deficiency, and α_1-antitrypsin Pittsburgh will be described. For the sake of completeness, the potential role of protein Z and the protein Z-dependent protease inhibitor deficiencies will be considered. While protein Z deficiencies were initially thought to be a cause of hemorrhage in humans, more recent animal data suggest that defects in protein Z and the protein Z inhibitor are more likely related to thrombotic phenomena.

The characteristics of these factors are important for their clinical understanding and are depicted in Table 5–1. They can best be classified as proenzymes, cofactors, structural proteins, and physiologic inhibitors as shown in Table 5–2. The information in these tables will aid the consultant in understanding the basis for the clinical condition as well as the diagnosis and possible treatment of each deficiency.

DISORDERS OF FIBRINOGEN

Congenital disorders of fibrinogen can be divided into afibrinogenemia and dysfibrinogenemia.

Afibrinogenemia

Congenital afibrinogenemia is a very rare disorder that occurs in patients who have no detectable circulating fibrinogen either in the plasma or in the blood platelets. It was first described in 1920, and since then more than 150 cases have been reported.[1] The heterozygous state of afibrinogenemia results in low circulating levels of normal fibrinogen. The hypofibrinogenemias will be considered under the dysfibrinogenemias.

Pathogenesis and Genetics

Three individual genes on chromosome 4 code for the α, β, and γ chains that constitute the fibrinogen molecule. Fibrinogen is a homodimer consisting of two identical pairs of α, β, and γ chains intertwined to form a trinodular fibrinogen structure. Several cases of afibrinogenemia have been reported with abnormalities in the genes for the α, β, and γ chains, suggesting that a gross defect in any one of the three fibrinogen genes may result in afibrinogenemia.[2,3]

Afibrinogenemia is inherited in an autosomal recessive pattern, and symptomatic individuals are homozygotes. Heterozygous individuals usually have mild hypofibrinogenemia and are asymptomatic unless the fibrinogen level is less than 50 mg/dL. The estimated incidence of congenital afibrinogenemia is approximately 1 to 2 per million of the population, and there is usually a history of consanguinity within the family. The disorder occurs in both sexes with no known racial predilection. The characteristics of two patients with afibrinogenemia are shown in Table 5–3.

Table 5-1 • SUMMARY OF LESS COMMON CLOTTING FACTOR DEFICIENCIES

Factor Deficiency	Biological Half-life	Estimated Incidence	Type of Bleeding	Screening Abnormalities Abnormal	Normal
I	2-4 days	1:1 million	None to severe	PT, PTT, TCT, BT	None
II	3 days	Very rare	Mild-moderate	PT, PTT	TCT, BT
V	36 hours	1:1 million	Moderate	PT, PTT, BT	TCT
VII	3-6 hours	1:500,000	Mild-severe	PT	PTT, TCT, BT
X	40 hours	1:500,000	Mild-severe	PT, PTT	TCT, BT
XI	80 hours	Rare	Mild-moderate	PTT	PT, TCT, BT
XII	50-70 hours	Unknown	No bleeding	PTT	PT, TCT, BT
XIII	9 days	1:5 million	Moderate-severe	None	PT, PTT, TCT, BT
PK	35 hours	Unknown	None	PTT	PT, TCT, BT
HK	150 hours	Very rare	None	PTT	PT, TCT, BT
α_2-PI	3 days	Unknown	Mild-moderate	None	PT, PTT, TCT, BT
α_1-ATP	—	Very rare	Variable-severe	PT, PTT, TCT, BT	None
Protein Z	2-3 days	Unknown	None	None	PT, PTT, TCT, BT
ZPI	Unknown	Unknown	None	None	PT, PTT, TCT, BT

PT, prothrombin time; PTT, partial thromboplastin time; TCT, thrombin clotting time; BT, bleeding time; PK, prekallikrein; HK, high-molecular-weight kininogen; α_2-PI, alpha-2-plasmin inhibitor; α_1-ATP, alpha-1-antitrypsin Pittsburgh; ZPI, protein Z-dependent protease inhibitor.

Clinical Manifestations

Individuals with congenital afibrinogenemia have a lifelong bleeding tendency of variable severity. Hemorrhagic manifestations usually start in the neonatal period with umbilical cord (approximately 75%) and postcircumcisional bleeding.[4] In infancy or childhood, intracerebral hemorrhage is a leading cause of death.[5] Easy bruising and mucosal, gastrointestinal, and genitourinary hemorrhage are also common. Hemopericardium, hemoperitoneum, and spontaneous splenic rupture have been reported rarely.[6] Hemarthroses occur in up to 20% of the patients, but chronic hemophilic arthropathy as seen in patients with classic hemophilia is surprisingly uncommon.[7] Affected women exhibit menometrorrhagia, first-trimester spontaneous abortions, abruptio placentae, and postpartum hemorrhage.[8-10] Occasionally patients with afibrinogenemia will show little physical evidence of their underlying chronic bleeding disorder, but they will always give a convincing history of lifelong easy bleeding.

Diagnosis

The diagnosis of afibrinogenemia can be made by careful history and coagulation screening tests. Patients give a long history of intermittent hemorrhagic episodes, usually in the soft tissues, and all screening tests of coagulation, including the prothrombin time (PT), partial thromboplastin time (PTT), and thrombin clotting time (TCT), exhibit infinite clotting times. These tests nor-

Table 5-2 • CLASSIFICATION OF LESS COMMON CLOTTING FACTORS

	Clotting Factor	Activator	Final Product
Structural protein	Fibrinogen	Thrombin	Fibrin
Zymogen	Prothrombin	Xa/Va/Ca/PL	Thrombin
	Factor VII	?Xa	Factor VIIa
	Factor X	TF/VIIa or IXa/Ca/PL	Factor Xa
	Factor XI	Thrombin	Factor XIa
	Factor XII	Factor XIa	Factor XIIa
	Factor XIII	Thrombin	Factor XIIIa
	Prekallikrein	Factor XIIa	Kallikrein
Co-factor	Factor V	Xa or thrombin	Factor Va
	HK	Factor XIIa	Bradykinin
	Protein Z	?	?
Inhibitors	ZPI	?	Xa inhibitors
	α_2-PI	—	Plasmin-α_2-PI complex
	α_1-ATP	—	Thrombin-α_1-ATP complex

Ca, calcium; PL, phospholipid (activated platelets); TF, tissue factor; HK, high-molecular-weight kininogen; ZPI, protein Z-dependent protease inhibitor; α_2-PI, alpha-2-plasmin inhibitor; α_1-ATP, alpha-1-antitrypsin Pittsburgh.

Table 5-3 • CHARACTERISTICS OF 2 PATIENTS WITH AFIBRINOGENEMIA

Location Defect	Genetic Defect	Symptoms	Consanguinity
α-chain	Deletion intron 1	Umbilical cord bleeding	No
β-chain	Missense mutations in exons 7 and 8	Umbilical cord bleeding Circumcisional bleeding Muscle hematoma Hemarthroses	Yes

malize in vitro with 1:1 mixing with normal plasma, thereby excluding an inhibitor.

To confirm the diagnosis of afibrinogenemia, specific fibrinogen assays must be used, including clotting and immunologic methods, both of which show no detectable fibrinogen. The bleeding time in afibrinogenemic patients is prolonged because of absent platelet fibrinogen.[11,12] Mild thrombocytopenia has also been reported in approximately 25% of patients with congenital afibrinogenemia, but platelet counts are usually not lower than 100,000/μL.[13]

Delayed-type hypersensitivity skin tests in individuals with afibrinogenemia typically will show only erythema but no induration because of the lack of fibrin deposition in the subcutaneous tissue.[14] The erythrocyte sedimentation rate is also very slow in these individuals since fibrinogen is one of the main determinants of this test.[15]

Differential Diagnosis

Acquired fibrinogen abnormalities must be excluded. Severe disseminated intravascular coagulation can result in severe hypofibrinogenemia, but other clotting factors and platelets are also usually markedly decreased. Acquired hypofibrinogenemia has been reported with liver disease and with the use of certain medications such as sodium valproate[16] and L-asparaginase,[17] both of which impair the hepatic synthesis of fibrinogen.

Treatment

The treatment of choice for individuals with afibrinogenemia and hypofibrinogenemia is cryoprecipitate, a rich source of fibrinogen. Solvent-detergent-treated products are preferred in order to inactivate the human immunodeficiency virus and hepatitis viruses. In European countries, purified, virally inactivated fibrinogen is available. Replacement treatment is indicated for episodes of active bleeding, preoperatively, and during pregnancy. To achieve hemostasis, increasing the fibrinogen level to 50 to 100 mg/dL is usually adequate. Prophylactic therapy is only recommended during pregnancy. To avoid miscarriages, a fibrinogen level above 60 mg/dL is necessary throughout the course of the pregnancy.[18]

Each bag of cryoprecipitate contains approximately 250 to 300 mg of fibrinogen. Thus, 5 to 10 bags are usually adequate for an individual who weighs 70 kg. Each bag of cryoprecipitate will raise the fibrinogen level by about 10 mg/dL, with an in vivo half-life of about 2 to 4 days. However, daily monitoring of fibrinogen levels is necessary to determine the fibrinogen dose, since the fibrinogen level can vary over time. For major surgical procedures (e.g., knee replacement) or severe trauma, the duration of treatment may be as long as 2 to 3 weeks of daily fibrinogen administration. For minor trauma, a single dose of fibrinogen sufficient to raise the level to 50 to 100 mg/dL is adequate. The administration of 1-desamino-8-D-arginine vasopressin (DDAVP) may decrease the bleeding time in certain patients, but it is not adequate for hemostasis.

Complications of replacement therapy include the risk of allergic reactions, transmission of viral diseases, and development of antifibrinogen antibodies.[19] Thrombotic phenomena have been reported in patients after normalization of the fibrinogen level. Some of the episodes have occurred in women on oral contraceptives, suggesting that they might have had an underlying hypercoagulable state.[20-22] Should thrombotic phenomena occur in the perioperative period, appropriate anticoagulation therapy should be used in combination with fibrinogen replacement.[23]

The Dysfibrinogenemias

The first case of dysfibrinogenemia was reported in 1964, but, since that time, numerous other cases have been described. Approximately 100 different genetic defects in fibrinogen that lead to dysfibrinogenemias have been detected.[24]

Pathogenesis and Genetics

Congenital dysfibrinogenemia is characterized by the synthesis of an abnormal fibrinogen molecule that does not function properly in the conversion of fibrinogen to fibrin. The functional defects include: (1) abnormal fibrinopeptide release; (2) defects in fibrin polymerization; (3) abnormal fibrin stabilization; and (4) resistance to fibrin lysis. The most common dysfibrinogenemias are those causing polymerization defects.[25] In most of the cases, congenital dysfibrinogenemia is inherited as an autosomal dominant trait with high levels of penetrance, but some patients exhibit an autosomal recessive inheritance. Patients may be homozygous or heterozygous for the defect. The majority of affected individuals are heterozygous with approximately 50% of normal fibrinogen, which is adequate for normal hemostasis unless the dysfunctional molecule disrupts the function of the normal component. Some individuals with dysfibrinogenemia will have fibrinogen levels well below normal.

Clinical Manifestations

Clinically, patients with dysfibrinogenemia will have one of the following phenotypes: no hemorrhagic manifestations; mild bleeding following trauma; thromboses; or both thrombotic and hemorrhagic manifestations. Approximately 43% of all individuals with congenital dysfibrinogenemia are asymptomatic, while about 20% have bleeding symptoms and 17% experience thrombotic manifestations. About 20% of patients have a combination of bleeding and thrombosis.[25,26] The bleeding tendency is variable, with most of the individuals having mild to moderate hemorrhages. Easy bruising, soft-tissue bleeding, menorrhagia, and intraoperative and postoperative bleeding are the most common events. Both venous and arterial thromboses have been associated with congenital dysfibrinogenemia, including deep-venous thrombosis of the lower extremities, pulmonary embolism, recurrent spontaneous abortions, and thrombosis of the carotid arteries and abdominal aorta.[25] The dysfibrinogenemias most likely associated with bleeding are associated with abnormalities in the amino-terminus of the α chain, although there are exceptions to this generality. Thrombotic manifestations, on the other hand, are most often associated with fibrinogen variants that, with a free cystine residue, permit disulfide linkage to albumin. These variants are resistant to lysis by plasmin, which probably accounts for the thrombotic tendencies. In many cases, however, thrombotic manifestations may be related to concurrent disorders (factor V Leiden mutation, protein C deficiency, etc.) rather than to the abnormal fibrinogen molecule, and clinicians should be aware of these possibilities. Since a normal fibrin clot is a necessary framework for normal wound healing, it is not surprising that poor healing and dehiscence of wounds is seen in certain dysfibrinogenemic patients.[27] Examples of the dysfibrinogenemias in the α, β, and γ chains are shown in Table 5–4.

Diagnosis

In most cases of dysfibrinogenemia, the screening tests of coagulation such as the PT, PTT, and TCT are usually prolonged and may or may not correct with 1:1 mixing with normal plasma. This is because some dysfibrinogenemias will interfere with normal fibrin formation. In some dysfibrinogenemias that are manifested by thrombotic episodes, the TCT may be shorter than normal. Fibrinogen levels are variable and can be relatively normal or low. One may encounter normal levels of fibrinogen by immunologic methods and at the same time reduced levels of fibrinogen by functional analysis. Other important diagnostic tests include the reptilase time and fibrinogen immunoelectrophoresis. The reptilase time is often prolonged and may be more sensitive than the TCT. Fibrinogen immunoelectrophoresis will sometimes show an abnormal migration in agarose gels. However, definitive diagnosis depends upon a biochemical characterization of the fibrinogen defect, which may require amino acid sequencing. More sophisticated diagnosis will require genetic characterization.

Differential Diagnosis

Dysfibrinogenemias can also be acquired, particularly in patients with liver disease of varied etiology. Frequently, the abnormality is due to an increase in sialic acid resi-

Table 5–4 • EXAMPLES OF DYSFIBRINOGENEMIA VARIANTS[a]

Variant	Clinical Effect	Functional Defect
Chapel Hill IV	Asymptomatic	Polymerization defect
Fukuoka II	Asymptomatic	Fibrinopeptide B release defect
Chapel Hill I	Bleeding	Polymerization defect
Christchurch II	Bleeding	Fibrinopeptide B release defect
Guarenas I	Bleeding	Fibrinopeptide A release and polymerization defect
Nijmegen	Thrombosis	Associated with disulfide-linked albumin and tPA binding defect
Naples II	Thrombosis	Fibrinopeptide A and B release defect
Paris V	Thrombosis	Polymerization defect, decreased binding of plasminogen, and decreased tPA-induced fibrinolysis
Marburg	Bleeding/thrombosis	Deletion of 150 aa with linkage to albumin

aa, amino acid; tPA, tissue plasminogen activator.
[a] See Lord[25] and Roberts and Bingham.[26]

dues.[28] In the dysfibrinogenemia of liver disease, other clotting proteins synthesized by the liver will be low. Autoantibodies against fibrinogen in nondeficient individuals should also be distinguished from dysfibrinogenemia, since they interfere with fibrinogen function and will mimic the abnormalities seen with the dysfibrinogenemias. Antifibrinogen antibodies have been associated with systemic lupus erythematosus, ulcerative colitis, liver cirrhosis, and other disorders. Fibrinogen degradation products seen in many diseases may also interfere with normal fibrinogen function and produce a condition resembling the dysfibrinogenemias.

Treatment

Therapy is not indicated in patients with congenital dysfibrinogenemia who are asymptomatic. To treat bleeding episodes or for preoperative procedures, fresh frozen plasma, cryoprecipitate, or fibrinogen concentrates should be administered. The guidelines outlined in the afibrinogenemia section can also be applied to the dysfibrinogenemias. Dysfibrinogenemic patients who have thrombotic episodes require anticoagulation with heparin followed by oral anticoagulants. Recurrent thrombotic episodes require prophylactic anticoagulation. Women with recurrent spontaneous abortions and dysfibrinogenemia can be treated with fibrinogen replacement therapy throughout the course of the pregnancy.

PROTHROMBIN DEFICIENCY (HYPOPROTHROMBINEMIA AND DYSPROTHROMBINEMIA)

The first reports of congenital prothrombin deficiency were described by Quick.[29,30] Fewer than 100 cases have been reported, and examples of these are listed in Table 5–5.

Pathogenesis and Genetics

A variety of mutations in the prothrombin gene have been discovered. They usually are caused by a missense mutation, i.e., the substitution of a single amino acid in regions that affect the function and/or structure of the prothrombin molecule.[31] These mutations result in dysprothrombinemia in which the prothrombin activity is reduced while the prothrombin antigen may be normal or decreased as shown in Table 5–5.

Prothrombin is normally converted to thrombin, which is necessary for the formation of a normal fibrin clot. The molecular defects in dysprothrombinemia may affect the amino-terminal pro-piece of prothrombin or the carboxyl-terminal thrombin portion of the molecule. Defects in the pro-piece usually result in delayed thrombin generation, but the thrombin that is generated functions normally. An example of a defect in the pro-piece of the molecule is prothrombin San Juan. Defects in the thrombin end of the molecule result in the generation of an abnormal thrombin such as seen in prothrombin Quick II. In some patients the dysprothrombinemia may be homozygous, while in others it may be heterozygous or compound heterozygous.

Dysprothrombinemia is inherited in an autosomal recessive pattern. There is no known predilection for race, although many patients seem to be of southern European ancestry.[32]

Clinical Manifestations

There is a weak correlation between functional prothrombin levels and the clinical picture of hemorrhage. All reported dysprothrombinemic patients have had measurable prothrombin activity, which supports the belief that complete deficiency is incompatible with life. This is corroborated in knockout mice, where complete deficiency of prothrombin results in fatal neonatal hemorrhage.[33,34]

In general, heterozygous patients are either asymptomatic or have minor bleeding symptoms, whereas homozygous or compound heterozygous individuals have more severe symptoms. Heterozygous individuals usually have prothrombin activity levels of 50%, with normal antigen levels.[32] These patients are usually asymptomatic, but can develop bleeding after surgical procedures. Individuals who are homozygous or compound heterozygous have mild to moderate bleeding symptoms, such as easy bruising, epistaxis, hematomas, and postoperative bleeding. In females, menorrhagia, postpartum hemorrhage, and miscarriages have been reported.[35] Hemarthroses as well as spontaneous subarachnoid and intracerebral hemorrhages occur rarely.[36]

Diagnosis

The diagnosis of dysprothrombinemia is suggested by a lifelong history of bleeding in patients with a prolonged PT and PTT that corrects when mixed 1:1 with normal plasma. The bleeding time and TCT are normal. Definitive diagnosis requires a specific assay for prothrombin functional activity. Immunologic assays of prothrombin may be helpful but sometimes are normal.

Differential Diagnosis

Hereditary prothrombin deficiency must be distinguished from other congenital deficiencies, which are characterized by a prolonged PT and PTT and normal TCT. The most common deficiencies with this pattern are factor V and factor X deficiencies, but they can be diagnosed by using specific assays for factors V and X, respectively. Acquired prothrombin deficiency is commonly seen in patients with liver disease, vitamin K deficiency, or ingestion of vitamin K antagonists such as warfarin or superwarfarins, both of which are found in rodenticides. In all of these conditions, all the vitamin K-dependent factors in addition to prothrombin, protein C, and protein S will be low. The surreptitious

Table 5–5 • PROTHROMBIN VARIANTS

Variant	Activity (%)	Antigen (%)	Bleeding Tendency
Homozygous			
Barcelona/Madrid	5–15	100	Yes
Carora	4	0	Yes
Denver	<1	13	Yes
Dharan	5	95	Yes
Frankfurt/Salatka	15	100	Yes/No
Marburg	3	100	Yes
Obihiro	18	100	Yes
Poissy	2	50	Yes
Perija	2	70	Yes
Segovia	7–20	100	Yes
Heterozygous			
Brussels	25–50	84	Yes
Cardeza	30–50	100	No
Clamart	50	100	No
Magdeburg	45	100	Yes
Padua	50	100	Yes
San Antonio	50	100	Yes
Compound Heterozygous			
Corpus Christi	2	25	No
Habana	1–10	50	Yes
Himi I	10	100	No
Himi II	10	100	No
Metz	10	50	Yes
Mexico City	<10	<10	Yes
Molise	10	45	Yes
Quick	<2	37–40	Yes
Quick II	<1	—	Yes
San Juan I & II	20	93	Yes
Tokushima	21	—	Yes
Uncharacterized genetics			
Gainesville	25	70	Yes
Houston	5–10	50	Yes

Data from Roberts and Bingham[26] and Roberts and Hoffman.[46]

use of warfarin or superwarfarins such as brodificoum should be suspected in individuals with a severe bleeding tendency who are otherwise apparently normal and without liver dysfunction. Such patients often ingest rodenticides and induce bleeding symptoms for secondary gain. Superwarfarins cannot be detected by simple warfarin assays, but specific testing is available at reference laboratories.

Dysprothrombinemias must also be distinguished from other causes of deficiency of vitamin K such as antibiotics containing the N-methyl-thio-tetrazole side chain present in the third generation cephalosporins. This side chain inhibits the vitamin K-dependent γ-carboxylation of glutamic acid residues that is required for the production of normal prothrombin and other vitamin K-dependent factors.[37]

Antibodies against prothrombin can be seen in patients with the lupus anticoagulant or the antiphospholipid syndrome and on rare occasions as isolated cases.[38] These antibodies usually result in a true prothrombin deficiency because of accelerated clearance of the antibody-prothrombin complex.[38,39] Patients with this type of acquired prothrombin deficiency will have similar symptoms to the dysprothrombinemias, but symptoms will not be lifelong.

Treatment

Pure prothrombin concentrates are not available for clinical use. Patients with minor bleeding episodes may not need replacement therapy but may require infusions of fresh frozen plasma. Major hemorrhages can be treated with fresh frozen plasma at a loading dose of 15 to 20 mL/kg of body weight, followed by 3 mL/kg of body weight every 12 to 24 hours, since the prothrombin half-life is approximately 3 days. Prothrombin levels of 20% to 40% are usually sufficient to maintain adequate hemostasis.[40] In patients with recurrent bleeding episodes, prophylactic plasma infusions every 3 to 5 weeks can be administered.[41]

An alternative treatment for dysprothrombinemia is the use of prothrombin complex concentrates (PCCs). Some of these contain significant amounts of prothrombin and other vitamin K-dependent factors. Care should be taken when using PCCs, since they have been associated with thromboembolic complications, presumably due to contamination with variable amounts of activated factors VIIa, Xa, and IXa.[42,43] There are several commercial PCCs on the market with variable levels of the vitamin K-dependent factors. Therefore, before using PCCs for replacement therapy of prothrombin deficiency, one should know the prothrombin level in a particular product. One regimen is to use an initial loading dose of 20 U of prothrombin per kilogram of body weight, followed by 5 U of prothrombin per kilogram of body weight every 24 hours.[44] Care should be taken not to exceed the 20-U/kg dose because of the danger of inducing disseminated intravascular coagulation or other thrombotic phenomena. Patients should be monitored for the development of disseminated intravascular coagulation during and after PCC use.[45] If one wishes to avoid the use of PCCs in patients who need surgery, plasma exchange can be performed before the operation to achieve near normal levels of prothrombin.[46]

FACTOR V DEFICIENCY

In 1943, Quick described a "labile factor" present in plasma that was required for a normal PT.[47] A few years later, Owren reported a patient with a lifelong history of bleeding who was found to be deficient in a "labile factor."[48] Both were describing an activity now known as factor V. Factor V deficiency is an uncommon disorder with an estimated incidence of less than one in 1 million of the population.

Pathogenesis and Genetics

Factor V is a glycoprotein that is found in plasma and the α granules of platelets. The origin of the factor V found in platelets is not known for certain. Most secretable platelet-derived factor V is thought to be derived from plasma, though this concept has been challenged.[49,50] Although hepatocytes synthesize most of the plasma factor V, megakaryocytes have been shown to contain factor V mRNA.[51] Platelet factor V accounts for about 20% of the total body pool of factor V and is released upon activation and degranulation of the platelets.[52] The relative roles of plasma and platelet factor V in hemostasis are not precisely known, although platelet factor V is known to be fully functional.

Congenital factor V deficiency is inherited as an autosomal recessive trait and is characterized by decreased or absent factor V activity in plasma and platelets. Consanguinity is common. The molecular genetics of factor V deficiency have not been well described, but it is known that several genetic variants of factor V exist.[53,54]

Clinical Manifestations

Factor V deficiency occurs in mild, moderate, and severe forms. Patients with severe deficiency (less than 1%) usually present with umbilical stump bleeding, easy bruising, epistaxis, menorrhagia, and postpartum and postoperative hemorrhage. Hemarthroses may occur, but they are usually traumatic in origin. In marked contrast to patients with less than 1% of factor VIII or IX who experience frequent spontaneous hemarthroses, patients with less than 1% factor V activity have few joint hemorrhages. This suggests that severely affected factor V-deficient patients are not completely deficient in the factor. Mice completely deficient in factor V, derived by gene knockout techniques, suffer neonatal death but can be rescued by the insertion of a minigene expressing less than 1% normal factor V activity.[55] There is clinical evidence that the bleeding tendency correlates more with the platelet factor V levels than with the plasma levels.[56] Mildly affected patients may be difficult to diagnose, and some may not be diagnosed until adulthood. Paradoxically, there have been several reports of patients with congenital factor V deficiency that present with thrombosis.[57] Inhibitors to factor V are very rare in patients with congenital factor V deficiency.[58]

Diagnosis

Laboratory evaluation reveals prolonged PT and PTT with a normal TCT. In severely affected patients who lack platelet factor V, the bleeding time is also prolonged, sometimes greater than 20 minutes. The definitive diagnosis for factor V deficiency requires a specific factor V assay.

Differential Diagnosis

Acquired factor V deficiency can be seen in patients with significant liver disease or in patients with disseminated intravascular coagulation. A syndrome of combined congenital deficiencies of factors V and VIII also exists and must be distinguished from simple factor V deficiency (see below).

Spontaneous inhibitors to factor V in patients without factor V deficiency have been frequently reported in postoperative patients and in association with antibiotics such as aminoglycosides and penicillin. Some of the inhibitors have been reported with infections (tuberculosis) and certain malignancies. In more than half of the patients with acquired inhibitors, the antibodies disappear spontaneously within a period of several weeks to months. Some patients have developed anti-factor V antibodies after being exposed to topical bovine thrombin that contains bovine factor V. Human antibodies to these bovine products have been shown to cross-react with both human thrombin and human factor V, and in some cases bleeding can be severe. The treatment of choice in these patients is corticosteroids and exchange transfusion.[59] Platelet factor V deficiency initially reported as factor V Quebec has now been shown to be due to proteolysis of factor V and several other proteins in platelet α granules.[60,61]

Treatment

No commercial factor V concentrates are available for replacement therapy. Minor bleeds like epistaxis or bleeding following dental extractions can be treated with local measures and antifibrinolytic therapy such as tranexamic acid and ε-aminocaproic acid. Fresh frozen plasma is the treatment of choice when more serious bleeding occurs. Mild to moderate hemorrhagic episodes can be treated with plasma at a loading dose of 15 to 20 mL/kg of body weight, followed by 3 to 6 mL/kg every 24 hours, to achieve a level of approximately 25% of normal. More frequent infusions are not necessary, given the long half-life of factor V (approximately 36 hours).[62] Higher levels can be achieved by plasma exchange in patients with severe hemorrhage, in preparation for surgery, or when fluid overload is a concern.[63] Platelet transfusions have been reported to correct the bleeding in some patients, since they are a source of factor V; but they are not always effective and are not recommended because of the potential for developing antiplatelet alloantibodies[64] (see Chapter 6).

FACTOR VII DEFICIENCY

Alexander and colleagues described the first case of congenital factor VII deficiency in 1951.[65] Over the years, many more cases have been described along with characterization of the specific genetic defects. Factor VII deficiency occurs with an estimated incidence of 1 in 500,000. There does not seem to be a racial or gender predilection for the defect.

Pathogenesis and Genetics

Since the factor VIIa/tissue factor complex is essential for the initiation of coagulation in vivo, a deficiency or structural defect in the factor VII molecule can lead to significant bleeding symptoms. More than 50% of the patients seem to have low functional activity and antigen, while others have a dysfunctional molecule (normal antigen and reduced activity). Factor VII deficiency is inherited in an autosomal recessive fashion with homozygotes and double heterozygotes exhibiting the majority of the bleeding symptoms. Numerous different genetic mutations have been described, many with a similar phenotypic expression of mild, moderate, or severe bleeding manifestations.[66] A detailed database of the mutations can be found on the World Wide Web at: http://193.60.222.13/.

Clinical Manifestations

The clinical presentation of factor VII deficiency varies widely from one patient to another, and there is a poor correlation between the plasma level of factor VII and bleeding symptoms. This may be explained by the fact that the in vitro factor VII activity is dependent upon the type of tissue factor used in the assay. The assay using human tissue factor seems to correlate best with the bleeding diathesis.[67] Some patients with less than 1% factor VII activity using rabbit tissue factor in the assay may have measurable factor VII activity when human tissue factor is used. These patients may have a mild or even negative history of hemorrhage.

In general, individuals with factor VII levels of less than 10% of normal are more likely to exhibit hemorrhagic episodes than patients with higher levels of the factor. Commonly, bleeding in factor VII-deficient patients includes easy bruising, epistaxis, and soft-tissue hemorrhage. Women can present with menorrhagia, menometrorrhagia, and postpartum bleeding. Postoperative bleeding is not rare but almost always occurs in severely affected patients. Patients with factor VII levels of less than 1% can have very severe bleeding, equivalent to that seen in hemophilia A and B, with hemarthroses, retroperitoneal bleeding, muscle hematomas, and fatal intracranial hemorrhage. However, occasional patients with less than 1% activity will have no history of bleeding. A high incidence of hemarthroses with mostly grade 3 and 4 arthropathy in 40 patients has been described from eight European hemophilia centers.[67] Central nervous system bleeding has been mostly reported in infants after vaginal delivery, with an incidence of up to 16%.[68] A few cases of thrombosis have been described in factor VII-deficient patients.[69] Inhibitory antibodies against exogenously administered factor VII have been reported in a very few patients with severe congenital deficiency of factor VII.[70]

Diagnosis

Individuals with factor VII deficiency will have an isolated, prolonged PT with normal PTT, TCT, and bleeding time. On rare occasions, the PTT can be prolonged and is usually due to unique genetic defects in the factor VII molecule. A specific factor VII assay is required to confirm the diagnosis; and the activity may vary, depending on the species from which the tissue factor is derived. Tissue factor from ox or rabbit brain may give results quite different from those obtained from tissue factor using human brain.

Differential Diagnosis

Acquired factor VII deficiency is the most common cause of a prolonged PT. Warfarin use, vitamin K deficiency and liver disease are the main causes of acquired factor VII deficiency. These individuals will have low levels not only of factor VII, but of all other vitamin K-dependent factors as well. Other less common causes of factor VII deficiency include the familial combined factor deficiencies (type III and IV), acquired factor VII inhibitors,[71] and association with homocystinuria[72] and aplastic anemia.[73] Seligsohn and colleagues described an association between hereditary factor VII deficiency and the Dubin-Johnson and Rotor syndromes.[74] There is also a possible association between Gilbert syndrome and factor VII deficiency.[75]

Treatment

For mild hemorrhage, factor VII levels of 5% to 10% of normal are sufficient to stop bleeding. For individuals undergoing surgery, levels of 15% to 25% of normal are recommended. In the United States products that are used for treatment include fresh frozen plasma, prothrombin complex concentrates and recombinant factor VIIa. Given the short half-life of factor VII (3 to 4 hours), it is difficult to administer plasma every 4 to 6 hours to maintain normal levels without producing volume overload. Recombinant factor VIIa (NovoSeven), which has been approved for use in the United States and other countries for individuals with hemophilia who have inhibitors, has been shown to be efficacious in factor VII deficiency, and is clearly the treatment of choice.[70] A dose of 20 to 30 μg/kg of body weight is sufficient for hemostasis. Frequency of dosing will depend on the severity of the bleeding episode. For mild to moderate bleeding one dose of factor VIIa may be sufficient. For more severe episodes, factor VIIa administered every 2 to 6 hours for several days may be required. Virally inactivated purified plasma-derived factor VII is available in some European countries.[76]

FACTOR X DEFICIENCY

In the 1950s two independent groups of investigators discovered factor X when they showed that two different patients lacked an identical factor that could be distinguished from all other known factor deficiencies.[77,78] Factor X deficiency occurs worldwide with an estimated incidence of 1 in 500,000. In countries where consanguineous marriages are more common, the relative frequency may be higher.

Pathogenesis and Genetics

Congenital factor X deficiency, which has been reported in over 50 kindred, is inherited as an autosomal recessive trait. The genetic and molecular defects resulting in factor X deficiency include small deletions, missense mutations, and frameshifts.[79] Individuals with factor X deficiency may synthesize abnormal factor X molecules in normal or reduced amounts. One of the original patients had no detectable factor X antigen, and the genetic defect in this patient probably resulted in intracellular destruction of the molecule. An absolute deficiency of factor X may be incompatible with life; in mice in which the factor X gene has been "knocked out," embryonic or neonatal death occurs regularly.[80] A registry of factor X variants can be found on the world wide web at www.hgmd.org

Clinical Manifestations

Hemorrhagic events in factor X-deficient patients may be mild, moderate, or severe. Bleeding symptoms seem to correlate with the level of factor X activity. Individuals with severe deficiency (less than 1% of normal) have bleeding episodes comparable to patients with severe classic hemophilia, including hemarthroses, soft tissue hemorrhages, retroperitoneal bleeding, central nervous system hemorrhages, hematuria, menorrhagia, and pseudotumors. In a study of 32 Iranian individuals with congenital factor X deficiency, 69% developed recurrent hemarthroses while 16% developed disabling joint disease.[81] In the same study, bleeding from the umbilical stump was described in 28% of infants. Patients with factor X activity of 15% or greater have fewer spontaneous bleeding episodes, although hemorrhage can occur in association with surgery or trauma. Neutralizing antibodies for factor X rarely occur in patients with a hereditary deficiency of the factor.

Diagnosis

In general, the diagnosis of inherited factor X deficiency is suggested by a lifelong history of excessive bleeding and laboratory studies showing prolonged PT and PTT that corrects with 1:1 mixing with normal plasma. The TCT and bleeding time are normal. The Russell's viper venom time, which measures the direct activation of factor X, is also prolonged. The definitive diagnosis of factor X deficiency requires a specific factor X assay since prolonged PT and PTT are also seen in other factor deficiencies (e.g., factor V, prothrombin).

Differential Diagnosis

Acquired factor X deficiency is most commonly seen in liver disease and vitamin K deficiency. In these settings, levels of the other vitamin K-dependent factors are also reduced. Isolated factor X deficiency has been reported in association with respiratory infections,[82,83] acute myeloid leukemia,[84] and other malignancies.[85] Acquired factor X inhibitors in patients without congenital factor X deficiency are rare, although cases have been described in patients with leprosy[86] and after antibiotic and agricultural chemical exposure, among others.[87,88] Factor X deficiency in association with amyloidosis is well described and is due to adsorption of factor X onto amyloid fibrils.[89] Factor X levels in these patients range from 2% to 50% of normal, and usually individuals have bleeding symptoms when factor levels drop below 10% of normal.

Treatment

Replacement therapy should be guided by the severity of the bleeding. Factor X levels of 10% to 15% should be sufficient to control mild hemorrhagic episodes, including hemarthroses and uncomplicated soft tissue bleeds. Given the long half-life of factor X (approximately 40 hours), plasma replacement therapy can be used with an initial loading dose of 15 to 20 mL/kg of fresh frozen plasma, followed by 3 to 6 mL/kg every 24 hours. For major bleeds, trauma, or surgical procedures, those PCCs containing significant amounts of factor X can be used to maintain a factor X level of about 50% of normal. Factor X levels persistently above 50% of normal are not recommended because of the concern for thromboembolic events. Administration of "factor X-rich" PCCs in doses of 20 to 30 U/kg of body weight every 24 hours is sufficient to maintain hemostasis.[76] Only products that are virally inactivated should be used. Factor X-deficient patients who develop inhibitors to the factor can be treated with larger than normal doses of factor X (using PCCs) or by exchange transfusion. Chronic treatment of patients with factor X inhibitors consists of immunosupression with alkylating agents and prednisone. Inhibitors that occur in patients without congenital factor X deficiency are usually transient and should be treated with steroids and intravenous gamma globulin preparations. In some cases, exchange transfusion and activated PCCs can be useful.[83,87]

Treatment of factor X deficiency due to amyloidosis is difficult since the half-life of factor X is shortened, most likely as a consequence of absorption of factor X by the amyloid fibrils. Factor X replacement therapy may thus be virtually useless in some patients.[89] In patients with amyloidosis and factor X deficiency, splenectomy, chemotherapy, and plasma exchange have all been tried, with variable results.[90-92]

FACTOR XI DEFICIENCY

The first report of congenital factor XI deficiency was described in 1953, when three related individuals were described who developed excessive bleeding after dental extractions.[93] Factor XI deficiency is more prevalent among Ashkenazi Jews, with a gene frequency of 4.3%, but the deficiency also occurs in non-Jewish populations.[94,95]

Pathogenesis and Genetics

Factor XI deficiency is inherited in an autosomal recessive fashion, with no gender predilection. Three different genotypes have been described, two of them with a higher frequency in the Ashkenazi Jewish population (types II and III).[95,96] Type I mutations occur at the intron-exon boundaries (splice junction mutations); type II mutations result from a premature stop codon (nonsense mutations); and type III mutations result from missense mutations. There is evidence that platelets have a factor XI-like activity, but the clinical significance of this finding is not known.[97]

Clinical Manifestations

Factor XI-deficient individuals have either a mild bleeding tendency or, in some cases, no bleeding tendency, even following surgery. The explanation that bleeding manifestations in factor XI-deficient patients are never as severe as those seen in severely affected hemophilia A and B patients is that the "tenase" and "prothrombinase" complexes leading to ultimate thrombin generation are intact in patients with factor XI deficiency. Thus, factor XI serves to "boost" thrombin generation in subjects who need boosting, but thrombin generation is never as impeded in factor XI-deficient patients as it is in other factor deficiencies. Some patients with factor XI deficiency have near normal thrombin generation, even in the complete absence of factor XI, an observation that explains why some severely affected factor XI-deficient patients exhibit normal hemostasis during surgery. The reason for this is not entirely clear, but may be related to the amount of factor XI-like activity on platelets.

Even though factor XI levels do not always correlate with the bleeding tendency, members of an affected family tend to have similar hemorrhagic symptoms. Individuals with factor XI activity less than 20% are most likely homozygotes or compound heterozygotes and can experience excessive bleeding. "Spontaneous" hemorrhagic episodes, including hemarthroses, are not features of factor XI deficiency. Increased bleeding may be seen after aspirin ingestion, prostatectomy, and oral cavity surgery and where there is increased fibrinolytic activity.[98,99] Common bleeding manifestations include hematomas, epistaxis, menorrhagia, postpartum bleeding, and hematuria. As a general rule, the best predictor of whether a factor XI-deficient patient will experience excessive hemorrhage is the presence or absence of a past history of significant bleeding.

Diagnosis

Individuals with factor XI deficiency will have a prolonged PTT with a normal PT and thrombin time. As opposed to hemophilia A and B, factor XI deficiency occurs in both males and females. Diagnosis requires a specific factor XI assay. Plasma from patients to be tested for factor XI deficiency should be collected fresh in plastic containers and processed rapidly, since results can be affected if the plasma is processed in a glass tube or is frozen and thawed before being assayed.

Differential Diagnosis

Congenital deficiency of factor XI can also be seen in individuals with familial combined factor deficiencies (types V and VI). It has also been associated with Noonan syndrome,[100] factor VIII deficiency,[101] factor IX deficiency,[102] von Willebrand disease,[103] and in patients with platelet defects.[104] Acquired factor XI inhibitors can be seen in patients with immunologic diseases (e.g., systemic lupus erythematosus).

Treatment

Mild bleeding episodes may not require treatment. A variety of successful surgical procedures have been performed under adequate replacement therapy in patients with factor XI deficiency,[105,106] even though it is not known what the ideal level of factor XI should be to maintain hemostasis. It seems safe to maintain a minimal level of 45% of normal for major surgery and of 30%

for minor surgery. Some clinicians have found that lower levels are adequate for hemostasis, while others believe that higher levels may occasionally be necessary. When therapy is required, fresh frozen plasma can be used at a loading dose of 15 to 20 mL/kg, followed by 3 to 6 mL/kg every 12 hours. The half-life of factor XI is approximately 50 ± 22 hours. On occasion, when an individual's bleeding cannot be controlled with plasma alone, plasma exchange may be helpful to maintain higher levels of factor XI. Patients with factor XI deficiency, even when severe, who have no past history of bleeding following significant trauma or surgery usually do not require replacement therapy.

Antifibrinolytic agents, such as ε-aminocaproic acid or tranexamic acid, can be used alone or in addition to plasma to control bleeding. Seligsohn and co-workers successfully treated 19 patients with severe factor XI deficiency who underwent dental surgery with tranexamic acid alone and without excessive bleeding.[107] Caution should be used in patients with hematuria when antifibrinolytic therapy is used, since ureteral or urethral obstruction from clots that are refractory to lysis can occur. Fibrin glue alone has also been used successfully for dental extractions.[108] Factor VIIa has also been used successfully to control hemorrhage in factor XI-deficient patients.

Inhibitors to factor XI have been described in several affected factor XI-deficient patients and are usually IgG alloantibodies. These inhibitors are rare but complicate replacement therapy and can prolong bleeding episodes in susceptible patients.[109,110] The treatment of choice for patients with inhibitors is recombinant factor VIIa. Commonly used doses of factor VIIa are 100 to 120 μg/kg of body weight adjusted every 2 to 4 hours until bleeding stops.[111] Eradication of factor XI inhibitor should be attempted by the administration of cyclophosphamide (100 to 200 mg/day) and prednisone (1 mg/kg/day) until the inhibitor disappears or side effects of therapy prohibit further treatment. Factor XI concentrates are not yet available in the United States, even though they are available in Europe.

DEFICIENCY OF THE CONTACT FACTORS

The physiologic role of the contact factors [factor XII (Hageman factor), prekallikrein, and high-molecular-weight kininogen] in coagulation is still not well understood. Interestingly, individuals with a deficiency of any of these contact factors do not have a bleeding tendency, even during major surgery. There is reasonable evidence to suggest that these factors play a role in host defense mechanisms and may contribute to the interaction between coagulation, fibrinolysis, the complement system, and other pathways of the inflammatory response.[112]

Factor XII Deficiency

Ratnoff and Colopy were the first to describe a patient with congenital factor XII deficiency (Mr. Hageman) after he was found to have a prolonged clotting time in a glass tube in a routine preoperative evaluation. He had no personal or family history of excessive bleeding.[113] Since then, hundreds of cases have been described, but in only a few of these cases has the structural defect in factor XII been recognized.

Pathogenesis and Genetics

In general, congenital factor XII deficiency is inherited in an autosomal recessive pattern, although autosomal dominant inheritance has been described in one family.[114] Homozygous individuals usually have undetectable factor XII activity levels, while heterozygotes have factor XII levels between 20% and 60% of normal. There are limited reports of specific genetic defects causing factor XII deficiency. The Asian population seems to have lower factor XII levels when compared to Caucasians.[115]

Clinical Manifestations

As mentioned previously, individuals with factor XII deficiency do not experience excessive bleeding, even after major surgical procedures or trauma. Various anecdotal case reports describing an association between factor XII deficiency and spontaneous abortion, premature delivery, arterial and venous thromboses, myocardial infarction, and pulmonary embolism have been published, but a definite cause-and-effect relationship has not been established.

Diagnosis

The characteristic of severe factor XII deficiency is a markedly prolonged PTT (greater than 100 seconds) with normal PT, TCT, and bleeding time in patients with no personal or family history of excessive bleeding. Diagnosis requires a specific factor XII assay.

Differential Diagnosis

Spontaneous autoantibodies (inhibitor) against factor XII occur rarely.[116] Sporadic case reports of patients with inhibitors have been described in patients with autoimmune disorders and in individuals treated with procainamide or chlorpromazine.[117,118] Congenital factor XII deficiency has also been described in association with other coagulation disorders, including von Willebrand disease and factor IX deficiency.[119,120] Low factor XII levels can also be seen in patients with liver disease. Prekallikrein and high-molecular-weight kininogen deficiencies must be distinguished from factor XII deficiency by specific assays.

Treatment

No treatment is necessary for individuals with factor XII deficiency.

Prekallikrein Deficiency

In 1965, Hathaway described deficiency of prekallikrein (PK; Fletcher factor) in a family with a prolonged PTT and no history of excessive bleeding.[121] PK deficiency is inherited in an autosomal recessive pattern. Homozygous individuals have less than 1% of activity, whereas heterozygotes have 20% to 60% of normal activity. Rare variants of abnormal prekallikrein molecules have been described. Paradoxically, some reports describe a possible association of PK deficiency and thromboembolic phenomena.[122] Individuals with this disorder will have a markedly prolonged PTT that corrects to normal with the addition of normal plasma. The PT, bleeding time, and TCT are normal. PK deficiency is clinically identical to factor XII and high-molecular-weight kininogen deficiency, and diagnosis requires a specific assay. No specific therapy is required for patients with PK deficiency since they do not have excessive bleeding. The differential diagnosis includes other contact factor deficiencies. Since PK is synthesized in the liver, acquired deficiency can occur in liver disease.[123]

High-Molecular-Weight Kininogen Deficiency

High-molecular-weight kininogen (HK), also known as Fitzgerald factor, Williams factor, and Flaujeac factor, was first described in 1979.[124] Its deficiency is an autosomal recessive transmitted disorder. Individuals with HK deficiency have a prolonged PTT with no bleeding abnormalities. Diagnosis requires a specific assay.

Factor XIII Deficiency

In 1960 Duckert and colleagues described the first case of congenital factor XIII deficiency in a patient with severe hemorrhage and poor wound healing.[125] Since then, more than 200 cases of congenital deficiency of this protein have been reported in the literature.

Pathogenesis and Genetics

In vivo, factor XIII acts as a *trans*-glutaminase that stabilizes the fibrin clot by cross-linking fibrin fibers by formation of peptide bonds between specific amino acid residues on adjacent α and γ chains of fibrin polymers. In the absence of factor XIII, clots are unstable and are held together only by weak hydrogen bonds and electrostatic forces. Such clots are permeable to blood, form a poor framework for wound healing, and are extremely sensitive to fibrinolysis.

Human factor XIII is found in plasma and platelets. In plasma it circulates as a tetramer consisting of two A chains and two B chains (A_2B_2). The B chains function as carriers for the A chains, which contain the active component of factor XIII. In platelets, factor XIII is a dimer composed of two A chains (A_2). Platelet factor XIII accounts for about 50% of the total body factor XIII activity.[126] Three forms of factor XIII deficiency have been described. In type I deficiency, there is absence of both A and B chains. Type II deficiency is characterized by lack of the A chain; in type III, the B chain is absent.[127] Most of the reported cases of factor XIII deficiency are due to the lack of A chains. Deficiency of factor XIII is an autosomal recessive disorder, with an estimated incidence of one in several million. Consanguinity is frequently found.

Clinical Manifestations

Symptomatic individuals with factor XIII deficiency have less than 1% of normal. Bleeding manifestations can present as early as the neonatal period, with umbilical stump hemorrhage in up to 80% of the cases. Hematomas, soft-tissue hemorrhage, pseudotumors, and poor wound healing are other manifestations of severely affected individuals. Children can present with severe hemorrhage after circumcision and recurrent gum bleeding while teething.[128] Females have recurrent spontaneous abortions,[129,130] while males can present with oligospermia and infertility.[131] Trauma is usually the triggering factor for most of the bleeding episodes, except for intracranial hemorrhage, which can be spontaneous. Intracranial hemorrhage occurs with an incidence of up to 30% of and is the leading cause of death in this disorder.[132] Some patients with congenital factor XIII deficiency develop alloantibodies against the factor following replacement therapy.

Diagnosis

The hallmark of patients with factor XIII deficiency consists of normal routine coagulation studies (PTT, PT, TCT, bleeding time, and platelet count) in a patient who is clearly a bleeder. Diagnosis can be made by a simple clot solubility test, using 5-M urea or 1% monochloroacetic acid. Plasma clots can be removed from thrombin-treated plasma samples and placed in one of the above solutions. Rapid dissolution of the clot within a few minutes will be seen in affected individuals, whereas normal clots remain insoluble for at least 24 hours. Patient's plasma mixed with normal plasma should also be tested to rule out an inhibitor to factor XIII. Factor XIII inhibitors will neutralize the factor XIII in normal plasma. Confirmation of the deficiency using a quantitative test should be done if the clot solubility test is abnormal. Quantitative tests are based on the amine-casein incorporation assay or ammonia production by the *trans*-amidase activity of factor XIII.[133]

Differential Diagnosis

Acquired factor XIII deficiency can be seen in patients without a congenital deficiency because of inhibitory antibodies that develop against factor XIII. Such antibodies have been reported in association with isoniazid, penicillin, and phenytoin.[134–136] In some patients, antibodies against factor XIII are idiopathic.[137–139] Decreased levels of factor XIII also have been described in patients with Henoch-Schönlein purpura,[140] Crohn's disease, and ulcerative colitis.[141]

Treatment

Since only low levels of factor XIII activity (approximately 5%) are needed to completely control bleeding and its half-life is long (9 to 10 days), prophylactic therapy is indicated, especially if intracranial bleeds are to be prevented.[142] For prophylaxis, fresh frozen plasma can be administered in doses of 2 to 3 mL of plasma per kilogram of body weight (approximately 1 to 2 units of plasma) every 4 to 6 weeks.[143] Cryoprecipitate is another source of factor XIII and can be given in doses of 1 bag per 10 to 20 kg of body weight every 3 to 4 weeks. Plasma-derived pasteurized factor XIII concentrates are available in Europe (Fibrogammin-P, Aventis Behring) and can be used prophylactically by intravenous administration every 5 to 6 weeks. Pregnancies in women with history of spontaneous abortions can be carried to term with the use of fresh frozen plasma every 14 days or with factor XIII concentrates every 21 days.[130] Complications from replacement therapy include bloodborne infections (hepatitis, human immunodeficiency virus, other viruses), allergic reactions to plasma, and the development of antibodies to factor XIII in individuals with congenital deficiency.[144] Patients with factor XIII deficiency who develop antibodies to exogenous factor XIII can be very difficult to manage. Administration of normal platelets containing factor XIII can be tried. Exchange transfusion may be necessary. Combined therapy using exchange transfusion and immunosupression using intravenous gamma globulin, cyclophosphamide, and steroids can also be tried.

FAMILIAL COMBINED FACTOR DEFICIENCIES

Multiple combined coagulation factor deficiencies have been described (Table 5–6). Type I (factor V-factor VIII deficiency) and type III deficiencies (combined factors II, VII, IX, and X deficiency) are well characterized. Familial combined deficiencies can be due to a single genetic defect, resulting in multiple factor deficiencies, or to different genetic defects associated with each deficient factor. The latter situation is usually associated with consanguinity.

Combined Factor V-Factor VIII Deficiency (Type I)

More than 30 affected families have been described in the literature. Affected individuals have factor V and factor VIII levels each between 5% and 15% of normal. These patients usually have bleeding symptoms after trauma and during or after surgery.

Pathogenesis and Genetics

Combined factor V-factor VIII deficiency is inherited in an autosomal recessive pattern. The gene for this combined deficiency has recently been identified in the long arm of chromosome 18 and corresponds to a marker of the endoplasmic reticulum-Golgi intermediate compartment, ERGIC-53. The ERGIC-53 gene product may serve as a "chaperon" for the transport of specific proteins like factor V and factor VIII[145,146] through the intracellular processing apparatus. Defects in the ERGIC-53 gene account for most, but not all, of these patients.

Treatment

Therapy consists of fresh frozen plasma (to replace factor V) and factor VIII concentrates. Before surgery, factor V levels should be raised to near normal by means of plasma exchange. Factor levels can then be maintained with infusions of plasma and factor VIII concentrates.

Combined Factor II, VII, IX, X, Protein C and S Deficiency (Type III)

Pathogenesis and Genetics

The combined deficiency of the vitamin K-dependent factors is transmitted in an autosomal recessive fashion. Genetic defects in either the vitamin K carboxylase or reductase genes have been identified in three patients.[147] Bleeding manifestations on occasions can be severe. In some patients, the use of high doses of oral vitamin K may be beneficial.[148,149] With excessive bleeding, PCCs can be used with caution. Care must be used to exclude the possibility of accidental or surreptitious administration of warfarin or "superwarfarin," but these patients will not give a lifelong history of bleeding and can be diagnosed by performing specific warfarin or superwarfarin assays on patients' plasma.

Table 5–6 • FAMILIAL COMBINED FACTOR DEFICIENCIES

Type	Deficient Factors	Genetic Defect
I	V and VIII	Defective ERGIC-53 gene
II	VIII and IX	Unknown
III	II, VII, IX, X	Vitamin K carboxylase or reductase deficiency
IV	VII and VIII	Unknown
V	VIII, IX, and XI	Unknown
VI	IX and XI	Unknown

Other Combined Familial Deficiencies

The other combined familial factor deficiencies listed in Table 5–6 are more rare. The genetic nature of these defects is largely unknown. When bleeding occurs, plasma or specific factor concentrates can be used for treatment.

α_2-PLASMIN INHIBITOR DEFICIENCY

α_2-Plasmin inhibitor (α_2-PI) deficiency was first described in 1976. Since then, more than 10 families with this disorder have been characterized.[150] These patients can be "missed" unless there is a high index of suspicion since routine tests of coagulation may be only slightly prolonged.

Pathogenesis and Genetics

Individuals with α_2-PI deficiency exhibit a hemorrhagic tendency caused by a reduced inhibition of plasmin, with resulting increased fibrinolytic activity. Deficiency is inherited in an autosomal recessive pattern with no predilection for gender or race. The gene is located on chromosome 17, and a variety of genetic defects, including additions, small deletions, and specific nucleotide substitutions, have been reported.

Clinical Manifestations

Bleeding manifestations are more pronounced in homozygous individuals and are characterized by easy bruising, epistaxis, hematuria, menorrhagia, and hemarthrosis. Bleeding after trauma or surgery can be severe and often is delayed. Heterozygous individuals usually have hemorrhagic symptoms only in association with trauma.

Differential Diagnosis

α_2-PI deficiency can also be acquired and may be seen in individuals with liver failure, amyloidosis, solid tumors, acute promyelocytic leukemia, and disseminated intravascular coagulation.[151] Decreased levels of α_2-PI have also been reported in patients receiving thrombolytic therapy and in other conditions associated with a hyperfibrinolytic state.[152]

Diagnosis

The diagnosis of α_2-PI deficiency requires a high degree of suspicion, since laboratory evaluation may exhibit completely normal PT, PTT, TCT, and bleeding time. Clots that are formed are not soluble in 5-M urea. However, the whole-blood and euglobulin lysis times are markedly accelerated. Definite diagnosis, however, requires a specific α_2-PI assay.

Treatment

Antifibrinolytics are the mainstay of treatment. During bleeding situations ε-aminocaproic acid can be used at a dose of 2 to 3 g orally or intravenously every 6 hours. Continuous intravenous infusion can also be administered at a dose of 1 g/h. The maximum recommended dose is 30 g a day in patients with normal renal function. Some clinicians find that lower doses, e.g., 4 to 6 g every 4 to 6 hours, are equally efficacious.

α_1-ANTITRYPSIN PITTSBURGH (Antithrombin III Pittsburgh)

To date only two individuals with this defect have been described.[153,154] Both patients had the same genetic mutation, even though the hemorrhagic manifestations were different. The bleeding manifestations in these patients occurred following trauma, which induced an increase in the level of the mutant enzyme, which is an acute phase reactant. The mutation in α_1-antitrypsin Pittsburgh (α_1-ATP) is characterized by the substitution of methionine for arginine at position 358 of the α_1-antitrypsin molecule. This substitution essentially converts α_1-antitrypsin into an antithrombin with both antithrombin and anti-factor Xa activity. One individual had severe bleeding episodes with soft tissue hematomas, hematuria, and melena. He died of massive hemorrhage. One individual had only mild bleeding symptoms. PT, PTT, TCT, and bleeding time were prolonged in both individuals. Low protein C (13%) was also seen in the second individual, but its etiology is not clear.

PROTEIN Z DEFICIENCY

Protein Z is a vitamin K-dependent protein that was first described in bovine plasma.[155] Human protein Z was discovered and purified by Broze and Miletich in 1984.[156] The plasma half-life is estimated to be 2 to 3 days. No correlation between age and gender has been found. Protein Z plasma concentration is variable. Since it is a vitamin K-dependent factor, its level is exquisitely sensitive to warfarin.[157] Protein Z is mentioned in this chapter because early studies suggested that patients with low protein Z levels have a mild bleeding tendency.[158] More recent reports, however, indicate that protein Z is a co-factor for a protein Z-dependent protease inhibitor (ZPI), a member of the serpin family of inhibitors.[159,160] ZPI, with protein Z as a co-factor, inhibits factor Xa (a serine protease) on phospholipid surfaces. Thus, deficiency of protein Z has been shown to predispose protein Z-deficient mice to thrombosis rather than hemorrhage. This suggests that protein Z deficiency in humans may be prothrombotic.[161] Reports suggesting that protein Z deficiency is associated with excessive bleeding may be inaccurate.

CONSULTATION CONSIDERATIONS

Although some of these factor deficiencies are rare, these are just the types of patients the hematologist will be consulted on, and therefore a broad differential diagnosis must be included. As many diseases are recessive in inheritance, a high degree of consideration must be given for consanguinity.

MEDICO-LEGAL ISSUES

It is important to have a firmly established diagnosis. It is not uncommon to see patients misdiagnosed with lupus anticoagulant or factor VIII or IX deficiency treated with concentrates, which was dubious, expensive, and perhaps dangerous, when they had an acquired inhibitor to a specific coagulation protein (i.e., factor VIII). On the other hand, we have also seen patients receive fresh frozen plasma indiscriminately, hoping that "a missing factor" can be replaced and the symptoms improved.

When an unusual diagnosis is made in a family member, consideration should be given to notifying and possibly testing other members of the family. Genetic counseling should always be part of the consultation when indicated.

COST-CONTAINMENT ISSUES

Once the right diagnosis has been established, one should treat with the most effective and safest material available. Cost consideration should not be the deciding factor in treatment but should always be considered. For example, some clinicians believe that recombinant products, though often more expensive than plasma-derived clotting factor concentrates, are preferred since they are less likely to be contaminated with potential transmissible agents not susceptible to currently used eradication techniques.

■ REFERENCES

References for Chapter 5

1. Rabe F, Salomon E. Uber Faserstoffmangel im Blut bei einem Falle von Hamophilie. Dtsch Arch Klin Med 1920;132:240–244.
2. Neerman-Arbez M, Honsberger A, Antonarakis SE, Morris MA. Deletion of the fibrinogen alpha-chain gene (FGA) causes congenital afibrinogenemia. J Clin Invest 1999;103(2):215–218.
3. Duga S, Asselta R, Santagostino E, et al. Missense mutations in the human beta fibrinogen gene cause congenital afibrinogenemia by impairing fibrinogen secretion. Blood 2000;95(4):1336–1341.
4. Al-Mondhiry H, Ehmann WC. Congenital afibrinogenemia. Am J Hematol 1994;46(4):343–347.
5. Menache D. Congenital fibrinogen abnormalities. Ann NY Acad Sci 1983;408:121–130.
6. Ehmann WC, al-Mondhiry H. Congenital afibrinogenemia and splenic rupture. Am J Hematol 1994;96:92–94.
7. Mammen EF. Fibrinogen abnormalities. Semin Thromb Hemost 1983;9(1):1–72.
8. Evron S, Anteby SO, Brzezinsky A, et al. Congenital afibrinogenemia and recurrent early abortion: a case report. Eur J Obstet Gynecol Reprod Biol 1985;19(5):307–311.
9. Goodwin TM. Congenital hypofibrinogenemia in pregnancy. Obstet Gynecol Surv 1989;44(3):157–161.
10. Ness PM, Budzynski AZ, Olexa SA, Rodvien R. Congenital hypofibrinogenemia and recurrent placental abruption. Obstet Gynecol 1983;61(4):519–523.
11. Weiss HJ, Rodgers J. Fibrinogen and platelets in the primary arrest of bleeding. Studies in two patients with congenital afibrinogenemia. N Engl J Med 1971;285(7):369–374.
12. Soria J, Soria C, Borg JY, et al. Platelet aggregation occurs in congenital afibrinogenemia despite the absence of fibrinogen or its fragments in plasma and platelets, as demonstrated by immunoenzymology. Br J Haematol 1985;60:503–514.
13. Flute PT. Disorders of plasma fibrinogen synthesis. Br Med Bull 1977;33(3):253–259.
14. Colvin RB, Mosesson MW, Dvorak HF. Delayed-type hypersensitivity skin reactions in congenital afibrinogenemia lack fibrin deposition and induration. J Clin Invest 1979;63(6):1302–1306.
15. Bithell TC. Hereditary coagulation disorders. In Lee GR, Bithell TC, Foerster J, et al. (eds): Wintrobe's Clinical Hematology, 9th ed. vol. 2. Philadelphia, Lea & Febiger, 1993, p 1439.
16. Dale BM, Purdie GH, Rischbieth RH. Fibrinogen depletion with sodium valproate [letter]. Lancet 1978;1(8077):1316–1317.
17. Gralnick HR, Henderson E. Hypofibrogenemia and coagulation factor deficiencies with L-asparaginase treatment. Cancer 1971;27(6):1313–1320.
18. Inanmoto Y, Terao T. First report of a case of congenital afibrinogenemia with successful delivery. Am J Obstet Gynecol 1985;153(7):803–804.
19. De Vries A, Rosenberg T, Kochwa S, Boss JH. Precipitating antifibrinogen antibody appears after fibrinogen infusions in a patient with congenital afibrinogenemia. Am J Med 1961;30:486–494.
20. Ingram GI, McBrien DJ, Spencer H. Fatal pulmonary embolus in congenital fibrinopenia. Report of two cases. Acta Haematol 1966;35(1):56–62.
21. MacKinnon HH, Fekete JF. Congenital afibrinogenemia. Vascular changes and multiple thromboses induced by fibrinogen infusions and contraceptive medication. Can Med Assoc J 1971;104(7):597–599.
22. Cronin C, Fitzpatrick D, Temperley I. Multiple pulmonary emboli in a patient with afibrinogenemia. Acta Haematol 1988;79(1):53–54.
23. Calenda E, Bor JY, Peillon C, et al. Perioperative management of a patient with congenital hypofibrinogenemia [letter]. Anesthesiology 1989;71(4):622–623.
24. Martinez J. Quantitative and qualitative disorders of fibrinogen. In Hoffman R, Benz EJ, Shattil SJ, et al. (eds): Hematology: Basic Principles and Practice, 3rd ed. New York, Churchill Livingstone, 2000, pp 1924–1936.
25. Lord ST. Fibrinogen. In High KA, Roberts HR (eds): Molecular Basis of Thrombosis and Hemostasis. New York, Marcel Dekker, Inc., 1995, pp 51–74.
26. Roberts HR, Bingham MD. Other coagulation deficiencies. In Loscalzo J, Schafer AI (eds): Thrombosis and Hemorrhage, 2nd ed. Baltimore: Williams & Wilkins, 1998, pp 773–802.
27. Forman WB, Ratnoff OD, Boyer MH. An inherited qualitative abnormality in plasma fibrinogen: fibrinogen Cleveland. J Lab Clin Med 1968;72(3):455–472.
28. Martinez J, Palascak JE, Kwasniak D. Abnormal sialic acid content of the dysfibrinogenemia associated with liver disease. J Clin Invest 1978;61:535–538.
29. Quick AJ. Congenital hypoprothrombinemia and pseudo-hypoprothrombinemia. Lancet 1947;2:379–382.
30. Quick AJ, Pisciotta AV, Hussey CV. Congenital hypoprothrombinemic states. Arch Int Med 1955;95:2–14.
31. Degen SJF. Prothrombin. In High KA, Roberts HR (eds): Molecular Basis of Thrombosis and Hemostasis. New York, Marcel Dekker, Inc., 1995, pp 75–99.
32. Girolami A, Scarano L, Saggiorato, G, et al. Congenital deficiencies and abnormalities of prothrombin. Blood Coagul Fibrinolysis 1998;9(7):557–569.

33. Xue J, Wu Q, Westfield LA, et al. Incomplete embryonic lethality and fatal neonatal hemorrhage caused by prothrombin deficiency in mice. Proc Natl Acad Sci USA 1998;95(13):7603–7607.
34. Sun WY, Witte DP, Degen JL, et al. Incomplete embryonic lethality and fatal neonatal hemorrhage caused by prothrombin deficiency in mice. Proc Natl Acad Sci USA 1998;95(13):7597–7602.
35. Catanzarite VA, Novotny WF, Cousins LM, Schneider JM. Pregnancies in a patient with congenital absence of prothrombin activity: case report. Am J Perinatol 1997;14(3):135–138.
36. Pool JG, Desai R, Kropatkin M. Severe congenital hypoprothrombinemia in a Negro boy. Thromb Diath Haemorr 1962;8:235–240.
37. Roberts HR, Liles D. Deficiencies of the vitamin K-dependent clotting factors. In Brain MC, Carbone PP (eds): Current Therapy in Hematology-Oncology, 5th ed. St. Louis, Mosby, 1995, pp 171–176.
38. Bajaj SP, Rapaport SI, Barclay S, Herbst KD. Acquired hypoprothrombinemia due to non-neutralizing antibodies to prothrombin: mechanism and management. Blood 1985;65(6):1538–1543.
39. Cote HC, Huntsman DG, Wu J, et al. A new method for characterization and epitope determination of a lupus anticoagulant-associated neutralizing antiprothrombin antibody. Am J Clin Pathol 1997;107(2):197–205.
40. Gill FM, Shapiro SS, Schwartz E. Severe congenital hypoprothrombinemia. J Pediatr 1978;93(2):264–266.
41. Owen CA, Jr., Hendriksen RA, McDuffie FC, Mann KG. Prothrombin Quick. A newly identified dysprothrombinemia. Mayo Clin Proc 1978;53(1):29–33.
42. White GC, Roberts HR, Kingdon HS, Lundblad RL. Prothrombin complex concentrates: potentially thrombogenic materials and clues to the mechanism of thrombosis in vivo. Blood 1977;49(2):159–170.
43. Philippou H, Adami A, Lane DA, et al. High purity factor IX and prothrombin complex concentrate (PCC): pharmacokinetics and evidence that factor IXa is the thrombogenic trigger in PCC. Thromb Haemost 1996;76(1):23–28.
44. Lechler E. Use of prothrombin complex concentrates for prophylaxis and treatment of bleeding episodes in patients with hereditary deficiency of prothrombin, factor VII, factor X, protein C, protein S, or protein Z. Thromb Res 1999;95(4 Suppl1):S39–S50.
45. Halbmayer WM. Rational, high quality laboratory monitoring before, during, and after infusion of prothrombin complex concentrates. Thromb Res 1999;95(4 Suppl 1):S25–S30.
46. Roberts HR, Hoffman M. Other clotting factor deficiencies. In Hoffman R, Benz EJ, Shattil SJ, et al. (ed): Hematology: Basic Principles and Practice, 3rd ed. New York, Churchill Livingstone, 2000, pp 1912–1924.
47. Quick AJ. On the constitution of prothrombin. Am J Physiol 1943;140:212–218.
48. Owren PA. The coagulation of blood. Investigations on a new clotting factor. Acta Med Scand 1947;194:11–41.
49. Camire RM, Pottak ES, Kaushansky K, Tracy, PB. Secretable human platelet-derived factor V originates from the plasma pool. Blood 1998;92(9):3035–3041.
50. Colman RW. Where does platelet factor V originate? [letter]. Blood 1999;93(9):3152–3153.
51. Gewirtz AM, Shapiro C, Shen YM, et al. Cellular and molecular regulation of factor V expression in human megakaryocytes. J Cell Phys 1992;153(2):277–287.
52. Breederveld K, Giddings JC, ten Cate JW, Bloom AL. The localization of factor V within normal human platelets and the demonstration of a platelet-factor antigen in congenital factor V deficiency. Br J Haemotol 1975;29(3):405–412.
53. Tracy PB, Mann KG. Abnormal formation of the prothrombinase complex: factor V deficiency and related disorders. Hum Pathol 1987;18(2):162–169.

54. Chiu HC, Whitaker E, Colman RW. Heterogeneity of human factor V deficiency. Evidence for the existence of antigen-positive variants. J Clin Invest 1983;72(2):493–503.
55. Yang TL, Cui J, Taylor JM, et al. Rescue of fatal neonatal hemorrhage in factor V deficient mice by low level transgene expression. Thromb Haemost 2000;83(1):70–77.
56. Miletich JP, Majerus DW, Majerus PW. Patients with congenital factor V deficiency have decreased factor Xa binding sites on their platelets. J Clin Invest 1978;62(4):824–831.
57. Manotti C, Quintavalla R, Pini M, et al. Thromboembolic manifestations and congenital factor V deficiency: a family study. Haemostasis 1989;19(6):331–334.
58. Fratantoni JC, Hilgartner M, Nachman RL. Nature of the defect in congenital factor V deficiency: study in a patient with an acquired circulating anticoagulant. Blood 1972;39(6):751–758.
59. Zehnder JL, Leung LL. Development of antibodies to thrombin and factor V with recurrent bleeding in a patient exposed to topical bovine thrombin. Blood 1990;76(10):2011–2016.
60. Tracy PB, Giles AR, Mann KG, et al. Factor V (Quebec): a bleeding diathesis associated with a qualitative platelet factor V deficiency. J Clin Invest 1984;74(4):1221–1228.
61. Janeway CM, Rivard GE, Tracy PB, Mann KG. Factor V Quebec revisited. Blood 1996;87(9):3571–3578.
62. Webster W, Roberts HR, Penick GD. Hemostasis in factor V deficiency. Am J Med Sci 1964;248:194–202.
63. Sallah AS, Angchaisuksiri P, Roberts HR. Use of plasma exchange in hereditary deficiency of factor V and factor VIII. Am J Hematol 1996;52(3):229–230.
64. Chediak J, Ashenhurst JB, Garlick I, Desser RK. Successful management of bleeding in a patient with factor V inhibitor by platelet transfusions. Blood 1980;56(5):835–841.
65. Alexander B, Goldstein R, Landwehr G, Cook CD. Congenital SPCA deficiency: a hitherto unrecognized coagulation defect with hemorrhage rectified by serum and serum fractions. J Clin Invest 1951;30:596–606.
66. Cooper DN, Millar DS, Wacey A, et al. Inherited factor VII deficiency: molecular genetics and pathophysiology. Thromb Haemost 1997;78(1):151–160.
67. Mariani G, Mazzucconi MG. Factor VII congenital deficiency. Clinical picture and classification of the variants. Haemostasis 1983;13(3):169–177.
68. Ragni MV, Lewis JH, Spero JA, Hasiba U. Factor VII deficiency. Am J Hematol 1981;10(1):79–88.
69. Gershwin ME, Gude JK. Deep vein thrombosis and pulmonary embolism in congenital factor VII deficiency. N Engl J Med 1973;288(3):141–142.
70. Lusher J, Ingerslev J, Roberts H, Hedner U. Clinical experience with recombinant factor VIIa. Blood Coagul Fibrinolysis 1998;9(2):119–128.
71. Delmer A, Horellou MH, Andreu G, et al. Life-threatening intracranial bleeding associated with the presence of an antifactor VII antibody. Blood 1989;74(1):229–232.
72. Dantzenberg MD, Saudubray JM, Girot R. Factor VII deficiency in homocysteinuria. Thromb Haemost 1983;50(abstract):409.
73. Weisdorf D, Hasegawa D, Fair DS. Acquired factor VII deficiency associated with aplastic anemia: correction with bone marrow transplantation. Br J Haematol 1989;71(3):409–413.
74. Seligsohn U, Shani M, Ramot B, et al. Hereditary deficiency of blood clotting factor VII and Dubin-Johnson syndrome in an Israeli family. Isr J Med Sci 1969;5(5):1060–1065.
75. Seligsohn U, Shani M, Ramot B. Gilbert syndrome and factor VII deficiency. Lancet 1970;1(7661):1398.
76. Peyvandi F, Mannucci PM. Rare coagulation disorders. Thromb Haemost 1999;82(4):1207–1214.
77. Hougie C, Barrow EM, Graham JB. Stuart clotting defect. I. Segregation of an hereditary hemorrhagic state from the heterogeneous group heretofore called "stable factor" (SPCA, proconvertin, factor VII) deficiency. J Clin Invest 1957;36:485–496.

78. Telfer TP, Denson KW, Wright DR. A "new" coagulation defect. Br J Haematol 1956;2:308–316.

79. Cooper DN, Millar DS, Wacey A, et al. Inherited factor X deficiency: molecular genetics and pathophysiology. Thromb Haemost 1997;78(1):161–172.

80. Dewerchin M, Liang Z, Moons L, et al. Blood coagulation factor X deficiency causes partial embryonic lethality and fatal neonatal bleeding in mice. Thromb Haemost 2000;83(2):185–190.

81. Peyvandi F, Mannucci PM, Lak M, et al. Congenital factor X deficiency: spectrum of bleeding symptoms in 32 Iranian patients. Br J Haematol 1998;102(2):626–628.

82. Currie MS, Stein AM, Rustagi PK, et al. Transient acquired factor X deficiency associated with pneumonia. NY State J Med 1984;84(11):572–573.

83. Smith SV, Liles DK, White GC, 2nd, Brecher ME. Successful treatment of transient acquired factor X deficiency by plasmaphereisis with concomitant intravenous immunoglobulin and steroid therapy. Am J Hematol 1998;57(3):245–252.

84. Caimi MT, Redaelli R, Cattaneo D, et al. Acquired selective factor X deficiency in acute nonlymphocytic leukemia. Am J Hematol 1991;36(1):65–66.

85. Nora RE, Bell WR, Noe DA, Sholar PW. Novel factor X deficiency. Normal partial thromboplastin time and associated spindle cell thymoma. Am J Med 1985;79(1):122–126.

86. Ness PM, Hymas PG, Gesme D, Perkins HA. An unusual factor X inhibitor in leprosy. Am J Hematol 1980;8(4):397–402.

87. Henson K, Files JC, Morrison FS. Transient acquired factor X deficiency: report of the use of activated clotting concentrate to control a life-threatening hemorrhage. Am J Med 1989;87(5):583–585.

88. Rao LV, Zivelin A, Iturbe I, Rapaport SI. Antibody-induced acute factor X deficiency: clinical manifestations and properties of the antibody. Thromb Haemost 1994;72(3):363–371.

89. Furie B, Greene E, Furie BC. Syndrome of acquired factor X deficiency and systemic amyloidosis in vivo studies of the metabolic fate of factor X. N Engl J Med 1977;297(2):81–85.

90. Greep PR, Kyle RA, Bowie EJ. Factor X deficiency in primary amyloidosis: resolution after splenectomy. N Engl J Med 1979;301(19):1050–1051.

91. Camoriano JK, Greipp PR, Bayer GK, Bowie EJ. Resolution of acquired factor X deficiency and amyloidosis with melphalan and prednisone therapy. N Engl J Med 1987;316(18):1133–1135.

92. Breadell FV, Varma M, Martinez J. Normalization of plasma factor X levels in amyloidosis after plasma exchange. Am J Hematol 1997;54(1):68–71.

93. Rosenthal RL, Dreskin OH, Rosenthal N. New hemophilia-like disease caused by deficiency of a third plasma thromboplastin factor. Proc Soc Exp Bio Med 1953;82:171–174.

94. Seligsohn U. High gene frequency of factor XI (PTA) deficiency in Ashkenazi Jews. Blood 1978;51(6):1223–1228.

95. Asakai R, Chung DW, Davie EW, Seligsohn U. Factor XI deficiency in Ashkenazi Jews in Israel. N Engl J Med 1991;325(3):153–158.

96. Fujikawa K, Chung DW. Factor XI. In High KA, Roberts HR (eds): Molecular Basis of Thrombosis and Hemostasis. New York, Marcel Dekker, Inc., 1995, pp 257–268.

97. Lipscomb MS, Walsh PN. Human platelets and factor XI. Localization in platelet membranes of factor XI-like activity and its functional distinction from plasma factor XI. J Clin Invest 1979;63(5):1006–1014.

98. Kitchens CS. Factor XI: a review of its biochemistry and deficiency. Semin Thromb Hemost 1991;17(1):55–72.

99. Sidi A, Seligsohn U, Jonas P, Many M. Factor XI deficiency: detection and management during urological surgery. J Urol 1978;119(4):528–530.

100. Kitchens CS, Alexander J. Partial deficiency of coagulation factor XI as a newly recognized feature of Noonan syndrome. J Pediatr 1983;102(2):224–227.

101. Lian EC, Deykin D, Harkness DR. Combined deficiencies of factor VIII (AHF) and factor XI (PTA). Am J Hematol 1976;1(3):319–324.

102. Soff GA, Levin J, Bell WR. Familial multiple coagulation factor deficiencies. II. Combined factor VIII, IX, and XI deficiency and combined factor IX and XI deficiency: two previously uncharacterized familial multiple factor deficiency syndromes. Semin Thromb Hemost 1981;7(2):149–169.

103. Tavori S, Brenner B, Tatarsky I. The effect of combined factor XI deficiency with von Willebrand factor abnormalities on haemorrhagic diathesis. Thromb Haemost 1990;63(1):36–38.

104. Peter MK, Meili EO, von Felton, A. Factor XI deficiency: additional hemostatic defects are present in patients with bleeding tendency. Thromb Haemost 1995;73:1442.

105. Vander Woude JC, Milam JD, Walker WE, et al. Cardiovascular surgery in patients with congenital plasma coagulopathies. Ann Thorac Surg 1988;46(3):283–288.

106. Blatt PM, McFarland DH, Eifrig DE. Ophthalmic surgery and plasma prothrombin antecedent (factor XI) deficiency. Arch Ophthalmol 1980;98(5):863–864.

107. Berliner S, Horowitz I, Martinowitz U, et al. Dental surgery in patients with severe factor XI deficiency without plasma replacement. Blood Coagul Fibrinolysis 1992;3(4):465–468.

108. Rakocz M, Mazar A, Varon D, et al. Dental extractions in patients with bleeding disorders. The use of fibrin glue. Oral Surg Oral Med Oral Pathol 1993;75(3):280–282.

109. Stern DM, Nossel HL, Owen J. Acquired antibody to factor XI in a patient with congenital factor XI deficiency. J Clin Invest 1982;69(6):1270–1276.

110. Ginsberg SS, Clyne LP, McPhedran P, et al. Successful childbirth by a patient with congenital factor XI deficiency and an acquired inhibitor. Br J Haemotol 1993;84(1):172–174.

111. Hedner U. NovoSeven as a universal haemostatic agent. Blood Coagul Fibrinolysis 2000;11(Suppl 1):S107–111.

112. Colman RW. Biologic activities of the contact favors in vivo—potentiation of hypotension, inflammation, and fibrinolysis, and inhibition of cell adhesion, angiogenesis and thrombosis. Thromb Haemost 1999;82(6):1568–1577.

113. Ratnoff OD, Colopy JE. A familial hemorrhagic trait associated with a deficiency of a clot-promoting fraction of plasma. J Clin Invest 1954;34:602–613.

114. Bennett B, Ratnoff OD, Holt JB, Roberts HR. Hageman trait (factor XII deficiency): a probably second genotype inherited as an autosomal dominant characteristic. Blood 1972;40(3):412–415.

115. Gordon EM, Donaldson VH, Saito H, et al. Reduced titers of Hageman factor (factor XII) in Orientals. Ann Intern Med 1981;95(6):697–700.

116. Criel A, Collen D, Masson PL. A case of IgM antibodies which inhibit the contact activation of blood coagulation. Thromb Res 1978;12(5):883–892.

117. Clyne LP, Farber LR, Chopyk RL. Procainamide-induced circulating anticoagulants in a congenitally-defective factor XI patient. Folia Haematol Int Mag Klin Morphol Blutforsch 1989;116(2):239–244.

118. Zucker S, Zarrabi MH, Romano GS, Miller F. IgM inhibitors of the contact activation phase of coagulation in chlorpromazine-treated patients. Br J Haematol 1978;40(3):447–457.

119. Bux-Gewehr I, Morgenschweis K, Zotz RB, et al. Combined von Willebrand factor deficiency and factor XII deficiency. Thromb Haemost 2000;83:514–516.

120. Mant MJ. Combined factor IX and XII deficiencies in both male and female members of a single family. Thromb Haemost 1979;42(2):816–818.

121. Hathaway WE, Belhasen LP, Hathaway HS. Evidence for a new plasma thromboplastin factor. I. Case report, coagulation studies and physicochemical properties. Blood 1965;26(5):521–532.

122. Saito H, Kojima T. Factor XII, prekallikrein, and high molecular weight kininogen. In High, KA, Roberts HR (eds): Molecular Basis of Thrombosis and Hemostasis. New York, Marcel Dekker, Inc., 1995, pp 269–285.

123. Wong PY, Talamo RC, Williams, GH. Kallikrein-kinin and renin-angiotensin systems in functional renal failure of cirrhosis of the liver. Gastroenterology 1977;73(5):1114–1118.

124. Saito H, Ratnoff OD, Waldmann R, Abraham JP. Deficiency of a hitherto unrecognized agent, Fitzgerald factor, participating in surface-mediated reactions of clotting, fibrinolysis, generation of kinins, and the property of diluted plasma enhancing vascular permeability (PF/DIL). J Clin Invest 1975;55:1082–1089.

125. Duckert F, Jung E, Shmerling DH. A hitherto undescribed congential haemorrhagic diathesis probably due to fibrin stabilizing factor deficiency. Thromb Diath Haemorrh 1960;5:179–186.

126. Lopaciuk S, Lovette KM, McDonagh J, et al. Subcellular distribution of fibrinogen and factor XIII in human blood platelets. Thromb Res 1976;8(4):453–465.

127. Lai T, Greenberg CS. Factor XIII. In High KA, Roberts HR (eds): Molecular Basis of Thrombosis and Hemostasis. New York, Marcel Dekker, Inc., 1995, pp 287–308.

128. Bouhasin JD, Altay C. Factor 13 deficiency: concentrations in relatives of patients and in normal infants. J Pediatr 1968; 72(3):336–341.

129. Fisher S, Rikover M, Naor S. Factor 13 deficiency with severe hemorrhagic diathesis. Blood 1966;28(1):34–39.

130. Kobayashi T, Terao T, Kojima T, et al. Congenital factor XIII deficiency with treatment of factor XIII concentrate and normal vaginal delivery. Gynecol Obstet Invest 1990;29(3):235–238.

131. Kitchens CS, Newcomb TF. Factor XIII. Medicine 1979; 58(6):413–429.

132. Duckert F. Documentation of the plasma factor XIII deficiency in man. Ann NY Acad Sci 1972;202:190–199.

133. Anwar R, Miloszewski KJ. Factor XIII deficiency. Br J Haemotol 1999;107(3):468–484.

134. Otis PT, Feinstein DI, Rapaport SI, Patch MJ. An acquired inhibitor of fibrin stabilization associated with isoniazid therapy: clinical and biochemical observations. Blood 1974;44(6): 771–781.

135. Lopaciuk S, Bykowska K, McDonagh JM, et al. Difference between type I autoimmune inhibitors of fibrin stabilization in two patients with severe hemorrhagic disorder. J Clin Invest 1978;61(5):1196–1203.

136. Godal HC, Ly B. An inhibitor of activated factor XIII, inhibiting fibrin cross-linking but not incorporation of amino acid into casein. Scand J Haemotol 1977;19(5):443–448.

137. Graham JE, Yount WJ, Roberts HR. Immunochemical characterization of a human antibody to factor XIII. Blood 1973; 41(5):661–669.

138. Lorand L, Velasco PT, Rinne JR, et al. Autoimmune antibody (IgG Kansas) against the fibrin stabilizing factor (factor XIII) system. Proc Natl Acad Sci USA 1988;85(1):232–236.

139. Tosetto A, Rodeghiero F, Gatto E, et al. An acquired hemorrhagic disorder of fibrin crosslinking due to IgG antibodies to FXIII, successfully treated with FXIII replacement and cyclophosphamide. Am J Hematol 1995;48(1):34–39.

140. Kamitsuji H, Tani K, Yasui M, et al. Activity of blood coagulation factor XIII as a prognostic indicator in patients with Henoch-Schönlein purpura. Efficacy of factor XIII substitution. Eur J Pediatr 1987;146(5):519–523.

141. Rasche H. Blood coagulation factor XIII and fibrin stabilization. Klin Wochenschr 1975;53(24):1137–1145.

142. Fear JD, Miloszewski KJ, Losowsky MS. The half life of factor XIII in the management of inherited deficiency. Thromb Haemost 1983;49(2):102–105.

143. Stenbjerg S. Prophylaxis in factor XIII deficiency [letter]. Lancet 1980;2(8188):257.

144. Godal HC. An inhibitor to fibrin stabilizing factor (FSF), factor XIII. Scand J Haemotol 1970;7(1):43–48.

145. Nichlos WC, Seligsohn U, Zivelin A, et al. Mutations in the ER-Golgi intermediate compartment protein ERGIC-53 cause combined deficiency of coagulation factors V and VIII. Cell 1998;93(1):61–70.

146. Moussalli M, Pipe SW, Hauri HP, et al. Mannose-dependent endoplasmic reticulum (ER)-Golgi intermediate compartment-53-mediated ER to Golgi trafficking of coagulation factors V and VIII. J Biol Chem 1999;274(46):32539–32542.

147. Wu SM, Stanley TB, Mutucumarana VP, Stafford DW. Characterization of the gamma-glutamyl carboxylase. Thromb Haemost 1997;78(1):599–604.

148. McMillan CW, Roberts HR. Congenital combined deficiency of coagulation factors II, VII, IX, and X. Report of a case. N Engl J Med 1966;274(23):1313–1315.

149. Goldsmith GH, Jr., Pence RE, Ratnoff OD, et al. Studies on a family with combined functional deficiencies of vitamin K-dependent coagulation factors. J Clin Invest 1982;69(6):1253–1260.

150. Aoki N. Alpha-2-plasmin inhibitor. In High KA, Roberts HR (eds): Molecular Basis of Thrombosis and Hemostasis. New York, Marcel Dekker, Inc., 1995, pp 545–559.

151. Meyer K, Williams EC. Fibrinolysis and acquired alpha-2-plasmin inhibitor deficiency in amyloidosis. Am J Med 1985; 79(3):394–396.

152. Collen D, Bounameaux H, De Cock F, et al. Analysis of coagulation and fibrinolysis during intravenous infusion of recombinant human tissue-type plasminogen activator in patients with acute myocardial infarction. Circulation 1986;73(3):511–517.

153. Owen MC, Brennan SO, Lewis JH, Carrell RW. Mutation of antitrypsin to antithrombin. Alpha 1-antitrypsin Pittsburgh (358 Met leads to Arg), a fatal bleeding disorder. N Engl J Med 1983;309(12):694–698.

154. Vidaud D, Emmerich J, Alhenc-Gelas M, et al. Met 358 to Arg mutation of alpha 1-antitrypsin associated with protein C deficiency in a patient with mild bleeding tendency. J Clin Invest 1992;89(5):1537–1543.

155. Prowse CV, Esnouf MP. The isolation of a new warfarin-sensitive protein from bovine plasma. Biochem Soc Trans 1977; 5(1):255–256.

156. Broze GJ, Jr., Miletich JP. Human protein Z. J Clin Invest 1984;73(4):933–938.

157. Miletich JP, Broze GK, Jr. Human plasma protein Z antigen: range in normal subjects and effect of warfarin therapy. Blood 1987;69(6):1580–1586.

158. Kemkes-Matthes B, Matthes KJ. Protein Z deficiency: a new cause of bleeding tendency. Thromb Res 1995;79(1):49–55.

159. Han X, Fiehler R, Broze GJ, Jr. Isolation of a protein Z-dependent plasma protease inhibitor. Proc Natl Acad Sci USA 1998;95(16):9250–9255.

160. Han X, Huang ZF, Fiehler R, Broze GJ, Jr. The protein Z-dependent protease inhibitor is a serpin. Biochemistry 1999; 38(34):11073–11078.

161. Yin ZF, Huang ZF, Cui J, et al. Prothrombotic phenotype of protein Z deficiency. Proc Natl Acad Sci USA 2000; 97(12):6734–6738.

dow
CHAPTER 6

Nonhemophilic Inhibitors of Coagulation

Bruce M. Ewenstein, M.D., Ph.D.
Kathleen G. Putnam, S.M.
Rhonda L. Bohn, M.P.H., Sc.D.

Although not often encountered in clinical practice, patients with acquired inhibitors of coagulation provide unique challenges to both medical personnel and institutional resources. Acquired inhibitors of coagulation are circulating immunoglobulins, usually of the immunoglobulin G (IgG) class, that neutralize the activity of a specific coagulation protein or accelerate its clearance from the plasma. These inhibitors are defined as *allo*antibodies when they arise following blood product exposure in individuals with congenital factor deficiencies, and as *auto*antibodies when they occur among patients without a pre-existent coagulation defect. Autoantibodies against coagulation factors are associated with a variety of clinical conditions in which there is a disturbance of immune function, but are also commonly found among patients whose only identifiable risk factor is advanced age. Nonhemophilic inhibitors are quite rare but are associated with significant morbidity and mortality and should be suspected in any patient who presents with signs and symptoms of bleeding in the absence of a personal or family history of a coagulation disorder.

The loss of tolerance to endogenously expressed coagulation proteins in affected patients is not fully understood, but is likely to involve dysregulated B- and T-cell responses. The most frequently affected coagulation protein is factor VIII, resulting in a condition that has been termed *acquired hemophilia*. Both factor VIII-specific CD4+ T cells and low levels of anti-factor VIII antibodies, including some with inhibitory activity, can be detected using immunologic methods in a significant number of apparently healthy subjects.[1-3] These findings suggest that inadequate tolerance of normal immune responses to factor VIII may play an important role in the development of clinically significant anti-factor VIII antibodies.[4] It remains possible that the pathogenic potential of autoantibodies recognizing factor VIII is also modulated through idiotypic determinants on these molecules.[5,6] The presence of anti-idiotypic antibodies may also be responsible, in part, for the ability of pooled IgG to suppress anti-factor VIII activity in some patients.[7,8]

In general, the clinical and laboratory manifestations of nonhemophilic inhibitors resemble the corresponding inherited coagulation disorder, although often with important differences. This chapter will focus principally on the natural history, diagnosis, and clinical management of patients with acquired hemophilia and then briefly review other inhibitors of coagulation. Lupus anticoagulants, antiphospholipid antibodies that interfere with coagulation-based laboratory assays but are principally associated with venous and arterial thrombosis, are discussed further in Chapter 18.

LABORATORY DIAGNOSIS

Screening Tests

In routine laboratory testing, both simple factor deficiencies and specific inhibitors result in prolongation of the activated partial prothrombin time (aPTT), prothrombin time (PT), or both. These conditions can be distinguished by mixing studies. In the presence of a simple factor deficiency, mixtures of equal volumes of patient and normal plasmas will correct the abnormality. In contrast, the presence of an inhibitor in the patient plasma will inactivate the target protein in the normal plasma, and the aPTT or PT remains prolonged.[9] The inactivation is time and temperature dependent[10] and may require several hours, especially in the case of weak inhibitors. Typically, the aPTT or PT is measured immediately following the mixture of normal and patient test plasma and after 1 and 2 hours of incubation at 37°C.

Because certain coagulation proteins, including factor VIII, are heat labile, the aPTT derived from mixtures of normal and patient plasmas must be compared to control mixtures of normal plasma and buffer incubated under the same conditions. A prolongation of greater than 10 seconds over the control is typically taken as a positive inhibitor screen. The sensitivity of the screening assay may be improved by increasing the proportion of patient to normal plasma to 4:1.[9]

Inhibitor Specificity

The next step in evaluating a patient with a prolonged screening test and a positive mixing study is to determine the specificity of the inhibitor. One goal is to distinguish inhibitors of specific coagulation pathway components from "lupus anticoagulants," antiphospholipid antibodies that may prolong the aPTT but that are not usually associated with clinical bleeding. This distinction is especially important in the evaluation of patients for whom there is no antecedent diagnosis of a factor deficiency. The second goal is to properly identify the specific coagulation protein that is being targeted.

Several methods are commonly employed for distinguishing lupus anticoagulants from inhibitors of factor VIII or other specific coagulation factors (Table 6-1).[11,12] The presence of a strong specific factor inhibitor may result in a more modest reduction in the measurement of other factors when the assays are performed at the standard dilutions, leading to the false impression that the inhibitor is not specific. When assays are performed on a series of increasingly more dilute patient plasma samples, the apparent concentrations of all factors except the one that is specifically inhibited will rise into the normal range. In contrast, progressive normalization of all factor levels will be observed with increasing dilution of the test plasma containing a lupus anticoagulant. Another commonly used technique, the Russell viper venom time (RVVT), makes use of an enzyme found in the venom of the Russell viper that promotes fibrin formation through the direct activation of factors V and X. The enzyme is dependent on the presence of phospholipid but not on factor VIII or other intrinsic pathway factors. The RVVT is thus prolonged in the presence of antiphospholipid antibodies but not inhibitors of the intrinsic pathway proteins.[13] A third technique makes use of the observations that the addition of platelet membranes or phospholipid (hexagonal-phase phosphatidylethanolamine) will shorten a prolonged aPTT due to a lupus anticoagulant, but will have little or no effect on prolongation of the aPTT due to specific factor inhibitors.[14] The diagnosis of a lupus anticoagulant is supported by the detection of antibodies to cardiolipin, β_2-glycoprotein I (β_2-GPI), or prothrombin (see below) using quantitative immunoassays. However, it should be recognized that not all lupus anticoagulant sera give positive results in these immunoassays.[15] Rarely, patients are encountered with both lupus anticoagulant and specific factor VIII inhibitors, producing complex laboratory test results.[16,17] The clinical presentation in such patients is primarily one of bleeding.

Quantitative Assays of Coagulation Factor Inhibitors

Once the presence of a specific factor inhibitor is established, it should be quantified because this will influence treatment strategies. The methodologies are best characterized for anti-factor VIII inhibitors. The most widely used assay today is the Bethesda method, which measures residual factor VIII activity after incubation of pooled normal plasma with dilutions of inhibitor patient plasma for 2 hours at 37°C.[18] Because factor VIII is labile, it is necessary to compare the residual factor (mixing control and patient plasmas) to the factor VIII activity remaining after mixing control plasma with buffer under identical conditions.[19] The quantity (in units) of inhibitor is defined as the reciprocal of the titer that produces 50% inhibition. The Bethesda assay may give false-positive results because of nonspecific loss of factor VIII activity. The Nijmegen modification, which includes the addition of buffers in the assay to minimize shifts in pH, permits more accurate measurements of low-titer inhibitors.[20]

The Bethesda assay methodology can be extended to assess the cross-reactivity of the inhibitor against porcine factor VIII (see below). Porcine factor concentrates, reconstituted into hemophilic plasma, are substituted for normal plasma in the assay test samples and standards. For both human and porcine factor VIII-based assays, inhibitor titers may be determined reliably only for antibodies that display second-order concentration dependence (type 1); the titer of antibodies with more complex kinetics (type 2) can only be approximated (Fig. 6-1). Particularly in the case of type 2 inhibitors, it is essential to use dilutions of patient plasma producing residual factor VIII activity as close to 50% as possible when calculating the inhibitor titer. These methodologies have been extrapolated to the detection and quantification of other factor inhibitors.

Other assays of factor inhibitors, which rely on immunologic rather than functional methodologies, are ex-

Table 6-1 • LABORATORY TESTS TO DISTINGUISH ANTIBODIES TO SPECIFIC COAGULATION FACTORS FROM LUPUS ANTICOAGULANTS

Method	Result	
	Specific inhibitor	Lupus anticoagulant
Normalization of all factor assays with increasing dilution of patient plasma	Negative	Positive
Kinetics of prolongation	Slow	Immediate
Prolonged RVVT	Negative[a]	Positive
Phospholipid neutralization procedure	Negative	Positive

[a] Except in the presence of inhibitors to factors in the "common pathway."

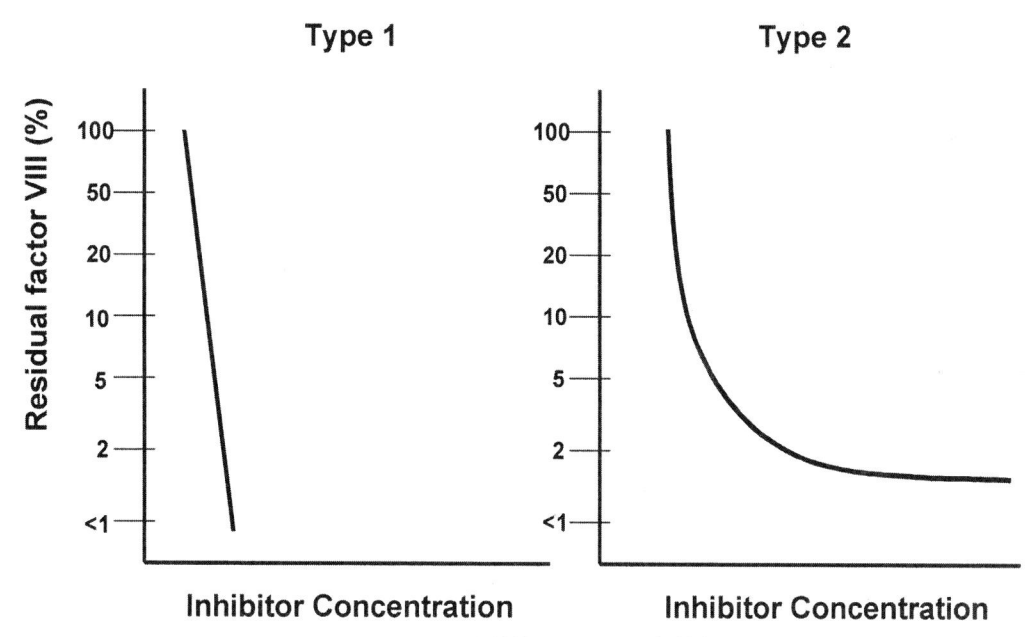

Figure 6–1 Inactivation of factor VIII by type 1 and type 2 inhibitors. Type 1 inhibitors, when present in excess, produce complete inactivation and a linear relationship exists between the concentration of inhibitor and the logarithm of residual factor VIII activity. Type 2 inhibitors, which are typical of nonhemophilic autoantibodies, do not produce complete inactivation of factor VIII. (Based on the work of Gawryl MS, Hoyer LW. Inactivation of factor VIII coagulant activity by two different types of human antibodies. Blood 1982;60:1103–1109, with permission.)

tremely sensitive, but are generally confined to research settings. These include immunodiffusion and enzyme-linked immunosorbent assay (ELISA).[21–23] Each method is able to detect antibodies that accelerate the clearance of the coagulation protein from the circulation without inhibiting its activity in vitro.[24] In the immunodiffusion assay, patient plasma is allowed to diffuse in an agarose gel containing citrated plasma that is then incubated with a calcium-containing solution to initiate the coagulation cascade in situ. Inhibition of fibrin formation, evident as a clear ring in the gel, provides a sensitive measure of factor inhibitors. The distinct advantage of this system is that the inhibitory activity is measurable even following factor replacement therapy. In the ELISA system, samples containing the inhibitor are applied to wells in which factor VIII previously has been immobilized. Monospecific antisera are then added to determine the immunoglobulin class and subclass and light-chain type of the inhibitor.

ACQUIRED INHIBITORS OF FACTOR VIII

Presentation and Natural History

The estimated incidence of acquired hemophilia is 0.1 to 1.0 per million, although it is likely that not all affected patients are reported.[25,26] Bleeding manifestations are often severe and can occur either spontaneously or following minor trauma. In contrast to patients with congenital factor VIII deficiency, where intra-articular bleeding is the archetypal manifestation, patients with acquired hemophilia principally experience soft tissue bleeding. Clinical features include intramuscular hemorrhage and bleeding in the gastrointestinal or urinary tract.[25–30] Retroperitoneal bleeding appears to be especially common and is sometimes fatal.[27,31]

The overall mortality in untreated patients is 8% to 22%,[25,28,32] with most hemorrhagic deaths occurring within the first few weeks after presentation. The median age at the time of diagnosis is 60 to 70 years old (Fig. 6–2A), a fact that, in part, may underscore the relatively high rates of morbidity and mortality.[25–31] Acquired inhibitors occur with similar frequency in males and females (Fig. 6–2B), although the age distribution for females is younger than for males because of postpartum inhibitor development.

Concomitant Conditions

In approximately half of the patients with inhibitors no concomitant disease can be found. In the remainder of patients, the conditions most commonly associated with factor VIII inhibitors include connective tissue disease, inflammatory bowel disease, the puerperium, malignancy, and certain dermatologic disorders[25,31] (Fig. 6–2C).

The development of a postpartum inhibitor to factor VIII is a serious and potentially life-threatening complication of an otherwise normal pregnancy. Symptoms generally appear at term or within 3 months of delivery and, less commonly, prior to parturition. Severe vaginal

Age at Diagnosis of Inhibitor

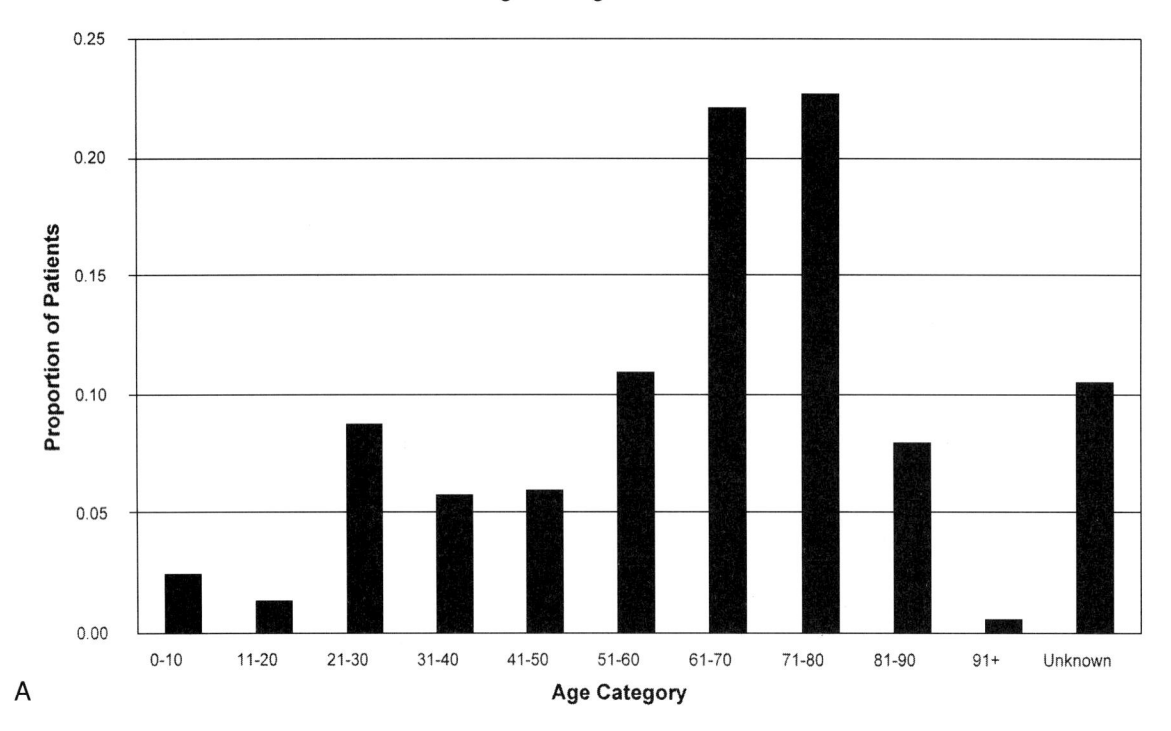

A

Gender Distribution of Patients with Acquired Inhibitors to Factor VIII

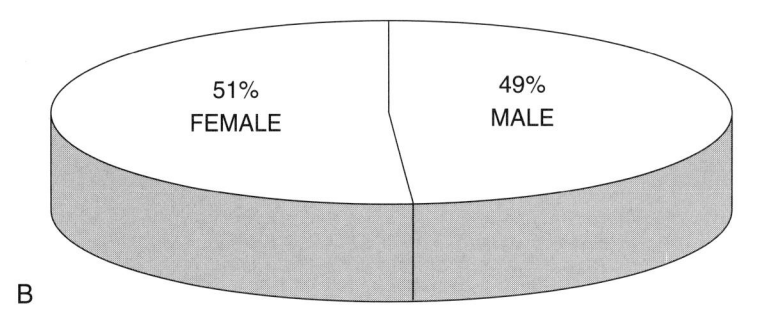

51% FEMALE
49% MALE

B

Figure 6–2 *See legend on opposite page*

bleeding is very common as are soft-tissue and intra-articular hemorrhages.[33] The vast majority of, if not all, postpartum inhibitors ultimately disappear but this may take up to 2 years, with or without the use of immunosuppressive drugs.[34] Among patients who have lost their inhibitors, the re-emergence of the inhibitor in subsequent pregnancies appears to be rare. Indeed, there are reports describing instances in which the inhibitor disappeared during a subsequent pregnancy.[35,36] Transplacental transfer of the inhibitor can be detected in the newborn and may lead to a severe, albeit transient, bleeding diathesis.[37,38]

Systemic lupus erythematosus (SLE) and rheumatoid arthritis are the most frequently encountered autoimmune disorders associated with factor VIII inhibitor development.[25,39–41] Moreover, several dermatologic conditions with a known autoimmune basis, such as psoriasis and pemphigus vulgaris, are also associated with acquired hemophilia.[25,39] Because these disorders are also associated with the development of antibodies to other coagulation factors and phospholipid-binding proteins (see below), special care must be taken to identify the specificity of the inhibitor in this group of patients.

Factor VIII inhibitors also arise among patients with a variety of solid tumors and hematologic malignancies. Perhaps the first reported case of acquired hemophilia, in 1940, was that of a 61 year-old man who died of hemorrhage following a lymph node excision.[42] In view of the relationship between factor VIII inhibitor formation and altered immune status, it is not surprising that the most common association is with lymphoproliferative disorders.[25,43–45] In rare instances, a IgA or IgM monoclonal paraprotein is identified as the factor VIII inhibitor.[46,47] Factor VIII inhibitors have been detected in association with numerous solid tumors, including neoplasms of the colon, pancreas, kidney, prostate, testes, brain, and lung.[25,29,31,44] As is often true in other

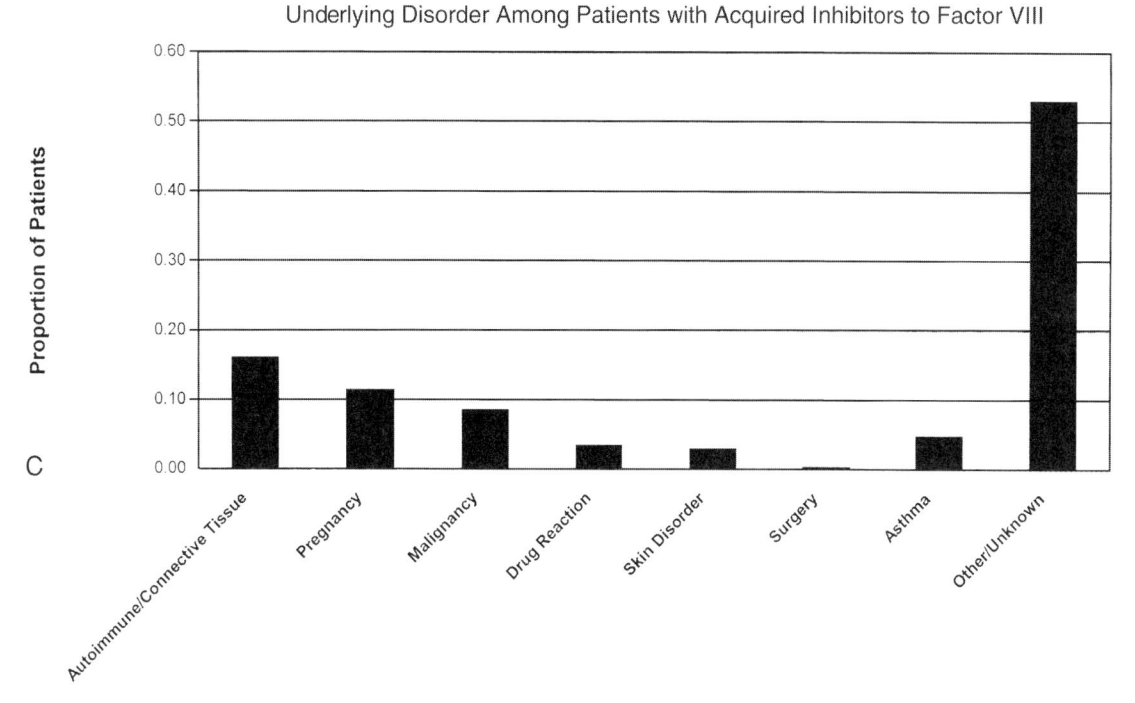

Figure 6–2 (*Continued*) Demographics of patients with nonhemophilic inhibitors to factor VIII. **A.** Age distribution. **B.** Gender. **C.** Underlying disorder. In the majority of patients, advanced age is the only identifiable risk factor. See text for references to primary data.

cases of rare disease associations, it is uncertain whether these reports represent chance occurrences or etiologically related events.[44] For example, the use of radiation therapy or systemic chemotherapy may induce generalized immunologic alterations predisposing to autoantibody formation.

Severe drug reactions, most commonly to penicillin, sulfa antibiotics, chloramphenicol, and phenytoin, have been associated with factor VIII inhibitor formation.[48] It appears likely that alterations in the immunologic state induced by the hypersensitivity reaction, rather than the drug-specific antibody itself, are responsible for the development of the inhibitor. Recent viral infections appear to be common among the rare nonhemophilic children who develop acquired inhibitors of coagulation.[49]

Immunochemistry of Factor VIII Inhibitors

Factor VIII circulates as cation-linked heterodimers in which heterogeneous 92 to 200-kD heavy chains (domains A1, A2, and B) are associated with 80-kD light chains (domains A3, C1 and C2).[50] In plasma, FVIII is noncovalently bound to von Willebrand factor (vWF), which serves to localize factor VIII to sites of vascular injury and to protect it from inactivation by activated protein C (APC).[51] Activation of factor VIII by thrombin results in its release from vWF and promotion of binding to phospholipid surfaces on the platelet.[52] Both the vWF and phospholipid binding regions of factor VIII are found on the light chain. Detailed studies using competitive binding and neutralization assays have demonstrated that the majority of factor VIII autoantibodies are directed against the C2 domain and other light chain sequences.[53–55] Antibodies recognizing the A2 domain of the heavy chain have also been described. Unexpectedly, allo- and autoantibodies bind to similar epitopes on factor VIII although the pattern of reactivity tends to be simpler in nonhemophilic patients with factor VIII inhibitors.[53,54] The further elucidation of the immunochemical complexity of factor VIII inhibitors ultimately may explain the observed differences between laboratory assays and clinical manifestations.

Anti-factor VIII antibodies exhibit a number of biochemical characteristics that are relevant to both their detection and clinical presentation. Almost all are high-affinity IgG immunoglobulins of restricted polyclonal origin.[56] There is a predominance of the IgG_4 subclass and both κ and λ light chains can be found with approximately equal frequency. IgG_4 antibodies do not fix complement and consequently patients will not develop renal or vascular complications even in the presence of endogenous factor VIII. Although the vast majority of inhibitors found in patients with acquired hemophilia are of the IgG class, isolated instances of IgM[47,57] or IgA[46] also have been reported. Progression from a predominantly IgM to IgG profile was observed on at least one occasion.[58]

Factor VIII inhibitors promote the increased catabolism of factor VIII or interfere with coagulation function through a variety of mechanisms. These include inhibition of the interaction of factor VIII with phospholipid,[59] or vWF,[56,60] or factor IX[61] and interference with thrombin-mediated factor VIII activation.[62,63] It is possible that some anti-factor VIII autoantibodies also interfere with vWF or platelet function, thus explaining their propensity to produce mucocutaneous bleeding.

The inactivation of factor VIII by acquired inhibitors is both time and temperature dependent.[40] Two types of inactivation patterns are described (see Fig. 6–1).[64,65] Type 1 antibodies, when present in excess, produce complete inactivation of factor VIII, and a linear relationship exists between the concentration of inhibitor and the (logarithm of) residual factor VIII activity. This pattern of inactivation permits accurate measurement of inhibitor potency using the Bethesda assay. In contrast, type 2 antibodies do not produce complete inactivation unless the factor VIII is first dissociated from the vWF with which it is normally complexed.[66]

Patients with acquired hemophilia almost always develop inhibitors that exhibit type 2 inactivation kinetics, and it is often possible to measure residual factor VIII levels even as the patients are experiencing severe bleeding complications. Factor VIII inhibitors in individuals with congenital hemophilia characteristically exhibit type 1 kinetics. The reason for partial inhibition of factor VIII by type 2 antibodies is unclear but may be related to the target epitope(s) or to the formation of immune complexes.[66,67]

Treatment

In considering treatment strategies, two objectives must be considered: the immediate control of bleeding manifestations and the long-term suppression of the inhibitor. In both instances, one must take into consideration a variety of factors, including the severity of the clinical symptoms, the patient's previous history of blood product exposure, the availability of therapeutic products, and the cost-effectiveness of such treatment.

Management of Acute Bleeding

When possible, optimal management of bleeding is achieved through the normalization of the plasma factor VIII level.[68] For patients with low-titer inhibitors (less than 5 BU), this goal can best be attained by the infusion of exogenous factor VIII in concentrations great enough to overwhelm the inhibitor so that hemostatic levels of factor VIII can be achieved and therapeutic efficacy assured. In the face of high-titer inhibitors (greater than 5 BU) this approach is not practical and strategies to bypass the inhibitor are required (Fig. 6–3).

Factor VIII Replacement Therapy

Porcine factor VIII concentrates have long been recognized for their effectiveness in treating hemophilic bleeding.[69] The single most important advantage of this

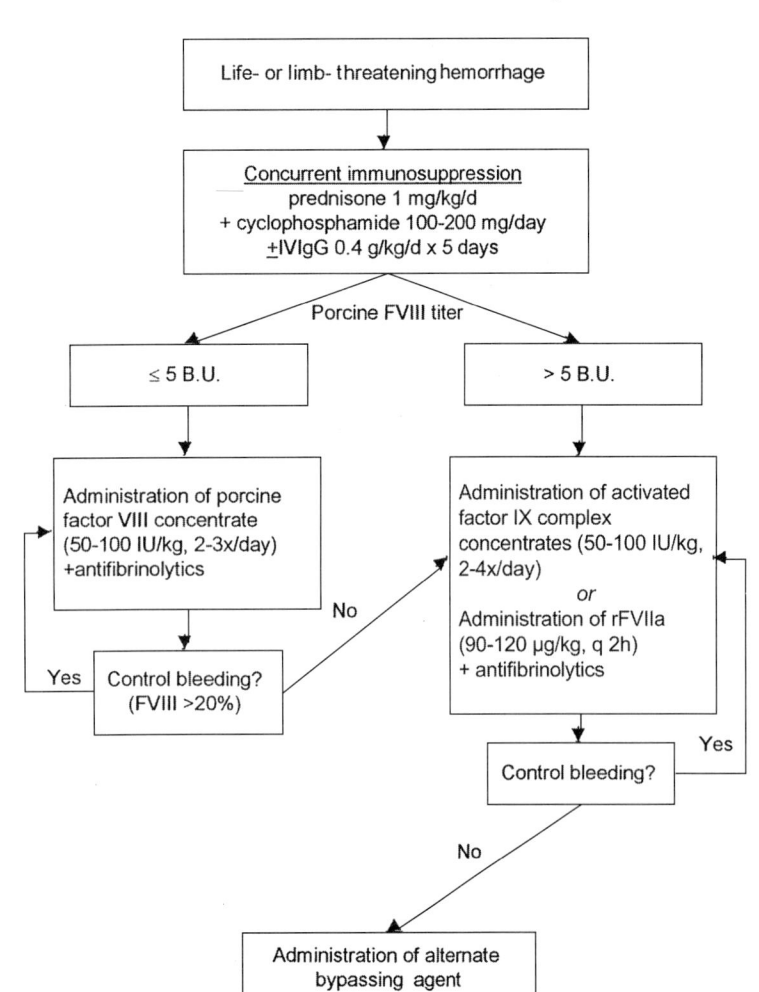

Figure 6–3 Suggested algorithm for the management of patients with nonhemophilic inhibitors to factor VIII experiencing a life- or limb-threatening hemorrhage. Treatment is directed at both suppression of the immune response and the correction of the hemostatic defect. Antifibrinolytic agents (e.g., ε-aminocaproic acid) should not be given concomitantly with activated factor IX complex concentrates and should be used with caution in other patients with risk factors for thromboembolic disease.

product lies in the fact that most autoantibodies, and some alloantibodies, neutralize porcine-derived factor VIII to a much lesser extent than factor VIII derived from human plasma.[70] The average degree of cross-reactivity between porcine and human factor VIII, measured as the ratio of porcine to human titers, is approximately 20% to 30%, and some patients have very little or no measurable inhibitory activity against porcine factor VIII[70-72] (Fig. 6–4). However, the variability in the ratio of human to porcine inhibitor titer is large, necessitating quantification of both on an individual basis. For some patients with human factor VIII inhibitor titers of less than 2 to 5 BU, human factor VIII concentrates may be the best choice for initial therapy, depending on the concurrent porcine factor VIII titer.

In treating hemophilia A patients, the initial dose of factor may be calculated roughly by the formula: 40 U factor VIII/kg plus 20 U factor VIII/kg per BU of inhibitor.[68] However, as mentioned previously, inhibitor titers among patients with acquired hemophilia are notoriously inaccurate and postinfusion factor VIII levels should be monitored closely as the measured Bethesda titer may not be predictive of the response. If the inhibitor has not yet been determined, one may consider the use of an empirically determined initial dose of 75 to 100 U/kg.[73] A particularly useful strategy when using either human or porcine factor VIII involves the administration of a bolus dose to neutralize the inhibitor, followed by a continuous infusion of factor to achieve hemostatic levels (30 to 50 U/dL).[73-75] This approach takes advantage of the fact that the kinetics of factor VIII inhibition are time dependent so that a steady state of uninhibited factor VIII can be achieved. The continuous availability of noncomplexed factor VIII may help to explain clinical improvement in response to factor VIII infusions even among patients in whom increases in the plasma factor VIII level cannot be demonstrated. Platelet activation induced by the porcine vWF present in the concentrate may also exert an important hemostatic effect.[76]

The principal drawbacks to the use of porcine factor VIII are anamnesis and transfusion reactions. In general, porcine factor VIII is less immunogenic than human plasma-derived product, although the development of antiporcine antibodies has been observed in 4% of patients with acquired hemophilia receiving a single treatment with this agent.[31] Transfusion reactions, including pyrexia, flushing, and urticaria, appear to be generally mild and were found to complicate only about 5% of porcine factor VIII infusions in several studies utilizing the currently available concentrate.[77-79] These reactions were most commonly seen during the initial infusion and were less frequent with continued treatment. Severe anaphylactoid reactions have been reported, but appear to be rare.[80] Modest postinfusion declines in platelet counts also have been observed in some patients[72,77,79,81] that are ascribed to platelet aggregation induced by the residual porcine vWF in the concentrate.[82] At least some of the observed complications of porcine factor VIII concentrates are likely to be dose related. For example, one study reported thrombocytopenia and/or transfusion reactions complicated the majority of infusions, however, relatively high doses of porcine factor were employed.[83] Nevertheless, it is rec-

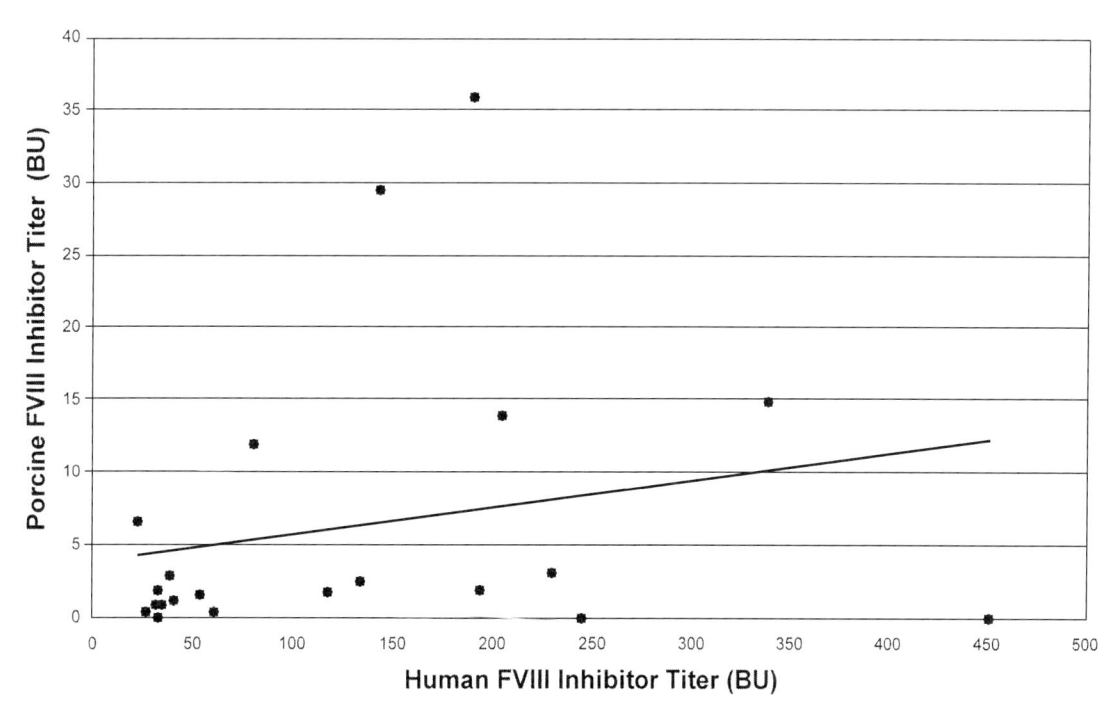

Figure 6–4 Relationship between human and porcine factor VIII inhibitor titers at the time of diagnosis. In many instances, the porcine titer is low (less than 5 BU) even in the presence of very high levels of anti-human factor VIII antibody. Only patients with anti-human titers greater than 20 BU are depicted. See text for references to primary data.

ommended that treatment with porcine factor VIII be initiated and continued for some months under the supervision of clinical personnel before considering home infusion of this product.[71] Although the currently available porcine factor VIII concentrate is not attenuated virally, it has not been associated with the transmission of viral infection during its 20 years of clinical use.

When the anti-human factor VIII titer is low (less than 5 BU), recombinant or plasma-derived human factor VIII may be used. The factor VIII present in intermediate-purity concentrates contains high concentrations of vWF, and therefore may be less susceptible to inactivation, especially by antibodies directed against the C2 domain.[84]

DDAVP

Intravenous administration of 1-deamino-8-D-arginine, abbreviated DDAVP (desmopressin) at a dose of 0.3 μg/kg results in the rapid increase of both vWF and factor VIII levels in normal individuals.[85] DDAVP may also increase the circulating factor VIII sufficiently to treat minor non-life-threatening bleeding in patients with acquired hemophilia.[86-88] Treatment is generally effective in cases where the inhibitor is low and the residual factor VIII level measurable. As might be predicted, DDAVP is associated with tachyphylaxis but does not produce anamnesis to factor VIII.

Hemostatic Agents That "Bypass" the Inhibitor

When the inhibitor titer is high, strategies to bypass the inhibitor may be employed. These strategies consist of infusing activators of the extrinsic or common coagulation pathways with the effect of generating thrombin in the absence of factor VIII.[89]

Factor IX complex concentrates (e.g., Proplex, Konyne, Profilnine), formerly designated prothrombin complex concentrates, are mixtures of partially activated vitamin K-dependent coagulation factors (factors VII, IX, X, and prothrombin) that are effective in the treatment of hemophilia A patients with inhibitors.[90] Additional factor IX complex concentrates in which coagulant factors are more fully activated (e.g., Autoplex, FEIBA) are also effective in arresting bleeding in hemophilia A patients with inhibitors, including those undergoing major surgery.[91] The mechanism(s) by which factor IX complex concentrates and the activated concentrates promote hemostasis are not fully understood. These products contain substantial quantities of factors VIIa, IXa, Xa, and thrombin.[92,93] The possible role of factor VIIa contained within these products has attracted particular attention (see below). In the only large, blinded study of the efficacy of the factor IX complex concentrates, single doses of each of two products infused at 50 to 75 U/kg were found to produce clinical improvement in approximately 50% of inhibitor patients with severe hemophilia with acute hemarthroses.[94] There is no comparable study among patients with acquired hemophilia. Nonetheless, factor IX complex concentrates are used widely for the treatment of non-life-threatening bleeding in this population.[95] In instances of serious bleeding, the fully activated concentrates usually are favored although whether these are more efficacious than their less activated counterparts remains unproven. The recommended dose of activated concentrate is 50 to 100 U/kg with a maximum daily dose of 200 U/kg.

Despite the usefulness of these concentrates in the treatment of acute bleeding episodes among patients with inhibitors to factor VIII, the products have certain limitations. The absence of laboratory measurements that accurately reflect the efficacy of factor IX complex concentrates among patients with factor VIII inhibitors means that only clinical endpoints can be used to monitor treatment. Even with repeated infusions, a substantial proportion of patients appears to gain little clinical benefit. In addition, patients may be exposed to infectious risks. Moreover the use of the concentrates is associated with occasional thrombotic events, including disseminated intravascular coagulation (DIC)[96] and myocardial infarction.[97] These risks appear to be greatest among patients receiving repeated doses of factor IX complex concentrates over short periods of time. Finally, although the concentrates are often used to avoid exposure to factor VIII and anamnestic immune responses, significant increases in factor VIII inhibitor titers have been reported in a small percentage of patients.[98] This is most likely due to the presence of small quantities of factor VIII in some products.[99]

Recombinant Factor VIIa

Recombinant human factor VIIa (rFVIIa) is a procoagulant protein concentrate developed to "bypass" factor VIII or IX inhibitors.[100] Several plausible mechanisms of action have been defined. At physiologic concentrations, the activity of rFVIIa is absolutely dependent on tissue factor (TF), a membrane protein expressed on cellular components of the vascular wall that is exposed only at times of injury. The FVIIa/TF complex activates factor X to Xa and thus promotes thrombin generation and fibrin formation. In the absence of the intrinsic pathway, tissue factor pathway inhibitor (TFPI) inhibits this activity and only small amounts of thrombin are generated. Pharmacologic concentrations of factor VIIa may escape this inhibition either by competing with zymogen factor VII for binding to TF[101] or by directly generating Xa and thus a burst of thrombin on the surface of activated platelets.[102] As may be expected, better results were obtained when rFVIIa was used as first-line therapy than in instances where hemorrhages were previously uncontrolled by alternative therapeutic agents. Typically, initial doses of 90 to 120 μg/kg every 2 hours have been used with a wide range of subsequent dosages, dose intervals, and durations. Importantly, rFVIIa, even when administered in high doses, appears not to produce systemic activation of coagulation,[103] nor have antibodies to factor VII or VIIa been observed in patients following repeated administration of these products.[104] Nonetheless, administration of rFVIIa should be undertaken with caution in older patients, especially in those with risk factors for atherosclerotic disease.[105] The feasibility of using rFVIIa by continuous infusion remains to be determined.[106,107]

Transient Reduction in Inhibitor Titer

The treatment of a life-threatening hemorrhage in a patient with a high-titer inhibitor who has not responded to bypass strategies is particularly difficult. In such circumstances, a temporary reduction of the inhibitor titer may be attempted in order to improve the efficacy of exogenous factor VIII infusions. This can be accomplished by exchange plasmapheresis,[108] with or without extracorporeal immunoadsorption.[109] Since most factor VIII inhibitors are of the IgG class, the extent of reduction in titer is limited by the inability of plasmapheresis to directly access the extravascular space, in which IgG is partly distributed. Nevertheless, it may be possible to achieve as much as a 90% reduction in the inhibitor titer.[110] Volume replacement usually consists of normal plasma followed by factor VIII infusion, although factor concentrate has also been used in the initial replacement fluid in a preoperative setting. Plasmapheresis cannot be used in patients who are hemodynamically unstable or in whom vascular access cannot be easily achieved.

The extracorporeal reduction in inhibitor titer can be improved dramatically by the addition of an immunoadsorption step.[111] Staphylococcal protein A, which binds with high affinity to the Fc portion of all IgG subclasses except IgG_3, is an effective means of selectively depleting plasma of a variety of auto- and alloantibodies. Since the predominant IgG subclass of factor VIII inhibitors is IgG_4 (see above), protein A appears to be ideally suited to the treatment of this disorder. For each plasma volume immunoadsorbed, the plasma level is reduced by approximately 50%, thus an 80% to 90% reduction in inhibitor titer is possible following the processing of three plasma volumes.[112] Following adsorption exchange plasmapheresis, patients are infused with immune globulin and human or porcine factor VIII. An even more specific immunoadsorption methodology has been demonstrated successfully in which inhibitor plasma is passed through a column of agarose coupled to monoclonal antihuman IgG_4 antibodies.[113] Despite the inherent logic of these approaches and the favorable outcomes reported in small groups of patients, technical difficulties with the adsorption columns have prevented their widespread application.

Intravenous Immune Globulin

Intravenous administration of immune globulin (2 g/kg total dose administered in either two or five daily fractions) results in at least partial suppression of factor VIII inhibitors in a subset of patients with acquired hemophilia.[6,114,115] In general, the best results are achieved in patients having low initial antibody titers. The rapid decline in measurable titer that is observed in patients[114,115] suggests that the success of intravenous IgG may be related to the presence of anti-idiotypic antibodies present in plasma pools derived from normal donors.[7,116]

Immunosuppression of Factor VIII Inhibitors

The long-term goal in the treatment of patients with acquired inhibitors of factor VIII is the eradication of the autoantibody. Despite the high rate of spontaneous remission in acquired hemophilia, the severity of bleeding and high mortality rate seen in this condition prompt most clinicians to employ immunosuppressive drugs to hasten the disappearance of the inhibitor. The most commonly used drugs are corticosteroids alone[117] or corticosteroids in combination with either azathioprine or cyclophosphamide.[118] In a large, multicenter retrospective study, clinical response was documented in 78 of 145 patients (54%) receiving immunosuppression with one or more of these drugs, whereas only 11 of 39 (28%) patients improved without specific treatment.[25] In the only prospective, randomized study on the subject, patients were treated initially with prednisone alone at a dose of 1 mg/kg daily for 3 weeks.[119] If antibody was still detectable, patients were then randomized to receive additional prednisone, prednisone with oral cyclophosphamide (2 mg/kg/d), or cyclophosphamide alone. Approximately one third of the patients responded to the initial prednisone course while approximately 50% of steroid-resistant patients responded to the cyclophosphamide-containing regimens. Combination of prednisone (50 to 80 mg/d) and oral cyclophosphamide (100 to 200 mg/d) was similarly effective in other small series of patients.[120,121] A prospective study reported a 91% response rate in 12 patients treated with repeated cycles of factor VIII concentrate, cyclophosphamide, vincristine, and prednisone, although none of the 11 good responders had initial antibody titers greater than 50 BU.[122] More favorable responses were also noted among patients with low-titer inhibitors in other studies.[118,119] It has been proposed that the addition of factor VIII to the regimen enhances responsiveness to immunosuppressive agents,[122] although this assertion has been disputed.[120] Cyclosporine may be useful for patients unresponsive to these agents[106] as may other newer immunosuppressive agents such as rituximab, a monoclonal antibody directed against CD20 antigen on B lymphocytes.[123]

INHIBITORS OF THE VITAMIN K-DEPENDENT PROTEINS

Inhibitors of Prothrombin and Thrombin

Antiprothrombin antibodies are commonly found in association with lupus anticoagulants and may be detected in up to 90% of patients diagnosed with the antiphospholipid syndrome.[124] Rarely, these antibodies produce a reduction in the level of prothrombin sufficient to elevate the PT and aPTT and to produce clinical bleeding.[125,126] Some antiprothrombin antibodies hamper prothrombin activation by coagulation factors Xa and Va and thus behave in vitro as acquired phospholipid-dependent inhibitors.[124] In many instances, antibodies are directed against nonfunctional epitopes on prothrombin (e.g., fragment 1) and thus promote accelerated clearance of the coagulation factor from the circulation but are not detectable in mixing studies.[127] Non-neutralizing antiprothrombin antibodies have also been described in a patient without evidence of a lupus anticoagulant.[128] Beneficial effects have been demonstrated following therapy with prednisone,[128] danazol,[129] and high-dose immunoglobulin.[130,131] Recombinant factor VIIa was successfully used to provide hemostatic coverage in a patient with acquired hypothrombinemia who required a minor surgical procedure.[126]

Some antiprothrombin antibodies are associated with lupus anticoagulant activity.[132] In certain groups of patients, such as those with SLE, the presence of antiprothrombin antibodies has been purported to increase the risk of thromboembolic events.[133] However, other studies have failed to confirm this finding[134] and the matter is at present unsettled.

Patients, both those who are asymptomatic and those with clinical bleeding diatheses, have also been described with neutralizing antibodies to thrombin.[135] The majority of patients were previously exposed to bovine thrombin or fibrin glue, a mixture of bovine thrombin and human fibrinogen used to promote local hemostasis.[136,137] There are also case reports, at least one with a fatal outcome, in which antibodies against thrombin arose in the setting of autoimmune disease or liver cirrhosis.[138,139] In the laboratory, one observes a prolonged PT, aPTT, and thrombin time, which do not correct in mixing studies.

Inhibitors of Factor IX

Inhibitors of factor IX arise in approximately 3% of patients with congenital factor IX deficiency following exposure to exogenous sources of the coagulation protein.[140] Factor IX inhibitors have also been reported in nonhemophilic patients in association with systemic autoimmune disorders.[141,142] In general, factor IX inhibitors are polyclonal immunoglobulins of the IgG class,[143] although there is at least one case report of a factor IX inhibitor due to a monoclonal gammopathy.[144] In the laboratory, factor IX inhibitors are first detected by the failure of normal plasma to correct the aPTT in mixing studies, and may be quantified by a modification of the Bethesda assay.[18] However, unlike the behavior of most factor VIII antibodies in vitro, anti-factor IX antibodies induce an immediate loss of factor IX activity that does not require prolonged incubation.[141]

Inhibitors of Factor X

Acquired factor X deficiency occurs in approximately 5% of patients with systemic amyloid disease.[145] In contrast to other acquired factor deficiencies, the bleeding diathesis in this instance arises not from a circulating inhibitor, but from the adsorption of the factor X on the amyloid fibrils, particularly in the spleen.[146] Bleeding into soft tissues is often severe.[145] Replacement therapy with factor X, using either fresh frozen plasma or factor IX complex concentrates, is often only partially effective because of the shortened half-life of the infused factor. Splenectomy may produce a rapid improvement in the factor X levels due to the physical removal of amyloid binding sites.[147] Chemotherapy drugs, such as melphalan and prednisone, may further limit amyloid deposition.[148] Recombinant factor VIIa was reported to be effective in achieving immediate hemostasis in a bleeding patient.[149]

INHIBITORS OF FACTOR XI

Factor XI inhibitors have been observed rarely among patients with congenital factor XI deficiency who have been exposed to exogenous factor XI.[150] Factor XI antibodies are also seen in association with a variety of autoimmune disorders, principally SLE.[151] Many of the older reports of factor XI antibodies among patients with SLE and thrombosis are likely to be misdiagnosed lupus anticoagulants.[152] Bleeding manifestations in this setting appear to be decidedly uncommon.

The laboratory diagnosis of factor XI inhibitors is usually made upon the discovery of a prolonged aPTT, normal PT, and lack of correction in mixing studies. Specific factor assays performed at progressive plasma dilutions will yield a persistently low factor XI level with normalization of the other factors, although factor XII levels may remain falsely low unless sufficient dilutions of patient plasma are made.

Although patients with congenital factor XI deficiency who develop inhibitors usually do not develop spontaneous hemorrhages, perioperative bleeding has been reported to be severe.[150,153] Since titers of factor XI inhibitors are generally low, adequate replacement therapy with fresh frozen plasma can sometimes be accomplished. Alternatively, factor IX complex concentrates, their active forms, or rFVIIa may be effective in achieving hemostasis.[100,154] High-dose prednisone, 60 to 80 mg/d, is often effective in suppressing the inhibitor.[151]

INHIBITORS OF FACTOR V

There are numerous reports of factor V inhibitors arising in individuals without a prior history of abnormal hemostasis.[155] The most common associations have been with the administration of aminoglycosides, such as streptomycin and gentamicin, and with recent surgical procedures. The occurrence of a factor V inhibitor was described following administration of a bovine topical thrombin preparation that was shown also to contain bovine factor V.[156] The immune response to the bovine protein generated antibodies that also cross-reacted with endogenous human factor V. Most of the inhibitors are composed of polyclonal IgG, although instances have been reported of IgG in association with IgM[157] or IgA.[158] Interference with the interaction of factor Va with phospholipid was demonstrated in the analysis of one such inhibitor.[159]

Factor V inhibitors initially are detected in routine laboratory evaluation by the prolongation of both the PT and aPTT, both of which fail to correct upon mixing with normal plasma. As in the case of lupus anticoagulants, the RVVT is prolonged, but factor V inhibitors can be distinguished from the latter by the failure to correct in the presence of excess phospholipid and by specific factor assays performed on progressive dilutions of patient plasma.

Bleeding in the setting of factor V inhibitors is variable, but is often severe and even fatal.[160] In general, the titer of the inhibitor correlates with the clinical severity. However, in some instances little if any clinical bleeding is observed even in surgical settings despite overtly abnormal in-vitro laboratory findings.[161] As in the case of congenital factor V deficiency, patients with acquired factor V inhibitors can usually be managed with fresh frozen plasma or platelet transfusion.[162,163] Platelet transfusion appears to be an especially useful means of "bypassing" the inhibitor since platelet factor V does not become accessible to the inhibitor until platelets are activated. The majority of factor V inhibitors appear to be of short duration, usually disappearing within 8 to 10 weeks. Some patients with newly discovered factor V inhibitors have been treated with immunosuppressive drugs, principally prednisone and cyclophosphamide,[163] but the effect of these agents on the natural history of the disorder is not known.

INHIBITORS OF FIBRINOGEN AND FACTOR XIII

Thrombin-mediated conversion of fibrinogen to fibrin, the formation of a fibrin mesh, and the cross-linking of the α and γ chains of fibrin by activated factor XIIIa comprise the final steps in blood coagulation.[164] Rare inhibitors to factor XIII, some specifically characterized as immunoglobulins, have been reported in congenitally deficient patients who have received exogenous factor XIII as well as in previously normal individuals. In the case of spontaneously acquired inhibitors, prior exposure to isoniazid[165] or procainamide[166] has also been implicated in the pathogenesis. It is known that isoniazid can be incorporated into protein by factor XIIIa, although the relationship of this action to inhibitor formation remains unclear.[167]

Inhibitors of factor XIII, principally immunoglobulins, act by a variety of molecular mechanisms to produce functional derangement. These include inhibition of thrombin activation, transamidase activity and fibrin cross-linking, and inhibition of factor XIIIa binding to fibrin.[166,168] In some cases, the antibody may exert the same effect by reacting with the cross-linking site on the fibrin substrate.[169] Other antibodies, both polyclonal and monoclonal, have been described that inhibit the conversion of fibrinogen to fibrin.[170,171] Generally, these antibodies can be detected in the laboratory by their effect on fibrin clot stability in dissociating agents such as 5M urea (urea clot solubility test).[166]

Clinically, patients with acquired defects in fibrin cross-linking often present with massive, and sometimes fatal, spontaneous hemorrhages. These patients exhibit high-titer inhibitors and are not easily treated by factor XIII replacement therapy. In one reported case, resolution of an acute bleeding episode was achieved after plasma immunoadsorption with staphylococcal protein A.[172] Fortunately, in many cases the inhibitors regress spontaneously over time or in response to immunosuppressive agents, such as cyclophosphamide.[173] Administration of a factor XIII concentrate can sometimes be sufficient to overwhelm the inhibitor and achieve transient hemostasis.[174]

INHIBITORS OF VON WILLEBRAND FACTOR

von Willebrand factor (vWF) is large, multimeric glycoprotein with two principal functions. It forms an essential bridge between platelets (via platelet glycoprotein Ib/IX) and subendothelial components (e.g., collagen) at sites of vascular injury and also serves as a carrier protein for circulating factor VIII.[175] von Willebrand syndrome (vWS), a collection of acquired disorders resembling congenital forms of von Willebrand disease (vWD) is described in association with numerous other diseases.[176,177] Most common among those are lymphoproliferative disorders, monoclonal gammopathies, autoimmune diseases, and myeloproliferative disorders.[178–181] vWS is also seen in association with acquired or congenital heart disease.[182] Two pathogenic mechanisms are described: adsorption of vWF, particularly the high-molecular-weight forms, by tumor cells or abnormal vasculature[179] and the presence of circulating anti-vWF immunoglobulins.[183] Most often, the latter represent true autoantibodies; less frequently, the paraprotein itself may be the offending agent. Acquired vWD can also be seen in some patients with hypothyroidism as a result of the decreased synthesis and/or release of the vWF protein. In the laboratory, factor VIII, vWF antigen and vWF ristocetin cofactor activity are reduced, though not always to the same extent. The absence of the largest multimeric forms of vWF and decreased ratio of vWF activity to antigen, a pattern resembling congenital type 2A vWD, is frequently seen in cases due to protein absorption. Among autoantibodies to vWF, less than 10% inhibit function (e.g., vWF binding to platelet glycoprotein Ib) and therefore can be demonstrated in mixing studies. Noninhibitory antibodies, which promote the accelerated clearance of vWF, can only be detected by immunoassays that are available only in research laboratories.[176]

The clinical manifestations of acquired vWS resemble those seen in the congenital vWD: spontaneous mucocutaneous bleeding and postsurgical hemorrhage. Bleeding from angiodysplastic lesions in the gastrointestinal tract is particularly common and often serious.[184] Overall, patients with autoantibodies to vWF are more severely affected than those individuals with other forms of the disease.[185] Treatment of the underlying pathology by surgical or medical means will often lead to improvement in the bleeding diathesis associated with vWS.[186,187] In instances where this is not possible, transient correction of the factor VIII and vWF activity levels and favorable hemostatic responses may be achieved with DDAVP or vWF/factor VIII concentrates.[188-190] Refractory patients have been successfully treated with rFVIIa.[191] Reduction in autoantibody titer can often be accomplished with immunoglobulin therapy or other immunosuppressive agents.[176,177,192]

■ REFERENCES

Chapter 6 References

1. Algiman M, Dietrich G, Nydegger U, et al. Natural antibodies to factor VIII (anti-hemophilic factor) in healthy individuals. Proc Natl Acad Sci USA 1992;89:3795-3799.
2. Gilles J, Saint-Remy J-M. Healthy subjects produce both anti-factor VIII and specific anti-idiotypic antibodies. J Clin Invest 1994;94:1496-1505.
3. Reding MT, Wu H, Krampf M, et al. CD4+ T cell response to factor VIII in hemophilia A, acquired hemophilia, and healthy subjects. Thromb Haemost 1999;82:509-515.
4. Reding MT, Wu H, Kramp FM, et al. Sensitization of CD4+ cells to coagulation factor VIII: response in congenital and acquired hemophilia patients and in healthy subjects. Thromb Haemost 2000;84:643-652.
5. Jerne NK. Towards a network theory of the immune system. Ann Immunol (Paris) 1974;125:373-389.
6. Sultan Y, Kazatchkine MD, Maisonneuve P, et al. Anti-idiotypic suppression of autoantibodies to factor VIII (anti-haemophilic factor) by high-dose intravenous gammaglobulin. Lancet 1984;2:765-768.
7. Rossi F, Dietrich G, Kazatchkine MD. Anti-idiotypes against autoantibodies in normal immunoglobulins: evidence for network regulation of human autoimmune responses. Immunol Rev 1989;110:135-149.
8. Moffat EH, Furlong RA, Dannatt AH, et al. Anti-idiotypes to factor VIII antibodies and their possible role in the pathogenesis and treatment of factor VIII inhibitors. Br J Haematol 1989;71:85-90.
9. Lossing TS, Kasper CK, Feinstein DI. Detection of factor VIII inhibitors with the partial thromboplastin time. Blood 1977;49:793-797.
10. Biggs R, Bidwell E. A method for the study of anti-haemophilic globulin inhibitors with reference to six cases. Br J Haematol 1959;5:379-395.
11. Goldsmith JC. Diagnosis of factor VIII versus nonspecific inhibitors. Semin Hematol 1993;30(suppl 1):3-6.
12. Brandt JT, Barna LK, Triplett DA. Laboratory identification of lupus anticoagulants: results of the second international workshop for identification of lupus anticoagulants. Thromb Haemost 1995;74:1597-1603.
13. Thiagarajan P, Pengo V, Shapiro SS. The use of the dilute Russell viper venom time for the diagnosis of lupus anticoagulants. Blood 1986;68:869-874.
14. Triplett DA, Barna LK, Unger GA. A hexagonal (II) phase phospholipid neutralization assay for lupus anticoagulant identification. Thromb Haemost 1993;70:787-793.
15. Triplett DA, Brandt JT, Musgrave KA, et al. The relationship between lupus anticoagulants and antibodies to phospholipid. JAMA 1988;259:550-554.
16. Saxena R, Dhot P, Saraya A, et al. Simultaneous occurrence of FVIII inhibitor and lupus anticoagulant. Am J Hematol 1993;42:232-233.
17. Triplett D. Simultaneous occurrence of lupus anticoagulant and factor VIII inhibitors. Am J Hematol 1997;56:195-196.
18. Kasper CK. Blood—its derivatives and its problems: factor IX. Ann NY Acad Sci 1975;240:172-180.
19. Triplett DA. New methods in coagulation. Crit Rev Clin Lab Sci 1981;15:25-84.
20. Verbruggen B, Novakova I, Wessels H, et al. The Nijmegen modification of the Bethesda assay for factor VIII:C inhibitors: improved specificity and reliability. Thromb Haemost 1995;73:247-251.
21. Ewing N, Kasper CK. In vitro detection of mild inhibitors to factor VIII in hemophilia. Am J Clin Pathol 1982;77:749-752.
22. Coots MC, Glueck HI, Miller MA. Agarose gel method: its usefulness in assaying factor VIII inhibitors, evaluating treatment and suggesting a mechanism of action for factor IX concentrates. Br J Haematol 1985;60:735-750.
23. Sanchez-Cuenca JM, Carmona E, Villaneava MJ, et al. Immunological characterization of factor VIII inhibitors by a sensitive micro-ELISA method. Thromb Res 1990;57:897-908.
24. Nilsson IM, Berntorp E, Zettervall O, et al. Non-coagulation inhibitory factor VIII antibodies after induction of tolerance to factor VIII in hemophilia A patients. Blood 1990;75:378-383.
25. Green D, Lechner K. A survey of 215 non-hemophilic patients with inhibitors to factor VIII. Thromb Haemost 1981;45:200-203.
26. Hoyer LW. Factor VIII inhibitors. Curr Opin Hematol 1995;2:365-371.
27. Lottenberg R, Kentro TB, Kitchens CS. Acquired hemophilia. A natural history study of 16 patients with factor VIII inhibitors receiving little or no therapy. Arch Intern Med 1987;147:1077-1081.
28. Kessler CM, Ludlam CA. The treatment of acquired factor VIII inhibitors: worldwide experience with porcine factor concentrate. Semin Hematol 1993;30 (suppl 1):22-27.
29. Di Bona E, Schiavoni M, Castaman G, et al. Acquired haemophilia: experience of two Italian centres with 17 new cases. Haemophilia 1997;3:183-188.
30. Bossi P, Cabane J, Ninet J, et al. Acquired hemophilia due to factor VIII inhibitors in 34 patients. Am J Med 1998;105:400-408.
31. Morrison AE, Ludlam CA, Kessler C. Use of porcine factor VIII in the treatment of patients with acquired hemophilia. Blood 1993;81:1513-1520.
32. Hay CR, Negrier C, Ludlam CA. The treatment of bleeding in acquired haemophilia with recombinant factor VIIa. Thromb Haemost 1997;78:1463-1467.
33. Solymoss S. Postpartum acquired factor VIII inhibitors: results of a survey. Am J Hematol 1998;59:1-4.
34. Hauser I, Schneider B, Lechner K. Post-partum factor VIII inhibitors. A review of the literature with special reference to the value of steroid and immunosuppressive treatment. Thromb Haemost 1995;73:1-5.
35. Voke J, Letsky E. Pregnancy and antibody to factor VIII. J Clin Pathol 1977;30:928-932.
36. Coller BS, Hultin MB, Hoyer LW, et al. Normal pregnancy in a patient with a prior postpartum factor VIII inhibitor: with observations on pathogenesis and prognosis. Blood 1981;58:619-624.
37. Vicente V, Alberca I, Gonzalez R, et al. Normal pregnancy in a patient with postpartum factor VIII inhibitor. Am J Hematol 1987;24:107-109.
38. Ries M, Wolfel D, Maier-Brandt B. Severe intracranial hemorrhage in a newborn infant with transplacental transfer of an acquired factor VIII:C inhibitor. J Pediatr 1995;127:649-650.
39. Margolius A, Jackson DP, Ratnoff OD. Circulating anticoagulants. a study of 40 cases and review of the literature. Medicine 1961;40:145-202.
40. Shapiro SS, Hultin MB. Acquired inhibitors to the blood coagulation factors. Semin Thromb Hemost 1975;1:336-385.

41. Soriano RM, Matthews JM, Guerado-Parra E. Acquired haemophilia and rheumatoid arthritis. Br J Rheumatol 1987;26:381–383.

42. Lozner EL, Jolliffe LS, Taylor FHL. Haemorrhagic diatheisis with prolonged coagulation time associated with a circulating anticoagulant. Am J Med Sci 1940;199:318–327.

43. Kesley PR, Leyland MJ. Acquired inhibitor to human factor VIII associated with paraproteinemia and subsequent development of chronic lymphocytic leukemia. Br J Med 1982;285:174–176.

44. Hultin MB. Acquired inhibitors in malignant and nonmalignant disease states. Am J Med 1991;91:9S–13S.

45. Sallah S, Nguyen NP, Abdallah JM, et al. Acquired hemophilia in patients with hematologic malignancies. Arch Pathol Lab Med 2000;124:730–734.

46. Gluck HI, Hong R. A circulating anticoagulant in IgA multiple myeloma: its modification of penicillin. J Clin Invest 1965;44:1866–1881.

47. Castaldi PA, Penny R. A macroglobulin with inhibitory activity against coagulation factor VIII. Blood 1970;35:370–376.

48. Green D. Cytotoxic suppression of acquired factor VIII: C inhibitors. Am J Med 1991;91:14S–19S.

49. Brodeur GM, O'Neill PJ, Willimas JA. Acquired inhibitors of coagulation in nonhemophiliac children. J Pediatr 1980;96:439–441.

50. Kaufman RJ, Wasley LC, Dorner AJ. Synthesis, processing and secretion of recombinant human factor VIII expressed in mammalian cells. J Biol Chem 1988;263:6352–6362.

51. Koedam JA, Meijers JCM, Sixma JJ, et al. Inactivation of human factor VIII by activated protein C. Cofactor activity of protein S and protective effect of von Willebrand factor. J Clin Invest 1988;82:1236–1243.

52. Hill-Eubanks DC, Parker CG, Lollar P. Differential proteolytic activation of factor VIII-von Willebrand factor complex by thrombin. Proc Natl Acad Sci USA 1989;86:6508–6512.

53. Scandella D, Mattingly M, de Graaf S, et al. Localization of epitopes for human factor VIII inhibitor antibodies by immunoblotting and antibody neutralization. Blood 1989;74:1618–1626.

54. Prescott R, Nakai H, Saenko EL, et al. The inhibitor antibody response is more complex in hemophilia A patients than in most nonhemophiliacs with factor VIII autoantibodies. Blood 1997;89:3663–3671.

55. Nogami K, Shima M, Giddings JC, et al. Circulating factor VIII immune complexes in patients with type 2 acquired hemophilia A and protection from activated protein C-mediated proteolysis. Blood 2001;97:669–677.

56. Hoyer LW, Gawryl MS, de la Fuente B. Immunochemical characterization of factor VIII inhibitors. In Hoyer L (Ed): Factor VIII Inhibitors. New York, Alan R. Liss, 1984, pp. 73–85.

57. Tiarks C, Pechet L, Humphreys RE. Development of anti-idiotypic antibodies in a patient with a factor VIII autoantibody. Am J Hematol 1989;32:217–221.

58. Marengo-Rowe AJ, Murff G, Leveson JE, et al. Hemophilia-like disease associated with pregnancy. Obstet Gynecol 1972;40:56–64.

59. Arai M, Scandella D, Hoyer LW. Molecular basis of factor VIII inhibition by human antibodies. Antibodies that bind to the factor VIII light chain prevent the interaction of factor VIII with phospholipid. J Clin Invest 1989;83:1978–1984.

60. Shima M, Nakai H, Scandella D, et al. Common inhibitory effects of human anti-C2 domain inhibitor alloantibodies on factor VIII binding to von Willebrand factor. Br J Haematol 1995;91:714–721.

61. Fulcher CA. Immunochemistry of factor VIII: C inhibitor antibodies. Am J Med 1991;91:6S–8S.

62. Lazarchick J, Ashby MA, Lazarchick JJ, et al. Mechanism of action of factor VIII inactivation by human antibodies. IV. Antibody binding prevents factor VIII proteolysis by thrombin. Ann Clin Lab Sci 1986;16:497–501.

63. Saenko EL, Shima M, Gilbert GE, et al. Slowed release of thrombin-cleaved factor VIII from von Willebrand factor by a monoclonal and a human antibody is a novel mechanism for factor VIII inhibition. J Biol Chem 1996;271:27424–27431.

64. Biggs R, Austen DEG, Denson KWE, et al. The mode of action of antibodies which destroy factor VIII. I. Antibodies which have second order concentration graphs. Br J Haematol 1972;23:125–135.

65. Biggs R, Austen DEG, Denson KWE, et al. The mode of action of antibodies which destroy factor VIII. II. Antibodies which give complex concentration graphs. Br J Haemotol 1972;23:137–155.

66. Gawryl MS, Hoyer LW. Inactivation of factor VIII coagulant activity by two different types of human antibodies. Blood 1982;60:1103–1109.

67. Nogami K, Shima M, Hosokawa K. et al. Factor VIII C2 domain contains the thrombin-binding site responsible for thrombin-catalyzed cleavage at Arg 1689. J Biol Chem 2000;275:25774–25780.

68. Kasper CK. Treatment of factor VIII inhibitors. Prog Hemost Thromb 1989;9:57–86.

69. Kernoff PB. Porcine factor VIII: preparation and use in treatment of inhibitor patients. Prog Clin Biol Res 1984;150:207–224.

70. Shulman NR, Hirschman RJ. Acquired haemophilia. Trans Assoc Am Physicians 1969;82:388–397.

71. Hay CRM, Laurian Y, Verroust F, et al. Induction of immune tolerance in patients with hemophilia A and inhibitors treated with porcine VIIIC by home therapy. Blood 1990;76:882–886.

72. Brettler DB, Levine PH. Factor concentrates for treatment of hemophilia: which one to choose? Blood 1989;73:2067–2073.

73. Inhibitor subcommittee of the association of hemophilia clinic directors of Canada. Suggestions for the management of factor VIII inhibitors. Haemophilia 2000;6 (suppl 1):52–59.

74. Bona RD, Riberio M, Klatsky AU, et al. Continuous infusion of porcine factor VIII for the treatment of patients with factor VIII inhibitors. Semin Hematol 1993;30:32–35.

75. Rubinger M, Houston DS, Schwetz N, et al. Continuous infusion of porcine factor VIII in the management of patients with factor VIII inhibitors. Am J Hematol 1997;56:112–118.

76. Chang H, Mody M, Lazarus AH, et al. Platelet activation induced by porcine factor VIII (Hyate:C). Am J Hematol 1998;57:200–205.

77. Kernoff PB, Thomas ND, Lilley PA, et al. Clinical experience with polyelectrolyte-fractionated porcine factor VIII concentrate in the treatment of hemophiliacs with antibodies to factor VIII. Blood 1984;63:31–41.

78. Brettler DB, Forsberg AD, Levine PH, et al. The use of porcine factor VIII concentrate (Hyate:C) in the treatment of patients with inhibitor antibodies to factor VIII. A multicenter US experience. Arch Intern Med 1989;149:1381–1385.

79. Hay CRM, Lozier JN, Lee CA, et al. Safety profile of porcine factor VIII and its use as hospital and home-therapy for patients with haemophilia A and inhibitors: the results of an international survey. Thromb Haemost 1996;75:25–29.

80. Morrison AE, Ludlam CA. The use of porcine factor VIII in the treatment of patients with acquired hemophilia: the United Kingdom experience. Am J Med 1991;91:23S–26S.

81. Gatti L, Mannucci PM. Use of porcine factor VIII in the management of seventeen patients with factor VIII antibodies. Thromb Haemost 1984;51:379–384.

82. Altieri DC, Capitanio AM, Mannucci PM. Von Willebrand factor contaminating porcine FVIII concentrate (Hyate:C) causes platelet aggregation. Br J Haematol 1986;63:703–711.

83. Gringeri A, Santagostino E, Tradati F, et al. Adverse effects of treatment with porcine factor VIII. Thromb Haemost 1991;65:245–247.

84. Suzuki T, Arai M, Amano K, et al. Factor VIII inhibitor antibodies with C2 domain specificity are less inhibitory to factor VIII

complexed with von Willebrand factor. Thromb Haemost 1996;76:749–754.
85. Mannucci PM. Desmopressin (DDAVP) in the treatment of bleeding disorders: the first 20 years. Blood 1997;90:2515–2521.
86. De la Fuente B, Kasper CK, Rickles FR, et al. Response of patients with mild and moderate hemophilia A and von Willebrand's disease to treatment with desmopressin. Ann Intern Med 1985;103:6–14.
87. Chistolini A, Ghirardini A, Tirindelli MC, et al. Inhibitor to factor VIII in a non-hemophilic patient: evaluation of the response to DDAVP and the in vitro kinetics of factor VIII. Nouv Rev Fr Hematol 1987;29:221–224.
88. Mudad R, Kane WH. DDAVP in acquired haemophilia A: case report and review of the literature. Am J Hematol 1993;43:295–299.
89. Sultan Y, Loyer F. In vitro evaluation of factor VIII–bypassing activity of activated prothrombin complex concentrate, prothrombin complex concentrate, and factor VIIa in the plasma of patients with factor VIII inhibitors: thrombin generation test in the presence of collagen-activated platelets. J Lab Clin Med 1993;121:444–452.
90. Abildgaard CF, Britton M, Harrison J. Prothrombin complex concentrate (Konyne) in the treatment of hemophilic patients with factor VIII inhibitors. J Pediatr 1976;88:200–205.
91. Hanna WT, Madigan RR, Miles MA, et al. Activated factor IX complex in treatment of surgical cases of hemophilia A with inhibitors. Thromb Haemost 1981;46:638–641.
92. Hultin MB. Activated clotting factors in factor IX concentrates. Blood 1979;54:1028–1038.
93. Lundblad RL, Bergstrom J, De Vreker R, et al. Measurement of active coagulation factors in Autoplex-T with colorimetric active site-specific assay technology. Thromb Haemost 1998;80:811–815.
94. Lusher JM, Blatt PM, Penner JA, et al. Autoplex versus proplex: a controlled, double-blind study of effectiveness in acute hemarthroses in hemophiliacs with inhibitors to factor VIII. Blood 1983;62:1135–1138.
95. Hay CRM, Baglin TP, Collins PW, et al. The diagnosis and management of factor VIII and IX inhibitors: a guideline from the UK Haemophilia Centre Doctors' Organization (UKHCDO). Br J Haemotol 2000;111:78–90.
96. Rodeghiero F. Castronovo S, Dini E. Disseminated intravascular coagulation after infusion of FEIBA (factor VIII inhibitor bypassing activity) in a patient with acquired haemophilia. Thromb Haemost 1982;48:339–340.
97. Sullivan DW, Purdy LJ, Billingham M, et al. Fatal myocardial infarction following therapy with prothrombin complex concentrates in a young man with hemophilia A. Pediatrics 1984;74:279–281.
98. Laurian Y, Girma JP, Lambert T, et al. Incidence of immune responses following 102 infusions of Autoplex in 18 hemophilic patients with antibody to factor VIII. Blood 1984;63:457–462.
99. Onder O, Hoyer LW. Factor VIII coagulant antigen in factor IX complex concentrates. Thromb Res 1979;15:569–572.
100. Hedner U, Glazer S, Falch J. Recombinant activated factor VII in the treatment of bleeding episodes in patients with inherited and acquired bleeding disorders. Transfus Med Rev 1993;7:78–83.
101. van't Veer C, Golden NJ, Mann KG. Inhibition of thrombin generated by the zymogen factor VII: implications for the treatment of hemophilia A by factor VIIa. Blood 2000;95:1330–1335.
102. Monroe DM, Hoffman M, Oliver J, et al. A possible mechanism of action of activated factor VII independent of tissue factor. Blood Coagul Fibrinol 1998;9 (Suppl 1):S15–20.
103. Gallistl S, Cvirn G, Muntean W. Recombinant factor VIIa does not induce hypercoagulability in vitro. Thromb Haemost 1999;81:245–249.
104. Nicolaisen EM. Antigenicity of activated recombinant factor VII followed through nine years of clinical experience. Blood Coagul Fibrinol 1998;9 (Suppl 1):S119–123.
105. Peerlinck K, Vermylen J. Acute myocardial infarction following administration of recombinant activated factor VII (Novo Seven) in a patient with haemophilia A and inhibitor. Thromb Haemost 1999;82:1775–1776.
106. Schulman S, Bech Jensen M, Varon D, et al. Feasibility of using recombinant factor VIIa in continuous infusion. Thromb Haemost 1996;75:432–436.
107. Mauser-Bunschoten E, de Goede-Bolder A, Rosendaal G, et al. Continuous infusion of recombinant factor VIIa in dental surgery: not as effective as bolus infusions? Thromb Haemost 1999;82 (Suppl):128–129.
108. Cobcroft R, Tamagnini G, Dormandy KM. Serial plasmapheresis in a haemophiliac with antibodies to FVIII. J Clin Pathol 1977;30:763–765.
109. Gjorstrup P, Watt RM. Therapeutic protein A immunoadsorption. A review. Trans Sci 1990;11:281–302.
110. Slocombe GW, Newland AC, Colvin MC, et al. The role of intensive plasma exchange in the prevention and management of haemorrhage in patients with inhibitors to factor VIII. Br J Haematol 1981;47:577–585.
111. Nilsson I, Sundqvist S-B, Freiburghaus C. Extracorporeal protein A sepharose and specific affinity chromatography for removal of antibodies. In Hoyer LW (Ed): Factor VIII Inhibitors. New York, Alan R. Liss, 1984; pp. 225–241.
112. Gjorstrup P, Berntorp E, Larsson L, et al. Kinetic aspects of the removal of IgG and inhibitors in hemophiliacs using protein A immunoadsorption. Vox Sang 1991;61:244–250.
113. Regnault V, Rivat C, Vallet JP, et al. A potential new procedure for removing anti-factor VIII antibodies from hemophilic plasma. Thromb Res 1987;45:51–57.
114. Sultan Y, Kazatchkine MD, Nydegger U, et al. Intravenous immunoglobulin in the treatment of spontaneously acquired factor VIII:C inhibitors. Am J Med 1991;91:35S–39S.
115. Schwartz RS, Gabriel DA, Aledort LM, et al. A prospective study of treatment of acquired (autoimmune) factor VIII inhibitors with high-dose intravenous gammaglobulin. Blood 1995;86:797–804.
116. Dietrich G, Algiman M, Sultan Y, et al. Origin of anti-idiotypic activity against anti-factor VIII autoantibodies in pools of normal human immunoglobulin G (IVIg). Blood 1992;79:2946–2951.
117. Spero JA, Lewis JH, Hasiba U. Corticosteroid therapy for acquired F VIII: C inhibitors. Br J Haematol 1981;48:635–642.
118. Green D. Suppression of an antibody to factor VIII by a combination of factor VIII and cyclophosphamide. Blood 1971;37:381–387.
119. Green D. Immunosuppression of factor VIII inhibitors in nonhemophilic patients. Semin Hematol 1993;30 (Suppl 1):28–31.
120. Shaffer LG, Phillips MD. Successful treatment of acquired hemophilia with oral immunosuppressive therapy. Ann Intern Med 1997;127:206–209.
121. Bayer RL, Lichtman SM, Allen SL, et al. Acquired factor VIII inhibitors—successful treatment with an oral outpatient regimen. Am J Hematol 1999;60:70–71.
122. Lian E C-Y, Larcada AF, Chiu A-Y. Combination immunosuppressive therapy after factor VIII infusion for acquired factor VIII inhibitor. Ann Intern Med 1989;110:774–778.
123. Gopal AK, Press OW. Clinical applications of anti-CD20 antibodies. J Lab Clin Med 1999;134:445–450.
124. Galli M, Barbui T. Antiprothrombin antibodies: detection and clinical significance in the antiphopholipid syndrome. Blood 1999;93:2149–2157.
125. Fleck RA, Rapaport SI, Rao LVM. Anti-prothrombin antibodies and the lupus anticoagulant. Blood 1988;72:512–519.
126. Holm M, Andreasen R, Ingerslev J. Management of bleeding using recombinant factor VIIa in a patient suffering from bleeding tendency due to a lupus anticoagulant-hypoprothrombinemia syndrome. Thromb Haemost 1999;82:1776–1778.

127. Bajaj SP, Rapaport SI, Fierer DS, et al. A mechanism for the hypoprothrombinemia of the acquired hypoprothrombinemia-lupus anticoagulant syndrome. Blood 1983;61:684–692.

128. Bajaj SP, Rapaport SI, Barclay S, et al. Acquired hypoprothrombinemia due to non-neutralizing antibodies to prothrombin: mechanism and management. Blood 1985;65:1538–1543.

129. Williams S, Linardic C, Wilson O, et al. Acquired hypoprothrombinemia: effects of danazol treatment. Am J Hematol 1996;53:272–276.

130. Pernod G, Arvieux J, Carpentier PH, et al. Successful treatment of lupus anticoagulant-hypoprothrombinemia syndrome using intravenous immunoglobulin. Thromb Haemost 1997;78:969–970.

131. Barbui T, Finazzi G, Falanga A, et al. Intravenous gammaglobulin, anti-phospholipid antibodies, and thrombocytopenia. Lancet 1988;2:969.

132. Horbach DA, van Oort E, Derksen RHWM, et al. The contribution of anti-prothrombin-antibodies to lupus anticoagulant activity. Discrimination between functional and non-functional anti-prothrombin-antibodies. Thromb Haemost 1998;79:790–795.

133. Horbach DA, van Oort E, Donders RCJM, et al. Lupus anticoagulant is the strongest risk factor for both venous and arterial thrombosis in patients with systemic lupus erythematosus—comparison between different assays for the detection of anti-phospholipid antibodies. Thromb Haemost 1996;76:916–924.

134. Galli M, Beretta G, Daldossi M, et al. Different anticoagulant and immunological properties of anti-prothrombin antibodies in patients with antiphopholipid antibodies. Thromb Haemost 1997;77:486–491.

135. Sie P, Bezeaud A, Dupouy D, et al. An acquired anti-thrombin autoantibody directed toward the catalytic center of the enzyme. J Clin Invest 1991;88:291–296.

136. Stricker RB, Lane PK, Leffert JD, et al. Development of anti-thrombin antibodies following surgery in patients with prosthetic cardiac valves. Blood 1988;72:1375–1380.

137. Banninger H, Hardegger T, Tobler A, et al. Fibrin glue in surgery: frequent development of inhibitors of bovine thrombin and human factor V. Br J Haematol 1993;85:528–532.

138. LaSpada AR, Skalhegg BS, Henderson R, et al. Brief report: fatal hemorrhage in a patient with an acquired inhibitor of human thrombin. N Engl J Med 1995;333:494–497.

139. Barthels M, Heimburger N. Acquired thrombin inhibitor in a patient with liver cirrhosis. Haemostasis 1985;15:395–401.

140. Briet E, Reisner HM, Roberts HR. Inhibitors in Christmas disease. In Hoyer LW (Ed): Factor VIII Inhibitors. New York, Alan R. Liss, 1984, pp. 123–139.

141. Lechner K. Factor IX inhibitors: report of two cases and a study of the biological, chemical and immunological properties of the inhibitors. Thromb Diath Haemorrh 1971;25:447–459.

142. Largo R, Sigg P, von Felten A, et al. Acquired factor IX inhibitor in a nonhaemophilic patient with autoimmune disease. Br J Haematol 1974;26:129–140.

143. Reisner HM, Roberts HR, Krumholz S, et al. Immunochemical characterization of a polyclonal human antibody to factor IX. Blood 1977;50:11–19.

144. Pike IM, Yount WJ, Puritz EM, et al. Immunochemical characterization of a monoclonal gamma G4-lambda human antibody to factor IX. Blood 1972;40:1–10.

145. Gertz MA, Lacy MQ, Dispenzieri A. Amyloidosis: recognition, confirmation, prognosis and therapy. Proc Mayo Clin 1999;74:490–494.

146. Furie B, Voo L, McAdam KPWJ, et al. Mechanism of factor X deficiency in systemic amyloidosis. N Engl J Med 1981:827–830.

147. Greipp PR, Kyle RA, Bowie EJ. Factor X deficiency in amyloidosis. Resolution after splenectomy. N Engl J Med 1979;301:1050–1051.

148. Camoriano JK, Greipp PR, Bayer GK, et al. Resolution of acquired factor X deficiency and amyloidosis with melphalan and prednisone therapy. N Engl J Med 1987;316:1133–1135.

149. Boggio L, Green D. Recombinant human factor VIIa in the management of amyloid-associated factor X deficiency. Br J Haematol 2001;112:1074–1075.

150. Schnall SF, Duffy TP, Clyne LP. Acquired factor XI inhibitors in congenitally deficient patients. Am J Hematol 1987;26:323–328.

151. Reece EA, Clyne LP, Romero R, et al. Spontaneous factor XI inhibitors. Seven additional cases and a review of the literature. Arch Intern Med 1984;144:525–529.

152. Triplett DA, Brandt JT, Maas RL. The laboratory heterogeneity of lupus anticoagulants. Arch Pathol Lab Med 1985;109:946–951.

153. Morgan K, Schiffman S, Feinstein D. Acquired factor XI inhibitors in two patients with hereditary factor XI deficiency. Thromb Haemost 1984;51:371–375.

154. Rolovic Z, Elezovic I, Obrenovic B, et al. Life-threatening bleeding due to an acquired inhibitor to factor XII-XI successfully treated with "activated" prothrombin complex concentrate (FEIBA) (letter). Br J Haematol 1982;51:659.

155. Feinstein D, Rapaport SI, McGehee WG, et al. Factor V anticoagulants: clinical, biochemical, and immunological observations. J Clin Invest 1970;49:1578–1588.

156. Zehnder JL, Leung LL. Development of antibodies to thrombin and factor V with recurrent bleeding in a patient exposed to topical bovine thrombin. Blood 1990;76:2011–2016.

157. Crowell EB Jr. Observations on a factor-V inhibitor. Br J Haematol 1975;29:397–404.

158. Lane TA, Shapiro SS, Burka ER. Factor V antibody and disseminated intravascular coagulation. Ann Intern Med 1978;89:182–185.

159. Ortel TL, Quinn-Allen MA, Charles LA, et al. Characterization of an acquired inhibitor to coagulation factor. J Clin Invest 1992;90:2340–2347.

160. Coots MC, Muhleman AF, Glueck HI. Hemorrhagic death associated with a high titer factor V inhibitor. Am J Hematol 1978;4:193–206.

161. Nesheim ME, Nichols WL, Cole TL, et al. Isolation and study of an acquired inhibitor of human coagulation factor V. J Clin Invest 1986;77:405–415.

162. Onuora CA, Lindenbaum J, Nossel HL. Massive hemorrhage associated with circulating antibodies to factor V. Am J Med Sci 1973;265:407–417.

163. Chediak J, Ashenhurst JB, Garlick I, et al. Successful management of bleeding in a patient with factor V inhibitor by platelet transfusions. Blood 1980;56:835–841.

164. McDonagh RPJ, McDonagh J, Duckert F. The influence of fibrin cross-linking on the kinetics of urokinase-induced clot lysis. Br J Haematol 1971;21:323–332.

165. Otis PT, Feinstein D, Rapaport SI, et al. An acquired inhibitor of fibrin stabilization associated with isoniazid therapy: clinical and biochemical observations. Blood 1974;44:771–781.

166. Fukue H, Anderson K, McPhedran P, et al. A unique factor XIII inhibitor to a fibrin-binding site on factor XIIIA. Blood 1992;79:65–74.

167. Lorand L, Campbell LK, Robertson BJ. Enzymatic coupling of isoniazid to proteins. Biochemistry 1972;11:434–438.

168. Lopaciuk S, Bykowska K, McDonagh JM, et al. Differences between type I autoimmune inhibitors of fibrin stabilization in two patients with severe hemorrhagic disorder. J Clin Invest 1978;61:1196–1203.

169. Rosenberg RD, Colman RW, Lorand L. A new haemorrhagic disorder with defective fibrin stabilization and cryofibrinogenaemia. Br J Haematol 1974;26:269–284.

170. Coleman M, Vigliano EM, Weksler ME, et al. Inhibition of fibrin monomer polymerization by lambda myeloma globulins. Blood 1972;39:210–223.

171. Marciniak E, Greenwood MF. Acquired coagulation inhibitor delaying fibrinopeptide release. Blood 1979;53:81–92.

172. Gailani D. An IgG inhibitor against coagulation factor XIII: resolution of bleeding after plasma immunoadsorption with staphylococcal protein A (letter). Am J Med 1992;92:110–112.

173. Nakamura S, Kato A, Sakata Y, et al. Bleeding tendency caused by IgG inhibitor to factor XIII, treated successfully by cyclophosphamide. Br J Haematol 1988;68:313–319.

174. Daly HM, Carson PJ, Smith JK. Intracerebral haemorrhage due to acquired factor XIII inhibitor—successful response to factor XIII concentrate. Blood Coagul Fibrinolysis 1991;2:507–514.

175. Sadler JE. von Willebrand factor. J Biol Chem 1991;266:22777–22780.

176. Veyradier A, Jenkins CSP, Fressinaud E, et al. Acquired von Willebrand syndrome: from pathophysiology to management. Thromb Haemost 2000;84:175–182.

177. Tefferi A, Nichols WL. Acquired von Willebrand disease: concise review of occurrence, diagnosis, pathogenesis and treatment. Am J Med 1997;103:536–540.

178. Mannucci PM, Lombardi R, Bader R, et al. Studies of the pathophysiology of acquired von Willebrand's disease in seven patients with lymphoproliferative disorders or benign monoclonal gammopathies. Blood 1984;64:614–621.

179. Richard C, Cuadrado MA, Prieto M, et al. Acquired von Willebrand disease in multiple myeloma secondary to absorption of von Willebrand factor by plasma cells. Am J Hematol 1990;35:114–117.

180. Simone JV, Cornet JA, Abildgaard CF. Acquired von Willebrand's syndrome in systemic lupus erythematosus. Blood 1968;31:806–812.

181. Carter C, Boughton BJ. Acquired von Willebrand's disease in myeloproliferative syndrome: spontaneous remission during pregnancy. Thromb Haemost 1992;67:387–388.

182. Warkentin TE, Moore JC, Morgan DG. Aortic stenosis and bleeding gastrointestinal angiodysplasia: is acquired von Willebrand's disease the link? Lancet 1992;340:35–37.

183. Handin RI, Martin V, Moloney WC. Antibody-induced von Willebrand's disease: a newly defined inhibitor syndrome. Blood 1976;48:393–405.

184. Fressinaud E, Meyer D. International survey of patients with von Willebrand disease and angiodysplasia. Thromb Haemost 1993;70:546 (letter).

185. Mohri H, Motomura S, Kanamori H, et al. Clinical significance of inhibitors in acquired von Willebrand syndrome. Blood 1998;91:3623–3629.

186. Scott JP, Montgomery RR, Tubergen DG, et al. Acquired von Willebrand's disease in association with Wilms' tumor: regression following treatment. Blood 1981;58:665–669.

187. Anderson RP, K M, Street A. Reversal of aortic stenosis, bleeding gastrointestinal angiodysplasia, and von Willebrand syndrome by aortic valve replacement. Lancet 1996;347:689–690.

188. Castaman G, Rodeghiero F, Di Bona E, et al. Clinical effectiveness of desmopressin in a case of acquired von Willebrand's syndrome associated with benign monoclonal gammopathy. Blut 1989;58:211–213.

189. Meyer D. Frommel D. Larrieu MJ, et al. Selective absence of large forms of factor VIII/von Willebrand factor in acquired von Willebrand's syndrome. Response to transfusion. Blood 1979;54:600–606.

190. Morris ES, Hampton KK, Nesbitt IM, et al. The management of von Willebrand's disease-associated gastrointestinal angiodysplasia. Blood Coagul Fibrinolysis 2001;12:143–148.

191. Meijer K, Peters FTM, van der Meer J. Recurrent severe bleeding from gastrointestinal angiodysplasia in a patient with von Willebrand's disease, controlled with recombinant factor VIIa. Blood Coagul Fibrinolysis 2001;12:211–213.

192. Macik BG, Gabriel DA, While GC 2nd, et al. The use of high-dose intravenous gammaglobulin in acquired von Willebrand syndrome. Arch Pathol Lab Med 1988;112:143–146.

CHAPTER 7

von Willebrand Disease

Margaret E. Rick, M.D.

von Willebrand disease (vWD) is an inherited autosomal dominant bleeding disorder that is found in approximately 1% of the population when random screening is carried out.[1] Only a fraction of these individuals are symptomatic, however, and the majority have mild or moderate manifestations that do not significantly affect daily living activities. Easy bruising, epistaxis, and oral bleeding with dental procedures are often the primary symptoms. In the majority of cases, the bleeding results from decreased von Willebrand factor (vWF)-mediated binding of platelets to the vascular subendothelium and decreased vWF-mediated platelet-platelet interactions that occur in areas of high shear (arterial circulation).[2]

Biochemical and physiologic information about vWF has aided in the understanding of the functions of this molecule and has allowed clarification of the terminology for its activities. vWF was originally thought to be a part of the same protein as coagulation factor VIII because these molecules circulate in plasma as a complex, the vWF acting as a carrier for factor VIII; vWF was called "factor VIII-related antigen" until the 1980s. (The current terminology and definitions are presented in Table 7–1). Genetic information has fostered the development of a new classification of vWD,[3] which is not only important for understanding the structure-function relationships of the protein, but also helps in the selection of optimal therapy for patients.

HISTORICAL OVERVIEW

Erik von Willebrand described the first patient with vWD in 1926, when he cared for a young patient and her extended family who lived on the Åland Islands in the Gulf of Bothnia. The proband was severely affected and died at the age of 13 years when she had uncontrollable menstrual bleeding; 4 of her 11 siblings were also severely affected. After evaluating 66 other family members and identifying the disease in 24, von Willebrand recognized that the inheritance pattern of this disease was autosomal dominant, different from that seen in hemophilia A (which is sex-linked recessive), and he named the disorder "hereditary pseudohemophilia." He also recognized that the patients' platelet counts were normal and that this disease was different from the other inherited bleeding disorders known at that time.[4]

When the laboratory test for factor VIII was developed in the 1950s, it was demonstrated that patients with vWD had decreased levels of factor VIII[5] and that the bleeding could be corrected with transfusion of plasma or partially purified preparations of factor VIII.[6] There was considerable debate about the nature of the von Willebrand protein until factor VIII and vWF were cloned in the 1980s[7–10]; prior to this there was uncertainty about whether one bifunctional protein or two different proteins carried out the platelet-related functions (vWF) and factor VIII functions. We now know that these are two entirely different molecules encoded by different genes and that factor VIII is bound to vWF in the blood, forming a noncovalent complex in the circulation.[11,12]

PHYSIOLOGY AND STRUCTURE-FUNCTION RELATIONSHIPS

vWF has two primary functions (Table 7–2): it binds to both platelets and subendothelial structures, acting as a bridging molecule for initial reactions during primary hemostasis,[2] and it binds factor VIII, protecting factor VIII from proteolysis in the circulation.[13,14] vWF is an extremely large multimeric glycoprotein that is synthesized in endothelial cells and megakaryocytes.[15,16] The largest multimers are created by the polymerization of

Table 7–1 • NOMENCLATURE

Designation	Function	Assay
von Willebrand factor (vWF)	Multimeric glycoprotein that promotes platelet adhesion and aggregation and is a carrier for factor VIII in plasma	See below
von Willebrand factor (vWF) activity	1. Binding activity of vWF that causes binding of vWF to platelets in the presence of ristocetin with consequent agglutination 2. Ability of vWF to bind to collagen	1. Ristocetin cofactor activity: quantitate platelet agglutination after addition of ristocetin and vWF 2. Collagen binding activity: quantitate binding of vWF to collagen-coated plates
von Willebrand factor (vWF) antigen	vWF protein as measured by immunologic assays; does not imply functional ability	Immunologic assays such as ELISA, RIA, Laurell electroimmunoassay
von Willebrand factor (vWF) multimers	Size distribution of vWF multimers as assessed by agarose gel electrophoresis	vWF multimer assay: electrophoresis in low-concentration agarose gel and visualization by monospecific antibody to vWF
Ristocetin-induced platelet aggregation (RIPA)	Test that measures the ability of patient vWF to bind to platelets in the presence of various concentrations of ristocetin	RIPA: aggregation of patient PRP to various concentrations of ristocetin

ELISA, enzyme-linked immunoabsorbent assay; RIA, radioimmunoassay; PRP, platelet-rich plasma.
From UpToDate, Rose BD (ed), UpToDate, Wellesley, Mass, 2001. Copyright 2001. UpToDate, Inc.

subunits that all contain the same binding sites (Fig. 7–1), and the repeated binding sites make vWF particularly well suited to act as a bridge between cells and other structures of the vasculature. Synthesis of vWF include the initial formation of a dimer between the basic subunits and subsequent multimerization of the dimers to form multimers of a magnitude greater than 20 million daltons. The newly synthesized vWF is either secreted constitutively or is targeted to storage granules, the Weibel-Palade bodies in endothelial cells or α-granules in megakaryocytes.[17] These storage granules contain the larger, more hemostatic forms of vWF that are released upon stimulation with agonists such as thrombin, epinephrine, and fibrin.[18–20] The vWF within storage granules comprises even larger multimers than are usually found in the circulation. It is thought that limited proteolysis occurs in plasma, cleaving these very large multimers,[17] and a protease has been described that appears to be responsible for this cleavage.[21,22] More recent evidence indicates that another protein, thrombospondin-1, may also reduce the size of these unusually large multimers by acting as a protein disulfide reductase.[22a] Also contained within the storage granules and released upon stimulation is von Willebrand antigen II, a propolypeptide containing a large sequence of the originally synthesized vWF that is cleaved near the time that multimerization takes place (Fig. 7–1).[17]

The gene for vWF is located on chromosome 12, and a number of polymorphisms and mutations have been identified in the gene sequence, the latter mostly in patients with qualitative defects of vWF (type 2 vWD) (reviewed in detail by Nichols and Ginsburg[23]). Many of the mutations responsible for type 2 vWD are located in areas of the gene responsible for the structure of important binding sites or cleavage sites in vWF (Fig. 7–1). The genetic abnormality(ies) responsible for the most common type of vWD (approximately 70%, type 1) are largely unknown.[23] A website containing reported mutations is administered by David Ginsburg, M.D., and a consortium of investigators (http://mmg2.im.med.umich.edu/vWF).

Platelet-related Functions of vWF

vWF circulates in a tangled coil configuration,[24] enclosing some of the subunits and binding sites; the molecule likely assumes a more linear configuration upon binding to a surface or when flowing through high-shear vessels in the arterial circulation.[25] The linear form allows the binding sites on many more of the subunits to become accessible for binding to receptors such as platelet glycoprotein Ib, (GPIb),[26] and subendothelial collagen, one of the important subendothelial molecules that binds vWF.[27] The binding of vWF to these ligands results in the tethering (adhesion) of platelets to the subendothelium in damaged blood vessels and in platelet-platelet interaction (aggregation) in high-shear vessels via a vWF bridge. The binding of vWF to platelet GPIb does not require prior activation of platelets and, in fact, initiates intrinsic platelet activation.[28] VWF contains a second binding site for another platelet receptor, platelet glycoprotein IIb/IIIa (GPIIbIIIa), and this binding does require prior activation of platelets for exposure of the receptor. It is thought to be important in the later, irreversible binding of platelets to the subendo-

Table 7–2 • FUNCTIONS OF vWF

Platelet-Subendothelial Binding
vWF binds to platelet receptor GPIb and to subendothelial collagen and other matrix molecules, binding platelets to damaged vessel

Platelet-Platelet Binding
vWF binds to platelet receptor GPIb in areas with high shear (arterial circulation), causing platelet aggregation

Carrier for Factor VIII in Plasma
vWF binds to factor VIII by a site in the amino-terminus of vWF, protecting factor VIII from proteolysis and prolonging its half-life

A. vWF mRNA

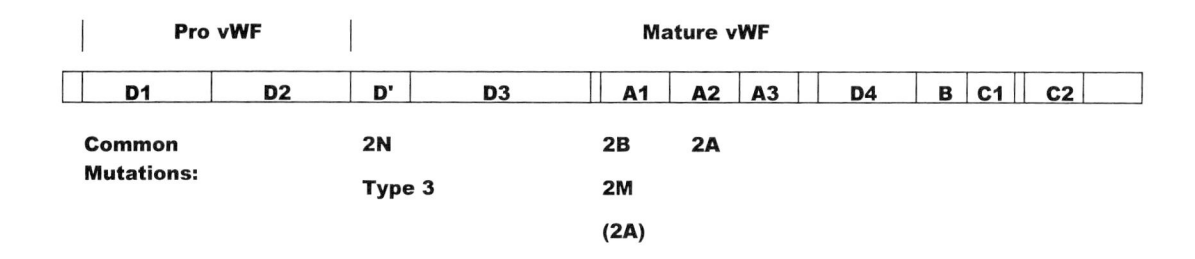

```
|   Pro vWF        |              Mature vWF
| D1 | D2 | D' | D3 | A1 | A2 | A3 | D4 | B | C1 | C2 |
```

Common Mutations:
- 2N (D')
- Type 3 (D')
- 2B (A1)
- 2M (A1)
- 2A (A2)
- (2A) (A1)

B. vWF Mature Subunit

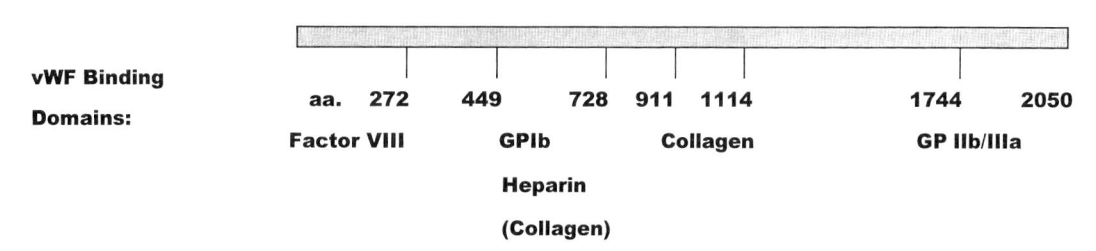

vWF Binding Domains:

aa. 272   449   728   911 1114   1744   2050
    Factor VIII GPIb   Collagen   GP IIb/IIIa
                 Heparin
                 (Collagen)

Figure 7–1 **A,** vWF mRNA is shown with the domain designations noted inside the figure. The different classification types of vWD are shown in the areas where the mutations that cause the particular type of vWD are most commonly found. **B,** The mature vWF subunit, aligned with the mRNA above, is depicted with amino acid numbering and binding sites shown below. (From UpToDate, Rose BD, (ed), UpToDate, Wellesley, Mass., 2001. Copyright 2001 UpToDate, Inc.)

thelium.[29] Other binding sites for heparin and sulfatides are also present in the vWF monomer.[30,31]

Factor VIII-Related Functions of vWF

vWF contains an important binding site for factor VIII that protects factor VIII from proteolysis in the circulation.[13] This noncovalent interaction of vWF with factor VIII prolongs the half-life of factor VIII in the circulation fivefold.[14] In addition to the platelet interactions described above, the binding and protection of factor VIII is the other important function of vWF. As one might anticipate, a defect in this part of the vWF molecule leads to a bleeding disorder in which there is a net decreased level of circulating factor VIII due to its brief, unprotected lifespan, but normal vWF-mediated platelet functions of vWD (see below, type 2 Normandy).

vWF Levels in Health and Disease

In addition to a broad normal range of vWF in plasma (50% to 200%), physiologic and pathologic conditions can alter the level of vWF in the circulation. Estrogen and thyroid hormone are important in regulating the synthesis of vWF,[32,33] and a low level of thyroid hormone can lead to clinically important decreases in levels of vWF.[34] Levels of vWF are at their baseline in women during the follicular phase of their menstrual cycle, and despite considerable day-to-day variation, they are generally higher during the late luteal phase.[35] During the second and third trimesters of pregnancy, vWF increases two- to threefold, often leading to "normal" levels of vWF in patients with mild vWD; the vWF levels fall within hours after delivery.[36] As an acute phase reactant, vWF (and factor VIII) levels are increased during physiologic changes that occur with inflammation.[37] There is also an important variation in the level of vWF in subjects with different blood groups: individuals with type O blood have circulating levels of vWF that are approximately 30% lower than those with type A, B, or AB.[38] The latter must be taken into account when trying to make a definitive diagnosis of vWD in a patient who presents with slightly low laboratory values for vWF.

The role of vWF in atherosclerosis and coronary artery syndromes is still being defined. Although markedly decreased levels of vWF play a protective role in preventing the development of coronary atherosclerosis in an animal model with type 3 vWD, there is not yet proof that extremely low vWF levels reduce atherosclerosis in humans.[39,40] However, studies that include more moderate (heterozygous) vWD animals and a few autopsy studes in humans with type 2 or type 3 vWD have shown that reduced vWF levels can prevent occlusive thrombi in atherosclerotic vessels.[41,42]

CLINICAL PRESENTATION

Patients with moderate and severe vWD present with bleeding symptoms in childhood or young adulthood; however, patients may present at any age because of the wide spectrum in the severity of bleeding symptoms.

Males and females are equally affected, and the majority of patients (type 1 and type 2) have mild or moderate disease. Since one of the primary functions of vWF is to support normal platelet function, the bleeding manifestations in patients with vWD are similar to those observed in platelet disorders: bruising and mucous membrane bleeding such as epistaxis, oral bleeding, menorrhagia, and gastrointestinal bleeding.[43] Patients may come to attention as a result of postsurgical bleeding (tooth extractions or tonsillectomy) or with the onset of menses. The most serious bleeding is generally gastrointestinal hemorrhage, and it can be life-threatening, particularly when it is associated with angiodysplasia.[44] The rare homozygous or doubly heterozygous (type 3) patients are severely affected and have low factor VIII levels (2% to 10%) associated with extremely low vWF levels; they have severe bleeding, which includes hemarthroses and soft tissue bleeding similar to the symptoms seen in hemophiliacs, in addition to the platelet-related symptoms. Homozygotes most likely represent the cases described by von Willebrand originally.

The severity of bleeding can vary modestly among affected family members and, to a much lesser degree, in an individual patient. There is also recent evidence that normal variation in the level of other unrelated platelet receptors, (e.g., collagen receptors) may affect the degree of bleeding in patients with mild vWD.[45] As mentioned above, levels of vWF (and hence bleeding) also vary with inflammatory processes, adrenergic stimulation, pregnancy, and during estrogen replacement therapy.

DIAGNOSIS

Laboratory Assays for vWF

Laboratory testing is essential for the diagnosis of vWD and includes (Table 7–3):

1. vWF antigen
2. vWF activity (usually measured as ristocetin cofactor activity)
3. Factor VIII activity (abnormal only in moderate or severe disease)
4. Bleeding time (prolonged only in moderate or severe disease).

Table 7–3 • ASSAYS FOR DIAGNOSIS OF vWD

Diagnostic Assays
vWF antigen
vWF activity (measured as ristocetin cofactor)
Factor VIII activity (abnormal only in moderate to severe vWD)
Bleeding time (prolonged only in moderate to severe vWD)
The aPTT is *not* recommended as a "rule-out" test as it is too insensitive and may be normal in vWD

Assays for Classification
RIPA (ristocetin-induced platelet aggregation)
vWF multimers

After the initial diagnosis of vWD, the following assays are used to classify the type of vWD:

1. Ristocetin-induced platelet aggregation (RIPA)
2. vWF multimer studies

The vWF antigen, activity, and multimer studies can also be performed on platelet vWF after it is isolated from platelets by separating platelets from plasma, washing, and lysing the platelets.[46] In rare cases of vWD, only the platelet vWF is decreased, while plasma levels are normal (designated "platelet-low" vWD).[47]

Currently the *vWF antigen* is generally assayed using an ELISA method, though electroimmunoassays and radioimmunoassays can be used.[48] An automated turbidometric test has also been introduced that uses latex particles coated with antibodies to vWF; addition of plasma dilutions containing vWF causes clumping of the particles, and the vWF can be thus quantified. False positives may be seen in patients with rheumatoid factors.[49]

The *vWF activity* can be measured in a number of different functional tests, including the *ristocetin cofactor* assay, which is the most commonly used assay and the "gold standard" despite the fact that it is difficult to standardize from laboratory to laboratory.[50] The test is performed by making dilutions of patient plasma (the source of vWF) and mixing the dilutions with normal platelets that have been washed to remove any adherent vWF; ristocetin, an antibiotic that binds to both vWF and platelets, is added at 1.0 to 1.2 mg/mL, and the time to platelet aggregation/agglutination is assessed either visually or in a platelet aggregometer. Lyophilized platelet membranes or platelets that have been fixed with formalin will also agglutinate and can be stored and used as convenient reagents rather than preparing fresh platelets for each test. A standard curve is established using dilutions of pooled normal plasma (PNP), and the patient results are compared with the standard curve from the PNP. The use of ristocetin for evaluation of vWF activity was first suggested by Howard and Firkin, who discovered that this antibiotic caused thrombocytopenia in individuals who had normal vWF.[51] Other functional tests, including *plasma vWF binding to collagen-coated plates*[52] and a more global assessment of platelet-vWF function measured in a *platelet function analyzer*[53,54] have also been introduced as newer and somewhat different functional assays for vWF.

Factor VIII activity is measured in a functional assay, usually using a modified activated partial thromboplastin time (aPTT) and clot end point. The aPTT itself is also used as a screening test, although it is less sensitive than the factor VIII assay. Both of these tests will be abnormal only when the patient has a sufficiently low level of vWF to cause a low factor VIII, or when the vWF has defective binding for factor VIII. Normal values for these tests cannot be used as exclusionary criteria for vWD.

The **bleeding time** is a global assessment for vascular integrity, platelet function, and plasma factors including vWF. It is helpful in the diagnosis of vWD if it is prolonged, but a normal bleeding time may be found in mild and even moderate vWD.[55,56] Quick reported a more marked prolongation of the bleeding time within 2 hours after aspirin ingestion in patients with mild type 1 vWD as compared to normal subjects.[57] Although the bleeding time often is prolonged more after aspirin ingestion in patients with vWD than in normals (and emphasizes to patients to avoid aspirin), many patients do not want to undergo multiple bleeding times, and this test is not widely used at present.

Ristocetin-induced platelet aggregation (RIPA) is different from the ristocetin cofactor test and is used to aid in classifying the type of vWD that the patient has. In the RIPA, the patient provides both the platelets and the vWF as platelet-rich plasma (PRP). PRP is prepared by low-speed centrifugation of citrated blood and several aliquots are placed in different cuvettes. Different concentrations of ristocetin are added to each (usually varying progressively from 0.4 to 1.2 mg/mL final concentration) and the presence or absence of platelet aggregation is assessed on the aggregometer. If the platelets aggregate with low concentrations of ristocetin (less than 0.8 mg/mL), the vWF may have a "gain-of-function" abnormality (see below).

vWF multimers are evaluated using electrophoresis of plasma in low-concentration agarose gels followed by detection with a specific antibody to vWF for visualization of the multimers.[58] These gels are utilized to detect the decrease or absence of high-molecular-weight multimers of vWF, which occurs in the more common subtypes within the type 2 vWD patients (type 2A and type 2B) (Fig. 7–2). The gels can also detect the unusually high-molecular-weight multimers of vWF that can be present in patients with thrombotic thrombocytopenic purpura and in the rare cases of an inherited defect where larger than normal multimers are present in the circulation (see type 2M, below).

The bleeding time, factor VIII, and aPTT are often normal in mild vWD, and the level of vWF varies in patients with vWD as well as normal subjects. The tests for vWF may be within the normal range at some timepoints in patients with mild vWD.[56] For this reason and also because there is an overlap of the normal and abnormal ranges, patients with borderline values should be tested on two or three occasions at 4 to 6-week intervals; it can also be very helpful to test family members and to evaluate the blood type of the persons undergoing evaluation, since people with type O blood have concentrations of vWF that are 25% to 30% lower than individuals with other blood types. Because vWF levels are at their baseline during the follicular phase in menstruating women, it is suggested that testing for vWD is best carried out during this time. It is reasonable to withhold a diagnosis in a patient with slightly low vWF levels if there is no personal or family bleeding history and family studies are negative. Conversely, a personal and family history consistent with vWD helps the clinician with interpretation of laboratory data. Additionally, it may not be possible to establish the diagnosis of vWD in women during the second or third trimester of pregnancy because of the physiologic increase in vWF and factor VIII levels; if test results are within the normal range, repeat testing may need to be delayed until several weeks after delivery.

CLASSIFICATION

vWD is classified into three types according to the results of laboratory testing and knowledge of mutations that cause some of the defects[3] (Table 7–4): *type 1*, a quantitative decrease in circulating vWF, comprising approximately 70% to 75% of vWD patients; *type 2*, a

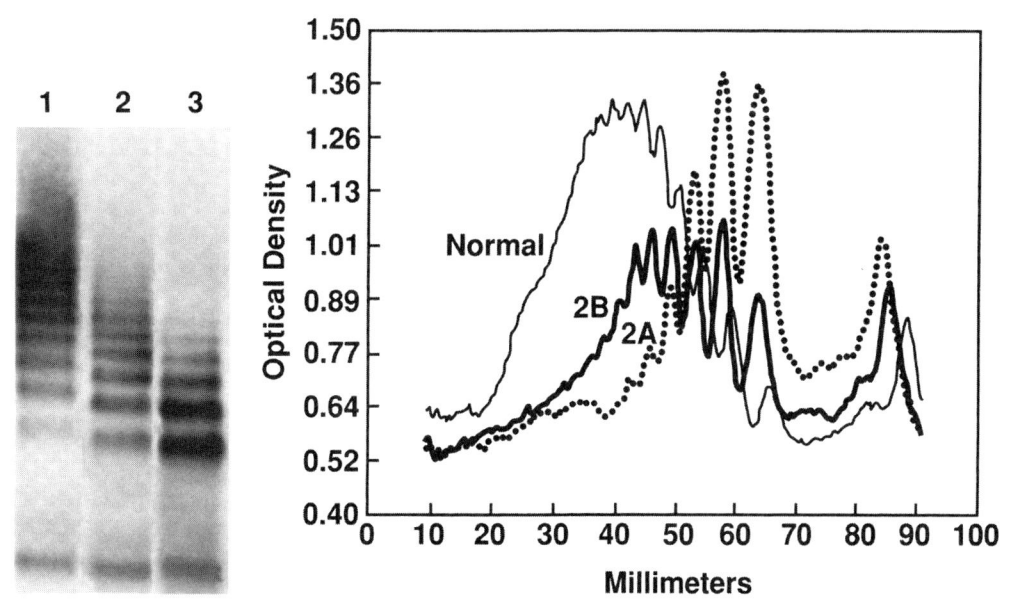

Figure 7–2 Left: Normal and variant vWF multimeric patterns. Lane 1: Normal vWF; Lane 2: Type 2B vWD showing decreased high-molecular-weight multimers; Lane 3: Type 2A vWD showing a decrease in both the high- and intermediate-molecular-weight multimers. **Right:** Densitometric tracing of lanes 1 to 3. (From Krizek DM, Rick ME. A rapid method to visualize von Willebrand factor multimers using agarose gel electrophoresis, immunolocalization and luminographic detection. Thromb Res 2000; 97:457–462, with permission from Elsevier Science.)

Table 7-4 • CLASSIFICATION OF vWD

Type	Inheritance	Frequency of VWD Type	vWF Activity	RIPA*	Multimer Pattern
Type 1 (Classic)	Autosomal dominant	70% to 75%	↓	↓	Uniform ↓ All multimers present
Type 2 (Variant)					
2A	Autosomal dominant (and recessive)	10% to 15%	↓	↓	↓ Large and intermediate multimers
2B	Autosomal dominant	5%	↓	↑	↓ Large multimers
2M	Autosomal dominant (and recessive)	Infrequent	↓	↓	Normal multimers
2N	Autosomal recessive	Infrequent	Normal	Normal	Normal multimers
Type 3 (Severe)	Autosomal recessive	Rare	↓↓	↓↓	Undetectable (usually cannot visualize)

* RIPA, ristocetin-induced platelet aggregation.
From UpToDate, Rose BD (Ed), UpToDate, Wellesley, Mass, 2001. Copyright 2001. UpToDate, Inc.

group of qualitative variants comprising approximately 20% to 25% of vWD patients; and *type 3*, a rare homozygous or doubly heterozygous group of patients, occurring in fewer than 1 in every 10^6 patients.

Type 1

This dominantly inherited common type of vWD is usually associated with mild or moderate bleeding symptoms, though occasionally bleeding can be quite severe, especially following aspirin administration. Childhood epistaxis is characteristic and may be "outgrown" following puberty. Its cause is unknown, with the exception of an uncommon mutation that may cause inhibition of multimer assembly and retention of monomers within the cell.[59] It is possible that the deficiency is due in some or many instances to increased clearance of vWF secondary to abnormal glycosylation, as was recently described in a mouse model of vWD.[60]

vWF antigen and activity (ristocetin cofactor) are usually decreased concomitantly, and factor VIII activity is decreased if the deficiency is sufficiently severe (Table 7-4). RIPA is decreased, and all vWF multimers are present ("normal distribution"). The bleeding time will be prolonged if the deficiency is severe enough.

Type 2

Type 2 vWD is divided into four subtypes:

Type 2A. This subtype is usually inherited as an autosomal dominant trait and accounts for 10% to 15% of vWD cases. It usually is associated with moderate to severe bleeding symptoms. A number of mutations have been identified in the region encoding the A2 domain of the vWF monomer where a normal cleavage site is situated (Fig. 7-1; see also internet vWF database). These mutations cause either a defect in the intracellular assembly and transport of vWF monomers (2A, type 1) or an increased suseptibility to proteolysis by the normal vWF-cleaving protease (2A, type 2).[61,62]

The vWF antigen is normal or decreased, the ristocetin cofactor activity is usually decreased out of proportion to the antigen, and the factor VIII activity may be normal or decreased (Table 7-4). The RIPA is decreased, and the *vWF multimers show an abnormal distribution with an absence of high- and intermediate-molecular-weight multimers* (*Fig. 7-2*). The bleeding time is usually prolonged.

Type 2B. This subtype is transmitted as an autosomal dominant trait and usually presents as moderate to severe disease; it accounts for approximately 5% of vWD cases. Mutations have been identified in an area of the gene that encodes the binding region for GPIb (Fig. 7-1), and they give rise to a vWF with a "gain-of-function" defect. These mutations cause the vWF to bind "spontaneously" to platelets in the circulation, which results in the removal of the largest multimers and thrombocytopenia in some instances[63,64]; the latter is likely due to the formation of small platelet aggregates and subsequent clearance. The vWF antigen is normal or decreased, and the ristocetin cofactor shows a more marked decrease, due to the absence of the more functional higher-molecular-weight multimers. On the other hand, the *RIPA is "increased"*; that is, there is aggregation of the patient's PRP with concentrations of ristocetin less than 0.6 to 0.8 mg/mL.[65] The factor VIII activity is normal or decreased, and the *vWF multimers show a decrease or absence of the high-molecular-weight forms,* usually less severe than seen in type 2A.

A platelet defect that causes the same phenotype (decreased high-molecular-weight multimers of vWF and decreased ristocetin cofactor) is called *"platelet-type"* or *"pseudo-von Willebrand disease."*[66,67] It is caused by an abnormal platelet GPIb receptor that binds normal vWF more readily than normal, removing the high-molecular-weight multimers of vWF from the circulation and often resulting in thrombocytopenia. Type 2B vWD and pseudo-vWD can be distinguished by a modification of the RIPA, using patient platelets mixed with normal plasma and separately, patient plasma mixed with normal platelets. In a research setting, type 2B vWD can be distinguished from pseudo-vWD by genetic studies.

Type 2M. This subtype of vWD is an uncommon disorder that is usually inherited in an autosomal dominant manner. It presents as moderate or moderately severe disease and is characterized by decreased binding of the abnormal vWF to GPIb; however, all multimers are present, thus differentiating it from type 2A vWD.[3] On gel electrophoresis the individual multimer bands may show abnormal patterns (formerly called types 1C and 1D)[68,69]; in other instances, larger than normal multimers are present in plasma ("Vicenza" variant),[70,71] or the variant vWF contains the propeptide in the multimers.[72] vWF antigen is variably decreased and ristocetin cofactor is decreased; factor VIII activity is reduced if the vWF is sufficiently low.

Type 2N. One of the first two patients with type 2N vWD was described in France (in Normandy) and presented with a low factor VIII level inherited in an autosomal pattern.[73,74] Patients with this subtype usually present with the constellation of autosomal inheritance and low factor VIII levels. The bleeding symptoms are moderate to moderately severe and include episodes of soft tissue bleeding and bleeding with invasive procedures that are more characteristic of factor VIII deficiency than the mucosal bleeding usually seen in vWD. This variant is characterized by mutations in the aminoterminus of the vWF monomer within the binding site for factor VIII, which leads to decreased binding and diminished protection of factor VIII in the circulation.[75–78] The half-life of the factor VIII is decreased from 8 to 12 hours to approximately 2 hours because of the lack of protection by vWF.[14] The platelet-related functions of vWF are usually intact unless (uncommonly) a second mutation has been inherited that causes another vWF defect such as those present in type 1 or other type 2 vWD. Because the concentration of vWF in plasma is so much higher that the concentration of factor VIII, the binding defect must be inherited in a homozygous fashion, or a second defect must be present that limits synthesis of vWF by the other allele. The factor VIII levels are low (usually 5% to 15%) and the vWF antigen, ristocetin cofactor, RIPA, and vWF multimers are normal.

Since the patients with type 2N vWD present with factor VIII deficiency, there is the potential that they will be misdiagnosed as having hemophilia A. The presence of an autosomal inheritance pattern and the presence or history of bleeding in females suggests that the patient should be tested for type 2N vWD. This is accomplished by testing the ability of the patient's vWF to bind factor VIII[73,74]; genetic studies are another way to establish this diagnosis.[75–78]

Type 3

Type 3 vWD is characterized by a severe deficiency of vWF and by a moderately severe deficiency of factor VIII. It is rare and is inherited in a homozygous or doubly heterozygous manner.[40] Patients present with both skin and mucous membrane bleeding (from decreased vWF) and with soft tissue and joint bleeding (from decreased factor VIII). Deletions, compound heterozygous mutations, and nondeletion defects leading to decreased mRNA expression have been identified in these patients.[3] Laboratory testing shows that vWF antigen is extremely low or unmeasurable, ristocetin cofactor is below the limits of detection, RIPA is absent, and vWF multimers usually cannot be visualized. Factor VIII is in the range of 2% to 10%.

ACQUIRED VON WILLEBRAND DISEASE

Acquired vWD may appear spontaneously or may be associated with diseases that lead to decreased levels of vWF by one of several mechanisms: antibodies to vWF, increased proteolysis of vWF, abnormal binding to cells (usually tumor cells), or decreased synthesis. Antibodies to vWF most often occur in autoimmune or lymphoproliferative diseases[79–81]; increased proteolysis occurs in patients with accelerated fibrinolysis and possibly myeloproliferative diseases[82,83]; binding and removal of vWF may occur in patients with noncyanotic congenital heart disease or high-grade aortic stenosis[84]; tumor adsorption has been described in Wilms' tumor[85]; and decreased synthesis has been described in hypothyroidism.[34,86] Some medications, such as valproic acid, dextrans, and hydroxyethyl starch, have also been associated with acquired vWD.[87–89]

TREATMENT

Inherited vWD

Selection of proper treatment for the patient depends on the type of vWD that the patient has, so a thorough laboratory evaluation should be completed before therapy if time permts. In addition, the patient's general medical condition, associated illnesses, and medications (particularly aspirin-containing medications, nonsteroidal anti-inflammatory agents, or other antiplatelet agents) should be taken into account. These factors may influence decisions about the duration of treatment and whether to give additional medication or replacement therapy such as platelet concentrates in cases of serious bleeding. The need for treatment in women with mild vWD may be minimized by scheduling elective minor surgical procedures during the latter half of their menstrual cycle, when slightly higher levels of vWF can be anticipated. In type 1 vWD patients with atherosclerotic heart disease who need heart catheterization for evaluation or treatment, the choice of a short-acting nonsteroidal anti-inflammatory agent over aspirin is prudent.

Since no laboratory tests predict or correlate well with the severity of bleeding in the patient, it is necessary to moniter the patient clinically.[90] However, as a general and empirical goal, therapy is usually given in the amount predicted to increase the level of vWF activity and factor VIII to 50% to 100% (Table 7–5).[91] In practice, it is often only the factor VIII level that may be available in a timely fashion for decision-making, and it can be followed safely in many patients to evaluate

Table 7–5 • TREATMENT OF vWD

Medication	Dose	Comments
DDAVP (desmopressin)	IV: 0.3 μg/kg in 50 mL saline over 20 min (maximum 20 μg) Nasal Spray: Weight >50 kg: 300 μg (1 spray in each nostril) <50 kg: 150 μg (1 spray in only one nostril)	Useful in most patients with type 1; variable in type 2*; not useful in type 3. Patient should have therapeutic trial before invasive procedure. May repeat dose after 12 h and q24 h. Tachyphylaxis and hyponatremia may occur; need to monitor patient.
vWF concentrates containing all vWF multimers	20–30 IU/kg q 12 h to keep vWF levels 50%–100% or to control clinical bleeding. Levels should be maintained 3–10 days for major surgery.	Dose and duration based on clinical experience.
Antifibrinolytic agents ε-aminocaproic acid Tranexamic acid	50 mg/kg (maximum 5 g/dose) qid 25 mg/kg tid	Use alone or in conjunction with other therapy. Especially useful for mucosal bleeding (often for dental procedures).
IVIg (for use in immune acquired inhibitors of vWF)	1 g/kg daily for 2 days—infusion over 8–12 h	Use after trial of DDAVP or other measures in patients with acquired vWD, particularly when associated with autoimmune diseases.

* Thrombocytopenia may worsen in some type 2B patients.
(Modified from Rick ME. Diagnosis and management of von Willebrand's syndrome. Med Clin North Am 1994; 78:609.)

therapy for adequate hemostasis as indicated by the clinical experience of experts who treat vWD.[92]

Treatment modalities include DDAVP (desmopressin), replacement therapy with vWF-containing plasma products, the use of antifibrinolytic and topical therapies, and estrogen (in women) (see Table 7–5).

DDAVP

DDAVP (desmopressin) is a synthetic analogue of antidiuretic hormone that causes release of vWF and factor VIII from the body stores by an indirect mechanism not yet understood.[93] DDAVP is the treatment of choice in the majority of patients with type 1 and in many with type 2 vWD.[94] It is administered in a much larger dose than the dose for antidiuretic hormone replacement therapy.

Although most patients with type 1 vWD respond to DDAVP, it is recommended that patients who will receive DDAVP for therapy undergo a trial prior to the first therapeutic use of the agent. DDAVP is given either as an intravenous infusion at a dose of 0.3 μg/kg (not to exceed 20 μg) or as an intranasal spray at a dose of 300 μg for patients over 50 kg or 150 μg for patients less than 50 kg. For intravenous infusion, it is diluted in 50 mL saline and administered over at least 20 minutes. The levels of ristocetin cofactor, vWF antigen, and factor VIII may be followed before infusion and at 2 to 4 hours, and some advocate measurement of bleeding times to assess whether prolonged values normalize or decrease significantly 2 or 4 hours after infusion. An increase in vWF and factor VIII levels of two- to fivefold is expected 30 to 60 minutes after infusion, and the values return to baseline in approximately 4 to 6 hours.[95] Side effects include flushing, hyper- or hypotension, headache, and rarely, tingling; these can usually be controlled by slowing the infusion of DDAVP. Although thrombosis has occurred following administration of DDAVP, it is uncertain whether it is causal.[96] Tachyphylaxis occurs after repeated administration and serious hyponatremia has also been observed, especially with concomitant intake of free water.[97] For these reasons, DDAVP is usually given 1 to 2 hours before a procedure and may be repeated 8 to 12 hours later and daily on the following 2 to 3 days if necessary.

DDAVP is useful in most patients with mild and moderate type 1 vWD, except those rare patients with type 1 who do not have normal levels of platelet vWF ("platelet-low" patients).[98] Patients with type 2A vWD respond variably to DDAVP,[99] and the patients with type 2B are problematic because thrombocytopenia may follow the increase in plasma levels of the abnormal 2B vWF.[100] Despite this possible drawback, a number of patients with type 2B vWD have undergone procedures after the administration of DDAVP, and any reduction in platelet count has usually normalized after 2 hours.[101] It is especially important to evaluate the effects of DDAVP in type 2B patients prior to surgery with a trial infusion. DDAVP is not helpful in patients with type 3 vWD, who rarely have sufficient stores of vWF.

Intranasal DDAVP has proven extremely useful and convenient for patients since they are able to administer the medication "on the spot" when bleeding occurs and not delay treatment. A good example is its use to control menstrual bleeding in women with vWD.[102] Oral bleeding and epistaxis have also been controlled by this method.

Replacement Therapy with vWF

Several preparations that contain vWF are available for use in patients with vWD. These include "intermediate-purity" factor VIII concentrates that contain vWF (*not* monoclonally purified or recombinant factor VIII concentrates, which lack vWF), more highly purified vWF concentrates, and cryoprecipitate. Most experts do not recommend cryoprecipitate unless no other vWF concentrate is available because of the possible transmission of viruses.[103] The other concentrates mentioned above undergo a step such as pasteurization to decrease the risk of viral transmission.

The vWF concentrate available in the United States that is labeled with the concentration of ristocetin cofactor units per vial is Humate P. Others are available in Europe.[104,105] The concentrates are usually administered as a short (approximately 15 minute) intravenous infusion, although studies have shown that when therapy is needed for several days, the total dose utilized is reduced by 20% to 50% when the concentrate is given by constant infusion.[106,107] The dose is estimated as the amount that will raise the ristocetin cofactor to 50% to 100% (20 to 30 units/kg) (Table 7-5). Repeat infusions may be necessary at 12-hour intervals for 3 to 10 days for major surgery or serious bleeding. If bleeding is not controlled by replacement therapy, patients may benefit from platelet transfusions in addition to the vWF.[108]

Replacement therapy as used to treat hemophilia is used for type 3 vWD patients, for type 2 patients who do not respond to DDAVP, and for the more severe type 1 patients who have either not responded to DDAVP or responded but need further long-range hemostatic support that cannot be accomplished with DDAVP.

Antifibrinolytic Therapy

Both ε-aminocaproic acid (EACA) and tranexamic acid have been used alone or as adjuncts to other therapy for patients with vWD, particularly for oral and other moderate mucous membrane bleeding. When given orally for this use, they are administered 3 or 4 times daily (Table 7-5) for 3 to 7 days.[91] Doses must be adjusted in patients with renal failure. These medications may also be given by the intravenous route. Prolonged use of either medication may lead to thrombosis in suseptible patients.

Topical Agents

These agents are usually used for oral or nasal bleeding and provide local therapy to the bleeding surface. Gelfoam or Surgicel may be soaked in topical thrombin before its application to the site. A micronized collagen (Avitene) and fibrin sealant have also been used topically[109] (see Chapter 26).

Estrogen

Estrogen can increase the synthesis of vWF, and women with mild to moderate vWD may benefit from therapy with estrogen. It is usually administered in doses equivalent to those used for hormone replacement therapy.[110]

Acquired vWD

There are different mechanisms leading to acquired vWD, and treatment may vary with the underlying pathophysiology. Treatment of an associated primary disease is usually undertaken in those cases where it can be identified; this is particularly important in the unusual cases where hypothyroidism is the underlying cause, since treatment with thyroid hormone will normalize vWF levels.[34,86] Many times selection of a treatment regimen is a process of empirical trials to find the treatment that is most useful: often a trial of DDAVP is given initially, followed by replacement therapy (if the DDAVP is unsuccessful in stopping the bleeding). If neither is successful, a trial of high-dose intravenous immune globulin (IVIg) is recommended (1 g/kg daily for 2 days), particularly if the cause is thought to be an acquired inhibitor associated with autoimmune disease or a monoclonal gammopathy.[111] In all situations, the response should be monitered by measuring vWF and factor VIII levels over the next hours after treatment as well as following any clinical response. Less commonly, plasmapheresis or extracorporeal immunoadsorption may be employed to remove an antibody, at least for a temporary period, if there is clinical bleeding.[112] Immunosuppressive medications used for the treatment of underlying disease may also decrease the antibody in some patients.[112]

vWD During Pregnancy

Since levels of vWF increase two- to three-fold over baseline during the second and third trimesters of pregnancy, treatment typically is not needed in many type 1 patients with vWD during delivery. Qualitative defects present in type 2 vWD do not correct, however, and increases in vWD levels can be variable in these patients.[113] Additionally, vWF levels fall rapidly after delivery, and excessive bleeding can occur in the weeks following delivery. DDAVP therapy is used after the initiation of labor in those patients who are responsive and have moderately severe disease with persisting lower levels of vWF in the third trimester; vWF replacement therapy is usually not required, but should be used in instances where patients are not responsive to DDAVP and bleeding occurs.[36,114]

Practical Considerations for Therapy

Because of an increased awareness and diagnosis of vWD, a number of patients present to emergency rooms with bleeding that requires urgent treatment who have an undocumented diagnosis of vWD. A careful past bleeding history and family history can be particularly helpful in deciding whether the patient should receive treatment for vWD. If the patient does require treatment, it is likely that DDAVP can be used successfully and the patient can be spared exposure to blood products. For serious bleeding (brisk gastrointestinal or central nervous system bleeding), replacement therapy should be given to keep the vWF between 50% and 100%, along with other therapy as indicated, until a more definitive diagnosis can be established. After the bleeding is controlled and the baseline health returns for 3 to 4 weeks, the patient should be asked to return for full evaluation and given a letter to carry with test results and recommendations for treatment in an emergency situation.

■ REFERENCES

Chapter 7 References

1. Rodeghiero F, Castaman G, Dini E. Epidemiological investigation of the prevalence of von Willebrand's disease. Blood 1987;69:454–459.
2. Ruggeri ZM, Ware J. von Willebrand factor. FASEB J 1993; 7:308–316.
3. Sadler JE. A revised classification of von Willebrand disease. For the Subcommittee on von Willebrand Factor of the Scientific and Standardization Committee of the International Society on Thrombosis and Haemostasis. Thromb Haemost 1994;71: 520–525.
4. Nilsson IM. Von Willebrand's disease—fifty years old. Acta Med Scand 1977;201:497–508.
5. Alexander B, Goldstein R. Dual hemostatic defect in pseudohemophilia. J Clin Invest 1953;32:551.
6. Nilsson IM, Blombäck M, Jorpes E, et al. V Willebrand's disease and its correction with human plasma fraction 1-0. Acta Med Scand 1957;159:179–188.
7. Ginsburg D, Handin RI, Bonthron DT, et al. Human von Willebrand factor (vWF): Isolation of complementary DNA (cDNA) clones and chromosomal localization. Science 1985;228:1401–1406.
8. Lynch DC, Zimmerman TS, Collins CJ, et al. Molecular cloning of cDNA for human von Willebrand factor: Authentication by a new method. Cell 1985;41:49–56.
9. Sadler JE, Shelton-Inloes BB, Sorace JM, et al. Cloning and characterization of two cDNAs coding for human von Willebrand factor. Proc Natl Acad Sci USA 1985;82:6394–6398.
10. Verweij CL, de Vries CJ, Distel B, et al. Construction of cDNA coding for human von Willebrand factor using antibody probes for colony-screening and mapping of the chromosomal gene. Nucleic Acids Res 1985;13:4699–4717.
11. Weiss HJ, Phillips LL, Rosner W. Separation of sub-units of antihemophilic factor (AHF) by agarose gel chromatography. Thromb Diath Haemorrh 1972;27:212–219.
12. Rick ME, Hoyer LW. Immunologic studies of antihemophilic factor (AHF, Factor VIII). V. Immunologic properties of AHF subunits produced by salt dissociation. Blood 1973;42:737–747.
13. Koedam JA, Meijers JC, Sixma JJ, Bouma BN. Inactivation of human factor VIII by activated protein C. Cofactor activity of protein S and protective effect of von Willebrand factor. J Clin Invest 1988;82:1236–1243.
14. Brinkhous KM, Sandberg H, Garris JB, et al. Purified human factor VIII procoagulant protein: Comparative hemostatic response after infusion into hemophilic and von Willebrand disease dogs. Proc Natl Acad Sci USA 1985;82:8752–8756.
15. Jaffe E, Hoyer L, Nachman R. Synthesis of antihemophilic factor antigen by cultured endothelial cells. J Clin Invest 1975;52:2757–2764.
16. Sporn L, Chavin S, Marder V. Biosynthesis of von Willebrand protein by human megakaryocytes. J Clin Invest 1985;76:1102–1106.
17. Wagner DD. Cell biology of von Willebrand factor. Annu Rev Cell Biol 1990;6:217–246.
18. Levine JD, Harlan JM, Harker LA, et al. Thrombin-mediated release of factor VIII-related antigen from human umbilical vein endothelial cells in culture. Blood 1982;60:531–534.
19. Rickles FR, Hoyer LW, Rick ME, Ahr DJ. The effects of epinephrine infusion in patients with von Willebrand's disease. J Clin Invest 1976;57:1618–1625.
20. Ribes JA, Francis CW, Wagner DD. Fibrin induces release of von Willebrand factor from endothelial cells. J Clin Invest 1987;79:117–123.
21. Tsai HM. Physiologic cleavage of von Willebrand factor by a plasma protease is dependent on its conformation and requires calcium ion. Blood 1996;87:4235–4244.
22. Furlan M, Robles R, Lamie B. Partial purification and characterization of a protease from human plasma cleaving von Willebrand factor to fragments produced by in vivo proteolysis. Blood 1996;87:4223–4234.
22a. Xie L, Chesterman CN, Hogg PJ. Control of von Willebrand factor multimer size by thrombospondin-1. J Exp Med 2001; 193:1341–1350.
23. Nichols WC, Ginsburg D. Reviews in Molecular Medicine: Von Willebrand disease. Medicine 1997;76:1–20.
24. Fowler WE, Fretto LJ, Hamilton KK, et al. Substructure of human von Willebrand factor. J Clin Invest 1985;76:1491–1500.
25. Siedlecki CA, Lestini BJ, Kottke-Marchant KK, et al. Shear-dependent changes in the three-dimensional structure of human von Willebrand factor. Blood 1996;88:2939–2950.
26. Mohri H, Fujimura Y, Shima M, et al. Structure of the von Willebrand factor domain interacting with glycoprotein Ib. J Biol Chem 1988;263:17901–17904.
27. Santoro SA. Adsorption of von Willebrand factor/factor VIII by the genetically distinct interstitial collagens. Thromb Res 1981;21:689–691.
28. De Marco L, Girolami A, Zimmerman TS, Ruggeri ZM. Interaction of purified type IIB von Willebrand factor with the platelet membrane glycoprotein Ib induces fibrinogen binding to the glycoprotein IIb/IIIa complex and initiates aggregation. Proc Natl Acad Sci USA 1985;82:7424–7428.
29. Savage B, Shattil SJ, Ruggeri ZM. Modulation of platelet function through adhesion receptors: A dual role for glycoprotein IIb-IIIa (integrin alpha IIb beta 3) mediated by fibrinogen and glycoprotein Ib-von Willebrand factor. J Biol Chem 1992; 267:11300–11306.
30. Mohri H, Yoshioka A, Zimmerman TS, Ruggeri ZM. Isolation of the von Willebrand factor domain interacting with platelet glycoprotein Ib, heparin, and collagen, and characterization of its three distinct functional sites. J Biol Chem 1989;264:17361–17367.
31. Roberts DD, Williams SB, Gralnick HR, Ginsburg V. von Willebrand factor binds specifically to sulfated glycolipids. J Biol Chem. 1986;26:3306–3309.
32. Harrison RL, McKee PA. Estrogen stimulates von Willebrand factor production by cultured endothelial cells. Blood 1984; 63:657–664.
33. Baumgartner-Parzer SM, Wagner L, Reining G, et al. Increase by tri-iodothyronine of endothelin-1, fibronectin and von Willebrand factor in cultured endothelial cells. J Endocrinol 1997; 154:231–239.
34. Dalton RG, Savidge GF, Matthews KB, et al. Hypothyroidism as a cause of acquired von Willebrand's disease. Lancet 1987; 1:1007–1009.
35. Kadir RA, Economides DL, Sabin CA, et al. Variations in coagulation factors in women: effects of age, ethnicity, menstrual cycle, and combined oral contraceptive. Thromb Haemost 1999; 82:1456–1461.
36. Ito M, Yoshimura K, Toyoda N, Wada H. Pregnancy and delivery in patients with von Willebrand's disease. J Obstet Gynaecol Res 1997;23:37–43.
37. Bennett B, Ratnoff OD. Changes in antihemophilic factor (AHF, factor 8) procoagulant activity and AHF-like antigen in normal pregnancy, and following exercise and pneumoencephalography. J Lab Clin Med 1972;80:256–263.

38. Gill JC, Endres-Brooks J, Bauer PJ, et al. The effect of ABO blood group on the diagnosis of von Willebrand disease. Blood 1987;69:1691–1695.
39. Fuster V, Bowie EJW, Lewis JC, et al. Resistance to arteriosclerosis in pigs with von Willebrand's disease: spontaneous and high cholesterol diet-induced arteriosclerosis. J Clin Invest 1978; 61:722–730.
40. Mannucci PM, Bloom AL, Larrieu MJ, et al. Atherosclerosis and von Willebrand factor. I. Prevalence of severe von Willebrand's disease in western Europe and Israel. Br J Haematol 1984; 57:163–169.
41. Nichols TC, Bellinger DA, Tate DA, et al. von Willebrand factor and occlusive arterial thrombosis. A study in normal and von Willebrand's disease pigs with diet-induced hypercholesterolemia and atherosclerosis. Arteriosclerosis 1990;10:449–461.
42. Federici AB, Mannucci PM, Fogato E, et al. Autopsy findings in three patients with von Willebrand disease type IIB and type III: presence of atherosclerotic lesions without occlusive arterial thrombi. Thromb Haemost 1993;70:758–761.
43. Miller CH, Graham JB, Goldin LR, Elston RC. Genetics of classic von Willebrand's disease. I. Phenotypic variation within families. Blood. 1979;54:117–136.
44. Ahr DJ, Rickles FR, Hoyer LW, et al. von Willebrand's disease and hemorrhagic telangiectasia: association of two complex disorders of hemostasis resulting in life-threatening hemorrhage. Am J Med 1977;62:452–458.
45. Di Paola J, Federici AB, Mannucci PM, et al. Low platelet alpha2beta1 levels in type I von Willebrand disease correlate with impaired platelet function in a high shear stress system. Blood. 1999;93:3578–3582.
46. Gralnick HR, Williams SB, McKeown LP, et al. Platelet von Willebrand factor: comparison with plasma von Willebrand factor. Thromb Res 1985;38:623–633.
47. Weiss HJ, Pietu G, Rabinowitz R, et al. Heterogeneous abnormalities in the multimeric structure, antigenic properties, and plasma-platelet content of factor VIII/von Willebrand factor in subtypes of classic (type I) and variant (type IIA) von Willebrand's disease. J Lab Clin Med 1983;101:411–425.
48. Ingerslev J. A sensitive ELISA for von Willebrand factor (vWf:Ag). Scand J Clin Lab Invest 1987;47:143–149.
49. Veyradier A, Fressinaud E, Sigaud M, et al. A new automated method for von Willebrand factor antigen measurement using latex particles [letter]. Thromb Haemost 1999;81:320–321.
50. Favaloro EJ, Smith J, Petinos P, et al. Laboratory testing for von Willebrand's disease: an assessment of current diagnostic practice and efficacy by means of a multi-laboratory survey. RCPA Quality Assurance Program (QAP) in Haematology Haemostasis Scientific Advisory Panel. Thromb Haemost 1999; 82:1276–1282.
51. Howard MA, Firkin BG. Ristocetin—a new tool in the investigation of platelet aggregation. Thromb Diath Haemorrh 1971; 26:362–369.
52. Favaloro EJ, Grispo L, Exner T, Koutts J. Development of a simple collagen based ELISA assay aids in the diagnosis of, and permits sensitive discrimination between type I and type II, von Willebrand's disease. Blood Coagul Fibrinolysis 1991;2:285–291.
53. Mammen EF, Comp PC, Gosselin R, et al. PFA-100 system: a new method for assessment of platelet dysfunction. Semin Thromb Hemost 1998;24:195–202.
54. Fressinaud E, Veyradier A, Truchaud F, et al. Screening for von Willebrand disease with a new analyzer using high shear stress: A study of 60 cases. Blood 1998;91:1325–1331.
55. Ratnoff OD, Bennett B. Clues to the pathogenesis of bleeding in von Willebrand's disease. N Engl J Med 1973;289:1182–1183.
56. Abildgaard CF. Diagnosis of von Willebrand disease. Prog Clin Biol Res 1990;324:263–268.
57. Quick AJ. Salicylates and bleeding: the aspirin tolerance test. Am J Med Sci 1966;252:265–269.
58. Krizek DM, Rick ME. A rapid method to visualize von Willebrand factor multimers using agarose gel electrophoresis, immunolocalization and luminographic detection. Thrombosis Res 2000;97:457–462.
59. Eikenboom JC, Matsushita T, Reitsma PH, et al. Dominant type 1 von Willebrand disease caused by mutated cysteine residues in the D3 domain of von Willebrand factor. Blood 1996;88:2433–2441.
60. Mohlke KL, Purkayastha AA, Westrick RJ, et al. MvWF, a dominant modifier of murine von Willebrand factor, results from altered lineage-specific expression of a glycosyltransferase. Cell 1999;96:111–120.
61. Lyons SE, Bruck ME, Bowie EJ, Ginsburg D. Impaired intracellular transport produced by a subset of type IIA von Willebrand disease mutations. J Biol Chem 1992;267:4424–4430.
62. Gralnick HR, Williams SB, McKeown LP, et al. In vitro correction of the abnormal multimeric structure of von Willebrand factor in type IIa von Willebrand's disease. Proc Natl Acad Sci USA 1985;82:5968–5972.
63. Cooney KA, Ginsburg D. Comparative analysis of type 2b von Willebrand disease mutations: implications for the mechanism of von Willebrand factor binding to platelets. Blood 1996; 87:2322–2328.
64. Gralnick HR, Williams SB, McKeown LP, et al. Von Willebrand's disease with spontaneous platelet aggregation induced by an abnormal plasma von Willebrand factor. J Clin Invest 1985;76:1522–1529.
65. Ruggeri ZM, Pareti FI, Mannucci PM, et al. Heightened interaction between platelets and factor VIII/von Willebrand factor in a new subtype of von Willebrand's disease. N Engl J Med 1980;302:1047–1051.
66. Weiss HJ, Meyer D, Rabinowitz R, et al. Pseudo-von Willebrand's disease. An intrinsic platelet defect with aggregation by unmodified human factor VIII/von Willebrand factor and enhanced adsorption of its high-molecular-weight multimers. N Engl J Med 1982;306:326–333.
67. Miller JL, Kupinski JM, Castella A, Ruggeri ZM. von Willebrand factor binds to platelets and induces aggregation in platelet-type but not type IIB von Willebrand disease. J Clin Invest 1983;72:1532–1542.
68. Ciavarella G, Ciavarella N, Antoncecchi S, et al. High-resolution analysis of von Willebrand factor multimeric composition defines a new variant of type I von Willebrand disease with aberrant structure but presence of all size multimers (type IC). Blood 1985;66:1423–1429.
69. Lopez-Fernandez MF, Gonzalez-Boullosa R, Blanco-Lopez MJ, et al. Abnormal proteolytic degradation of von Willebrand factor after desmopressin infusion in a new subtype of von Willebrand disease (ID). Am J Hematol 1991;36:163–170.
70. Mannucci PM, Lombardi R, Castaman G, et al. Von Willebrand disease "Vicenza" with larger-than-normal (supranormal) von Willebrand factor multimers. Blood 1988;71:65–70.
71. Schneppenheim R, Federici AB, Budde U, et al. Von Willebrand disease type 2M "Vicenza" in Italian and German patients: identification of the first candidate mutation (G3864A; R1205H) in 8 families. Thromb Haemost 2000;83:136–140.
72. Montgomery RR, Dent J, Schmidt W, et al. Hereditary persistence of circulating pro von Willebrand factor (pro-vWF) [Abstract]. Circulation 1986;74(Suppl 2):406.
73. Nishino M, Girma J-P, Rothschild C, et al. New variant of von Willebrand disease with defective binding to factor VIII. Blood 1989;74:1591–1599.
74. Mazurier C, Dieval J, Jorieux S, et al. A new von Willebrand factor (vWf) defect in a patient with factor VIII (fVIII) deficiency but normal levels and multimeric patterns of both plasma and platelet vWF. Characterization of abnormal vWf/fVIII interaction. Blood 1990;75:20–26.
75. Cacheris PM, Nichols WC, Ginsburg D. Molecular characterization of a unique von Willebrand disease variant. A novel muta-

tion affecting von Willebrand factor/factor VIII interaction. J Biol Chem 1991;266:13499–13502.

76. Gaucher C, Mazurier B, Jorieux S, et al. Identification of two point mutations in the von Willebrand factor gene of three families with the 'Normandy' variant of von Willebrand disease. Br J Haematol 1991;78:506–514.

77. Kroner PA, Friedman KD, Fahs SA, et al. Abnormal binding of factor VIII is linked with the substitution of glutamine for arginine 91 in von Willebrand factor in a variant form of von Willebrand disease. J Biol Chem 1991;266:19146–19149.

78. Rick ME, Krizek, DM. Identification of a His54Gln substitution in von Willebrand factor from a patient with defective binding of factor VIII. Am J Hematol 1996;51:302–306.

79. Handin RI, Martin V, Moloney WC. Antibody-induced von Willebrand's disease: A newly defined inhibitor syndrome. Blood 1976;48:393–405.

80. Wautier, JL Levy-Toledano S, Caen JP. Acquired von Willebrand's syndrome and thrombopathy in a patient with chronic lymphocytic leukaemia. Scand J Haematol 1976;16:128–134.

81. Mohri H, Motomura S, Kanamori H, et al. Clinical significance of inhibitors in acquired von Willebrand syndrome. Blood 1998;91:3623–3629.

82. Eikenboom JCJ, van der Meer FJM, Briet E. Acquired von Willebrand's disease due to excessive fibrinolysis. Br J Haematol 1992;81:618–620.

83. Budde U, Schaefer G, Mueller N, et al. Acquired von Willebrand's disease in the myeloproliferative syndrome. Blood 1984;64:981–985.

84. Gill JC, Wilson AD, Endres-Brooks J, Montgomery RR. Loss of the largest von Willebrand factor multimers from the plasma of patients with congenital cardiac defects. Blood 1986;67:758–761.

85. Bracey AW, Wu AH, Aceves J, et al. Platelet dysfunction associated with Wilms tumor and hyaluronic acid. Am J Hematol 1987;24:247–257.

86. Aylesworth CA, Smallridge RC, Rick ME, Alving BA. Acquired von Willebrand's disease: A rare manifestation of postpartum thyroiditis. Am J Hematol 1995;50:217–219.

87. Kreuz W, Linde R, Funk M, et al. Valproate therapy induces von Willebrand disease type I. Epilepsia 1992;33:178–184.

88. Aberg M, Hedner U, Bergentz SE. Effect of dextran on factor VIII (antihemophilic factor) and platelet function. Ann Surg 1979;189:243–247.

89. Sanfelippo MJ, Suberviola PD, Geimer NF. Development of a von Willebrand-like syndrome after prolonged use of hydroxyethyl starch. Am J Clin Pathol 1987;88:653–655.

90. Ratnoff, OD, Saito, H. Bleeding in von Willebrand's disease. N Engl J Med 1974;290:1089.

91. Scott JP, Montgomery RR. Therapy of von Willebrand disease. Semin Thromb Hemost 1993;19:37–47.

92. Lusher JM. Clinical guidelines for treating von Willebrand disease patients who are not candidates for DDAVP—a survey of European physicians. Haemophilia 1998;4 Suppl 3:11–14.

93. Moffat EH, Giddings JC, Bloom AL. The effect of desamino-D-arginine vasopressin (DDAVP) and naloxone infusions on factor VIII and possible endothelial cell (EC) related activities. Br J Haematol 1984;57:651–662.

94. Mannucci PM. Treatment of von Willebrand's disease. J Intern Med 1997;(suppl)740:129–132.

95. Aledort LM. Treatment of von Willebrand's disease. Mayo Clin Proc 1991;66:841–846.

96. Mannucci PM, Lusher JM. Desmopressin and thrombosis [letter]. Lancet 1989;2:675.

97. Mannucci PM, Bettega D, Cattaneo M. Patterns of development of tachyphylaxis in patients with haemophilia and von Willebrand disease after repeated doses of desmopressin (DDAVP). Br J Haematol 1992;82:87–93.

98. Mannucci PM, Lombardi R, Bader R, et al. Heterogeneity of type I von Willebrand disease: Evidence for a subgroup with an abnormal von Willebrand factor. Blood 1985;66:796–802.

99. Sutor AH. DDAVP is not a panacea for children with bleeding disorders. Br J Haematol 2000;108:217–227.

100. Holmberg L, Nilsson EM, Borge L, et al. Platelet aggregation induced by 1-desamino-8-D-arginine vasopressin (DDAVP) in type 2 von Willebrand's disease. N Engl J Med 1983;309:816–821.

101. Casonato A, Pontara E, Dannhaeuser D, et al. Re-evaluation of the therapeutic efficacy of DDAVP in type IIB von Willebrand's disease. Blood Coagul Fibrinolysis 1994;5:959–964.

102. Lethagen S, Ragnarson Tennvall G. Self-treatment with desmopressin intranasal spray in patients with bleeding disorders: effect on bleeding symptoms and socioeconomic factors. Ann Hematol 1993;66:257–260.

103. Chang AC, Rick ME, Pierce LR, Weinstein, MJ. Summary of a workshop on potency and dosage of von Willebrand factor concentrates. Haemophilia 1998;4 Suppl 3:1–6.

104. Pasi KJ, Williams MD, Enayat MS, Hill FG. Clinical and laboratory evaluation of the treatment of von Willebrand's disease patients with heat-treated factor VIII concentrate (BPL 8Y). Br J Haematol 1990;75:228–233.

105. Goudemand J, Negrier C, Ounnoughene N, Sultan, Y. Clinical management of patients with von Willebrand's disease with a VHP vWF concentrate: the French experience. Haemophilia 1998;4 Suppl 3:48–52.

106. Varon D, Martinowitz U. Continuous infusion therapy in haemophilia. Haemophilia 1998;4:431–435.

107. Lubetsky A, Schulman S, Varon D, et al. Safety and efficacy of continuous infusion of a combined factor VIII-von Willebrand factor (vWF) concentrate (Haemate-P) in patients with von Willebrand disease. Thromb Haemost 1999;81:229–233.

108. Castillo R, Escolar G, Monteagudo J, et al. Hemostasis in patients with severe von Willebrand disease improves after normal platelet transfusion and normalizes with further correction of the plasma defect. Transfusion 1997;37:785–790.

109. Hemophilia and von Willebrand's disease: 2. Management. Association of Hemophilia Clinic Directors of Canada. CMAJ 1995;153:147–157.

110. Alperin JB. Estrogens and surgery in women with von Willebrand's disease. Am J Med 1982;73:367–371.

111. Federici AB, Rand JH, Castaman G, et al. Treatment of acquired von Willebrand syndrome in patients with monoclonal gammopathy of uncertain significance: comparison of three different therapeutic approaches. Blood 1998;92:2707–2711.

112. Viallard JF, Pellegrin JL, Vergnes C, et al. Three cases of acquired von Willebrand disease associated with systemic lupus erythematosus. Br J Haematol 1999;105:532–537.

113. Conti M, Mari D, Conti E, et al. Pregnancy in women with different types of von Willebrand disease. Obstet Gynecol 1986;68:282–285.

114. Walker ID, Walker JJ, Colvin BT et al. Investigation and management of haemorrhagic disorders in pregnancy. Haemostasis and Thrombosis Task Force. J Clin Pathol 1994;47:100–108.

CHAPTER 8

General Aspects of Thrombocytopenia, Platelet Transfusions, and Thrombopoietic Growth Factors

Anne Angiolillo, M.D.
Amal M. Abu-Ghosh, M.B.B.S.
Virginia Davenport, R.N.
Mitchell S. Cairo, M.D.

HISTORICAL PERSPECTIVE

In the 1870s, both Osler and Jayem described and illustrated blood platelets.[1] Julius Bizzorzero in 1882 was the first to use the term *platelet* (*Blutplättchen*) and to note their involvement in hemostasis.[1] In 1890, Howell identified the megakaryocyte (Mk) and in 1906, Wright recognized that this large cell in the bone marrow produces blood platelets.[2] Since the 1970s, a number of major insights have been achieved: recognition of different stages of normal and abnormal megakaryocytopoiesis, discovery and cloning of cytokines acting on megakaryocytic lineage, and delineation of functions of megakaryocytes (Mks) and platelets. In 1993, Wendling and Vainchenker's group identified the c-*mpl* proto-oncogene as the receptor for thrombopoietin, a major regulator of thrombocytopoiesis.[3] Subsequently, several groups simultaneously isolated and cloned c-*mpl* ligand or thrombopoietin.[4–8] Identification of c-*mpl* and its ligand, thrombopoietin, represents one of the most important recent advances in megakaryocytopoiesis.[2]

PHYSIOLOGIC THROMBOPOIESIS

Megakaryocytopoiesis and platelet production represent complex processes whose regulation remains incompletely understood.[9] Mks grow to a size 10 times the diameter of most other bone marrow cells and contain up to 128 times the normal chromosomal content, yet represent less than 0.5% of the cells in the bone marrow. Ultimately, they give rise to blood platelets, the cells responsible for re-establishing vascular integrity following injury (primary hemostasis).[10,11] Mk differentiation can artificially be divided into three developmental stages: progenitor cells, immature Mks (promegakaryoblasts; PMkBs), and mature Mks.[1]

Mks arise from pluripotent hematopoietic stem cells that develop into progenitor cells, Mk-HPP-CFCs (megakaryocyte high-proliferative-potential colony-forming cells), BFU-Mks (burst-forming units of Mks), and CFU-Mks (colony-forming units of Mks) that have a proliferative capacity and are committed to Mk lineage in response to a number of mitotic signals.[10] The most primitive progenitor cell of this lineage is the Mk-HPP-CFC. In-vitro studies show that Mk progenitor cells progressively lose proliferative potential and that the most differentiated of the progenitor cells is the CFU-Mk. The Mk-HPP-CFC, BFU-Mk, and CFU-Mk generate a few thousand, few hundred, and several Mks, respectively.[1]

The PMkBs are transitional cells that serve as bridges between the progenitor cells and the more mature Mks.[1] The Mks undergo endomitosis, a process by which DNA synthesis is uncoupled from mitosis, resulting in cells that display up to 128 times the normal chromosomal complement.[11] Mks and their precursors express a variety of developmentally regulated antigenic determinants. As the cell develops a highly polyploid nucleus,

---

Supported in part from a grant from the Pediatric Cancer Research Foundation.

it expresses platelet-specific proteins: platelet glycoproteins IIb/IIIa (CD41), GPIb-IX, platelet factor 4 (PF 4), thrombospondin, and thrombomodulin. These cell surface glycoproteins are involved in platelet adhesion or aggregation. In addition, cytoplasmic granules contain ADP, factor V, fibrinogen, PF 4, von Willebrand factor (vWF), serotonin, β-thromboglobulin, and other substances critical for platelet function. Finally, the highly polyploid Mk undergoes cytoplasmic partitioning (demarcation membranes form), giving rise to thousands of normal platelets.[1,11]

Megakaryocytopoiesis is a complex biological process regulated by numerous cytokines, hormones, stromal cells, and extracellular matrix proteins. Regulation of human megakaryocytopoiesis is controlled by several thrombopoietic growth factors: IL-3, IL-6, IL-11, granulocyte-macrophage colony-stimulating factor (GM-CSF), and thrombopoietin. The identification and cloning of thrombopoietin, the major regulator of platelet production, represents one of the most important recent advances in enhancing our understanding of the physiology of megakaryocytopoiesis.[12]

PATHOPHYSIOLOGY AND CLASSIFICATION

Thrombocytopenia is defined as a platelet count less than 150,000/μL. Because platelets are essential for primary hemostasis, the clinical manifestations of thrombocytopenia typically involve skin or mucous membranes. Classic signs of thrombocytopenia include petechiae, ecchymoses, epistaxis, gingival bleeding, hematuria, menorrhagia, and hematochezia. Hematomas are rare.[13] Is there a particular platelet count below which physicians should be concerned about the possibility of bleeding? The criteria are well established: the patient with a platelet count 10,000 to 20,000/μL is severely thrombocytopenic and is at risk for life-threatening hemorrhage; the patient with a platelet count less than 50,000/μL is moderately thrombocytopenic with bleeding in response to surgery or trauma; and the patient with a count less than 100,000/μL (but greater than 50,000/μL) is mildly thrombocytopenic and is usually asymptomatic.[13] (See platelet transfusion therapy section for further discussion on this subject.)

The evaluation of a patient with thrombocytopenia includes a careful history, complete physical exam, review of the blood smear, and selected laboratory tests. Thrombocytopenia may be suspected in the patient with signs or symptoms of bleeding or it may be an incidental finding in a complete blood count (CBC). Approximately 0.1% of blood samples contain EDTA-dependent platelet agglutinins which cause a low platelet count to be recorded. Examination of the peripheral blood smear for platelet clumping allows recognition of this phenomenon, which is known as "pseudothrombocytopenia."

Thrombocytopenia is the result of one of three main pathophysiologic processes: platelet sequestration, decreased platelet production, or increased platelet destruction. A review of the differential diagnosis of thrombocytopenia is given in Table 8–1, with a more detailed discussion of specific entities in other chapters.

Table 8–1 • DIFFERENTIAL DIAGNOSIS OF THROMBOCYTOPENIA

Platelet Sequestration
Hypersplenism
Hypothermia
Venous stasis
Heat stroke

Decreased Production
Congenital
  Thrombocytopenia—absent radius syndrome
  Fanconi anemia
  Wiskott-Aldrich syndrome
  May-Hegglin anomaly
  Bernard-Soulier syndrome
  Alport syndrome
  Neonatal rubella/cytomegalovirus
  Maternal thiazides
Acquired
  Aplastic anemia
  Myeolophthisic processes
  Ionizing radiation
  Myelosuppressive drugs
  Drug suppression
  Cyclic thrombocytopenia
  Nutritional deficiency
  Viral infection
  Paroxsymal nocturnal hemoglobinuria (PNH)
  Renal failure

Increased Destruction
Immune-based
  Neonatal alloimmune thrombocytopenia
  Neonatal idiopathic thrombocytopenic purpura (ITP)
  Drug-induced ITP
  Post-transfusion
  Anaphylaxis
  Acute ITP
  Chronic ITP
  Autoimmune disease (systemic lupus erythematosus, Evans syndrome, Graves disease)
  Secondary ITP (hepatitis B, sarcoidosis, mononucleosis)
  Viruses (human immunodeficiency virus [HIV]), hepatitis C
  Heparin-induced thrombocytopenia
Nonimmune
  Kasabach-Merritt syndrome (giant cavernous hemangioma)
  von Willebrand disease (type IIB and platelet T-type)
  Sepsis/infection
  Snake bite (crotalid)
  Burn (body surface area 10% or greater)
  Fat embolism
  Aortic valve dysfunction (natural valve or mechanical)
  Thrombotic thrombocytopenic purpura (TTP)
  Hemolytic uremic syndrome (HUS)
  Hemolysis, elevated liver enzymes, low platelets (HELLP)/eclampsia
  Disseminated intravascular coagulation (DIC)

Platelet Sequestration

Under normal circumstances, two thirds of the platelets are distributed in plasma and one third in the spleen.[13]

The fraction of platelets that is located in the spleen increases in proportion to spleen size. Splenic enlargement will cause thrombocytopenia despite normal rates of platelet production and destruction.[13] Thus, the presence of splenomegaly should be considered in interpreting the platelet count. With splenomegaly, platelet counts rarely fall below 20,000/μL; consequently, bleeding is rare.[13] Most commonly in practice, the platelet count is 60,000 to 100,000/μL. Other clinical conditions that may cause sequestration are listed on Table 8–1.

Decreased Production

Platelet production defects can be classified into two general categories: congenital and acquired (Table 8–1). One of the primary congenital platelet production defects is the syndrome of thrombocytopenia with absent radii (TAR). Children with TAR have low platelet counts at birth and roentgenographically demonstrated associated skeletal anomalies of the radial bone, but not the thumb.[14] Another rare congenital defect is congenital amegakaryocytic thrombocytopenia. Thrombocytopenia is present at an early age and the patient may or may not have other physical anomalies.[14] Children with Fanconi anemia have thrombocytopenia and macrocytosis associated with skin pigmentation, thumb defects, and renal or eye abnormalities. These patients usually do not present with thrombocytopenia in the neonatal period.[14] Usually, the hematologic abnormalities worsen with time and there is a high risk of hematologic malignancies. The Wiskott-Aldrich syndrome is diagnosed by the presence of the classic triad of thrombocytopenia, immunodeficiency, and eczema.[14] Additional hereditary thrombocytopenias exist and are very rare (Table 8–1).

Acquired diminished platelet production may be secondary to new-onset aplastic anemia, marrow infiltration by malignancy, irradiation, myelosuppressive drugs, viral infection, and nutritional deficiencies (Table 8–1).[13] Thrombocytopenia is a common finding in patients with neoplastic diseases. Whether the patient has a malignancy originating in the bone marrow (e.g., acute leukemia) or has marrow infiltration from metastatic disease (e.g., breast cancer, lung cancer, or lymphoma), the end result is new-onset thrombocytopenia. The thrombocytopenia is secondary to either abnormal stem cell differentiation or decreased Mk production as the malignant cells usurp normal hematopoiesis.[15] A CBC from a patient with leukemia will often show thrombocytopenia, anemia, and leukocytosis, whereas pancytopenia will be present in a patient with metastatic malignancy to the bone marrow.[15] Nucleated red cells are commonly encountered.

Acquired thrombocytopenia may also result from the use of certain cytotoxic drugs. Myelosuppressive drugs include cytosine arabinoside, carboplatin, topotecan, and cyclophosphamide, among others.[13] Some drugs cause isolated suppression of platelet production. There is an association between the ingestion of either thiazide diuretics or diethylstilbestrol and thrombocytopenia.[16]

Two toxins, ethanol and cocaine, have been associated with decreased platelet production.[16]

Decreased thrombopoiesis can also be caused by viruses since Mks are prime sites for viral replication. Rubella, cytomegalovirus (CMV), Epstein-Barr virus, mumps, varicella, and parvovirus are among the most common viruses that cause thrombocytopenia.[13]

Finally, deficiencies of vitamin B_{12} or folate can cause diminished Mk production sufficiently severe to cause bleeding as the presenting feature.[13]

Increased Destruction

Thrombocytopenia secondary to increased destruction may be divided into two general categories: immune mediated and nonimmune mediated (Table 8–1). In immune-mediated thrombocytopenia, antibody (usually IgG) bound to the platelet surface causes premature removal from the circulation by the phagocytic cells of the reticuloendothelial system or by complement-mediated lysis. The spleen is the major site of immune destruction.[13] Immune thrombocytopenia includes a number of disorders. If the antibody is autoimmune in nature, the condition may be either idiopathic thrombocytopenic purpura (ITP) or associated with other conditions (e.g., systemic lupus erythematosus, Graves disease) or infection (e.g., human immunodeficiency virus; HIV).[16] If the antibody is alloimmune it occurs either in the neonatal period (neonatal alloimmune thrombocytopenia) or in patients who have received repeated transfusions.[14]

In nonimmune-mediated thrombocytopenia, platelets are consumed together with coagulation factors when the coagulation cascade is initiated (disseminated intravascular coagulation) or platelets aggregate within the microvasculature (thrombotic thrombocytopenia purpura; TTP).[16] Kasabach-Merritt syndrome causes platelet destruction secondary to mechanical entrapment by a cavernous hemangioma.[16] Other nonimmune-mediated platelet-destructive conditions include hemolytic-uremic syndrome (HUS), hemolysis, elevated liver enzymes, low platelets (HELLP), eclampsia, and aortic value dysfunction (Table 8–1).[13] These conditions are discussed in detail in other chapters.

THROMBOCYTOPENIA AND PLATELET TRANSFUSION THERAPY

Over the last several decades much effort has been expended determining the relationship between the risk of bleeding episodes and the patient's platelet count in order to establish a prophylactic platelet transfusion "trigger point." In 1962, Gaydos et al., in a study of adult leukemia patients, demonstrated there was an inverse relationship between major hemorrhagic episodes and the circulating platelet count, especially if the platelet count was less than 20,000/μL.[17] Although many patients in this study were concomitantly being treated with acetylsalicylic acid (ASA), thus increasing the risk of bleeding, the "trigger point" for prophylactic platelet transfusions was established at less than 20,000/μL. Studies over the last 10 years have re-examined the trigger point for prophylactic platelet transfusions in the absence of ASA administration to determine the minimum platelet count that is associated with the least risk of major hemorrhage.

Gmur et al. reported in 1991 on a 10-year prospective, nonrandomized study of 102 newly diagnosed adult acute leukemia patients with platelet counts of 5000, 10,000, or 20,000/μL based on bleeding risk factors.[18] All patients without bleeding risks were transfused at 5000/μL, 6000 to 10,000/μL with fever over 38°C or minor bleeding, 11,000 to 20,000/μL prior to bone marrow biopsy/lumbar puncture, heparin therapy, or coagulation disorders, and over 20,000/μL with major bleeding complications or prior to minor surgical procedures. There were 31 major hemorrhagic episodes, 28 nonfatal and 3 fatal, occurring in 23 patients. The severity of bleeding was assessed using the WHO grading scale (0 = none, 1 = petechiae, 2 = mild bleeding, 3 = gross bleeding, and 4 = debilitating blood loss). The nonfatal major bleeding episodes included epistaxis, hemoptysis, gastrointestinal hemorrhage, macrohematuria, and retinal hemorrhage. Fatal episodes involved subdural hematoma, cerebral hemorrhage with rupture into the ventricular system, and epidural and subdural hematoma of the spinal cord. This study showed a definite correlation between the degree of thrombocytopenia and the risk of bleeding episodes. There was a 20% risk for minor bleeding on the days the circulating platelet count ranged between 6000 and 10,000/μL and a risk of 0.7% for major bleeding. Patients were at risk for minor bleeding episodes 84% of the days the circulating platelet count decreased to below 5000/μL and were at risk for major bleeding 9% of the days. Minor and major bleeding episodes were noted in fewer than 1% of the days when the platelet count was 11,000/μL or higher (Table 8–2).

In 1997, Heckman et al. reported on a 4-year prospective, randomized, single-institution trial comparing platelet counts of 10,000/μL and 20,000/μL as the prophylactic platelet transfusion threshold in 78 newly diagnosed or relapsed adult leukemia patients.[19] Patients were randomized to receive prophylactic platelet transfusions at either 10,000/μL (n = 37) or 20,000/μL (n = 41) and were assessed for bleeding complications and platelet utilization. There was no statistical difference in the median number of total bleeding episodes per patient for the 10,000/μL group vs. the 20,000/μL group. All bleeding episodes (major and minor) were analyzed and no patient mortality was noted. The total number of platelet transfusions per patient in the 10,000/μL arm was 7 as compared to 11 in the 20,000/μL arm. There was slightly higher platelet utilization in the 10,000/μL arm for therapeutic reasons (1 vs. 0), and higher utilization in the 20,000/μL arm for prophylactic reasons (10 vs. 6) This study concluded that 10,000/μL was a more reasonable prophylactic platelet threshold during induction chemotherapy for newly diagnosed or relapsed adult leukemia and was safe and comparable to the trigger of 20,000/μL. Additionally, limited platelet resources are greatly spared.

A multicenter prospective nonrandomized study by Wandt et al.[20] of 105 newly diagnosed adult acute myeloid leukemia patients undergoing induction and consolidation chemotherapy evaluated 216 cycles of therapy and 3843 days of platelet counts below 25,000/μL for the safety of platelet transfusion thresholds at platelet counts of 10,000/μL and 20,000/μL. Each of the 17 participating institutions decided whether to use 10,000/μL or 20,000/μL as the transfusion threshold prior to study entry (8 used 10,000/μL and 9 used 20,000/μL). There were 58 patients enrolled in group A (10,000/μL) and 47 patients in group B (20,000/μL). Grade 2–4 hemorrhagic complications, assessed by the WHO criteria, were noted in 19 of 58 patients in group A and 13 of 47 in group B, not statistically significant. There was a one-third cost reduction between using 10,000/μL (group A) and 20,000/μL (group B) as the platelet transfusion threshold per chemotherapy cycle. There was no patient mortality due to bleeding complications. A longer duration of thrombocytopenia was noted in group A, thought to reflect this group's lower platelet count at study entry, yet was not associated with increased bleeding episodes. This study supported the use of a platelet count of 10,000/μL as the trigger point for prophylactic platelet transfusions in patients with acute myeloid leukemia undergoing induction and consolidation chemotherapy.

In 1999, Slichter et al.[21] measured chromium-labeled stool blood loss to assess clinical bleeding during a randomized study using triggers of 5000, 10,000, and 20,000/μL for prophylactic platelet transfusions. There were 81 adult patients undergoing either chemotherapy (72%) or peripheral blood stem cell transplant (28%) for malignant disorders. Patients were randomized to the 5000/μL (n = 31), 10,000/μL (n = 26), or 20,000/μL (n = 24) prophylactic platelet trigger arms. Gastrointestinal tract bleeding was the predictor of overall bleeding risk assessed by chromium-labeled stool blood loss. Autologous red cells were labeled with chromium and

Table 8–2 • CIRCULATING PLATELET COUNT AND RISK OF HEMORRHAGE

Platelet Count	<5000/μL n[a] = 280	6–10,000/μL n = 687	11–15,000/μL n = 805	16–20,000/μL n = 642	>20,000/μL n = 3588
Minor bleeding (%) (average)	84%	20%	<1%	<1%	<1%
Major bleeding (%) (average)	9%	0.7%	<1%	<1%	<1%

[a] n = Days at risk.
Data from Gmur J, Burger J, Schanz U, et al. Safety of stringent prophylactic platelet transfusion policy for patients with acute leukemia. Lancet 1991;338:1123–1126, with permission.

Table 8-3 • RECOMMENDATIONS FOR PROPHYLACTIC PLATELET TRANSFUSION THERAPY

Platelet Count	Indications
<10,000/μL	All patients
11,000–19,000/μL	Febrile >38° and/or
	Minor bleeding and/or presumed sepsis
>20,000–50,000/μL	Bone marrow and/or spinal tap procedures, minor surgical procedures, and/or major hemorrhage

reinjected at study entry, and subsequent daily stool specimens and blood samples analyzed for radioactivity. There was a significantly greater number of platelet transfusions per thrombocytopenic days in the 20,000/μL arm when compared to either of the other two arms. This study reported no difference between the trigger points in terms of bleeding risks. These data suggested that a prophylactic platelet transfusion trigger of 5000/μL is safe in patients with malignancy undergoing chemotherapy.

In summary, the study of Heckman and co-workers[19] reported a median of four bleeding episodes per 37 patients (11%) with platelet counts at 10,000/μL and a median of two episodes per 41 patients at 20,000/μL (5%). Wandt et al.[20] reported 19 bleeding episodes in 58 patients (32.8%) at 10,000/μL and 13 episodes in 47 patients (27.7%) at 20,000/μL. These two studies showed safety in using a threshold of 10,000/μL or less for prophylactic platelet transfusion. The Slichter study[21] reported no difference in the risk of bleeding episodes at 5000, 10,000, or 20,000/μL. Determining a safe, lower platelet "trigger point" will decrease platelet transfusion risks and cost. We therefore propose a new classification for the platelet trigger point for prophylactic platelet transfusions based on the above-mentioned studies (Table 8-3).

PLATELET COLLECTIONS AND TRANSFUSIONS

Most platelet transfusion therapy is given prophylactically prior to the onset of moderate or major hemorrhage. To decrease the morbidity and mortality associated with platelet transfusions, especially in immunosuppressed patients, donor platelets may be filtered, irradiated, and/or selected to be CMV negative. Platelets may be obtained from multiple donors, "pooled," or obtained from a single donor by apheresis.

In 1995, Wallace et al. published a survey of the practices for collection and transfusion of blood and blood components at American Association of Blood Banks member hospitals (n = 1936), nonmember hospitals (n = 1299), and regional blood centers (n = 157).[22] The results showed a 14.8% increase in platelet transfusions from 1989 (7,258,000) to 1992 (8,330,000). The transfusion of single-donor platelets increased by 72.4% (352,000 in 1989 vs. 607,000 in 1992), while the use of platelet concentrates in 1989 (5,146,000) decreased by 8.9% in 1992 (4,688,000).

The majority of platelets for transfusions are typed to be ABO/Rh compatible with the recipient. During severe platelet alloimmunization, platelets may also be HLA A, B, DR matched between donor and recipient. Random-donor platelet concentrates consist of platelets from 4 to 10 donors pooled for administration. Multiple donors expose the recipient to multiple HLA antigens, which may increase the risk of platelet refractoriness or alloimmunization. There is also a greater risk of viral and bacterial contamination when platelets are pooled from numerous donors. The average number of platelets in a single platelet concentrate (one donor) is 7×10^{10}. Single-donor apheresed platelets may be more effective than pooled platelets because of the reduction of platelet alloimmunization. Single-donor platelets are harvested by continuous or semicontinuous flow centrifugation devices; the average platelet yield is 5×10^{11} in an apheresed concentrate.[11, 17] HLA-matched platelets are obtained from an HLA-compatible single donor and are usually necessary when the recipient is refractory to single- or random-donor platelets.

RISKS OF PLATELET TRANSFUSION THERAPY

While in selected cases the use of prophylactic platelet transfusion therapy may decrease the risk of hemorrhagic morbidity and mortality, the increased use of platelet transfusions comes with potential risks of morbidity and mortality. The transmission of bacterial and viral infections, alloimmunization, nonhemolytic transfusion reactions, and transfusion-related graft-versus-host disease (GVHD) are potential risks of platelet transfusions (Table 8-4).

Gram-positive organisms are the most frequent cause of bacteremia. Platelets must to be stored in a warm environment (20° to 24°C) with gentle agitation to prevent aggregation and to maintain good gas exchange

Table 8-4 • POTENTIAL RISKS OF PLATELET TRANSFUSIONS

Risk	Incidences
Infection	
Bacterial	1 : 12,000
Viral	
Hepatitis A	1 : 1,000,000
Hepatitis B	1 : 30,000–1 : 250,000
Hepatitis C	1 : 30,000–1 : 1,150,000
Non A,B,C	Unknown
CMV	Variable
HIV	1 : 200,000–1 : 2,000,000
Alloimmunization	1%–50%
Nonhemolytic reactions	1%
Graft vs. host disease	<1%

Data from Herman and Kamel,[23] Menitove,[24] Goodnough et al,[27] and Murphy.[28]

and proper pH (above 6.0).[23] Since platelets must be stored at room temperature, the risk of bacterial contamination significantly increases compared to other blood products. In 1986 the U.S. Food and Drug Administration (FDA) required a maximum allowable room-temperature platelet storage interval of 5 days.[24]

In 1993, Yomtovian et al. reported on a 1-year prospective surveillance program executing Gram staining and microbiologic cultures of platelets at the time of transfusion.[25] A total of 3141 random-donor platelet units and 2467 single-donor apheresis units were cultured. Contamination was found in six (0.19%) of the random-donor platelet units and in none of the apheresis units. *Staphylococcus epidermidis* (four cases), *Bacillus cereus* (one case), and *Staphylococcus aureus* (one case) were isolated. The incidence of bacterial contamination was six times as high in platelets stored 5 days as in those stored for less than 4 days.

A prospective study to determine the risk of symptomatic bacteremia following platelet transfusion in 161 patients undergoing bone marrow transplantation was reported by Chiu et al. in 1994.[26] A total of 3584 random-donor platelet concentrates were transfused, with each patient receiving a median of 21 transfusions (range 6 to 72). The median storage time was 5 days (range 3 to 5). A post-transfusion temperature rise of more than 2°C initiated an evaluation for sepsis. There were 37 febrile events (1% of all transfusions), with 10 episodes of bacteremia resulting from transfusion. Septic shock was reported in 4 of those 10 cases. The bacteria isolated were *S. epidermidis* (four cases), *Staphylococcus enteritidis* (two cases), *Staphylococcus warneri* (one case), *B. cereus* (one case), and coagulase-negative staphylococcus (two cases).

Bacterial infections remain a significant risk of platelet transfusions. One of the first clinical symptoms is an unexpected severe febrile reaction, rigors, or hypotension, often accompanied by shock, soon after initiation of the transfusion.[23,24] Asymptomatic bacteremia of the donor, microabscess at the venipuncture site, breaks in antiseptic techniques at collection or infusion, and length of storage time are possible sources of contamination. Clinical treatment for bacterial sepsis increases the cost incurred for a platelet transfusion.

Improvements in routine screening and volunteer donor collection have helped to decrease the risks of transfusion-related viral infections. Hepatitis virus (A, B, C, and others), CMV, and human immunodeficiency virus (HIV) remain a problem with platelet transfusions (Table 8–4). Blood is routinely screened for hepatitis B surface antigen and antibody to B core antigen, antibody to hepatitis C, p24 antigen and antibody to HIV, and antibody to human T-cell leukemia/lymphoma virus (HTLV).

Hepatitis A is rarely seen as a transfusion-transmitted occurrence. Transmission of this virus is usually by the fecal-oral route and chronic hepatitis usually does not occur following blood transfusions. The risk of contracting hepatitis B following blood transfusions is estimated at 1:30,000 to 1:250,000 transfusion events. Hepatitis B has a 1% to 10% risk of inducing chronic hepatitis.[24,27]

The most common transfusion-transmitted viral infection is hepatitis C. Ninety percent of post-transfusion hepatitis cases are hepatitis C. The risk of contracting hepatitis C through transfusions is estimated at 1:30,000 to 1:150,000. Hepatitis C has an incubation period of 6 to 7 weeks and has a greater than 85% chance of inducing chronic hepatitis, a 2% chance of inducing cirrhosis, and a 1% to 5% chance of inducing hepatocellular carcinoma.[24,27]

Transfusion-related CMV infection is a major concern following blood transfusions, with a high rate of morbidity in the immunocompromised patient. A large portion of the general population is unaware they are CMV positive because they are usually asymptomatic. All blood products can be screened for CMV. The immunosuppressed patient who is CMV seronegative and has a CMV-seronegative allogeneic donor should always receive CMV-negative blood products. Preparation of platelets for transfusion may be filtered to remove leukocytes, further reducing the risk of CMV infection.

In 1995, the Centers for Disease Control and Prevention reported that approximately 1% of all reported HIV cases were transfusion related. The FDA licensed the first test to screen blood donors for HIV-1 p24 antigen in March 1996, and the use of this antigen has decreased the antibody-negative window from a median of 51 to 55 days in 1985 to 16 days.[24] The risk of contracting HIV-1 infection from screened blood products has since declined and currently occurs in approximately 1:200,000 to 1:2,000,000 transfusions.[27]

Alloimmunization is the development of HLA-A or HLA-B antibodies following HLA-disparate platelet transfusions. This syndrome usually develops within 4 to 8 weeks of the initiation of HLA-disparate platelet transfusions.[23] Decreased responsiveness to platelet transfusions can be the first indication and may occur in as many as 50% of patients receiving multiple HLA-disparate platelet transfusions.[28] Decreasing the contamination of leukocytes with the use of leukocyte filtration devices and ultraviolet B irradiation of platelets destroys lymphocytes, decreasing alloantibody-mediated refractoriness. When the patient becomes refractory to random- and single-donor platelets, HLA-compatible donors are required.

In 1997, Slichter et al. published the results of a multicenter randomized, blinded trial conducted to determine the benefit of leukocyte reduction (filtration) and ultraviolet B irradiation of platelets in preventing alloimmunization and refractoriness following platelet transfusions.[29] Five hundred and thirty patients receiving induction chemotherapy for acute myeloid leukemia were enrolled on this study. Patients were randomized to receive one of four types of platelet transfusions for 8 weeks following the first transfusion of assigned platelets: (A) unmodified, pooled platelets (control); (B) filtered, pooled platelets; (C) ultraviolet B irradiated, pooled platelets, and (D) apheresed, filtered, single-donor platelets. The rate of platelet transfusion refractoriness and antibody development was 16%/45% in the control, 7%/18% in group B, 10%/21%, in group C, and 8%/17% in group D, respectively. In comparison to the control group, the treated groups (B, C, D) experienced significantly reduced development of alloimmune refractoriness ($p = <0.03$) and lymphocytotoxic antibodies ($p = <0.001$). There was no significant difference in the development of refractoriness or lymphocytotoxic antibodies among the treated groups. Therefore, ultraviolet B irradiation and leukocyte reduction by filtration were equivalent in reducing the development of platelet refractoriness and alloimmunization.

Allergic and febrile nonhemolytic transfusion reactions are common risks, with mild symptoms usually occurring during or shortly after completion of infusion. Nonhemolytic reactions occur in approximately 1% of transfused patients and are due to antileukocytic antibodies of the recipient.[23] Filtering and irradiation to remove leukocytes reduces the risks of these side effects. Premedicating patients with either antihistamines or acetaminophen can also help to reduce the symptoms of these reactions.

Graft-versus-host disease (GVHD) is a rare platelet transfusion risk but is a major concern for the immunocompromised patient. Irradiation of all blood products with 1500 to 3000 cGy, especially for immunosuppressed patients, significantly reduces the risk of GVHD following platelet transfusions.[23]

Although improvements in donor screening, collection, and storage techniques, the development of leukocyte-depleted, ultraviolet B irradiated blood products, and the use of single-donor platelets have reduced the risks associated with platelet transfusions, decreasing the number of transfusions by employing the lowest transfusion threshold may be the greatest factor in decreasing the risks of complications associated with platelet transfusions.

The costs involved with platelet transfusion therapies vary depending on the source of the platelets, the manipulation of the donor platelets, the duration of platelet transfusion therapy, and the occurrence of any transfusion risk that requires treatment. The cost of a platelet transfusion includes the platelet component, the collection and treatment of the component, and the time of the medical and nursing personnel, and the cost varies with each institution.

In 1998, Bernstein et al. reported on a multicenter observational study of 789 patients receiving myeloablative therapy and hematopoietic stem cell transplantation (allogeneic vs. autologous and peripheral blood stem cell [PBSC] vs. bone marrow[BM]) to assess platelet recovery.[30] This study also reported on the financial impact of platelet transfusion therapy. The trigger point for prophylactic platelet transfusions varied among institutions (up to 10,000 μL in 4 institutions; up to 15,000 μL in 1; up to 20,000 μL in 12; up to 30,000 μL in 1). There were 10,626 platelet transfusions: 8794 (83%) single donor and 1832 (17%) random donor. The estimated cost of $592 for each single apheresis unit included apheresis ($413), irradiation ($13), transport and handling ($10), tubing ($15), and hospital charges ($141). The cost for each six-unit random donor platelet concentrate of $475 included $276 for the concentrate and the above transport, handling, tubing, and hospital charges. The median number of platelet transfusions following autologous PBSC varied between a low of 4 for patients with breast cancer and a high of 10.5 for those with acute lymphocytic leukemia. Similarly, the median number of platelet transfusion events following allogeneic bone marrow transplantation varied between a low of 9 for patients with lymphoma and a high of 14.5 for those with acute myelogenous leukemia. The percentage of patients requiring platelet transfusion after transplantation varied significantly between autologous PBSC and allogeneic bone marrow transplantation. While 90% of patients required a platelet transfusion on day 7 in both the autologous PBSC group and the allogeneic bone marrow transplantation group, at day +28, only 15% of the autologous PBSC group vs. 50% of the allogeneic bone marrow transplantation group still required platelet transfusions. The study concluded the estimated average 60-day platelet transfusion cost per patient was approximately $4000 for autologous PBSC and $11,000 for allogeneic bone marrow transplantation.

While the perceived need for platelet transfusions has decreased over the past 10 years, as the intensity of chemoradiotherapy increases, the need for platelet transfusions will increase. Although some risks of platelet transfusion therapy have lessened, there is still a significant risk of serious morbidity. Alternatives include decreasing the dose intensity of chemoradiotherapy, which could result in decreased disease-free survival, and reducing the number of platelet transfusions, which could increase the risk of serious hemorrhagic complications. New approaches are required to both maintain dose intensity of chemoradiotherapy and decrease the need for platelet transfusions. New thrombopoietic growth factors, some approved and some in development, could serve in this capacity. A general review of thrombopoietic growth factors will be discussed in the next section of this chapter.

THROMBOPOIETIC GROWTH FACTORS

Interleukin-3

Interleukin-3 (IL-3) is a monomeric glycoprotein with a weight of 28kD.[31] The IL-3 gene was cloned in 1986[32] and maps to chromosome 5q23.31 in proximity to the GM-CSF (granulocyte-macrocyte colony-stimulating factor) gene.[33] IL-3 is synthesized and produced by activated T lymphocytes, marrow stroma cells, and mast cells (Table 8–5). IL-3 is an early-acting cytokine, stimulating the proliferation of hematopoietic progenitor stem cells, including Mks, erythrocytes, granulocytes and macrophages, eosinophils, and basophils. In addition, IL-3 modifies the sensitivity of marrow cells to late-acting cytokines and thus affects the proliferation and differentiation of more committed hematopoietic lineages.[34,35] The use of IL-3 in murine models demonstrated a multilineage response in the peripheral blood and spleen, with stimulation of bone marrow megakaryopoiesis.[36] The combination of IL-3 with other hematopoietic growth factors in murine and human models has

Table 8–5 • THROMBOPOIETIC GROWTH FACTORS

Thrombokine	Size (kD)	Chromosome	Cell Source	Current Phase of Investigation
IL-3	28	5q23.31	Activated T cells, marrow stroma cells, mast cells	No in-vivo trials Ex-vivo use only
IL-6	26	7q21	Monocytes, T cells, B cells, fibroblasts, endothelial cells, several tumor cell lines	No in-vivo trials Ex-vivo use only
IL-11	19.14	19q13.3–q13.4	Hematopoietic, central nervous system, testis, bone, connective tissues, thymus, lung, uterus, skin	FDA approved for chemotherapy-induced thrombocytopenia
Rh-TPO	80–100	3q27–28	Liver, kidney (constitutive) Bone marrow (decreased platelets)	Adult/phase III Pediatric/phase I
Rh-MGDF	80–100	3127–28	Liver, kidney (constitutive) Bone marrow (decreased platelets)	Ex-vivo use only

shown synergistic effects on hematopoiesis. The use of IL-3 with GM-CSF stimulated megakaryocyte progenitors,[37] and the combination of IL-3 with IL-6 stimulated cell cycling and thrombopoiesis in both murine and primate models.[38,39] The use of IL-3 alone or in combination with IL-6 in animal studies following chemotherapy has also shown an improved platelet and neutrophil recovery compared to controls.[40]

Several phase I/II clinical trials have evaluated the toxicity and efficacy of IL-3 following chemotherapy in cancer patients. Higher doses of IL-3 provided greater platelet protection, with reduction of the duration of thrombocytopenia and increased platelet count nadirs when used in patients with ovarian tumors following chemotherapy. However, higher IL-3 dosages (greater than 10 μg/kg/d) were associated with dose-limiting toxicities such as headaches, diarrhea, fatigue, fever, chills, and myalgias.[41–47] The stimulatory effects of IL-3 on hematopoiesis were seen in patients with normal bone marrow as well as patients with prolonged severe cytopenias.[48]

A phase II trial investigated the role of IL-3 following chemotherapy in patients with small cell lung carcinoma.[49] The use of IL-3 significantly elevated the platelet count nadir, shortened the duration of thrombocytopenia (less than 75,000/μL), and shortened the mean time to platelet recovery (greater than 100,000/μL) as compared to the control group. Neutrophil count nadir was also increased and the time of neutropenia (less than 1000/μL) was significantly reduced.[49]

IL-3 has also been used in combination with other hematopoietic growth factors such as granulocyte colony-stimulating factor (G-CSF) and GM-CSF following autologous bone marrow transplantation in patients with malignant lymphoma or breast cancer.[50–52] The sequential or combined administration of IL-3 with G-CSF or GM-CSF has enhanced platelet recovery and reduced the frequency of platelet transfusion when compared to the recovery time in clinical trials using a single hematopoietic growth factor (IL-3, G-CSF, or GM-CSF).[51–55] Enhanced recovery of neutrophils and reduced infectious complications were also noted.

The efficacy of a genetically engineered IL-3/GM-CSF fusion protein (PIXY 321) has been investigated in a phase III trial for patients with lymphoma undergoing autologous bone marrow transplantation. There was no improvement in platelet or neutrophil recovery in patients receiving PIXY 321 when compared to patients receiving GM-CSF.[50] Another trial was done following moderate doses of chemotherapy in breast cancer patients. Although a significant reduction of grade III and IV neutropenia was seen, thrombocytopenia was more common in the PIXY 321 group when compared to patients receiving placebo.[56] However, the use of PIXY 321 in children with relapsed solid tumors treated with ifosfamide/carboplatin/etoposide (ICE) chemotherapy has shown an improved platelet recovery time when compared to earlier studies using the same regimen and G-CSF following ICE chemotherapy.[57]

Interleukin-6

Interleukin-6 (IL-6) is a pleiotropic cytokine consisting of 184 amino acids, with a weight of 26 kD. IL-6 was initially cloned from T lymphocytes as a B-cell differentiation factor.[58] However, IL-6 is a multifunctional cytokine with activity on B cells, T cells, hepatocytes, hematopoietic progenitor cells, Mks, and many other nonhematopoietic cells.[59,60] IL-6 is produced by monocytes, T and B cells, fibroblasts, and endothelial cells, as well as several tumor cell lines (Table 8–5).[59]

Several in-vitro studies have demonstrated the effects of recombinant human IL-6 (rhIL-6) to induce the maturation of megakaryocytes.[37,61–63] The addition of IL-3 and GM-CSF to IL-6 has shown a synergistic effect in vitro and augmented the proliferation of Mk progenitors as well as the proliferation of other hematopoietic progenitor cells.[61,64–67] Several in-vivo studies done in mice and nonhuman primates have shown that IL-6 induced thrombocytosis and when administered following chemotherapy or radiation-induced thrombocytopenia, IL-6 enhanced platelet recovery.[62,68–72] The use of IL-6 prior to bone marrow collection in donor Balb/C mice resulted in increased platelet count nadir in lethally irradiated mice recipients and accelerated platelet recovery when compared to recipients of unstimulated marrow. Similarly, the use of IL-6 following transplantation of normal marrow cells has resulted in an increased platelet nadir and accelerated platelet reconstitution.[73]

Therefore, these in-vitro and in-vivo studies have led to several clinical trials testing the effects of IL-6 in patients with chemotherapy-induced thrombocytopenia, aplastic anemia, and myelodysplastic syndrome. IL-6 therapy was given to patients with advanced cancer in several phase I/II clinical trials.[74-78] Most patients responded with a substantial increase in platelet count and leukocyte count. Higher doses were associated with increased toxicities that included flu-like symptoms, fever, anemia, fatigue, myalgia, headaches, nausea and vomiting, and elevated levels of serum transaminases. Dose-limiting toxicities included atrial fibrillation, neurologic toxicity, and hepatic toxicity that were reversible upon discontinuation of therapy. The use of IL-6 was also studied in phase I/II clinical trials for patients with ovarian cancer, breast cancer, and non-small cell lung cancer following chemotherapy, and has shown enhanced platelet recovery with variable effects on neutrophil counts.[79,80] These studies have also shown no increase in Mk numbers or Mk progenitor cells, but have shown an increase in Mk ploidy, thus supporting the preclinical studies that have shown the maturational effect of IL-6 on Mks when used as a single hematopoietic growth factor.[80,81] Anemia was seen with high frequency in patients receiving IL-6 and was shown to be secondary to plasma volume expansion.[82] The use of IL-6 in patients with myelodysplastic syndrome or marrow failure resulted in limited platelet response and increased toxicity that precluded the use of IL-6 as a single agent in patients with myelodysplastic syndrome.[81-83] Results from pediatric clinical trials using IL-6 in combination with G-CSF following ICE chemotherapy have shown an enhanced platelet and neutrophil recovery when compared to the use of G-CSF alone. However, an increase in grade III/IV constitutional toxicities was also observed.[84,85] Further clinical trials with IL-6 have been suspended secondary to excessive constitutional toxicity.

Interleukin-11

Recombinant human interleukin-11 (rhIL-11) was first cloned in 1990 from a primate stromal cell line PU-34,[86] was mapped to chromosome 19q13.3-q13.4,[87] and has a molecular weight of 19.144 kD.[88] IL-11 is expressed in a wide variety of mesenchymal tissues, including hematopoietic cells, central nervous system cells, testis, bone, connective tissue, thymus, lung, uterus, and skin (Table 8–5).[89-93] IL-11 is a multifunctional hematopoietic growth factor that acts synergistically with other growth factors, such as IL-3, stem cell factor (SCF), or IL-4 to support the growth and formation of blast cell colonies derived from human or murine bone marrow stem cells.[94-96] In-vitro studies have shown the effects of IL-11 when combined with IL-3 in the absence of erythropoietin on promoting the expansion of erythroid burst-forming units (BFU-E).[97] The effects of IL-11 on megakaryopoiesis has been extensively studied. IL-11 synergizes with IL-3 to stimulate bone marrow Mk progenitor cells, and increases both the size and ploidy in the absence of other growth factors.[98,99] In-vivo studies have also demonstrated the effects of IL-11 on stimulating megakaryopoiesis, increasing Mk progenitor cells, and increasing peripheral platelet counts in normal mice as well as mice treated with sublethal chemoradiotherapy.[100-102] IL-11 therapy has resulted in a multilineage proliferative effect on the bone marrow and spleen, causing proliferation of megakaryocytic, erythroid, granulocytic, and macrophage progenitor cells and an acceleration of platelet and neutrophil recovery when compared to controls.[101,102] Similar effects were observed in humans with normal bone marrow function treated with chemotherapy for breast cancer and IL-11.[103] An inverse correlation has been shown between circulating platelet counts and serum levels of IL-11 in children undergoing myeloablative chemotherapy.[104]

Phase I/II clinical trials have tested the efficacy and safety of rhIL-11 in patients undergoing intensive chemotherapy for breast cancer. A phase I clinical trial by Gordon et al.[105] using an escalating dose of IL-11 (10, 25, 50, 75, and 100 μg/kg/d) following administration of cyclophosphamide and doxorubicin showed a reduction of chemotherapy-induced thrombocytopenia at dosages of 25 μg/kg/d or greater. IL-11 was well tolerated and was associated with grade II constitutional symptoms (fatigue, myalgias, or arthralgias) at higher dosages (75 μg/kg/d). Grade III neurologic toxicity was reported in one patient receiving a 100-μg/kg dose and dose escalation was stopped at 75 μg/kg in this trial.[105]

A randomized, placebo-controlled phase II trial of IL-11 at 25 and 50 μg/kg/d was performed in adults with solid tumors or lymphomas.[106] IL-11 or placebo was administered daily subcutaneously beginning 1 day after completion of chemotherapy and continuing for 14 to 21 days or until the platelet count rose above 100,000/μL. The most significant side effects were transient atrial arrhythmias, edema, and headache. This pivotal study demonstrated that IL-11 significantly increases the likelihood that platelet transfusions can be avoided during the subsequent cycle of chemotherapy. Thirty percent of the patients randomized to IL-11 at 50 μg/kg/d avoided platelet transfusion as compared with 4% of the patients randomized to receive placebo ($p < 0.05$).[106]

In another randomized, placebo-controlled study in women with breast cancer receiving dose-intensive cyclophosphamide and doxorubicin and G-CSF, IL-11 was administered subcutaneously at a dosage of 50 μg/kg/d for 10 to 17 days or until the platelet count had risen above 50,000/μL.[107] Sixty-eight percent of the patients randomized to IL-11 did not require platelet transfusions compared to 41% of the patients randomized to placebo. IL-11 significantly reduced the frequency of platelet transfusions and time to platelet recovery when compared to the control group, allowing maintenance of planned doses over repeated cycles.[107] IL-11 was well tolerated, with only mild to moderate reversible side effects.

The preliminary results of a phase I/II study of IL-11 and G-CSF following ICE chemotherapy in pediatric patients with solid tumors or lymphoma have been recently reported.[108] IL-11 was administrated subcutaneously once a day at escalating dosages of 25, 50, 75, and 100 μg/kg/d. IL-11 was well tolerated and has shown no evidence of grade III/IV toxicity at double (100 μg/kg/d) the recommended adult dosage of 50 μg/kg/d. In comparison to historical controls utilizing G-CSF (5 μg/kg/d) alone, the combination of IL-11 (100 μg/kg/d) and G-CSF appeared to decrease the median time of platelet and neutrophil recovery following ICE chemotherapy. Platelet recovery decreased from an average of 27 to 19 days and neutrophil recovery decreased from 22 to 17 days.[109,110] The percentage of patients recovering from their thrombocytopenia by day 21 and the median number of platelet transfusions following ICE chemotherapy also compared favorably to the historical control with G-CSF alone: 67% vs. 25% and six vs. two platelet transfusions. The combination of IL-11 and G-CSF significantly increased the subsets of early (CD34+, CD34+/38+, CD34+/38-, CD34+/DR+) and committed (CD34+/41+) progenitor cells. In addition, the cells expressing IL-3 and GM-CSF receptors in peripheral blood at the time of myeloid recovery following ICE chemotherapy were significantly increased compared to baseline values.[108]

Recently, IL-11 (Neumega) has been approved by the FDA for the prevention of chemotherapy-induced thrombocytopenia. The recommended adult dosage is 50 μg/kg/d and the recommended pediatric dosage is 75 μg/kg/d. Current recommendations include the use of IL-11 in patients experiencing severe chemotherapy-induced thrombocytopenia in a previous cycle of chemotherapy (20,000/μL or lower), starting IL-11 immediately after the last dose of chemotherapy and continuing its use until the platelet count has recovered to 50,000/μL or higher untransfused from its nadir after chemotherapy.

Thrombopoietin

The cloning and characterization of the proto-oncogene c-*mpl* by Vigon in 1992 subsequently provided a unique opportunity for the identification of the chief regulator of Mk production, the c-*mpl* ligand, or thrombopoietin (TPO), by five independent groups in 1994.[4–8,111] TPO is encoded by a single-copy gene located on chromosome 3q 27-28.[112] The major site of TPO production is in the liver and kidney.[10] Expression also occurs in muscle and stromal cells of the bone marrow and spleen.[113] TPO is a 60 to 70-kDa polypeptide of 332 amino acids with two distinct domains (*Epo-like* domain and *glycan* domain) (Table 8–5). The N–terminal domain shares significant homology with erythropoietin and it has been suggested that the biological activity of the cytokine resides in this domain.[114] The c-terminal region is heavily glycosylated, thus possibly facilitating secretion of the cytokine.

To determine the relationship of endogenous TPO levels with circulating platelet counts, we measured the circulating levels of TPO in patients with significant thrombocytopenia secondary to both marrow hypoplasia and increased platelet destruction.[104] TPO levels were elevated in patients with severe thrombocytopenia following myeloablative therapy; conversely, TPO levels remained undetectable in patients with severe thrombocytopenia secondary to a destructive process, namely, ITP.[104] Together, these results suggest that in patients with normal liver function, TPO production is constitutive and that the absolute number of circulating platelets may not be the sole regulator of endogenous TPO levels. Instead, TPO levels may be regulated by the total Mpl proto-oncogene receptor-expressing cellular mass.[104] Thus, patients with bone marrow hypoplasia have low amounts of total Mpl receptor-expressing cellular mass, causing an increase in TPO levels, and, in contrast, patients with ITP have an increased total number of Mpl receptor and TPO catabolism, resulting in low levels of TPO.[104]

TPO is a potent thrombopoietic stimulus and acts predominantly on cells of the Mk lineage.[115] The biological effects of TPO are mediated via binding to its specific surface receptor, c-*mpl* protein.[115] The thrombopoietic effect of TPO is through activation of intracellular signaling pathways, including the Janus kinase (JAK) signal transducers and activators of transcription (STAT) and Ras cascades.[116]

TPO affects all stages of Mk and platelet development and has proved to be the most potent platelet production cytokine to date.[9] Along with other cytokines (IL-3 and GM-CSF), TPO induces Mk colony formation. IL-6 and IL-11 potentiate the action of IL-3 and GM-CSF by acting primarily on Mk maturation.[112] It is known that TPO is the most potent stimulator of endomitosis and polyploidy in Mks. TPO also acts on the final stages of Mk maturation, leading to platelet shedding.[113]

The isolation of TPO has been a major advance in the understanding of megakaryocytopoiesis. Two recombinant thrombopoietic growth factors have been developed: a polyethylene glycol-conjugated, recombinant truncated polypeptide, PEG-rHuMGDF; and the full-length, glycosylated recombinant protein, rHuTPO.[117] Preclinical studies in animal models have revealed the safety of and efficacy of TPO to overcome thrombocytopenia associated with chemo/radiotherapy.[112,114,116] One study demonstrated that the administration of single-bolus subcutaneous PEG-rHuMGDF to healthy human volunteers doubled the peripheral platelet count on day 12 and that platelets exhibited normal function and viability during the ensuing 10 days.[117]

Clinical trials of TPO therapy in humans are ongoing and to date have shown TPO to enhance platelet recovery in cancer patients receiving myelosuppressive chemotherapy.[112,115,116] In contrast, other clinical studies evaluating PEG-rHuMGDF in patients receiving more intensive chemotherapy (acute myeloid leukemia patients) have not shown clinically meaningful benefit.[118] Patients receiving PEG-rHuMGDF achieved higher platelet counts after remission, yet there was no effect on the duration of severe thrombocytopenia or the platelet transfusion requirement with the schedule and dose of PEG-rHuMGDF administered in one study.[118] The data suggest that future trials of TPO in patients with acute myeloid leukemia should consider different doses and schedule strategies.

Thrombocytopenia is a significant complication of myeloablative chemotherapy for hematopoietic stem cell transplantation (HSCT). Nash et al. conducted a multicenter, phase I dose-escalation study to evaluate the safety and tolerance level of rhTPO in patients after HSCT.[119] No significant adverse effects were observed but the study could not answer the question of whether the recoveries of platelet counts observed in some patients were spontaneous or influenced by rhTPO.[119]

The Children's Cancer Group is currently conducting a phase I study (CCG-09717) of rHuTPO plus G-CSF in children receiving ICE chemotherapy for recurrent or refractory solid tumors. This dose-escalation phase I trial will determine the pharmacokinetics and toxicity of rHuTPO in children receiving this regimen of myelosuppressive chemotherapy. CCG-09717 will also evaluate the depth and duration of thrombocytopenia as well as the number of platelet transfusion events during each cycle of chemotherapy.

REFERENCES

Chapter 8 References

1. Long MW. Megakaryocyte differentiation events. Semin Hematol 1998;35:192–199.
2. Caen JP, Han ZC. Preface. Baillieres Clin Haematol 1997;10:ix.
3. Methia N, Louache F, Vainchenker W, et al. Oligodeoxynucleotides antisense to the proto-oncogene c-mpl specifically inhibit in vitro megakaryocytopoiesis. Blood 1993;82:1395–1401.
4. Sohma Y, Akahori H, Seki N, et al. Molecular cloning and chromosomal localization of the human thrombopoietin gene. FEBS Lett 1994;353:57–61.
5. Lok S, Kaushansky K, Holly RD, et al. Cloning and expression of murine thrombopoietin cDNA and stimulation of platelet production in vivo. Nature 1994;369:565–568.
6. Kuter DJ, Beeler DL, Rosenberg RD. The purification of megapoietin: A physiological regulator of megakaryocyte growth and platelet production. Proc Natl Acad Sci USA 1994;91:11104–11108.
7. deSauvage FJ, Hass PE, Spencer SD, et al. Stimulation of megakaryocytopoiesis and thrombocytopoiesis by the c-mpl ligand. Nature 1994;369:553–558.
8. Bartley TD, Bogenberger J, Hunt P, et al. Identification and cloning of a megakaryocyte growth and development factor that is a ligand for the cytokine receptor mpl. Cell 1994;77:1117–1124.
9. Wendling F, Han Z-C. Positive and negative regulation of megakaryocytopoiesis. Baillieres Clin Haematol 1997;10:29–45.
10. Nurden P, Poujol C, Nurden AT. The evolution of megakaryocytes to platelets. Baillieres Clin Haematol 1997;10:1–27.
11. Kaushansky K. The enigmatic megakaryocyte gradually reveals its secrets. Bioessays 1999;21:353–360.
12. Caen JP, Han ZC, Bellucci S, et al. Regulation of megakaryocytopoiesis. Haemostasis 1999;29:27–40.
13. Goebel RA. Thrombocytopenia. Emerg Med Clin North Am 1993;11:445–464.
14. Homans A. Thrombocytopenia in the neonate. Pediatr Clin North Am 1996;43:737–756.
15. Doyle B, Porter D. Thrombocytopenia. AACN Clin Issues 1997;8:469–480.
16. Rutherford C, Frenkel EP. Thrombocytopenia. Issues in diagnosis and therapy. Med Clin North Am 1994;78:555–575.
17. Kruskall MS. The perils of platelet transfusions. N Engl J Med 1997;337:1914–1915.
18. Gmur J, Burger J, Schanz U, et al. Safety of stringent prophylactic platelet transfusion policy for patients with acute leukemia. Lancet 1991;338:1123–1126.
19. Heckman K, Weiner G, Davis C, et al. Randomized study of prophylactic platelet transfusion threshold during induction therapy for adult acute leukemia: 10,000/μL versus 20,000/μL. J Clin Oncol 1997;15:1143–1149.
20. Wandt H, Frank M, Ehninger G, et al. Safety and cost effectiveness of a 10×10^9/L trigger: a prospective comparative trial in 105 patients with acute myeloid leukemia. Blood 1998;91:3601–3606.
21. Slichter SJ, LeBlanc R, Jones MK, et al. Quantitative analysis of bleeding risk in cancer patients (PTS) prophylactically transfused at platelet (PLT) counts (CTS) of 5,000, 10,000, or 20,000 PLTS/μL. Blood 1999 (abstract);94:376a.
22. Wallace EL, Churchill WH, Surgenor DM, et al. Collection and transfusion of blood and blood components in the United States, 1992. Transfusion 1995;35:802–812.
23. Herman JH, Kamel HT. Platelet transfusion current techniques, remaining problems, and future prospects. Am J Pediatr Hematol/Oncol 1987;9:272–286.
24. Menitove JE. Transfusion-transmitted infections: Update. Semin Hematol 1996;33:290–301.
25. Yomtovian R, Lazarus HM, Goodnough LT, et al. A prospective microbiologic surveillance program to detect and prevent the transfusion of bacterially contaminated platelets. Transfusion 1993;33:902–909.
26. Chiu EKW, Yuen KY, Lie AKW, et al. A prospective study of symptomatic bacteremia following platelet transfusion and of its management. Transfusion 1994;34:950–954.
27. Goodnough LT, Brecher ME, Kanter MH, et al. Transfusion Medicine. N Engl J Med 1999;340:438–447.
28. Murphy MF. Clinical aspects of platelet transfusion therapy. Infusionsther Transfusionsmed 1994;21 Suppl 3:34–38.
29. Slichter SJ. Leukocyte reduction and ultraviolet B irradiation of platelets to prevent alloimmunization and refractoriness to platelet transfusions. N Engl J Med 1997;337:1861–1869.
30. Bernstein SH, Nademanee AP, Vose JM, et al. A multicenter study of platelet recovery and utilization in patients after myeloablative therapy and hematopoietic stem cell transplantation. Blood 1998;91:3509–3517.
31. Ihle JN, Keller J, Oroszalan S, et al. Biologic properties of homogeneous interleukin 3. I. Demonstration of WEHI-3 growth factor activity, mast cell growth factor activity, p cell-stimulating factor activity, colony-stimulating factor activity, and histamine-producing cell-stimulating factor activity. J Immunol 1983;131:282–287.
32. Yang Y-C, Ciarletta AB, Temple PA, et al. Human IL-3 (multi-CSF): Identification by expression cloning of a novel hematopoietic growth factor related to murine IL-3. Cell 1986;47:3–10.
33. Yang Y-C, Kovacic S, Kriz R, et al. The human genes for GM-CSF and IL-3 are closely linked in tandem on chromosome 5. Blood 1988;71:958–961.
34. Stahl CP, Winton EF, Monroe MC, et al. Differential effects of sequential, simultaneous, and single agent interleukin-3 and granulocyte-macrophage colony-stimulating factor on megakaryocyte maturation and platelet response in primates. Blood 1992;80:2479–2485.

35. Ganser A, Lindemann A, Seipelt G, et al. Clinical effects of recombinant human interleukin-3. Am J Clin Oncol 1991; 14:S51–S63.
36. Metcalf D, Begley CG, Johnson GR, et al. Effects of purified bacterially synthesized murine multi-CSF (IL-3) on hematopoiesis in normal adult mice. Blood 1986;68:46–57.
37. Bruno E, Hoffman R. Effect of interleukin 6 on in vitro human megakaryocytopoiesis: Its interaction with other cytokines. Exp Hematol 1989;17:1038–1043.
38. Geissler K, Valent P, Bettelheim P. In vivo synergism of recombinant human interleukin-3 and recombinant human interleukin-6 on thrombopoiesis in primates. Blood 1992;79:1155–1160.
39. Bodine DM, Karlsson S, Nienhuis AW. Combination of interleukins 3 and 6 preserves stem cell function in culture and enhances retrovirus-mediated gene transfer into hematopoietic stem cells. Proc Natl Acad Sci USA 1989;86:8897–8901.
40. Gillio AP, Gasparetto C, Laver J, et al. Effects of interleukin-3 on hematopoietic recovery after 5-fluorouracil or cyclophosphamide treatment of cynomolgus primates. J Clin Invest 1990;85:1560–1565.
41. Yamamoto K, Yajima A, Terashima Y, et al. Phase II clinical study on the effects of recombinant human interleukin-3 on thrombocytopenia after chemotherapy for advanced ovarian cancer. SDZ ILE 964 [IL-3] Study Group. J Immunother 1999;22:539–545.
42. Veldhuis GJ, Willemse PH, van Gameren MM, et al. Recombinant human interleukin-3 to dose-intensify carboplatin and cyclophosphamide chemotherapy in epithelial ovarian cancer: a phase I trial. J Clin Oncol 1995;13:733–740.
43. Speyer JL, Mandeli J, Hochster H, et al. A phase I trial of cyclophosphamide and carboplatinum combined with interleukin-3 in women with advanced-stage ovarian cancer. Gynecol Oncol 1995;56:387–394.
44. Rinehart J, Margolin KA, Triozzi P, et al. Phase I trial of recombinant interleukin 3 before and after carboplatin/etoposide chemotherapy in patients with solid tumors: a Southwest Oncology Group study. Clin Cancer Res 1995;1:1139–1144.
45. Hofstra LS, Kristensen GB, Willemse PH, et al. Randomized trial of recombinant human interleukin-3 versus placebo in prevention of bone marrow depression during first-line chemotherapy for ovarian carcinoma. J Clin Oncol 1998;16:3335–3344.
46. Bukowski RM, Olencki T, Gunn H, et al. Phase I trial of subcutaneous interleukin 3 in patients with refractory malignancy: hematological, immunological, and pharmacodynamic findings. Clin Cancer Res 1996;2:347–357.
47. Biesma B, Willemse PH, Mulder NH, et al. Effects of interleukin-3 after chemotherapy for advanced ovarian cancer. Blood 1992;80:1141–1148.
48. Ganser A, Lindemann A, Seipelt G, et al. Effects of recombinant human interleukin-3 in patients with normal hematopoiesis and in patients with bone marrow failure. Blood 1990;76:666–676.
49. Kudoh S, Sawa T, Kurihara N, et al. Phase II study of recombinant human interleukin 3 administration following carboplatin and etoposide chemotherapy in small-cell lung cancer patients. SDZ ILE 964 (IL-3) Study. Cancer Chemother Pharmacol 1996;38:S89–S95.
50. Vose JM, Pandite AN, Beveridge RA, et al. Granulocyte-macrophage colony-stimulating factor/interleukin-3 fusion protein versus granulocyte-macrophage colony-stimulating factor after autologous bone marrow transplantation for non-Hodgkin's lymphoma: results of a randomized double-blind trial. J Clin Oncol 1997;15:1617–1623.
51. Lemoli RM, Rosti G, Visani G, et al. Concomitant and sequential administration of recombinant human granulocyte colony-stimulating factor and recombinant human interleukin-3 to accelerate hematopoietic recovery after autologous bone marrow transplantation for malignant lymphoma. J Clin Oncol 1996; 14:3018–3025.
52. Fay JW, Bernstein SH. Recombinant human interleukin-3 and granulocyte-macrophage colony-stimulating factor after autologous bone marrow transplantation for malignant lymphoma. Semin Oncol 1996;23:22–27.
53. Sheridan WP, Morstyn G, Wolf M, et al. Granulocyte colony-stimulating factor and neutrophil recovery after high-dose chemotherapy and autologous bone marrow transplantation. Lancet 1989;2:891–895.
54. Nemunaitis J, Rabinowe SN, Singer JW, et al. Recombinant granulocyte-macrophage colony-stimulating factor after autologous bone marrow transplantation for lymphoid cancer. N Engl J Med 1991;324:1773–1778.
55. Nemunaitis J, Appelbaum FR, Singer JW, et al. Phase I trial with recombinant human interleukin-3 in patients with lymphoma undergoing autologous bone marrow transplantation. Blood 1993;82:3273–3278.
56. Jones SE, Khandelwal P, McIntyre K, et al. Randomized, double-blind, placebo-controlled trial to evaluate the hematopoietic growth factor PIXY 321 after moderate-dose fluorouracil, doxorubicin, and cyclophosphamide in stage II and III breast cancer. J Clin Oncol 1999;17:3025–3032.
57. Cairo MS, Krailo MD, Weinthal JA, et al. A Phase I study of granulocyte-macrophage-colony stimulating factor/interleukin-3 fusion protein (PIXY 321) following ifosfamide, carboplatin, and etoposide therapy for children with recurrent or refractory solid tumors: a report of the Children's Cancer Group. Cancer 1998;83:1449–1460.
58. Hirano T, Yasukawa K, Harada H, et al. Complementary DNA for a novel human interleukin (BSF-2) that induces B lymphocytes to produce immunoglobulin. Nature 1986;324:73–76.
59. Weber J: Interleukin-6: Multifunctional cytokine, in Devita VT, Hellman S, Rosenberg SA (eds): Biologic Therapy of Cancer Updates. J.B. Lippincott Philadelphia, 1993, pp 1.
60. Olencki T, Budd GT, Murthy S, et al. Immunoregulatory and hematopoietic effects of interleukin-6 (rhIL-6) in cancer patients. Proc ASCO 1993 (abstract);12:292.
61. Lotem J, Shabo Y, Sachs L. Regulation of megakaryocyte development by interleukin-6. Blood 1989;74:1545–1551.
62. Ishibashi T, Kimura H, Uchida T, et al. Human interleukin 6 is a direct promoter of maturation of megakaryocytes in vitro. Proc Natl Acad Sci USA 1989;86:5953–5957.
63. Ishibashi T, Kimura H, Shikama Y, et al. Interleukin-6 is a potent thrombopoietic factor in vivo in mice. Blood 1989;74:1241–1244.
64. Williams N, De Giorgio T, Banu N, et al. Recombinant interleukin 6 stimulates immature murine megakaryocytes. Exp Hematol 1990;18:69–72.
65. Quesenberry PJ, McGrath HE, Williams ME, et al. Multifactor stimulation of megakaryocytopoiesis: effects of interleukin 6. Exp Hematol 1991;19:35–41.
66. Leary AG, Ikebuchi K, Hirai Y, et al. Synergism between interleukin-6 and interleukin-3 in supporting proliferation of human hematopoietic stem cells: comparison with interleukin-1 alpha. Blood 1988;71:1759–1763.
67. Bot FJ, van Eijk L, Broeders L, et al. Interleukin-6 synergizes with M-CSF in the formation of macrophage colonies from purified human marrow progenitor cells. Blood 1989;73:435–437.
68. Zeidler C, Kanz L, Hurkuck F, et al. In vivo effects of interleukin-6 on thrombopoiesis in healthy and irradiated primates [see comments]. Blood 1992;80:2740–2745.
69. Takatsuki F, Okano A, Suzuki C, et al. Interleukin 6 perfusion stimulates reconstitution of the immune and hematopoietic systems after 5-fluorouracil treatment. Cancer Res 1990;50:2885–2890.
70. Suzuki C, Okano A, Takatsuki F, et al. Continuous perfusion with interleukin 6 (IL-6) enhances production of hematopoietic stem cells (CFU-S). Biochem Biophys Res Commun 1989; 159:933–938.
71. Laterveer L, van Damme J, Willemze R, et al. Continuous infusion of interleukin-6 in sublethally irradiated mice accelerates platelet reconstitution and the recovery of myeloid but not of

71. ...megakaryocytic progenitor cells in bone marrow. Exp Hematol 1993;21:1621–1627.
72. Asano S, Okano A, Ozawa K, et al. In vivo effects of recombinant human interleukin-6 in primates: stimulated production of platelets. Blood 1990;75:1602–1605.
73. Laterveer L, Zijlmans JM, Liehl E, et al. Accelerated platelet reconstitution following transplantation of bone marrow cells derived from IL-6-treated donor mice. Ann Hematol 1996; 73:239–245.
74. Weber J, Yang JC, Topalian SL, et al. Phase I trial of subcutaneous interleukin-6 in patients with advanced malignancies. J Clin Oncol 1993;11:499–506.
75. Weber J, Gunn H, Yang J, et al. A phase I trial of intravenous interleukin-6 in patients with advanced cancer. J Immunother Emphasis Tumor Immunol 1994;15:292–302.
76. van Gameren MM, Willemse PH, Mulder NH, et al. Effects of recombinant human interleukin-6 in cancer patients: a phase I-II study. Blood 1994;84:1434–1441.
77. Sosman JA, Aronson FR, Sznol M, et al. Concurrent phase I trials of intravenous interleukin 6 in solid tumor patients: reversible dose-limiting neurological toxicity. Clin Cancer Res 1997; 3:39–46.
78. Schuler M, Bruntsch U, Spath-Schwalbe E, et al. Lack of efficacy of recombinant human interleukin-6 in patients with advanced renal cell cancer: results of a phase II study. Eur J Cancer 1998;34:754–756.
79. Veldhuis GJ, Willemse PH, Sleijfer DT, et al. Toxicity and efficacy of escalating dosages of recombinant human interleukin-6 after chemotherapy in patients with breast cancer or non-small-cell lung cancer. J Clin Oncol 1995;13:2585–2593.
80. D'Hondt V, Weynants P, Humblet Y, et al. Dose-dependent interleukin-3 stimulation of thrombopoiesis and neutropoiesis in patients with small-cell lung carcinoma before and following chemotherapy: a placebo-controlled randomized phase Ib study [see comments]. J Clin Oncol 1993;11:2063–2071.
81. Gordon MS, Nemunaitis J, Hoffman R, et al. A phase I trial of recombinant human interleukin-6 in patients with myelodysplastic syndromes and thrombocytopenia. Blood 1995;85:3066–3076.
82. Atkins MB, Kappler K, Mier JW, et al. Interleukin-6-associated anemia: determination of the underlying mechanism. Blood 1995;86:1288–1291.
83. Schrezenmeier H, Marsh JC, Stromeyer P, et al. A phase I/II trial of recombinant human interleukin-6 in patients with aplastic anaemia. Br J Haematol 1995;90:283–292.
84. Shen V, Bergeron S, Krailo M, et al. Enhanced hematological recovery but a high incidence of grade (GD) III/IV toxicities attributed to interleukin-6 (IL-6) in children with recurrent/refractory solid tumors treated with rIL-6 and G-CSF following ifosfamide, carboplatin, and etoposide (ICE). Proc ASCO 1997 (abstract);16:110a.
85. Bracho F, Krailo M, Blazar B, et al. Clinical and hematological recovery in children with recurrent/refractory solid tumors treated with ifosfamide, carboplatin, and etoposide (ICE) followed by sequential trials of IL11/G-CSF, IL-6/G-CSF, PIXY321, or G-CSF: Children's Cancer Group (CCG) and Genetics Institute experience. Proc ASCO 1999 (abstract);18:43a.
86. Paul SR, Bennett F, Calvetti JA, et al. Molecular cloning of a cDNA encoding interleukin 11, a stromal cell-derived lymphopoietic and hematopoietic cytokine. Proc Natl Acad Sci USA 1990;87:7512–7516.
87. McKinley D, Wu Q, Yang-Feng T, et al. Genomic sequence and chromosomal location of human interleukin-11 gene (IL11). Genomics 1992;13:814–819.
88. Ohsumi J, Miyadai K, Kawashima I, et al. Adipogenesis inhibitory factor. A novel inhibitory regulator of adipose conversion in bone marrow. FEBS Lett 1991;288:13–16.
89. Zheng T, Nathanson MH, Elias JA. Histamine augments cytokine-stimulated IL-11 production by human lung fibroblasts. J Immunol 1994;153:4742–4752.
90. Morris JC, Neben S, Bennett F, et al. Molecular cloning and characterization of murine interleukin-11. Exp Hematol 1996; 24:1369–1376.
91. Maier R, Ganu V, Lotz M. Interleukin-11, an inducible cytokine in human articular chondrocytes and synoviocytes, stimulates the production of the tissue inhibitor of metalloproteinases. J Biol Chem 1993;268:21527–21532.
92. Elias JA, Tang W, Horowitz MC. Cytokine and hormonal stimulation of human osteosarcoma interleukin-11 production. Endocrinology 1995;136:489–498.
93. Du X, Everett ET, Wang G, et al. Murine interleukin-11 (IL-11) is expressed at high levels in the hippocampus and expression is developmentally regulated in the testis. J Cell Physiol 1996; 168:363–372.
94. Musashi M, Yang YC, Paul SR, et al. Direct and synergistic effects of interleukin 11 on murine hemopoiesis in culture. Proc Natl Acad Sci USA 1991;88:765–769.
95. Musashi M, Clark SC, Sudo T, et al. Synergistic interactions between interleukin-11 and interleukin-4 in support of proliferation of primitive hematopoietic progenitors of mice. Blood 1991;78:1448–1451.
96. Leary AG, Zeng HQ, Clark SC, et al. Growth factor requirements for survival in G0 and entry into the cell cycle of primitive human hemopoietic progenitors. Proc Natl Acad Sci USA 1992;89:4013–4017.
97. Quesniaux VF, Clark SC, Turner K, et al. Interleukin-11 stimulates multiple phases of erythropoiesis in vitro. Blood 1992; 80:1218–1223.
98. Yonemura Y, Kawakita M, Masuda T, et al. Synergistic effects of interleukin 3 and interleukin 11 on murine megakaryopoiesis in serum-free culture. Exp Hematol 1992;20:1011–1016.
99. Teramura M, Kobayashi S, Hoshino S, et al. Interleukin-11 enhances human megakaryocytopoiesis in vitro. Blood 1992; 79:327–331.
100. Neben TY, Loebelenz J, Hayes L, et al. Recombinant human interleukin-11 stimulates megakaryocytopoiesis and increases peripheral platelets in normal and splenectomized mice. Blood 1993;81:901–908.
101. Leonard P, Quinto CM, Kozitza MK, et al. Recombinant human interleukin-11 stimulates multilineage hematopoietic recovery in mice after a myelosuppressive regimen of sublethal irradiation and carboplatin. Blood 1994;83:1499–1506.
102. Du XX, Neben T, Goldman S, et al. Effects of recombinant human interleukin-11 on hematopoietic reconstitution in transplant mice: acceleration of recovery of peripheral blood neutrophils and platelets. Blood 1993;81:27–34.
103. Orazi A, Cooper RJ, Tong J, et al. Effects of recombinant human interleukin-11 (Neumega rhIL-11 growth factor) on megakaryocytopoiesis in human bone marrow. Exp Hematol 1996;24:1289–1297.
104. Chang M, Suen Y, Meng G, et al. Differential mechanisms in the regulation of endogenous levels of thrombopoietin (TPO) and interleukin-11 (IL-11) during thrombocytopenia: insight into the regulation of platelet production. Blood 1996;88:3354–3362.
105. Gordon MS, McCaskill-Stevens WJ, Battiato LA, et al. A phase I trial of recombinant human interleukin-11 (Neumega rhIL-11 growth factor) in women with breast cancer receiving chemotherapy. Blood 1996;87:3615–3624.
106. Tepler I, Elias L, Smith JW, 2nd, et al. A randomized placebo-controlled trial of recombinant human interleukin-11 in cancer patients with severe thrombocytopenia due to chemotherapy. Blood 1996;87:3607–3614.
107. Isaacs C, Robert NJ, Bailey FA, et al. Randomized placebo-controlled study of recombinant human interleukin-11 to prevent chemotherapy-induced thrombocytopenia in patients with breast cancer receiving dose-intensive cyclophosphamide and doxorubicin. J Clin Oncol 1997;15:3368–3377.
108. Kirov I, Goldman S, Blazar B, et al. Recombinant human interleukin 11 (Neumega) is tolerated at double the adult dose

and enhances hematopoietic recovery following ifosfamide, carboplatin, and etoposide (ICE) chemotherapy in children: Correlation with rapid clearance, lack of induction of inflammatory cytokines and mobilization of early progenitor cells. Blood 1997 (abstract);90:581a.

109. Cairo MS, Shen W-P, Miser J, et al. A randomized trial of two doses of G-CSF (5.0 vs. 10.0 μg/kg/d) following ifosfamide, carboplatin, and etoposide (ICE) chemotherapy in children with recurrent solid tumors (RST): significant clinical activity but no improvement in hematopoietic recovery (HR) with increased dose of G-CSF. Proc ASCO 1995 (abstract);14:255.

110. Ali-Nazir A, Davenport V, Reaman G, et al. A phase I/II trial of rh IL-ii following ifosfamide, carboplatin, and etoposide (ICE) chemotherapy in pediatric patients (pts) with solid tumors (ST) or lymphoma (L): Enhancement of hematological reconstitution. Proc ASCO 1996 (abstract);15:274.

111. Vigon I, Mornon JP, Cocault L, et al. Molecular cloning and characterization of *MPL*, the human homolog of the *V-mpl* oncogene: identification of a member of the hematopoietic growth factor receptor superfamily. Proc Natl Acad Sci USA 1992; 89:5640–5644.

112. Wendling F. Thrombopoietin: its role from early hematopoiesis to platelet production. Haematologica 1999;84:158–166.

113. Prow D, Vadhan-Raj S. Thrombopoietin: Biology and potential clinical applications. Oncology 1998;12:1597–1604.

114. Kaushansky K. Thrombopoietin. N Engl J Med 1998;339: 746–754.

115. Miyazaki H, Kato T. Thrombopoietin: biology and clinical potentials. Int J Hematol 1999;70:216–225.

116. Alexander WS. Mini review. Thrombopoietin. Growth Factors 1999;17:13–24.

117. Harker LA, Roskos LA, Marzec UM, et al. Effects of megakaryocyte growth and development factor on platelet production, platelet life span, and platelet function in healthy human volunteers. Blood 2000;95:2514–2522.

118. Schiffer CA, Miller KB, Larson RA, et al. A double-blind, placebo-controlled trial of pegylated recombinant human megakaryocyte growth and development factor as an adjunct to induction and consolidation therapy for patients with acute myeloid leukemia. Blood 2000;95:2530–2535.

119. Nash RA, Kurzrock R, DiPersio J, et al. A phase I trial of recombinant human thrombopoietin in patients with delayed platelet recovery after hematopoietic stem cell transplantation. Biol Blood Marrow Transplant 2000;6:25–34.

# CHAPTER 9

Immune Thrombocytopenic Purpura

James N. George, M.D.
Kiarash Kojouri, M.D.

Immune thrombocytopenic purpura (ITP) is defined as isolated thrombocytopenia with no clinically apparent associated conditions or other causes of thrombocytopenia.[1] No specific criteria establish the diagnosis of ITP; the diagnosis requires the exclusion of other causes of thrombocytopenia.[1] ITP can be an acute disorder, with the abrupt onset of bleeding symptoms and spontaneous resolution in several weeks or months. These clinical features may occur in adults[2] but they are more common in young children, less than 10 years old, in whom acute and spontaneously resolving ITP is the rule.[3] ITP can also be a chronic disorder, with an insidious onset of minor bleeding symptoms and persistent, perhaps even permanent, thrombocytopenia. This is the more common clinical course in adults. This chapter will focus on the issues of diagnosis and management of ITP in adults.

The incidence of ITP in adults was estimated by a recent study from Denmark to be 27 newly diagnosed patients per million population per year.[4] Since ITP is a very persistent disorder, and since the mortality is negligible, the prevalence is certainly much greater. This study presented several important observations: (1) The incidence increased over the 22 years of observations, principally because of increased detection of asymptomatic patients with mild thrombocytopenia, an inevitable result of the wider use of routine platelet counts. Currently, as many as one third of ITP patients may be discovered incidentally. (2) A surprising observation was that the incidence rate increased with age, reaching 46 per million per year in patients over 60 years old, compared to 19 per million per year for patients less than 60. (3) The female predominance, so characteristically present in previous case series and present in this study among patients less than 60 years old, was not present in patients more than 60 years of age. Therefore the common assumption that ITP in adults is primarily a disease of young women may be incorrect; ITP is being recognized with increasing frequency among older patients of either sex.

HISTORICAL ASPECTS OF UNDERSTANDING THE PATHOGENESIS OF ITP

The etiology of ITP is increased platelet destruction caused by antiplatelet autoantibodies. However, some studies have also demonstrated a concomitant lack of appropriate increased marrow production of platelets, even decreased platelet production in patients with clinically typical ITP.[5] The interpretation of both of these observations, autoantibody-mediated platelet destruction and relative marrow failure, is difficult because the methods required to document these abnormalities are complex and difficult to reproduce. Measurement of antiplatelet antibodies is not a routine clinical laboratory test, and has not been validated by comparison with clinical parameters to establish sensitivity and specificity. Estimates of platelet kinetics to document platelet production rates are dependent on radioisotope labeling of autologous platelets, and these studies are technically difficult. For example, the use of autologous platelets, though perhaps preferred to avoid alloantibody sensitization,[5] has the risk that the patient's platelets remaining in the circulation may be younger and relatively less susceptible to destruction, and may therefore have a longer survival. This would be interpreted as indicating less platelet turnover and therefore less platelet production than would kinetic studies using isotope-labeled donor platelets from a normal subject which may have a shorter survival.

In spite of these technical issues, the principal etiology is increased platelet destruction, supported by in-vivo studies in human volunteers demonstrating the presence

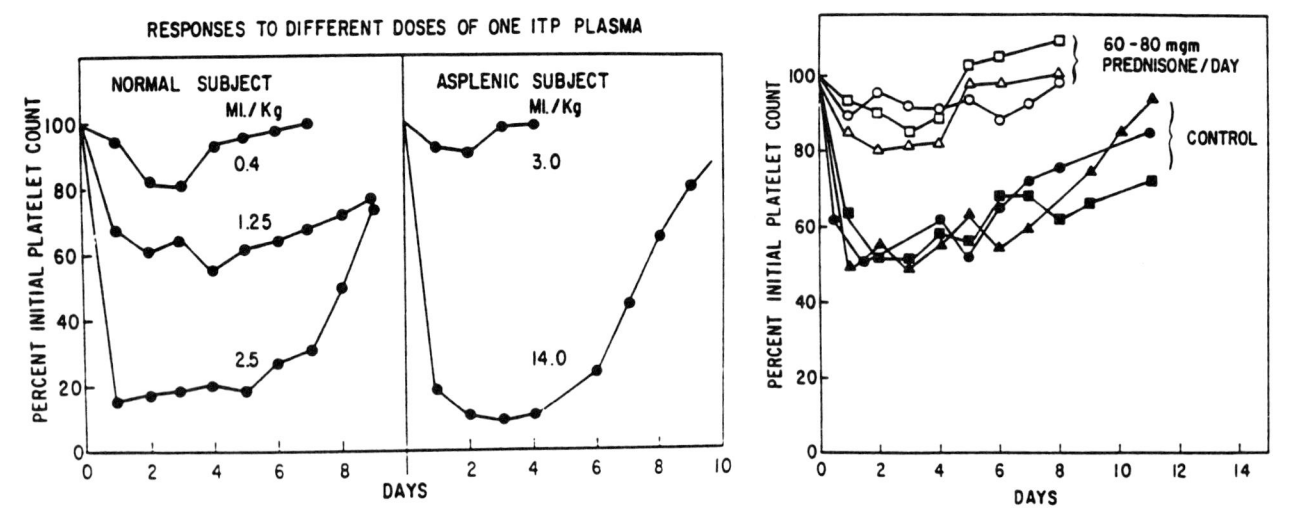

Figure 9–1 Response to infusions of plasma from ITP patients into normal subjects. The *left* two panels illustrate the occurrence of thrombocytopenia in a normal subject following different doses of plasma from a patient with ITP, and the results of infusion of the same ITP plasma into a splenectomized subject. Note that the ITP plasma dose that did not produce thrombocytopenia in the splenectomized subject was greater than the dose that produced marked thrombocytopenia in the normal subject. The *right* panel illustrates the effect of prednisone on the response to ITP plasma. Plasma from one ITP patient was infused into three normal subjects without and with treatment with prednisone, 60 to 80 mg/d. Prednisone was begun 3 h, 1 day, or 3 days before the plasma infusion and continued for a minimum of 7 days. The control infusions were given 1 and 2 months prior to, and 3 weeks after, the treatment with prednisone. (Adapted from Shulman NR, Weinrach RS, Libre EP, Andrews HL. The role of the reticuloendothelial system in the pathogenesis of idiopathic thrombocytopenic purpura. Trans Assoc Am Physicians 1965;78:374–390, with permission.)

of antiplatelet antibodies in the plasma of patients with ITP. The initial classic report of Harrington, Hollingsworth, and others, in which they described infusing themselves with plasma from a woman with acute, severe ITP and the resulting prompt, profound thrombocytopenia,[6] has been retold in graphic detail.[7] Shulman and others subsequently extended these studies with quantitative assessment of infusions of ITP plasma into normal and asplenic subjects (Fig. 9–1).[8] Increasingly larger volumes of plasma from an ITP patient transfused into a normal recipient caused increasingly severe thrombocytopenia. Higher doses of ITP plasma were required to cause the same degree of thrombocytopenia in an asplenic subject, documenting the role of the spleen in removing antibody-sensitized platelets. Glucocorticoids administered to the recipient also diminished the ability of ITP plasma to cause thrombocytopenia when infused into a normal subject (Fig. 9–1). In this series of investigations, an estimate of the titer of antiplatelet antibody could be deduced by the infusion studies in normal subjects: Table 9–1 demonstrates that the patients with higher titers of antiplatelet antibodies were patients with more severe ITP and who were less responsive to treatment.

Table 9–1 • CORRELATION BETWEEN IN VIVO ASSESSMENT OF THE TITER OF ANTIPLATELET ANTIBODY AND RESPONSE TO TREATMENT

ITP Patient	Titer of Antiplatelet Antibody	Platelet Count (per µL) Before Treatment	After Prednisone	After Splenectomy
1	<1:3	12,000	70,000	200,000
2	<1:3	5000	200,000	400,000
3	<1:3	<1000	200,000	—
4	<1:3	2000	200,000	—
5	1:3	5000	100,000	—
6	1:20	5000	25,000	30,000
7	1:20	3000	10,000	10,000
8	1:20	9000	12,000	15,000
9	1:40	<1000	2000	2000
10	1.50	1500	2000	2000

Antiplatelet antibody titer was determined as the dilution of each ITP patient's plasma that caused an approximately 50% decrease of the platelet count in a normal recipient, similar to the dose of 1.25 mL/kg in Fig. 9–1 (left). Assuming a plasma volume of 40 mL/kg, this plasma would have an estimated titer of 1:32. Plasma from patients with estimated titers of less than 1:3 did not cause a 50% decrease in a normal recipient's platelet count even when 15 mL/kg (approximately 1 liter) was infused. Patients 3, 4, and 5 did not undergo splenectomy. (Adapted from Shulman NR, Weinrach RS, Libre EP, Andrews HL. The role of the reticuloendothelial system in the pathogenesis of idiopathic thrombocytopenic purpura. Trans Assoc Am Physicians 1965;78:374–390, with permission).

EVALUATION OF A PATIENT PRESENTING WITH ISOLATED THROMBOCYTOPENIA

An algorithm for a diagnostic approach to isolated thrombocytopenia is illustrated in Figure 9–2. The history, physical examination, and examination of the peripheral blood smear are sufficient to exclude other possible etiologies of thrombocytopenia and establish the diagnosis of ITP in most patients. Certainly these time-honored activities are sufficient in patients with incidentally discovered asymptomatic thrombocytopenia, and they may also be the only essential items for evaluation of patients who present with severe, symptomatic thrombocytopenia. Response to treatment and the clinical course of symptomatic patients provide additional diagnostic confirmation.

Several features of peripheral blood morphology are critical for the diagnosis of ITP (Table 9–2). First, actual thrombocytopenia should be confirmed. There should be no abnormalities of red cell or white cell number or morphology, other than expected associated conditions such as iron deficiency from chronic bleeding or incidental conditions such as thalassemia minor. Platelet morphology should be normal, though some reports describe larger size of platelets in ITP, postulated to represent younger, "stress" platelets produced in response to the accelerated peripheral platelet destruction.[9] However, the presence of truly giant platelets, approaching or exceeding the size of red blood cells, is not consistent with the diagnosis of ITP but suggests the presence of congenital thrombocytopenia.[10]

Table 9–2 • THE PERIPHERAL BLOOD SMEAR IN ITP

Features Consistent with the Diagnosis of ITP
1. Thrombocytopenia, with normal platelet size and morphology, or slightly larger than normal platelets.
2. Normal red cell number and morphology. Exceptions may be abnormalities from expected associated conditions, such as iron deficiency from chronic bleeding, or incidental conditions, such as thalassemia minor.
3. Normal white cell number and morphology.

Features Not Consistent with the Diagnosis of ITP
1. Predominance of giant platelets, similar to the diameter of red cells.
2. Red cell abnormalities such as schistocytes, oval macrocytes, teardrop cells, and nucleated red cells.
3. Leukocytosis or leukopenia with immature or abnormal cells.

Tests for antiplatelet antibodies are not recommended for the diagnostic evaluation of patients with suspected ITP.[1] Measurements of platelet-associated IgG merely reflect the plasma IgG concentration and platelet α-granule content of plasma proteins.[11] In one small study, both the sensitivity and specificity of two commonly used commercial tests for antiplatelet antibody detection were poor.[12] Furthermore, results with multiple assays for antiplatelet antibodies on the same samples in multiple research laboratories were inconsistent in one study.[13] Therefore the possibility of disinformation is high.

Contrary to the opinion of some physicians, splenomegaly is rarely present in ITP. One large study reported palpable spleens in only 7 of 271 (2.6%) patients,[14] a

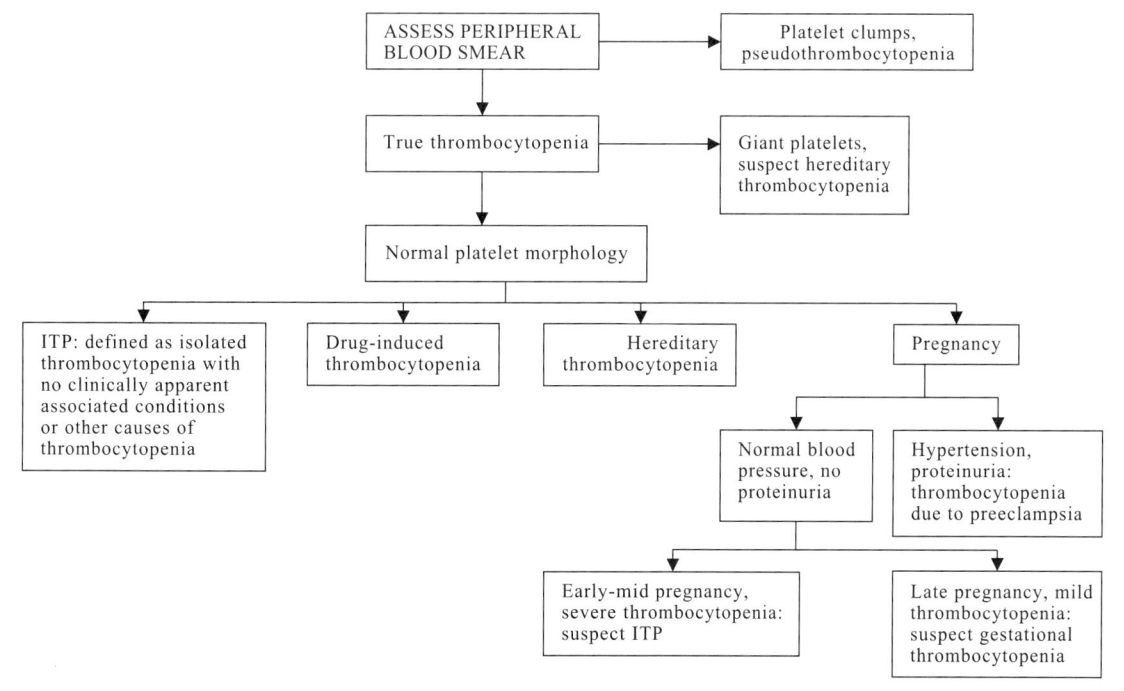

Figure 9–2 Algorithm for evaluation of isolated thrombocytopenia in an otherwise healthy person. (From George JN. Platelets. Lancet 2000;355:1531–1539, with permission from Elsevier Science.)

frequency similar to the 2.9% incidence of palpable spleens in healthy college students.[15] Enlargement of the spleen should broaden the differential diagnosis to include thrombocytopenia that may be part of immune disorders characterized by enlarged spleens, notably lupus erythematosus and chronic lymphocytic leukemia. Additionally, the spleen may be enlarged when patients have concomitant Coombs'-positive hemolytic anemia (so-called Evan syndrome) or when patients actually have myelodysplasia or hypersplenism rather than ITP.

The role of bone marrow aspiration is controversial. Some hematologists believe that it is necessary in all patients who present with a new observation of thrombocytopenia; other hematologists believe it is inappropriate.[1] Guidelines for the evaluation of patients with suspected ITP have suggested that bone marrow aspiration may be appropriate in patients over age 60 to exclude the possibility of myelodysplasia.[1] A bone marrow aspiration may also be appropriate when splenectomy is considered.[1] However, in most patients a bone marrow aspiration is not helpful in the differential diagnosis. For example, other than in myelodysplasia and acquired pure megakaryocytic aplasia, bone marrow aspiration would not be helpful for the differential diagnostic possibilities listed in Table 9–3. Systematic studies of the diagnostic value of bone marrow aspiration have not been conducted in adults as they have been in children; in children with presumed ITP, bone marrow aspiration provided an alternative diagnosis only when there were abnormalities present in the initial evaluation by history, physical examination, and examination of the peripheral blood smear.[16]

Table 9–3 • DIFFERENTIAL DIAGNOSIS OF ITP

Disorders	Clinical Features
Pseudothrombocytopenia	
EDTA-dependent clumping	Actual platelet count normal but falsely low on laboratory report because platelets are clumped in vitro and on blood smear
Platelet satellitism	Actual platelet count normal; in vitro platelets adhere to granulocytes or monocytes
Common Causes of Thrombocytopenia	
Drug-induced thrombocytopenia	Initially indistinguishable from ITP. Diagnosis established by prompt recovery upon withdrawal of the drug and, in some circumstances, rechallenge. May also be caused by nutrition products, herbal remedies, foods.
Pregnancy	Asymptomatic, mild thrombocytopenia common near term and may actually be an exacerbation of subclinical ITP. More severe thrombocytopenia may accompany pre-eclampsia/HELLP syndrome.
Hypersplenism	Asymptomatic, mild thrombocytopenia may be the initial clue to occult liver disease
Infection	Asymptomatic mild thrombocytopenia may occur with HIV infection, viral immunizations, EBV infection. More severe thrombocytopenia may be prominent with rickettsial infections, *Ehrlichia*, leptospirosis.
Less Common Causes of Thrombocytopenia	
Congenital thrombocytopenias	Typically mistaken for ITP and inappropriately treated.
Bernard-Soulier syndrome	Giant platelets. Autosomal recessive, therefore consanguinity common. Bleeding symptoms greater than expected because of GP Ib-IX abnormality and defective vWF binding.
May-Hegglin anomaly	Giant platelets, granulocyte inclusions. Autosomal dominant. Typically mild bleeding symptoms.
Alport syndrome variants	Giant platelets, sensorineural deafness and nephritis; may have leukocyte inclusions.
Fanconi syndrome	Autosomal recessive, short stature. May present in adults with isolated thrombocytopenia but typically progresses to aplasia or myelodysplasia.
Wiskott-Aldrich syndrome	X-linked. Small platelets. Typically associated with eczema and immunodeficiency, but may present as isolated thrombocytopenia.
Thrombocytopenia with absent radius	Autosomal recessive, associated with multiple skeletal anomalies. Typically presents as severe thrombocytopenia in infancy, but may cause mild thrombocytopenia in adults.
Other uncharacterized congenital thrombocytopenias	May be autosomal dominant, recessive, or X-linked. A family history is the key to diagnosis.
von Willebrand disease, type 2B	Autosomal dominant thrombocytopenia due to in-vivo platelet clumping and clearance caused by abnormal vWF. Bleeding symptoms greater than expected because of associated vWF deficiency.
Myelodysplasia	May present as isolated thrombocytopenia in older patients.
Chronic disseminated intravascular coagulation	May initially be detected because of thrombocytopenia.
Thrombotic thrombocytopenic purpura-hemolytic uremic syndrome	Typically acute onset with multiple organ dysfunction, but may have a prodrome of isolated thrombocytopenia
Acquired pure megakaryocytic	Indistinguishable from ITP until a marrow aspirate is done because of poor response to treatment.

DIFFERENTIAL DIAGNOSIS OF ITP

The differential diagnosis of ITP includes all disorders that can present with an unexpected observation of a low platelet count or purpura. Since the diagnosis of ITP requires the exclusion of other causes of thrombocytopenia, the conditions listed in Table 9-3 must be considered.

Pseudothrombocytopenia

Pseudothrombocytopenia is consistently observed in 1 in 1000 subjects and is not related to the presence or absence of any disease[17-22] (Table 9-4). The most common cause of pseudothrombocytopenia is a "naturally occurring" autoantibody against a neo-epitope on GPIIb-IIIa, exposed by the EDTA anticoagulant used for routine blood counts.[23] In EDTA, these autoantibodies cause platelet clumping and falsely low platelet counts in vitro. Platelet counts in citrate-anticoagulated blood are usually, but not always, normal, as calcium chelation by citrate is not strong enough to alter the configuration of the GPIIb-IIIa molecule. The EDTA-dependent platelet agglutinins are of no clinical importance,[24] except that they may be responsible for the acute thrombocytopenia that can occur with initial administration of the new class of antithrombotic agents, which block fibrinogen binding to GPIIb-IIIa and may cause structural alteration similar to EDTA.[25] Pseudothrombocytopenia may also result from in-vitro platelet adherence to leukocytes, typically granulocytes.[26] This phenomenon may also only occur in EDTA-anticoagulated blood.[26] Either cause of pseudothrombocytopenia will be clearly demonstrated by examination of the peripheral blood smear.

Drug-Induced Thrombocytopenia

Drug-induced thrombocytopenia cannot initially be distinguished from ITP. A careful history not only of drugs[27] but also of foods,[28] herbal remedies,[29] and nutrition products[30] must be obtained. The critical reason for the investigation of drug-induced thrombocytopenia is to emphasize to the patient that not only prescription drugs may be involved. For example, quinine is the second most commonly reported cause of drug-induced thrombocytopenia,[27] but patients may not recognize quinine as a "drug," and therefore they may continue it even after they have been advised to discontinue all medications.[30] Furthermore quinine is present in tonic water[31] as well as in over-the-counter nutrition supplements[30] in sufficient concentration to cause profound thrombocytopenia. Drug-dependent antibodies are not demonstrable in all patients with drug-induced thrombocytopenia.[32] The only effective diagnostic strategy is to observe recovery from thrombocytopenia within 7 days after discontinuing all drugs and other potentially causative compounds.[27] Patients with symptomatic thrombocytopenia are typically treated with prednisone, and therefore even platelet count recovery may not allow a distinction from ITP. Some "complete remissions" of ITP following prednisone may actually be due to occult drug-induced thrombocytopenia. A recent systematic review, updated through December 31, 1999, evaluated all published case reports with standardized criteria for assessing the causal relationship of drugs to thrombocytopenia (*http://moon.ouhsc.edu/jgeorge*).[27]

Pregnancy

Mild thrombocytopenia, typically with platelet counts above 70,000/μL, occurs in 5% of women as pregnancy approaches term, resolving spontaneously after delivery.[33] This abnormality has been termed "gestational thrombocytopenia" or "incidental thrombocytopenia of pregnancy," and has been thought to be a pregnancy-related syndrome, distinct from ITP.[1] The diagnostic features include (1) asymptomatic, mild thrombocytopenia with (2) no past history of thrombocytopenia (except possibly during a previous pregnancy), (3) occurring during late gestation, that is (4) not associated with fetal thrombocytopenia, and that (5) resolves spontaneously after delivery.[1] However, several observations suggest that gestational thrombocytopenia may be only a common, mild, and transient presentation of ITP, perhaps an exacerbation of platelet destruction normally compensated by increased platelet production.[9] First, multiple different methods for detecting antiplatelet antibodies could not distinguish patients with a clinical diagnosis of ITP from patients with gestational thrombocytopenia who were diagnosed by the above criteria.[34] Second, patients with ITP and mild or moderate thrombocytopenia may have lower platelet counts toward the end of pregnancy that return to their previous level following delivery.[35] This is consistent with clinical observations in other autoimmune disorders that can exacerbate during pregnancy. For example, hemolysis increased in 18 of 19 patients with autoimmune hemolytic anemia during the third trimester of pregnancy, resolving during the first 3 months postpartum.[36] Third, the risk of neonatal thrombocytopenia is related to the se-

Table 9-4 • FREQUENCY OF PSEUDOTHROMBOCYTOPENIA CAUSED BY EDTA-DEPENDENT PLATELET AGGLUTININS

Study	Frequency
Payne and Pierre[17]: all platelet counts for 1 year at Mayo Clinic	124/143,000; 0.09%
Savage[18]: all platelet counts for 9 months at Cleveland Clinic	154/135,806; 0.11%
Vicari et al.[19]: all platelet counts for 1 year at Istituto S. Raffaele, Milan	43/33,623; 0.13%
Garcia Suarez et al.[20]: ambulatory patients, Asturias Hospital, Madrid	23/20,760; 0.11%
Sweeney et al.[21]: healthy blood donors, Norfolk, VA	2/945; 0.21%
Bartels et al.[22]: hospital and clinic patients in The Netherlands	46/45,000; 0.10%

verity of maternal thrombocytopenia,[37] consistent with the early observations on higher titers of antiplatelet antibodies in patients with severe ITP (Table 9–1).[8] Therefore it may be anticipated that women whose ITP only becomes clinically apparent during pregnancy, but who otherwise have normal platelet counts, would not be expected to have thrombocytopenic infants at birth.

Hypersplenism Due to Chronic Liver Disease

Perhaps the most common cause of thrombocytopenia among hospitalized patients is the mild thrombocytopenia caused by splenic pooling due to portal hypertension and congestive splenomegaly. In these patients, thrombocytopenia is typically mild, with platelet counts rarely below 40,000/μL, with most being in the range of 50,000 to 90,000/μL. Total body platelet counts are actually normal, as is platelet survival; the only abnormality is passive pooling of most platelets in the congested, enlarged spleen.[38] Patients with more severe thrombocytopenia associated with liver disease may also have decreased platelet production due to decreased thrombopoietin synthesis in the liver.[39]

Infections

Human immunodeficiency virus (HIV) can commonly cause thrombocytopenia due to infection of marrow stromal cells;[40] this may be indistinguishable from ITP (see Chapter 33). Other viral infections and even immunizations[41] commonly cause a decreased platelet count, though rarely to levels that are symptomatic. In some infections, such as Rocky Mountain spotted fever and erlichiosis,[42] severe and symptomatic thrombocytopenia may occur, but other systemic signs and symptoms distinguish these disorders from ITP.

Congenital Thrombocytopenias

Adults with newly recognized congenital thrombocytopenia are almost always initially diagnosed and treated as having ITP.[43] There are many well-described syndromes of congenital thrombocytopenias (Table 9–3), but perhaps more common are disorders that fit no described syndrome.[10] The key diagnostic feature is a family history of a low platelet count, which is often not initially known. The key problem with the misdiagnosis of ITP is the unfortunate intervention with glucocorticoids or even splenectomy, which is not efficacious.[43] Congenital thrombocytopenia should be considered in patients who are unresponsive to initial prednisone treatment, who have unusually large platelets on their peripheral blood smear, who have other inherited anomalies such as skeletal deformities, or who have a family history of consanguinity, which increases the opportunity for expression of autosomal recessive traits.

The presence of truly giant platelets, similar to the diameter of red cells, should suggest congenital thrombocytopenia (Table 9–2). Inherited giant platelet disorders are heterogeneous, typically are associated with minimal bleeding symptoms, and are often initially misdiagnosed as ITP.[44–48] In some inherited syndromes, there may be associated abnormalities such as skeletal deformities, nephritis, and sensorineural deafness (Table 9–3). In some syndromes bleeding may be greater than expected for the degree of thrombocytopenia because of an associated platelet function defect, as in Bernard-Soulier syndrome, or an associated hemostatic disorder, as in von Willebrand disease, type 2B (Table 9–3). However, most patients with congenital thrombocytopenia have no distinguishing clinical features other than moderate thrombocytopenia.[43,49,50]

Myelodysplasia

Myelodysplasia may present as isolated thrombocytopenia,[51] but this is uncommon. Since myelodysplastic syndromes are much more frequent among older patients, a bone marrow aspiration and biopsy is appropriate when patients present with apparent ITP at age over 60.[1] This was, of course, a consideration in the recent epidemiologic study on the incidence of ITP[4] that documented a higher than expected occurrence among older men. However, in this study most older patients had bone marrow examinations that were normal, and no ITP patient from the study period subsequently developed a myelodysplastic syndrome.[4]

Disseminated Intravascular Coagulation

Although it is very rare for disseminated intravascular coagulation (DIC) to occur in the absence of an overt clinical cause, and even more rare for chronic, indolent DIC to present as isolated thrombcytopenia, this has been observed.[52] Patients with large hemangiomas may have localized intravascular coagulation, which may first be recognized in adulthood as asymptomatic thrombocytopenia. A comparable but more severe disorder presenting infancy is the Kasabach-Merritt syndrome.[53] Recognition of this possibility is important simply to emphasize the broad spectrum of abnormalities that can mimic ITP and can lead to inappropriate treatment (see Chapter 12).

Thrombotic Thrombocytopenic Purpura-Hemolytic Uremic Syndrome

Thrombotic thrombocytopenic purpura-hemolytic uremic syndrome (TTP-HUS) typically presents as an acute severe illness with symptoms and signs of multiple organ dysfunction. However, patients may have a syndrome of isolated, asymptomatic thrombocytopenia, which is indistinguishable from ITP. This is increasingly apparent with close follow-up of patients who have recovered from TTP-HUS. In these patients, incidentally discovered thrombocytopenia may, or may not, predict a relapse of acute TTP-HUS (see Chapter 22).

Acquired Pure Megakaryocytic Aplasia

Autoantibodies to thrombopoietin or megakaryocytes may cause severe thrombocytopenia indistinguishable from ITP until a bone marrow aspiration is done. These patients may not respond to prednisone and IVIg but can achieve durable remissions with cyclosporine and antithymocyte globulin, the more intensive immunosuppressive regimen used for aplastic anemia.[54]

Thrombocytopenia Associated with Other Autoimmune Disorders

Patients in whom thrombocytopenia is part of a clinically overt autoimmune disorder are considered to be distinct from ITP because the clinical course is determined by the primary disease. For example, in patients with Graves disease and thrombocytopenia, the thrombocytopenia often resolves with effective treatment of the hyperthyroidism.[55] However, isolated abnormalities of serologic tests for antinuclear antibodies or antiphospholipid antibodies are frequently encountered in patients with typical ITP and do not influence the management or clinical course.[56–58]

MANAGEMENT

The single goal of management of patients with ITP is to prevent major bleeding. Therefore the practical goal is maintenance of a safe platelet count. Cure is not a goal. Although simple in concept, this principle of management is essential to prevent the common occurrence of making the side effects of treatment worse than the symptoms of the disease.

What Is a Safe Platelet Count?

The consistent clinical observation is that most patients with ITP never have clinically important bleeding even when their platelet counts are very low. Easy bruising may be common; petechiae may be numerous; but truly extensive purpura with innumerable petechiae and extensive ecchymoses are very rare. These cutaneous bleeding symptoms are often referred to as "dry purpura",[59] to distinguish them from overt mucous membrane bleeding, such as persistent epistaxis or gingival bleeding, referred to as "wet purpura." Wet purpura is less common but more alarming, and may be associated with greater risk for major bleeding. The feared complication of ITP is intracranial hemorrhage. Intracranial hemorrhage is too rare to have a documented incidence among patients with ITP. Suggestions have been made that the incidence may be 0.1% to 1.0%,[1] but this high frequency, if true, would only be relevant to patients with severe and symptomatic thrombocytopenia.

Few platelets are required to provide adequate hemostasis. Clinical studies in other disorders, such as aplastic anemia[60] and thrombocytopenia following chemotherapy for acute leukemia,[61,62] suggest that spontaneous, clinically important bleeding does not occur with platelet counts above 5000 to 10,000/μL. Since younger platelets are assumed to have greater hemostatic ability than older platelets,[63] patients with ITP may have even less risk for bleeding at comparable platelet counts than patients with thrombocytopenia caused by marrow failure. Therefore the analogy may be made to patients with hemophilia, where the presence of any measurable factor VIII or factor IX transforms the disease from one of severe bleeding risk to a clinically occult disorders.[64]

Initial Management of ITP in Children

The conservative management of children with ITP has important lessons for management of adults. Because a spontaneous remission will occur in most children within several weeks to months, some pediatric hematologists believe that careful observation without specific treatment is sufficient.[65] Although the platelet count in children will recover more quickly with glucocorticoid or intravenous immune globulin (IVIg) treatment,[66] no studies have demonstrated that a more rapid recovery results in less bleeding. Although many pediatric hematologists treat children initially with IVIg,[67] it is expensive, not always promptly available, may require hospitalization, and has frequent side effects of headache with nausea and vomiting.[68] These side effects can mimic intracranial hemorrhage, causing severe alarm and thus requiring further diagnostic studies.

For children whose ITP who does not spontaneously resolve, conservative management without specific treatment still remains a common practice. In a recent audit of 427 children with ITP in the United Kingdom, only 3 had undergone splenectomy.[3] The avoidance of splenectomy is in part related to the high rate of spontaneous remissions in children even after many years,[69] but it is also because of concern for subsequent severe sepsis, particularly when splenectomy is performed before age 5.[70]

Although bleeding risks may be greater in older adults than in children, because of comorbidities such as hypertension,[71,72] adults have the advantage of moderating their activity and avoiding trauma, difficult assignments for young children.

Initial Management of Adult Patients Who Have Incidentally Discovered Asymptomatic Thrombocytopenia

If the patient is asymptomatic, probably no specific therapy is indicated. However, in standard practice, treatment of ITP is linked to the level of thrombocytopenia. If it is assumed that a platelet count above 10,000/μL is safe,[60–62] then a reasonable approach would be that treatment is unnecessary for patients with platelet counts above 20,000/μL. This is, in fact, a common standard of care for children presenting with a new diagnosis of acute ITP.[65] However, in adults, because of the uncertainty regarding the stability of persistent thrombocytopenia and because of the simplicity of initial prednisone therapy, initial treatment with prednisone is inevitably prescribed unless the platelet count is significantly higher than 10,000 to 20,000/µL.

Two case series have followed adult patients with newly diagnosed ITP and platelet counts above 30,000[72] and 50,000/µL[73] who have had no specific treatment. In these case series, with follow-up for 3 to 8 years, there were no reported adverse outcomes of major bleeding. A few of these patients may develop more severe thrombocytopenia and require treatment; also, in a few patients the platelet count may spontaneously return to normal.[73] However, it appears that in most patients, incidentally detected mild thrombocytopenia is persistent for the duration of follow-up. Another large case series supports the clinical practice of no specific therapy for patients with initial platelet counts over 30,000/µL.[73a] If no specific treatment is prescribed, then the interval for measuring the platelet count becomes an issue. If the interval between platelet counts seems too long, the patient becomes apprehensive and the physician may appear unconcerned. On the other hand, platelet counts done too frequently also cause patient apprehension by obsessively focusing on clinically unimportant variations. The resolution of this issue requires thorough patient education about the nature of ITP, its clinical course, its risks, and the goals of treatment. After several platelet counts to establish the consistency of the thrombocytopenia, the patient must be gradually weaned from dependence on knowing their current platelet count.

Initial Management of Adult Patients Who Present with Severe Thrombocytopenia and Symptomatic Purpura

Adults with symptomatic purpura are always treated initially with prednisone. The dosage is empirical, but 1 mg/kg/d given as a single dose is a common, standard regimen; lower doses may be as effective.[74] Most, but not all, patients respond, and then the dose is gradually tapered. The case for more rapid tapering of prednisone is to determine if the severe, symptomatic thrombocytopenia at presentation was perhaps a transient, reversible occurrence in the course of more mild ITP, or perhaps occult drug-induced thrombocytopenia. If severe thrombocytopenia recurs upon tapering prednisone, this becomes an indication for splenectomy. The patient himself may urge withdrawal of prednisone, because of the misery from symptoms of emotional liability, inability to concentrate, tremulousness, difficulty sleeping, and the inevitable depressing "moon facies." Of greater concern is that prednisone doses that are equivalent to or even less than physiologic cortisol secretion (2.5 to 5.0 mg of prednisone per day) can cause bone loss within several months by impairing normal diurnal cortisol secretion.[75,76]

In spite of these reasons for more quickly tapering prednisone, some hematologists believe that there is a greater opportunity to achieve a durable remission and to avoid splenectomy if a more prolonged course of prednisone and a more gradual tapering regimen is carried out.

Treatment of Acute Bleeding Due to Severe Thrombocytopenia

Patients must be alert for the symptoms and signs of acute bleeding, and physicians must be prepared for emergency care. For a bleeding emergency, in addition to conventional critical care measures, appropriate treatments include platelet transfusions, high-dose parenteral glucocorticoids, and IVIg.[1] Emergency splenectomy may also be important to provide more durable recovery from severe thrombocytopenia.[77] Despite presumably having a short platelet survival, platelet transfusions can provide substantial platelet count increments in some patients.[78,79] Continuous infusion of platelets to provide continual hemostatic support has been suggested.[80] High-dose glucocorticoids, such as 1 g/d of methylprednisolone given by intravenous infusion and repeated daily for 2 additional days, can rapidly increase the platelet count. IVIg, given as 1 g/kg/d for 2 days, will increase the platelet count in most patients within 3 days. Furthermore, IVIg given before a platelet transfusion may increase the platelet count increment and prolong the duration of response.[81]

IVIg may cause systemic symptoms of myalgias, fever, nausea, and headache in one third of patients.[68] Actual aseptic meningitis may occur,[82] with signs mimicking intracranial hemorrhage. Acute renal failure has also been reported, which appears to be related to osmotic injury to proximal renal tubules associated with the sucrose content of the IVIg product.[83,84] Therefore older patients, patients with pre-existing renal insufficiency, and patients who are receiving concomitant nephrotoxic drugs should be given IVIg only with caution. A newer product, WinRho-SDF, was developed based on the hypothesis that hemolysis caused by alloantibodies in IVIg may be the mechanism for blocking sequestration of autoantibody-coated platelets. This product is a preparation of anti-Rh(D) alloantibodies, often referred to simply as anti-D. Anti-D is easier to administer than IVIg (a 15- to 30-minute infusion) but it is only effective in patients whose red cells are D positive and appears to be effective only in nonsplenectomized patients.[85] It causes fewer systemic symptoms; the major and dose-limiting side effect is alloimmune hemolytic anemia, and severe, life-threatening intravascular hemolysis has been reported.[86] Although the typical regimen of anti-D (50 to 75 µg/kg given once) costs less than IVIg (an approximate cost for a course of IVIg in an adult is $10,000 to $15,000; for anti-D, $5000 to $8000), these are both very expensive treatments. Much less expensive is the use of intravenous methylprednisolone, which may have efficacy comparable to IVIg and anti-D.

Splenectomy

In adult patients who continue to have severe and symptomatic thrombocytopenia following an initial course of prednisone treatment, splenectomy is the next treatment consideration. Although splenectomy is far from universally effective (or else it would be recommended sooner and more often), the relative efficacy and risks of splenectomy are better than for any other treatment of ITP. The response to splenectomy may be prompt, supporting experimental observations (Fig. 9–1) that the spleen is the principal source of removal of autoantibody-coated platelets. The response to splenectomy may also be durable, consistent with the spleen as the major source of autoantibody production.

Historically, splenectomy was the first effective treatment for ITP, established long before glucocorticoid therapy was introduced in 1950. Many case series describe the results of splenectomy, but many of these reports include patients from decades ago, when splenectomy was often performed as initial therapy at diagnosis and also routinely performed in children as well as adults.[14] Therefore these earlier studies included patients who would be expected to have spontaneous recoveries and therefore consistently report better outcomes. Even among adults, younger patients appear to respond better to splenectomy than older patients. One report suggested that response to IVIg correlated with response to subsequent splenectomy,[87] but others have not confirmed this correlation.[88] Most case series suggest that approximately two thirds of patients achieve and sustain a normal platelet count after splenectomy, requiring no additional therapy.[1] However, the duration of follow-up in most case series is limited, and optimism for good outcomes must be balanced by the regular observations of recurrent thrombocytopenia in patients many years after splenectomy. One preliminary report suggested that relapses of ITP following splenectomy continually occur, with complete remissions persisting in fewer than 25% of patients after more than 5 years of follow-up.[89]

The morbidity and mortality from splenectomy is thought to be minimal, but data are sparse. In a review of 36 case series, operative mortality rates were less than 1%, an impressive figure because these data include reports before the advent of platelet transfusions, IVIg, and effective antibiotics to manage postoperative infections.[1] Most operative deaths occur in older patients with coexisting illnesses.[71] Postoperative morbidity may be related to the extent of previous glucocorticoid therapy.[14]

Because splenectomy will often be considered in adult patients who present with severe and symptomatic thrombocytopenia, it is appropriate to immunize these patients upon diagnosis, in anticipation of possible splenectomy. Earlier immunization may be more effective, before immunosuppression with prednisone becomes established. Although the occurrence of overwhelming sepsis in adults following splenectomy is too rare to describe an incidence, and most reports of this lethal complication data from the era prior to pneumococcal immunization contain and modern antibiotic treatment, anecdotes of overwhelming sepsis continue to be reported. Therefore immunization at least 2 weeks prior to elective splenectomy is appropriate, not least because the potential benefits of immunization outweigh the risks in all subjects. Current recommendations are that patients should be immunized with pneumococcal polysaccharide vaccine, *Hemophilus influenzae* b vaccine, and quadrivalent meningococcal polysaccharide vaccine.[1] Most cases of overwhelming sepsis in asplenic subjects are due to pneumococci.[90,91] Five years after splenectomy, patients should be revaccinated with pneumococcal vaccine. Children are routinely placed on daily oral prophylactic penicillin following splenectomy, at least up until age 5 years, but often into adolescence; this is not routine care for adults in the United States. However, in the United Kingdom, prophylaxis with daily oral penicillin is recommended for all subjects, both children and adults, following splenectomy.[91] Splenectomized patients must be instructed to seek medical attention immediately when they have symptoms of fever and chills; this may be the single most important aspect of education for patients prior to splenectomy and management of patients following splenectomy.

Management of Patients Who Have Failed to Respond to Prednisone and Splenectomy

The management of patients with chronic, refractory thrombocytopenia, defined as those who do not respond to initial treatment with prednisone followed by splenectomy, is a dilemma. There is no clear priority of treatment strategies following splenectomy. There is no evidence that any treatment is more effective than another, or for assessing which treatments result in more good than harm.[1,92]

But perhaps this dilemma is overstated, as many patients are safe and relatively asymptomatic with no specific treatment. Whereas initial treatment of adults with newly diagnosed ITP is guided by the platelet count, with initial prednisone prescribed for essentially all patients with platelet counts below 20,000 to 30,000/μL, the indications for treatment intervention in patients following failure of prednisone and splenectomy must be more stringent. For these patients, the chance for success is less and the risk that the side effects of treatment will be worse than the symptoms of bleeding is great. It may be appropriate to only carefully observe patients who have negligible bleeding symptoms, even if their platelet counts are very low, even less than 10,000/μL. But in practice, patients with such low platelet counts are inevitably believed to be at risk for major bleeding and therefore receive some form of immunosuppressive treatment, often a sequence of several different treatments. Perhaps too often sufficient motivation to merely observe the patient without treatment only occurs when the doctor and patient become frustrated because the platelet count fails to increase despite intolerable side effects. For some patients, the quality of life on no treatment is far better than with any of the commonly prescribed treatments for chronic refractory ITP.[2]

Treatment decisions are traditionally based solely on the severity of thrombocytopenia, but consideration of other factors is critical. The absence of overt bleeding should make physicians cautious about recommending aggressive immunosuppressive therapy. Treatment decisions must also include assessment of lifestyle and other medical conditions that could influence the risk of bleeding and immunosuppressive treatment. Older patients, with greater frequency of hypertension and greater risk of intracerebral hemorrhage,[71,72] may require higher platelet counts, but these patients are also more vulnerable to the side effects of treatment.[71] Younger patients with a more vigorous lifestyle may also require higher platelet counts. But most patients, after experiencing the limited efficacy and major problems with immunosuppressive regimens, will comfortably adapt to low platelet counts and minor bleeding symptoms. These issues emphasize the need for the physician and patient to discuss and decide together future management, based on the best estimates of the benefits and risks of treatment compared to the risks of no specific treatment.[93]

An algorithm for managing patients with chronic refractory ITP is presented in Table 9–5. Even this algorithm may overemphasize the need for treatment interventions. The most important consideration is to not base treatment decisions solely on the platelet count, but to measure treatment intensity against actual bleeding symptoms. This rule was stated succinctly in Gilbert and Sullivan's *Mikado*: "Let the punishment fit the crime."

Once a decision for intervention is made, the choice is often among the following regimens.

Glucocorticoids

In some patients, a safe platelet count can be maintained on very low doses, or even intermittent doses, of prednisone that do not cause the disturbing side effects. However, even very low doses of prednisone may cause or contribute to osteoporosis.[75,76] One report describes success in 10 selected patients with a regimen adapted from the management of multiple myeloma: dexamethasone, 40 mg/d for 4 days, repeated every 4 weeks.[94] Six of these patients had failed to respond to splenectomy and all apparently responded with normal platelet counts sustained after treatment was discontinued.[94] However, others have been unable to confirm these results and have reported serious adverse events with this regimen.[95,96]

Cyclophosphamide

Uncontrolled and selected case series have reported complete responses to cyclophosphamide in 20% to 40% of patients who failed previous treatment with prednisone and splenectomy.[97–99] Complete responses have occurred after 1 to 6 months of treatment with daily oral cyclophosphamide, typically given in a dosage of 1 to 2 mg/kg/d, adjusted for leukopenia. Intermittent intravenous doses of 1000 mg/m^2, repeated at 4 week intervals for one to five doses, have also been recommended.[99] The risks from cyclophosphamide therapy include dose-related marrow suppression, which may exacerbate thrombocytopenia and may actually increase risk for bleeding. Other potential risks include teratogenicity in pregnant women, infertility, alopecia, and bothersome hemorrhagic cystitis.

Vinca Alkaloids

Vinblastine and vincristine have been administered either by intravenous bolus injection or by intravenous infusion; results are comparable with both agents by both methods of administration. A common regimen is to give vincristine by intravenous bolus, 2 mg once

Table 9–5 • SEQUENCE OF MANAGEMENT OPTIONS FOR PATIENTS WITH CHRONIC, REFRACTORY ITP

Intervention	Indication	Outcome
Observation with supportive care	No bleeding symptoms; platelet count >20,000/μL	Stable asymptomatic thrombocytopenia may persist. Morbidity of treatment may exceed risk of bleeding. Some patients with greater risk for bleeding may require treatment.
Glucocorticoid	Bleeding symptoms; platelet count <20,000/μL	Goal is a safe platelet count with a minimal dose, such as: (1) prednisone, 10 mg every other day, or (2) dexamethasone, 10–40 mg/day for 4 days, repeated every 4 weeks or as needed.
Immunosuppressive agents/combinations	Bleeding symptoms unresponsive to glucocorticoid	Goal is a safe platelet count with control of bleeding symptoms.
Investigational protocols	Severe bleeding symptoms unresponsive to conventional immunosuppressive combination regimens	Goal is a safe platelet count with control of bleeding symptoms.
Observation with supportive care	Unresponsive to treatment	Some patients may have minimal or no bleeding in spite of persistent severe thrombocytopenia.

This sequence is empirical and has not been validated by controlled clinical observations. The goal of management is to prevent major bleeding, which rarely occurs unless the platelet count is below 10,000/μL, and minimize risks from treatment. Aggressive immunosuppressive treatment is appropriate only for patients with severe symptomatic thrombocytopenia. For patients with major bleeding unresponsive to conventional regimens, investigational treatment is appropriate. Finally, some patients refractory to all treatments may actually have minimal or no bleeding symptoms in spite of prolonged, severe thrombocytopenia. (Adapted from George JN, Kojouri K, Perdue JJ, Vesely SK. Management of patients with chronic refractory idiopathic thrombocytopenic purpura. Semin Hematol 2000;37:1–10, with permission.)

weekly for up to 3 to 6 weeks, until the dose-related side effect of peripheral neuropathy inevitably occurs. A platelet count response may occur within several days, although in most responding patients the platelet count returns to the pretreatment level in several weeks. As may be expected in reports from uncontrolled and selected case series, the reports of success vary greatly, with durable responses reported in as few as 3% or as many as 30% of patients.[100-102]

Azathioprine

Uncontrolled and selected case series have reported approximately 20% complete responses with azathioprine given at a daily oral dose of 1 to 2 mg/kg.[98,103] The average time required for response is 4 months, and most patients require continued treatment to sustain a remission.[103] As with cyclophosphamide, marrow suppression may occur with worsening of thrombocytopenia, actually increasing the risk for hemorrhage.

Danazol

The recommended dosages of danazol for ITP vary greatly, from 50 mg/d[104] to 800 mg/d.[105] Also the reported efficacy varies from no response[106,107] to sustained responses for as long as danazol treatment is continued.[104,105] Side effects include headache, nausea, breast tenderness, skin rash, and liver function abnormalities. Hirsuitism and a deeper voice may occur in women.[107] Particularly disturbing are the reports of drug-induced thrombocytopenia in five patients given danazol for endometriosis or to stimulate erythropoiesis; in two of these patients, acute thrombocytopenia recurred with readministration of danazol.[108,109]

Removal of Accessory Spleens

Accessory spleens are found and removed at the time of splenectomy in 15% to 20% of patients. Additional accessory spleens may be found at a later time in as many as 10% of patients who are refractory to splenectomy or who relapse following splenectomy.[110] In spite of frequent suggestions of efficacy of surgical removal of accessory spleens in patients with refractory or recurrent ITP, durable remissions are rarely reported. As with all treatment modalities, children may have a higher frequency of responses.[110]

Combination Therapy

One report described the use of several different regimens, adapted from the treatment of patients with malignant lymphoma, in 10 patients with severe chronic refractory ITP; 5 had a complete response.[111] More recent reports have described 10 patients treated with even more intensive chemotherapy, either with[112-114] or without[115] peripheral blood stem cell support. Of these 10 patients, 4 had sustained remissions,[112,114] 5 had no response,[113,114] and 1 died.[115]

Other Treatments

Multiple other treatments have been used in patients with chronic refractory ITP. All are supported by anecdotal reports of success in a few patients but none can be advised for routine use. One case series reported on 14 patients treated with colchicine, 3 of whom had partial responses.[116] Vitamin C was studied following a serendipitous observation of an increased platelet count in a patient who took vitamin supplements;[117] later, multiple small case series reported a few patients with limited responses but most had no response.[1] One report of 72 patients treated with immunoadsorption by ex vivo perfusion of plasma through a protein A column reported that 22% of patients had a transient response;[118] others have reported much less favorable results and significantly greater toxicity, including debilitating vasculitis.[119,120] Seven patients treated with 2-chlorodeoxyidensine had no response.[121] Several reports have described success with interferon, but higher platelet counts were not sustained after treatment was discontinued.[122] Interferon may also exacerbate thrombocytopenia.[123] Other reports have suggested benefit from treatment with cyclosporine[124] and dapsone.[125]

Investigational Treatment

Early reports have described successful treatment in a few patients with rituxan,[126,126a] a murine monoclonal antibody to the surface CD20 antigen on B lymphocytes that is approved for treatment of low-grade lymphoma. A murine monoclonal antibody to a surface antigen on activated T cells, CD40 ligand, has also been reported to have success in a few patients with severe chronic refractory ITP.[127]

MANAGEMENT OF ITP IN PREGNANT WOMEN AND THEIR NEWBORN INFANTS

The diagnostic distinction between ITP and gestational thrombocytopenia, described above, is not relevant to management decisions. Mild thrombocytopenia, whatever the cause, requires no treatment; it can be expected to resolve following delivery. The indications for treatment during pregnancy are not different from treatment of any other patients with ITP, except for greater caution for any intervention. Treatment with prednisone and intermittent IVIg are considered safe and appropriate when severe, symptomatic thrombocytopenia is present.[1] Splenectomy may also be appropriate for severe, symptomatic thrombocytopenia unresponsive to prednisone and IVIg, though there is risk for inducing miscarriage early during pregnancy and premature labor later during pregnancy; there is also greater technical difficulty with splenectomy late during pregnancy because of the gravid uterus. Other than possibly exacerbating the severity of thrombocytopenia, pregnancy itself does not cause risk for the patient with ITP.

The major concern for a woman with ITP considering pregnancy is the risk for the newborn infant, who may be thrombocytopenic at birth from passive transfer of maternal antiplatelet antibodies and therefore may be at risk for bleeding. This risk occurs at delivery and during the first week of life; there is no risk for thrombocytopenic bleeding in utero, distinct from alloimmune thrombocytopenia, which can cause severe intrauterine fetal hemorrhage. Two recent reports have documented a correlation between the severity of maternal ITP and fetal platelet counts.[37,128] Maternal characteristics that predicted the occurrence of severe thrombocytopenia in the infant (platelet count below 50,000/μL) were a history of prior splenectomy and severe maternal thrombocytopenia (platelet count below 50,000/μL) during the pregnancy. If neither of these criteria were present, none of 23 infants had severe thrombocytopenia at birth; if one or both of these criteria were present, 8 of 41 infants had severe thrombocytopenia at birth.[129] In a review of all reports describing 10 or more women with ITP and the platelet counts of their infants at birth, 10% of infants had platelet counts below 50,000/μL at birth; 4% had platelet counts below 20,000/μL.[129]

In spite of the risk for neonatal thrombocytopenia, reports of intracranial hemorrhage among newborn infants are rare. Most intracranial hemorrhages may occur during the first several days after birth, not at birth.[129] This is because the platelet counts in infants born to mothers with ITP characteristically fall during the first few days following birth,[130] due to the rapid development of splenic function following birth. Hyposplenism at birth is documented by the appearance of pitted red cells and Howell-Jolly bodies in the circulation;[131] these signs correlate with the degree of prematurity of the infant and disappear within the first 2 months of life. Decreasing platelet counts following birth in infants born to mothers with ITP are similar to observations of infants born with hereditary spherocytosis, whose hemoglobin values are usually normal at birth but may decrease sharply during the first several weeks.[132] The important lesson from these observations is that most neonatal hemorrhage is preventable by careful observation of the infant's platelet count during the first weeks of life, with treatment of thrombocytopenia with glucocorticoids and IVIg as needed. These observations also support the current recommendation that caesarean section offers no advantage to the infant over routine vaginal delivery.[1,133]

■ REFERENCES

Chapter 9 References

1. George JN, Woolf SH, Raskob GE, et al. Idiopathic thrombocytopenic purpura: A practice guideline developed by explicit methods for the American Society of Hematology. Blood 1996;88:3–40.
2. George JN, Rizvi MA. Management issues in idiopathic thrombocytopenic purpura. In Alving BM (ed.): Blood Components and Pharmacologic Agents in the Treatment of Congenital and Acquired Bleeding Disorders. Bethesda, AABB Press, 2000, pp. 263–288.
3. Bolton-Maggs PHB, Moon I. Assessment of UK practice for management of acute childhood idiopathic thrombocytopenic purpura against published guidelines. Lancet 1997;350:620–623.
4. Frederiksen H, Schmidt K. The incidence of ITP in adults increases with age. Blood 1999;94:909–913.
5. Ballem PJ, Segal GM, Stratton JR, et al. Mechanisms of thrombocytopenia in chronic autoimmune thrombocytopenic purpura. Evidence for both impaired platelet production and increased platelet clearance. J Clin Invest 1987;80:33–40.
6. Harrington WJ, Minnich V, Hollingsworth JW, Moore CV. Demonstration of a thrombocytopenic factor in the blood of patients with thrombocytopenic purpura. J Lab Clin Med 1951;38:1.
7. Altman LK. Black and blue at the flick of a feather. Who Goes First? New York, Random House, 1987, pp. 273–282.
8. Shulman NR, Weinrach RS, Libre EP, Andrews HL. The role of the reticuloendothelial system in the pathogenesis of idiopathic thrombocytopenic purpura. Trans Assoc Am Physicians 1965;78:374–390.
9. Karpatkin S. Autoimmune (idiopathic) thrombocytopenic purpura. Lancet 1997;349:1531–1536.
10. Najean Y, Lecompte T. Hereditary thrombocytopenias in childhood. Semin Thromb Hemost 1995;21:294–304.
11. George JN. Platelet immunoglobulin G: Its significance for the evaluation of thrombocytopenia and for understanding the origin of alpha-granule proteins. Blood 1990;76:859–870.
12. Raife TJ, Olson JD, Lentz SR. Platelet antibody testing in idiopathic thrombocytopenic purpura. Blood 1997;89:1112–1113.
13. Berchtold P, Müller D, Beardsley D, et al. International study to compare antigen-specific methods used for the measurement of antiplatelet autoantibodies. Br J Haematol 1997;96:477–483.
14. Doan CA, Bouroncle BA, Wiseman BK. Idiopathic and secondary thrombocytopenic purpura: clinical study and evaluation of 381 cases over a period of 28 years. Ann Intern Med 1960;53:861–876.
15. McIntyre OR, Ebaugh FG Jr. Palpable spleens in college freshmen. Ann Intern Med 1967;66:301–306.
16. Calpin C, Dick P, Poon A, Feldman W. Is bone marrow aspiration needed in acute childhood idiopathic thrombocytopenic purpura to rule out leukemia? Arch Pediatr Adolesc Med 1998;152:345–347.
17. Payne BA, Pierre RV. Pseudothrombocytopenia: A laboratory artifact with potentially serious consequences. Mayo Clin Proc 1984;59:123–125.
18. Savage RA. Pseudoleukocytosis due to EDTA-induced platelet clumping. Am J Clin Pathol 1984;81:317–322.
19. Vicari A, Banfi G, Bonini PA. EDTA-dependent pseudothrombocytopaenia: A 12-month epidemiological study. Scand J Clin Lab Invest 1988;48:537–542.
20. Garcia Suarez J, Calero MA, Ricard MP, et al. EDTA-dependent pseudothrombocytopenia in ambulatory patients: Clinical characteristics and role of new automated cell-counting in its detection. Am J Hematol 1992;39:146–147.
21. Sweeney JD, Holme S, Heaton WAL, et al. Pseudothrombocytopenia in plateletpheresis donors. Transfusion 1995;35:46–49.
22. Bartels PCM, Schoorl M, Lombarts AJPF. Screening for EDTA-dependent deviations in platelet counts and abnormalities in platelet distribution histograms in pseudothrombocytopenia. Scand J Clin Lab Invest 1997;57:629–636.
23. Fiorin F, Steffan A, Pradella P, et al. IgG platelet antibodies in EDTA-dependent pseudothrombocytopenia bind to platelet membrane glycoprotein IIb. Am J Clin Pathol 1998;110:178–183.
24. Bizzaro N. EDTA-dependent pseudothrombocytopenia: A clinical and epidemiological study of 112 cases, with 10-year follow-up. Am J Hematol 1995;50:103–109.

25. George JN. Platelets. Lancet 2000;355:1531–1539.
26. Kjeldsberg CR, Swanson J. Platelet satellitism. Blood 1974;43: 831–836.
27. George JN, Raskob GE, Shah SR, et al. Drug-induced thrombocytopenia: A systematic review of published case reports. Ann Intern Med 1998;129:886–890.
28. Arnold J, Ouwehand WH, Smith G, Cohen H. A young woman with petechiae. Lancet 1998;352:618.
29. Azuno Y, Yaga K, Sasayama T, Kimoto K. Thrombocytopenia induced by *Jui*, a traditional Chinese herbal medicine. Lancet 1999;354:304–305.
30. Kojouri K, Perdue JJ, Medina PJ, George JN. Occult quinine-induced thrombocytopenia. Oklahoma State Med J 2000;93: 519–521.
31. Siroty RR. Purpura on the rocks—with a twist. JAMA 1976; 235:2521–2522.
32. Gentilini G, Curtis BR, Aster RH. An antibody from a patient with ranitidine-induced thrombocytopenia recognizes a site on glycoprotein IX that is a favored target for drug-induced antibodies. Blood 1998;92:2359–2365.
33. Burrows RF, Kelton JG. Fetal thrombocytopenia and its relation to maternal thrombocytopenia. N Engl J Med 1993;329:1463–1466.
34. Lescale KB, Eddleman KA, Cines DB, et al. Antiplatelet antibody testing in thrombocytopenic pregnant women. Am J Obstet Gynecol 1996;174:1014–1018.
35. Moise KJ. Autoimmune thrombocytopenic purpura in pregnancy. Clin Obstet Gynecol 1991;34:51–63.
36. Chaplin H, Cohen R, Bloomberg G, et al. Pregnancy and idiopathic autoimmune haemolytic anaemia: a prospective study during 6 months gestation and 3 months post-partum. Br J Haematol 1973;24:219–229.
37. Valat AS, Caulier MT, Devos P, et al. Relationships between severe neonatal thrombocytopenia and maternal characteristics in pregnancies associated with autoimmune thrombocytopenia. Br J Haematol 1998;103:397–401.
38. Aster RH. Pooling of platelets in the spleen: Role in the pathogenesis of "hypersplenic" thrombocytopenia. J Clin Invest 1966;45:645–657.
39. Martin TG III, Somberg KA, Meng YG, et al. Thrombopoietin levels in patients with cirrhosis before and after orthotopic liver transplantation. Ann Intern Med 1997;127:285–288.
40. Bahner I, Kearns K, Coutinho S, et al. Infection of human marrow stroma by human immunodeficiency virus-1 (HIV-1) is both required and sufficient for HIV-1-induced hematopoietic suppression in vitro: Demonstration by gene modification of primary human stroma. Blood 1997;90:1787–1798.
41. Oski FA, Naiman JL. Effect of live measles vaccine on the platelet count. N Engl J Med 1966;275:352–356.
42. Standaert SM, Dawson JE, Schaffner W, et al. Ehrlichiosis in a golf-oriented retirement community. N Engl J Med 1995; 333:420–425.
43. Drachman JG, Jarvik GP, Mehaffey MG. Autosomal dominant thrombocytopenia: incomplete megakaryocyte differentiation and linkage to human chromosome 10. Blood 2000;96:118–125.
44. Mhawech P, Saleem A. Inherited giant platelet disorders—classification and literature review. Am J Clin Pathol 2000; 113:176–190.
45. Noris P, Spedini P, Belletti S, et al. Thrombocytopenia, giant platelets, and leukocyte inclusion bodies (May-Hegglin anomaly): Clinical and laboratory findings. Am J Med 1998; 104:355–360.
46. Heyns A duP, Lotter MG, Badenhorst PN, et al. Kinetics of distribution and sites of destruction of ^{111}In-labeled human platelets. Br J Haematol 1980;44:269.
47. Young G, Luban NLC, White JG. Sebastian syndrome: Case report and review of the literature. Am J Hematol 1999;61:62–65.
48. Rocca B, Ranelletti FO, Maggiano N. Inherited macrothrombocytopenia with distinctive platelet ultrastructural and functional features. Thromb Haemost 2000;83:35–41.
49. Iolascon A, Perrotta S, Amendola G, et al. Familial dominant thrombocytopenia: Clinical, biologic, and molecular studies. Pediatr Res 1999;46:548–552.
50. Tonelli R, Strippoli P, Grossi A, et al. Hereditary thrombocytopenia due to reduced platelet production—report on two families and mutational screening of the thrombopoietin receptor gene (*c-mpl*). Thromb Haemost 2000;83:931–936.
51. Menke DM, Colon-Otero G, Cockerill KJ, et al. Refractory thrombocytopenia: A myelodysplastic syndrome that may mimic immune thrombocytopenic purpura. Am J Clin Pathol 1992; 98:502–510.
52. Mosesson MW, Colman RW, Sherry S. Chronic intravascular coagulation syndrome. Report of a case with special studies of an associated plasma cryoprecipitate ("cryofibrinogen"). N Engl J Med 1968;278:815–821.
53. Enjolras O, Wassef M, Mazoyer E, et al. Infants with Kasabach-Merritt syndrome do not have "true" hemangiomas. J Pediatr 1997;130:631–640.
54. Leach JW, Hussein KK, George JN. Acquired pure megakaryocytic aplasia: Report of two cases with long-term responses to antithymocyte globulin and cyclosporine. Am J Hematol 1999; 62:115–117.
55. Aggarwal A, Doolittle G. Autoimmune thrombocytopenic purpura associated with hyperthyroidism in a single individual. South Med J 1997;90:933–936.
56. Kurata Y, Miyagawa S, Kosugi S, et al. High-titer antinuclear antibodies, anti-SSA/Ro antibodies and antinuclear RNP antibodies in patients with idiopathic thrombocytopenic purpura. Thromb Haemost 1994;71:184–187.
57. Stasi R, Stipa E, Masi M, et al. Prevalence and clinical significance of elevated antiphospholipid antibodies in patients with idiopathic thrombocytopenic purpura. Blood 1994;84:4203–4208.
58. Lipp E, Von Felten A, Sax H, et al. Antibodies against platelet glycoproteins and antiphospholipid antibodies in autoimmune thrombocytopenia. Eur J Haematol 1998;60:283–288.
59. Crosby WH. Wet purpura, dry purpura. JAMA 1975;232: 744–745.
60. Slichter SJ, Harker LA. Thrombocytopenia: Mechanisms and management of defects in platelet production. Clin Haematol 1978;7:523–539.
61. Wandt H, Frank M, Ehninger G, et al. Safety and cost effectiveness of a 10×10^9/L trigger for prophylactic platelet transfusions compared with the traditional 20×10^9/L trigger: A prospective comparative trial in 105 patients with acute myeloid leukemia. Blood 1998;91:3601–3606.
62. Rebulla P, Finazzi G, Marangoni F, et al. The threshold for prophylactic platelet transfusions in adults with acute myeloid leukemia. N Engl J Med 1997;337:1870–1875.
63. Alberio L, Safa O, Clemetson KJ, et al. Surface expression and functional characterization of alpha-granule factor V in human platelets: effects of ionophore A23187, thrombin, collagen, and convulxin. Blood 2000;95:1694–1702.
64. Kitchens CS. Occult hemophilia. Johns Hopkins Med J 1980; 146:255–259.
65. Lilleyman JS. Management of childhood idiopathic thrombocytopenic purpura. Br J Haematol 1999;105:871–875.
66. Blanchette VS, Luke B, Andrew M, et al. A prospective, randomized trial of high-dose intravenous immune globulin G therapy, oral prednisone therapy, and no therapy in childhood acute immune thrombocytopenic purpura. J Pediatr 1993;123:989–995.
67. Vesely S, Buchanan GR, George JN, et al. Self-reported diagnostic and management strategies in childhood idiopathic thrombocytopenic purpura: Results of a survey of practicing pediatric hematology/oncology specialists. Am J Pediatr Hematol Oncol 2000;22:55–61.

68. Kattamis AC, Shankar S, Cohen AR. Neurologic complications of treatment of childhood acute immune thrombocytopenic purpura with intravenously administered immunoglobulin G. J Pediatr 1997;130:281–283.
69. Reid MM. Chronic idiopathic thrombocytopenic purpura: incidence, treatment, and outcome. Arch Dis Child 1995;72:125–128.
70. Gaston MH, Verter JI, Woods G, et al. Prophylaxis with oral penicillin in children with sickle cell anemia: a randomized trial. N Engl J Med 1986;314:1593–1599.
71. Guthrie TH, Brannan DP, Prisant LM. Idiopathic thrombocytopenic purpura in the older adult patient. Am J Med Sci 1988;296:17–21.
72. Cortelazzo S, Finazzi G, Buelli M, et al. High risk of severe bleeding in aged patients with chronic idiopathic thrombocytopenic purpura. Blood 1991;77:31–33.
73. Stasi R, Stipa E, Masi M, et al. Long-term observation of 208 adults with chronic idiopathic thrombocytopenic purpura. Am J Med 1995;98:436–442.
73a. Portielje JEA, Westendorp RGJ, Kluin-Nelemans HC, et al. Morbidity and mortality in adults with idiopathic thrombocytopenic purpura. Blood 2001;97:2549–2554.
74. Bellucci S, Charpak Y, Chastang C, Tobelem G. Low doses v conventional doses of corticoids in immune thrombocytopenic purpura (ITP): Results of a randomized clinical trial in 160 children, 223 adults. Blood 1988;71:1165–1169.
75. Lukert BP, Raisz LG. Glucocorticoid-induced osteoporosis: Pathogenesis and management. Ann Intern Med 1990;112:352–364.
76. Reid IR. Glucocorticoid osteoporosis—mechanisms and management. Eur J Endocrinol 1997;137:209–217.
77. Wanachiwanawin W, Piankijagum A, Sindhvananda K, et al. Emergency splenectomy in adult idiopathic thrombocytopenic purpura. A report of seven cases. Arch Intern Med 1989;149:217–219.
78. Carr JM, Kruskall MS, Kaye JA, Robinson SH. Efficacy of platelet transfusions in immune thrombocytopenia. Am J Med 1986;80:1051–1054.
79. Abrahm J, Ellman L. Platelet transfusion in immune thrombocytopenic purpura. JAMA 1976;236:1847.
80. McMillan R. Therapy for adults with refractory chronic immune thrombocytopenic purpura. Ann Intern Med 1997;126:307–314.
81. Baumann MA, Menitove JE, Aster RH, Anderson T. Urgent treatment of idiopathic thrombocytopenic purpura with single-dose gammaglobulin infusion followed by platelet transfusion. Ann Intern Med 1986;104:808–809.
82. Sekul EA, Cupler EJ, Dalakas MC. Aseptic meningitis associated with high-dose intravenous immunoglobulin therapy: Frequency and risk factors. Ann Intern Med 1994;121:259–262.
83. Windrum P, Bharucha C, Desai ZR. Intravenous immunoglobulin therapy and renal dysfunction. Br J Haematol 1998;101:592–592.
84. Epstein JS, Zoon KC. FDA Important Drug Warning: Acute renal failure associated with the administration of immune globulin intravenous (Human IGIV) products. FDA Warning Letter to Physicians 1998.
85. Scaradavou A, Woo B, Woloski BMR, et al. Intravenous anti-D treatment of immune thrombocytopenic purpura: Experience in 272 patients. Blood 1997;89:2689–2700.
86. Gaines AR. Acute onset hemoglobinemia and/or hemoglobinuria and sequelae following RHo(D) immune globulin intravenous administration in immune thrombocytopenic purpura patients. Blood 2000;95:2523–2529.
87. Law C, Marcaccio M, Tam P, et al. High-dose intravenous immune globulin and the response to splenectomy in patients with idiopathic thrombocytopenic purpura. N Engl J Med 1997;336:1494–1498.
88. Schneider P, Wehmeier A, Schneider W. High-dose intravenous immune globulin and the response to splenectomy in patients with idiopathic thrombocytopenic purpura. N Engl J Med 1997;337:1087–1088.
89. Rovo A, Penchasky D, Korin J, et al. Splenectomy in idiopathic thrombocytopenic purpura (ITP). Effective, yes, but for how long? Blood. 1998;92:177a.
90. Schilling RF. Estimating the risk for sepsis after splenectomy in hereditary spherocytosis. Ann Intern Med 1995;122:187–188.
91. Lortan JE. Management of asplenic patients. Br J Haematol 1993;84:566–569.
92. George JN, Kojouri K, Perdue JJ, Vesely SK. Management of patients with chronic, refractory idiopathic thrombocytopenic purpura. Semin Hematol 2000;37:1–10.
93. Woolf SH. Shared decision-making: the case for letting patients decide which choice is best. J Fam Prac 1997;45:205–208.
94. Andersen JC. Response of resistant idiopathic thrombocytopenic purpura to pulsed high-dose dexamethasone therapy. N Engl J Med 1994;330:1560–1564.
95. Caulier MT, Rose C, Roussel MT, et al. Pulsed high-dose dexamethasone in refractory chronic idiopathic thrombocytopenic purpura: A report on 10 cases. Br J Haematol 1995;91:477–479.
96. Demiroglu H, Dündar S. High-dose pulsed dexamethasone for immune thrombocytopenia. N Engl J Med 1997;337:425–426.
97. Verlin M, Laros RK, Penner JA. Treatment of refractory thrombocytopenic purpura with cyclophosphamide. Am J Hematol 1976;1:97–104.
98. Pizzuto J, Ambriz R. Therapeutic experience on 934 adults with idiopathic thrombocytopenic purpura: multicentric trial of the cooperative Latin American group on hemostasis and thrombosis. Blood 1984;64:1179–1183.
99. Reiner A, Gernsheimer T, Slichter SJ. Pulse cyclophosphamide therapy for refractory autoimmune thrombocytopenic purpura. Blood 1995;85:351–358.
100. Ahn YS, Harrington WJ, Mylvaganam R, et al. Slow infusion of vinca alkaloids in the treatment of idiopathic thrombocytopenic purpura. Ann Intern Med 1984;100:192–196.
101. Fenaux P, Quiquandon I, Caulier MT, et al. Slow infusions of vinblastine in the treatment of adult idiopathic thrombocytopenic purpura: a report on 43 cases. Blut 1990;60:238–241.
102. Facon T, Caulier MT, Wattel E, et al. A randomized trial comparing vinblastine in slow infusion and by bolus i.v. injection in idiopathic thrombocytopenic purpura: A report on 42 patients. Br J Haematol 1994;86:678–680.
103. Quiquandon I, Fenaux P, Caulier MT, et al. Re-evaluation of the role of azathioprine in the treatment of adult chronic idiopathic thrombocytopenic purpura: a report on 53 cases. Br J Haematol 1990;74:223–228.
104. Ahn YS, Mylvaganam R, Garcia RO, et al. Low-dose danazol therapy in idiopathic thrombocytopenic purpura. Ann Intern Med 1987;107:177–181.
105. Ahn YS, Harrington WJ, Simon SR, et al. Danazol for the treatment of idiopathic thrombocytopenic purpura. N Engl J Med 1983;308:1396–1399.
106. McVerry BA, Auger M, Bellingham AJ. The use of danazol in the management of chronic immune thrombocytopenic purpura. Br J Haematol 1985;61:145–148.
107. Ambriz R, Pizzuto J, Morales M, et al. Therapeutic effect of danazol on metrorrhagia in patients with idiopathic thrombocytopenic purpura (ITP). Nouv Rev Fr Hematol 1986;28:275–279.
108. Arrowsmith JB, Dreis M. Thrombocytopenia after treatment with Danazol. N Engl J Med 1986;314:585–585.
109. Rabinowe SN, Miller KB. Danazol-induced thrombocytopenia. Br J Haematol 1987;65:383–384.
110. Facon T, Caulier MT, Fenaux P, et al. Accessory spleen in recurrent chronic immune thrombocytopenic purpura. Am J Hematol 1992;41:184–189.
111. Figueroa M, Gehlsen J, Hammond D, et al. Combination chemotherapy in refractory immune thrombocytopenic purpura. N Engl J Med 1993;328:1226–1129.

112. Lim SH, Kell J, Al-Sabah A, et al. Peripheral blood stem-cell transplantation for refractory autoimmune thrombocytopenic purpura. Lancet 1997;349:475–475.
113. Skoda RC, Tichelli A, Tyndall A, et al. Autologous peripheral blood stem cell transplantation in a patient with chronic autoimmune thrombocytopenia. Br J Haematol 1997;99:56–57.
114. Nakamura R, Huhn RD, Read EJ, et al. Intensive immunosuppression with high-dose cyclophosphamide and autologous CD34+ selected hematopoietic cell support for chronic refractory autoimmune thrombocytopenia (AITP): interim report. Blood 1999;94:646a.
115. Brodsky R, Petri M, Smith BD, et al. Immunoablative high-dose cyclophosphamide without stem cell rescue for refractory, severe autoimmune disease. Ann Intern Med 1998;129:1031–1035.
116. Strother SV, Zuckerman KS, LoBuglio AF. Colchicine therapy for refractory idiopathic thrombocytopenic purpura. Arch Intern Med 1984;144:2198–2200.
117. Brox AG, Howson-Jan K, Fauser AA. Treatment of idiopathic thrombocytopenic purpura with ascorbate. Br J Haematol 1988; 70:341–344.
118. Snyder HW, Cochran SK, Balint JP, et al. Experience with protein A-immunoadsorption in treatment-resistant adult immune thrombocytopenic purpura. Blood 1992;79:2237–2245.
119. Cahill MR, Macey MG, Cavenagh JD, Newland AC. Protein A immunoadsorption in chronic refractory ITP reverses increased platelet activation but fails to achieve sustained clinical benefit. Br J Haematol 1998; 100:358–364.
120. Kabisch A, Kroll H, Wedi B, et al. Severe adverse effects of protein A immunoadsorption. Lancet 1994;343:116.
121. Figueroa M, McMillan R. 2-chlorodeoxyadenosine in the treatment of chronic refractory immune thrombocytopenic purpura. Blood 1993;81:3484–3485.
122. Fujimura K, Takafuta T, Kuriya S, et al. Recombinant human interferon α-2b (rh IFNα-2b) therapy for steroid resistant idiopathic thrombocytopenic purpura (ITP). Am J Hematol 1996;51:37–44.
123. Vianelli N, Tazzari PL, Baravelli S, et al. Interferon-alpha2b is not effective in the treatment of refractory immune thrombocytopenic purpura. Haematologica 1998;83:761–763.
124. Shirota T, Yamamoto H, Fujimoto H, et al. Cyclic thrombocytopenia in a patient treated with cyclosporine for refractory idiopathic thrombocytopenic purpura. Am J Hematol 1997; 56:272–276.
125. Godeau B, Durand JM, Roudot-Thoraval F, et al. Dapsone for chronic autoimmune thrombocytopenic purpura: A report of 66 cases. Br J Haematol 1997;97:336–339.
126. Perotta A, Sunneberg TA, Scott J, et al. Rituxan in the treatment of chronic idiopathic thrombocytopenic purpura (ITP). Blood 1999;94:14a.
126a. Stasi R, Pagano A, Stipa E, et al. Rituximab chimeric anti-CD20 monoclonal antibody treatment for adults with chronic idiopathic thrombocytopenic purpura. Blood 2001;98:952–957.
127. George JN, Raskob GE, Bussel J, et al. Safety and effect on platelet count of repeated doses of monoclonal antibody to CD40 ligand in patients with chronic ITP. Blood 1999;94:19a.
128. Payne SD, Resnik R, Moore TR, et al. Maternal characteristics and risk of severe neonatal thrombocytopenia and intracranial hemorrhage in pregnancies complicated by autoimmune thrombocytopenia. Am J Obstet Gynecol 1997;177:149–155.
129. Burrows RF, Kelton JG. Pregnancy in patients with idiopathic thrombocytopenic purpura: Assessing the risks for the infant at delivery. Obstet Gynecol Surv 1993;48 (12):781–788.
130. Burrows RF, Kelton JG. Low fetal risks in pregnancies associated with idiopathic thrombocytopenic purpura. Am J Obstet Gynecol 1990;163:1147–1150.
131. Holroyde CP, Oski FA, Gardner FH. The "pocked" erythrocyte. Red cell alterations in reticuloendothelial immaturity of the neonate. N Engl J Med 1969;281:516–520.
132. Delhommeau F, Cynober T, Schischmanoff PO, et al. Natural history of hereditary spherocytosis during the first year of life. Blood 2000;95:393–397.
133. Silver RM, Branch DW, Scott JR. Maternal thrombocytopenia in pregnancy: Time for a reassessment. Am J Obstet Gynecol 1995;173:479–482.

CHAPTER 10

Disorders of Platelet Function

A. Koneti Rao, M.D.

Hemostasis encompasses a series of inter-related and simultaneously occurring events involving the blood vessel, platelets, and coagulation system. Defects affecting any of these major participants may lead to a hemostatic defect and a bleeding disorder. This chapter will focus on the disorders related to impairment in platelet function.

OVERVIEW OF PHYSIOLOGY

Following injury to the blood vessel, platelets adhere to exposed subendothelium by a process (adhesion) that involves the interaction of a plasma protein, von Willebrand factor (vWF), and a specific glycoprotein complex on the platelet surface, glycoprotein Ib-IX-V (GPIb-IX-V) (Fig. 10–1). Adhesion is followed by recruitment of additional platelets, which form clumps, a process called aggregation (cohesion). This involves binding of fibrinogen to specific platelet surface receptors—a complex composed of glycoproteins IIb-IIIa (GPIIb-IIIa). Activated platelets release contents of their granules (secretion or release reaction), such as adenosine diphosphate (ADP) and serotonin from the dense granules, which causes recruitment of additional platelets. In addition, platelets play a major role in coagulation mechanisms; several key enzymatic reactions occur on the platelet membrane lipoprotein surface. A number of physiologic agonists interact with specific receptors on platelet surface to induce responses, including a change in platelet shape from discoid to spherical (shape change), aggregation, secretion, and thromboxane A_2 (TxA_2) production. Other agonists, such as prostacyclin, inhibit these responses. Ligation of the platelet receptors initiates the production or release of several intracellular messenger molecules, including Ca^{2+} ions, products of phosphoinositide (PI) hydrolysis by phospholipase C (diacylglycerol [DAG], and inositol 1,4,5-triphosphate [InP_3]), TxA_2, and cyclic nucleotides (cAMP) (Fig. 10–1). These induce or modulate the various platelet responses of Ca^{2+} mobilization, protein phosphorylation, aggregation, secretion, and liberation of arachidonic acid. The interaction between the agonist receptors and the key intracellular effector enzymes (e.g., phospholipases A_2 and C, adenylyl cyclase) is mediated by a group of GTP-binding proteins which are modulated by GTP. As in most secretory cells, platelet activation results in a rise in cytoplasmic ionized calcium concentration; $InsP_3$ functions as a messenger to mobilize Ca^{2+} from intracellular stores. Diacylglycerol activates protein kinase C (PKC) and this results in the phosphorylation of a 47-kD protein pleckstrin. PKC activation is considered to play a major role in platelet secretion and in the activation of GP IIb-IIIa. Numerous other mechanisms, such as activation of tyrosine kinases and phosphatases, are also triggered by platelet activation but are beyond the scope of this chapter. Either inherited or acquired defects in the above platelet mechanisms may lead to impaired platelet function in hemostasis.

DISORDERS OF PLATELET FUNCTION

Disorders of platelet function are characterized by highly variable mucocutaneous bleeding manifestations and excessive hemorrhage following surgical procedures or trauma. A majority of patients, but not all, have a prolonged bleeding time. Platelet aggregation and secretion studies provide evidence for the defect but are not always predictive of the severity of clinical manifestations. Defects in platelet function may be inherited or acquired, with the latter being far more commonly encountered. The platelet dysfunction in these patients arises by diverse mechanisms.[1–3]

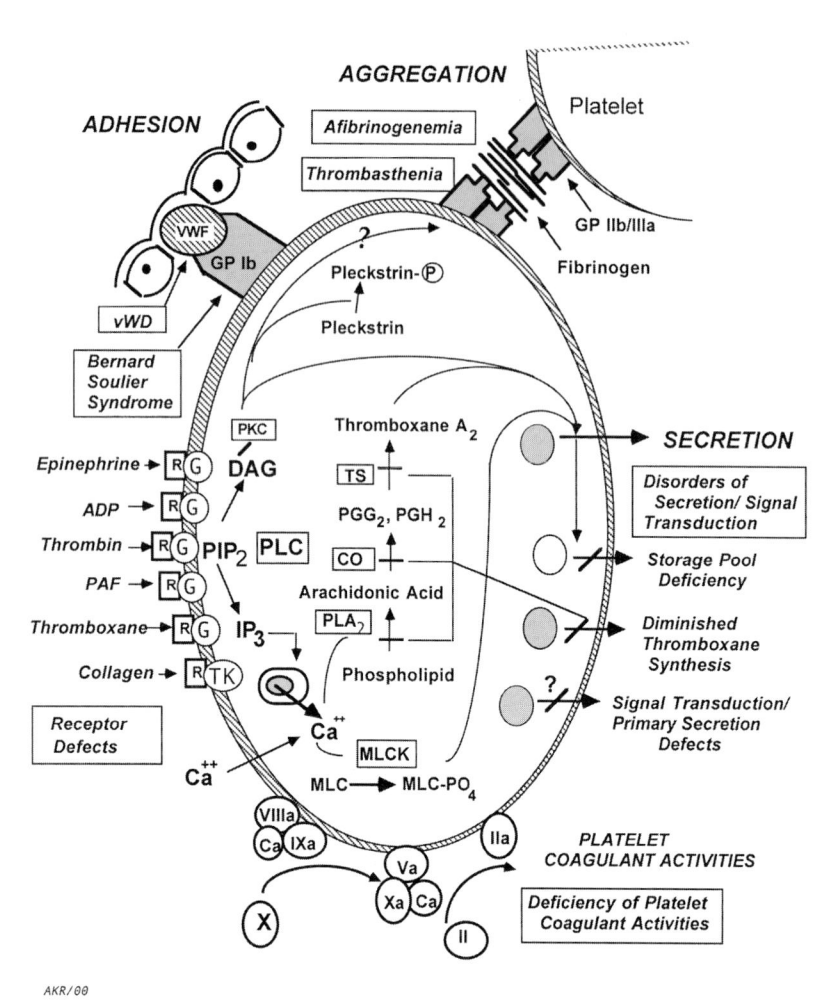

Figure 10–1 A schematic representation of the normal platelet responses and the congenital disorders of platelet function. CO, cyclo-oxygenase; DAG, diacylglycerol; IP₃, inositoltrisphosphate; MLC, myosin light chain; MLCK, myosin light chain kinase; PAF, platelet activating factor; PIP₂ phosphatidylinositol bisphosphate; PKC, protein kinase C; PLC, phospholipase C; PLA₂, phospholipase A₂; TS, thromboxane synthase; vWF, von Willebrand factor; vWD, von Willebrand disease.

Congenital Disorders of Platelet Function

Table 10–1 provides a classification based on abnormality of any of the multiple platelet functions or responses that are depicted in Figure 10–1. Although some of these disorders are rare, studies leading to the discovery of their defects have shed enormous light on platelet physiology. In patients with defects in platelet–vessel wall interactions, adhesion of platelets to subendothelium is abnormal. The two disorders in this group are von Willebrand disease (vWD), due to a deficiency or abnormality in plasma vWF,[4] and the Bernard-Soulier syndrome, in which platelets are deficient in GPIb (and GPV and IX) and thus the binding of vWF to platelets is abnormal.[5] Disorders characterized by abnormal platelet–platelet interactions (aggregation) arise because of a severe deficiency of plasma fibrinogen (congenital afibrinogenemia) or because of a quantitative or qualitative abnormality of the platelet membrane GPIIb-IIIa complex (Glanzmann thrombasthenia).[6] Patients with defects in platelet secretion and signal transduction are a heterogeneous group lumped together for convenience of classification rather than on the basis of an understanding of the specific underlying abnormality. The major common characteristic in these patients, as currently perceived, is an inability to release intracellular granule (dense) contents upon activation of platelet-rich plasma with agonists such as ADP, epinephrine, and collagen. In aggregation studies the second wave of aggregation is blunted or absent. A small proportion of these patients have a deficiency of dense-granule stores (storage pool deficiency). In some of the other patients, the impaired secretion results from aberrations in the signal transduction events that govern end responses such as secretion and aggregation. Lastly are the patients who have an abnormality in interactions of platelets with proteins of the coagulation system; the best described is the Scott syndrome.[7] In addition to the above groups, there are patients who have abnormal platelet function associated with systemic disorders such as Down syndrome and the May-Hegglin anomaly where the specific aberrant platelet mechanisms are still unclear.

Disorders of Platelet Adhesion

Bernard-Soulier Syndrome. The Bernard-Soulier syndrome is a rare autosomal recessive platelet function disorder resulting from an abnormality in platelet GPIb-IX-V complex which normally mediates the binding of

Table 10-1 • CLASSIFICATION OF CONGENITAL DISORDERS OF PLATELET FUNCTION

1. Defects in platelet–vessel wall interaction (disorders of adhesion)
   a. von Willebrand disease (deficiency or defect in plasma vWF)
   b. Bernard-Soulier syndrome (deficiency or defect in GPIb)
2. Defects in platelet–platelet interaction (disorders of aggregation)
   a. Congenital afibrinogenemia (absence of plasma fibrinogen)
   b. Glanzmann thrombasthenia (deficiency or defect in GPIIb-IIIa)
3. Disorders of platelet secretion and signal transduction
   a. Abnormalities of granules
      i. Storage pool deficiency
      ii. Quebec platelet disorder
   b. Signal transduction defects (primary secretion defects)
      i. Defects in platelet–agonist interaction (receptor defects)
         Receptor defects: thromboxane A$_2$, collagen, ADP, epinephrine
      ii. Defects in G-protein activation
         Gαq deficiency
      iii. Defects in phosphatidylinositol metabolism
         Phospholipase C-β2 deficiency
      iv. Defects in calcium mobilization
      v. Defects in protein phosphorylation (pleckstrin)
   c. Abnormalities in arachidonic acid pathways and thromboxane A$_2$ synthesis
      i. Impaired liberation of arachidonic acid
      ii. Cyclo-oxygenase deficiency
      iii. Thromboxane synthase deficiency
   d. Defects in cytoskeletal regulation
      Wiskott-Aldrich syndrome
4. Disorders of platelet coagulant–protein interaction
   a. Defect in factor Va–Xa interaction on platelets (Scott syndrome)

vWF to platelets and thus plays a major role in platelet adhesion to the subendothelium, especially at the higher shear rates.[5] GPIb exists in platelets as a complex consisting of GPIb, GPIX, and GPV. There are 25,000 copies of GPIb-IX-V on platelets and these are reduced or abnormal in the Bernard-Soulier syndrome. Although GPV is also decreased in platelets of patients with the Bernard-Soulier syndrome, it is not required for GPIb-IX expression. The bleeding time is markedly prolonged in patients with the Bernard-Soulier syndrome. The platelet counts are moderately decreased, and on the peripheral smear, the platelets are markedly increased in size. In platelet aggregation studies, the responses to the commonly used agonists ADP, epinephrine, thrombin, and collagen are normal. Characteristically, the aggregation in platelet-rich plasma in response to ristocetin is decreased or absent, a feature shared with patients with vWD.

Disorders of Platelet Aggregation

Glanzmann Thrombasthenia. Glanzmann thrombasthenia is a rare autosomal recessive disorder characterized by markedly impaired platelet aggregation, a prolonged bleeding time, and relatively more severe mucocutaneous bleeding manifestations than most platelet function disorders.[8] It has been reported in clusters in populations in which consanguinity is common.

Normal resting platelets possess approximately 80,000 GPIIb-IIIa complexes on the surface. The primary abnormality in thrombasthenia is a quantitative or qualitative defect in the GPIIb-IIIa complex on platelets. GPIIb-IIIa complex is a heterodimer consisting of GPIIb and GPIIIa whose synthesis is governed by distinct genes located on chromosome 17. The primary abnormality leading to thrombasthenia may be a defect in GPIIb or GPIIIa genes resulting in decreased expression of the complex on the platelet surface. A variety of distinct mutations involving GPIIb and GPIIIa have been described in patients with thrombasthenia.[9] Because of this, fibrinogen binding to platelets on activation and aggregation are impaired. Moreover, the spreading of platelets along the subendothelium, mediated by GPIIb-IIIa binding to fibronectin and vWF, is also decreased. Clot retraction, a function of the interaction of the GPIIb-IIIa with the platelet cytoskeleton, is also impaired.

The diagnostic hallmark of thrombasthenia is absence or marked decrease of platelet aggregation in response to various platelet agonists with absence of both the primary and secondary wave of aggregation, while aggregation in response to ristocetin is preserved. The shape change response is preserved; platelet size and number are normal. Heterozygotes have approximately half the number of platelet GPIIb-IIIa complexes and platelet aggregation responses are normal. Although congenital afibrinogenemia is also characterized by absence of platelet aggregation, in this disorder both prothrombin time (PT) and activated partial thromboplastin time (aPTT) are markedly prolonged, while they are normal in thrombasthenia.

Disorders of Platelet Secretion and Signal Transduction

As an unifying theme, patients lumped in this heterogeneous group generally manifest impaired secretion of granule contents and absence of the second wave of aggregation upon stimulation of platelet-rich plasma with ADP and epinephrine; responses to collagen, thromboxane analog (U46619), arachidonic acid, and platelet-activating factor (PAF) may also be impaired. Platelet function is abnormal in these patients either when the granule contents are diminished (storage pool deficiency, SPD) or when there is an aberration in the activation mechanisms governing aggregation and secretion (Table 10–1).

Deficiency of Granule Stores. The term *storage pool deficiency* (SPD) refers to a deficiency in platelet content of dense granules (δ-SPD), α-granules (α-SPD), or both types of granules ($\alpha\delta$-SPD).[3,10] The Quebec platelet disorder is an autosomal dominant disorder associated with abnormal proteolysis of α-granule proteins, deficiency of platelet α-granule multimerin (a factor V binding protein), and markedly impaired aggregation with epinephrine as a striking feature.[10]

Defects in Platelet Signal Transduction (Primary Secretion Defects). Signal transduction mechanisms encompass processes that are initiated by the interaction of agonists with specific platelet receptors and include responses such as G-protein activation and activation of effector enzymes such as phospholipase C and phospholipase A_2. If the key components in signal transduction are the surface receptors, the G proteins, and the effectors, evidence now exists for specific platelet abnormalities at each of these levels.

Defects in Platelet-Agonist Interaction: Receptor Defects. These patients have impaired responses because of an abnormality in the platelet surface receptor for a specific agonist. Such receptor defects have been documented for epinephrine[11] collagen,[12–15] ADP,[16–18] and thromboxane A_2.[19–22] Hirata et al.[19] have described an Arg 60 to Leu mutation of the human TxA_2 receptor in a dominantly inherited bleeding disorder. Patients described by Cattaneo et al.[16,18] and Nurden et al.[17] have a defect in the interaction of ADP with one of its receptors. Because ADP and TxA_2 play a synergistic role in platelet responses to several agonists, patients with these receptor defects manifest abnormal responses to multiple agonists. A few patients have been described in whom platelet responses to only collagen are blunted which are associated with deficiencies in membrane glycoproteins including GPIa and GPVI.[12–15] GPVI deficient platelets have been reported to have impaired collagen activation of Syk but not c-Src.[23]

Defects in G-Protein Activation. G proteins are a heterogeneous group of proteins that link surface receptors and intracellular effector enzymes, and constitute an important potential aberrant locus leading to platelet dysfunction. Convincing evidence for such a defect has been provided by Gabbeta et al.[24] in a patient with a mild bleeding disorder, abnormal aggregation and secretion responses to a number of agonists, and diminished GTPase activity (a reflection of G-protein α-subunit function) on activation. This patient had a selective decrease in platelet membrane $G\alpha q$ subunit with normal levels of Gi_2, $G\alpha_{12}$, $G\alpha_{13}$, and $G\alpha_z$. She has been reported to have impaired Ca^{2+} mobilization[25] and diminished release of free arachidonic acid from phospholipids on platelet activation.[26] Essentially identical abnormal platelet findings have been reported in $G\alpha q$ deficient knock-out mice.[27] Impaired G-protein activation has also been reported in patients with the TxA_2 receptor defect.[20, 21]

Defects in Phospholipase C Activation, Calcium Mobilization and Pleckstrin Phosphorylation. Several patients have been identified who have a relatively mild bleeding diathesis and impaired dense-granule secretion, although their platelets have normal granule stores and, in general, synthesize substantial amounts of TxA_2.[28,29] On laboratory testing, these patients have abnormal aggregation and secretion, particularly in response to weaker agonists (ADP, epinephrine, PAF); the response to relatively stronger agonists such as arachidonate and high concentrations of collagen may be normal. Such patients are far more common than those with SPD or defects in TxA_2 synthesis. Lages and Weiss[28] have described eight such patients who had decreased initial rates and extents of aggregation in response to ADP, epinephrine, and U44069. Defects in early platelet activation events were postulated in these patients. These investigators subsequently demonstrated a defect in phosphatidylinositol hydrolysis and phosphatidic acid formation,[30] and in pleckstrin phosphorylation[31] in one patient.

An early response to platelet stimulation is the rise in cytoplasmic Ca^{2+} concentration. Therefore, attention has been focused on this process to explain the impaired aggregation and secretion. In several patients, defects in calcium mobilization have been proposed based on impaired platelet responses to the calcium ionophore $(A23187)^1$; however, this evidence is indirect, at best. Direct evidence has been provided that some of these patients have impaired Ca^{2+} mobilization upon platelet activation.[25,32] Detailed studies in two patients with impaired aggregation and secretion revealed that resting cytoplasmic Ca^{2+} concentration was normal, but the peak Ca^{2+} concentrations following activation with ADP, collagen, PAF, or thrombin were diminished[32] with abnormalities in both the release of Ca^{2+} from intracellular stores and in the influx of extracellular Ca^{2+}.[25] Further studies showed a defect in platelet formation of InP_3 (the key intracellular mediator of Ca^{2+} release) and diacylglycerol, and in pleckstrin phosphorylation,[33] indicating a defect in phospholipase C (PLC) activation. Human platelets contain at least seven PLC isozymes in the quantitative order PLC-γ2> PLC-β2> PLC-β3> PLC-β1> PLC-γ1> PLC-δ1>PLC-β4.[34] Studies in one of these patients revealed a selective deficiency in PLC-β2 with normal levels of other PLC isoforms.[34] These studies provide strong evidence that PLC-β2, a G protein-linked PLC isozyme, plays a major physiologic role in platelet responses to activation. In line with these studies, the knock-out mice deficient in PLC-β2 have impaired Ca^{2+} mobilization in neutrophils.[35]

Several other studies provide evidence for defects in signaling mechanisms, phosphatidylinositol metabolism, and protein phosphorylation in patients with abnormal platelet aggregation and secretion.[30,31,36,37] Another patient has been described with impaired platelet responses and diminished phosphoinositide metabolism in whom the altered stimulus–response coupling has been attributed to abnormal membrane phospholipid composition.[38] Fuse et al.[21] have reported a patient with a mild bleeding disorder whose platelets had impaired aggregation, secretion, InP_3 formation, and Ca^{2+} mobilization in response to a TxA_2 mimetic (STA_2) associated with normal TxA_2 formation. Interestingly, GTPase activity upon activation with STA_2 was also impaired, leading to the conclusion that the platelets had an abnormality in coupling between TxA_2 receptor and PLC. In the patient described by Mitsui et al.,[37] the abnormal platelet aggregation was associated with decreased TxA_2-induced InP_3 formation but with normal TxA_2 receptors and GTPase activity on stimulation with TxA_2 analog U46619, suggesting an abnormality in PLC activity downstream of the receptor. In an analysis of five patients with absent TxA$_2$-induced aggregation, Fuse et al.[22] found evidence for a receptor defect in three patients; in the other two the primary abnormality appeared distal to the receptor. Together, the above studies provide evidence for abnormalities in signal transduction pathways in patients with diminished platelet aggregation and secretion responses.

Yang et al.[29] have summarized detailed studies on signaling mechanisms in eight patients with abnormal aggregation and secretion in response to several different surface receptor-mediated agonists despite presence of normal dense-granule contents. Both PKC-induced pleckstrin phosphorylation and cytoplasmic Ca^{2+} mobilization play a major role in aggregation secretion on activation. Receptor-mediated Ca^{2+} mobilization and/or pleckstrin phosphorylation were abnormal in seven of the patients. Combined platelet activation with a cell-permeable direct PKC activator DiC$_8$ and ionophore A23187, which possibly bypass two major intracellular mediators (InP$_3$, diacylglycerol), induced normal secretion in platelet-rich plasma in all patients, suggesting that the ultimate process of exocytosis or secretion per se is intact and impaired secretion in these patients results from abnormalities in early signal transduction events.

Signal Transduction Defects and Activation of GPIIb-IIIa Complex. Activation of GPIIb-IIIa and platelet fibrinogen binding, a prerequisite for aggregation, is a signal transduction-dependent process and has been linked to PKC activation. Therefore, it is likely that abnormalities in signaling mechanisms may impair the activation of GPIIb-IIIa on platelets. Evidence that this is indeed the case is provided by the decreased activation of otherwise normal platelet GPIIb-IIIa complexes in a patient with markedly abnormal platelet aggregation and impaired pleckstrin phosphorylation.[39] The number and ligand-binding capacity of the GPIIb-IIIa complex were intact. A similar abnormality in GPIIb-IIIa activation has been observed in platelets with the Gαq deficiency,[24] attesting to the role of Gαq in GPIIb-IIIa activation. Moreover, the defect in GPIIb-IIIa activation provides a cogent explanation for abnormalities in initial aggregation responses noted by Lages and Weiss[28] in a number of their patients. Diminished activation of GPIIb-IIIa secondary to upstream signal transduction defects may be a more common mechanism than defects in the GPIIb-IIIa complex per se in patients with blunted aggregation.[24]

Abnormalities in Arachidonic Acid Pathways and Thromboxane Production. A major platelet response to activation is liberation of arachidonic acid from phospholipids and its subsequent oxygenation to TxA$_2$. TxA$_2$ production plays a synergistic role in the response to several agonists. Patients have been described with impaired liberation of arachidonic acid from membrane phospholipids during platelet stimulation.[24,26,36] Several patients have been described with platelet dysfunction associated with congenital deficiencies of cyclo-oxygenase and thromboxane synthase.[1]

Defects in Cytoskeletal Assembly. The Wiskott-Aldrich syndrome (WAS) is an X-linked inherited disorder affecting T lymphocytes and platelets and characterized by thrombocytopenia, immunodeficiency, and eczema.[40] Several platelet abnormalities, including dense-granule deficiency, have been reported in WAS. WAS arises from mutations in the gene coding for a novel protein of 502 amino acids that binds to several other signaling proteins, including Cdc42 (a GTPase) and p47nck (a SH3-containing adapter protein).[40,41] This protein constitutes a link between the cytoskeleton and signaling pathways, and is a key regulator of cytoskeletal assembly.[41]

Disorders of Platelet Procoagulant Activities

Platelets play a major role in blood coagulation by providing the surface on which several specific key enzymatic reactions occur.[42,43] In resting platelets, there is an asymmetry in the distribution of some of the phospholipids such that phosphatidylserine (PS) and phosphatidylethanolamine (PE) are located predominantly on the inner leaflet, while phosphatidylcholine (PC) has the opposite distribution. The asymmetry is maintained by an aminophospholipid translocase. Platelet activation results in a redistribution with expression of PS on the outer surface, mediated by an enzyme, phospholipid scramblase.[42] The exposure of PS on the outer surface is an important event in the expression of platelet procoagulant activities. A few patients have described in whom the platelet contribution to blood coagulation is impaired, and this is referred to as the Scott syndrome.[42,44] In these patients, who have a bleeding disorder, the bleeding time and platelet aggregation responses have been normal along with a normal PT and PTT. However, the *serum* PT has been abnormally short. In the patient described by Weiss et al.,[44] platelet factor Xa binding sites as well as the binding of factors IXa and VIIIa were diminished associated with a decreased surface expression of PS following platelet activation. Interestingly, erythrocytes also revealed a parallel abnormality. In platelets, erythrocytes, and lymphocytes scramblase activity was decreased. Although the conventional markers of a platelet defect (bleeding time, platelet aggregation studies) are normal in patients with the Scott syndrome, the management of these patients would require platelet transfusions.

Relative Frequencies of Various Congenital Platelet Abnormalities

Thrombasthenia and the Bernard-Soulier syndrome are rare disorders. Although there are no published data, patients currently classified in the heterogenous category of defects in platelet secretion and signal transduction probably constitute the most frequently encountered inherited platelet function abnormalities, excluding vWD. In our experience, the SPD is present in less than 10% to 15% of patients with congenital platelet defects. Abnormalities in thromboxane production occur in about 20% of patients. A large proportion of the remaining patients with abnormal aggregation and secretion demonstrate adequate dense-granule stores and produce substantial amounts of TxA_2. In some of these patients there is evidence for defects in the signaling mechanisms. In this heterogeneous group, the underlying mechanisms still need to be established.

Consultation Considerations

Diagnosis of Congenital Platelet Function Defects. The bleeding manifestations in patients with inherited platelet function defects are highly variable. The usual reasons for referral for evaluation include mucocutanteous bleeding manifestations, excessive bleeding following a procedure or surgery, or a prolonged bleeding time with a reasonable platelet count. In patients suspected to have a platelet function defect, the main clinically available laboratory studies include a platelet count, the bleeding time, and studies to assess platelet aggregation and secretion responses in vitro. The platelet studies are usually performed using platelet-rich plasma harvested from anticoagulated blood and responses are monitored to various agonists, including ADP, epinephrine, collagen, thromboxane A_2 analog U46619, thrombin receptor peptides and ristocetin. The patterns of responses observed may often provide clues to the nature of the underlying platelet defect, although specific techniques, chiefly available only in research laboratories, are required to delineate the precise platelet mechanisms that are altered (Fig. 10–2). Classical thrombasthenia is characterized by the absence of both the primary and the secondary waves of aggregation in response to all of the commonly used agonists excepting ristocetin; the shape change response is normal. Impaired or absent response to ristocetin but with normal aggregation response to other agonists suggests vWD or the Bernard-Soulier syndrome. In the latter disorder, the platelet counts are decreased and the platelet size is increased. Although these findings may occur in some variants of vWD (e.g., type IIb), plasma levels of vWF and factor VIII, as well as the multimeric pattern of vWF are normal in the Bernard-Soulier syndrome but abnormal in vWD. Patients with impaired granule

Inherited Disorders of Platelet Function

Platelet Aggregation and Secretion Studies

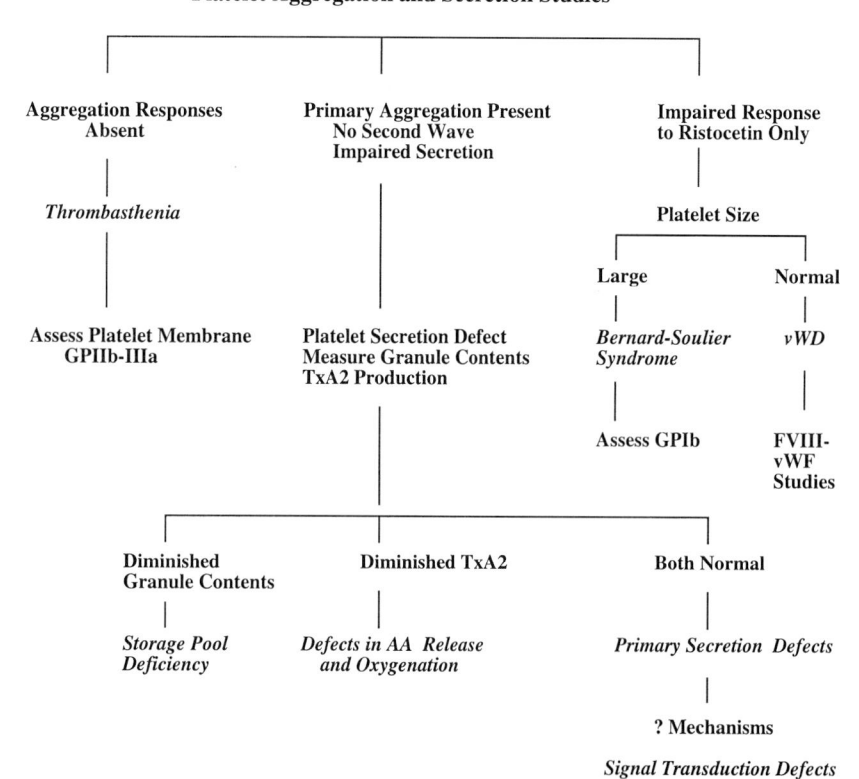

- Aggregation Responses Absent
  - *Thrombasthenia*
  - Assess Platelet Membrane GPIIb-IIIa
- Primary Aggregation Present No Second Wave Impaired Secretion
  - Platelet Secretion Defect Measure Granule Contents TxA2 Production
    - Diminished Granule Contents
      - *Storage Pool Deficiency*
    - Diminished TxA2
      - *Defects in AA Release and Oxygenation*
    - Both Normal
      - *Primary Secretion Defects*
      - ? Mechanisms
      - *Signal Transduction Defects*
      - **Studies on Platelet Activation Mechanisms**
- Impaired Response to Ristocetin Only
  - Platelet Size
    - Large
      - *Bernard-Soulier Syndrome*
      - Assess GPIb
    - Normal
      - *vWD*
      - FVIII-vWF Studies

Figure 10–2 Inherited disorders of platelet function. AA, arachidonic acid; GP, glycoprotein; vWF, von Willebrand factor; vWD; von Willebrand disease; TxA_2, thromboxane A_2.

secretion or diminished dense-granule contents (SPD) generally show a diminished or absent second wave of aggregation in response to ADP, epinephrine, and PAF, and blunted responses to other agonists (collagen, U46619) associated with markedly decreased release of granule contents.

Therapy of Congenital Platelet Function Defects. Patients with vWD and afibrinogenemia are managed during bleeding episodes and surgical procedures by methods aimed at elevating the deficient factor levels in plasma and are discussed in Chapters 7 and 5, respectively. Platelet transfusions and 1-desamino-8D-arginine vasopressin (DDAVP) administration are the mainstays of therapy of patients with inherited platelet defects. Because of the wide disparity in bleeding manifestations, therapeutic approaches need to be individualized. Platelet transfusions are effective in controlling the bleeding manifestations but come with potential risks associated with blood products, including alloimmunization. Patients with thrombasthenia may develop antibodies[8,45] against GPIIb-IIIa that may compromise the efficacy of subsequent platelet transfusions. A viable alternative to platelet transfusions is intravenous administration of DDAVP, which shortens the bleeding time in a substantial number of patients with platelet function defects.[46-49] The effect on the bleeding time lasts about 4 to 5 hours. This response appears to be dependent on the abnormalities leading to the platelet dysfunction.[46,48,49] Most patients with thrombasthenia have not responded to DDAVP infusion with a shortening of the bleeding time[46,48-50] but exceptions exist.[51] However, it is unknown whether DDAVP improves clinical hemostasis in these patients despite a lack of shortening of the bleeding time. Responses in patients with SPD have been variable, with a shortening of the bleeding time in some patients[49,52,53] but not others.[46,48] In uncontrolled studies it has been feasible to manage selected patients with congenital platelet defects undergoing surgical procedures with DDAVP alone.[46,48] However, this approach needs to be individualized based on the nature of the surgery and the intensity of bleeding symptoms, and platelet transfusions need to be readily available for use in the event excess hemorrhage. The mechanisms by which DDAVP enhances hemostasis in patients with platelet defects are unclear.[47,54] Its administration induces a rise in plasma vWF, factor VIII, and tissue plasminogen activator. The abnormal in vitro platelet aggregation or secretion responses in patients with platelet defects are not corrected by DDAVP.[48]

The other approaches that have been utilized to improve hemostasis in patients with inherited platelet defects include a short 3 to 4-day course of prednisone (20 to 50 mg/d)[55] and the administration of antifibrinolytic agents ε-aminocaproic acid (EACA) or tranexamic acid, which have been successfully used in patients with coagulation disorders.[47,56,57] Although allogeneic bone marrow transplantation has been successfully performed with complete correction in patients with thrombasthenia[58] and the Wiskott-Aldrich syndrome,[40,59] such a drastic therapy is rarely required in patients with congenital platelet function disorders.

Acquired Disorders of Platelet Function

Alterations in platelet function occur in many acquired disorders of diverse etiologies (Table 10-2).[3] In most, the specific biochemical and pathophysiologic aberrations leading to platelet dysfunction in hemostasis are poorly understood. In several disorders, abnormalities have been described in multiple aspects of platelet function, including adhesion, aggregation, and secretion, and in the platelet coagulant activities. Acquired platelet dysfunction arises by different mechanisms. In some, such as the myeloproliferative disorders, there is production of intrinsically abnormal platelets by the bone marrow. In others the dysfunction results from interaction of platelets with exogenous factors such as pharmacologic agents, artificial surfaces (cardiopulmonary bypass), compounds that accumulate in plasma due to impaired renal function, and antibodies. Some of the acquired causes of platelet dysfunction (liver disease, cardiopulmonary bypass) are described in Chapters 31 and 30, respectively.

Myeloproliferative Diseases

Bleeding tendency, thromboembolic complications, and qualitative platelet defects are recognized in all myeloproliferative disorders (MPDs), which include essential thrombocythemia (ET), polycythemia vera (PV), agnogenic myeloid metaplasia (AMM), and chronic myelogenous leukemia (CML).[60-63] The platelet abnormalities most likely result from their development from an abnormal clone of stem cells but some may be secondary to enhanced platelet activation in vivo. The clinical impact of the in-vitro qualitative platelet defects is often unclear. Platelet defects are demonstrable even in asymptomatic patients, and bleeding and thrombotic

Table 10–2 • DISORDERS IN WHICH ACQUIRED DEFECTS IN PLATELET FUNCTION ARE RECOGNIZED

Uremia
Myeloproliferative disorders
   Essential thrombocythemia
   Polycythemia vera
   Chronic myelogenous leukemia
   Agnogenic myeloid metaplasia
Acute leukemias and myelodysplastic syndromes
Dysproteinemias
Cardiopulmonary bypass
Acquired von Willebrand disease
Acquired storage-pool deficiency
Antiplatelet antibodies
Liver disease
Drugs and other agents

Modified from Rao AK, Carvalho A. Acquired qualitative platelet defects. In: Colman RW, Hirsh J, Marder VJ, Salzman GW (eds.): Hemostasis and thrombosis: Basic Principles and Clinical Practice, 3rd Ed. Philadelphia, J.B. Lippincott, 1994, pp. 685–704, with permission.

events may occur in the same patient. Overall, platelet abnormalities likely contribute to the excessive morbidity and mortality of these disorders.

Clinical Features. Although both hemorrhagic and thrombotic complications occur in MPD patients, the impact of the latter is greater on the resulting morbidity.[60,61] Both bleeding and thrombosis are less frequent in CML compared to other MPDs. Bleeding appears more prevalent in AMM, while patients with other MPD are more prone to thrombosis. Bleeding is chiefly mucocutaneous, with particular involvement of the gastrointestinal and genitourinary tracts. The risk of spontaneous hemorrhage may be increased with platelet counts in excess of 2 million/μL. Moreover, ingestion of aspirin or other drugs that decrease platelet function is an important contributing factor to the hemorrhagic events.

Thrombotic events encompass both arterial and venous events and may occur at unusual sites, such as the splenic, hepatic, and mesenteric vessels, and cerebral venous sinuses (see Chapter 15). Deep venous thrombosis and pulmonary embolism, and arterial events involving the peripheral, coronary, and cerebral vessels have been documented. In addition to the often underestimated large-vessel thrombosis, MPDs are associated with microcirculatory arterial events resulting in erythromelalgia and neurologic symptoms. Erythromelalgia is characterized by intense burning or throbbing pain in the extremities, predominantly the feet, and is associated with warmth and mottled erythema.[64] Erythromelalgia occurs predominantly in ET and may progress to digital ischemia and necrosis. The arterial pulses in the extremities are generally normal in these patients. Histologically, erythromelalgia is characterized by fibromuscular intimal proliferation, endothelial swelling, and thrombotic occlusions. Platelet survival is decreased in patients with ET and erythromelalgia compared to patients with asymptomatic ET and reactive thrombocytosis.[64] Aspirin relieves the symptoms of erythromelalgia effectively and reverses the shortened platelet survival. Neurologic symptoms are frequently noted in MPD patients and span a wide spectrum from nonspecific headaches and dizziness to focal neurologic events, such as transient ischemic events, seizures, and monocular blindness.[61,62,65] The transient neurologic events are also highly responsive to aspirin therapy.[65]

Risk factors for thrombosis identified in patients with ET include increasing age, a prior thrombotic event, inadequate control of thrombocytosis, presence of risk factors for atherosclerotic cardiovascular disease, and in-vitro occurrence of spontaneous megakaryocyte colony formation.[66-69] Neither the degree of thrombocytosis nor the abnormal in-vitro platelet responses[66,67,70] correlate with risk of thrombosis in MPD patients. However, the degree of erythrocytosis in PV correlates with an increased risk of thrombosis. Hepatic vein and/or portal vein thrombosis may be an initial presentation of patients with MPDs, especially PV. Other abnormalities reported in MPDs include an increased risk of recurrent spontaneous abortions, fetal growth retardation, premature deliveries, and abruptio placentae in patients with ET.[62]

In assessing the impact of hemorrhagic and thrombotic events it needs to be noted that life expectancy in patients with ET is normal.[71] The incidence of thrombosis in ET has been estimated to be 6.6 episodes per 100 patient-years of observation.[68] In different studies, 20% to 50% of the ET patients have had thrombotic events.[61] In CML the prognosis is primarily determined by progression to blast crisis. The incidence of thrombotic and hemorrhagic complications is low in the chronic phase[61]; bleeding increases in the accelerated phase, largely due to thrombocytopenia. Survival in AMM is determined by the progression of the hematologic disease; bleeding is common in the advanced thrombocytopenic stage. Patients with PV have a prolonged survival and, as in ET, morbidity and mortality are influenced by vascular events. In two large trials[72,73] in PV patients, thrombotic events occurred in 34% and 41% of patients, respectively.

Morphologic and Functional Abnormalities in MPDs. A large number of studies have examined platelet function and morphology in patients with MPD.[60-63,74] The bleeding time is prolonged in a minority (approximately 17%) of patients with MPD, and appears to be more often prolonged in AMM than in other MPDs[60] yet does not correlate with an increased risk of bleeding symptoms. Platelet aggregation responses are also highly variable and often vary in the same patient over time. Decreased platelet responses are more common, although some patients demonstrate enhanced responses to agonists or even spontaneous aggregation without addition of an agonist.[75,76] In one analysis[60] responses to ADP, collagen, and epinephrine were decreased in 39%, 37%, and 57% of patients, respectively. The impairment in aggregation in response to epinephrine has been more commonly encountered than with other agonists; however, a diminished response to epinephrine is not pathognomonic of an MPD. Numerous alterations have been described in MPD platelets, including diminished platelet α_2-adrenergic receptors, impaired dense-granule secretion, diminished membrane surface glycoproteins, and blunted agonist-induced Ca^{2+} mobilization, thromboxane formation, and lipo-oxygenase products. A decrease in plasma vWF, particularly in the large vWF multimers, has been described in MPDs (and in reactive thrombocytosis); as diverse as they are, these changes have been inversely related to the platelet counts and have improved following cytoreduction.

Therapy. Guidelines for the therapy of MPD patients are still evolving. The two major pharmacologic approaches are cytoreduction and platelet inhibition. However, it is still somewhat unclear which MPD patients require therapy—an uncertainty arising because of a lack of adequate data on efficacy, and the recognition of potential side effects of the agents (hemorrhage and leukemogenesis). Patients with PV are clearly benefited by reduction in red cell mass. The prognosis in patients with AMM is dictated by the effects of increasing fibrosis. Much of the discussion here revolves around patients with ET who have a normal life span, but thrombohemorrhagic events occur in a substantial number of patients. There is general consensus that treatment is indicated in ET patients with a history of a thromboembolic event. These patients have an increased risk of recurrent thrombosis. Lowering of platelet counts (target 600,000/μL) with hydroxyurea prevents recurrence of events. In addition to patients with a previous thrombotic event, patients with cardiovascular risk factors are at high risk and are candidates for specific therapy. In asymptomatic patients without the above risk factors the role of cytoreduction remains to be established. In patients with life-threatening hemorrhage or thrombosis, plateletpheresis is an effective measure to rapidly lower the count and reduces morbidity.

The various pharmacologic agents for cytoreduction in MPDs have included hydroxyurea, anagrelide, interferon-α, alkylating agents (busulfan), and radioactive phosphorus. Hydroxyurea has been widely used. Contrary to earlier beliefs, hydroxyurea also confers a leukemogenic risk on prolonged use,[77] at least in the MPD population. This finding becomes an important consideration in its use in asymptomatic patients or young patients. The use of busulfan and ^{32}P in ET has been abandoned because of enhanced leukemogenic potential.

Anagrelide is a nonmutagenic quinazoline derivative that is orally active and inhibits maturation of megakaryocytes.[78] Over 90% of ET patients respond to anagrelide with a decline in platelet counts. The side effects of anagrelide include palpitations, fluid retention, nausea, diarrhea, anemia, headache, dizziness, confusion, and, in a small number of patients, congestive heart failure. The selective reduction in platelet counts without effecting the white cell count is an advantage of this agent over hydroxyurea, although the side effects may restrict its use in some elderly patients. Anagrelide is not recommended for use in pregnancy. Another agent shown to be effective in reducing platelet counts, as well as splenomegaly, in ET and other MPD patients is interferon-α (IFN-α), which has a potent antiproliferative effect on the hematopoietic stem cells. It is nonmutagenic and nonleukemogenic but its widespread use has been limited because of the cost and side effects of fever and flu-like symptoms.[79]

The role of aspirin in MPD patients is not well defined. Its use has been associated with serious bleeding, particularly at high doses.[60,63] On the other hand, aspirin is effective in controlling microvascular complications, digital ischemia, erythromelalgia, and neurologic events.[64,65] At present aspirin is indicated in patients with arterial thrombotic events and microvascular events but with recognition of the potential for hemorrhage. Its role in asymptomatic patients is unclear. It is considered to be relatively contraindicated in patients with previous bleeding episodes and those with platelet counts higher than 1.5 million/μL.[62]

Acute Leukemias, Myelodysplastic Syndromes, and Dysproteinemias

The most common cause of bleeding in these conditions is thrombocytopenia. However, in patients with normal or elevated platelet counts, bleeding complications may be associated with platelet dysfunction. Acquired platelet defects associated with clinical bleeding are more commonly found in acute myelogenous leukemia, but have been reported in acute lymphoblastic and myelomonoblastic leukemias, hairy cell leukemia, and myelodysplastic syndromes (MDSs).

Excessive clinical bleeding may occur in patients with dysproteinemias, and this appears to be related to multiple mechanisms, including platelet dysfunction, specific coagulation abnormalities (e.g., factor X deficiency), hyperviscosity, and alterations in blood vessels due to amyloid deposition. An acquired form of vWD has been described in some patients. The impaired platelet function appears to correlate with the serum paraprotein levels.[80,81] Acute bleeding episodes can be managed by lowering the paraprotein levels by plasmapheresis, and chronic bleeding may be controlled by chemotherapy aimed at reducing the concentration of the abnormal protein.

Uremia

Bleeding has been a frequent and sometimes fatal complication of uremia in the past, but its incidence has clearly declined, possibly because of earlier and better treatment of the underlying disorders. In uremic patients undergoing surgery or invasive procedures hemorrhage remains a serious concern. Bleeding in uremia is generally mucocutaneous, but rarely may be intracranial or pericardial. It is well recognized that the bleeding time is prolonged in uremia. The pathogenesis of the hemostatic defect in uremia remains unclear, but platelet dysfunction and impaired platelet–vessel wall interaction are considered the major causes of the bleeding tendency. Reduced blood coagulation factors and thrombocytopenia occur infrequently in uremia and are not a major factor in the uremic hemostatic defect.

Multiple platelet abnormalities have been recognized in uremia.[74] Adhesion of platelets to the subendothelium is an initial step in normal hemostasis and involves the interaction of vWF with platelets and the subendothelium. Adhesion of platelets from uremic whole blood perfused over de-endothelialized rabbit aorta has been reported to be impaired; platelet adhesion was decreased when perfusions were carried out with mixtures containing either washed uremic platelets and normal plasma or normal platelets and uremic plasma.[82] This may be related to an unknown component in uremic plasma directly inhibiting the platelet interaction with artery segments. It is relevant to note that vWF levels are normal in uremic plasma; although in some, vWF activity was consistently lower than the antigen level. The multimeric structure of vWF has been shown to be normal in some studies and abnormal in others. It remains unclear whether the vWF–platelet interaction is modified in vivo by the high levels of prostacyclin reported in uremic patients.[83,84] The number of GPIb and GPIIb/GPIIIa sites per platelet has also been shown to be normal in uremia. The reduced number of red blood cells in uremia also influences both the platelet adhesion and bleeding time, and the prolonged bleeding time in such patients is corrected by the transfusion of washed packed red blood cells or administration of recombinant human erythropoietin.[82,85,86]

Platelet aggregation responses to agonists (ADP, epinephrine, and collagen) are impaired in uremia, with sometimes conflicting results. In general, in these studies there was no correlation between the severity or cause of the renal disease and the platelet aggregation defects. Thrombin- and ristocetin-induced platelet aggregation have more often been shown to be normal. Platelet aggregation can be inhibited in vitro by dialyzable substances such as guanidinosuccinic acid, phenols, urea, and "middle molecules" at concentrations found in uremia.[87,88]

Therapy. Many therapeutic modalities have been tried in an attempt to correct the hemostatic defect in uremia, with varying success. There is general agreement that aggressive dialysis is an important component of management of these patients. Intensive dialysis improves the bleeding diathesis in some patients but is only partially effective in others. Both hemo- and peritoneal dialysis are effective. Other modalities (see below) are generally indicated only for clinically significant bleeding or in relation to surgical procedures. Improvement of the hematocrit with transfusion of packed red blood cells or therapy with recombinant erythropoietin has been shown to shorten the bleeding time, improve platelet adhesion, and correct mild bleeding in uremic patients.[85,86] A simplistic explanation for this is that the repletion of red blood cells leads to a mechanical displacement of platelets toward the vessel wall and facilitates the platelet–vessel wall interaction. Although preferable to blood transfusions, therapy with recombinant erythropoietin may be associated with an increased risk of thrombosis and worsening of hypertension.[86] Other treatments for uremic patients with significant bleeding include administration of platelets, DDAVP, cryoprecipitate, or conjugated estrogens. The role of platelet transfusions in uremia is limited largely because of the availability of other modalities, the transfusion-related risks, and the probability that transfused platelets rapidly acquire the uremic defects in vivo. Intravenous infusion of DDAVP induces the release of vWF from endothelial cells and shortens the bleeding time in 75% of uremic patients.[47] The effect of DDAVP correlates with a rise in circulating vWF, including its largest multimeric forms, which are believed to mediate platelet adhesion. DDAVP is commonly administered as an intravenous infusion (0.3 μg/kg) over 20 to 30 minutes, but is also effective if given subcutaneously or intranasally. The effect of DDAVP on the bleeding time occurs within an hour and lasts up to 4 hours. The intranasal route requires 10-fold higher dosages and has variable absorption. DDAVP does not appear to affect the quantity or quality of the patient's platelets. The side effects of DDAVP include reduction of arterial pressure, facial flushing, water retention, hyponatremia, and rarely cerebral thrombosis.

Cryoprecipitate transfusions in uremic patients shorten the bleeding time and improve clinical bleeding.[89] This effect occurs within 1 to 24 hours and may last up to 36 hours. However, some patients fail to correct the bleeding time or stop bleeding. Moreover, cryoprecipitate administration has the same risks inherent in all blood-product transfusions.

Conjugated estrogens shorten the bleeding time and prevent clinical bleeding in uremic patients.[90,91] In these studies a single intravenous infusion of 0.6 mg/kg of Emopremarin (Ayerst, NY) shortened the bleeding time within 6 hours, and this effect disappeared within 72 hours.[91] Repeated daily infusions for 5 days shortened the bleeding time by 50%, an effect that lasted 14 days. Oral conjugated estrogens (Premarin 10 to 50 mg/d) have also corrected the bleeding time to normal.[90] The mechanism by which estrogens shorten the bleeding time remains unknown. The side effects of estrogens include hot flashes, fluid retention, elevation of blood pressure, and abnormal liver function tests. Estrogen therapy may be particularly useful in uremic patients who need longer-lasting hemostatic control, such as those with gastrointestinal telangiectases or intracranial bleeding or those undergoing major surgery.[47,91]

Acquired von Willebrand Disease

von Willebrand disease is a heterogeneous bleeding disorder characterized by a prolonged bleeding time, quantitative or qualitative abnormalities of vWF, and low factor VIII procoagulant activity (FVIIIC) (see Chapter 7). While most cases of vWD are inherited, there are several reports of patients with a mild to moderate bleeding disorder in whom this disease appears to be acquired. Most patients have been over age 40 years without previous manifestations of a bleeding diathesis; the associated disorders in these patients have included MPDs, reactive thrombocytosis, collagen vascular diseases, lymphoproliferative disorders, including monoclonal gammopathy of unknown significance, gastrointestinal angiodysplasia, Wilms tumor, and congenital cardiac defects.[74]

Acquired Storage Pool Disease

Several patients have been reported in whom the dense-granule SPD appears to be acquired. In general, this defect probably reflects in vivo release of platelet dense-granule contents due to activation or a hematopoietic abnormality with abnormal platelets being produced by the marrow. Acquired SPD may, therefore, occur in diverse clinical states, including in patients with antiplatelet antibodies, collagen vascular disease, disseminated intravascular coagulation, idiopathic thrombocytopenic purpura, thrombotic thrombocytopenic purpura, multiple congenital cavernous hemangioma, and MPDs.

Antiplatelet Antibodies and Platelet Function

Binding of an antibody to platelets may induce several effects, including accelerated destruction, cell lysis, aggregation, secretion of granule contents, and expression of platelet factor-3 activity. Platelet–antibody interaction may lead to impaired function, both as a consequence of such an activation and due to interaction of the antibodies with specific platelet glycoproteins on the surface (see below). The overall impact of the antibodies may be thrombocytopenia or impaired platelet function, as noted in a wide range of autoimmune disorders, including idiopathic thrombocytopenic purpura, collagen vascular diseases, and acquired immunodeficiency syndrome.

Drugs That Inhibit Platelet Function

Many drugs affect platelet function (Table 10–3). While some drugs are administered specifically to inhibit platelet function, others do so as an unintentional side effect. For several drugs the effects have been established largely in vitro, and the relevance of such findings to the drug levels achieved in clinical practice is not well established. Even when they have been shown to alter platelet responses, information regarding the impact on hemostasis is unavailable for many drugs. Effects of some of the major groups of drugs are presented here. Details regarding others is reviewed elsewhere.[74]

Aspirin and Nonsteroidal Anti-inflammatory Agents. Aspirin ingestion results in inhibition of platelet aggregation and secretion upon stimulation with ADP, epinephrine, and low concentrations of collagen. Aspirin irreversibly acetylates and inactivates the platelet cyclo-oxygenase, leading to the inhibition of endoperoxide (PGG_2 and PGH_2) and $TX-A_2$ synthesis. The overall result is a mild impairment of hemostasis in otherwise normal individuals. Aspirin prolongs the bleeding time in many normal individuals. Ingestion of aspirin during pregnancy has been reported to result in excessive bleeding at delivery in both the neonate and the mother. Preoperative ingestion of aspirin increases blood loss in patients undergoing cardiac surgery. Long-term aspirin antithrombotic therapy is associated with a significantly higher incidence of easy bruising, mucosal bleeding (including gastrointestinal bleeding), and blood transfusion requirement.[92]

Gastrointestinal (GI) bleeding is a major adverse effect of aspirin.[93–95] Aspirin-induced gastrointestinal toxicity, but not its antithrombotic effect, is dose related in the range 30 to 1300 mg daily.[93,96] However, even at low doses (30 to 50 mg daily) aspirin may be associated with serious GI bleeding. The overall relative risks of GI complications with the use of nonsteroidal antiinflammatory drugs (NSAIDs) (including aspirin) have been estimated to be between 3.0 and 5.0 as compared to nonusers.[95] Subjects who may develop considerable postoperative or even spontaneous bleeding during aspirin ingestion are those with underlying hemostatic

Table 10–3 • DRUGS THAT AFFECT PLATELET FUNCTION[a]

Drugs that inhibit thromboxane synthesis
  Cyclo-oxygenase inhibitors
    Aspirin
    Nonsteroidal anti-inflammatory agents
      Indomethacin, phenylbutazone, ibuprofen, sulfinpyrazone, sulindac, meclofenamic acid
ADP receptor antagonists
  Ticlopidine, clopidogrel
GPIIb-IIIa receptor antagonists
  c7E3 (abciximab), tirofiban, eptifibatide
Drugs that increase platelet cyclic AMP or cyclic GMP
  Adenylate cyclase activators
    Prostaglandins I_2, D_2, E_1 and analogs
  Phosphodiesterase inhibitors
    Dipyridamole
    Cilostazol
    Methyl xanthines
    Caffeine, theophylline, aminophylline
Nitric oxide and nitric oxide donors
Antimicrobials
  Penicillins
  Cephalosporins
  Nitrofurantoin
  Hydroxychloroquine
Cardiovascular drugs
  β-Adrenergic blockers (propranolol)
  Vasodilators (nitroprusside, nitroglycerin)
  Diuretics (furosemide)
  Calcium channel blockers
  Quinidine
  Angiotensin converting enzyme inhibitors
Anticoagulants
  Heparin
Thrombolytic agents
  Streptokinase, tissue plasminogen activator, urokinase
Psychotropics and anesthetics
  Tricyclic antidepressants
    Imipramine, amitryptyline, nortriptyline
  Phenothiazines
    Chlorpromazine, promethazine, trifluoperazine
  Local anesthetics
  General anesthesia (halothane)
Chemotherapeutic agents
  Mithramycin
  BCNU
  Daunorubicin
Miscellaneous agents
  Dextrans
  Lipid lowering agents (clofibrate, halofenate)
  ε-Aminocaproic acid
  Antihistaminics
  Ethanol
  Vitamin E
  Radiographic contrast agents
  Food items and alternative medications (onions, garlic, ginger, cumin, tumeric, clove, black tree fungus)

[a] For most of the drugs, there is little evidence that their impact on platelet aggregation responses or on the bleeding time is associated with a clinically significant hemostatic defect.

defects such as vWD, hemophilia, or mild platelet function defects, and those receiving oral anticoagulant therapy. In these patients aspirin ingestion may lead to a striking increase in the bleeding time and bleeding manifestations, and should be avoided. In otherwise normal subjects on aspirin who need to undergo elective surgery, aspirin may ideally be discontinued 7 to 10 days prior to the procedure. However, this may often not be feasible in many patients. If excessive perioperative hemorrhage is encountered, it is generally responsive to platelet transfusions, but DDAVP infusion, which shortens the prolongation in bleeding time with aspirin,[47] may be preferable.

Several other NSAIDs also impair platelet function by inhibiting the enzyme cyclo-oxygenase which may prolong the bleeding time and increase the risk of GI bleeding. These include indomethacin, ibuprofen, sulfinpyrazone, meclofenamic acid, phenylbutazone, and sulindac. Compared with aspirin, the inhibition of cyclo-oxygenase by these agents is generally short lived and reversible. The relative risk of upper GI bleeding appears to be lowest for ibuprofen and diclofenac; intermediate for aspirin, indomethacin, naproxen, and sulindac; and higher for azapropazone, tolmetin, ketoprofen, and piroxicam.[94] Like aspirin, most NSAIDs inhibit both forms of cyclo-oxygenase (cyclo-oxygenase-1 and -2). The two selective cyclo-oxygenase-2 inhibitors, celexocib (Celebrex) and rececoxib (Vioxx), have no antiplatelet activity and appear to lead to fewer gastrointestinal ulcers than NSAIDs.

Ticlopidine and Clopidogrel: ADP Receptor Antagonists. Ticlopidine and its analog clopidogrel are orally administered thienopyridine derivatives that inhibit platelet function by inhibiting the binding of ADP to one of its receptors.[97,98] Platelet aggregation responses to several agonists, including ADP, collagen, epinephrine, and thrombin, are inhibited to various extents depending on agonist concentrations. Inhibition of platelet aggregation is observed after 2 to 3 days of therapy, with a maximal effect at 4 to 7 days.[97] The platelet inhibitory effect persists for 7 to 10 days after therapy is discontinued. Neither ticlopidine nor clopidogrel prolong the bleeding time. Recent reports have associated ticlopidine and clopidogrel with thrombotic thrombocytopenic purpura.[99,100]

Glycoprotein IIb-IIIa Receptor Agonists. GPIIb-IIIa receptor antagonists are a class of compounds that inhibit fibrinogen binding and platelet aggregation.[93,101,102] These include the monoclonal antibody against the GPIIb-IIIa receptor c7E3 (Abciximab, Reopro) and several peptides, such as eptifibatide (Integrilin), and tirofiban (Aggrastat). These agents are used in acute coronary syndromes and in the context of percutaneous coronary interventions.[93,101,102] They are potent inhibitors of aggregation (both primary and secondary) in response to all of the usual agonists; they all prolong the bleeding time, are more potent than aspirin, yet are often used concomitantly with aspirin. Bleeding is a potential complication with these agents and platelet transfusions are indicated in management of this situation, although the transfused platelets may acquire the same drug-induced defect. Thrombocytopenia is another potential feature with many of the GPIIb-III antagonists.[93,102,103]

Antimicrobial Agents. β-Lactam antibiotics, including penicillins and cephalosporins, inhibit platelet aggregation responses, and some induce a bleeding diathesis at high doses. These include carbenicillin, penicillin G, ticarcillin, ampicillin, nafcillin, cloxacillin, mezlocillin, oxacillin, and piperacillin.[74,104] The platelet inhibition appears to be dose dependent, taking about 2 to 3 days to manifest and 3 to 10 days to abate after discontinuation of the drug. Cephalosporins may also impair platelet function.[105–107] Moxalactam has been reported to induce platelet dysfunction associated with prolonged bleeding times and clinical hemorrhage. However, other third-generation cephalosporins appear to show little effect on normal platelet function.

A number of generalizations can be made regarding the overall effects of β-lactam antibiotics. First, the effects on platelet function and hemostasis appear to be dose dependent and time dependent, with effects becoming discernible over several days.[104,105,108–110] Second, the patients at particular risk of bleeding appear to be those with concurrent illnesses, including sepsis, malnourishment, thrombocytopenia, and malignancy; the typical setting is the intensive care unit. Third, the impairment in hemostasis noted with some of the β-lactam antibiotics (e.g., moxalactam, cefamandole, cefoperazone) is related to a concomitant inhibitory effect on synthesis of vitamin K-dependent coagulation. From a management point of view, the general context in which the bleeding events are encountered in patients on antibiotics prevents identification of the precise role played by the antimicrobials, because of the presence of concomitant factors (thrombocytopenia, disseminated intravascular coagulation, infection, vitamin K deficiency). Discontinuation of a specifically indicated antibiotic is usually not an option or necessary. Supportive measures using blood products and other interventions (correcting metabolic abnormalities, vitamin K deficiency) are indicated in the overall management.

Cardiovascular Drugs, Anticoagulants, and Thrombolytic Agents. Propranolol and other β-blockers are weak inhibitors of platelet function and do not influence the bleeding time. The interaction of heparin with platelets may result in effects ranging from potentiation or impairment of in-vitro platelet responses to severe thrombocytopenia and extensive arterial thromboses.[111] The major complication of thrombolytic agents (streptokinase, urokinase, and tissue plasminogen activator (rt-PA)) is hemorrhage, which arises from multiple mechanisms, including the effect of plasmin on the plasma coagulation system and platelets, and the dissolution of blood clots providing hemostasis at the site of vascular breach; the bleeding time in patients receiving rt-PA may be prolonged.[112,113] In-vitro plasmin induces several effects in platelets; these include initial platelet activation followed by inhibition. Several other factors may also contribute to platelet inhibition in patients receiving thrombolytic therapy, including radiographic contrast media, and other medications (e.g., aspirin, nitrates, heparin).

Miscellaneous Agents. Several other drugs, including dextrans, psychotropic drugs, and anesthetics, also affect platelet function, but the clinical significance remains to be defined.[74] Ethanol inhibits platelet responses in vitro and, although by itself ethanol does not prolong the bleeding time, acute ingestion of 50 g of ethanol potentiates aspirin-induced prolongation of bleeding time even in otherwise normal subjects.[114] Some of the other agents reported to inhibit platelet function, including food items, are shown in Table 10-3.

CONSULTATION CONSIDERATIONS

Given the large number of medications and diseases affecting platelet function, it is not uncommon to encounter platelet dysfunction in the clinical setting. In the acute setting, there is often concomitant thrombocytopenia. In a patient with unexplained bleeding the potential contribution of platelet dysfunction secondary to either underlying disease states (e.g., renal failure, MPD) or medications needs to be considered. In some instances administration of platelet transfusions or DDAVP may be beneficial.

A vexing problem not infrequently encountered in the nonacute setting is the patient who is found to have a prolonged bleeding time obtained in relation to an elective procedure. In general, an isolated mildly prolonged bleeding time in a patient without a history of abnormal hemostasis may not accurately predict bleeding. The evaluation should encompass a detailed history including regarding the nature and intensity of bleeding manifestations, family history of such symptoms, presence of other disorders (such as MPD, renal insufficiency) and, most importantly, exposure to medications or agents known to alter platelet function. Withdrawal of such a substance may be required. It is essential that medications and other agents be discontinued for several days before expensive platelet function tests are obtained. This would include all over-the-counter medications and food supplements. Demonstration of an underlying platelet function defect would require specific management based on the underlying cause, as described earlier.

ACKNOWLEDGMENTS

The excellent secretarial assistance of Ms. JoAnn Hamilton is gratefully acknowledged. This work is supported by Grant HL 056724 from the National Heart, Lung and Blood Institute.

■ REFERENCES

Chapter 10 References

1. Rao AK. Congenital disorders of platelet function: disorders of signal transduction and secretion. Am J Med Sci 1998;316:69–76.
2. Rao AK. Congenital disorders of platelet secretion and signal transduction. In Colman RW, Marden VJ, Clowes P, George JN (eds.): Hemostasis and Thrombosis: Basic Principles and Clinical Practice, 4th ed. Philadelphia, Lippincott, Williams & Wilkens, 2001; pp. 893–904.
3. Rao AK. Acquired qualitative platelet defects. In Colman RW, Marder VJ, Clowes P, George JN (eds.): Hemostasis and Thrombosis: Basic Principles and Clinical Practice, 4th ed. Philadelphia, Lippincott, Williams & Wilkens, 2001; pp. 905–920.
4. Nichols WC, Ginsberg D. von Willebrand's disease. Medicine 1997;76:1–20.
5. Lopez JA, Andrews RK, Afshar-Kharghan V, et al. Bernard-Soulier syndrome. Blood 1998;91:4397–4418.
6. Nurden AT, George JN. Inherited disorders of the platelet membrane: Glanzmann thrombasthenia, Bernard-Soulier syndrome, and other disorders. In: Colman RW, Hirsh J, Marder VJ, Clowes P, George JN (eds.): Hemostasis and Thrombosis. Basic Principles and Clinical Practice, 4th ed. Philadelphia, Lippincott, Williams & Wilkes, 2001; pp. 921–943.
7. Weiss HJ. Scott syndrome. A disorder of platelet coagulant activity. Semin Hematol 1994;31:301–311.
8. George JN, Caen JP, Nurden AT. Glanzmann's thrombasthenia: the spectrum of clinical disease. Blood 1990;75:1383–1395.
9. French DL, Seligsohn U. Platelet glycoprotein IIb/IIIa receptors and Glanzmann's thrombasthenia. Arterioscler Thromb Vasc Biol 2000;20:607–610.
10. Hayward CPM. Inherited disorders of platelet alpha-granules. Platelets 1997;8:197–209.
11. Rao AK, Willis J, Kowalska MA, et al. Differential requirements for epinephrine induced platelet aggregation and inhibition of adenylate cyclase. Studies in familial alpha$_2$-adrenergic receptor defect. Blood 1988;71:494–501.
12. Nieuwenhuis HK, Akkerman JWN, Houdijk WPM, et al. Human blood platelets showing no response to collagen fail to express surface glycoprotein Ia. Nature (London) 1985;318:470–472.
13. Moroi M, Jung SM, Okuma M, et al. A patient with platelets deficient in glycoprotein VI that lack both collagen-induced aggregation and adhesion. J Clin Invest 1989;84:1440–1445.
14. Kehrel B, Balleisen L, Kokott R, et al. Deficiency of intact thrombospondin and membrane glycoprotein Ia in platelets with defective collagen-induced aggregation and spontaneous loss of disorder. Blood 1988;71:1074–1078.
15. Ryo R, Yoshida A, Sugano W, et al. Deficiency of P62, a putative collagen receptor, in platelet from a patient with defective collagen-induced platelet aggregation. Am J Hematol 1992;38:25–31.
16. Cattaneo M, Lecchi A, Randi AM, et al. Identification of a new congenital defect of platelet function characterized by severe impairment of platelet responses to adenosine diphosphate. Blood 1992;80:2787–2796.
17. Nurden P, Savi P, Heilmann E, et al. An inherited bleeding disorder linked to a defective interaction between ADP and its receptor on platelets. Its influence on glycoprotein IIb-IIIa complex function. J Clin Invest 1995;95:1612–22.
18. Cattaneo M, Lombardi R, Zighetti ML, et al. Deficiency of (^{33}P-2MeS-ADP binding sites on platelets with secretion defect, normal granule stores and normal thromboxane A$_2$ production. Thromb Haemost 1997;77:986–990.
19. Hirata T, Kakizuka A, Ushikubi F, et al. Arg60 to Leu mutation of the human thromboxane A2 receptor in a dominantly inherited bleeding disorder. J Clin Invest 1994;94:1662–1667.
20. Ushikubi F, Ishibashi T, Narumiya S, et al. Analysis of the defective signal transduction mechanism through the platelet thromboxane A$_2$ receptor in a patient with polycythemia vera. Thromb Haemost 1992;67:144–146.
21. Fuse I, Mito M, Hattori A, et al. Defective signal transduction induced by thromboxane A2 in a patient with a mild bleeding disorder: impaired phospholipase C activation despite normal phospholipase A2 activation. Blood 1993;81:994–1000.

22. Fuse I, Hattori A, Mito M, et al. Pathogenetic analysis of five cases with a platelet disorder characterized by the absence of thromboxane A2 (TXA2)-induced platelet aggregation in spite of normal TXA2 binding activity. Thromb Haemost 1996; 76:1080–1085.
23. Ichinohe T, Takayama H, Ezumi Y, et al. Collagen-stimulated activation of Syk but not c-Src is severely compromised in human platelets lacking membrane glycoprotein VI. J Biol Chem 1997;272:63–68.
24. Gabbeta J, Yang X, Kowalska MA, et al. Platelet signal transduction defect with Galpha subunit dysfunction and diminished Galphaq in a patient with abnormal platelet responses. Proc Natl Acad Sci USA 1997;94:8750–8755.
25. Rao AK, Disa J, Yang X. Concomitant defect in internal release and influx of calcium in patients with congenital platelet dysfunction and impaired agonist-induced calcium mobilization: thromboxane production is not required for internal release of calcium. J Lab Clin Med 1993;121:52–63.
26. Rao AK, Koike K, Willis J, et al. Platelet secretion defect associated with impaired liberation of arachidonic acid and normal myosin light chain phosphorylation. Blood 1984;64:914–921.
27. Offermanns S, Toombs CF, Hu YH, et al. Defective platelet activation in Gaq-deficient mice. Nature 1997;389:183–186.
28. Lages B, Weiss HJ. Heterogeneous defects of platelet secretion and responses to weak agonists in patients with bleeding disorders. Br J Haematol 1988;68:53–62.
29. Yang X, Sun L, Gabbeta J, et al. Platelet activation with combination of ionophore A23187 and a direct protein kinase C activator induces normal secretion in patients with impaired receptor mediated secretion and abnormal signal transduction. Thromb Res 1997;88:317–328.
30. Lages B, Weiss HJ. Impairment of phosphatidylinositol metabolism in a patient with a bleeding disorder associated with defects of initial platelet responses. Thromb Haemost 1988;59:175–179.
31. Speiser-Ellerton S, Weiss HJ. Studies on platelet protein phosphorylation in patients with impaired responses to platelet agonists. J Lab Clin Med 1990;115:104–111.
32. Rao AK, Kowalska MA, Disa J. Impaired cytoplasmic ionized calcium mobilization in inherited platelet secretion defects. Blood 1989;74:664–672.
33. Yang X, Sun L, Ghosh S, et al. Human platelet signaling defect characterized by impaired production of 1,4,5 inositol triphosphate and phosphatic acid, and diminished pleckstrin phosphorylation. Evidence for defective phospholipase C activation. Blood 1996;88:1676–1683.
34. Lee SB, Rao AK, Lee K-H, et al. Decreased expression of phospholipase C-$\beta 2$ isozyme in human platelets with impaired function. Blood 1996;88:1684–1691.
35. Jiang H, Kuang Y, Wu Y, et al. Roles of phospholipase C $\beta 2$ in chemoattractant-elicited responses. Proc Natl Acad Sci USA 1997;94:7971–7975.
36. Holmsen H, Walsh PN, Koike K, et al. Familial bleeding disorder associated with deficiencies in platelet signal processing and glycoproteins. Br J Haematol 1987;67:335–344.
37. Mitsui T. Defective signal transduction through the thromboxane A$_2$ receptor in a patient with a mild bleeding disorder. Deficiency of the inositol 1,4,5-triphosphate formation despite normal G-protein activation. Thromb Haemost 1997;77:991–995.
38. Cartwright J, Hampton KK, Macneil S, et al. A haemorrhagic platelet disorder associated with altered stimulus-response coupling and abnormal membrane phospholipid composition. Br J Haematol 1994;88:129–136.
39. Gabbeta J, Yang X, Sun L, et al. Abnormal inside-out signal transduction-dependent activation of GPIIb-IIIa in a patient with impaired pleckstrin phosphorylation. Blood 1996;87:1368–1376.
40. Remold-ODonnell E, Rosen FS, Kenney DM. Defects in Wiskott-Aldrich syndrome blood cells. Blood 1996;87:2621–2631.
41. Featherstone C. The many faces of WAS protein [news]. Science 1997;275:27–28.
42. Solum NO. Procoagulant expression in platelets and defects leading to clinical disorders. Arterioscler Thromb Vasc Biol 1999;19:2841–2846.
43. Walsh PN. Platelet-coagulant protein interactions. In: Colman RW, Hirsh J, Marder VJ (eds.): Hemostasis and Thrombosis. Basic Principles and Clinical Practice. Philadelphia, J.B. Lippincott, 1994; pp. 629–651.
44. Weiss HJ. Scott syndrome: a disorder of platelet coagulant activity. Semin Hematol 1994;31:312–319.
45. Degos L, Dautigny A, Brouet JC, et al. A molecular defect in thrombasthenic platelets. J Clin Invest 1975;56:235.
46. Mannucci PM. Desmopressin (DDAVP) in the treatment of bleeding disorders; the first 20 years. Blood 1997;90:2515–2521.
47. Mannucci PM. Hemostatic drugs. N Engl J Med 1998;339:245–253.
48. Rao AK, Ghosh S, Sun L, et al. Effect of mechanism of platelet dysfunction on response to DDAVP in patients with congenital platelet function defects. A double-blind placebo-controlled trial. Thromb Haemost 1995;74:1071–1078.
49. Kobrinsky NL, Israels ED, Gerrard JM, et al. Shortening of bleeding time by 1-deamino-8-D-arginine vasopressin in various bleeding disorders. Lancet 1984;1:1145–1148.
50. Schulman S, Johnson H, Egberg N, et al. DDAVP-induced correction of prolonged bleeding time in patients with congenital platelet function defects. Thromb Res 1987;45:165–174.
51. DiMichele DM, Hathaway WE. Use of DDAVP in inherited and acquired platelet dysfunction. Am J Hematol 1990;33:39–45.
52. Mannucci PM. Desmopression (DDAVP) for treatment of disorders of hemostasis. In: Progress in Hemostasis and Thrombosis. Orlando, FL, Grune & Stratton, 1986, pp. 19–44.
53. Nieuwenhuis HK, Sixma JJ. 1-Desamino-8-d-arginine vasopressin (Desmopressin) shortens the bleeding time in storage pool deficiency. Ann Intern Med 1988;108:65–67.
54. Mannucci PM, Vicente V, Vianello L, et al. Controlled trial of desmopressin in liver cirrhosis and other conditions associated with a prolonged bleeding time. Blood 1986;67:1148–1153.
55. Mielke CH, Jr., Levine PH, Zucker S. Preoperative prednisone therapy in platelet function disorders. Thromb Res 1981;21:655–662.
56. Berliner S, Horowitz I, Martinowitz U, et al. Dental surgery in patients with severe factor XI deficiency without plasma replacement. Blood Coagul Fibrinolysis 1992;3:465–468.
57. Sindet-Pedersen S, Ramstrom G, Bernvil S, et al. Hemostatic effect of tranexamic acid mouthwash in anticoagulant-treated patients undergoing oral surgery. N Engl J Med 1989;320:840–843.
58. Bellucci S, Devergie A, Gluckman E, et al. Complete correction of Glanzmann's thrombasthenia by allogeneic bone-marrow transplantation. Br J Haematol 1985;59:635–641.
59. Mullen CA, Anderson KD, Blaese RM. Splenectomy and/or bone marrow transplantation in the management of the Wiskott-Aldrich syndrome: long-term follow-up of 62 cases. Blood 1993;82:2961–2966.
60. Schafer AI. Bleeding and thrombosis in myeloproliferative disorders. Blood 1984;64:1–12.
61. Wehmeier A, Sudhoff T, Meierkord F. Relation of platelet abnormalities to thrombosis and hemorrhage in chronic myeloproliferative disorders. Semin Thromb Hemost 1997;23:391–402.
62. Ravandi-Kashani F, Schafer AI. Microvascular disturbances, thrombosis, and bleeding in thrombocythemia: current concepts and perspectives. Semin Thromb Hemost 1997;23:479–488.
63. Landolfi R, Marchioli R, Patrono C. Mechanisms of bleeding and thrombosis in myeloproliferative disorders. Thromb Haemost 1997;78:617–621.
64. van Genderen PJ, Michiels JJ. Erythromelalgia: a pathognomonic microvascular thrombotic complication in essential throm-

bocythemia and polycythemia vera. Semin Thromb Hemost 1997;23:357–363.
65. Koudstaal PJ, Koudstaal A. Neurologic and visual symptoms in essential thrombocythemia: efficacy of low-dose aspirin. Semin Thromb Hemost 1997;23:365–370.
66. Tefferi A, Hoagland HC. Issues in the diagnosis and management of essential thrombocythemia. Mayo Clin Proc 1994;69:651–655.
67. Colombi M, Radaelli F, Zocchi L, et al. Thrombotic and hemorrhagic complications in essential thrombocythemia. A retrospective study of 103 patients. Cancer 1991;67:2926–2930.
68. Cortelazzo S, Viero P, Finazzi G, et al. Incidence and risk factors for thrombotic complications in a historical cohort of 100 patients with essential thrombocythemia. J Clin Oncol 1990; 8:556–562.
69. Lahuerta-Palacios JJ, Bornstein R, Fernandez-Debora FJ, et al. Controlled and uncontrolled thrombocytosis. Its clinical role in essential thrombocythemia. Cancer 1988;61:1207–1212.
70. Fenaux P, Simon M, Caulier MT, et al. Clinical course of essential thrombocythemia in 147 cases. Cancer 1990;66:549–556.
71. Rozman C, Giralt M, Feliu E, et al. Life expectancy of patients with chronic nonleukemic myeloproliferative disorders. Cancer 1991;67:2658–2663.
72. Berk PD, Wasswerman LR, Fruchtman SM, et al. Treatment of polycythemia vera: A summary of clinical trials conducted by the Polycythemia Vera Study Group. In: Wasserman LR, Berk PD, Berlin NI (eds.): Polycythemia Vera and the Myeloproliferative Disorders. Philadelphia, WB Saunders, 1995, pp. 166–194.
73. Policitemia GIS. Polycythemia vera: the natural history of 1213 patients followed for 20 years. Ann Intern Med 1995;123: 656–654.
74. Rao AK, Carvalho A. Acquired qualitative platelet defects. In: Colman RW, Hirsh J, Marder VJ, Salzman EW (eds.): Hemostasis and Thrombosis: Basic Principles and Clinical Practice, 3rd Ed. Philadelphia, J.B. Lippincott, 1994, pp. 685–704.
75. Waddell CC, Brown JA, Repinecz YA. Abnormal platelet function in myeloproliferative disorders. Arch Pathol Lab Med 1981; 105:432–435.
76. Wu KK. Platelet hyperaggregability and thrombosis in patients with thrombocythemia. Ann Intern Med 1978;88:7–11.
77. Sterkers Y, Preudhomme C, Lai JL, et al. Acute myeloid leukemia and myelodysplastic syndromes following essential thrombocythemia treated with hydroxyurea: high proportion of cases with 17p deletion [see comments]. Blood 1998;91:616–622.
78. Tefferi A, Silverstein MN, Petitt RM, et al. Anagrelide as a new platelet-lowering agent in essential thrombocythemia: mechanism of action, efficacy, toxicity, current indications. Semin Thromb Hemost 1997;23:379–383.
79. Elliott MA, Tefferi A. Interferon-alpha therapy in polycythemia vera and essential thrombocythemia. Semin Thromb Hemost 1997;23:463–472.
80. Perkins HA, McKenzie MR, Fudenberg HH. Hemostatic defects in dysproteinemias. Blood 1970;35:695–707.
81. McGrath KM, Stuart JJ, Richards FD. Correlation between serum IgG, platelet membrane IgG, and platelet function in hypergammaglobulinaemic states. Br J Haematol 1979;42:585–591.
82. Castillo R, Lozano T, Escolar G, et al. Defective platelet adhesion on vessel subendothelium in uremic patients. Blood 1986;68:337–342.
83. Remuzzi GD, Marchesi M, Livio AE, et al. Altered platelet and vascular prostaglandin-generation in patients with chronic renal failure and prolonged bleeding times. Thromb Res 1978; 13:1007–1015.
84. Sinzinger H, Leithner C. Eicosanoids of platelets and vascular wall in chronic renal insufficiency. Am J Nephrol 1987;7:212–220.
85. Livio M, Gotti E, Marchesi D, et al. Uraemic bleeding: role of anemia and beneficial effect of red cell transfusions. Lancet 1982;II:1013–1015.

86. Moia M, Mannucci PM, Vizzotto L, et al. Improvement in the haemostatic defect of uraemia after treatment with recombinant human erythropoietin. Lancet 1987;8570:1227–1229.
87. Horowitz HI, Stein IM, Cohen BD, et al. Further studies on the platelet inhibitory effect of guanidinosuccinic acid: its role in uremic bleeding. Am J Med 1970;49:336–345.
88. Rabiner SF, Molinas F. The role of phenol and phenolic acids on the thrombocytopathy and defective platelet aggregation of patients with renal failure. Am J Med 1970;49:346–351.
89. Janson PA, Jubelirer SJ, Weinstein MJ, et al. Treatment of the bleeding tendency in uremia with cryoprecipitate. N Engl J Med 1980;303:1318–1322.
90. Liu Y, Kosfeld RE, Marcum SG. Treatment of uraemic bleeding with conjugated oestrogen. Lancet 1984;II:887–890.
91. Livio M, Mannucci PM, Vigano G, et al. Conjugated estrogens for the management of bleeding associated with renal failure. N Engl J Med 1986;315:731–735.
92. Steering Committee of the Physicians' Health Study Research Group. Final report on the aspirin component of the ongoing Physicians' Health Study. N Engl J Med 1989;321:129–135.
93. Patrono C, Coller B, Dalen JE, et al. Platelet-active drugs: the relationships among dose, effectiveness, and side effects. Chest 1998;114:470S–488S.
94. Garcia Rodriguez LA, Cattaruzzi C, Troncon MG, et al. Risk of hospitalization for upper gastrointestinal tract bleeding associated with ketorolac, other nonsteroidal anti-inflammatory drugs, calcium antagonists, and other antihypertensive drugs. Arch Intern Med 1998;158:33–39.
95. Henry D, Lim LL, Garcia Rodriguez LA, et al. Variability in risk of gastrointestinal complications with individual non-steroidal anti-inflammatory drugs: results of a collaborative meta-analysis [see comments]. BMJ 1996;312:1563–1566.
96. Roderick PJ, Wilkes HC, Meade TW. The gastrointestinal toxicity of aspirin: an overview of randomised controlled trials. Br J Clin Pharmacol 1993;35:219–226.
97. Sharis PJ, Cannon CP, Loscalzo J. The antiplatelet effects of ticlopidine and clopidogrel. Ann Intern Med 1998;129:394–405.
98. Coukell AJ, Markham A. Clopidogrel. Drugs 1997;54:745–50; discussion 751.
99. Bennett CL, Weinberg PD, Rozenberg-Ben-Dror K, et al. Thrombotic thrombocytopenic purpura associated with ticlopidine. A review of 60 cases. Ann Intern Med 1998;128:541–544.
100. Bennett CL, Connors JM, Carwile JM, et al. Thrombotic thrombocytopenic purpura associated with clopidogrel [see comments]. N Engl J Med 2000;342:1773–7.
101. Coller BS. Platelet GPIIb/IIIa antagonists: the first anti-integrin receptor therapeutics. J Clin Invest 1997;100:S57–60.
102. Topol EJ, Byzova TV, Plow EF. Platelet GPIIb–IIIa blockers. Lancet 1999;353:227–231.
103. Berkowitz SD, Harrington RA, Rund MM, et al. Acute profound thrombocytopenia after C7E3 Fab (abciximab) therapy [see comments]. Circulation 1997;95:809–813.
104. Johnson GJ. Platelets, penicillins, and purpura: what does it all mean? J Lab Clin Med 1993;121:531–533.
105. Sattler FR, Weitekamp MR, Ballard JO. Potential for bleeding with the new beta-lactam antibiotics. Ann Intern Med 1986; 105:924–931.
106. Natelson EA, Brown CH, III, Bradshaw MW, et al. Influence of cephalosporin antibiotics on blood coagulation and platelet function. Antimicrob Agents Chemother 1976;9:91–93.
107. Weitekamp MR, Aber RC. Prolonged bleeding times and bleeding diathesis associated with moxalactam administration. JAMA 1983;249:69–71.
108. Brown CH, III, Natelson EA, Bradshaw MW, et al. The hemostatic defect produced by carbenicillin. N Engl J Med 1974;291:265–270.
109. Fass RJ, Copelan EA, Brandt JT, et al. Platelet mediated bleeding caused by broad spectrum penicillins. J Infect Dis 1987;155:1242–1248.

110. Brown CH, III, Natelson EA, Bradshaw MW. A study of the effects of ticarcillin on blood coagulation and platelet function. Antimicrob Agents Chemother 1975;7:652–657.
111. Warkentin TE. Heparin-induced thrombocytopenia: a clinicopathologic syndrome. Thromb Haemost 1999;82:439–442.
112. Gimple LW, Gold HK, Leinbach RC, et al. Correlation between template bleeding times and spontaneous bleeding during treatment of acute myocardial infarction with recombinant tissue-type plasminogen activator. Circulation 1989;80:581–588.
113. Coller BS. Platelets and thrombolytic therapy. N Engl J Med 1990;322:33–42.
114. Deykin D, Janson P, McMahon L. Ethanol potentiation of aspirin-induced prolongation of the bleeding time. N Engl J Med 1982;306:852–854.

CHAPTER 11

Purpura and Related Hematovascular Lesions

Craig S. Kitchens, M.D.

Purpura is a general term that describes either small punctate lesions called petechiae or larger lesions called ecchymoses (see Table 11–1 for terminology). *Purpura* is derived from the Latin term for purple, the color generated by the extravasation of red cells into the skin. Extravasation may result from coagulation disorders, physical trauma, or systemic conditions that lead to alterations of the microvasculature. Purpura is due to extravasation of blood from the microcirculation, which consists of the smallest arterioles, capillaries, and postcapillary venules. Purpura is thus a disorder of the microcirculation.

The hematologist is often asked to evaluate patients with purpura because the differential diagnosis of disorders that may result in purpura includes many hematologic processes. Because purpuric disorders require careful consideration of both hematologic and dermatologic etiologies, the hematologist should be familiar with hematologic purpura as well as its imitators. One may wish to consult with a dermatologist on many patients. The differential diagnosis of disorders leading to purpuric lesions encompasses a considerable range of processes, from mild chronic dermatologic disorders to rapidly progressive, life-threatening illnesses such as meningococcemia with disseminated intravascular coagulation.

Although Osler-Weber-Rendu (OWR) syndrome (also known as hereditary hemorrhagic telangiectasia (HHT)) is not truly a purpuric disorder as blood is not extravasated, discussion of OWR syndrome traditionally is placed among discussions of purpura. We will address other hematovascular perturbations of skin that are included in the differential diagnosis of purpura.

HISTORICAL PERSPECTIVE

Because of their ready visibility, purpuric lesions have been described throughout history. Victims of the bubonic plague, which circled the globe in the Middle Ages killing untold millions of people, often were purpuric (hence "Black Death"), which led to the rapid recognition of the affliction and banishment by others. Typhus is claimed to have killed more soldiers throughout history than all battles combined.[1] Scurvy, particularly the prevention of scurvy, which was appreciated and practiced by the British Navy, was highly instrumental in England's defeat of Napoleon's navy, which did not practice scurvy prevention. Prior to the British Navy's adoption of antiscorbutic measures, 1500 cases of scurvy were admitted to the main naval hospital in England each year. After institution of antiscorbutic policies, scurvy was essentially eliminated from the British Navy and extant records reveal only two cases in the 5-year period following Alfred Lord Nelson's destruction of the French Navy in 1805. This story has been delightfully recounted in the medical literature.[2]

Although purpura had been known for centuries, scientific interest in purpura was established in the 18th century when Werlhof, then serving as Court Physician to King George II of England, accurately described what we now call acute idiopathic thrombocytopenic purpura (ITP).[3] At the very beginning of the 19th century Willan[4] reviewed purpura, establishing five categories in the first rudimentary attempt to understand purpura as a rightfully circumscribed area of clinical science. His five subtypes of purpura were (1) purpura simplex, (2) purpura haemorrhagica, (3) purpura urticans, (4) purpura senilis, and (5) purpura contagiosa. More likely than not, the five subtypes of purpura that he was illustrating 200 years ago would now be regarded as, respectively, purpura simplex, acute ITP, Henoch-Schönlein purpura, senile purpura, and meningococcemia as well as other acute bacterial infections related to purpura. Approximately 100 years later, at the turn of the 19th century, purpura was reviewed by Austin Flint in his textbook.[5] The understanding of purpura had not substantially ad-

Table 11-1 • TERMINOLOGY USED IN THIS CHAPTER

Purpura	A general term for nonblanching, bluish-purple lesions due to extravasated blood fading over time to greenish-yellow lesions as those extravasated cells deteriorate.
Petechiae	A specific type purpura being macular pinpoint lesions (≤ 3 mm) with well-demarcated borders.
Ecchymosis	A specific type purpura being a larger macular purpuric lesion due to either confluence of petechiae or more commonly a larger hemorrhagic lesion. Borders are not sharply defined.
Palpable purpura	Purpuric lesions that appear to be raised (i.e., papular) and occasionally are palpable due to infiltration of lesions with leukocytes.
Bruise	A lay term without specific meaning but a frequent chief complaint.
Hematoma	A palpable mass ≥ 1 cm usually due to bleeding into or between tissue planes.
Vasculitis	Palpable purpura due to infectious, inflammatory, or immunologic mechanisms with white cell infiltration.
Necrotizing vasculitis	Infarctive necrosis of the skin due to vasculitis. Subsequent to necrosis, lesions may turn from purple to "gun-metal gray" or black.
Erythema	Reddened skin due to increased cutaneous blood flow from vasodilation secondary to fever, exercise, or emotional factors. Ill-defined borders. Readily blanchable.
Telangiectases	Pleural term for 1- to 4-mm dark-red masses of capillaries without extravasation which blanch to pressure. May be macular or somewhat papular.
Cherry angiomas	Very papular 1- to 4-mm cherry-red "hard" hemangiomas that compress only with difficulty. A normal finding in middle-aged and older persons, particularly in the lower chest and upper abdominal area.
Spiders	Appropriately named lesions with a central 1- to 2-mm visible arteriole ("body") with "legs" branching centrifugally for 1 to 3 cm. Gentle pressure on the body occludes the arteriole and the legs rapidly disappear.
Livedo reticularis	Purplish, faint, ill-defined reticular network of small vessels on legs and occasionally arms.
Purple (or blue) toes	Ischemic toes and extremities from arteriolar infarction due to arteriolar emboli, especially from cholesterol embolization or thrombosis in the setting of heparin induced thrombocytopenia.
Warfarin skin necrosis	Ischemic skin over fatty tissue resulting from capillary and venular infarction due to fibrin deposition.

vanced since Willan's review. Flint did clearly separate clinical purpura from hemophilia and traumatic hemorrhage. His description of purpura simplex is more reminiscent of benign dermatologic types of purpura such as the progressive pigmented purpura of Schamberg and perhaps mild cases of primary cutaneous vasculitis. He preferred the term *purpura rheumatica* to purpura urticans and clearly described what we now refer to as Henoch-Schönlein purpura (HSP). He did not like Willan's term, *purpura haemorrhagica*, recognizing that all purpura was indeed hemorrhagic. He preferred to revert to the older European name for ITP, namely *morbus maculosus Werlhofii*, or Werlhof disease. Although he did not use a separate descriptive category for scurvy, he correctly described the two primary differences between ITP and scurvy: the lack of gum swelling and hemorrhage characteristic of advanced scurvy and the fact that ITP did not respond to dietetic manipulation as did scurvy. William Osler in the major textbook of medicine in that era competing with that of Flint gave a similar account of purpura.[6] He again clearly separated hemophilia from the purpuric disorders. Demonstrating his strength in observational medicine, he was the first to accurately describe petechiae, differentiating them from ecchymoses. He described cases of purpura following iodine administration, which were probably the result of iodine-induced cutaneous vasculitis. He preferred the term *cachectic purpura* to senile purpura. Osler also clearly distinguished HHT (now one of the several diseases bearing his name, OWR syndrome) from hemophilia while recognizing that both were hereditary hemorrhagic diatheses.[7]

That thrombocytopenia was causally related to the petechiae of ITP was recognized by the end of the 19th century. The existence of nonthrombocytopenic purpura received a large boost in credibility when Wolbach[8] in 1919 described that the purpura in Rocky Mountain spotted fever was associated with the infestation of rickettsiae in the walls of microcirculatory vessels. In 1942, Wintrobe opined that although thrombocytopenia was characteristic in ITP, there were many purpuric diseases in which the platelet counts were normal and therefore concluded that "some obscure change in the capillary endothelium" must account for at least some cases of nonthrombocytopenic purpura.[9] In 1948, Haden and colleagues[10] demonstrated that cutaneous hemorrhage could occur with a normal platelet count and normal clotting system. They promulgated the concept of "increased capillary fragility," a term that by virtue of its accuracy has continued to be used until today. In 1952 Spaet[11] and in 1953 Ackroyd[12] clearly, convincingly, and permanently established vascular damage as a primary cause of nonthrombocytopenic purpura. The study of the microcirculation and endothelial biology in particular became possible with electron microscopy, endothelial cell culture, and other modern biomedical techniques.

MICROVASCULAR STRUCTURE–FUNCTION INTERRELATIONS

The study of the fine structure of the microcirculation was pioneered by Majno.[13] The microcirculation is defined as terminal arterioles, capillaries, and postcapillary venules. Figure 11–1 depicts a normal capillary. The capillary will be used as the model of the basic microvascular structural unit. The primary anatomic difference between capillaries and arterioles as well as postcapillary venules is that both of the latter have an investiture of smooth muscle cells in order to control blood flow. The capillary, by anatomic definition, lacks smooth muscle investiture, as its function is not to regulate traffic; rather, as the "business end" of the circulation, it is the site of unimpeded gas, fluid, and nutrient exchange. Accordingly, its structue is simple. The primary structural unit is a series of two to five endothelial cells that are joined by tight junctions. Endothelial cells are now known to be extremely influential, providing a great deal of secretory activity on both luminal and abluminal surfaces and assuming, under appropriate stimulation, a neutral, antithrombotic, or prothrombotic stance. The subendothelial basement membrane is immediately beneath the closed circle of endothelial cells. This ill-defined material probably affords some degree of structural integrity but chiefly is highly procoagulant in the event that blood makes contact with it by virtue of a breach in the endothelial membrane. Liberally scattered both longitudinally and circumferentially around capillaries are collagen bundles, which offer resilience against mechanical stresses. Around capillaries are pericytes, whose function is probably largely one of support. Accordingly, the four chief functioning members of the structure of the capillary circulation that keep the circulatory system closed are (1) the endothelium, (2) the subendothelial basement membrane, (3) collagen, and (4) pericytes.

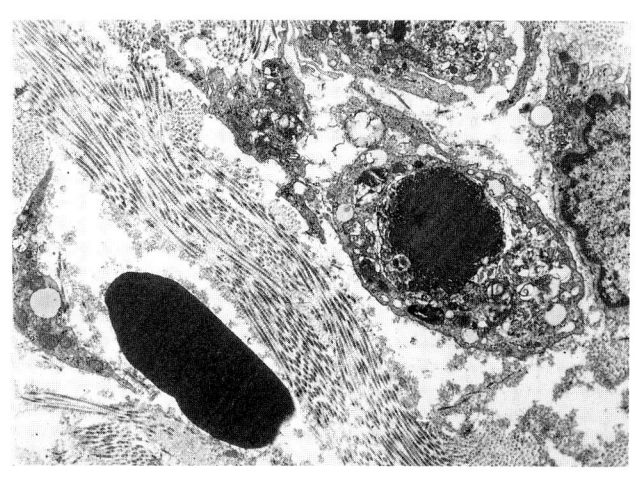

Figure 11–2 Electron micrograph of a petechia. Two extravasated red cells are apparent. The one on the bottom left is in the interstitial space surrounded by bundles of collagen. The one on the right has been phagocytized by a macrophage and is being degraded. The cytoplasm of the macrophage contains residual material from previous red cell ingestion.

The histologic hallmark of purpura is extravasation of red blood cells from the microcirculation. Color Plate 11–1 shows a light-microscopic examination of a biopsy of a single petechia in which red cells have extravasated from a nearby capillary. In Figure 11–2, extravasated red cells abound, with at least one phagocytized by a tissue macrophage. Iron from the heme in red cell remains in the skin, causing hemosiderin deposition characteristic of the extremities of patients who have had long-standing purpura. In Figure 11–3, one sees a red cell that has found its way into a lymphatic and will be returned to the general circulation via lymphatic drainage.

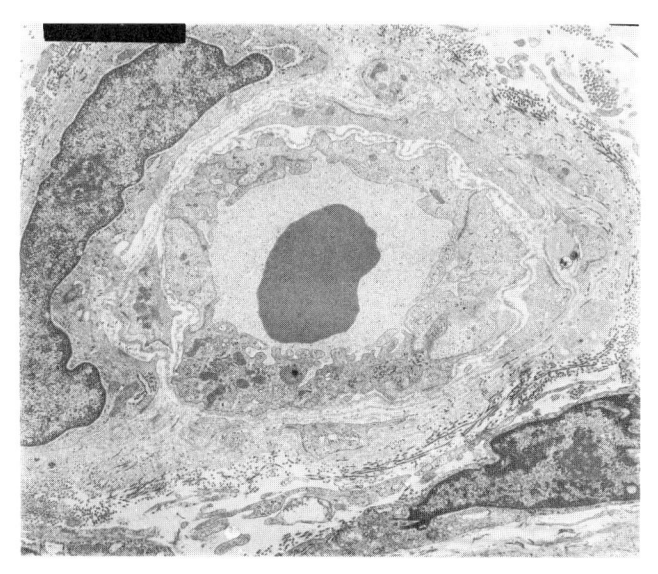

Figure 11–1 Electron micrograph of a normal capillary. This capillary consists of parts of five endothelial cells. A red cell is in the lumen. The thickness of the endothelium is approximately 2500 μm. Supporting tissue includes the basement membrane immediately on the ablumenal side of the endothelium. Darker bands of collagen are seen both longitudinally and circumferentially around the capillary. The two large nuclei are those of pericytes.

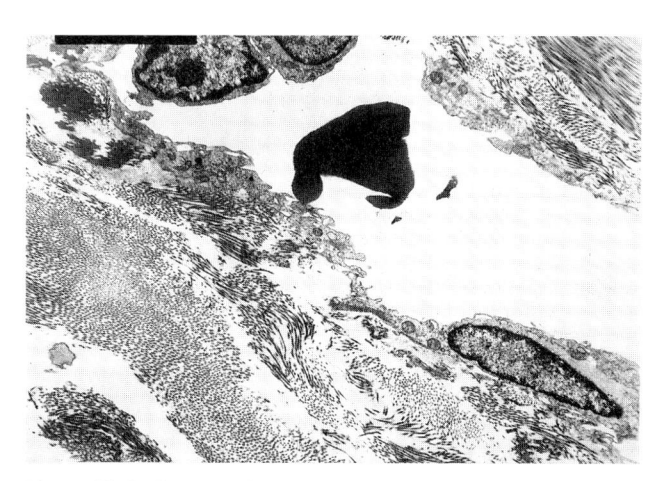

Figure 11–3 Electron micrograph of an extravasated red cell in a lymphatic vessel. This red cell has regained entry into the circulation via this lymphatic. Lymphatic channels are characterized by large nuclei that bulge into the lumen as well as by their extremely thin wall. There is a relative lack of electron density in the lumen owing to the low protein concentration of lymph.

PATHOPHYSIOLOGIC CATEGORIES OF PURPURA

Table 11-2 presents a classification of purpura and hematovascular lesions.

Purpura Not Associated with Known Microvascular Pathology

Frequently purpura is found in which there is no known anatomic aberration of the microcirculation. These are truly purpuric in that if one chooses to biopsy such lesions, extravasated red cells are seen.

Mechanical Purpura

The mechanical strength of the capillary unit is finite and thus any pressure that exceeds that limit could well lead to the extravasation of red cells. Elliott[14] has determined that a vacuum of 200 mmHg over normal skin will extravasate red cells. That the human mouth can generate this suction is exemplified by lesions about the neck known as "hickeys." Petechiae on the face and neck may result from increased venous pressure following vomiting or seizures, or even from prolonged hanging upside down by one's feet in order to alleviate back pain. Purpura found on the palms and soles of the feet may result from leisure activities such as weight-lifting or traumatic blows from one's avocation or occupation.[15] The chief diagnostic criterion is the history of activities prior to the appearance of purpura.

Factitious Purpura

When patients with purpura provide a history that is vague or not credible, one should suspect factitious purpura. A variety of suction devices have been applied to every imaginable part of the body in order to produce purpura for whatever gain the patient may seek. Color Plate 11-2 shows a pattern of purpura that clearly suggests the patient's raking reachable parts of his body with a gardening implement. Factitious purpura is more common than one may at first appreciate but can be suspected when the patient has been seen repeatedly by multiple physicians without any hemostatic abnormalities being found. This purpura tends to be well circumscribed and found only in areas that can be readily reached by the patient.

Psychogenic Purpura

This is an unusual form of purpura that is increasingly regarded as factitious in origin.[16] It is indisputable that patients having this type of purpura harbor major deep emotional disturbances and a great deal of unresolved emotional conflict. Lesions of this purpura usually begin with bruises that are heralded after a variable lead time by a feeling of warmth, stinging, or swelling. Later an ecchymotic lesion might appear. These bruises can vary from small to rather large. They still have many of the features of factitious purpura in that they are often linear, have well-demarcated edges, and chiefly occur in areas that can be reached (Color Plate 11-3). The relationship of this disorder to autoerythrocyte sensitization as described by Gardner and Diamond[17] is uncertain.

Purpura Simplex

This vascular phenomenon is nonpathologic and is a normal process. Many people have small bruises that

---

Table 11-2 • PURPURA AND HEMATOVASCULAR LESIONS

Purpura Not Associated with Known Microvascular Pathology
Mechanical purpura
Factitious purpura
Psychogenic purpura
Purpura simplex
Hematomas
Progressive pigmented purpuras (PPPs)

Purpura Associated with Abnormalities of Platelets
Thrombocytopenic purpura
Purpura associated with abnormal platelet function

Cutaneous Vasculitis (CV)
Primary
    Hypersensitivity vasculitis
    Henoch-Schönlein purpura
Secondary (see Table 11-3)

Purpura Associated with Microbial Endothelial Damage
Rickettsial diseases
Leptospiral diseases
Parvovirus B19
Viral hemorrhagic diseases

Purpura Associated with Decreased Microvascular Mechanical Strength
Scurvy
Hypercortisolism
Senile or atrophic purpura
Heritable disorders of connective tissue
Amyloidosis
Osler-Weber-Rendu Disease (OWR)

Purpura Associated with Microthrombi
Disseminated intravascular coagulation (DIC)
Warfarin skin necrosis
Fat embolism syndrome
Myeloblastemia
Thrombotic thrombocytopenic purpura (TTP)
Heparin-induced thrombocytopenia (HIT)
Purple (blue) toe syndrome and cholesterol emboli

Purpura Associated with Vascular Malignancy

Nonpurpuric Hematovascular Disorders
Livedo reticularis
Hemangiomas
Angiomas
Spiders
Erythema

are associated with trauma of daily living. Women do bruise or complain of bruising more than men.[18] Color Plate 11-4 shows an ecchymotic area on the lateral surface of the thigh. It is striking how frequently these bruises are about 30 inches above the floor—the height of most furniture, cabinets, and tables about the house or at work. Purpura simplex may result from being pinched; such lesions are also referred to as "devil's pinches" if there is no recall of being pinched. As this purpura is not of pathologic origin, further evaluation is not necessary. Such patients may undergo surgery or invasive procedures safely.

Bruises and Hematomas

Bruises (including purpura simplex) are not palpable (i.e., not true hematomas) but are flat within the surface of the skin. Bruises result from trauma but of course can be exacerbated by platelet or coagulation defects to become larger bruises or even hematomas. Simple bruises have been somewhat arbitrarily defined as being smaller than 3 cm in diameter and not palpable; they usually number no more than four to six over the body. If larger and more multiple, consideration may be given to a hemostatic defect, especially if they are palpable masses (i.e., true hematomas). Color Plate 11-5 shows a large hematoma of the shin following an athletic incident that served as the diagnostic event for a teenager with heretofore undiagnosed mild hemophilia A with 7% of normal factor VIII activity. Large ecchymotic areas with hematoma formation (Color Plate 11-6) is the typical presentation of factor VIII inhibitors, as discussed in Chapter 6.

Progressive Pigmented Purpuras

A variety of dermatologic diseases have no known underlying cause but are characterized by long periods of progressive crops of purpuric lesions about the legs. Dermatologists have subdivided these progressive pigmented purpural (PPPs) into a variety of categories, such as progressive pigmented purpura of Schamberg, telangiectodes of Majocchi, lichen aureus, or Gougerot-Blum purpura.[19] These disorders on skin biopsy are similar, with the specific absence of leukocytoclastic vasculitis, but many of them do display mononuclear pericapillaritis. Laboratory examinations such as the complete blood count (CBC) and immunologic tests are normal. Electron microscopic studies in these disorders have failed to show any abnormalities in the capillaries. These disorders have no major sequelae and therapy is primarily cosmetic.

Purpura Associated with Abnormalities of Platelets

Thrombocytopenic purpura results most commonly from mild trauma with profound thrombocytopenia (30,000/dL or less) but may also be found in patients with qualitative platelet defects.

Thrombocytopenic Purpura

Spontaneous purpura and epistaxis are most frequently seen in severe thrombocytopenia (10,000/dL or less) and as such sudden, spontaneous petechial hemorrhage is the clinical hallmark of acute ITP. Purpura probably results from two closely related but separate pathophysiologic events. Clearly platelets do serve a reparative function in the microcirculation, being called upon to bridge breaches in the endothelium by adhesion to disrupted endothelium and subendothelial tissues with subsequent aggregation. However, lack of this reparative process does not readily explain the concept of increased capillary fragility. Petechiae, ecchymosis, and epistaxis occur during severe thrombocytopenia even without any trauma. Examples of capillary fragility include the ring of petechiae around the arm under a blood pressure cuff following blood pressure determination (Color Plate 11-7) and petechiae following simply scratching one's self. More likely than not this is due to intense capillary fragility resulting from severe thrombocytopenia. In experimental animals and humans with severe thrombocytopenia, the microvascular endothelium undergoes morphologic changes, including extreme thinning of the endothelium from its normal 2000 to 3000 μm to 20 to 50 μm, or even in some places to only narrow fenestrations composed of only the endothelial cell membranes (Fig. 11-4). Clearly such endothelial lesions afford virtually no strength against mechanical stresses or pressure and in fact may spontaneously leak red cells. Of interest, the capillary membrane thickness revert toward normal even without a quantitative improvement of

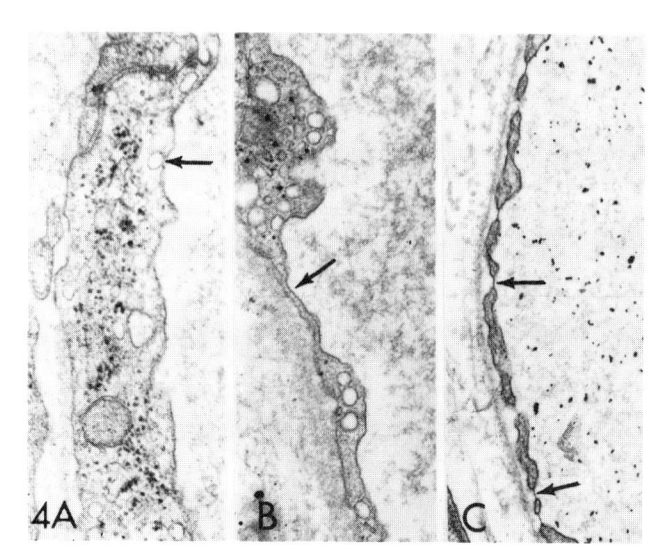

Figure 11-4 Electron micrograph of capillaries in experimental thrombocytopenia. A. A capillary from a nonthrombocytopenic control animal. The endothelial membrane has a thickness of approximately 2000 to 2500 μm. The arrow points to a normal vesicle. B. Thinning of the endothelium in experimental thrombocytopenia. The endothelium has been thinned (*arrow*) nearly to the same size as the normal vesicle. C. Even further thinning (*arrows*) to the point where the endothelium has become fenestrated, an anatomic finding not characteristic of cutaneous capillaries. The lumen of the capillary is oriented to the right in all three panels. (From Kitchens CS. Ameliorization of endothelial abnormalities by prednisone in experimental thrombocytopenia in the rabbit. J Clin Invest 1977;60:1129-1134, with permission.)

platelets following the administration of glucocorticosteroids.[20,21] A recent study suggests that platelets provide the endothelium with growth factor(s). The absence of growth factor(s) may explain, in part, endothelial morphologic alterations in severe thrombocytopenia.[22]

Purpura Associated with Abnormal Platelet Function

Occasionally platelets are sufficient in number but their quality is such that hemostatic failure manifested as purpura or epistaxis may occur. Theoretically this can be seen with antiplatelet agents such as aspirin or any of the newer agents that are being increasingly used in the treatment of ischemic heart disease. Whether or not there is an accompanying endothelial morphologic disturbance by virtue of qualitative platelet defects as there is in quantitative defects is not known. Congenital defects of platelet function that cause purpura, such as Bernard-Soulier syndrome or Glanzmann thrombasthenia, are discussed in Chapter 10.

Cutaneous Vasculitis

Cutaneous vasculitis (CV) is a common cause of nonthrombocytopenic purpura and because of its frequent association with significant underlying medical diseases is of interest to the hematologist and internist. That CV is often associated with diseases of rheumatic origin led early investigators such as William Osler and Austin Flint to refer to this as *purpura rheumatica*. We now frequently refer to CV also by its chief clinical attribute (*palpable purpura*) or its histologic hallmark (*leukocytoclastic vasculitis*). In leukocytoclastic vasculitis (LCV), the smallest vessels in the skin are encased by sheets of neutrophils in various stages of disintegration, often referred to as "nuclear dust" (Color Plate 11–8). The heavy infiltration by the leukocytes is what actually gives rise to the perception of palpability in palpable purpura (Color Plate 11–9). It is hypothesized that this pathologic event results from leakage of immune complexes through the vessel wall into the subendothelial area. These complexes then induce the egress of leukocytes. Subsequently, the neutrophils disintegrate, releasing their proteolytic enzymes into the area around the adjacent vessel, causing digestion and disruption of the endothelial membrane with subsequent egress of red cells (Fig. 11–5). When LCV is acutely severe, it is termed *necrotizing vasculitis*.

The list of disorders associated with CV is long and varied (Table 11–3). These are best categorized as rheumatic in origin and associated with requisite immune complexes. Table 11–4 demonstrates the appreciated etiologic differences between adult and childhood CV. The predominance of CV in children is termed *primary CV* because no obvious chronic underlying cause can be found. The majority (89%) of pediatric primary cases are associated with some combination of palpable pur-

Table 11–3 • DISORDERS ASSOCIATED WITH CUTANEOUS VASCULITIS (CV)

Primary CV	Secondary CV
Idiopathic	
Hypersensitivity reaction*	Systemic lupus erythematosus
Upper respiratory tract infection, viral, or bacterial	Chronic hepatitis B
	Chronic hepatitis C
	Cryoglobulinemia
Drugs:	Sjögren's syndrome
Penicillin	Polyarteritis nodosa
Iodine	Rheumatoid arthritis
Aspirin	Mixed connective tissue syndrome
Antibiotics	Subacute bacterial endocarditis
Analgesics	Wegner granulomatosis
NSAIDs	Churg-Strauss syndrome
Thiazides	Hypergrammaglobulinemic purpura of Waldenstrom
Colchicine	Myelodysplastic syndromes
	Malignancies

* Hypersensitivity reactions may be termed Henoch-Schönlein purpura (HSP) if the patient has colicky gastrointestinal symptoms, gastrointestinal bleeding, hematuria or other evidence of nephritis, and large-joint arthralgias or swelling *and* not on medication known to be associated with hypersensitivity vasculitis.
Adapted from Blanco R, Martinez-Taboada VM, Rodriguez-Valverde V, et al. Cutaneous vasculitis in children and adults. Associated diseases and etiologic factors in 303 patients. Medicine 1998;77;403–418.

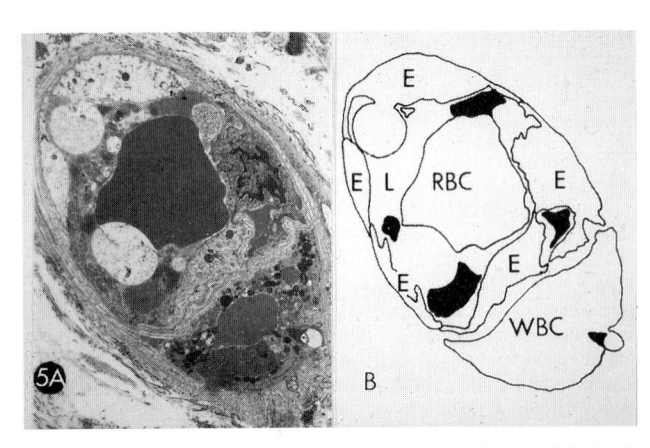

Figure 11–5 Electron micrograph of leukocytoclastic vasculitis. A. A capillary with an extravasated granulocyte (*WBC*) at the lower pole. The endothelial cell (*E*) on the top has become ballooned and is nonviable. B. A key with RBC representing a red blood cell, L, the lumen, and the blackened areas representing electron-dense immune complexes.

Table 11–4 • CUTANEOUS VASCULITIS BY AGE GROUPS

	Children (<20 years)	Adults (>20 years)
Primary	99%	63%
Hypersensitivity vasculitis	11%	64%
Henoch-Schönlein purpura	89%	36%
Secondary	1%	37%

Adapted from Blanco R, Martinez-Taboada VM, Rodriguez-Valverde V, et al. Cutaneous vasculitis in children and adults. Associated diseases and etiologic factors in 303 patients. Medicine 1998;77;403–418.

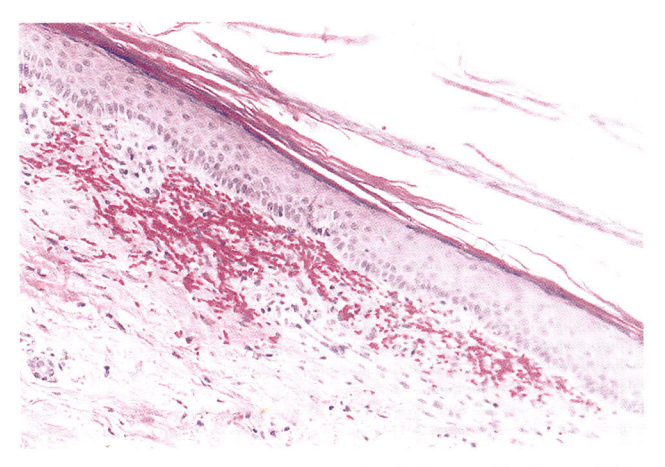

Color Plate 11–1 Light micrograph of a single petechia. Beneath the skin one sees the longitudinal cut of a capillary from which innumerable red cells have extravasated and are trapped in the interstitial connective tissue. The diameter of the entire field is roughly that of a petechia, namely on the order of 1 mm.

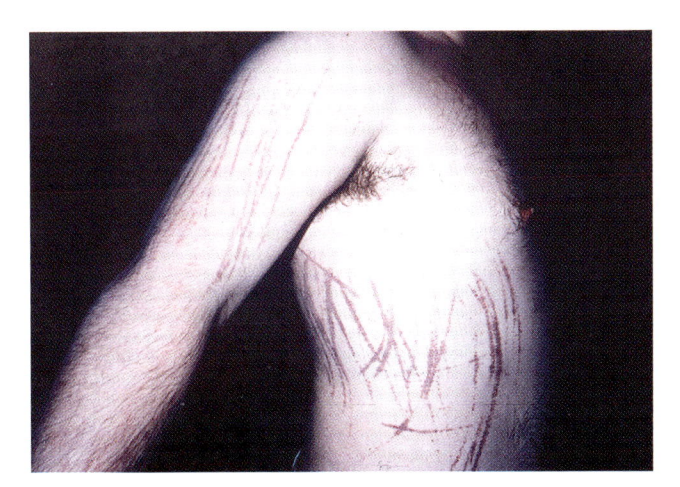

Color Plate 11–2 Factitious purpura. These long linear lesions with very sharply demarcated borders appear only in places that the patient can reach. All hemostatic tests were normal and there was no evidence of any underlying medical disorder. These lesions were probably produced by traumatizing his skin with a gardening implement.

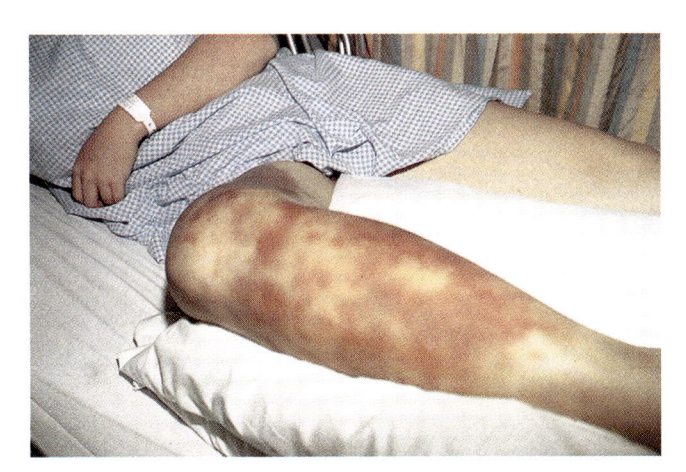

Color Plate 11–3 Factitious purpura. This patient has diffuse purpura on one leg without true hematoma formation while the other leg has no lesions at all. All hemostatic studies were normal. She had underlying psychological problems and she later admitted to causing these lesions by beating her leg with a hairbrush.

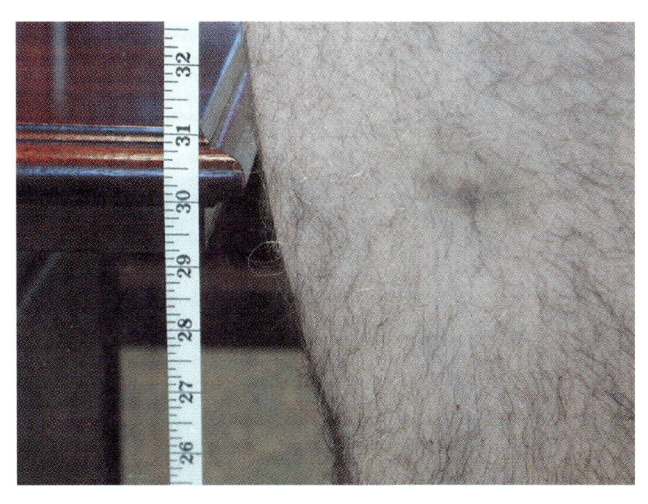

Color Plate 11–4 Simple bruise due to day-to-day trauma. Such bruises are caused by encounters with objects on a daily basis. As demonstrated, these lesions occur on the external surface of the thigh and are typically 30 inches above the ground as this is the height of most American furniture, desks, and countertops.

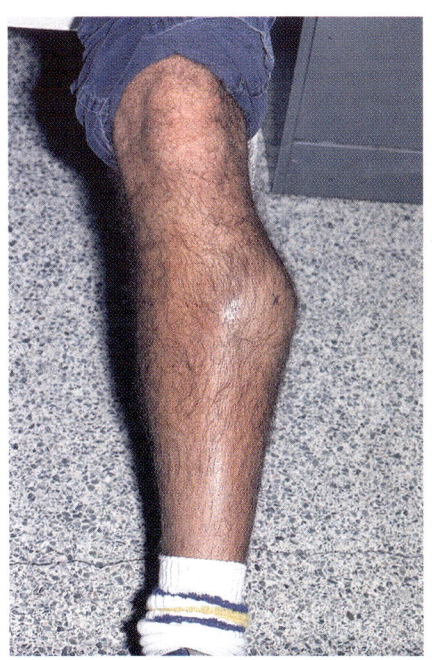

Color Plate 11–5 True hematoma in a previously undiagnosed hemophiliac. This 22-year-old college athlete developed a large hematoma over the external surface of his leg following a baseball game in which his leg was stepped upon by another player. The patient was found to have 7% of normal factor VIII activity.

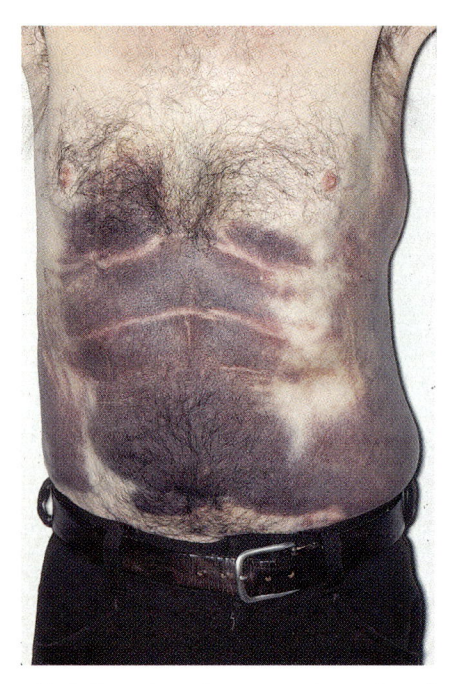

Color Plate 11–6 Extensive subcutaneous hemorrhage in a patient with acquired hemophilia. This patient's extrathoracic hematoma occurred following mild trauma to the skin over his left scapula. Over the next several days he bled several units of blood and was found to have a high titer antibody against factor VIII.

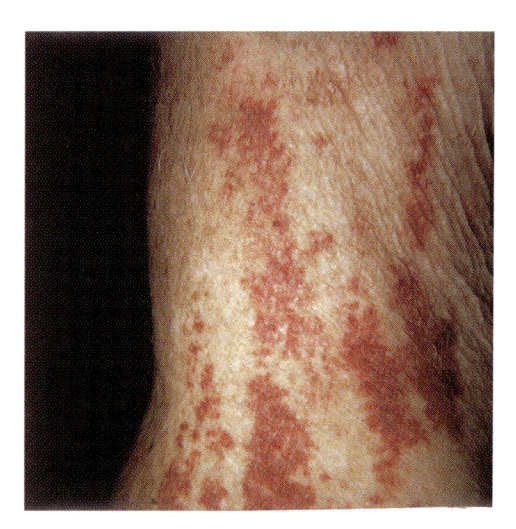

Color Plate 11–7 Capillary fragility. This man developed petechiae on his upper arm in the area underneath a blood pressure cuff following determination of his blood pressure. His platelet count was found to be 5000/μL and he was diagnosed as having ITP.

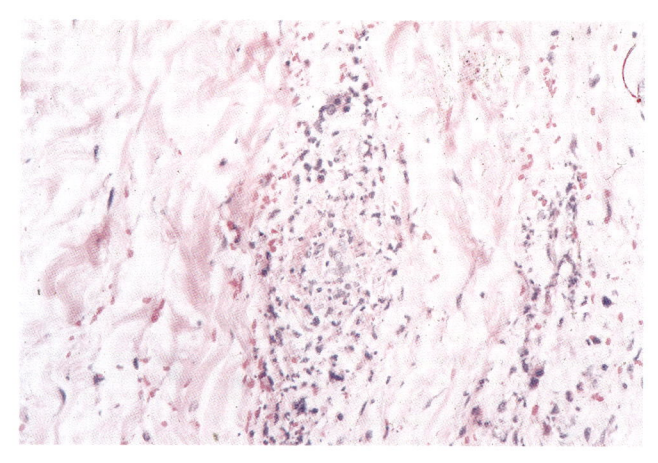

Color Plate 11–8 Leukocytoclastic vasculitis. This photomicrograph shows a central capillary surrounded by extravasated red cells and neutrophils in various grades of disintegration ("nuclear dust"). This infiltrative process gives rise to the notion of "palpable purpura."

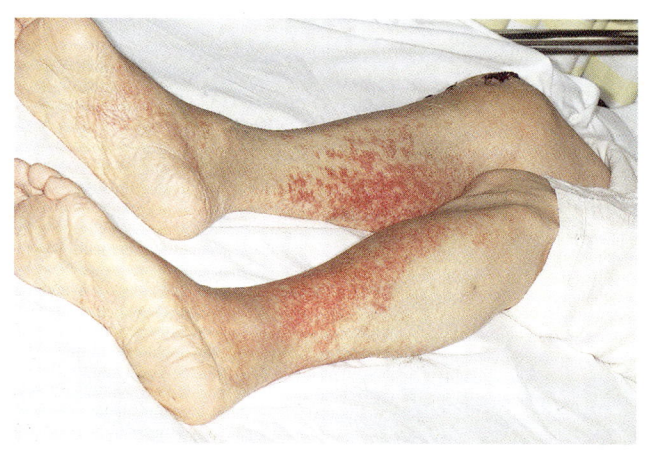

Color Plate 11–9 Palpable purpura. This man had an upper respiratory tract infection, received antibiotics, and several days later developed cutaneous vasculitis typical of palpable purpura.

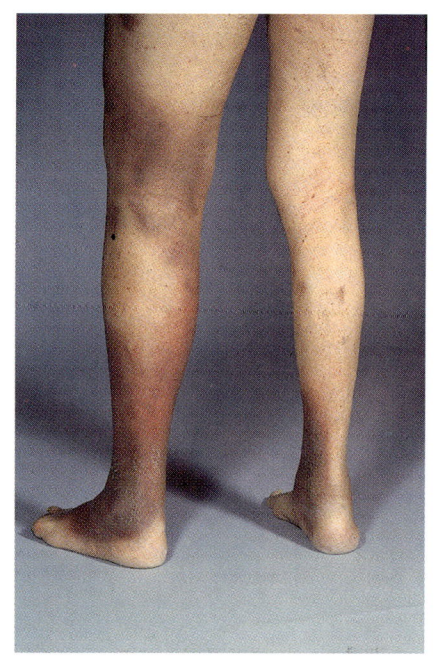

Color Plate 11–10 Scurvy. These large plate-like ecchymotic areas are characteristic of scurvy. They promptly resolved following resumption of a normal diet.

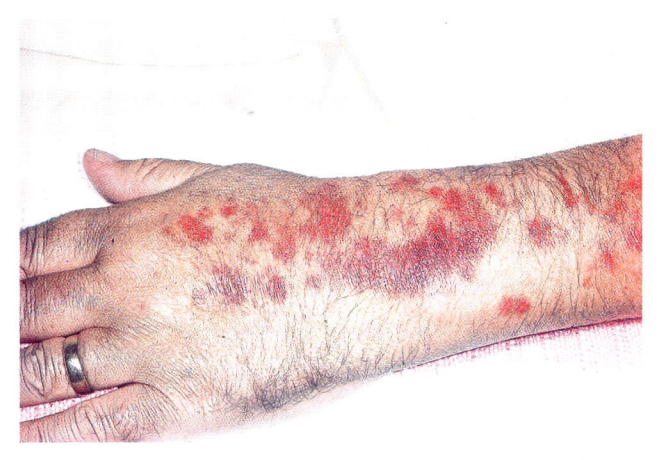

Color Plate 11–11 Hypercortisolism. Subcutaneous purpura is seen in this man's arm as well as slight edema consistent with his hypercortisolism due to long-term, high-dose glucocorticosteroid therapy.

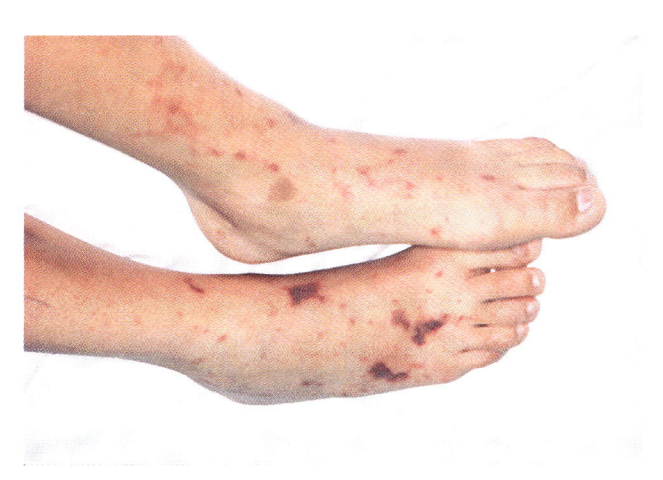

Color Plate 11–14 Meningococcal purpura. This young woman presented with fever and headache. Her early bright red petechiae rapidly became darker, with the characteristic "gun-metal gray" necrosis.

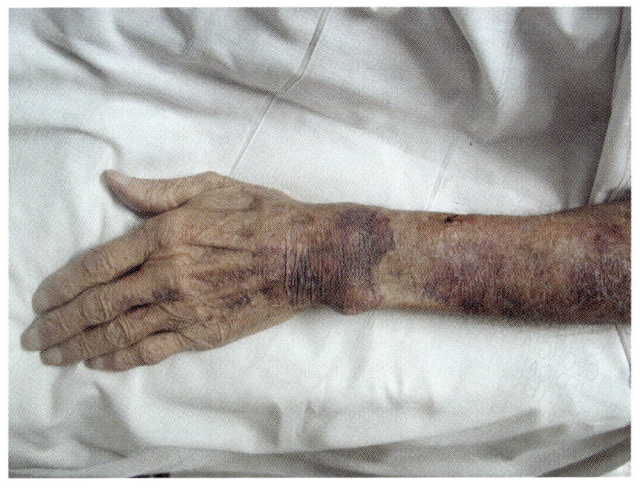

Color Plate 11–12 Actinic or solar purpura. The skin of this man's forearm is very thin; the tendons of the hand are visible. The skin can easily be torn away. The purpura consists of sheets of extravasated red cells. It is not palpable.

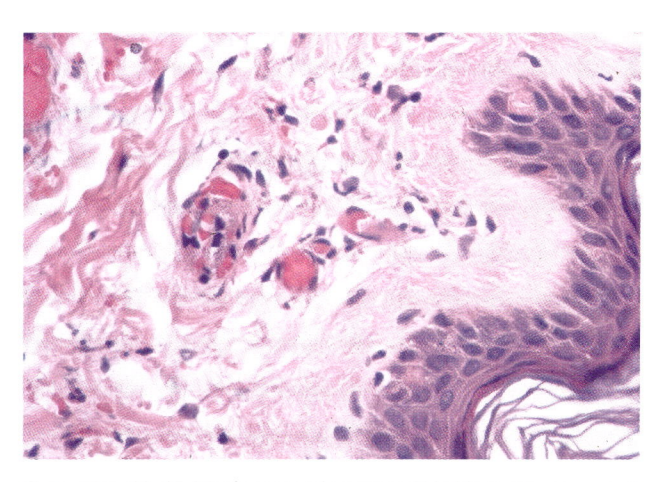

Color Plate 11–15 Meningococcal purpura. Skin biopsy shows several capillaries tensely engorged with fibrin deposition (DIC), which can lead to rupture of the microcirculation as well as ischemic infarction of the skin.

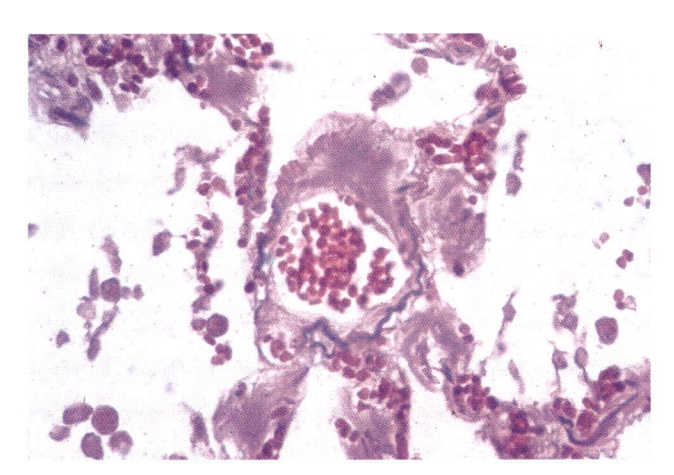

Color Plate 11–13 Amyloidosis. This small vessel is encased in amorphous material between the endothelial wall and the basement membrane, resulting in increased capillary fragility.

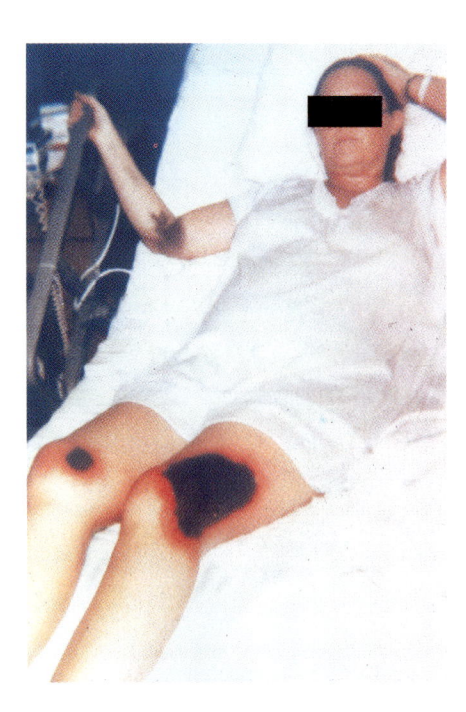

Color Plate 11–16 Warfarin skin necrosis. This woman was administered warfarin and developed painful infarctive lesions a few days later, which are shown here as necrotic eschars.

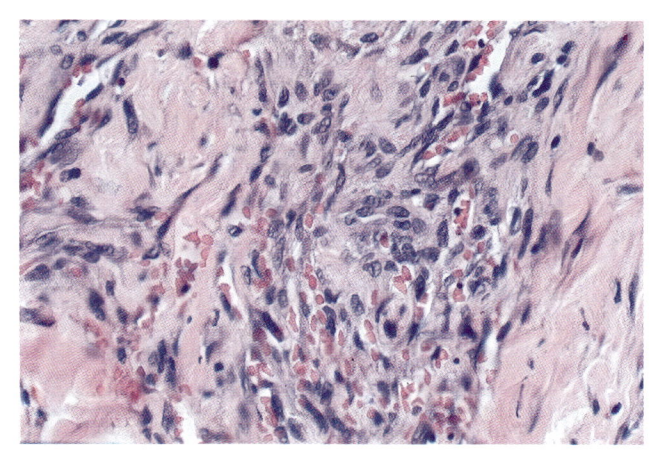

Color Plate 11–19 Kaposi sarcoma. Biopsy shows disorganized entanglement of neoplastic endothelial cells with occasional "vascular slits" and extravasated red blood cells.

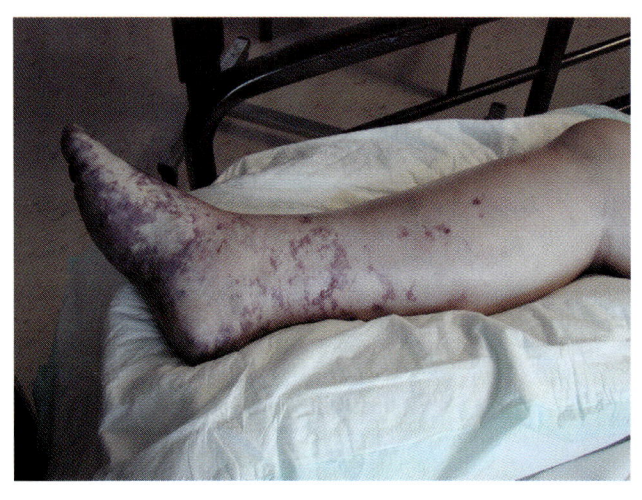

Color Plate 11–17 Cholesterol embolization. This man had severe peripheral vascular disease and had recently undergone cardiac catheterization. The lesions resemble livido reticularis but are painful and darker, and the margins are more easily delineated. Additionally ischemic blisters are seen in this case near the Achilles tendon.

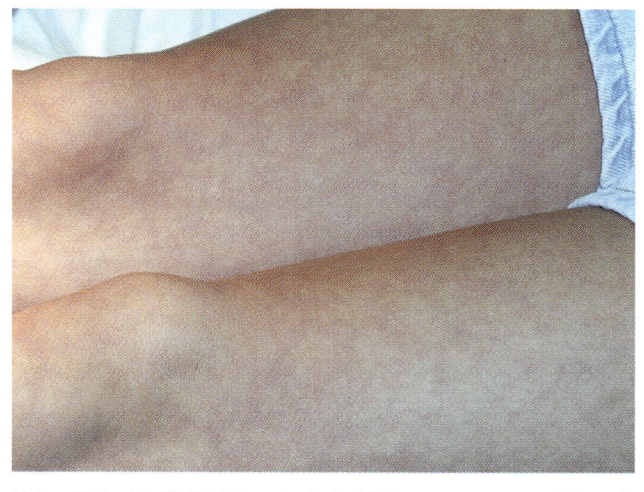

Color Plate 11–20 Livido reticularis. This young woman with antiphospholipid syndrome has the lacy, evanescent-appearing web-like pattern characteristic of this skin disorder.

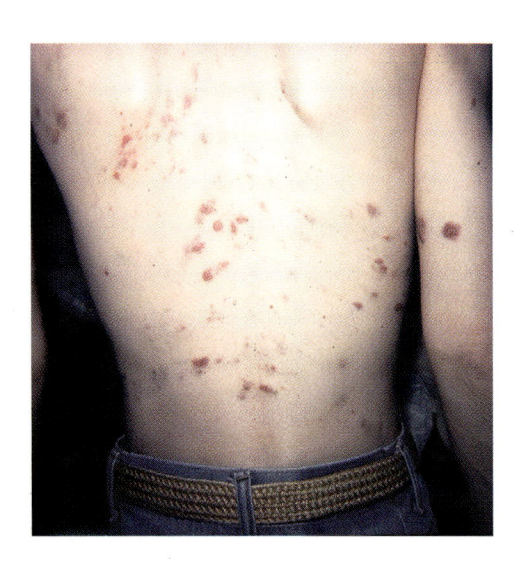

Color Plate 11–18 Kaposi sarcoma. These fleshy tumors are purpuric as a result of extravasated blood cells yet are most purpuric only in their early stages.

pura, arthralgias, colicky abdominal pain, or evidence of nephritis and are commonly referred to as Henoch-Schönlein purpura (HSP). In a large series[23] these findings occurred in 100%, 70%, 70%, and 50%, respectively, of patients who were deemed to have HSP. There is no underlying disease. The other 11% of pediatric cases represent acute hypersensitivity reactions. Only about 1% of CV in children and young adults is determined to be secondary to some underlying more serious chronic disease.

In adults, again the majority (63%) are deemed primary CV, but two thirds are labeled acute hypersensitivity vasculitis, with only one third meeting criteria for HSP. Roughly one third of all adult CV is found to be secondary, with the causes as listed in Table 11–3 the most common ones being lupus erythematosus, cryoglobulinemia, chronic hepatitis B or C, Sjögren syndrome, polyarteritis nodosa, rheumatoid arthritis, and subacute bacterial endocarditis.[24]

As mentioned previously, CV is often referred to by its historical name of Henoch-Schönlein purpura (HSP) when it is associated with any two or three of the following four cardinal features: symmetrical petechial process, abdominal pain, large-joint arthralgias or swelling, and evidence of nephritis. Others have found the diagnosis of HSP is facilitated by ultrasound of the abdomen, which can frequently show edematous bowel walls but with visible blood flow.[25] Indeed, the line between the disease classically referred to as HSP, especially when adult and childhood variation is taken into account, and the increasingly used term CV has blurred,[26] and in fact some[27] have questioned why we still use the term HSP as the distinction occasionally is quite arbitrary, especially if one uses preemptory criteria such as an age cutoff and whether or not microvascular deposition of immunoglobulin IgA is found. If a specific chronic underlying disease is not encountered and the patient has arthralgias, nephritis, or abdominal pain, perhaps the more narrow term HSP is best. If no cause can be found and criteria for HSP are not met, primary hypersensitivity vasculitis is the term used, denoting that there may be a hypersensitivity reaction to some commonly occurring viral infection, medications used to treat such upper respiratory tract infections, or other drugs.

Primary CV is indicated not only by the lack of an obvious underlying disease but also by the normal results of almost all routine laboratory studies, with the exception of the sedimentation rate, which is greatly elevated in 69% of cases. Studies that return normal include the CBC, coagulation profile, serum studies for cryoglobulins and serologic studies for antinuclear antibodies (ANA), serum complement levels, and antineutrophil cytoplasmic antibodies (ANCA).[28] A proposed guideline for the evaluation of palpable purpura[26] includes studies shown in Table 11–5. More specific studies are guided by one's clinical index of suspicion for a specific underlying disorder.

The diagnosis of secondary CV is not difficult to make when one notices palpable purpura in a patient known to have a disorder such as lupus erythematosus, subacute bacterial endocarditis, or other immune complex illness. On the other hand, the evaluation of CV may lead to

Table 11–5 • LABORATORY EVALUATION FOR CUTANEOUS VASCULITIS

All Ages
History and physical examination
Complete blood count
Erythrocyte sedimentation rate
Urinalysis
Stool guaiac testing
Routine serum biochemical profile
Skin biopsy

For Adults
Studies for hepatitis B and C
Cryoglobulins
Antinuclear antibodies (ANA)
Antineutrophilic cytoplasmic antibody (ANCA)
Rheumatoid factor (RF)
Serum protein electrophoresis (SPEP)
Chest x-ray

Additional Studies Pursued as a Function of Index of Suspicion (Examples)
Blood cultures (for subacute bacterial endocarditis)
Bone marrow examination (for myelodysplastic syndrome)
Otolaryngoscopic exam (for Wegner granulomatosis)
Lip biopsy (for Sjögren syndrome)

the discovery of an important underlying disease first manifested by palpable purpura.

The prognosis for CV is excellent; a complete recovery occurs in 90% of the cases in adults and children with primary CV. Frequently, especially in childhood, the process will spontaneously resolve over weeks. The prognosis in the secondary types depends on the prognosis of the underlying disease, particularly the presence or absence of nephropathy, which determines the outcome in many adults.[29]

Purpura Associated with Microbial Endothelial Damage

The endothelium may be the site of residence and proliferation of microorganisms or can be directly attacked by microorganisms. Either situation may lead to destruction of the endothelial membrane with resultant extravasation of red cells.

Rickettsial Diseases

The best-studied rickettsial disease involving purpura is Rocky Mountain spotted fever (RMSF), due to *Rickettsia rickettsii*. This agent is an obligate endothelial cell organism the endothelial presence of which was demonstrated as early as 1919 by Wolbach.[8] The petechial rash may be first detectable on the first day of illness but generally is not clearly manifest until the third or fourth day. These spots become larger than most petechiae, growing up to 5 to 6 mm in diameter, and may have vague borders blending into erythema.

One of the unusual features is that the spots also may appear on the palms and soles. The seriousness of the disease is brought about by the invasion of the vasculature of all organs by the organism and intense increase in vascular permeability brought about by destruction of endothelial cell integrity. This results in simultaneous edema and intravascular hypovolemia with characteristic increases in serum concentrations of blood urea nitrogen and creatinine. Although mild thrombocytopenia occurs, it is not thought to be the genesis of hemorrhage. True disseminated intravascular coagulation (DIC) is rare. The hematologist may be asked to consult for evaluation of mild thrombocytopenia in a febrile patient having multiorgan failure who is not improving despite antibiotics. The hematologist may be the first practitioner to suspect RMSF. Other rickettsial diseases may be associated with petechial rashes, but not to the extent of RMSF.

Leptospiral Diseases

Leptospirosis is due to systemic invasion by the spirochete genus *Leptospira*. In the severe form, often known as Weil disease, nearly all tissues are invaded by this microbe. Endothelial damage gives rise to the vasculitis, capillary leak syndrome, and petechial rash characteristic of the disorder. Other hemorrhagic phenomena may be abetted by the modest thrombocytopenia and DIC that may occur. The penicillins are usually the antibiotic group of choice for therapy.

Parvovirus B19

This virus may cause a variety of hematologic disorders, such as pure red cell aplasia or hypoplastic pancytopenia. It is also the agent of "fifth disease." Recently it is reported to cause a peculiar "socks and gloves" petechial rash that is self limited.[30] On skin biopsy no evidence for vasculitis is found so endothelial damage is speculated to be the cause of the extravasation of blood.

Viral Hemorrhagic Fevers

Several viruses have been incriminated as destroying endothelial cells, resulting in various hemorrhagic fevers. Owing in part to the global distribution of these illnesses, typically in remote areas, detailed investigation into the diseases has been severely limited. Whereas bleeding may also be in part due to accompanying thrombocytopenia or even DIC, petechial manifestations of these hemorrhagic fevers are thought to represent endothelial damage by direct invasion and destruction. These hemorrhagic fevers include Lassa fever, Rift Valley fever, dengue, and yellow fever. The mortality of these diseases varies from rather low to extremely high.[31] A periodically discovered and rediscovered hemorrhagic fever with a mortality as high as 90% is Ebola hemorrhagic fever, which directly causes endothelial cell damage.[32] Hemorrhage in all these disorders not only is cutaneous in the way of purpura but involves multiple organs, the dysfunction of which results from hemorrhage and is the ultimate cause of death. Unfortunately, treatment is nonexistent. If any of these viral hemorrhagic diseases is seriously considered in the different diagnosis, especially in persons having recently been abroad, rapid consultation with infectious disease experts and the Centers for Disease Control in Atlanta is mandatory.

Purpura Associated with Decreased Microvascular Mechanical Strength

The following disorders have in common that the structural integrity of the microvascular unit, shown in Figure 11–1, has been compromised. Many investigators have tried to ascribe platelet defects and mild coagulation disorders as causative or additive in this classification of purpura, but none of these theories has stood the test of time.

Scurvy

We have alluded to scurvy previously in the Historical Perspective section of this chapter. Scurvy was the first hemorrhagic disease to have a specific cure following Lind's study of this disabling bleeding disorder. Scorbutic bleeding is characterized by perifollicular hemorrhage, large if not even huge, flat plate-like ecchymoses (Color Plate 11–10), and hypertrophic spongy, bleeding gums. The disease is only rarely seen now because of improved dietary habits, with severe chronic inveterate alcoholics with poor nutrition representing nearly all current patients with scurvy.

The disease is diagnosed clinically by its appearance. One may send serum samples for vitamin C level determination in equivocal cases. The response to vitamin C administration either pharmacologically or dietarily is gratifying and rapid. The disorder is due to the inability to cross-link fibers of collagen at proline sites, as vitamin C is necessary to convert proline into hydroxyproline in order to participate in the cross-linking of the helical structure of collagen. Microvascular strength and structure is enormously compromised by virtue of weakened collagen synthesis.

Hypercortisolism

Hypercortisolism, whether exogenous or endogenous, also results in decreased collagen strength. Cortisol is known to decrease collagen synthesis and since collagen catabolism is not affected, collagen becomes scarce, resulting in capillary fragility. The purpura is seen primarily on the extensor surface of the forearms (Color Plate 11–11). The skin is thin, which accounts for the superficial appearance of extravasated blood. Treatment involves cessation of cortisone administration in exogenous hypercortisolism or correction, if possible, of endogenous sources resulting in the increased production of cortisol. Vitamin C administration has not been shown to help in management of these patients.

"Senile," "Atrophic," or "Actinic" Purpura

This purpura is quite common in older and debilitated patients, but is hardly limited to the elderly as any extremely ill patient exhibiting weight loss and negative nitrogen balance is subject to this process. It is also seen in fairly healthy patients who have excessive solar exposure, which increases breakdown of collagen. Accordingly the extensor surfaces of the forearms are characteristic locations of this purpura, particularly in those who work outdoors with short or no sleeves. The skin has the appearance on close examination of being extremely thin across the extensor surface of the arms and backs of the hands (Color Plate 11–12). Should the skin be biopsied, the dermal–epidermal junction is found to be thin with characteristically flattened rete pegs. Patients often report that just the slightest trauma or stretching of the skin can cause the skin to physically rupture, with subcutaneous bleeding. There is no specific treatment. Vitamin C is not efficacious in this disorder.

Heritable Disorders of Connective Tissue

These are rare inherited metabolic disorders of connective tissue. Subcutaneous hemorrhage may be encountered yet essentially is never of diagnostic importance as these heritable disorders are usually quite obvious to all. These include the Ehlers-Danlos syndromes,[33] pseudoxanthoma elasticum, osteogenesis imperfecta, and Marfan syndrome. These disorders are heralded primarily by the extreme joint laxity and skin stretching, resulting in the so-called India rubber man syndrome; the "plucked chicken" appearance of the skin, particularly in the neck; multiple bone fractures and deformities; and the tall, gangly appearance with lens dislocation and tendency toward dissecting aneurysm characteristic of each of these four disorders, respectively. Bleeding in these disorders is usually more of a result of tearing of fragile subcutaneous tissues and skin rather than spontaneous purpuric lesions. Bleeding, especially purpura, can be noticeable and bothersome, however. No persistent coagulation or platelet abnormality has been elucidated. No specific treatment is available. Surgical hemostasis is normal but healing is impaired.

Amyloidosis

In this purpuric disorder, bleeding may very well be one of the initial findings that leads to the correct diagnosis. Purpuric bleeding was found in 15% of all cases of amyloidosis in one large review.[34] Amyloid material is deposited between the endothelium and the basement membrane (Color Plate 11–13) and therefore can be found in the vasculature of any organ. Amyloid not only leads to probable increased capillary fragility but also, for arterioles, impedes the ability of those vessels to constrict, thereby failing to limit regional flow and bleeding from injured vessels. The hallmark of the diagnosis is the finding of material that stains consistent with amyloid in vessels from nearly any organ or from subcutaneous fat. There is no highly effective treatment for amyloidosis unless the disorder is associated with a plasma cell dyscrasia, the treatment of which may slow the progress of this disorder. Coagulation abnormalities are frequent, multiple, and of variable patterns in amyloidosis and may confuse the diagnostician away from true cause of the purpura, which is the deposition of amyloid. The distribution of the purpura is somewhat unusual in that it is not nearly as dependent as most purpuric lesions are but seems to occur more along pressure points, with a peculiar periorbital predilection.

Osler-Weber-Rendu Syndrome

This disorder is also referred to as hereditary hemorrhagic telangiectasia (HHT), which is a quite accurate term as it describes the key elements of the disease. However, the historical significance of the eponym prevails. OWR syndrome is not truly a purpuric disorder as there is no extravasation of red cells as they remain in the intravascular space until the lesions rupture. Because of this, telangiectases blanch easily on external pressure. This disorder is discussed under purpuric diseases as it is traditionally classified in such reviews. The hemorrhagic component of the disorder is due to decreased mechanical strength of the microvasculature.

The microanatomy of OWR syndrome has recently been elucidated by Braverman and colleagues.[35] Probably owing to genetic lack of a normal structural protein referred to as endoglin, the structural anatomy is abnormal in that the defect somehow allows the normal capillary anastomosis between dermal arterioles and venules to become grossly enlarged. This results in huge dilations of the capillaries such that they are the size of venules, thus creating a small arteriolar-venous malformation (AVM). The process continues throughout life, worsening as the microscopic AVM becomes visible in the form of a telangiectasis. Arterialization of the descending limb of the venule occurs.

As shown in Figure 11–6, the anatomy of these vessels represents an altered structure–function relationship. Whereas each segment of the capillary wall has the vascular architecture and integrity of a capillary, the enormous diameter of the aberrant vessel shows that it is in fact functioning as a capacitance venule. According to the law of Laplace, a force required to rupture any vessel is a function of the radius of that vessel; accordingly, these vessels very easily rupture with even slight force. Additionally, since these large pseudovenules are anatomically in fact capillaries, they lack smooth muscle investiture and therefore are unable to constrict; this

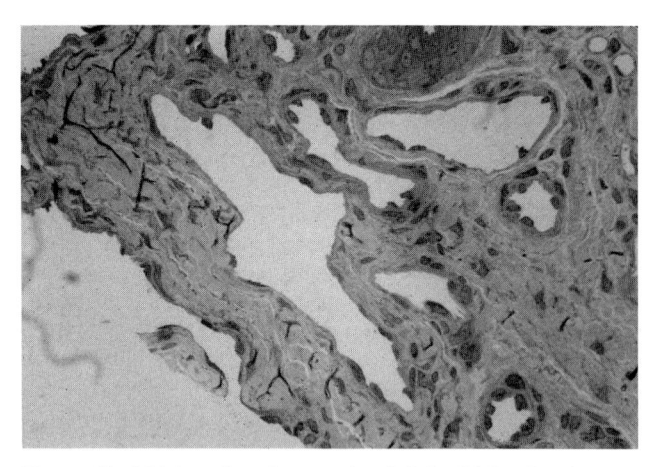

Figure 11–6 Light microphotograph of Osler-Weber-Rendu syndrome. This section has been made through a telangiectasis. There are no extravasated red cells. Red cells have been washed out of the lumen of these vessels during preparation. Toward the top and also on the right-hand edge are seen several normal capillaries. Toward the center are several larger vessels and in the extreme lower left corner is the lumen of an even larger vessel. The wall of all these vessels is anatomically that of capillary, being thin-walled consisting only of an endothelial cell. These anatomic characteristics give insufficient strength to vessels larger than capillaries, which leads to increased hemorrhage.

probably accounts for the prolonged slow ooze that is both problematic and characteristic of this disorder.

Numerous attempts to demonstrate coagulation defects have usually not been borne out on a consistent basis. There are individual case reports of concomitant von Willebrand disease and OWR syndrome.

Telangiectases are seen most often on the hands, fingernail beds, lips, tongue and about the mucosa and surface of the face. They become progressively more apparent as the patient ages. This autosomal dominant disease is most commonly first manifest by epistaxis that begins in the second or third decade and slowly worsens. This is in contradistinction to von Willebrand disease, which also often starts with epistaxis in the first decade that usually ceases or abates by the end of the second decade.[36] Although the telangiectases are scattered about the skin, skin bleeding is very unusual with most of the bleeding being from the mucosa, particularly the nose. The most troublesome bleeding is chronic gastrointestinal bleeding. This hemorrhage is due to multiple telangiectases that often enlarge to rather discrete AVMs, which can be found and cauterized on endoscopy. One of the most common causes eventually found to explain chronic occult gastrointestinal hemorrhage is OWR syndrome.[37] Although rarer, central nervous system and pulmonary AVMs can become quite large and cause bleeding or can be associated with brain abscesses. If such are found, they can be ligated or therapeutically embolized. Most but not all patients who have troublesome AVMs of their lung or brain have a family history of such and therefore patients in such kindreds should probably be screened with appropriate imaging, including magnetic resonance imaging. In a large review of pulmonary AVMs, OWR syndrome was found to be the most common underlying disorder, accounting for 56% of all cases.[38] Hepatic involvement with OWR syndrome may lead to portal hypertension and biliary tract disease.[39]

Molecular genetics has had its impact on OWR syndrome as several subtypes have been described having unique alterations of the endoglin gene.[40] It is possible that specific genomes may be found to represent those subtypes of OWR syndrome with the most aggressive manifestations such as troublesome pulmonary or brain AVMs. A surgical approach should not be discounted for fear of bleeding as OWR syndrome is not a primary hemostatic defect. Patients undergo surgery for these AVMs or other procedures not related to their OWR syndrome without risk of excessive bleeding.

The troublesome bleeding from the nose is best handled by an otolaryngologic approach such as cauterization, septal dermatoplasty, or laser ablation. The gastrointestinal bleeding can be very difficult to manage but is clearly best approached by routine and vigorous iron therapy, which can essentially negate the use of transfusions as large quantities of iron can be given intravenously, keeping the patient in positive iron balance. This is important because in previous decades, transfusion reactions and other complications of transfusion were actually a leading cause of death. The majority of OWR syndrome patients can be maintained with iron infusions as needed and determined by the progressive anemia and microcytosis characteristic of their iron deficiency. Few patients can maintain iron balance simply by oral intake.

Estrogen therapy has been advocated by some[41,42] but may have significant side effects. Male patients do not generally comply with such therapy.

Telangiectases are not limited to OWR syndrome. Many otherwise normal persons have a few telangiectases while having no family history of characteristic hemorrhage. The lesions may become even more prominent during pregnancy. Telangiectases are seen in some other disorders, particularly as part of the CREST syndrome of scleroderma. They may also result from actinic damage or be secondary to therapeutic radiation.

Purpura Associated with Microthrombi

The microcirculation may become obstructed by emboli, which may cause microinfarction and disruption of the endothelial membrane with subsequent extravasation of red cells. These dermal emboli cause purpuric lesions. In its most expressive form, the process is termed *purpura fulminans*. Because microthrombi are often simultaneously occurring in other organs, end organ damage may occur and lead to multiorgan dysfunction syndrome (MODS).

Disseminated Intravascular Coagulation

Multiple causes give rise to the syndrome called disseminated intravascular coagulation (DIC). Tissue samples or autopsy specimens frequently show occlusive deposition of fibrin, particularly in the microcirculation. These emboli lead to purpuric skin lesions and frank purpura fulminans. One of the foremost causes of the latter is meningococcemia, which results in characteristic rapidly progressive necrotizing purpura fulminans (Color Plates 11–14 and 11–15). Fibrin deposition is not limited to the skin; MODS is the most frequent cause of death in DIC. Recognition and treatment of orders associated with DIC are more thoroughly discussed in Chapter 12, while purpura fulminans is discussed in Chapter 15.

Warfarin Skin Necrosis

This is a special cause of fibrin deposition that appears limited to the dermal microcirculation.[43,44] This process was previously thought to be due to an idiosyncratic toxic reaction to warfarin. It is now thought to be due to the precipitous drop in levels of protein C following initiation of warfarin administration. The half-life of protein C is only 4 to 5 hours; therefore, the rapid decrease in this anticoagulant occurs prior to the decrease in the procoagulant factors II, VII, IX, and X. This is thought to induce an early hypercoagulable state. Levels of protein C may already be low for genetic reasons and/or because of further consumption during the thrombotic process. A further decrease in protein C levels allows for relative localized hypercoagulability in the microcirculation, the site of protein C's primary action.

As protein S is the cofactor of protein C, congenital or acquired protein S deficiency is also a risk factor for warfarin skin necrosis. This process is normally heralded first by a stinging or burning sensation about 2 to 4 days after the initiation of warfarin therapy. The site becomes hemorrhagic a day or two later. For some reason warfarin skin necrosis occurs more frequently in women than men (9:1 ratio) and usually develops in areas where there is generous adipose tissue such as the thighs, buttocks, or breasts. If the condition is not recognized and treated promptly, the site becomes necrotic and assumes the appearance of a large burn eschar, usually requiring subsequent skin grafting (Color Plate 11–16). On biopsy, fibrin deposition is prominent in the microcirculation. This process is not as common as it used to be when large doses of warfarin (up to 1 mg/kg) were used as a "loading dose." It is best prevented by not loading patients with warfarin but starting with a dose that approximates the estimated maintenance dose. It may also be rarer now as patients with active thromboses are first aggressively administered heparin. If warfarin skin necrosis is entertained, prompt initiation of heparin therapy and cessation of warfarin is considered the best treatment. A similar pattern of unopposed decrease of protein C levels may be seen with the intermittent stopping and then restarting of warfarin and nearly certainly explains warfarin skin necrosis occurring in patients thought to have been continually on long-term warfarin therapy. Initiation of warfarin therapy should follow heparin therapy and overlap 4 to 5 days in patients known to have either protein C or S deficiency or those with a personal or family history of warfarin skin necrosis. Warfarin skin necrosis is extremely unlikely following initiation of warfarin for treatment of stroke or for prophylaxis in atrial fibrillation as a large, fresh clot is not present and that population is not thought to harbor patients with congenital deficiency of protein C or S. Accordingly, heparin therapy is not routinely given first to such patients unless there is a prior history to suggest an underlying thrombophilia. Warfarin skin necrosis may complicate warfarin therapy in patients with heparin-induced thrombocytopenia (see Chapter 23).

Fat Embolism Syndrome

Fat embolism[45–47] occurs in up to 2% of patients with traumatic long-bone fractures, particularly fractures of the femur. The incidence or at least the manifestations may be enhanced by the coexistence of shock. It may occur in 1% of manipulations of the medullary canal such as with prosthetic hip and knee surgery or the insertion of various nails or other hardware. This peculiar syndrome usually is first noted on day one but no later than day three following surgery or trauma, i.e., several days prior to the typical presentation of postoperative pulmonary embolism. The syndrome includes pulmonary distress with hypoxia, reduced levels of consciousness, tachycardia, fever, and the appearance of petechiae. The appearance of petechiae is often the seminal observation that alerts one to fat embolism given that other symptoms are somewhat nonspecific, particularly in the trauma patient. The petechiae have an unusual distribution, occurring around the neck and on the shoulders, axillary folds, upper chest, and conjunctivae. The mechanism of microcirculatory extravasation is not clear but probably is a combination of the simple ischemic mechanical obstruction of capillaries due to embolism by large fat globules and the direct hemorrhagic toxic effect due to local release of free fatty acids from hydrolysis of the embolized neutral fat. The morbidity appears to be quite high, ranging from 30% to 50%. There is no specific treatment other than general support.

Myeloblastemia

Leukostasis syndromes typically are manifest by central nervous system dysfunction and hypoxia when the cerebral and pulmonary capillary beds are involved.[48] Leukostasis is most typically seen with a large number of circulating myeloblasts and promyelocytes such as in blast crisis of chronic myelogenous leukemia. These may also embolize in the dermal microcirculation and cause infarctive lesions far in excess of the degree of thrombocytopenia that may accompany leukemia and its treatment. The most appropriate therapy is cytoreduction of the malignant cells.

Thrombotic Thrombocytopenic Purpura (TTP)

This interesting disease is discussed thoroughly in Chapter 22. Although platelet aggregates induce thrombosis in many tissues, there is a paucity of cutaneous purpura despite its name. Nonetheless, petechial purpuric and infarctive lesions are occasionally present but are often overshadowed by the other manifestations of this disorder.

Heparin-Induced Thrombocytopenia with Thrombosis (HIT)

Purpura and embolic ischemia but rarely petechiae are characteristic of this disorder. Ischemia of the extremities in patients receiving heparin and who are thrombocytopenic should alert the practitioner to this possibility. HIT is discussed in Chapter 23.

Blue Toe Syndrome, Purple Toe Syndrome, and Cholesterol Emboli Syndrome

These are different terms for what most likely are variations of the same process.[44,49] Whether they occur during heparin administration, during warfarin administration, following abdominal trauma, following cardiac catheterization, or even spontaneously, the two unifying points are that all these patients have significant underlying atherosclerosis and the histologic picture is one of cholesterol crystals in the arterioles of biopsied lesions.

In the past the purple (or blue) discoloration of the toes that occurred when patients were administered either an oral or a parenteral anticoagulant was thought to be a reaction to the anticoagulants. Far more likely than not, the lesions are due to the underlying process for which the anticoagulants were indicated. Use of anticoagulants does result in remodeling of the clots that commingle among large atherosclerotic plaques, allowing either bleeding into the atherosclerotic plaques or the freeing up of cholesterol crystals, which then embolize distally.

The process resembles livedo reticularis but differs in that it is usually significantly bluer and is quite painful because of the ischemia. This appears to be strictly an arteriolar embolization syndrome as deposition of fibrin that one sees in the venules in warfarin fat necrosis is not encountered. The process may progress to involve not only purple or blue toes but through-and-through necrosis of the toes and feet as well as significant parts of the soft tissue, usually of the legs and sometimes into the lower flank and back (Color Plate 11–17).

Occasionally the differential diagnosis is not straightforward unless there has been a recent history of manipulation or trauma of the arterial system. When it occurs spontaneously one can often be led astray by many findings that suggest a vasculitis, including weight loss, anorexia, fever, anemia, eosinophilia, and a very high erythrocyte sedimentation rate. There may be coexistent calf muscle tenderness with elevations of the serum creatine kinase level, both of which can broaden the differential diagnosis; however, this is thought to be due to an ischemic myositis from infarcts that are simultaneously taking place in the calf muscles.

Assessment should be focused on the arterial system. Echocardiography including the aortic arch is indicated, as is imaging of the entire aorta. An ankle-to-brachial pressure index may be helpful but sometimes arterial pulses are palpable and half the time even described as bounding. There is usually a very high probability of finding cholesterol crystal deposition on skin biopsy of appropriate material.

These conditions are serious, not necessarily because of the ischemia but because of the underlying atherosclerosis. Treatment probably is best done by minimizing or totally avoiding any further invasive procedures of the arterial system, or if catheterization studies are necessary, consideration should be given to using the upper extremity.

Purpura Associated with Vascular Malignancy

Endothelial cells, like any cells, may become malignant. Although multiple rare endothelial malignancies exist, the prototypical and most common form is Kaposi sarcoma (KS).[50] Whereas this disease in the past used to be very rare it is now more common because of its association with acquired immunodeficiency syndrome (AIDS).

The hematologist from time to time will be asked to see a patient with a purpuric lesion that proves to be KS (Color Plate 11–18). KS typically starts as an ecchymotic-appearing macular lesion that then progresses to a plaque or nodular lesion. KS has become more common in the AIDS pandemic and is thought to be due to the opportunistic coinfection of human immunodeficiency virus (HIV) positive patients with Kaposi sarcoma herpes virus (KSHV), which is also known as human herpes virus type 8 (HHV8). Although KS is seen chiefly in homosexual men and at one time was the AIDS-defining illness in approximately half of such patients, there has been a dramatic decrease over the last decade, with KS being found in only about 15% of AIDS patients and in 1% of newly diagnosed HIV-positive patients.[51] A variety of dermal processes are included in the differential diagnosis but a very important clue, typical of all the purpuric lesions, is that the early KS lesion does not blanch on external pressure. As the lesions become larger, more plaque-like, and nodular they are clearly distinguished from purpura. The diagnosis may ultimately depend on biopsy, which can be undertaken without excessive risk of hemorrhage despite the vascular nature of the tumor.

Research of this tumor has created a wealth of information on angiogenesis.[52] The sarcomatous tissue produces vascular endothelial growth factor (VEGF), which greatly stimulates further proliferation of endothelial cells. This accounts for the massing of endothelial cells in an attempt to make channels, referred to as "vascular slits," which is the histologic hallmark of this lesion (Color Plate 11–19). Also found is a swirling arrangement of spindle-shaped cells admixed with the angiogenic component. The spindle cells stain for smooth muscle actin, which suggests their relation to vascular cells. These cells also produce matrix metalloproteinase 2 (MMP-2), as well as a collagenase and other enzymes that tend to degrade the hemostatic membrane and may very well facilitate both migration of endothelial cells among the growing lesion as well as extravasation of red cells.

The lesions rarely cause severe morbidity and mortality but often do cause cosmetic and other less life-threatening burdens. As KS progresses, lesions may become internalized, particularly in the respiratory tract, mouth, and gastrointestinal tract.[53]

Nonpurpuric Hematovascular Findings of Hematologic Interest

For completeness, several disorders of interest and germane to this topic will be presented.

Livedo Reticularis

Livedo reticularis is commonly seen and in the correct clinical setting is indicative of antiphospholipid syndrome. Livedo reticularis is dusky, ill-defined violaceous reticular pattern that is seen primarily on the legs and occasionally on the arms (Color Plate 11–20). It vaguely resembles a pair of blue or purple fishnet stockings. It may be seen transiently in normal people, especially if they are in a cool environment. Anticardiolipin antibodies were found in roughly half of 65 patients with livedo reticularis studied by Asherson and colleagues.[54] It can also be seen in lupus without antiphospholipid syndrome and in other rheumatic disorders. Sneddon recognized the association of livedo reticularis with cerebrovascular accidents; this disorder was referred to as Sneddon syndrome although it appears he was recording two manifestations of antiphospholipid syndrome.[55]

Histopathologic samples of livedo reticularis show a slight endotheliitis usually without necrotizing features. Should necrotic lesions be encountered, the process may be termed *livedoid vasculitis*. Following necrotization, small cutaneous porcelain-white ulcerations, called *atrophia blanche*, result.[56]

Livedo reticularis serves as one of the minor diagnostic criteria for antiphospholipid syndrome (see Chapter 18). Therapy is not indicated other than the treatment of underlying disease. Other dermal manifestations of antiphospholipid syndrome have been recently reviewed by Gibson and colleagues.[57]

Hemangiomas

These soft bluish tumors are common in infancy and usually spontaneously regress.[58] Persistent huge cavernous hemangiomas have a worse prognosis and may require aggressive treatment. The Kasabach-Merritt syndrome is thrombocytopenic hemorrhage from either DIC or hyperfibrinolysis or both when occurring in a patient with a giant hemangioma. The hemostatic defect is thought to result from activation of the coagulation and fibrinolytic systems from stagnation of blood creeping through the maze of entangled vessels in these large lesions.

Cherry Angiomas

These appear as cherry-red small 1- to 3-mm domed papules over the upper abdomen and lower chest and occur in the second half of life. They consist of proliferated capillaries but vessels not as large as those in OWR syndrome and do not blanch nearly as easily or completely as the telangiectases of OWR syndrome. At one time they were also known as de Morgan spots and were thought to herald internal malignancy, but this is no longer held as true.

Spiders

These vascular lesions are noted by their 1- to 3-cm "legs" that radiate out from a 1- to 2-mm central body. The body of the spider is a dermal arteriole with anastomoses to the legs. Gentle pressure on the head causes collapse of the spider and disappearance of the legs. Spiders are seen in aging, cirrhosis, and pregnancy and require no specific therapy. Vascular spiders are occasionally of cosmetic concern.

Erythema

Simple increased supply of blood to the skin dilates normal dermal vessels with resultant reddening of the skin, especially the skin of the face. Erythema has no clear-cut borders but blanches with pressure or application of cold to decrease cutaneous blood flow. Erythema may result from a hot environment, hyperthermia, fever, mild viral infections ("slapped cheeks" of fifth disease), or emotional phenomena.

CONSULTATION CONSIDERATIONS

In hospitalized patients with purpura, high probabilities exist for CV, DIC, amyloidosis, and livedo reticularis, as well as the above-mentioned classic hemostatic diatheses. Essentially all patients in the category of purpura due to microthrombi will be hospitalized because of their underlying illness.

In healthy ambulatory patients, the most commonly encountered processes are senile purpura, purpura simplex, PPPs, OWR syndrome, CV, and factitious purpura.

Clues exist in the distribution of purpura. Postictal petechiae, petechiae secondary to fat embolization, the telangiectases of OWR syndrome, and the purpura associated with amyloidosis occur about the head and face. Mouth bleeding from boggy gums should signal the possibility of scurvy.

Body and trunk ecchymoses in purpura are seen with hemophilia, factor VIII inhibitors, concomitant anticoagulant use, amyloidosis, and even purpura simplex, especially if the patient's activities involve leaning over and bearing weight on the lower rib cage.

Dependent purpura is seen in acute and chronic ITP, PPPs, CV, and scurvy. Livedo reticularis is seen most commonly on the legs. Painful acral purpuric lesions are indicative of ischemia from emboli such as seen in subacute bacterial endocarditis, cholesterol embolization, or cardioembolization from atrial myxoma or nonbacterial thrombotic emboli (marantic endocarditis).[59]

The nearly mirror-image, symmetrical involvement of the legs and trunk in the palpable purpura of CV is noteworthy. A high degree of asymmetry should increase the index of suspicion for a factitious process.

Acute-onset purpura will generally have a worse prognosis than chronic purpura and haste must be used to evaluate for and rule out infectious causes, DIC, cholesterol embolism, and other catastrophic processes in the microthrombotic category. Long-standing purpuric lesions may well be OWR syndrome, PPPs, purpura simplex, purpura secondary to heritable connective tissue disorders, or chronic ITP. Hemosiderin deposits in the dependent portions of the legs connotes chronicity due to accumulation of heme iron retained in the cutaneous macrophages. Both senile (atrophic or actinic) purpura and the purpura secondary to hypercortisolism are essentially limited to the extensor surfaces of the forearms, a pattern that essentially is diagnostic for one of these two disorders.

LABORATORY EVALUATION

The hematologist will nearly always order a CBC with a platelet count and differential white cell count as well as a prothrombin time and a partial thromboplastin time for screening purposes. Such practice is both understandable and defensible. Otherwise the laboratory should be used primarily to rule out and or rule in other specific disorders in a manner not unlike those listed in Table 11–5 used to specifically evaluate for secondary causes of CV.

The bleeding time is normal except in qualitative and quantitative platelet disorders. The normal bleeding time is consistent with the fact that the other purpuric disorders do not primarily interfere with the platelet–endothelial interaction as is tested by the bleeding time.

Skin biopsy is frequently helpful and is usually ordered in collaboration with a dermatologist. It is particularly useful in establishing CV, PPPs, amyloidosis, KS, and senile purpura if these diagnostic considerations are not otherwise straightforward, thus justifying further testing.

COST CONTAINMENT

The modest laboratory evaluation just described will considerably curtail costs. A reasonable knowledge base of purpura with a good history and physical examination are typically all that are needed to establish the diagnosis in the majority of patients with purpura. This approach leads to the accurate diagnosis of mechanical purpura, factitious purpura, purpura simplex, PPPs, many causes of CV, RMSF, scurvy, hypercortisolism, senile purpura, heritable disorders of connective tissue, OWR syndrome, DIC, warfarin skin necrosis, fat embolism syndrome, cholesterol emboli, and the associated nonpurpuric hematovascular disorders such as livedo reticularis, angiomas, and spiders.

TREATMENT ISSUES

Clearly treatment begins with a correct diagnosis. No treatment is necessary for many patients (e.g., purpura simplex, PPPs, or cases of primary CV), while hematologic treatment is indicated for others (e.g., ITP, TTP, DIC, OWR). Nonhematologic treatment is indicated for a third group (e.g., psychiatric evaluation in factitious purpura; rheumatologic evaluation in many cases of secondary CV; antibiotics for RMSF, subacute bacterial endocarditis, or meningococcemia; or dietary management for scurvy). This review does not cover all treatment aspects for all causes of purpura.

With the obvious exceptions of patients with a qualitative or quantitative platelet defect, hemophilia, or an acquired coagulation factor inhibitor and those on anticoagulants, purpuric patients do not harbor a systemic hemorrhagic diathesis. Accordingly, those patients with OWR syndrome, senile purpura, purpura simplex, PPPs, CV, scurvy, heritable disorders of connective tissue, and KS may undergo invasive and operative procedures without fear of hemostatic failure. Patients with amyloidosis fall in between these two groups and may require special consideration before an elective invasive procedure.

MEDICAL-LEGAL CONSIDERATIONS

In patients with bruising and hematomas, consideration must always be given to the possibility of trauma due to abuse. While abused patients may present with bruising as their sole complaint, nonabused patients may be falsely accused of being abused simply by the presence of purpuric lesions. Parents of a child unknowingly having von Willebrand disease or mild hemophilia may be accused of abuse.

■ REFERENCES

Chapter 11 References

1. Jones HW, Tocantins LM. The history of purpura hemorrhagica. Ann Med Hist 1933;5:349–359.
2. Bullet AJ. How Lind, as much as Nelson, broke the power of Napoleon. Resident Staff Physician 1993;39:85–88.
3. Werlhof PG, Wichmann JE. Opera Medica. Hamnoverae, imp fractorem, 1775–1776, p. 748.

4. Willan, R. On cutaneous diseases. London, J. Johnson, 1808, as referenced by Jones and Tocantins (ref 92). Ann Med Hist 1933;5:349.
5. Flint A. A Treatise in the Principles and Practice of Medicine, 6th 6d. Philadelphia, Lea Brothers, 1886, pp. 1130–1134.
6. Osler W. The Principles and Practice of Medicine, 2nd Ed. New York, Appleton, 1896, pp. 343–350.
7. Osler W. On a family form of recurring epistaxis, associated with multiple telangiectases of skin and mucous membranes. Bull Johns Hopkins Hosp 1901;12:333–337.
8. Wolbach SB. Studies on Rocky Mountain spotted fever. J Med Res 1919;41:1–197.
9. Wintrobe MM. Clinical Hematology, 1st ed. Philadelphia, Lea & Febiger, 1942, pp. 154.
10. Haden RL, Schneider RH, Underwood LC. Abnormal hemorrhage with normal platelet count and normal clotting. Ann NY Acad Sci 1948;49:641–646.
11. Spaet TH. Vascular factors in the pathogenesis of hemorrhagic syndromes. Blood. 1952;7:641–652.
12. Ackroyd JF. Allergic purpura, including purpura due to foods, drugs, and infections. Am J Med 1953;14:605–632.
13. Majno G. Ultrastructure of the vascular membrane. In Hamilton WF (ed.). Handbook of Physiology, sec 2, vol III. Washington, D.C., American Physiological Society, 1965, p. 2293.
14. Elliott RHE. The suction test for capillary resistance in thrombocytopenic purpura. JAMA 1938;110:1177–1179.
15. Rashkovsky I, Safadi R, Zlotogorski A. Black palmar macules. Palmar petechiae ("black palm"). Arch Dermatol 1998;134: 1020, 1023–1024.
16. Ratnoff OD. Psychogenic bleeding. Chapter 20 In Ratnoff OD, Forbes CD (eds.). Disorders of Hemostasis, 3rd Ed. W.B. Philadelphia, Saunders, 1996.
17. Gardner FH, Diamond LK. Autoerythrocyte sensitization: A form of purpura producing painful bruising following autosensitization to red blood cells in certain women. Blood 1955;10:675–690.
18. Lackner H, Karpatkin S. On the "easy bruising" syndrome with normal platelet count. Ann Intern Med 1975;83:190–196.
19. Kim HJ, Skidmore RA, Woosley JT. Pigmented purpura over the lower extremities. Purpura annularis telangiectodes of Majocchi. Arch Dermatol 1998;134:1477, 1480.
20. Kitchens CS. Amelioration of endothelial abnormalities by prednisone in experimental thrombocytopenia in the rabbit. J Clin Invest 1977;60:1129–1134.
21. Kitchens CS, Pendergast JF. Human thrombocytopenia is associated with structural abnormalities of the endothelium which are ameliorated by glucocorticosteroid administration. Blood 1986;67:203–206.
22. Li J-J, Huang Y-Q, Basch R, et al. Thrombin induces the release of angiopoietin-1 from platelets. Thromb Haemost 2001;83:204–206.
23. Kraft DM, McKee D, Scott C. Henoch-Schönlein purpura: A review. Am Fam Physician 1998;58:405–411.
24. Dispenzieri A, Gorevic PD. Cryoglobulinemia. Hematol Oncol Clin North Am 1999;13:1315–1349.
25. Shirahama M, Umeno Y, Tomimasu R, et al. The value of colour Doppler ultrasonography for small bowel involvement of adult Henoch-Schönlein purpura. Br J Radiol 1998;71:788–791.
26. Blanco R, Martinez-Taboada VM, Rodriguez-Valverde V, et al. Cutaneous vasculitis in children and adults. Associated diseases and etiologic factors in 303 patients. Medicine 1998;77:403–418.
27. Piette WW. What is Schönlein-Henoch purpura, and why should we care? Arch Dermatol 1997;133:515–518.
28. Martinez-Taboada VM, Blanco R, Garcia-Fuentes M, et al. Clinical features and outcome of 95 patient with hypersensitivity vasculitis. Am J Med 1997;102:186–191.
29. Blanco R, Martinez-Taboada VM, Rodriguez-Valverde V, et al. Henoch-Schönlein purpura in adulthood and childhood: Two different expressions of the same syndrome. Arthrit Rheum 1997;40:859–864.
30. Halasz CLG, Cormier D, Den M. Petechial glove and sock syndrome caused by parvovirus B19. J Am Acad Dermatol 1992; 27:835–838.
31. Peters CJ. Infections caused by arthropod- and rodent-borne viruses. Chapter 200 In Fauci AS, Braunwald E, Isselbacher KJ, Wilson JD, Martin JB, Kasper DL, Hauser SL, Longo DL (eds.). Harrison's Principles of Internal Medicine, 14th Ed. New York, McGraw-Hill, 1998.
32. Connolly BM, Steele KE, Davis KJ, et al. Pathogenesis of experimental Ebola virus infection in guinea pigs. J Infect Dis 1999; 179(suppl 1): S203–S217.
33. de Paepe A. The Ehlers-Danlos syndrome: A heritable collagen disease as a cause of bleeding. Thromb Haemost 1996;75:379–386.
34. Gertz MA, Lacy MQ, Dispenzieri A. Amyloidosis. Hematol Oncol Clin North Am 1999;13:1211–1233.
35. Braverman IM, Keh A, Jacobson BS. Ultrastructure and three-dimensional organization of the telangiectases of hereditary hemorrhagic telangiectasia. J Invest Dermatol 1990;95:422–427.
36. Guttmacher AE, Marchuk DA, White RI. Hereditary hemorrhagic telangiectasia. N Engl J Med 1995;333:918–924.
37. Rockey DC. Occult gastrointestinal bleeding. N Engl J Med 1999;341:38–46.
38. Swanson KL, Prakash UBS, Stanson AW. Pulmonary arteriovenous fistulas: Mayo Clinic experience, 1982–1997. Mayo Clin Proc 1999;74:671–680.
39. Garcia-Tsao G, Korzenik R, Young L, et al. Liver disease in patients with hereditary hemorrhagic telangiectasia. N Engl J Med 2000;343:931–936.
40. Shovlin CL. Molecular defects in rare bleeding disorders: Hereditary haemorrhagic telangiectasia. Thromb Haemost 1997;78: 145–150.
41. van Cutsem E, Rutgeerts P, Vantrappen G. Treatment of bleeding gastrointestinal vascular malformations with oestrogen-progesterone. Lancet 1990;335:953–954.
42. Barkin JS, Ross BS. Medical therapy for chronic gastrointestinal bleeding of obscure origin. Am J Gastroenterol 1998;93:1250–1254.
43. McKnight JT, Maxwell AJ, Anderson RL. Warfarin necrosis. Arch Fam Med 1992;1:105–108.
44. Sallah S, Thomas DP, Roberts HR. Warfarin and heparin-induced skin necrosis and the purple toe syndrome: Infrequent complications of anticoagulant treatment. Thromb Haemost 1997;78: 785–790.
45. Muller C, Rahn BA, Pfister U, et al. The incidence, pathogenesis, diagnosis and treatment of fat embolism. Orthopaedic Rev 1994;23:107–117.
46. Pell ACH, Hughes D, Keating J, et al. Fulminating fat embolism syndrome caused by paradoxical embolism through a patent foramen ovale. N Engl J Med 1993;329:926–929.
47. Fabian TC. Unraveling the fat embolism syndrome. N Engl J Med 1993;329:961–963.
48. McKee LC Jr., Collins RD. Intravascular leukocyte thrombi and aggregates as a cause of morbidity and mortality in leukemia. Medicine 1974;53:463–478.
49. O'Keefe ST, Woods BO'B, Breslin DJ, et al. Blue toe syndrome. Causes and management. Arch Intern Med 1992;152:2197–2202.
50. Antman K, Chang Y. Kaposi's sarcoma. N Engl J Med 2000; 342:1027–1038.
51. Samet JH, Muz P, Cabral P, et al. Dermatologic manifestations in HIV-infected patients. A primary care perspective. Mayo Clin Proc 1999;74:658–660.
52. Kroll MH, Shandera WX. AIDS-associated Kaposi's sarcoma. Hospital Practice 1998;April:85–102.

53. Dezube BJ. Clinical presentation and natural history of AIDS-related Kaposi's sarcoma. Hematol Oncol Clin North Am 1996;10:1023–1029.
54. Asherson RA, Mayou SC, Merry P, et al. The spectrum of livedo reticularis and anticardiolipin antibodies. Br J Dermatol 1989;120:215–221.
55. Sneddon JB. Cerebrovascular lesions and livedo reticularis. Br J Dermatol 1965;77:180–185.
56. Bard JW, Winkelmann RK. Livedo vasculitis: segmental hyalinizing vasculitis of the dermis. Arch Dermatol 1967;96:489–499.
57. Gibson GE, Su WPD, Pittelkow MR. Antiphospholipid syndrome and the skin. J Am Acad Dermatol 1997;36:971–982.
58. Drolet BA, Esterly NB, Frieden IJ. Hemangiomas in children. N Engl J Med 1999;341:173–181.
59. McAllister SM, Bornstein AM, Callen JP. Painful acral purpura. Arch Dermatol 1998;134:789–791.

CHAPTER 12

Disseminated Intravascular Coagulation

Craig S. Kitchens, M.D.

An enormous amount has been written about disseminated intravascular coagulation (DIC). During the 1970 and 1980s, it was rather fashionable to report on yet another "cause" of DIC. In the last two decades, however, it has become increasingly clear that DIC, rather than being a specific disease, is really the pathophysiologic final common pathway of the coagulation system gone awry. That single understanding brings into focus that DIC is an "intermediary mechanism of disease"[1] and collapses the nearly infinite list of causes into an understandable and functional process. Less time is now spent on indexing new and unique causes of DIC, with the thrust toward recognizing the underlying and initiating process of DIC and directing therapy toward that cause. The central role of tissue factor and various cytokines in the initiation and continuation of coagulation up to and including DIC has been elucidated.

Even the terminology has been controversial. DIC has been called *defibrination syndrome, acquired afibrinogenemia, consumptive coagulopathy,* and *consumptive thrombohemorrhagic disorder.* Although each term certainly has its advocates and rationale for use, the term *disseminated intravascular coagulation,* and "DIC" in particular, seems to be rooted in our medical vocabulary and so DIC will be used in this chapter. Additionally, microvascular thrombosis appears to be a major pathologic mechanism resulting in multiorgan dysfunction syndrome (MODS). MODS is the actual cause of death among patients suffering processes associated with DIC. Hence there is an association between DIC and MODS.

HISTORICAL OVERVIEW

The end result of DIC has been long known. The "Black Death" refers to the intense peripheral gangrene and bleeding resulting from thrombosis and defibrination of the plague that scourged the Earth over the first millennium. That fatal bleeding could occur with various obstetric emergencies has been known also for centuries.[2] In 1834 de Blainville[3] was able to induce fatal massive intravascular thrombosis in animals by the rapid infusion of brain tissue. Nauyn[4] 40 years later observed similar manifestations when animals were infused with hemolyzed red cells. In 1884 Foa and Pellacani[5] elaborated on de Blainville's experiment by showing that extracts of several organs when infused could cause both thrombosis and hemorrhage. In further studying de Blainville's model, Wooldridge[6] in 1893 infused brain tissue slowly rather than rapidly as did de Blainville and demonstrated that the animals did not die of massive intravascular thrombosis but rather their blood became unclottable and, further, after this state had been achieved, that rapid infusions of more brain tissue did not cause any outward harm to the animal. It was Mills[7] in 1921 who observed that the latter findings were in fact due to selective defibrination that occurred with slow infusion of brain tissue and that the secondary rapid infusion failed to cause thrombosis as the animal had been defibrinated. In 1957, Krevans and colleagues[8] studied defibrination following hemolytic transfusion reactions in humans and made seminal observations regarding what we would now call DIC. At about that same time, Schneider[9] infused placental tissue into rabbits and was able to induce hemorrhage in these animals, thus offering a peek into the mechanism of DIC characteristic of obstetric catastrophes. In the late 1960s, Merskey's[10] laboratory developed a test to detect serum fibrin degradation products (FDPs) and thus opened the door to laboratory investigation of DIC. Further studies into the fate of fibrinogen and mechanism of FDP production in DIC were made by Marder's group.[11] Corrigan and colleagues[12] made rapid advances in the elucidation of DIC associated with septicemia, focusing on meningococcemia. McKay[1] catalogued the knowledge base regarding DIC in 1965, making it a distinct clinical entity. In 1968 microangiopathic hemolysis to include that seen in DIC was described.[13] The rapid growth in experience and knowledge was again thoroughly reviewed by Colman in 1972.[14] The notion of a pristine laboratory approach to diagnosing DIC was dismantled when Merskey[15] pointed out that not everything that appears to be DIC by laboratory criteria may be DIC, while sometimes true DIC may not "fit" if the primary criteria are laboratory findings rather than the underlying illness and overall clinical picture. Mant and King[16] appropriately argued that DIC may be severe and acute, while Sack and colleagues[17] clearly and accurately described chronic DIC associated with neoplasia. Causes of DIC are heterogeneous and signs and symptoms variable.[18]

During the next 20 years and up to the present, innumerable papers have been written on the initiation and control of both normal hemostasis and the pathologic end result, DIC. These discoveries will be covered in more detail in the following pages.

PHYSIOLOGY AND PATHOPHYSIOLOGY

Coagulation is initiated by either interruption of the endothelial lining of the vascular system or entry of tissue factor (TF) into the blood. With the former mechanism, the intrinsic clotting system may be activated by interaction of blood with subendothelial tissue and collagen, while with the latter, TF, which is within all or most cells with the exception of unperturbed endothelial and peripheral blood cells and is released with cellular disruption,[19] causes activation of the tissue factor (extrinsic) clotting system. It appears that the extrinsic TF-driven system is the predominant force in hemostasis. Provided that the impetus is durable or protracted enough to sustain a procoagulant force, thrombin will be generated. During this cascade of activation, each step must pass physiologic hurdles, be they potential inactivation of activated serine proteases (factors XIa, Xa, IXa, VIIa, and IIa) by antithrombin III (ATIII) or degradation of activated cofactors (factors Va and VIIIa) by the protein C system. Should thrombin be eventually generated, it must continue to evade ATIII as well as endothelial-bound thrombomodulin (TM) to finally convert fibrinogen to fibrin. All of this is quite physiologic following a surgical incision or other event for which we regard hemostasis as desirable. When a breach in the circulatory system has been corrected, it is then appropriate for any remaining procoagulants, but especially thrombin, to be neutralized by these physiologic inhibitors. By virtue of the fact that a clot begets its own dissolution by incorporation of plasminogen, which is then activated by the fibrinolytic system, the clot remains in place for a while until it eventually is cleared by the action of plasmin. Any excess plasmin is neutralized by its inhibitor, α_2-plasmin inhibitor (α_2PI). This all physiologically happens continually. One could arguably claim that events that could lead to DIC occur every day but DIC does not routinely happen because these are tightly regulated events.

What separates the pathophysiologic process of DIC from physiologic clotting is the combination of nonphysiologic, sustained, and excessive initiation of coagulation (obstetric catastrophes, sepsis, cancer, trauma) and the inability to neutralize circulating activated products of coagulation because of deficiencies in the inhibitory system (congenital deficiencies, hepatic insufficiency, or impaired circulation) such that the initiating stimulus for coagulation is not neutralized. If the stimulus is massive, sustained, and/or not neutralized, the resultant procoagulant wave soon inundates physiologic inhibitors, resulting in free, circulating, unopposed thrombin and plasmin, the two key agents responsible for DIC. Table 12–1 lists the inhibitors that are overcome in the genesis of DIC. Each inhibitor system is in place to neutralize a key hemostatic force listed on the left, each of which is key in the initiation and sustainment of DIC. Any attempt to hold these in check by their individual inhibitors will be overwhelmed by the continued massing of procoagulants. The pathologic consequence of overwhelming the inhibitors is listed to the right. In fact, the clinical and laboratory manifestations of DIC can be explained by pathologic circulation of thrombin and plasmin. Thrombin will result in the pathologic intravascular clotting of fibrinogen, especially in the microcirculation, and deposition of platelets in nonphysiologic areas as well as consumption of coagulation factors, while plasmin degrades fibrinogen, fibrin, and multiple coagulation factors generating FDPs and D-dimer characteristic of DIC (Fig. 12–1). Of interest in profound DIC, circulating levels of plasminogen activator inhibitor-1 (PAI-1) paradoxically increase by virtue of

Table 12–1 • HEMOSTATIC CONSEQUENCES OF LOSS OF INHIBITORS IN DIC

Key Hemostatic Forces	Inhibitor	Consequence of Loss of Inhibitor
Tissue factor (TF)	Tissue factor pathway inhibitor (TFPI)	Enhanced thrombin generation
Activated factors V and VIII	Protein C and protein S	Enhanced thrombin generation
Activated coagulation factors, especially thrombin	Antithrombin III (ATIII)	Enhanced fibrin formation and platelet activation
Tissue plasminogen activator (tPA)	Plasminogen activator inhibitor, type 1 (PAI-1)	Enhanced fibrinolytic activation with decrease in PAI-1 and enhanced thrombosis with increase in PAI-1 (see text)
Plasmin	α_2-antiplasmin (α_2-AP)	Unopposed fibrinolysis

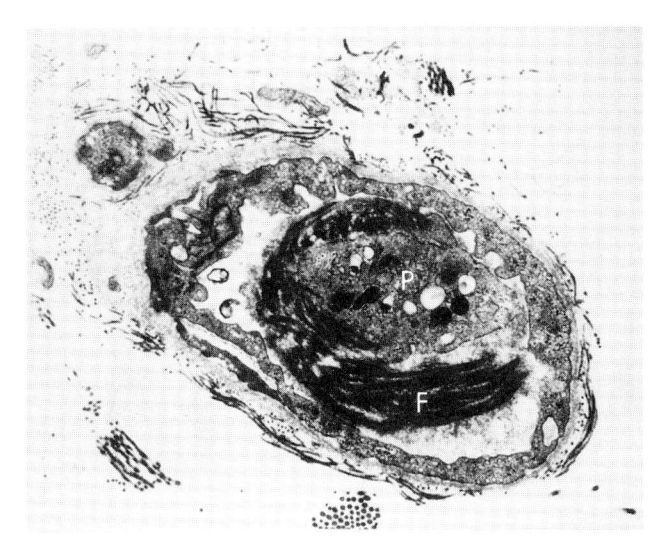

Figure 12-1 Electron micrograph of a capillary in experimental DIC. The intact capillary contains both a network of fibrin (*F*) and an occluded platelet (*P*) (×13,000).

being an acute phase reactant greatly intensified by cytokines.[20] This increase in PAI-1 efficiently downregulates the fibrinolytic system, which correlates with more massive thrombosis, MODS, and death.[21] During infusion of *Escherichia coli* endotoxin into normal human subjects, circulating levels of tissue plasminogen activator (tPA) initially increase and fibrinolysis is promoted; however, with continual infusion, levels of PAI-1 greatly increase, resulting in a total loss of tPA functional activity.[22] D-dimer is a specific FDP generated by plasmin lysis of two γ-chain fragments of fibrin that have been crosslinked by the action of activated factor XIII. Since factor XIII activation requires the presence of thrombin and the only initiator of fibrinolysis is plasmin, this D-dimer complex serves as a "footprint" proving the prior dual existence of thrombin and plasmin in the circulation.[23,24]

CAUSES OF DIC

Whereas DIC was previously regarded as a specific disorder, we now hold that DIC, much as fever, hyponatremia, or abdominal pain, is a manifestation of a pathologic process. These are all abnormalities but are not recognized diseases. Rather, these are always due to some underlying cause. Accordingly, recognizing DIC in a patient implies that an underlying process is becoming such a burden on the patient's hemostatic system that the patient's situation is becoming increasingly unstable. DIC should be regarded as an indicator of a severe disease process or injury that is blatantly obvious (burns, trauma, cardiopulmonary collapse, carcinomatosis, sepsis), yet occasionally DIC will serve as part of the original diagnosis and may help establish the presence of an underlying process. Common examples include recognition of DIC as distinguishing meningococcemia from viral headache and fever in a young healthy patient, establishing acute promyelocytic leukemia (APL) in a previously uncertain type of leukemia, and appreciating an obstetric catastrophe such as abruptio placentae or placenta previa from an otherwise mildly complicated labor and delivery. Table 12-2 lists several processes that may induce DIC.

INITIATION OF DIC

Following is a brief outline of the physiologic activation of coagulation that may help to explain how continued and unchecked activation results in the clinical syndrome known as DIC.

Figure 12-2 is a crude attempt to pictorialize key events in DIC. Any graphic attempting to exhaustively demonstrate all the on-going reactions, interactions, and counteractions would be unfathomable and thus this chart admittedly greatly simplifies seminal points of DIC. For instance, the direct infusion of substances (snake venoms) that activate directly either prothrombin or factor X[25] are not portrayed by this simplification. The key role of the liver in holding in check DIC by the clearance of activated factors is also not satisfactorily addressed. The importance of the liver was revealed by the pioneering works of Deykin.[26] Key inhibitors of coagulation are represented by letters at proposed control points, although they too are greatly simplified. For example, Sanset and colleagues[27] demonstrated that elimination of TF pathway inhibitor (TFPI) from experimental animals proved that TFPI was an important governor of experimental DIC.

Nonetheless Figure 12-2 does depict the general flow of events. Effects of vascular injuries that occur are not as neatly divided into activation of the extrinsic (TF-driven) clotting system or the intrinsic (contact system–driven) system as previously held. Accordingly, in the

Table 12-2 • PROCESSES THAT MAY INDUCE DIC

Tissue Damage	*Infections*
Trauma	Gram-positive bacteria
Crush injuries	Gram-negative bacteria
CNS injuries	Spirochetes
Heat stroke	Rickettsiae
Burns	Protozoa
Hemolytic transfusion reaction	Fungi
Acute transplant rejection	Viruses
Neoplasia	*Obstetric Conditions*
Cancers	Abruptio placentae
Leukemias	Placenta previa
Cancer chemotherapy	Retained dead fetus syndrome
Tumor lysis syndrome	Amniotic fluid embolism
	Uterine atony
Miscellaneous	Therapeutic abortion
Shock	Toxemia of pregnancy
Cardiac arrest	
Near drowning, especially in fresh water	
Fat embolism	
Aortic aneurysm	
Giant hemangiomas	
Snake bites	

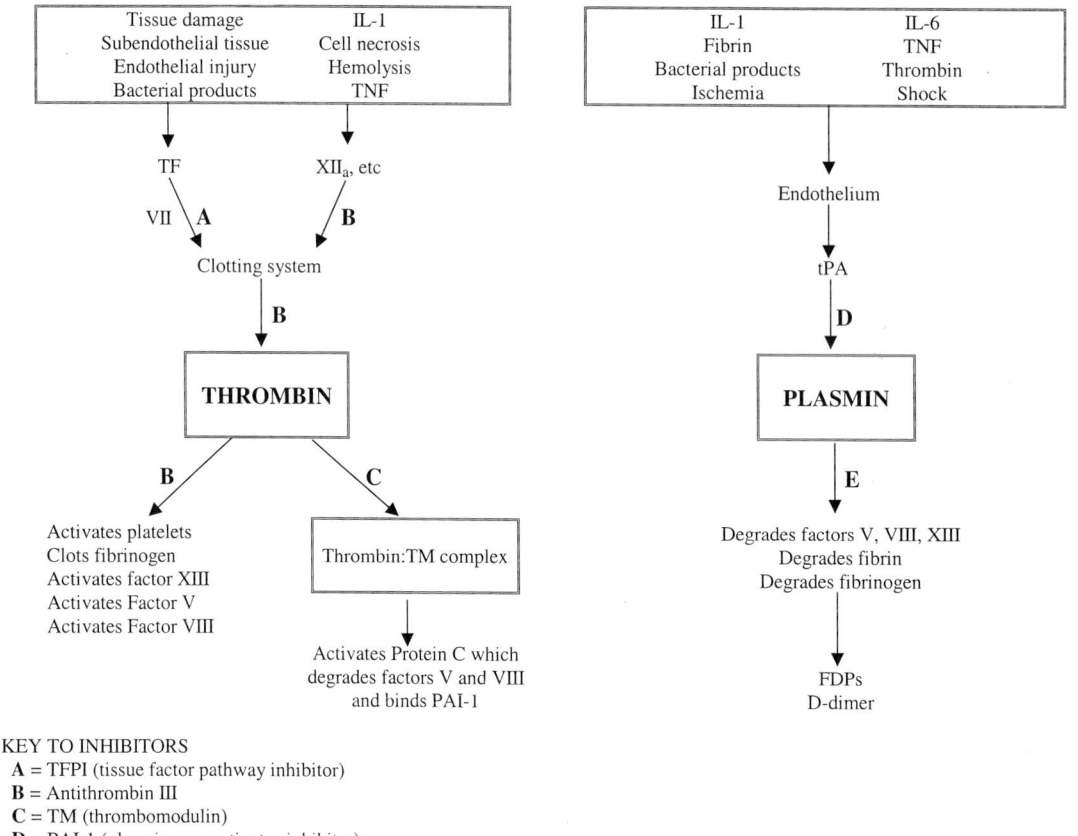

168 PART II Hemorrhagic Processes

```
Tissue damage        IL-1
Subendothelial tissue  Cell necrosis
Endothelial injury     Hemolysis
Bacterial products     TNF
         |                |
         ↓                ↓
        TF            XII_a, etc
    VII \ A          / B
         Clotting system
              |
              B
              ↓
          THROMBIN
         /        \
        B          C
       ↓            ↓
Activates platelets   Thrombin:TM complex
Clots fibrinogen              |
Activates factor XIII         ↓
Activates Factor V      Activates Protein C which
Activates Factor VIII   degrades factors V and VIII
                        and binds PAI-1
```

```
IL-1         IL-6
Fibrin         TNF
Bacterial products  Thrombin
Ischemia       Shock
         ↓
      Endothelium
         |
         ↓
        tPA
         |
         D
         ↓
      PLASMIN
         |
         E
         ↓
Degrades factors V, VIII, XIII
Degrades fibrin
Degrades fibrinogen
         ↓
        FDPs
       D-dimer
```

KEY TO INHIBITORS
A = TFPI (tissue factor pathway inhibitor)
B = Antithrombin III
C = TM (thrombomodulin)
D = PAI-1 (plasminogen activator inhibitor)
E = α_2 PI (α_2 plasmin inhibitor)

Figure 12–2 A brief overview outlining forces initiating coagulation that could lead to DIC. Key in the generation of DIC is circulating thrombin and plasmin free of physiologic inhibition.

box on the left, initiation by tissue damage, endothelial injury, and exposure of blood to bacterial products, necrotic cells, and subendothelial tissue are probably correctly depicted as activating both the intrinsic and extrinsic systems. However, the intrinsic system's role appears to actually be less important than that of the TF-driven extrinsic system in initiating DIC.[28,29] Endotoxin and other bacterial products can activate the contact system.[30] Those systems result in the generation of thrombin, which is absolutely essential to either normal or perturbed hemostasis. Thrombin then activates platelets, clots fibrinogen, and actives factors V, VIII, and XIII. All these result in a profound prothrombotic force. When their inhibitors as depicted by A (TFPI) and B (ATIII) are overwhelmed, thrombin generation becomes pathologic and DIC starts.

Circulating thrombin binds to TM. When thrombin binds to TM to make a thrombin:TM complex, thrombin metamorphoses from a powerful procoagulant to powerful anticoagulant by virtue of it activating proteins C and S, which in turn enhance the fibrinolytic system by neutralizing PAI-1. The product of the fibrinolytic system is the conversion of plasminogen to circulating plasmin. Other enhancers of fibrinolysis include endotoxin, interleukin-1 (IL-1), IL-6, factor XIIa, and fibrin, as well as tissue necrosis factor (TNF) which release endothelial tPA and uPA (urokinase-like plasminogen activator). Just as important as the keystone role of thrombin in DIC is the role of plasmin, as it causes degradation not only of fibrin but also of fibrinogen and factors V, VIII, and XIII. Degradation of fibrinogen and fibrin results in the characteristic "footprints" of circulating FDPs and D-dimer. Attempting to check plasminogen activation is PAI-1, whose concentration is greatly increased in the inflammatory reaction. If levels of PAI-1 greatly increase, the fibrinolytic system totally shuts down, potentiating catastrophic thrombosis. The inhibitor of plasmin, α_2PI also attempts to keep plasmin activity under control but is overwhelmed in DIC.

Table 12–3 lists a variety of newer discoveries in both human and experimental DIC, the importance and exact prioritization of which have yet to be determined. Some observations conflict with others. This listing is offered to indicate newer intricacies and nuances of DIC.

DIC may be characterized along three different axes representing tempo, extent, and clinical manifestation (Table 12–4). While recognizing that this simplistic approach may represent some degree of overlap, it offers a glimpse into the multiple and varied ways that DIC can present. The tempo axis distinguishes DIC as either acute or chronic. The classic diseases representing acute DIC include most of the sepsis syndromes, DIC secondary to trauma, and cardiopulmonary collapse. Chronic

Table 12-3 • MEDIATORS, CYTOKINES, AND THEIR RESPONSES IN DIC

Human DIC

TFPI, a major inhibitor of coagulation, is stored in endothelial cells and released by heparin treatment.[27, 31]

Cytokines (particularly TNF, IL-1, IL-6, and IL-10) have a central stimulatory role in DIC.[32, 33]

In human DIC, levels of TFPI and TF double.[34, 35]

TF is increased in DIC and decreases as patients improve.[36]

Severe depletion of antithrombin III and plasminogen predict death.[37]

High levels of PAI-1 do not predict lethality.[37]

High levels of PAI-1 were the best predictor of lethality.[21]

Serum levels of TM and neutrophil elastase are increased in trauma patients, more so in trauma-induced DIC, and even more so in fatal cases, all with good correlation with Injury Severity Score.[38]

In trauma patients with DIC, the cytokines TNF and IL-1 are greatly increased, more so in patients who develop MODS/ARDS/DIC, and yet more so in nonsurvivors.[39]

PAI-1 increases in progressive DIC, resulting in fibrinolytic shutdown, microvascular thrombosis, and MODS.[32]

ATIII levels are decreased in DIC and infusion of ATIII in DIC may be rational.[35]

Experimental DIC

Endothelial cells are normally antithrombotic but stimulation, especially with TNF, can cause the release of TF, TFPI, tPA, PAI-1, and TM from endothelial cells, thus changing endothelial cells from antithrombotic to prothrombotic.[40]

TFPI plays a key role in down-modulation of TF activity. Animals depleted of TFPI are extremely sensitive to induction of experimental DIC, whereas animals infused with TFPI prior to the experimental induction of DIC have increased survival.[35]

Compared to controls, volunteers infused with TFPI experience less DIC but similar cytokine response when challenged with infused endotoxin.[41]

Cultured endothelial cells do not elaborate TF but when cultured endothelial cells are infected with *Rickettsia rickettsii*,[42] or various respiratory viruses,[43] TF is released.

Endothelial cells and monocytes normally do not release TF but can be induced to release TF by *Rickettsia*,[44] bacteria, and endotoxin.[35]

Human volunteers infused with endotoxin release tPA with subsequent fibrinolysis, yet with continual infusion PAI-1 increases such that fibrinolysis is blocked.[22]

Infusion of antibodies against TF in experimental animals prevents induction of experimental DIC, demonstrating the central role of TF in initiation of DIC.[19]

High doses of IL-6 increase plasma fibrinogen, tPA, and PAI-1.[45]

DIC can be experimentally induced in baboons by infusion of X_a and phospholipids, which releases large amounts of tPA in a dose-dependent fashion. PAI-1 is not released at low infusion rates but is released at high rates.[45]

DIC is represented by the retained dead fetus syndrome, large intra-abdominal aortic aneurysms, and Trousseau syndrome.

Regarding extent, localized causes of DIC include abdominal aortic aneurysm (AAA), an empyema or necrotic gall bladder, or an obstetric catastrophe such as placenta previa or abruptio placentae. Systemic causes include most leukemias and lymphomas, carcinomatosis, sepsis, heat stroke, and burns.

The third axis to consider is clinical manifestation, which can be thrombotic, hemorrhagic, or, occasionally, both. An example of the thrombotic arm is Trousseau syndrome, whereas examples of almost pure hemorrhagic DIC would include abruptio placentae or hemolytic transfusion reaction.

COMMENTS ABOUT TWO REPRESENTATIVE CAUSES OF DIC

Closed head injury is a model for acute, severe DIC.[46] In experimental head injury in rats, fixed amounts of head trauma result in reproducible amounts of fibrin deposition in the microcirculation.[47] The same investigators[48] found that among patients with head injury, there was a correlation between extent of head injury, hemostatic defects, and worsening clinical outcome. Olson et al.[49] confirmed these findings in a large series of patients with head injuries. Head injuries not only lead to neurologic damage, paralysis, and venous stasis, but cause coagulation activation, as damaged brain tissue serves as the source of tissue thromboplastin released into the circulation. Selladurai and colleagues[50] prospectively studied 204 patients with acute closed head injury using readily available coagulation tests and found that 38% had either moderate or severe alterations of such global tests supporting the diagnosis of DIC. They noticed an increasing incidence of DIC with decreasing Glasgow coma scores ($p < 0.0001$). Patients whose laboratory data suggested DIC had a worse overall outcome than those without such findings. The DIC associated with closed head injury is usually rather brisk and self-limited because the spillage of the brain tissue into the circulation usually ceases. On the other hand, closed head injury often has such a high mortality that the patient may expire from the primary injury.

Abdominal aortic aneurysm (AAA) serves as a model for chronic compensated DIC in that the platelet count can either be low, high, or normal, as can the fibrinogen concentration. Most frequently, DIC in AAA is recognized when the platelet count is somewhat low, in the 40,000 to 80,000/μL range, and analysis for serum FDP is positive. It is thought that the rough saccular nature of the aneurysm allows for pockets of clotting to take place and therefore some degree of localized DIC oc-

Table 12-4 • THE THREE AXES OF DIC, WITH CLINICAL EXAMPLES

Axis	Example
Tempo	
Acute	Meningococcemia
Chronic	Retained dead fetus syndrome
Extent	
Localized	Abdominal aortic aneurysm
Systemic	Acute promyelocytic leukemia
Manifestation	
Hemorrhagic	Abruptio placentae
Thrombotic	Trousseau syndrome

curs. Of interest, microangiopathic hemolytic anemia changes of the red cells may be seen as well as laboratory evidence of intravascular hemolysis, including decreased levels of serum haptoglobin and the presence of urine hemosiderin. Low-dose heparin, such as 5000 units administered subcutaneously twice daily, has been advocated to attenuate the chronic DIC and allow the platelet count to increase so that the patient is a better surgical candidate. The platelet count may increase yet fluctuate on its own. Oba and colleagues[51] opine that, since the cause of the DIC is the aneurysm itself, rather than spend days to weeks administering heparin to such patients and waiting for results, the aneurysm should be surgically approached as soon as possible. Aboulafia and Aboulafia[52] reportedly found evidence of such chronic DIC in 2 of 67 consecutive cases of AAA. They reviewed reports of 34 cases of DIC associated with AAA and concluded that DIC was a variable process and that often the platelet count improved whether heparin was administered or not. They also suggested that the best approach was surgical correction of the AAA. It is not clear whether the presence of DIC added to the overall surgical morbidity of AAA.

Diagnosis of DIC

The most common clinical manifestations of DIC are bleeding, thrombosis, and concomitant bleeding and thrombosis, often with resultant dysfunction of either one or many organs. This is what the clinician sees. Bleeding will be manifest from all incisions, mildly traumatized mucosal membranes, and IV sites, and in the urine. Occasionally thrombosis will be the first clinical observation. This can be in the form of ecchymoses, which may rapidly progress into purpura fulminans (the manifestation of subdermal microthrombosis with skin necrosis), a cold pulseless limb, or the sudden loss of vision or some other neurologic catastrophe from thrombosis.

The diagnosis of DIC is, indeed, a clinical diagnosis (Table 12–5).[16] Because such patients are already at such high clinical suspicion for DIC, only a few simple and readily available laboratory tests are necessary to confirm the diagnosis. These include the prothrombin time (PT), partial thromboplastin time (aPTT), thrombin time (TT), platelet count, FDP level, and blood smear.

Table 12–5 • CLINICAL DIAGNOSTIC CRITERIA FOR DIC

- Patient bleeding, thrombosing, or both, typically with progressive organ dysfunction.
- An underlying illness or process that may cause tissue damage, cell death, or production/release of tissue factor.
- Usually some pertubation exists of simple, readily available tests such as thrombin time (TT), prothrombin time (PT), partial thromboplastin time (aPTT), fibrin degradation products (FDP)/D-dimer, or platelet count. These values may markedly change as the clinical situation changes.

Table 12–6 • REASONS WHY LABORATORY FINDINGS ARE OF SECONDARY IMPORTANCE IN THE DIAGNOSIS OF DIC

- There is always an underlying problem that presents its own varied pertubations of many tests.
- Tests represent static "snapshots" of a highly dynamic situation.
- Special tests frequently are esoteric and results arrive long after the dynamic situation has changed.
- Diagnostic test results rarely direct or redirect therapy and may confuse the clinical picture.

The PT and aPTT, in clinically severe and life-threatening DIC, are prolonged in approximately 50% to 75% of cases by virtue of consumption of many coagulation factors. The TT is significantly prolonged in approximately 70% to 80% of cases because levels of fibrinogen will be low while FDPs will be high, both of which serve to prolong the TT. The platelet count will be moderately reduced, or at least lower than a previous pre-DIC observation about 80% to 90% of the time. Usually the initial platelet count will not be lower than 30,000 to 40,000/μL. Analysis for FDPs will be abnormal 95% of the time (i.e., high sensitivity); when FDPs are increased and D-dimers (i.e., high specificity) are concomitantly present in patients for whom the clinical suspicion for DIC is high, virtually 100% will indeed have DIC.[23] Examination of the blood smear confirms the thrombocytopenia as well as demonstrates schistocytic hemolysis in about half the cases.

Some have written extensively on more detailed laboratory evaluations of DIC. Because various factors are consumed, measurement of any of the classic coagulation factors may reveal reduced levels, as well as reduced levels of ATIII, plasminogen, and α_2PI. The difficulties with a pure laboratory approach are several (Table 12–6). First, it implies that the initiation of the consideration of a diagnosis of DIC should be in the laboratory, whereas it is, in fact, at the bedside. Second, DIC is an extremely dynamic situation in which its initiation may be extremely brisk, yet brief, such as with an intermittent sepsis from a necrotic gallbladder, empyema, or abscess. This initiating force for DIC may be so rapid that by the time the clinical manifestations of DIC are observed, laboratory parameters may already have been righted by reparative mechanisms before the tests are ordered, samples collected, tests performed, reported, and interpreted. These more sophisticated tests require a considerable amount of time, laboratory expertise, and expense and in the author's opinion are unlikely to add more clinically useful information than the simple tests described.

Others[21,37,53,54] have advocated a more aggressive incorporation of laboratory data to support a diagnosis of DIC. Bick has evaluated and ranked over 20 tests that could be used in formulating such a diagnosis.[53] These tests arguably are frequently but not always altered in DIC. One might object that availability of many of these tests is much more restricted than the tests that we have favored, which are readily available in almost any clinical setting. Using elaborate laboratory data,

Reister and colleagues[54] have formulated four different levels of DIC (DIC I to DIC IV), claiming that progression of DIC through these phases is supported by progressive pertubations of eleven laboratory tests. Gando and colleagues[21] have established a score using four laboratory tests and three clinical situations. They also state that by following this score that they were able to separate patients into survivors (those whose scores decreased over the next 5 days) and nonsurvivors (those whose scores remained high for the 5-day period). They also noted that higher scores correlated not only with clinical deterioration of the patient but with progressive organ failure until MODS developed. Gando's report[21] parenthetically noted that an increase in the PAI-1 level was their best predictor for lethality of DIC, whereas Wada and colleagues[37] found that there was no correlation between the PAI-1 levels and the prediction of outcome of their patients. Not only may laboratory data in DIC be confusing but results may show trends in opposing directions when one compares either acute vs. chronic DIC or compensated vs. decompensated DIC.[55] Accordingly, unless and until such interesting laboratory findings prove both more predictive and cost-effective, the conservative usage of inexpensive and rapidly available tests seems most prudent.

DIFFERENTIAL DIAGNOSIS OF DIC

Several situations should be considered in the differential diagnosis of DIC because their clinical manifestations or laboratory abnormalities may mimic DIC. Most common among these is severe hepatic cirrhosis, the laboratory coagulation abnormalities of which mimic DIC (see Chapter 31). In patients with hepatic cirrhosis, decreased levels of hemostatic factors, including fibrinogen, ATIII, protein C, protein S, and plasminogen, are due to impaired production and not enhanced activation, as would be found in DIC. Because the liver clears the small amount of FDPs due to physiologic production, decreased clearance with hepatic disease results in an accumulation of FDPs in the serum. Portal hypertension with hypersplenism is also characteristic of advanced cirrhosis, hence thrombocytopenia is frequently encountered. Bleeding varices and gastritis in these patients are due not to DIC but to hepatic failure.

Measurable decreases in plasma fibrinogen (typically elevated in pregnancy) and increases in serum FDP are found in the immediate postpartum period even in uncomplicated deliveries. These measurable changes should be viewed not as pathologic but as physiologic. However, in an appropriate clinical setting such as massive hemorrhage, these changes may support a diagnosis of DIC.

The differential diagnosis of DIC may include the HELLP (*H*emolysis, *E*levated *L*iver function tests, and *L*ow *P*latelets) syndrome, which is discussed thoroughly in Chapter 28.[56] Indeed, distinguishing among DIC, massive thrombosis, thrombotic thrombocytopenic purpura (TTP) and the HELLP syndrome[57] can represent a challenge. Table 12–7 lists some differences among these presentations. Treatment of the HELLP syndrome centers around delivery of the child and placenta as soon as feasible. Delivery is timed closely with the obstetrician. If possible, waiting a few extra days will increase the viability of the fetus as this syndrome often comes into light in the beginning of the third trimester.[58] Paradoxically, the HELLP syndrome frequently deteriorates 2 to 4 days before or after delivery. One must be on guard at that time for the possibility of overt thrombosis. In fact, one can justify prophylactic administration of heparin immediately postpartum if the platelet count is not less than 20,000/μL. Distinguishing between the HELLP syndrome and DIC can be difficult or impossible as it is clear that the HELLP syndrome can degenerate to DIC. Van Dam and colleagues[58] and De Boer and colleagues[59] studied this transition and found that laboratory manifestations heralding a worsening of the HELLP syndrome into probable DIC included progression of the PT and aPTT from normal to abnormal, the progressive appearance of serum FDPs, and a decrease in the serum ATIII level.

While TTP (discussed in Chapter 22) is clearly a thrombotic process with major organ damage resulting from pathologic intravascular deposition of large aggregates of platelets, it is not regarded as being representative of DIC. The PT, aPTT, TT, and FDP level are nearly always normal. Microangiopathic hemolysis is a hallmark.

A thrombin-like enzyme, crotalase, found in the venom of the Eastern diamondback rattlesnake (*Crotalus adamantus*), partially clots fibrinogen.[25] However, it does not activate platelets or bind to ATIII, which distinguishes its actions from those of thrombin. Although the laboratory findings after envenomation by the Eastern diamondback rattlesnake are highly reminiscent of those of DIC, neither thrombotic nor hemorrhagic complications usually occur.

It has been long known that there was an association between thromboembolic disease and carcinoma. If thromboembolism occurs as described by Trousseau over 100 years ago,[60] the process is appropriately known as Trousseau syndrome. The approximate two- to three-fold incidence of bland deep venous thrombosis (DVT) found in cancer patients is not Trousseau syndrome. Rather, Trousseau syndrome is a subset of the hypercoagulability associated with carcinoma and is recognized by specific characteristics (Table 12–8). Trousseau syndrome is now regarded as chronic DIC as elaborated by Sack and colleagues.[17] The syndrome is particularly associated with adenocarcinoma and frequently the tumor is occult. It is thought to be due to the release of procoagulant products from tumors, one of which is TF.[61] Indeed, these authors showed an association between malignant tissue TF concentrations and hypercoagulability. The metastatic potential of a tumor may be related to TF expression in the malignant cells.[62]

There have been many studies to find laboratory abnormalities that would be sensitive and specific enough to establish the diagnosis of Trousseau syndrome but these have not gained much popularity because of their inherent variability. Situations such as Trousseau syn-

Table 12-7 • DIFFERENTIAL DIAGNOSIS OF DIC

Feature	Acute DIC (e.g., sepsis)	Chronic DIC (e.g., Trousseau Syndrome)	Thrombotic Storm[57]	HELLP	TTP	Primary Hyperfibrinolysis
Patient population	Patients with severe obstetric, medial, or surgical illnesses	Patients with cancer	Patients with hypercoagulability	Pregnant patients	Usually otherwise healthy	Prostate cancer, post-CAB
Mechanism	Tissue damage and release of thromboplastins and cytokines	Tumor cell release of procoagulants or cell death	Uncontrolled hypercoagulability	Placental factors?	Platelet microthrombi	Direct plasminogen activation
Course	Usually acute	Subacute	Subacute	Subacute	Acute	Acute
Thrombosis[a]	Usually microcirculation	Arteries, veins, and microcirculation	Multiple veins and arteries	Nil	Microvascular	Nil
Hemorrhage	Frequent	Nil	Nil	Nil	Microvascular	Massive
Coagulation parameters	Usually abnormal	Usually normal	Normal	Normal	Normal	Abnormal
Platelet count	Low	Variable	Normal	Low	Low	Normal
Response to heparin	Nil	Fair	Good	NA	NA	NA
Response to warfarin following heparin	Nil	Nil	Good	NA	NA	NA
Prognosis with aggressive therapy	Good if underlying cause corrected	Poor	Good	Improved following delivery	Improved with plasma therapy	May be self-limited; consider EACA
Hemolysis	Microangiopathic	Microangiopathic	None	Microangiopathic	Microangiopathic	None

[a] Without anticoagulant therapy.

Table 12–8 • FEATURES OF TROUSSEAU SYNDROME

Clinical
Recurrent migratory thrombophlebitis
Unusual sites of thrombosis: axillary/subclavian veins; superficial veins of the neck, thorax, or abdomen; visceral or cerebral veins
Failure to respond clinically to warfarin
Usually respond clinically to heparin but may relapse immediately after discontinuation
May simultaneously experience arterial thrombosis and hemorrhage
Associated with nonbacterial thrombotic endocarditis
Tumor typically small or occult adenocarcinoma

Laboratory
No laboratory test sensitive or specific
Platelets and ATIII levels are usually decreased
Red blood cells may show changes consistent with microangiopathic hemolysis

drome have been referred to as *chronic compensated DIC* by Mammen,[55] who observed that the simplest tests such as the platelet count, PT, aPTT, and fibrinogen level can be low, normal, or high. Typically, but not always, the ATIII level will be decreased and the concentration of FDPs will be increased in Trousseau syndrome.

Trousseau syndrome is recognized by its features as listed in Table 12–8. A particularly useful diagnostic criterion is the recurrent nature of DVT, which is usually controlled by heparin but then recurs almost as soon as heparin therapy is withdrawn after the initiation of warfarin therapy regardless of the INR achieved. The vessels involved may be veins, particularly those in unusual places such as superficial veins in the thorax and abdomen, subclavian veins, and especially the cerebral veins.[63] Arterial thromboses also occur and can be sudden, catastrophic, life-threatening, or fatal.[17] Therapy is challenging. Warfarin therapy fails. Heparin, often in very large doses, is required to keep the aPTT at target levels or at least to maintain the heparin concentration at therapeutic levels such as 0.3 to 0.8 U/mL, which can be achieved using large doses of standard unfractionated heparin even on an outpatient basis. Whether low-molecular-weight heparin (LMWH) is more efficacious than standard heparin in this situation is not certain. However, if one does use LMWH, measurement of heparin levels by anti-Xa activity to validate sufficient concentration for chronic ambulatory therapy appears rational. The patient may succumb either to uncontrolled venous and arterial thrombosis of Trousseau syndrome or to the therapy, as metastases may hemorrhage. The thrombohemorrhagic syndrome is as lethal as the primary tumor.[64,65]

The fibrinolytic system may be activated independent of the coagulation system. Activation of the fibrinolytic system in the overwhelming majority of cases of DIC is the secondary physiologic result of thrombosis. In some circumstances the fibrinolytic system may be activated in a primary fashion. The existence of primary hyperfibrinolysis has been debated for some time and probably does exist in selected instances. Of interest, an enzyme in the venom of the Western diamondback rattlesnake (*Crotalus atrox*) directly activates plasminogen and causes primary hyperfibrinolysis.[25] In this situation bleeding may be significant, but thrombosis is not a feature. Primary hyperfibrinolysis may also result in some cases of carcinoma[65a] or acute promyelocytic leukemia as such cells may elaborate plasminogen activators.[66] The late phases of cardiopulmonary bypass (rewarming) and orthotopic liver transplant (wash-out of the donor liver) also are associated with a brisk release of endogenous tPA, resulting in probably the most common cause of bleeding following cardiopulmonary bypass and liver transplantation.[67,68] In keeping with that hypothesis, use of aprotinin is clearly associated with decreased hemorrhage in those procedures. Obviously, infusion of pharmacologic plasminogen activators, such as streptokinase or tPA, causes a primary hyperfibrinolytic state. Hemorrhage may be brisk but often is self-limited, especially following cardiovascular surgery or liver transplantation. Coagulation tests reflect the very low fibrinogen level and high levels of FDPs and include prolonged TT, PT, and aPTT. The platelet count and ATIII level will be normal or near normal and microangiopathic hemolytic anemia is conspicuously absent. If not self-limited and DIC (thrombosis) can be excluded, treatment with antifibrinolytic agents such as ε-aminocaproic acid (EACA) or tranexamic acid can be carefully attempted.

CONSEQUENCES OF DIC

The consequences, often life-threatening or fatal, of DIC involve multiorgan failure, resulting in what is now termed *multiorgan dysfunction syndrome* (MODS) (Table 12–9). At autopsy, target organs are found to be damaged and rendered ineffective by both hemorrhage into the organ and thromboses. Both events tend to be more at the microcirculatory level than the macrocirculatory level. Liver function tests can deteriorate at an alarming rate. This may be due not only to the hemorrhage and infarction of the organ, but also to circulatory collapse with so-called shock liver. Clearly, pre-existing liver disease will make this syndrome worse. Because of the liver's key role in clearance of activated factors and its role in synthesizing hemostatic factors, sustained liver function is key for survival. Additionally, the liver

Table 12–9 • MULTIORGAN DYSFUNCTION SYNDROME (MODS) AS A CONSEQUENCE OF DIC

- Pertubation of liver function tests
- Leakage of cardiac enzymes indicating ischemia
- Cardiac rhythm disturbances
- Central nervous system abnormalities
- Oliguria
- Decreased renal function
- Acute respiratory distress syndrome (ARDS)
- Gastrointestinal tract mucosal ulceration with bleeding
- Adrenal insufficiency
- Purpura fulminans

has been shown to be central in the host's survival in sepsis.

Cardiac abnormalities are demonstrated by either the appearance of elevated levels of serum cardiac enzymes, such as creatine kinase (CK), or cardiac rhythm disturbances due to destruction of the cardiac conduction system. Central nervous system abnormalities include seizures, mental status alterations, and behavioral abnormalities that may appear to be psychiatric in origin. Decreased renal function often occurs because of microinfarction of the filtering and collecting tubular apparatus. Usually oliguria is the harbinger of renal insufficiency and is quickly followed by elevation of the serum creatinine and/or BUN. Adult respiratory distress syndrome (ARDS) is a very common and frequently lethal manifestation of sepsis with shock and occurs especially in situations severe enough to result in DIC. Gastrointestinal manifestations are chiefly mucosal ulcerations with subsequent bleeding. Adrenal glands may infarct and then necrose, leaving the patient adrenally insufficient. Skin manifestations include petechiae from bleeding and infarctive necrosis, with the prime example being purpura fulminans. The onset of MODS, especially with progressive and sequential organ failure despite therapeutic efforts, accurately forecasts lethality.

It is impossible to accurately predict lethality of DIC for two reasons. The first of these is that by its very definition, DIC may include a range of patients, from those who will have no immediate mortality (those with liver disease presenting with laboratory data mimicking DIC), to those who have a long-range mortality (such as those with AAA or chronic DIC from neoplasia), to those with a relatively high acute mortality (such as those with acute leukemias, crush injuries, and shock), and finally to those with exceedingly high mortality (such as those with septic shock or meningococcemia). Second, each initiating process will be recognized and treated in a different fashion and the overall approach to the patient and his or her morbidity hinges on those factors. The process of DIC is less important regarding lethality than the host, the disease, and its treatment. Mant and King[16] showed that 85% of their patients with acute, severe DIC expired. Most expired, in their opinion, from the underlying disease and not DIC itself. Wada and colleagues[37] showed that of their 395 patients with DIC, a total of 25% died. Their patients comprised 154 leukemics (of whom 21% died) and 241 patients who did not have leukemia but cancer, sepsis, and other infectious diseases (of whom 28% died).

Predictors of death using laboratory criteria are even more difficult to establish. Some have claimed specific laboratory data did[21] or did not[37] predict death. The more laboratory abnormalities present and the greater the degree of alteration, the more likely the patient is to expire. Additionally, hepatic insufficiency is an effective predictor of mortality as is shock. At autopsy many patients who die of DIC will have ARDS and MODS. Multiple interrelationships exist between DIC, ARDS, MODS, and systemic inflammatory response syndrome (SIRS).[69] These are either separate factors that indicate a very ill patient with processes that are progressively killing the patient or, more likely, are all different manifestations of an evolving fatal process.[21,27,55,69,70] From a clinical point of view, one may predict at least a 25% to 50% mortality if the presenting syndrome of a very ill patient is any one of DIC, MODS, ARDS, or SIRS and the patient fails to rapidly improve. The mortality is even higher if the presenting syndrome is conjoined by or progresses to another of the DIC, MODS, SIRS, or ARDS group.

TREATMENT OF DIC

As DIC is a grave consequence of a grave underlying disease, it would seem reasonable that primary treatment should be directed at control of that disease. Such has become increasingly accepted although stating this fact is easier than accomplishing it. This approach is so successful that, when it can be accomplished, recognition of DIC in a patient sanctions use of aggressive therapy directed toward the primary process. The author knows of no clinical setting in which this is more successful than in DIC from obstetric emergencies. Women may present in labor with massive bleeding, having all the laboratory and clinical manifestations of DIC. The appropriate treatment is now recognized by obstetricians to be evacuation of the uterus. Time should not be spent in studying or trying to analyze in great depth the individual parameters of DIC; rather, the patient should be taken to the delivery suite, with resuscitation of blood pressure and volume by appropriate fluids, and the uterus evacuated. It is remarkable that a patient who is severely hemorrhaging can become hemostatically normal within a few hours of evacuation of the uterus. The success of this situation additionally underscores the marked restorative ability of an otherwise healthy person with normal hepatic function and a normal circulatory system to rectify these hemostatic abnormalities.

DIC may occur from bacterial sepsis as a complication of an empyema, necrotic gall bladder, or other abscess.[32] Again, time should not be spent analyzing various patterns and parameters of laboratory data in attempts to stratify, stage, or correct the DIC; rather, this situation is a medical and surgical emergency, neither of which will get better until the abscess is drained. Too frequently, surgical colleagues request "correction of the coagulopathy" prior to drainage of the abscess, when it is precisely drainage of the abscess that will lead to correction of the coagulopathy. It is far more likely the patient will die from bleeding and/or thrombosis from the DIC while one vainly attempts to correct the DIC rather than the minimal amount of bleeding that may occur from prompt drainage of the abscess to which the DIC will respond.

Table 12–10 represents a treatment schema for DIC. First, treating the underlying cause is the mainstay of treatment of DIC. Second, and almost equally important, is resuscitation of the patient's circulatory system. It would be difficult to overestimate the value of the liver in both neutralizing activated coagulation products and reconstitution of normal procoagulant and inhibitory proteins.[71] Hepatic circulation will not be maximal

Table 12-10 • TREATMENT OF DIC

Treatment	Example	Rationale
Treat underlying cause	Abruptio placentae	Interrupt cause of DIC
Resuscitation	Maintain blood pressure, correct acid/base balance	Maximize blood flow from areas of activation to clearance by liver
Replacement	Fresh frozen plasma and platelet transfusions	Provide enough procoagulant materials to control hemostasis
Antithrombin III	Severe liver disease with concomitant DIC	Replace severely decreased levels of ATIII
Heparin therapy	Trousseau syndrome, purpura fulminans, abdominal aortic aneurysm	May decrease on-going thrombosis
Antifibrinolytic therapy	Kasabach-Merritt syndrome, prostate cancer	Occasionally used to control fibrinolysis, but only after administration of heparin

and hence correction of blood abnormalities will not be maximal until hepatic perfusion is normalized by correction of volume, electrolyte, and blood pressure abnormalities. Failure to correct the initiating process and pre-existing hepatic hypoperfusion are harbingers of a bad outcome.

The role of fresh frozen plasma (FFP) and/or platelet transfusions appears to be simultaneously uncertain yet necessary. In order for thrombocytopenia to be a key potentiator of hemorrhage in patients, the platelet count is usually substantially below 50,000/μL. Similarly, in order for depletion of fibrinogen and other coagulation factors to be clinically significant, their levels must be below approximately 50 to 60 mg/dL and below 25% of normal levels, respectively. Otherwise, administration of fibrinogen, FFP or platelet transfusions is not indicated as these pertubations are the result of DIC and not the cause of bleeding. However, if the patient is hemorrhaging and the platelet count is less than 50,000/μL, transfusing platelets in order to keep the platelet count in the range of 50,000 to 75,000/μL seems quite reasonable. Equally, in a patient who is bleeding and the fibrinogen concentration is less than 50 to 60 mg/dL, fibrinogen may be infused in the form of FFP or preferably cryoprecipitate in amounts to raise the fibrinogen level to that minimal level. Usually 10 "units" of cryoprecipitate (each containing about 200 mg of fibrinogen) will suffice. Rarely are other blood coagulation factor levels lower than 25% of normal and accordingly FFP is rarely recommended for the replacement of other coagulation factors.

If ATIII is considered to be the primary inhibitor of the circulating thrombin, it would seem that ATIII infusion would be efficacious in treating DIC. ATIII is available in FFP but has more recently become available as a purified concentrate. Infusion in DIC has not been rigorously established, but its use certainly is rational. In experimental models, ATIII infusions blunt lethality, DIC, and SIRS in response to infusion of lethal amounts of *E. coli*.[72] Preliminary studies[73,74] have indicated the safety and efficacy of ATIII concentrates, particularly in septic shock syndromes and in patients whose liver insufficiency is such that an acquired ATIII deficiency state exists. ATIII may be administered in amounts to support the ATIII level in the range of 100% of normal. This may be approximated by the infusion of 100 units of ATIII per kilogram of body weight. This formula is complicated by the variable and often brief half-life of ATIII in DIC. For clinical purposes, ATIII has an overall half-life of approximately 24 hours; in DIC it may be as brief as 3 or 4 hours. Should ATIII concentrates be employed, frequent measurement of ATIII levels is indicated to help regulate the infusion. At this time, infusion of ATIII concentrates generally is not recommended.[75]

Activated protein C infusion has shown some initial success in decreasing mortality in patients with severe sepsis.[75a]

Direct thrombin inhibitors such as hirudin have the theoretical advantage of neutralizing thrombin, a key participant in DIC, while not being a direct anticoagulant. In preliminary human DIC studies, several laboratory markers improved but overall survival is uncertain using this evolving treatment modality.[76]

Heparin therapy remains extremely controversial. In some studies, the infusion of heparin has seemed to increase not only death, but particularly hemorrhagic death.[16] It is intellectually attractive to administer heparin in order to decrease thrombotic events; its use may be even more reasonable when the clinical axis of thrombosis vs. hemorrhage is more toward the thrombotic end. Accordingly, its use in Trousseau syndrome is quite established as not only rational but life-saving.[64] It may also be useful in purpura fulminans, acute promyelocytic leukemia (APL), and AAA, all of which represent a subacute thrombotic form of DIC. When heparin is used in situations in which coagulation tests are abnormal, one cannot monitor it by the usual coagulation tests so it must be given empirically. One commonly recommended method is to administer approximately 8 to 10 units/kg of standard heparin per hour by constant intravenous infusion. In more chronic DIC such as Trousseau syndrome, one may monitor heparin administration by the aPTT or plasma heparin levels.

Antifibrinolytic inhibitors such as EACA are occasionally advocated in patients who are on the extreme hemorrhagic end of the thrombotic–hemorrhagic axis. Such agents are very effective in blocking fibrinolysis and therefore must be used with caution. Patients with massive fibrinolysis may be considered candidates for EACA therapy; however, EACA should not be administered unless heparin has previously been infused in order to block the prothrombotic arm of DIC before the antifibrinolytic arm is blocked. A 4-g intravenous loading dose followed by 1 g every 2 hours intravenously for 24 hours may be tried. If bleeding does not decrease by 24 hours, it is unlikely to do so.

Treatment of APL with all-trans-retinoic acid (ATRA) has prevented the majority of hemorrhagic complications of that disease.[77] Heparin and antifibrinolytic agents are now held in reserve for exceptional cases.

CONSULTATION CONSIDERATIONS

Patients who are consulted upon usually fall into two groups, with one being rather typical severe acute DIC in which bleeding, hypotension, and organ failure generate the consultation. On the other hand, consultations for DIC are occasionally generated by a stable patient having laboratory data making the referring practitioner consider the possibility of DIC.

Promptness in consultation is in order. Because of the great utility of the readily available and inexpensive global tests such as PT, aPTT, TT, FDP level, and CBC, it is strongly advisable to order those tests to be repeated immediately in one's preparation to see the patient. One should insist that the blood samples be drawn through a fresh venipuncture and not through intra-arterial or intravenous lines that may contain blood, saline, or heparin. Very frequently one finds that a new, fresh, reliable set of data is of more use than a set that may have been performed 1 or 2 days in the past let alone any disinformation generated from an incorrectly obtained sample. The consultant should have an open dialog with the coagulation laboratory technicians since discussion heightens the hematology technician's involvement in the patient's problem. The technician's expertise frequently generates data or observations not immediately available to the consultant that would be helpful. The laboratory technician may be the first to observe schistocytes on the blood smear, signifying microangiopathic hemolysis; vacuolization of white cells, signifying sepsis; or spontaneous lysis of a test-tube clot, signifying high plasmin activity.

During the consultation, one must think extremely broadly as an internist rather than just as a subspecialist, a comment justified by the extraordinarily broad range of differential diagnoses and initiating processes in DIC. The consultant may be the first to recognize either petechiae on a febrile patient, thus securing a working diagnosis of meningococcemia and justifying rapid, aggressive antibiotic treatment, or the peripheral stigmata of chronic liver disease, which, heretofore not appreciated, would indicate the patient's laboratory data are more consistent with chronic liver insufficiency than with acute DIC.

Should it be determined that an invasive procedure such as drainage of an abscess or evacuation of the uterus may be needed, the surgeon, obstetrician, or invasive radiologist must appreciate that the necessity of the procedure overrides concern regarding "coagulopathy" as the cure of the coagulopathy is the procedure itself.

COST-CONTAINMENT ISSUES

These patients are typically so ill that they are usually in an intensive care unit, so hospital costs are truly considerable. Blood replacement costs can escalate if one does elect to use large amounts of FFP or platelet transfusions. Blood products should probably be used in moderation, perhaps as indicated in the section entitled Treatment, with the aim of keeping the platelet count higher than 25,000 to 50,000/μL and/or the fibrinogen higher than 50 mg/dL with active bleeding. Most practitioners would not transfuse either platelets or FFP unless such critical levels are reached, while transfusion at levels above these cutoffs have not been proven to improve clinical outcome.

Probably the most prudent area concerning cost containment in DIC is the use of the laboratory. The routine laboratory tests advocated in this chapter such as the CBC, TT, PT, aPTT, and FDP level are generally available and quite useful in making a diagnosis in the current clinical setting. Their rapid turnaround and low cost justifies their use. Selected tests such as the ATIII, D-dimer, and fibrinogen levels may be of intermittent use. Not only are most of the other tests that some have advocated extremely expensive, but also, because of their relative nonavailability, more often than not, the results are returned to the practitioner too late to be of clear use in daily bedside decision-making.

MEDICAL-LEGAL CONSIDERATIONS

As DIC may be difficult to diagnose, is typically associated with a wide variety of dire clinical circumstances, and has a high mortality, one might expect medical-legal concerns to arise periodically. On the other hand, there are no clear standards of care or practice guidelines established for recognition or treatment of DIC. Physicians will be held to practice in a manner consistent with good medical care and to approach the patient as any reasonable and prudent physician would do. As in any dire clinical situation, frank and open discussion with the patient and family is in order.

Potential areas of controversy would include failure to obtain a sufficiently detailed history or physical examination, documentation of facts, and interpretation of the myriad of laboratory data. This may be another reason to limit laboratory data, focusing on those tests one is accustomed to ordering, reviewing, and interpreting. Treatment is sharply focused on the initiating cause of DIC; therefore, treatment of DIC itself would hardly be expected to be a standard of care issue as it is anecdotal and controversial. It is not even established whether one should use heparin or how much FFP or platelet transfusion support patients require. Use of antifibrinolytics is extremely controversial and one should probably not employ those agents unless heparin or some other antithrombotic agent is first administered.

■ REFERENCES

Chapter 12 References

1. McKay DG. DIC: An Intermediary Mechanism of Disease. New York, Harper-Hoeber, 1965, p. 493.
2. Hunter J. A Treatise on the Blood, Inflammation, and Gun-Shot Wounds. Philadelphia, Webster, 1817.
3. DeBlainville HMD. Injection de matiere cerebrale dans les veins. Gaz Med Paris (ser. 2) 1834;2:524–567.
4. Nauyn B. Unterschungen Ober Blutgirinnung Im Lebenden Tiere und Ihre Folgen. Arch Exp Pathol Pharmak 1873;1:1.
5. Foa P, Pellacani P. Sul Fermento Fibrinogeno: Sulle Azioni Tossiche, Escercitate da Alcuni Organi Fresch. Arch Sci Med (Torino) 1884;7:113.
6. Wooldridge LD. In: Horsley V, Starling E (eds): On the Chemistry of the Blood and Other Scientific Papers. London, Kegan, Paul, Trench, Trubner, and Co., 1893.
7. Mills CA. The action of tissue extracts in the coagulation of blood. J Biol Chem 1921;46:167–192.
8. Krevans JR, Jackson DP, Conley CL, et al. The nature of the hemorrhagic disorders accompanied by hemolytic transfusions in man. Blood 1957;12:834–843.
9. Schneider C. Etiology of fibrinopenia: fibrination defibrination. Ann NY Acad Sci 1959;75:634–675.
10. Mersky C, Kleiner GJ, Johnson AJ. Quantitative estimation of split products of fibrinogen in human serum, relation to diagnosis and treatment. Blood 1966;28:1–18.
11. Marder VJ, Shulman HR, Carroll WR. High molecular weight derivatives of human fibrinogen produced by plasmin. I. Physicochemical and immunological characterization. J Biol Chem 1969;244:2111–2119.
12. Corrigan JJ. Changes in the blood coagulation system associated with septicemia. N Engl J Med 1968;279:851–856.
13. Bull B, Rubenberg M, Dacie J, et al. Microangiopathic haemolytic anemia: mechanisms of red-cell fragmentation. Br J Haematol 1968;14:643–652.
14. Colman RW, Robboy SJ, Minna JD. DIC: An approach. Am J Med 1972;52:679–689.
15. Merskey C. Defibrination syndrome or. . .? Blood 1973;41:599–603.
16. Mant MJ, King EG. Severe acute DIC. Am J Med 1979;67:556–563.
17. Sack GH, Levin J, Bell WR. Trousseau's syndrome and other manifestations of chronic disseminated coagulopathy in patients with neoplasms: Clinical, pathologic and therapeutic features. Medicine (Baltimore) 1977;56:1–37.
18. Okajima K, Sakamoto Y, Uchiba M. Heterogeneity in the incidence and clinical manifestations of disseminated intravascular coagulation. Am J Hematol 2000;65:215–222.
19. Semeraro N, Colucci M. Tissue factor in health and disease. Thromb Haemost 1997;78:759–764.
20. Gabay C, Kushner J. Acute-phase proteins and other systemic responses to inflammation. N Engl J Med 1999;340:448–454.
21. Gando S, Kameve T, Nanzaki S, et al. Disseminated intravascular coagulation is a frequent complication of systemic inflammatory response syndrome. Thromb Haemost 1996;75:220–228.
22. Suffredini AF, Harpel PC, Parrillo JE. Promotion and subsequent inhibition of plasminogen activation after administration of intravenous endotoxin to normal subjects. N Engl J Med 1989;320:1165–1172.
23. Carr JM, McKinney M, McDonagh J. Diagnosis of disseminated intravascular coagulation. Role of D-dimer. Am J Clin Pathol 1989;91:280–287.
24. Mombelli G, Fiori G, Monotto R, et al. Fibrinopeptide A in liver cirrhosis: evidence against a major contribution of disseminated intravascular coagulation to coagulopathy of chronic liver disease. J Lab Clin Med 1993;121:83–90.
25. Kitchens CS. Hemostatic aspects of envenomation by North American snakes. Hematol Oncol Clin NA 1992;6:1189–1195.
26. Deykin D. The role of the liver in serum-induced hypercoagulability. J Clin Invest 1966;45:256–263.
27. Sandset PM, Warn-Cramer BJ, Maki SL, et al. Immunodepletion of extrinsic pathway inhibitor sensitizes rabbits to endotoxin-induced intravascular coagulation and the generalized Shwartzman reaction. Blood 1991;78:1496–1502.
28. Pixley RA, De La Cadena R, Page JD et al. The contact system contributes to hypotension but not disseminated intravascular coagulation in lethal bacteremia: In vivo use of a monoclonal anti-factor XII antibody to block contact activation in baboons. J Clin Invest 1993;92:61–68.
29. Levi M, ten Cate H. Disseminated intravascular coagulation. N Engl J Med 1999;341:586–592.
30. Tapper H, Herwald H. Modulation of hemostatic mechanisms in bacterial infectious diseases. Blood 2000;96;2329–2337.
31. Sandset PM, Bendy B. Tissue factor pathway inhibitor: Clinical deficiency states. Thromb Haemost 1997;78:467–470.
32. Levi M, van der Poll T, ten Cate H, et al. The cytokine-mediated imbalance between coagulant and anticoagulant mechanisms in sepsis and endotoxaemia. Eur J Clin Invest 1997;27:3–9.
33. Ten Cate JW, van der Poll T, Levi M et al. Cytokines: Triggers of clinical thrombotic disease. Thromb Haemost 1997;78:415–419.
34. Takahashi H, Sato N, Shibata A. Plasma tissue factor pathway inhibitor in disseminated intravascular coagulation: comparison of its behavior with plasma tissue factor. Thromb Res 1995;80:339–348.
35. Fourrier F, Jourdain M, Tournois A, et al. Coagulation inhibitor substitution during sepsis. Intensive Care Med 1995;21:S264–268.
36. Vervloet MG, Thijs LG, Hack CE. Derangements of coagulation and fibrinolysis in critically ill patients with sepsis and septic shock. Semin Thromb Hemost 1998;24:33–44.
37. Wada H, Wakita Y, Nakase T, et al. Outcome of disseminated intravascular coagulation in relation to the score when treatment was begun. Thromb Haemost 1995;74:848–852.
38. Gando S, Nakanishi Y, Kameue T, et al. Soluble thrombomodulin increases in patients with disseminated intravascular coagulation and in those with multiple organ dysfunction syndrome after trauma: role of neutrophil elastase. J Trauma 1995;39:660–664.
39. Asakura H, Kamikubo Y, Goto A, et al. Role of tissue factor in disseminated intravascular coagulation. Thromb Res 1995;80:217–224.
40. Endo S, Inada K, Nakae H, et al. Blood levels of endothelin-1 and thrombomodulin in patients with disseminated intravascular coagulation and sepsis. Res Commun Mol Pathol Pharmacol 1995;90:277–288.
41. de Jonge E, Dekkers PEP, Creasey AA, et al. Tissue factor pathway inhibitor dose-dependently inhibits coagulation activations without influencing the fibrinolytic and cytokine response during human endotoxemia. Blood 2000;95:1124–1129.
42. Sporn LA, Haidaris PJ, Shi R-J, et al. Rickettsia rickettsii infection in cultured endothelial cells induces tissue factor expression. Blood 1994;83:1527–1534.
43. Visseren FLJ, Bouwman JJM, Bouter KP, et al. Progcoagulant activity of endothelial cells after infection with respiratory viruses. Thromb Haemost 2000;874:319–324.
44. Behl R, Klein MB, Dandelet L, et al. Induction of tissue factor procoagulant activity in myelomonocytic cells inoculated by the agent of human granulocytic ehrlichosis. Thromb Haemost 2000;83:114–118.

45. Kruithof EK, Mestries JC, Gascon MP, Ythier A. The coagulation and fibrinolytic responses of baboons after in vivo thrombin generation—effect of interleukin 6. Thromb Haemost 1997;77:905–910.
46. Goodnight SH. Defibrination after brain-tissue destruction: A serious complication of head injury. N Engl J Med 1974;290:1043–1047.
47. Van der Sande JJ, Emiss JJ, Lindeman J. Intravascular coagulation: A common phenomenon in minor experimental head injury. J Neurosurg 1981;54:21–25.
48. Van der Sande JJ, Veltkamp JJ, Boekhout-Mussert RJ et al. Hemostasis and computerized tomography in head injury: Their relationship to clinical features J. Neurosurg 1981;55:718–724.
49. Olson JD, Kaufman HH, Moake J, et al. The incidence and significance of hemostatic abnormalities in patients with head injuries. Neurosurgery 1989;24:825–832.
50. Selladurai BM, Vickneswaran M, Duraisamy S, et al. Coagulopathy in acute head injury—a study of its role as a prognostic indicator. Br J Neurosurg 1997;11:398–404.
51. Oba J, Shiiya N, Matsui Y, et al. Preoperative disseminated intravascular coagulation (DIC) associated with aortic aneurysm—does it need to be corrected before surgery? Surg Today 1995;25:1011–1014.
52. Aboulafia DM, Aboulafia ED. Aortic aneurysm-induced disseminated intravascular coagulation. Ann Vasc Surg 1996;10:396–405.
53. Bick RL. Disseminated intravascular coagulation: Pathophysiological mechanisms and manifestations. Semin Thromb Hemost 1998;24:3–18.
54. Reister F, Heyl W, Rath W. Coagulation disorders in pregnancy. Biomed Prog 1997;10:62–67.
55. Mammen EF. The haematological manifestations of sepsis. J Antimicrob Chemother 1998;41:17–24.
56. Stone JH. HELLP syndrome: hemolysis, elevated liver enzymes, and low platelets. JAMA 1998;280:559–562.
57. Kitchens CS. Thrombotic storm: When thrombosis begets thrombosis. Am J Med 1998;104:381–385.
58. Van Dam PA, Renier M, Baekelandt M, et al. Disseminated intravascular coagulation and the syndrome of hemolysis, elevated liver enzymes, and low platelets in severe preeclampsia. Obstet Gynecol 1989;73:97–102.
59. De Boer K, Buller HR, ten Cate JW, et al. Coagulation studies in the syndrome of haemolysis, elevated liver enzymes and low platelets. Br J Obstet Gynaecol 1991;98:42–47.
60. Trousseau A. Phlegmasia alba dolens. Clinique Medicale de l'Hotel-Dieu de Paris. London, The New Sydenham Society 3:94, 1865.
61. Callander NS, Varki N, Mohan LV. Immunohistochemical identification of tissue factor in solid tumors. Cancer 1992;70:1194–1201.
62. Shigemori C, Wada H, Matsumoto K, et al. Tissue factor expression and metastatic potential of colorectal cancer. Thromb Haemost 1998;80:894–898.
63. Hickey WF, Garnick MB, Henderson IC, et al. Primary cerebral venous thrombosis in patients with cancer: A rarely diagnosed paraneoplastic syndrome. Am J Med 1982;73:740–750.
64. Bell WR, Starksen NF, Tong S, et al. Trousseau's syndrome: Devastating coagulopathy in the absence of heparin. Am J Med 1985;79:423–430.
65. Woerner EM, Rowe RL. Trousseau's syndrome. Am Fam Phys 1988;38:195–201.
65a. Meijer K, Smid WM, Geerards S, et al. Hyperfibrinogenolysis in disseminated adenocarcinoma. Blood Coagul Fibrinolysis 1998;9:279–283.
66. Menell JS, Cesarman GM, Jacovina AT, et al. Annexin II and bleeding in acute promyelocytic leukemia. N Engl J Med 1999;340:994–1004.
67. Kalus P, Tooze JA, Talbot S, et al. Aprotinin inhibits fibrinolysis, improves platelet adhesion and reduces blood loss. Eur J Cardiothorac Surg 1994;8:315–323.
68. Boylan JF, Klinck JR, Sandler AN, et al. Tranexamic acid reduces blood loss, transfusion requirements, and coagulation factor use in primary orthotopic liver transplantation. Anesthesiology 1996;85:1043–1048.
69. Rangel-Frausto MS, Pittet D, Costigan M, et al. The natural history of the systemic inflammatory response syndrome (SIRS). JAMA 1995;273:117–123.
70. Gando S, Nakanishi Y, Tedo I. Cytokines and plasminogen activator inhibitor-1 in posttrauma disseminated intravascular coagulation: relationship to multiple organ dysfunction syndrome. Crit Care Med 1995;23:1835–1842.
71. Wells MJ, Sheffield WP, Blajchman MA. The clearance of thrombin-antithrombin and related serpin-enzyme complexes from the circulation: Role of various hepatocyte receptors. Thromb Haemost 1999;81:325–327.
72. Minnema MC, Chang CK, Jansen PM, et al. Recombinant human antithrombin III improves survival and attenuates inflammatory responses in baboons lethally challenged with *Escherichia coli*. Blood 2000;95:1111–1123.
73. Baudo F, Caimi Tk deCataldo F, et al. Antithrombin II (ATIII) replacement therapy in patients with sepsis and/or postsurgical complications: a controlled double-blind, randomized, multicenter study. Intensive Care Med 1998;24:336–342.
74. Inthorn D, Hoffmann JN, Hartl WH, et al. Antithrombin III supplementation in severe sepsis: beneficial effects on organ dysfunction. Shock 1997;8:328–334.
75. Wheeler AP, Bernard GR. Treating patients with severe sepsis. N Engl J Med 1999;340:207–214.
75a. Bernard GR, Vincent J-L, Laterre P-F, et al. Efficacy and safety of recombinant human activated protein C for severe sepsis. N Engl J Med 2001;344:699–709.
76. Saito M, Asakura H, Jokaji H, et al. Recombinant hirudin for the treatment of disseminated intravascular coagulation in patients with haematological malignancy. Blood Coagul Fibrinolysis 1995;6:60–64.
77. Tallman MS. The thrombophilic state in acute promyelocytic leukemia. Semin Thromb Hemost 1999;25:209–215.

PART III

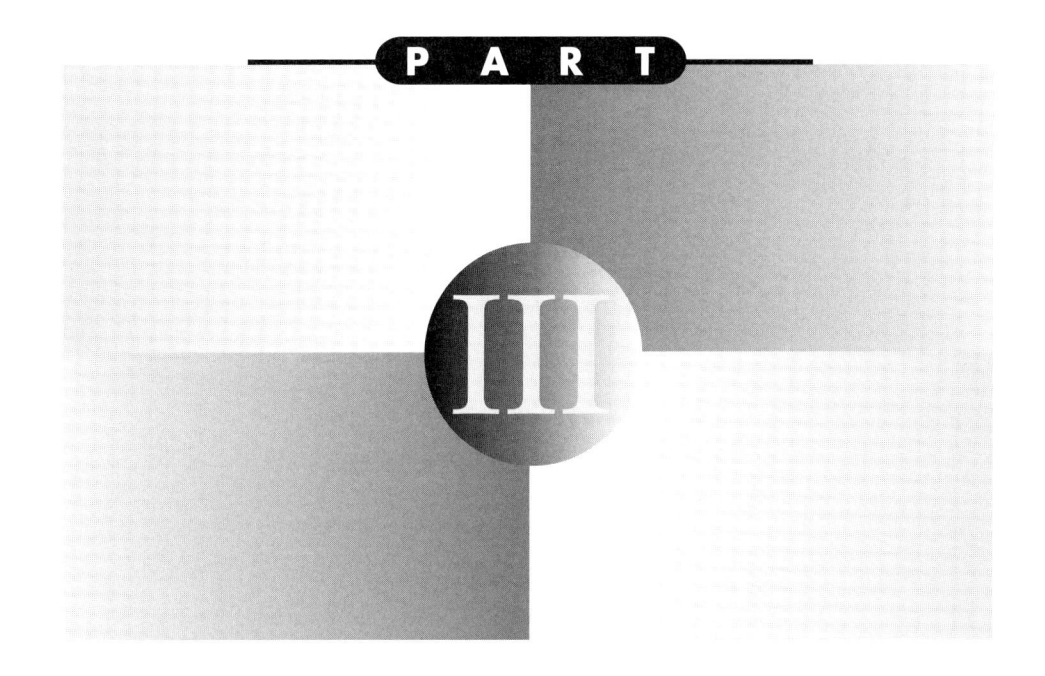

THROMBOTIC PROCESSES

CHAPTER 13

Thrombophilia

Jeffrey Zwicker, M.D.
Kenneth A. Bauer, M.D.

Unusual patterns of thrombosis have long been suspected as being familial in origin. In fact, John Briggs in 1905 aptly reasoned that in the absence of a clearer understanding of the "intimate nature" of these events, they should be described as *idiopathic recurrent thrombophlebitis*.[1] For the next century, the term *idiopathic* remained frustratingly apropos. Only recently, as our understanding of the basic mechanisms underlying thrombosis has advanced, so too has our ability to identify defects responsible for thrombophilic disorders. Currently there are several hereditary defects known to be associated with venous thromboembolic disease, including deficiencies of antithrombin, protein C, and protein S, the factor V Leiden mutation, and the prothrombin G20210A mutation. Although these hereditary defects are responsible for a significant percentage of idiopathic thrombotic events, numerous diagnostic and therapeutic issues remain unresolved. This chapter details our current understanding of these hereditary defects, including clinical and laboratory assessment and management. Hyperhomocysteinemia, which results from the interaction of genetic as well as environmental factors, is also included here. The antiphospholipid syndrome is discussed in Chapter 18.

BACKGROUND, PREVALENCE, AND DIAGNOSIS

Antithrombin Deficiency

Antithrombin, initially designated *antithrombin III*, is a plasma protein synthesized by the liver that binds and neutralizes thrombin and factors IXa, Xa, XIa, and XIIa. Inhibition of these coagulation serine proteinases by antithrombin is relatively slow, but is markedly enhanced by heparin. Antithrombin has two major active functional sites: the reactive center and the heparin-binding site located at the amino terminus of the molecule. Thrombin cleaves the reactive site followed by the formation of an inactive complex which is rapidly cleared from the circulation.[2]

Antithrombin deficiency was the first hereditary hypercoagulable disorder identified. In 1965, Egeberg investigated a Norwegian family with a strong history of thrombosis and found that affected individuals had plasma antithrombin concentrations that were 40% to 50% of normal.[3] Subsequent studies described families with similar clinical and laboratory abnormalities.[4,5] Heterozygosity for antithrombin deficiency can be found in approximately 4% of families with inherited thrombophilia and in 1% of consecutive patients with an initial episode of deep venous thrombosis (Table 13–1).[6,7] Original estimates of the prevalence of antithrombin deficiency in the general population using an immunoassay were 1 in 2000 to 5000.[8,9] Subsequently, studies using functional assays identified the prevalence to be 1 in 250 to 500[10]; however, as discussed below, the functional assays identify antithrombin variants less likely to result in thromboembolic disease.

Antithrombin deficiency is inherited as an autosomal dominant trait and can be classified into two general categories: decreased synthesis (type I) and dysfunctional activity (type II). Over 80 distinct mutations have been described in individuals with type I deficiency and more than 35 in type II deficiency.[11] Type II deficiencies can be further subcategorized on the basis of two different functional assays of antithrombin activity. The first is the antithrombin-heparin cofactor assay, which measures the ability of heparin to bind lysyl residues on antithrombin and catalyze the neutralization of coagulation enzymes such as factor Xa. The second test is the progressive antithrombin assay, which quantifies the ca-

Supported in part by the Medical Research Service of the Department of Veterans Affairs.

Table 13-1 • PREVALENCE OF DEFECTS IN PATIENTS WITH IDIOPATHIC DEEP VENOUS THROMBOSIS

Factor V Leiden	12%–40%
Prothrombin G20210A mutation	6%–18%
Deficiencies of antithrombin, protein C, or protein S	5%–15%
Hyperhomocysteinemia	10%–20%
Antiphospholipid syndrome	10%–20%

Data from Heijboer H, Brandjes DPM, Büller HR, et al. Deficiencies of coagulation-inhibiting and fibrinolytic proteins in outpatients with deep venous thrombosis. N Engl J Med 1990; 323:1512–1516; and Lane DA, Mannucci PM, Bauer KA, et al. Inherited thrombophilia: part 1. Thromb Haemost 1996; 76:651–662.

pacity of antithrombin to neutralize the enzymatic activity of thrombin in the absence of heparin. The distinction between the different type II defects is clinically relevant because variants with heparin-binding defects are associated with only a mild increase in thrombotic risk, except when present in the homozygous state.[12] Homozygosity for type I deficiency is thought to be lethal in utero.

In plasma samples from normal individuals, the range of antithrombin concentrations is reasonably narrow. Most laboratories report a normal range between 75% and 120% of a normal plasma pool for antithrombin-heparin cofactor activity.[13] The antithrombin-heparin cofactor assay will detect type I and type II deficiencies and is, therefore, the best single laboratory screening test for the disorder. The assay should employ factor Xa or bovine thrombin as the target enzyme because heparin cofactor II (see below) can elevate the apparent level of antithrombin when human thrombin is used as the reagent.[14]

A variety of pathophysiologic conditions can reduce the concentration of antithrombin in the blood (Table 13-2). Antithrombin levels can drop substantially in disseminated intravascular coagulation, sepsis, burns, and severe trauma but less commonly in the setting of acute thrombosis.[15,16] Reduced levels can also be seen in liver disease owing to decreased synthesis or in nephrotic syndrome as a consequence of urinary protein loss.[17,18] Modest reductions are also found in users of oral contraceptives or estrogens.[19,20] In addition, the administration of heparin decreases plasma antithrombin levels presumably by accelerated clearance of the heparin-antithrombin complex.[21] Thus, evaluation of plasma samples from individuals during a period of heparinization can potentially lead to an erroneous diagnosis of antithrombin deficiency.

Due to the number of clinical disorders that can be associated with reductions in the plasma concentration of antithrombin, definitive diagnosis of the hereditary state is often difficult. Whereas an antithrombin level in the normal range is usually sufficient to exclude the disorder, low levels should be confirmed at a later date. This determination ideally is performed when the individual is no longer receiving warfarin because plasma antithrombin concentrations occasionally can be elevated into the normal range in individuals with the deficiency state. In such situations, clinical assessment of the individual's risk of recurrent thrombosis will determine if discontinuation of warfarin is feasible. In most antithrombin-deficient subjects, however, this effect of oral anticoagulants is not of sufficient magnitude to obscure the diagnosis.[22] Confirmation of the hereditary nature of the disorder requires the investigation of other family members. Diagnosis of other affected family members also allows for appropriate counseling regarding the need for prophylaxis against venous thrombosis.

Protein C Deficiency

Protein C is a vitamin K-dependent protein synthesized by the liver and circulates as a zymogen. It exerts its anticoagulant function after activation to the serine protease, activated protein C (APC). This process can be mediated by thrombin alone but occurs more efficiently when thrombin is bound to thrombomodulin on endothelial cells.

In 1981, Griffin et al.[23] first described low levels of protein C in a family with recurrent thrombotic events. In subsequent large cohort studies, protein C deficiency was documented in 2% to 9% of individuals with a history of venous thrombosis.[24] From these cohorts, estimates placed the prevalence of protein C deficiency between 1 in 16,000 and 1 in 32,000 of the general population. These estimates were based on the assumption that protein C was an autosomal dominant disorder with high penetrance and at least half the individuals with the deficiency would demonstrate symptomatic thrombosis.[25] Curiously, parents of neonates with purpura fulminans, in association with the homozygous or doubly heterozygous form of protein C deficiency, infrequently report any history of thrombosis. This led Miletich and others to screen healthy blood donors; they found a much higher prevalence of heterozygosity for protein C deficiency, ranging from 1 in 200 to 500, in the general population.[25,26] Similar to other inherited thrombophilias, this variability in phenotypic expression of protein C deficiency is not yet explained by differences in the particular genetic defect alone and likely represents a complex interaction with other modulating factors.

Table 13-2 • COMMON CAUSES OF ACQUIRED DEFICIENCIES IN ANTITHROMBIN, PROTEIN C, AND PROTEIN S

Antithrombin	Protein C	Protein S
Neonatal period	Neonatal period	Neonatal period
Pregnancy	Liver disease	Pregnancy
Liver disease	Sepsis	Liver disease
Sepsis	Acute thrombosis	Sepsis
Acute thrombosis	DIC	Acute thrombosis
Disseminated intravascular coagulation (DIC)		DIC
Nephrotic syndrome		Nephrotic syndrome
Medications		
Heparin	Warfarin	Warfarin
L-asparaginase	L-asparaginase	L-asparaginase
Estrogens		Estrogens

Two major subtypes of heterozygous protein C deficiency have been identified using immunologic and functional assays (Table 13–3). The classic or type I deficiency state is the most common form and is characterized by a reduction in both the immunologic and biologic activity of protein C to approximately 50% of normal. More than 160 different mutations have been identified, most commonly missense or nonsense mutations.[27] The functional or type II deficiency state is characterized by normal synthesis of an abnormal protein. The functional capacity of protein C most often is assessed using a snake venom protease (Protac)-based assay to directly activate the protein. Following activation, an amidolytic assay can assess the functionality of the catalytic site of the protein.[28] Several individuals have been described with normal levels of protein C antigen and amidolytic activity, but who have substantial reductions in protein C anticoagulant activity.[29] Consequently, protein C anticoagulant activity can be measured using a clotting assay (based upon prolongation of the activated partial thromboplastin time [aPTT]) and abnormalities presumably reflect reduced ability of activated protein C to interact with the platelet membrane or its substrates such as factor Va and factor VIIIa. The coagulant assay thus has the highest sensitivity in screening patients for hereditary protein C deficiency.[30]

The levels of protein C antigen in the heterozygous deficiency state overlap with those in the normal population, thus making it difficult to define the diagnosis in some patients. In general, antigen levels of 60% to 70% represent borderline values and warrant repeat testing. Protein C antigen levels can also vary depending on age. Protein C levels in newborns are 20% to 40% of normal adult levels,[31] and preterm infants have even lower levels.[32] Neonates with significant perinatal thrombosis can have levels suggestive of homozygous deficiency.[33] In adults, protein C levels typically increase 4% per decade.[25]

Acquired protein C deficiency is found in numerous disease states, including liver disease, disseminated intravascular coagulation (DIC), and sepsis (see Table 13–2). A particularly severe form of acquired protein C deficiency has been reported in association with purpura fulminans and DIC in individuals with acute meningococcal infections.[34,35] In contrast to antithrombin, the antigenic concentrations of vitamin K-dependent plasma proteins, including protein C, are often elevated in individuals with nephrotic syndrome.[36] Most individuals with uremia have low levels of protein C anticoagulant activity, but normal levels of protein C amidolytic activity and antigen.[37] This is attributable to a dialyzable moiety in uremic plasma that interferes with most clotting assays for protein C activity.[38]

Warfarin therapy reduces functional and to a lesser extent immunologic measurements of protein C, thus complicating the diagnosis of the deficiency state.[29] Several researchers have proposed that based on the ratios of protein C antigen to factor II or factor X antigen, the diagnosis can be made. However, type II deficiency will not be detected with this method and it can only be used in subjects in a stable phase of oral anticoagulation.[39] Other groups have used protein C activity assays in conjunction with functional measurements of factor VII, a vitamin K-dependent zymogen with a similar plasma half-life.[40] In practice, it is preferable to investigate individuals suspected of having the deficiency state after oral anticoagulation has been discontinued for at least one week and to perform family studies. If it is not possible to discontinue warfarin because of the severity of the thrombotic diathesis, such individuals can be studied while receiving heparin therapy, which does not alter plasma protein C levels.

Protein S Deficiency

Protein S is a vitamin K-dependent protein that enhances the anticoagulant effect of activated protein C. Primarily synthesized by hepatocytes but also by endothelial cells, megakaryocytes, and brain cells,[30] protein S serves as a cofactor for APC, which then inactivates factor Va and factor VIIIa. Factor Va inactivation occurs by an ordered series of peptide bond scissions in the molecule's heavy chain: there is first a rapid cleavage at Arg 506 followed by slower cleavages at Arg 306 and then Arg 679.[41] Protein S interaction with APC results in both an increased affinity for negatively charged phospholipids and a 20-fold enhancement of the slower phase of factor Va inactivation. In plasma, only 40% of protein S is available in the "free" form, whereas the remainder is bound to C4b-binding protein and cannot interact with APC.

Protein S deficiency is an autosomal dominant disorder originally described in 1984 in several kindreds with low levels of protein S and a striking history of recurrent thrombosis.[42] There is a reported frequency of approximately 10% in families with inherited thrombophilia[43,44]; however, the prevalence is much lower (around 1%) among consecutive patients with a first deep venous thrombosis.[45] Three types of protein S deficiency states can be identified based on measurements of total and free antigen as well as functional activity. The type I deficiency state is associated with approximately 50% of the normal total S antigen level[46] and greater reductions in free protein S antigen and protein S functional activity.[47] This defect is most often secondary to missense mutations and base pair insertions or deletions. The type II qualitative deficiency state (normal total and free protein S antigen levels but abnormal functional activity) has been identified infrequently, sug-

Table 13–3 • ASSAY MEASUREMENTS IN HETEROZYGOUS PROTEIN C DEFICIENCY

Types	Antigen	Amidolytic Activity	Anticoagulant Activity
I	Low	Low	Low
II[a]	Normal	Low	Low
	Normal	Normal	Low

[a] For type II, some individuals have a deficiency of protein C only when anticoagulant activity is measured.

gesting that current functional assays may not screen for all such defects. Type III deficiency has normal total protein S antigen levels with disproportionately decreased free protein S antigenic and functional activity.

The biologic basis and clinical implications of the type III deficiency state are unclear. Mutations have been identified in only 44% of these individuals, raising the possibility that some cases represent acquired abnormalities.[48] Among French individuals with the low free protein S phenotype, 82% of the genetic defects identified were a single mutation thought to result in abnormal binding of protein S to C4b-binding protein. It is not clear that this mutation results in an increased thrombotic risk as it has been identified at a similar frequency in individuals with thrombosis (0.7%) as in the general population (0.5%).[49] In addition, a study documented the coexistence of the type I and III deficiencies, leading the authors to propose that these two defects can result from the same genotype.[50]

There are multiple causes of acquired protein S deficiency, including pregnancy and oral contraceptive use (see Table 13–2). Protein S levels are commonly low in inflammatory states, including DIC and acute thrombosis, largely due to increased levels of C4b-binding protein complexing with protein S. C4b-binding protein is an acute phase reactant and shifts the protein to the complexed, inactive form, leading to decreased free protein S activity.[51] The levels of total and free protein S are significantly reduced in men with HIV infection.[52] Although total protein S antigen measurements are generally increased in individuals with nephrotic syndrome, functional assays are often reduced due to the loss of free protein S in the urine and elevations in C4b-binding protein levels.[36]

The lower limit of normal total and free protein S in plasma is approximately 65%; however, there is a considerable overlap between the heterozygous deficiency state and "low normals." This is largely due to the influence of age, which leads to an increase in protein S levels, and gender, since females have a normal range of plasma protein S level lower than males. Thus it is difficult to diagnose heterozygous protein S deficiency by performing a single assay; repeat sampling and family studies are usually required to establish the diagnosis.

Factor V Leiden

Prior to 1993, hereditary deficiencies were infrequently identified in patients with familial thromboembolic disease. Dahlbäck et al.[53] identified a proband and family that appeared resistant to activated protein C in an aPTT-based clotting assay. In comparison to controls, most of the family members had a blunted anticoagulant response to APC. The following year, Bertina et al.[54] identified the genotype underlying most cases of APC resistance as a single point mutation in the factor V gene leading to substitution of an arginine-506 by glutamine. This mutation at an APC cleavage site renders factor Va relatively resistant to inactivation by APC.[41,54]

Following Dahlbäck's description of APC resistance, several small studies revealed that this defect was relatively common among individuals with venous thrombosis. Svensson and Dahlbäck[55] screened 104 consecutive Swedish individuals referred for evaluation of venous thrombosis and found that 33% of the subjects demonstrated APC resistance. In a U.S. referral population of individuals younger than 50 with unexplained venous thromboembolic disease, Griffin et al.[56] found that approximately 50% had APC resistance.

Dutch investigators had previously initiated the Leiden Thrombophilia Study to identify risk factors for a first episode of venous thrombosis in unselected patients. Excluding patients with known malignancies, 345 consecutive outpatients with a confirmed deep venous thrombosis under the age of 70 were initially reported.[57] Using a screening aPTT-based assay, investigators identified APC resistance in 21% of individuals with thrombosis and 5% of age- and sex-matched healthy controls. The factor V-Arg506Gln (or factor V Leiden) mutation was found in more than 80% of the patients who had been found to be APC-resistant.[54] The lower frequency of APC resistance seen in the Leiden Thrombophilia Study in comparison to previous studies is attributable to differences in selection criteria and referral cohorts. Following the observation that factor V Leiden was prevalent among the general Dutch population, genetic studies confirmed the high frequency of factor V Leiden heterozygosity among Northern Europeans (5% to 10%). However, the defect was found to be extremely rare in Asian and African populations.[58]

The initial observation by Dahlbäck facilitated the development of an aPTT-based assay that serves as a screening test for APC resistance. The aPTT is performed with the addition of a standardized amount of APC, and clotting times are converted to an APC ratio (aPTT with APC divided by aPTT without APC). The results can be interpreted by comparing the ratio to that of the normal range, or by normalizing it to the APC resistance ratio obtained using normal pooled plasma (APC ratio of patient divided by APC ratio of normal plasma) and comparing this to the normal range. Whereas these "first-generation" APC resistance assays were conceptually quite simple and easy to perform, they required careful standardization and determination of the normal range in at least 50 controls. The level of APC, the aPTT reagent, and the instrumentation used for clot detection affected the performance characteristics of the assay. Some assays using this format therefore had inadequate sensitivity and specificity for the factor V Leiden mutation. Also, individuals receiving anticoagulants or with an abnormal aPTT due to other coagulation defects could not be investigated with this assay, and the test was not validated in individuals with acute thrombotic events or in pregnant women.

With the finding that the factor V Leiden mutation was responsible for most cases of APC resistance, "second-generation" coagulation assays were developed by diluting an individual's plasma with factor V-deficient plasma. Consequently, the influence of the levels of other coagulation factors on clotting time determinations was minimized. With proper standardization, the modified APC resistance test can give very high sensitivity and specificity for the factor V Leiden mutation.

At present, the most cost-effective approach to diagnosing individuals with the factor V Leiden mutation is to test for APC resistance using a "second-generation" coagulation assay. Individuals with low APC resistance ratios should then be genotyped for the mutation, although it can be argued that such confirmatory testing is unnecessary in laboratories having perfect concordance between the results of their APC resistance assay and factor V Leiden genotype. If the "first-generation" aPTT-based assay for APC resistance is used, a small number of individuals with APC resistance without the factor V Leiden mutation can be identified. Even though de Visser et al.[59] have shown that this abnormality is associated with an increased risk of venous thrombosis, this assay is not recommended as part of the routine laboratory evaluation since the commercially available APC resistance assays using undiluted plasma do not replicate the performance characteristics of the assay used in this study.

Prothrombin G20210A Mutation

Prothrombin (factor II) is the precursor of thrombin, the end product of the coagulation cascade. It is a vitamin K-dependent protein that is synthesized in the liver and has a half-life of approximately 3 to 5 days. The gene spans 21 kb on chromosome 11 and consists of 14 exons and 13 introns.

A single base-pair mutation in the prothrombin gene has recently been identified as a independent risk factor for hereditary venous thromboembolic disease and is the second most common hereditary thrombophilic defect after factor V Leiden. Originally described by Poort et al.[60] in 1996, a G to A substitution in the 3'-untranslated region at position 20210 was identified in 18% of individuals among 28 probands with a personal and familial history of venous thrombosis. Studies have shown that individuals with the prothrombin 20210A mutation have higher plasma prothrombin activity than those with a normal genotype. Linkage studies in 397 individuals from 21 Spanish families suggest that prothrombin G20210A is a functional polymorphism responsible for elevated prothrombin antigen levels and activity.[61]

The prothrombin G20210A mutation has been documented at significantly higher frequency in patients with venous thrombosis than healthy controls in numerous studies. Large population studies have shown an overall prevalence about 2% in the general Caucasian population, with significant geographic variation. Among southern Europeans the prevalence was about 3%, but it was only very rarely identified in individuals of Asian or African descent.[62] In the Leiden Thrombophilia Study, which investigated individuals with an idiopathic first deep venous thrombosis the prevalence of the prothrombin G20210A mutation was 6.2% versus 2.3% in healthy matched controls. Similar frequencies were confirmed in a Swedish study of 99 consecutive outpatients in which 7.1% of individuals were identified with the prothrombin G20210A allele versus 1.8% of controls.[63]

Polymerase chain reaction (PCR) methods have been used to detect the prothrombin G20210A mutation in genomic DNA.[60] In addition, methods are available to detect both the prothrombin G20210A mutation and factor V Leiden in the same reaction.[64] Although plasma prothrombin activity and antigen levels are significantly higher in individuals with the prothrombin G20210A mutation, concentrations cannot be used to screen for the defect owing to significant overlap with the normal population.[60,61]

Hyperhomocysteinemia

Homocysteine is a sulfur-containing amino acid involved in metabolic pathways leading to the formation of other amino acids. As shown in Figure 13–1, methionine is generated through the remethylation of homocysteine or metabolized to cysteine via trans-sulfuration. Elevated levels of homocysteine are seen in a variety of disorders that affect either the concentration of substrates or the activity of enzymes involved in its metabolism (Table 13–4).

The association between severe hyperhomocysteinemia and premature atherosclerosis was initially described in children with homocystinuria. Homocystinuria results from several rare inborn errors of metabolism and is most frequently seen in cases of homozygous cystathionine β-synthase deficiency. Other clinical manifestations include venous thromboembolism as well as mental retardation, ectopic lenses, and skeletal abnormalities. In 1969, McCully[65] reported an infant with severe homocystinuria secondary to an inborn error of cobalamin metabolism with advanced atherosclerotic disease similar in nature to that seen with cystathionine

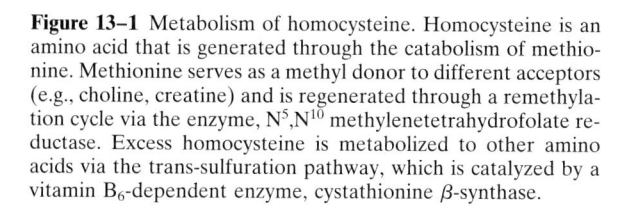

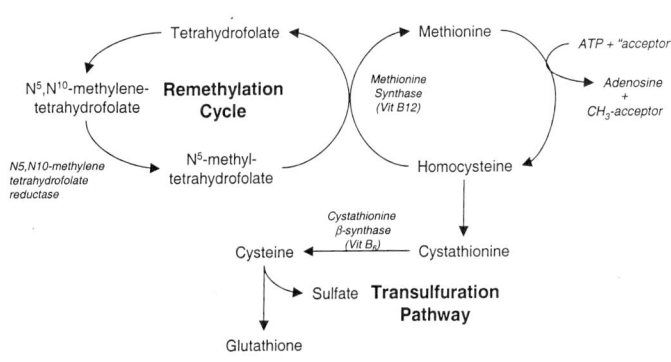

Figure 13–1 Metabolism of homocysteine. Homocysteine is an amino acid that is generated through the catabolism of methionine. Methionine serves as a methyl donor to different acceptors (e.g., choline, creatine) and is regenerated through a remethylation cycle via the enzyme, N^5,N^{10} methylenetetrahydrofolate reductase. Excess homocysteine is metabolized to other amino acids via the trans-sulfuration pathway, which is catalyzed by a vitamin B_6-dependent enzyme, cystathionine β-synthase.

Table 13–4 • GENETIC AND ACQUIRED CAUSES OF HYPERHOMOCYSTEINEMIA

Genetic
Cystathionine β-synthase deficiency
Methylenetetrahydrofolate reductase (MTHFR deficiency or thermolabile variant)
Enzymatic disorders of vitamin B_{12} metabolism

Acquired
Folate, vitamin B_{12}, or vitamin B_6 deficiency
Age
Smoking
Alcohol
Renal failure
Liver failure
Medications:
    Methotrexate
    Trimethoprim
    Cholestyramine
    Carbamezpine

β-synthase deficiency. The accumulation of plasma homocysteine provided the common link between these two metabolic abnormalities. Subsequent case-control and cross-sectional studies noted an association between even mild elevations in serum or plasma homocysteine and atherosclerotic or venous thromboembolic disease.[66–69]

Several genetic and acquired abnormalities can lead to mild or moderate elevations in serum homocysteine concentrations. The most common genetic defects include heterozygous cystathionine β-synthase deficiency, which occurs in approximately 0.3% of the population, and homozygosity for a methylenetetrahydrofolate reductase (MTHFR) mutation, which is present in approximately 20% of Italian and U.S. Hispanic populations but less than 1% of African Americans.[70] The MTHFR variant is due to an alanine-for-valine substitution at amino acid 677, which causes thermolability of the enzyme and a 50% reduction in its activity.[71]

The most common causes of acquired hyperhomocysteinemia include mild to moderate deficiencies in vitamin B_{12}, folate, or vitamin B_6, which act as cofactors in homocysteine metabolism. There is a strong inverse correlation between hyperhomocysteinemia and folate levels and, to a lesser degree, vitamin B_{12} and B_6.[72] Other acquired causes of hyperhomocysteinemia include advanced age, smoking, and disease states such as liver or renal failure. Chronic alcoholism causes elevations in homocysteine concentrations, possibly due to coexisting vitamin deficiencies. Medications can also affect homocysteine levels through vitamin malabsorption (i.e., bile acid sequestrants) or through direct enzymatic effects such as methotrexate inhibition of dihydrofolate reductase leading to deficiencies of the methyl-donor tetrahydrofolate (see Table 13–4).

There are several proposed mechanisms by which hyperhomocysteinemia leads to atherosclerotic or thromboembolic disease. In vitro studies have shown that homocysteine can induce vascular injury directly through free-radical formation, impaired vasodilation due to decreased levels of nitric oxide, or its accumulation with LDL-cholesterol in vascular macrophages.[73,74] The thrombogenic effects of hyperhomocysteinemia have been attributed to the inhibition of heparan sulfate expression, tissue-type plasminogen activator binding, or factor V activation.[75–77]

Hyperhomocysteinemia is usually diagnosed by measuring fasting plasma levels of homocysteine by high-pressure liquid chromatography. Normal homocysteine levels range between 5 and 15 μmol/L, and hyperhomocysteinemia has been classified as mild (15 to 30 μmol/L), moderate (30 to 100 μmol/L), or severe (more than 100 μmol/L). Fasting homocysteine levels have been regarded as representative of the remethylation pathway (dependent on folate, vitamin B_{12}, and MTHFR), whereas homocysteine levels 4 hours after an oral methionine load reflect the integrity of the trans-sulfuration pathway (dependent on vitamin B_6 and cystathionine β-synthase). Because individuals with heterozygous cystathionine β-synthase deficiency may have normal levels of fasting homocysteine, the methionine oral load has been used to diagnose these heterozygous individuals. However, recent studies indicate that abnormal results from loading tests are not specific for heterozygous cystathionine β-synthase deficiencies.[78]

Heparin Cofactor II Deficiency

Heparin cofactor II is a heparin-dependent glycoprotein that acts as a thrombin inhibitor. In contrast to antithrombin, this inhibitor does not inhibit factor Xa or other coagulation serine proteases. Several families have been described with quantitative deficiency of this protein, which is inherited as an autosomal dominant trait. Heterozygous individuals have plasma heparin cofactor II concentrations that are approximately 50% of normal values.

It is uncertain whether heparin cofactor II deficiency is a risk factor for thrombosis.[79] In one series of 305 patients with juvenile thromboembolic episodes, two patients had heparin cofactor II deficiency. However, each of these patients had a second defect: the factor V Leiden mutation or protein C deficiency.[80]

Plasminogen Deficiency

Congenital plasminogen deficiency is inherited as an autosomal dominant trait. There are both quantitative defects and functional defects. Thrombosis has been reported in young patients when the plasminogen concentration is less than 40% of control values. The development of ligneous conjunctivitis, hyperviscosity of tracheobronchial secretions, and hydrocephalus has been reported in a patient with homozygous plasminogen deficiency.[81] Replacement therapy with lysine-conjugated plasminogen resulted in marked improvement.

Despite this observation, the clinical importance of plasminogen deficiency as a risk factor for thrombosis is uncertain. In a Spanish study of 2132 consecutive patients with thrombosis, plasminogen deficiency was seen in 0.75% versus 0.29% of healthy blood donors.[82]

Dysfibrinogemia

The dysfibrinogemias are a heterogeneous group of disorders that cause alterations in the conversion of fibrinogen to fibrin. Approximately 300 abnormal fibrinogens have been reported, with a wide variation in phenotypic expression ranging from asymptomatic to a bleeding diathesis to recurrent thromboembolic disease.[83] Fewer than 20 cases of variant fibrinogens have been reported to be associated with thrombotic complications.

Factor XII Deficiency

Factor XII is the zymogen of a serine protease that initiates the contact activation reactions and intrinsic blood coagulation in vitro. Subjects with severe factor XII deficiency (less than 1% of normal) have markedly prolonged aPTTs but do not exhibit a bleeding diathesis[84]; however, there have been a number of cases of venous thromboembolism or myocardial infarction in factor XII-deficient individuals.[85] This thrombophilic tendency has been attributed to reduced plasma fibrinolytic activity.[86] The frequency with which severe factor XII deficiency leads to thrombosis is uncertain. One review found that 8% had a history of thromboembolism.[84] However, interpretation is difficult considering complications are more likely to be reported than asymptomatic patients. This led to cross-sectional analyses of thromboembolic events in larger numbers of unselected families with factor XII deficiency. In a study of 14 Swiss families with factor XII deficiency, 2 of 18 homozygous or doubly heterozygous patients had sustained deep venous thrombosis; however, each episode occurred in association with predisposing thrombotic risk factors. Only 1 of the 45 heterozygotes in these families had a possible history of venous thrombosis.[87] However, other groups have found a more pronounced association with thrombosis.[88,89] Thus it remains unproven if factor XII deficiency is associated with an increased risk of thrombosis.

Elevated Factors VIII, IX, and XI and Thrombin-Activatable Fibrinolysis Inhibitor

Recently, investigators have focused on the presence of supranormal levels of clotting factors and their role in venous thrombosis. In the Leiden Thrombophilia Study, 25% of patients with a first episode of venous thrombosis and 11% of healthy controls had factor VIII coagulant activity (VIII:C) greater than 150% of normal (greater than 150 IU/dL). Individuals with VIII:C levels greater than 150 IU/dl had a five-fold increased risk of thrombosis when compared to individuals with lower VIII:C levels (less than 100 IU/dL).[90] Several studies confirmed this association of factor VIII activity and venous thrombosis after adjustment for other possible influences such as von Willebrand factor and blood type. Similarly, researchers examined the possible role of VIII:C as an acute phase reactant and found that the association between elevated VIII:C levels and thrombosis was independent of immediate versus delayed testing or C-reactive protein and fibrinogen levels.[90–93] An Austrian study prospectively followed 360 patients for an average of 30 months and found that among the 38 patients who developed recurrent thromboembolism, the mean VIII:C level was greater than among those without recurrence.[94] Among those individuals with levels above the 90th percentile, the likelihood of recurrence at 2 years was 37% versus 5% with lower VIII:C levels (relative risk 6.7).[94] Elevated antigenic levels of several other coagulation factors, including factor XI, factor IX, and thrombin-activatable fibrinolysis inhibitor (TAFI), also confer a modest, albeit significantly increased risk for an initial episode of deep venous thrombosis.[95–97] The mechanisms for high levels of VIII:C and these other factors have yet to be elucidated, but family studies suggest that high factor VIII levels are likely to be genetically determined.[98] Corroborating studies are required prior to recommending routine measurement of VIII:C levels in patients with a prior venous thrombotic event.

CLINICAL IMPLICATIONS OF INHERITED THROMBOPHILIA

Risk of Initial Thrombosis

Deficiencies of Antithrombin, Protein C, and Protein S

Initial investigations estimating the risk of thrombosis of a particular inherited thrombophilia were largely based on familial cohort studies. Typically, a deficiency state was identified in a proband with an unusual propensity for recurrent thrombosis. After investigating the proband's family, risk estimates were generated based on its association with thrombosis. Commonly, the incidence of thrombosis in these families was large, with frequencies greater than 50%.[50,99] It is also possible that other known or even unknown thrombophilic genetic defects could coexist among members of sentinel families having a high prevalence of venous thromboembolism. Recent studies have examined the prevalence of thrombosis in large numbers of families with hereditary deficiencies of antithrombin, protein C, or protein S. In a study of 150 Italian families, the lifetime relative risk of developing thrombosis in subjects with antithrombin, protein C, or protein S deficiency (compared to their normal relatives) was 8.1, 7.3, and 8.5, respectively.[43] Such estimates likely still overstate the risk of thrombosis as the cohorts were selected for their remarkable tendency toward thrombotic events (thus warranting the initial investigation). Therefore, risk estimates generated from familial studies may not be applicable to the general population. This was highlighted in a study by Miletich et al.,[25] in which the plasmas from 5422 healthy blood donors were analyzed; surprisingly, heterozygous protein C deficiency was identified in 79 patients without any history of thrombosis. This led the researchers to postulate that a protein C deficiency state was not an important risk factor for thrombosis in the absence of concomitant defects. However, the data were collected from healthy individuals and thus also suffer from selection bias, thereby underestimating the true risk of thrombosis. In an attempt to generate risk estimates more applicable to the general population, case-control studies such as the Leiden Thrombophilia Study were conducted in consecutive patients with a first episode of deep venous thrombosis.

The Leiden Thrombophilia Study investigated 474 unselected consecutive patients following an initial episode of deep venous thrombosis matched with an equal number of healthy controls.[100] Subjects were excluded if they were older than 70 years or had evidence of malignancy. The odds ratio for thrombosis associated with these genetic defects was considerably lower than previously identified in familial studies: antithrombin (2.2), protein S (1.6) and protein C deficiencies (3.1) (Table 13–5).[45] It should be noted, however, that the thrombotic risk attributed to the various deficiencies was based on a small number of patients with the deficiency states.

Factor V Leiden

Prior to the discovery of the factor V Leiden mutation and prothrombin G20210A mutation, inherited deficiencies were identified infrequently; approximately 12% of individuals with thrombosis were identified as deficient in antithrombin, protein C, or protein S.[82] Dahlbäck's description of hereditary resistance to APC led to several small clinical studies that classified APC resistance as fairly ubiquitous, with deficiencies identified in over 30% of individuals with a first episode of venous thrombosis.[55,56] The Physicians' Health Study confirmed the high incidence of heterozygous factor V Leiden.[101] In this nested case-control study of 14,916 healthy men older than age 40, heterozygosity for the factor V Leiden mutation was identified in 12% of men with a first episode of deep venous thrombosis or pulmonary embolism and in 6% of controls. The relative risk of venous thromboembolism was 3.5-fold in those with factor V Leiden without concomitant risk factors. Similar results were generated by the Leiden Thrombophilia Study, where 21% of patients with deep venous thrombosis were classified as having resistance to APC versus 5% of controls (odds ratio of 6.6).[57] Individuals who were homozygous for the mutation experienced an even higher risk thromboembolism (odds ratio of 80), usually occurring at a younger age than heterozygotes (31 versus 44 years old).[102]

Interestingly, factor V Leiden has been shown to be a prevalent risk factor among elderly individuals with idiopathic deep venous thrombosis. The Physicians' Health Study found that 26% of men over 60 years of age with a first episode of deep venous thrombosis or pulmonary embolism were heterozygous for factor V Leiden.[101] Similarly, 16.4% of individuals over 50 in the Leiden Thrombophilia Study were heterozygous for factor V Leiden.[102]

Prothrombin G20210A Mutation

The prothrombin G20210A gene mutation is also a common genetic risk factor for venous thrombosis. Based on data from the Leiden Thrombophilia Study, 6.2% of individuals with thrombosis and 2.3% of controls had the prothrombin G20210A allele.[60] This resulted in a 2.8-fold increased risk of thrombosis for carriers of the mutation, an effect that was seen in both sexes and all age groups. A similar four-fold increased risk was demonstrated in a Swedish study of consecutive outpatients with deep venous thrombosis.[63]

Hyperhomocysteinemia

Mild or moderate hyperhomocysteinemia is an independent risk factor for myocardial infarction, stroke, and carotid artery disease.[103–105] Data from the Framingham Heart Study showed that elderly subjects with mild hyperhomocysteinemia (greater than 14.4 μmol/L) were twice as likely to have significant carotid artery stenosis than those with lower homocysteine levels.[105] In a large cohort study, over 5000 British men were prospectively followed for evidence of stroke or myocardial infarction. Among the 107 subjects who suffered a stroke, there was a graded increase in relative risk based on increasing homocysteine concentrations.[104] There have also been numerous cross-sectional and case-control studies documenting an association between hyperhomocysteinemia and coronary disease; however, prospective studies have been less predictive and pooled analysis of seven prospective studies found a smaller association between homocysteine levels and coronary artery disease.[69]

After establishing an association between mild hyperhomocysteinemia and atherosclerotic disease, several

Table 13–5 • DATA FROM THE LEIDEN THROMBOPHILIA STUDY: RISK OF A FIRST IDIOPATHIC DEEP VENOUS THROMBOSIS IN CONSECUTIVE OUTPATIENTS

Defect	Odds Ratio	95% CI
Antithrombin deficiency	2.2	1.0–4.7
Factor V Leiden:		
Heterozygous	6.6	3.6–12.0
Homozygous	80	22–289
Elevated homocysteine level	2.5	1.2–5.2
Protein S deficiency	1.6	0.6–4.0
Protein C deficiency	3.1	1.4–7.0
Prothrombin G20210A	2.8	1.4–5.6

Data from Koster T, Rosendaal FR, Briët E, et al. Protein C deficiency in a controlled series of unselected outpatients: an infrequent but clear risk factor for venous thrombosis (Leiden Thrombophilia Study). Blood 1995;85:2756–2761.

case-control studies confirmed the role of homocysteine in venous thrombosis. The Leiden Thrombophilia Study showed that individuals with plasma homocysteine levels above the 95th percentile (greater than 18.5 μmol/L) were 2.5 times more likely to suffer an initial episode of deep venous thrombosis.[66] Similarly, a meta-analysis of 10 case-control studies generated a pooled estimate of the odds ratio at 2.5.[68] Curiously, although homozygosity for the thermolabile MTHFR variant has been documented in a significant percentage of individuals with hyperhomocysteinemia, several studies have shown that the corresponding genotype is not an independent risk factor for deep venous thrombosis.[78] This paradox may be explained by the prothrombotic effect of hyperhomocysteinemia being attributable to the interplay of environmental (such as relative vitamin deficiencies) and genetic factors.

Combined Thrombophilic Defects

Hereditary defects such as factor V Leiden or the prothrombin G20210A mutation can be identified in a significant percentage of the general population (2% to 6%). Although such defects confer an increased risk of thrombosis, the actual incidence of thrombosis remains quite low. In a study of 150 thrombophilic families, the annual incidence of thrombosis was only 0.29% in individuals carrying the factor V Leiden mutation.[43] One explanation is that the phenotypic expression of hereditary thrombophilia is complicated and depends on the presence of multiple genetic defects.

Because factor V Leiden is common, many studies have documented this mutation in combination with other hereditary defects. In studies of families with other hereditary defects, the percentage of individuals experiencing thrombosis was significantly higher in the presence of factor V Leiden versus those with another hereditary defect alone[106–108] (Table 13–6). Data from the Physicians' Health Study showed that men with both factor V Leiden and hyperhomocysteinemia had a 10-fold increase in risk for any first episode of deep venous thrombosis and a 20-fold increased risk of an idiopathic event.[67] Similar results have also been documented in patients with double defects involving the prothrombin G20210A gene mutation.[109]

Table 13–6 • RISK OF THROMBOSIS IN SELECTED FAMILIES WITH DEFICIENCIES OF ANTITHROMBIN, PROTEIN C, AND PROTEIN S IN COMBINATION WITH FACTOR V LEIDEN

	%Thrombosis Isolated Defect	%Thrombosis + Factor V Leiden
Protein S deficiency	4/21 (19%)	13/18 (72%)
Protein C deficiency	12/34 (36%)	16/23 (73%)
Antithrombin deficiency	4/7 (57%)	11/12 (92%)

Data from refs 57, 60, 66, and 106.

APPROACH TO THROMBOSIS

History, Physical Examination, and Routine Laboratory Testing

In approaching individuals with a suspected prothrombotic disorder, it is useful clinically to distinguish patients with acquired from those likely to have hereditary hypercoagulable states. As previously described, hereditary thrombophilic disorders often are attributed to a single mutation of a protein in a critical anticoagulant pathway. In contrast, the acquired hypercoagulable states consist of a heterogeneous group of disorders that are associated with an increased tendency toward thrombotic complications (Table 13–7). In a case-control study of 1272 outpatients with deep venous thrombosis, pregnancy was associated with the greatest risk of thrombosis (OR 11.41) followed by muscle trauma (7.59), immobilization (5.61), venous insufficiency (4.45), chronic heart failure (2.93), and long-distance travel (2.35).[110] Although commonly considered a risk factor, the issue of extended travel is controversial; a recent study of 788 patients found no association with deep venous thrombosis following travel greater than 5 hours.[111]

A complete history and physical examination is mandatory in evaluating individuals with a recent or remote history of thrombosis, with special attention given to age of onset, location of prior thromboses, and results of objective diagnostic studies documenting thrombotic episodes. Screening for provocation should include questions regarding surgical procedures, trauma, or immobility. Women should be questioned carefully regarding use of oral contraceptives or hormone replacement therapy and obstetric history. A family history is particularly important, especially in first-degree relatives. Thrombosis can be the initial manifestation of a malignancy so it is important to inquire about constitutional symptoms, pain, hematochezia, hemoptysis, or

Table 13–7 • ACQUIRED CONDITIONS AND DISORDERS ASSOCIATED WITH HYPERCOAGULABLE STATES

Pregnancy
Immobilization
Trauma
Postoperative state
Advancing age
Estrogen therapy
Antiphospholipid syndrome
Malignancy
Nephrotic syndrome
Heparin-induced thrombocytopenia
Thrombotic thrombocytopenic purpura
Myeloproliferative disorders
Paroxysmal nocturnal hemoglobinuria
Hyperlipidemia
Diabetes mellitus
Hyperviscosity
Congestive heart failure

hematuria. Ethnic background should be considered given the extremely low prevalence of the most common hereditary defects, factor V Leiden and the prothrombin G20210A mutation, in individuals of African, American Indian, and Asian populations.[58,62]

The physical examination should be directed toward the extremities for signs of superficial or deep venous thrombosis and skin examination for evidence of necrosis, hemosiderin deposition, varicosities, or livedo reticularis. Considering the high association of malignancy and thrombosis, rectal examination and stool testing for occult blood is necessary, as are breast and pelvic examinations in women.

The laboratory evaluation for individuals with thrombosis should begin with a complete blood count and review of the peripheral smear. Elevations in hematocrit or platelet count may indicate the presence of a myeloproliferative disorder, which can be associated with either venous or arterial thrombosis. Secondary polycythemia can also provide evidence of an underlying occult malignancy. Leukopenia and thrombocytopenia can be found in paroxysmal nocturnal hemoglobinuria, which is characterized by intravascular hemolysis along with thrombotic sequelae. The development of thrombosis and thrombocytopenia concurrent with heparin administration should always prompt consideration of heparin-induced thrombocytopenia. The peripheral smear should be reviewed for evidence of red cell fragmentation that would indicate microangiopathic hemolytic anemia such as occurs with disseminated intravascular coagulation (DIC). In individuals with malignancy, chronic DIC can result in either venous or arterial thrombosis. A leukoerythroblastic picture with nucleated red cells or immature white cells suggests the possibility of marrow infiltration by tumor.

Serum chemistries such as liver and renal function also are important. Individuals with thrombosis of the hepatic venous circulation (Budd-Chiari syndrome) usually have abnormalities in liver function tests. Nephrotic syndrome is characterized by large amounts of protein in the urine and may be complicated by thrombosis, especially in the renal veins (see Chapter 15).

Baseline coagulation tests can also serve as a screen for a lupus anticoagulant. Some individuals with lupus anticoagulants have elevated titers of cardiolipin antibodies, which should be identified in those suspected of carrying this acquired defect. Abnormal tests for lupus anticoagulants or cardiolipin antibodies should be re-evaluated over time as they are only considered thrombotic risk factors if they are persistently abnormal over several months (see Chapter 18).

Arterial versus Venous Thrombosis

In contrast to lupus anticoagulants and hyperhomocysteinemia, hereditary deficiencies of antithrombin, protein C, and protein S have not clearly been shown to predispose to arterial thrombosis. Several case reports have described young patients with arterial thrombosis and protein C or S deficiencies, but larger studies have not convincingly demonstrated an association. In one series of 127 young individuals with ischemic stroke, abnormal protein C or S levels were found in 9.[112] However, 7 of these patients had an acquired risk factor for thrombosis, such as estrogen use. Similarly, an association between factor V Leiden and arterial disease has not been established[113] and conflicting data exist regarding the role of the prothrombin G20210A mutation as a risk factor for cerebrovascular ischemic disease in the young. In a study of 72 patients with documented stroke before 50 years of age, 7.6% had the gene mutation versus 1.2% of controls.[114] However, another series of 131 unselected patients with ischemic stroke and transient ischemic attacks found that the prevalence of the prothrombin G20210A mutation similar to that of a control population.[115] Based on current data, our general recommendation in patients with idiopathic arterial thrombosis is to screen for markers of the antiphospholipid syndrome or hyperhomocysteinemia and avoid screening for hereditary thrombophilic defects. In addition, appropriate tests for hyperlipidemia would be performed.

Recurrent Thrombosis

Standard therapy for patients with deep venous thrombosis typically includes anticoagulation with warfarin for 3 to 6 months. However, following this period of anticoagulation, there is a high rate of recurrent thrombotic events of approximately 5% to 10% per year.[116] A study by Kearon et al.[117] investigated 3 months versus extended therapy for an initial episode of deep venous thrombosis. The study was terminated early because of a very high recurrence rate; among those receiving placebo after 3 months of warfarin therapy, there was a 27.4% recurrence rate per year versus 1.3% in those receiving indefinite treatment. Considering the high rate of recurrent events, it would be particularly helpful to identify those individuals who are especially prone to subsequent thrombosis.

Although multiple studies have documented that the presence of dual hereditary defects significantly increases the likelihood of recurrent thrombosis,[118,119] studies of isolated defects have yielded conflicting results.[120] In the Physicians' Health Study, individuals with a first spontaneous deep venous thrombosis and factor V Leiden had a significantly higher rate of recurrence at 4 years (29%) than those without the mutation (11%).[121,122] An Austrian study also showed a higher incidence of subsequent venous thromboembolism in individuals with hyperhomocysteinemia, 18% versus 8% of controls (OR 2.7).[123] However, several studies have shown that recurrence rates in individuals with factor V Leiden or the prothrombin G20210A mutation alone were not significantly higher than in unaffected individuals.[118,124,125] Further investigation is necessary to firmly establish an association between isolated hereditary defects and recurrent deep venous thrombosis (see Treatment of Thrombotic Events).

Evaluation of Hereditary Thrombophilia

Although studies have not shown conclusively that the factor V Leiden or prothrombin G20210A mutations alone result in higher rates of recurrent thrombosis, a number of arguments can be advanced in favor of screening for hereditary defects. For instance, such knowledge could lead to antithrombotic prophylaxis during temporary periods of increased thrombotic risk such as surgery or during pregnancy. Additionally, the information can help to identify other family members with a similar predisposition toward thrombotic events given the autosomal dominant transmission of these thrombophilias. In older individuals, such diagnoses might mitigate concern regarding an underlying malignancy, which in some studies is subsequently diagnosed in over 10% of individuals after an initial episode of idiopathic deep venous thrombosis.[126]

Given the lack of consensus regarding the optimal treatment for hereditary thrombophilia coupled with the cost of performing a complete laboratory evaluation, a targeted approach to the laboratory diagnosis of thrombophilic disorders seems prudent. In general, laboratory investigation is not routinely recommended in instances of acquired causes of hypercoagulability such as major surgery, malignancy, systemic lupus erythematosus, and myeloproliferative disorders. In contrast, acquired states such as oral contraception, the puerperium, and pregnancy frequently trigger thrombotic events in women with hereditary thrombophilia and thus warrant further investigation.[127]

In order to guide laboratory evaluation, it is useful to classify patients as *strongly* or *weakly* thrombophilic (Fig. 13–2). An individual can be labeled *strongly* thrombophilic based on three historical features:

- First thromboembolic event occurring prior to age 50
- History of recurrent thrombotic episodes
- A first-degree relative with a documented venous thromboembolic event prior to age 50

In those individuals who meet any of the above criteria, full laboratory investigation is warranted, including testing for the factor V Leiden and prothrombin G20210A mutations and deficiencies of antithrombin, protein C, and protein S. On the other hand, a more focused diagnostic approach should be conducted in *weakly* thrombophilic patients. The frequency of the factor V Leiden or prothrombin G20210A mutations in older individuals remains significant and thus screening for these defects is reasonable. Both *strongly* and *weakly* thrombophilic patients should also undergo laboratory testing for the presence of antiphospholipid syndrome and hyperhomocysteinemia. As previously described, these last two defects should also be investigated in those individuals with unexplained arterial thrombosis.

Distinguishing between *weakly* and *strongly* thrombotic individuals can increase the diagnostic yield of uncommon deficiencies. In one study of 2132 consecutive patients with venous thromboembolism, approximately 30% of those individuals with two *strongly* thrombophilic clinical characteristics had a deficiency of antithrombin, protein C, or protein S as compared to less than 8% without historical risk factors.[82] Likewise, the prevalence of prothrombin G20210A can reach 20% and factor V Leiden almost 50% in selected populations.[55,60]

In cases of thrombotic events in unusual locations such as portal, cerebral, and retinal veins, a complete evaluation is generally warranted. However, these episodes often are attributed to acquired risk factors such as myeloproliferative disorders, oral contraceptives, or recent surgical procedures.[128–133] In addition, the prevalence of familial coagulation defects in these individuals does not differ significantly from the *weakly* thrombotic population. For instance, in an uncontrolled study of 36 individuals with portal vein thrombosis, the factor V Leiden mutation was identified only once (2.8%), prothrombin G20120 mutation in five individuals (14%), and MTHFR in four (11%).[132] Only one case of antithrombin deficiency was confirmed by familial testing. In another study comparing the prevalence of inherited defects in 92 individuals with portal vein thrombosis and 474 healthy controls, the incidence of protein S and antithrombin deficiencies did not differ significantly from the control population.[128] Six individuals (6.5%) were found to be protein C deficient, although these results were not confirmed in family studies. In the same study, factor V Leiden was found to be the predominant inherited defect in patients with hepatic vein thrombosis, occurring in 11 of 43 individuals. Again, several cases of protein C deficiency (4 of 43) were identified but none of protein S or antithrombin deficiencies. In other unusual sites of venous thrombosis such as the retinal or cerebral veins, the abnormalities most commonly identified were factor V Leiden, hyperhomocysteinemia, and antiphospholipid antibodies, whereas protein C, protein S, and antithrombin deficiencies remain rare.[130,133,134]

There are several other clinical circumstances that deserve special diagnostic consideration. Approximately one third of individuals who sustain the rare complication of warfarin-induced skin necrosis will have hereditary protein C deficiency. However, this syndrome has also been reported in individuals with protein S deficiency and the factor V Leiden mutation.[135,136] In

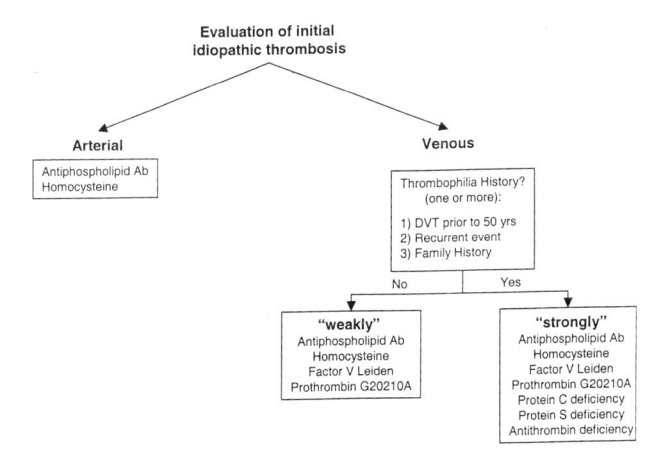

Figure 13–2 A targeted approach to the evaluation of initial idiopathic thrombosis based on thrombophilia history. *"Strongly" thrombophilic* refers to the presence of any of the following historical features: a deep venous thrombosis (DVT) prior to age 50 years, a history of two or more thrombotic episodes, or a family history of DVT.

newborn infants, the development of skin necrosis and visceral thrombosis (neonatal purpura fulminans) is usually associated with severe hereditary protein C deficiency, although one case has been reported in association with homozygous protein S deficiency.[137]

Timing of Diagnostic Testing

An important consideration in the evaluation of hereditary thrombophilia is the timing of testing. As discussed previously, the levels of antithrombin, protein C, or protein S can be affected by acute thrombosis, anticoagulation, or disease states. Acute thrombosis can transiently reduce the levels of antithrombin and occasionally proteins C and S. Anticoagulation with heparin leads to a decline in antithrombin levels, whereas warfarin produces a drop in the antigenic and functional levels of protein C and protein S. Rarely, warfarin has also been shown to elevate antithrombin levels into the normal range in individuals with a hereditary deficiency. Although "first-generation" coagulation assays for APC resistance cannot be reliably interpreted while patients are receiving anticoagulants, the "second-generation" assays are sensitive and specific for the factor V Leiden mutation even in individuals taking anticoagulants. Genetic tests for the factor V Leiden and prothrombin G20210A mutations are not affected by the timing of testing.

Optimally, evaluation for a hereditary abnormality should be done at least 2 weeks after completing the initial 3- to 6-month course of anticoagulation. If, upon acute presentation of the patient, levels of antithrombin, protein C, or protein S are obtained and are within normal range, then the diagnosis of deficiency can be reliably excluded. However, a low value will require confirmation after anticoagulation is discontinued. In those in whom temporary discontinuation of anticoagulation is not practical, heparin can be substited for warfarin. Additionally, confirmation in first-degree relatives can be helpful.

TREATMENT OF THROMBOTIC EVENTS

Acute Thrombosis

The initial management of acute thromboembolic disease is generally not affected by the presence of inherited risk factors for thrombosis. The usual treatment consists of unfractionated heparin or low-molecular-weight heparin (LMWH) followed by anticoagulation with warfarin. Heparin or LMWH should be administered in adequate dosage because failure to reach a therapeutic level of anticoagulation within the first 24 hours increases the risk of recurrent thromboembolism.[138] Heparin should be continued for at least 5 days. This includes a 2-day overlap with warfarin when the prothrombin time reaches the therapeutic range, typically an INR of 2 to 3.

Special attention may occasionally be needed for patients with deficiencies of antithrombin or protein C. Some patients with antithrombin deficiency are heparin resistant and may require large doses of unfractionated heparin to obtain an adequate anticoagulant effect as measured by the aPTT. Antithrombin concentrate can be used in special circumstances such as recurrent thrombosis despite adequate anticoagulation, unusually severe thrombosis, or difficulty achieving adequate anticoagulation.[139] It is also reasonable to treat antithrombin-deficient patients with concentrate before major surgeries or in obstetric situations when the risks of bleeding from anticoagulation are unacceptable.

Hereditary protein C deficiency can be associated with warfarin-induced skin necrosis due to a transient hypercoagulable state. The initiation of warfarin at standard doses leads to a decrease in protein C anticoagulant activity to approximately 50% of baseline within 1 day. Consequently, treatment with warfarin should be started only after the individual is fully heparinized and the dose of the drug should be increased gradually, after starting from a relatively low dose (e.g., 2 mg). Individuals with a history of warfarin-induced skin necrosis can be anticoagulated after receiving a source of exogenous protein C either via fresh frozen plasma or an investigational protein C concentrate. This offers a bridge until a stable level of anticoagulation can be achieved.

Long-Term Therapy

The risk of recurrent thrombosis must be weighed against the inherent risk of prolonged anticoagulation. On average, the annual risk of major bleeding events in patients on warfarin therapy is approximately 3% and of those episodes about one in five (i.e., overall 0.6%) is fatal.[117] Considering the annual risk of thrombosis is only 1.5% for asymptomatic individuals with antithrombin, protein C, or protein S deficiencies[140] and even lower for carriers of the factor V Leiden or prothrombin G20210A mutations,[141] it is generally recommended that asymptomatic patients with hereditary thrombophilia identified through family studies or screening not receive chronic anticoagulation. They should, however, receive counseling regarding their diagnosis, the need for prophylaxis during high-risk situations, and symptoms that require immediate medical attention.

Unfortunately no controlled trials have studied the duration of therapy in hereditary thrombophilia and thus long-term treatment following a thrombotic event must be determined on an individual basis. In patients with a first thrombotic event in the setting of a transient triggering factor, anticoagulation can be discontinued after 3 to 6 months. Patients with venous thromboembolism in the absence of triggering factors should be treated for 6 months. Criteria for indefinite anticoagulation include:

- Presence of more than one genetic defect
- Initial life-threatening thrombosis (e.g., massive pulmonary embolism)

- Cerebral, mesenteric, portal, or hepatic vein thrombosis
- Two or more spontaneous thrombotic episodes

The potential benefit of chronic anticoagulation in high-risk patients was addressed in a controlled trial that evaluated the efficacy of long-term warfarin therapy (INR 2 to 2.85) for 6 months or indefinitely in 227 patients with a second venous thrombotic episode, but not specifically inherited thrombophilia. Long-term warfarin was highly effective in preventing recurrences as compared to 6 months of therapy (2.6% versus 21% at 4 years, respectively). This benefit was partially counterbalanced by an increased incidence of major hemorrhage (8.6% versus 2.3%, respectively). The mortality did not differ significantly between the two groups.[142]

As previously discussed, at a yearly rate of recurrence of approximately 5%, individuals with the factor V Leiden or prothrombin G20210A mutations may not be at significantly higher risk than those without such defects. Despite the high recurrence rates, several studies argue against long-term warfarin therapy after a first thromboembolic episode. In one study, the median time to recurrence after discontinuation of oral anticoagulant therapy was 9 years.[143] The period was significantly shorter (3.5 years) among patients who suffered an idiopathic rather than a provoked first event. It was estimated that, even in the latter group, death from hemorrhage would probably exceed the number of fatal pulmonary emboli prevented with chronic warfarin therapy. Thus, prolonged anticoagulation after a single episode of thromboembolism cannot be recommended unless the event was life threatening or in an unusual location, or if more than one genetic defect exists. Many clinicians also recommend indefinite anticoagulation for patients with symptomatic antithrombin deficiency as they appear more thrombosis prone than patients with other single heritable defects. Some also recommend such an approach for symptomatic patients with heterozygous deficiencies of protein C or protein S.

■ REFERENCES

Chapter 13 References

1. Briggs JB. Recurring phlebitis of obscure origin. Johns Hopkins Hosp Bull 1905;16:228–233.
2. Perry D. Antithrombin and its inherited deficiencies. Blood Rev 1994;8:37–55.
3. Egeberg O. Inherited antithrombin deficiency causing thrombophilia. Thromb Diath Haemorrh 1965;13:516–530.
4. Gruenberg JC, Smallridge RC, Rosenberg RD. Inherited antithrombin-III deficiency causing mesenteric venous infarction: a new clinical entity. Ann Surg 1975;181:791–794.
5. Marciniak E, Farley CH, DeSimone PA. Familial thrombosis due to antithrombin III deficiency. Blood 1974;43:219–231.
6. Heijboer H, Brandjes DPM, Büller HR, et al. Deficiencies of coagulation-inhibiting and fibrinolytic proteins in outpatients with deep venous thrombosis. N Engl J Med 1990;323:1512–1516.
7. Lane DA, Mannucci PM, Bauer KA, et al. Inherited thrombophilia: part 1. Thromb Haemost 1996;76:651–662.
8. Rosenberg RD. Actions and interaction of antithrombin and heparin. N Engl J Med 1975;292:146–151.
9. Odegard OR, Abildgaard U. Antithrombin III: critical review of assay methods. Significance of variations in health and disease. Haemostasis 1978;7:127–134.
10. Meade TW, Dyer S, Howarth DJ, et al. Antithrombin III and procoagulant activity; sex differences and effects of the menopause. Br J Haematol 1990;74:77–81.
11. Lane DA, Bayston T, Olds RJ, et al. Antithrombin mutation database: 2nd (1997) update. Thromb Haemost 1997;77:197–211.
12. Finazzi G, Caccia R, Barbui T. Different prevalence of thromboembolism in the subtypes of congenital antithrombin deficiency: review of 404 cases (letter). Thromb Haemost 1987;58:1094.
13. Odegard OR, Lie M, Abildgaard U. Heparin cofactor activity measured with an amidolytic method. Thromb Res 1975;6:287–294.
14. Demers C, Henderson P, Blajchman MA, et al. An antithrombin III assay based on factor Xa inhibition provides a more reliable test to identify congenital antithrombin III deficiency than an assay based on thrombin inhibition. Thromb Haemost 1993;69:231–235.
15. de Boer AC, van Riel LAM, den Ottolander GJH. Measurement of antithrombin III, α_2-macroglobulin and α_1-antitrypsin in patients with deep venous thrombosis and pulmonary embolism. Thromb Res 1979;15:17–25.
16. Damus PS, Wallace GA. Immunologic measurement of antithrombin III-heparin cofactor and α_2-macroglobulin in disseminated intravascular coagulation and hepatic failure coagulapathy. Thromb Res 1989;6:27–38.
17. von Kaulla E, von Kaulla KN. Antithrombin III and diseases. Am J Clin Pathol 1967;48:69–80.
18. Kauffman RH, Vetlkamp JJ, Van Tilburg NH, et al. Acquired antithrombin III deficiency and thrombus in the nephrotic syndrome. Am J Med 1978;65:607–613.
19. Weenink GH, Kahle LH, Lamping RJ, et al. Antithrombin III in oral contraceptive users and during normotensive pregnancy. Acta Obstet Gynecol Scand 1984;63:57–61.
20. Caine YG, Bauer KA, Barzegar S, et al. Coagulation activation following estrogen administration to postmenopausal women. Thromb Haemost 1992;68:392–395.
21. Marciniak E, Gockermen JP. Heparin-induced decrease in circulating antithrombin III. Lancet 1978;2:581–584.
22. Kitchens CS. Amelioration of antithrombin III deficiency by coumarin administration. Am J Med Sci 1987;293:403–406.
23. Griffin JH, Evatt B, Zimmerman TS, et al. Deficiency of protein C in congenital thrombotic disease. J Clin Invest 1981;68:1370–1373.
24. Horellou MH, Conard J, Bertina RM, et al. Congenital protein C deficiency and thrombotic disease in nine French families. Br Med J 1984;289:1285–1287.
25. Miletich JP, Sherman L, Broze GJ, Jr. Absence of thrombosis in subjects with heterozygous protein C deficiency. N Engl J Med 1987;317:991–996.
26. Tait RC, Walker ID, Reitsma PH, et al. Prevalence of protein C deficiency in the healthy population. Thromb Haemost 1995;73:87–93.
27. Reitsma PH, Bernardi F, Doig RG, et al. Protein C deficiency: a database of mutations, 1995 update. Thromb Haemost 1995;73:876–879.
28. Francis RB, Jr., Seyfert U. Rapid amidolytic assay of protein C in whole plasma using an activator from the venom of *Agkistrodon contortrix*. Am J Clin Pathol 1987;87:619–625.
29. D'Angelo SV, Comp PC, Esmon CT, et al. Relationship between protein C antigen and anticoagulant activity during oral anticoagulation and in selected disease states. J Clin Invest 1986;77:416–425.
30. Lane DA, Mannucci PM, Bauer KA, et al. Inherited thrombophilia: part 2. Thromb Haemost 1996;76:824–834.
31. Manco-Johnson MJ, Marlar RA, Jacobson LJ, et al. Severe protein C deficiency in newborn infants. J Pediatr 1988;113:359–363.

32. Karpatkin M, Mannucci PM, Bhogal M, et al. Low protein C in the neonatal period. Br J Haematol 1986;62:137–142.
33. Polack B, Pouzol P, Amiral J, et al. Protein C level at birth. Thromb Haemost 1984;52:188–190.
34. Auletta MJ, Headington JT. Purpura fulminans. A cutaneous manifestation of severe protein C deficiency. Arch Dermatol 1988;124:1387–1391.
35. Gerson WT, Dickerman JD, Bovill EG, et al. Severe acquired protein C deficiency in purpura fulminans associated with disseminated intravascular coagulation: treatment with protein C concentrate. Pediatrics 1993;91:418–422.
36. Vigano-D'Angelo S, D'Angelo A, Kaufman CE, Jr., et al. Protein S deficiency occurs in the nephrotic syndrome. Ann Intern Med 1987;107:42–47.
37. Sorensen PJ, Knudsen F, Nielsen AH, et al. Protein C activity in renal disease. Thromb Res 1985;38:243–249.
38. Faioni EM, Franchi F, Krachmalnicoff A, et al. Low levels of the anticoagulant activity of protein C in patients with chronic renal insufficiency: an inhibitor of protein C is present in uremic plasma. Thromb Haemost 1991;66:420–425.
39. Pabinger I, Kyrle PA, Speiser W, et al. Diagnosis of protein C deficiency in patients on oral anticoagulant treatment: comparison of three different functional protein C assays. Thromb Haemost 1990;63:407–412.
40. Jones DW, Mackie IJ, Winter M, et al. Detection of protein C deficiency during oral anticoagulant therapy—use of the protein C:factor VII ratio. Blood Coagul Fibrinol 1991;2:407–411.
41. Kalafatis M, Bertina RM, Rand MD, et al. Characterization of the molecular defect in factor V R506Q. J Biol Chem 1995; 270:4053–4057.
42. Comp PC, Esmon CT. Recurrent venous thromboembolism in patients with a partial deficiency of protein S. N Engl J Med 1984;311:1525–1528.
43. Martinelli I, Mannucci PM, DeStefano V, et al. Different risks of thrombosis in four coagulation defects associated with inherited thrombophilia: a study of 150 families. Blood 1998;92:2353–2358.
44. Gandrille S, Borgel D, Ireland H, et al. Protein S deficiency: a database of mutations. For the Plasma Coagulation Inhibitors Subcommittee of the Scientific and Standardization Committee of the International Society on Thrombosis and Haemostasis. Thromb Haemost 1997;77:1201–1214.
45. Koster T, Rosendaal FR, Briët E, et al. Protein C deficiency in a controlled series of unselected outpatients: an infrequent but clear risk factor for venous thrombosis (Leiden Thrombophilia Study). Blood 1995;85:2756–2761.
46. Schwarz HP, Fischer M, Hopmeier P, et al. Plasma protein S deficiency in familial thrombotic disease. Blood 1984;64:1297–1300.
47. Comp PC, Doray D, Patton D, et al. An abnormal plasma distribution of protein S occurs in functional protein S deficiency. Blood 1986;67:504–508.
48. Borgel D, Gandrille S, Aiach M. Protein S deficiency. Thromb Haemost 1997;78:351–356.
49. Bertina RM, Ploos van Amstel HK, van Wijngaarden A, et al. Heerlen polymorphism of protein S, an immunologic polymorphism due to dimorphism of residue 460. Blood 1990;76:538–548.
50. Zöller B, de Frutos PG, Dahlback B. Evaluation of the relationship between protein S and C4b-binding protein isoforms in hereditary protein S deficiency demonstrating type I and type III deficiencies to be phenotypic variants of the same genetic disease. Blood 1995;85:3524–3531.
51. D'Angelo A, Vigano-D'Angelo S, Esmon CT, et al. Acquired deficiencies of protein S. Protein S activity during oral anticoagulation, in liver disease, and in disseminated intravascular coagulation. J Clin Invest 1988;81:1445–1454.
52. Stahl CP, Wideman CS, Spira TJ, et al. Protein S deficiency in men with long-term human immunodeficiency virus infection. Blood 1993;81:1801–1807.
53. Dahlbäck B, Carlsson M, Svensson PJ. Familial thrombophilia due to a previously unrecognized mechanism characterized by poor anticoagulant response to activated protein C: prediction of a cofactor to activated protein C. Proc Natl Acad Sci USA 1993;90:1004–1008.
54. Bertina RM, Koeleman BPC, Koster T, et al. Mutation in blood coagulation factor V associated with resistance to activated protein C. Nature 1994;369:64–67.
55. Svensson PJ, Dahlback B. Resistance to activated protein C as a basis for venous thrombosis. N Engl J Med 1994;330:517–522.
56. Griffin JH, Evatt B, Wideman C, et al. Anticoagulant protein C pathway defective in majority of thrombophilic patients. Blood 1993;82:1989–1993.
57. Koster T, Rosendaal FR, de Ronde H, et al. Venous thrombosis due to poor anticoagulant response to activated protein C: Leiden Thrombophilia Study. Lancet 1993;342:1503–1506.
58. Rees DC, Cox M, Clegg JB. World distribution of factor V Leiden. Lancet 1995;346:1133–1134.
59. de Visser MCH, Rosendaal FR, Bertina RM. A reduced sensitivity for activated protein C in the absence of factor V Leiden increases the risk of venous thrombosis. Blood 1999;93:1271–1276.
60. Poort SR, Rosendaal FR, Reitsma PH, et al. A common genetic variation in the 3′-untranslated region of the prothrombin gene is associated with elevated prothrombin levels and an increase in venous thrombosis. Blood 1996;88:3698–3703.
61. Soria J, Almasy L, Souto J, et al. Linkage analysis demonstrates that the prothrombin G20210A mutation jointly influences plasma prothrombin levels and risk of thrombosis. Blood 2000;95:2780–2785.
62. Rosendaal FR, Doggen CJM, Zvelin A, et al. Geographic distribution of the 20210 G to A prothrombin variant. Thromb Haemost 1998;79:706–708.
63. Hillarp A, Zöller B, Svensson P, et al. The 20210 A allele of the prothrombin gene is a common risk factor among Swedish outpatients with verified deep vein thrombosis. Thromb Haemost 1997;78:990–992.
64. Gomez E, van der Poel S, Jansen J, et al. Rapid simutaneous screening of factor V Leiden and G20210A prothrombin variant by multiplex polymerase chain reaction on whole blood (letter). Blood 1995;91:2208–2209.
65. McCully KS. Vascular pathology of homocysteinemia: implications for the pathogenesis of arteriosclerosis. Am J Pathol 1969;56:111–128.
66. Den Heijer M, Koster T, Blom HJ, et al. Hyperhomocysteinemia as a risk factor for deep-vein thrombosis. N Engl J Med 1996; 334:759–762.
67. Ridker PM, Hennekens CH, Selhub J, et al. Interrelation of hyperhomocyst(e)inemia, factor V Leiden, and risk of future venous thromboembolism. Circulation 1997;95:1777–1782.
68. Den Heijer M, Rosendaal F, Blom H, et al. Hyperhomocysteinemia and venous thrombosis: a meta-analysis. Thromb Haemost 1998;80:874–877.
69. Christen W, Ajani U, Glynn R, et al. Bloods levels of homocysteine and increased risks of cardiovascular disease. Arch Intern Med 2000;160:422–434.
70. Botto L, Yang Q. 5, 10 Methylenetetrahydrofolate reductase gene variants and congenital anomalies. Am J Epidemiol 2000;151:862–877.
71. Frosst P, Blom HJ, Milos R, et al. A candidate genetic risk factor for vascular disease: a common mutation in methylenetetrahydrofolate reductase. Nat Genet 1995;10:111–113.
72. Selhub J, Jacques PF, Wilson PWF, et al. Vitamin status and intake as primary determinants of homocysteinemia in an elderly population. JAMA 1993;270:2693–2698.
73. Stamler JS, Osborne JA, Jaraki O, et al. Adverse vascular effects of homocysteine are modulated by endothelium-derived relaxing factor and related oxides of nitrogen. J Clin Invest 1993; 91:308–318.

74. Starkebaum G, Harlan JM. Endothelial cell injury due to copper-catalyzed hydrogen peroxide from homocysteine. J Clin Invest 1986;77:1370–1376.
75. Fryer RH, Wilson BD, Gubler DB, et al. Homocysteine, a risk factor for premature vascular disease and thrombosis, induces tissue factor activity in endothelial cells. Arterioscler Thromb Vasc Biol 1993;13:1327–1333.
76. Nishinaga M, Ozawa T, Shimada K. Homocysteine, a thrombogenic agent, suppresses heparan sulfate expression in cultured porcine aortic endothelial cells. J Clin Invest 1993;92:1381–1386.
77. Hajjar KA. Homocysteine-induced modulation of tissue plasminogen activator binding to its endothelial cell membrane receptor. J Clin Invest 1993;91:2873–2879.
78. Kluijtmans LA, den Heijer M, Reitsma PH, et al. Thermolabile methylenetetrahydrofolate reductase and factor V Leiden in the risk of deep-vein thrombosis. Thromb Haemost 1998;79:254–258.
79. Bertina RM, van der Linden IK, Engesser L, et al. Hereditary heparin cofactor II deficiency and the risk of development of thrombosis. Thromb Haemostas 1987;57:196–200.
80. Bernardi F, Legnani C, Micheletti F, et al. A heparin cofactor II mutation (HCII Rimini) combined with factor V Leiden or type I protein C deficiency in two unrelated thrombophilic subjects. Thromb Haemost 1996;76:505–509.
81. Schott D, Dempfle C-E, Beck P, et al. Therapy with a purified plasminogen concentrate in an infant with ligneous conjuctivitis and homozygous plasminogen deficiency. N Engl J Med 1998;339:1679–1686.
82. Mateo J, Oliver A, Borrell M, et al. Laboratory evaluation and clinical characteristics of 2,132 consecutive unselected patients with venous thromboembolism—results of the Spanish multicentric study on thrombophilia (EMET Study). Thromb Haemost 1997;77:444–451.
83. McDonagh J. Dysfibrinogenemia and other disorders of fibrinogen structure or function. In: Colman RW, Hirsh J, Marder VJ, Clowes AW, George JN, (eds): Hemostasis and Thrombosis: Basic Principles and Clinical Practice, 4th ed. Philadelphia, Lippincott Williams & Wilkins, 2001; pp. 856–892.
84. Saito H. Contact factors in health and disease. Semin Thromb Hemost 1987;13:36–49.
85. Goodnough LT, Saito H, Ratnoff OD. Thrombosis or myocardial infarction in congenital clotting factor abnormalities and chronic thrombocytopenias: a report of 21 patients and a review of 50 previously reported cases. Medicine 1983;62:248–255.
86. Lodi S, Isa L, Pollini E, et al. Defective intrinsic fibrinolytic activity in a patient with severe factor XII deficiency and myocardial infarction. Scand J Haematol 1984;33:80–82.
87. Lammle B, Wuillemin WA, Huber I, et al. Thromboembolism and bleeding tendency in congenital factor XII deficiency—a study on 74 subjects from 14 Swiss families. Thromb Haemost 1991;65:117–121.
88. Rodeghiero F, Castaman G, Ruggeri M, et al. Thrombosis in subjects with homozygous and heterozygous factor XII deficiency (letter). Thromb Haemost 1992;67:590.
89. Mannhalter C, Fischer M, Hopmeier P, et al. Factor XII activity and antigen concentrations in patients suffering from recurrent thrombosis. Fibrinolysis 1987;1:259–263.
90. Koster T, Blann AD, Briët E, et al. Role of clotting factor VIII in effect of von Willebrand factor on occurrence of deep-vein thrombosis. Lancet 1995;345:152–155.
91. Kraaijenhagen RA, in't Anker PS, Koopman MMW, et al. High plasma concentration of factor VIIIc is a major risk factor for venous thromboembolism. Thromb Haemost 2000;83:5–9.
92. Kamphuisen PW, Eikenboom JCJ, Vos HL, et al. Increased levels of factor VIII and fibrinogen in patients with venous thrombosis are not caused by acute phase reactions. Thromb Haemost 1999;81:680–683.
93. O'Donnell J, Tuddenham EGD, Manning R, et al. High prevalence of elevated factor VIII levels in patients referred for thrombophilia screening: role of increased synthesis and relationship to the acute phase reaction. Thromb Haemost 1997;77:825–828.
94. Kyrle PA, Minar E, Hirschl M, et al. High plasma factor VIII and the risk of recurrent venous thromboembolism. N Engl J Med 2000;343:457–462.
95. van Tilburg NH, Rosendaal FR, Bertina RM. Thrombin activatable fibrinolysis inhibitor and the risk for deep vein thrombosis. Blood 2000;95:2855–2859.
96. Meijers JCM, Tekelenberg W, Bouma BN, et al. High levels of coagulation factor XI as a risk factor for venous thrombosis. N Engl J Med 2000;342:696–701.
97. van Hylckama A, van der Linden IK, Bertina RM, et al. High levels of factor IX increase the risk of venous thrombosis. Blood 2000;95:3678–3682.
98. Kamphuisen PW, Lensen R, Houwing-Duistermaat JJ, et al. Heritability of elevated factor VIII antigen levels in factor V Leiden families with thrombophilia. Br J Haematol 2000;109:519–522.
99. Engesser L, Broekmans AW, Briet E, et al. Hereditary protein S deficiency: clinical manifestations. Ann Intern Med 1987;106:677–682.
100. van der Meer FJM, Koster T, Vandenbroucke JP, et al. The Leiden Thrombophilia Study (LETS). Thromb Haemost 1997;78:631–635.
101. Ridker PM, Hennekens CH, Lindpaintner K, et al. Mutation in the gene coding for coagulation factor V and the risk of myocardial infarction, stroke, and venous thrombosis in apparently healthy men. N Engl J Med 1995;332:912–917.
102. Rosendaal FR, Koster T, Vandenbroucke JP, et al. High-risk of thrombosis in patients homozygous for factor V Leiden (APC-resistance). Blood 1995;85:1504–1508.
103. Stampfer MJ, Malinow MR, Willett WC, et al. A prospective study of plasma homocyst(e)ine and risk of myocardial infarction in US physicians. JAMA 1992;268:877–881.
104. Perry IJ, Refsum H, Morris RW, et al. Prospective study of serum total homocysteine concentration and risk of stroke in middle-aged British men. Lancet 1995;346:1395–1398.
105. Selhub J, Jacques PF, Bostom AG, et al. Association between plasma homocysteine concentrations and extracranial carotid-artery stenosis. N Engl J Med 1995;332:286–291.
106. van Boven HH, Reitsma PH, Rosendaal FR, et al. Factor V Leiden (R506Q) in families with inherited antithrombin deficiency. Thromb Haemost 1996;75:417–421.
107. Koeleman BPC, Reitsma PH, Allaart CF, et al. Activated protein C resistance as an additional risk factor for thrombosis in protein C-deficient families. Blood 1994;84:1031–1035.
108. Zöller B, Berntsdotter A, de Frutos G, et al. Resistance to activated protein C as an additional risk factor in hereditary deficiency of protein S. Blood 1995;12:3518–3523.
109. Makris M, Preston FE, Beauchamp NJ, et al. Co-inheritance of the 20210A allele of the prothrombin gene increases the risk of thrombosis in subjects with familial thrombophilia. Thromb Haemost 1997;78:1426–1429.
110. Samama M. An epidemiologic study of risk factors for deep vein thrombosis in medical outpatients. Arch Interm Med 2000;160:3415–3420.
111. Kraaijenhagen R, Haverkamp D, Koopman M, et al. Travel and risk of venous thrombosis. Lancet 2000;356:1492–1493.
112. Douay X, Lucas C, Caron C, et al. Antithrombin, protein C and protein S levels in 127 consecutive young adults with ischemic stroke. Acta Neurol Scand 1998;98:124–127.
113. Price DT, Ridker PM. Factor V Leiden mutation and the risks for thromboembolic disease: a clinical perspective. Ann Intern Med 1997;127:895–903.
114. De Stefano V, Chiusolo P, Paciaroni K, et al. Prothrombin G20210A mutant genotype is a risk factor for cerebrovascular ischemic disease in young patients. Blood 1998;91:3562–3565.

115. Reuner KH, Ruf A, Grau A, et al. Prothrombin gene G20210A transition is a risk factor for cerebral venous thrombosis. Stroke 1998;29:1765–1769.
116. Prandoni P, Lensing AWA, Cogo A, et al. The long-term clinical course of acute deep venous thrombosis. Ann Intern Med 1996;125:1–7.
117. Kearon C, Gent M, Hirsh J, et al. A comparison of three months of anticoagulation with extended anticoagulation for a first episode of idiopathic venous thromboembolism. N Engl J Med 1999;340:901–907.
118. De Stefano V, Martinelli I, Mannucci PM, et al. The risk of recurrent deep venous thrombosis among heterozygous carriers of both factor V Leiden and the G20210A prothrombin mutation. N Engl J Med 1999;341:801–806.
119. Margaglione M, D'Andrea G, Colaizzo D, et al. Coexistence of factor V Leiden and factor II A20210 mutations and recurrent venous thromboembolism. Thromb Haemost 1999;82:1583–1587.
120. Lensing AWA, Prins MH. Recurrent deep vein thrombosis and two coagulation factor gene mutations: Quo vadis? Thromb Haemost 1999;82:1564–1566.
121. Ridker PM, Miletch JP, Stampfer MJ, et al. Factor V Leiden and risks of recurrent idiopathic venous thromboembolism. Circulation 1995;92:2800–2802.
122. Simioni P, Prandoni P, Lensing AWA, et al. The risk of recurrent venous thromboembolism in patients with an Arg506→Gln mutation in the gene for factor V (factor V Leiden). N Engl J Med 1997;336:399–403.
123. Eichinger S, Stumpflen A, Hirschl M, et al. Hyperhomocysteinemia is a risk factor of recurrent venous thromboembolism. Thromb Haemost 1998;80:566–569.
124. Eichinger S, Pabinger I, Schneider B, et al. The risk of recurrence of venous thromboembolism in patients with and without factor V Leiden. Thromb Haemost 1997;77:624–628.
125. Lindmarker P, Schulman S, Sten-Linder M, et al. The risk of recurrent venous thromboembolism in carriers and non-carriers of the G1691A allele in the coagulation factor V gene and the G20210A allele in the prothrombin gene. Thromb Haemost 1999;81:684–690.
126. Schulman S, Lindmarker P. Incidence of cancer after prophylaxis with warfarin against recurrent venous thromboembolism. N Engl J Med 2000;342:1953–1958.
127. Vandenbroucke JP, Koster T, Briet E, et al. Increased risk of venous thrombosis in oral-contraceptive users who are carriers of factor V Leiden mutation. Lancet 1994;344:1453–1457.
128. Janssen H, Meinardi J, Vleggaar F, et al. Factor V Leiden mutation, prothrombin gene mutation, and deficiencies in coagulation inhibitors associated with Budd-Chiari syndrome and portal vein thrombosis: results of a case-control study. Blood 2000;96:2364–2368.
129. Amitrano L, Brancaccio V, Guardascione M, et al. High prevalence of thrombophilic genotypes in patients with acute mesenteric vein thrombosis. Am J Gastroenterol 2001;96:146–149.
130. Backhouse O, Parapia L, Mahomed I, et al. Familial thrombophilia and retinal vein occlusion. Eye 2000;14:13–17.
131. Egesel T, Buyukasik Y, Dunder SV, et al. The role of natural anticoagulant deficiencies and factor V Leiden in the development of idiopathic portal vein thrombosis. J Clin Gastroenterol 2000;30:66–71.
132. Denninger M, Chait Y, Casadevall N, et al. Cause of portal or hepatic venous thrombosis in adults: the role of multiple concurrent factors. Hepatology 2000;31:587–591.
133. Stolz E, Kemkes-Matthes B, Potzsch B, et al. Screening for thrombophilic risk factors among 25 German patients with cerebral venous thrombosis. Acta Neurol Scand 2000;102:31–36.
134. Hansen L, Kristensen H, Bek T, et al. Markers of thrombophilia in retinal vein thrombosis. Acta Ophthalmol Scand 2000;78:523–526.
135. Friedman KD, Marlar RA, Houson JG, et al. Warfarin-induced skin necrosis in a patient with protein S deficiency (abstract). Blood 1986;68(suppl 1):333a.
136. Makris M, Bardhan G, Preston FE. Warfarin induced skin necrosis associated with activated protein C resistance (letter). Thromb Haemost 1996;75:523–524.
137. Mahasandana C, Suvatte V, Chuansumrit A, et al. Homozygous protein S deficiency in an infant with purpura fulminans. J Pediatr 1990;117:750–753.
138. Hull RD, Raskob GE, Hirsh J, et al. Continuous intravenous heparin compared with intermittent subcutaneous heparin in the initial treatment of proximal vein thrombosis. N Engl J Med 1986;315:1109–1114.
139. Bucur SZ, Levy JH, Despotis GJ, et al. Uses of antithrombin III concentrate in congenital and acquired deficiency states. Transfusion 1998;38:481–498.
140. Sanson B, Simioni P, Tormene D, et al. The incidence of venous thromboembolism in asymptomatic carriers of a deficiency of antithrombin, protein C, or protein S: a prospective cohort study. Blood 1999;94:3702–3706.
141. Simioni P, Sanson B, Prandoni P, et al. Incidence of venous thromboembolism in families with inherited thrombophilia. Thromb Haemost 1999;81:198–202.
142. Schulman S, Granqvist S, Holmström M, et al. The duration of oral anticoagulant therapy after a second episode of venous thromboembolism. N Engl J Med 1997;336:393–398.
143. Baglin C, Brown K, Luddington R, et al. Risk of recurrent thromboembolism in patients with the factor V Leiden (FVR506Q) mutation: effect of warfarin and prediction by precipitating factors. East Anglian Thrombophilia Study Group. Br J Haematol 1998;100:764–768.

CHAPTER 14

Deep Venous Thrombosis and Pulmonary Embolus

William D. Haire, M.D.

INTRODUCTION: THE CONCEPT OF VENOUS THROMBOEMBOLISM (VTE)

Deep venous thrombosis (DVT) of the legs and pulmonary thromboembolism (PE) are common disorders that complicate a wide spectrum of diseases. Consequently, they are encountered by virtually all medical practitioners. Indeed, practitioners of most specialties are quite adept at dealing with the more common aspects of these disorders—particularly as they present in their specialty—and seek consultation only for assistance in making decisions with rarer or more complex aspects of these cases. Rather than attempt to provide exhaustive coverage of all aspects of DVT/PE in all of their presentations—an attempt that would be doomed to failure in anything smaller than an entire book—this chapter will provide background concepts and suggest diagnostic and therapeutic approaches that will allow the hematology consultant to be clinically helpful to patients and practitioners faced with problems that are not routinely encountered in their specialty or that do not have generally accepted solutions.

While often presenting clinically as one syndrome or the other, DVT and PE usually coexist. Pulmonary emboli do not arise de novo by blood turning from a liquid to a solid form in the pulmonary arteries, they arrive in the pulmonary circulation after physically breaking away from their origins in the venous circulation, generally the veins of the legs. Portions of thrombi forming in the veins of the legs often break loose and travel through the venous circulation where they are filtered out in the pulmonary arterial tree, larger venous thrombi generating larger embolic fragments. Clinically, for reasons not always apparent, one component of the DVT/PE spectrum is often asymptomatic. Venography done on patients presenting with symptoms of PE shows an incidence of DVT of up to 82%, almost half of which are asymptomatic.[1,2] The lack of venographically defined DVT in some of these patients may be due to the fact that virtually all of the original thrombus broke free from its attachment to the vein wall and embolized, a phenomenon that can be induced in experimental settings.[3] Almost half of patients presenting with symptomatic DVT of the thigh but no syndrome suggestive of PE are found to have lung scans that are read as high probability for PE.[4,5] Since DVT and PE are so frequently found to coexist, it is currently thought that they are two clinically distinct components of a larger syndrome, known as *venous thromboembolism* (VTE). The etiologic components and mechanisms of pathogenesis of the syndrome of VTE confer a risk of both DVT and PE and their sequelae. Which component of the syndrome is more clinically apparent in any given patient is presumably dependent on patient-specific variables, most of which are poorly understood.

ETIOLOGY AND PATHOGENESIS

Well over a century ago, Virchow proposed that VTE was caused by alteration of one or more of the following: (1) the rate of flow of blood through the vein, or "stasis," (2) the "coagulability" of the blood flowing through the vein, and (3) the viability of the venous tissue, or venous "injury." These factors have become known as "Virchow's triad" and the triad has been widely quoted as an explanation for the development of most, if not all, episodes of VTE. This model is still a valid concept when the components of the triad are viewed with a modern biochemical perspective (Table 14–1). Stasis due to physical immobility appears to contribute to the genesis of VTE based on studies of stoke victims

Table 14–1 • INTERPRETATION OF VIRCHOW'S TRIAD USING MODERN UNDERSTANDING OF THE PHYSIOLOGIC MECHANISMS OF THROMBOSIS

Virchow's Triad	Modern Interpretation
Stasis	Immobility: of minor importance except that it may indicate underlying disease activity
	Paralysis induces "microtears" in the venous endothelium
Blood coagulability	Impaired inhibition of coagulation
	Deficiencies of ATIII, PC, PS
	Factor V Leiden, prothrombin 20210
	Effects of inflammatory cytokines
	Increased monocyte tissue factor
	Increased plasminogen activator inhibitor
Venous injury	Direct trauma
	Torsion during surgery
	Hydrodynamic trauma from tourniquet use
	Effects of inflammatory cytokines
	Endothelial cell apoptosis
	Increased endothelial cell tissue factor
	Decreased thrombomodulin expression

wherein the incidence of DVT was found to be higher in the paralyzed limb than the unaffected limb.[6,7] Having said that, it must be recognized that: (1) paralysis with immobility may do more to venous tissue than simply slow the rate of blood flow through the vein (2) the degree of immobility short of complete paralysis necessary to predispose to DVT is not known, and (3) most clinical states associated with nonparalytic immobility (bed rest) are caused by systemic illnesses with their own potentially additive risk factors for VTE beyond simple stasis of venous blood. Intraoperative paralysis, for instance, induces dilation of the veins of the leg that results in "microtears" in the venous endothelium, exposing components of the flowing blood to injured endothelial cells and subendothelial collagen and other thrombogenic substances.[8] Consequently, even in the "cleanest" of clinical experimental models, it is impossible to quantitate the contribution of stasis to the predisposition to VTE relative to the concurrent venous endothelial damage and systemic alterations in blood coagulability induced by the disease necessitating the immobility. Presumably for these reasons, no study has causally related stasis *alone* to the development of VTE.[8] Consequently, where mild to moderate immobility is the sole apparent reason for the development of VTE, such as prolonged airplane or car travel in an otherwise apparently healthy person, other additive causes should be sought to explain the clinical event.

It is becoming increasingly apparent that the coagulability of the blood is a major component of Virchow's triad, if this term is taken in its broadest context to include not only altered activation of hemostatic mechanism but also impairment or inhibition of the hemostatic mechanisms and interference with the processes of thrombolysis. An increasing number of congenital abnormalities, generally resulting in impaired inhibition of hemostatic activation, have shown that they predispose to VTE in the apparent absence of other components of the triad (see Chapter 5). In addition, a number of pathologic conditions known to be associated with VTE have been shown to alter blood coagulability temporarily in otherwise apparently normal individuals. The common denominator of these acquired clinical conditions is the presence of an inflammatory response—a response to either sterile (surgery, trauma, chemotherapy, etc.) or septic (bacterial, viral, parasitic, etc.) stimuli. Poorly understood components of this inflammatory response, notably tumor necrosis factor and other proinflammatory cytokines, can activate components of the hemostatic system of the flowing blood,[9] possibly in part by exposing tissue factor on circulating monocytes,[10] and impair fibrinolysis by increasing levels of plasminogen activator inhibitor 1 (PAI-1).[11] The final component of Virchow's triad, venous injury, must also be taken to include more than direct physical injury. In addition to physical trauma, such as that induced during surgical procedures—especially during joint replacement procedures (from traction/torsion during manipulation of the joint[12] and hydrodynamic effects from tourniquet use)—components of the inflammatory reaction can downregulate thrombomodulin,[13] promote the expression of tissue factor on the endothelial cell surface,[14] and, ultimately, induce apoptosis of the endothelial cells, thus rendering them thrombogenic.[15]

The understanding that physiologic responses to exogenous inflammatory stimuli can alter the components of Virchow's triad and predispose to thrombosis can be helpful in predicting outcomes in patients with VTE. Given that a wide spectrum of pathologic conditions (surgery, infection, trauma, cancer chemotherapy, pancreatitis, etc.) can induce a strong inflammatory response, it is conceivable that such a response could alter all three components of the triad sufficiently to induce VTE in an otherwise normal individual. Such a person could be considered as having VTE secondary to the inflammatory disorder. Once such individuals had recovered from the inflammatory stimulus they might revert to their normal state and not have a significant risk for recurrent VTE in the absence of subsequent proinflammatory stimuli. This concept has been borne out in clinical studies demonstrating patients whose VTE occurred in association with reversible risk factors (surgery, major medical illness, pregnancy, etc.) have a low risk (approximately 2% per year) of recurrent VTE after a few months' course of anticoagulant therapy.[16–19] On the other hand, patients who suffer VTE without clinically obvious, significant venous stasis and endothelial cell dysfunction (due to trauma or biochemical alteration) might be inferred to have an underlying abnormality of blood coagulability (congenital, acquired, or both). Such an abnormality might not be reversible. Without knowledge of such an abnormality, an episode of VTE would be considered idiopathic and such patients seem to have a higher risk of recurrent VTE after cessation of a short course of anticoagulant therapy. This concept has been substantiated in clinical studies demonstrating that patients whose VTE occurs without obvious, clinically detectable reversible risk factors for altered blood coagulability (i.e., without surgery, major medical illness, pregnancy, etc.) have a rate of recurrent VTE of approximately 10% per year for up to 2 years after completing a 6-month course of anticoagulant therapy.[16-19] These observations suggest that alterations of the components of Virchow's triad can be either temporary or of long duration. The greater the extent of alteration in venous blood flow and endothelial cell injury due to clinically apparent causes, the more likely the alterations are be to be temporary. Such patients may need secondary thromboprophylaxis for only such time as required for them to recover from their provoking insult. However, those patients whose VTE occurred in the absence of any clinically apparent reason for significant alteration of venous blood flow in conjunction with alteration in venous endothelial physiology may be more likely to have an endogenous defect in blood coagulability that may not be readily reversible. Such patients may require protracted secondary thromboprophylaxis to prevent recurrent VTE. The clinical significance of the concepts of idiopathic and secondary VTE will be discussed to a greater extent in the Treatment component of this chapter.

PREVENTION

Background

The concept of prevention is based on three premises: (1) that VTE is an adverse clinical event, (2) that there exist definable groups of patients with a significantly higher than normal rates of VTE, and (3) that there exist effective and safe means to lower the incidence of VTE in these populations. The last two premises are facts borne out by extensive clinical and experimental evidence and really are not open to much question in an academic forum. However, the first of these premises is an opinion and, as such, is subject to varying intensity of acceptance by different individuals. While it is vanishingly rare that anyone openly suggests that fatal pulmonary emboli are not adverse experiences, some raise the question that a low postoperative pulmonary embolism mortality rate of 0.2% to 0.3% may not "outweigh the risk (and, nowadays, justify the financial cost)" of prophylaxis,[20] especially given the results of an audit of postoperative outcomes of hip replacement procedures with and without "chemical thromboprophylaxis" (not further defined) that demonstrated no difference in PE mortality at 42 days between the groups.[21] The clinical significance of other, nonfatal manifestations of VTE are questioned with some frequency, especially those manifestations associated with minimal immediately apparent symptoms. This is especially true when the patients in question are thought to be at risk for adverse outcomes from prophylactic interventions, such as the risk of bleeding from prophylactic anticoagulant therapy in postoperative patients. Since most of the studies of incidence and prevention of VTE in various patient populations have asymptomatic VTE as endpoints, the first premise is often called into question since neither the patient nor the practitioner is aware of the VTE and, consequently, cannot ascribe any subsequent adverse event to it. Also, because many of the studies on which the second premise is based involve the detection of asymptomatic VTE and since the individual practitioner never sees asymptomatic VTE, he has a tendency to think that the frequency of VTE in his patient population is not significantly higher than the general population (in whom he rarely sees symptomatic VTE as well). Since no therapeutic intervention is perfect, some patients experience clinically evident VTE despite the use of prophylactic measures, calling into question the first component of the third premise, especially if the practitioner has had this occur in one of his or his colleagues' patients. Finally, the groups of patients at highest risk for VTE (postoperative patients and those with major trauma; or victims of severe medical disease) are also at higher risk of bleeding, a complication widely regarded as an unacceptable outcome, particularly of elective surgery. Bleeding in patients who have been given anticoagulant agents is too often perceived as being caused by the anticoagulant rather than the underlying disease, calling into question the latter component of the third premise. The consulting hematologist must be aware that not all practitioners are truly convinced that the premises on which the concept of prophylaxis are based are valid in the population of patients that they personally treat. Consequently, the concept and use of prophylaxis will be found to be embraced to varying degrees by individual practitioners and groups of specialists; occasionally, the concept of prophylaxis will be greeted with overt animosity.[22] These concepts may help to explain why, after a generation of intense study, thromboprophylaxis is still underused[23] and why formal education processes have only marginal benefit in increasing its utilization.[24] Unless the consulting hematologist is aware of these often unstated mindsets among many practitioners and uses this awareness in interactions with them, personal experience suggests that effectiveness as a consultant will be limited.

In approaching both the patient's bedside as well as the voluminous literature on the subject of primary thromboprophylaxis, several points must been borne in mind:

1. Most patients with fatal pulmonary emboli have such massive emboli as to cause cardiac arrest and die despite medical intervention[25] or to cause death within 30 minutes or so from the onset of symptoms—too short a period of time to allow therapy to be given.[26,27]
2. Most pulmonary emboli in high-risk patients arise from asymptomatic DVT.[26] Hence, most fatal emboli have no symptoms of VTE until shortly before death.
3. Therefore, to prevent fatal pulmonary emboli one has to prevent asymptomatic DVT.
4. By inference, then, anything that lowers the incidence of asymptomatic DVT will lower the incidence of fatal PE to a similar extent (recognizing this is a reasonable, though unproven, concept).

The consulting hematologist must have the concept firmly understood: The primary goal of thromboprophylaxis is prevention of fatal PE by the prevention of the absolute requirement for fatal PE—DVT, generally asymptomatic DVT of the leg.

General Medical and Surgical Patients

Generally, prospective studies evaluating the incidence of VTE and methods of prevention of VTE in various patient populations have considered primarily the effect of various pathologic states on diverse groups of individuals (surgery, stroke, myocardial infarction, acute infectious disease, etc.) without prospectively considering patient-specific risk factors (obesity, varicose veins, estrogen treatment, prior history of VTE, etc.) in analyzing the outcome. Consequently, practitioners dealing with specific procedures or diseases that have been widely studied are generally conversant with techniques of thromboprophylaxis in the pathologic states seen in their specialty and do not seek help from consultants for their routine patients. These techniques are periodically reviewed in great depth and these reviews are used by many practitioners to update their practice.[26] However, many of these specialists will seek consultation to help with patients they perceive as having an unusually high risk of thrombosis due to patient-specific abnormalities, generally when that patient is scheduled for an elective operation or suffers acute medical or surgical illness. It is the outcomes of these patients that is of greatest concern for the consulting hematologist.

The list of patient-specific risk factors for VTE is fairly extensive: age (starting at 40), immobility/paralysis, prior VTE, cancer, varicose veins, obesity, congestive heart failure, myocardial infarction, stroke, bone fractures, inflammatory bowel disease, nephrotic syndrome, and estrogen use.[26] While it is fairly certain that patients with these entities are at higher than normal risk for VTE, most of the data from which that determination is derived come from patients in clinical circumstances different from the postoperative state or the presence of acute illness,[28] areas that generally encountered by the consultant. The data that state that these patients are at unusual risk for thrombosis in these situations are often limited, coming from extrapolation from nonacutely ill populations or from post-hoc analyses of limited numbers of studies in which all relevant variables have not been prospectively taken into consideration. For instance, patients undergoing various surgical procedures for malignancy are found to have higher rates of postoperative VTE than patients undergoing surgery for nonmalignant conditions.[28] However, the extent and duration of the surgical procedures in the malignant and nonmalignant groups are rarely compared, as are other potentially additive patient-specific risk factors. When analyzed in a multivariate model, many of these risk factors, such as malignancy, age, estrogen use, and obesity, end up not being significant in many studies. Importantly for the consultant, the contribution of these risk factors to the subsequent development of VTE is difficult to quantitate, making a precise risk : benefit ratio determination difficult, if not impossible. However, as a practical rule of thumb, the older and sicker the patient is, the more likely he or she is to develop VTE under any circumstance of acute medical/surgical illness. The categories of risk range from low (less than 0.01% fatal PE) to very high (up to 5% risk of fatal PE). These categories and examples of patients generally thought to fall within these categories are listed in Table 14–2. While it has not frequently been subjected to prospective clinical study, it is also reasonable to assume that the greater an individual's risk for VTE, the more likely he or she is to fail in response to standard methods of thromboprophylaxis. Consequently, in these patients it is generally reasonable to intensify and/or prolong the efforts at thromboprophylaxis—greater risk of VTE justifies the greater risk of more intense prophylaxis. Typical thromboprophylaxis regimens generally recommended for the various risk categories are listed in Table 14–2.

Recent studies have tried to quantify the contribution of a large number of clinical abnormalities to the development of a patient's first episode of symptomatic VTE using multivariate logistic regression analysis to control for the existence of many potential prothrombotic states in one person.[27] These investigators confirmed that many of the classically regarded risk factors, such as age, obesity, estrogen therapy, and congestive heart failure, while being associated with clinically apparent VTE on univariate analysis, are not significantly associated on multivariate analysis. The odds ratios for the various risk factors that stood out on multivariate analysis are shown in Figure 14–1. As expected, the greatest risks were associated with surgery, trauma, and in-patient hospitalization, with lesser risks being conferred by malignancy, neurologic disease, varicose veins, and superficial venous thrombosis. While this information is helpful in understanding the pathophysiology of VTE, it is impossible to use in estimating the risk : benefit ratio of VTE prophylaxis in a given patient without knowing the baseline risk of VTE in the population being studied. By assuming the baseline risk is approximately 250 cases per 1,000,000 persons per year, somewhat lower for those of Hispanic, Asian, or Pacific Island descent,[29] these data can be used to estimate the absolute risk of first episode of VTE in the patient populations studied. For instance, using the 95th percentile of the confidence interval for the odds of developing symptomatic first episode of VTE in patients with malignancy undergoing chemotherapy (an odds ratio of approximately 20), the absolute risk may be as high as approximately 5000 cases per 1,000,000 patient-years, or 0.5% per patient-year. It should be pointed out that this rate is the "tip of the iceberg"—the rate of symptomatic VTE. The actual rate, including asymptomatic VTE (which poses a risk of fatal PE), is probably much higher. If, for instance, the absolute rate of all VTE is assumed to be 10 times that of the symptomatic rate (as it appears to be in patients dismissed from the hospital after total hip replacement—see below), then the rate could be as high as 5% per patient-year, a rate that probably exceeds the rate of medical complications of pharmacologic prophylaxis under these circumstances.[30] This type of data can be helpful when trying to determine the wisdom of using

Table 14-2 • **THE FOUR STRATA OF RISK FOR POSTOPERATIVE VTE WITH EXAMPLES OF PATIENTS THOUGHT TO FALL WITHIN EACH STRATUM AND PROPHYLACTIC MANEUVERS THOUGHT TO BE SUCCESSFUL FOR THEM**

	Low	Moderate	High	Highest
Examples	Uncomplicated minor surgery in patients <40 yrs with no clinical risk factors	Any surgery (major and minor) in patients 40–60 yrs but no additional risk factors; major surgery in patients <40 yrs but no additional risk factors; minor surgery in patients with risk factors	Major surgery in patients >60 yrs without additional risk factors; major surgery in patients 40–60 yrs who have additional risk factors; patients with MI and medical patients with risk factors	Major surgery in patients >40 yrs plus prior VTE or malignant disease or hypercoagulable state; patients with elective major lower extremity orthopedic surgery, or hip fracture, or stroke, or multiple trauma, or spinal cord injury
Calf vein thrombosis, %	2	10–20	20–40	40–80
Proximal vein thrombosis, %	0.4	2–4	4–8	10–20
Clinical PE, %	0.2	1–2	2–4	4–10
Fatal PE, %	0.002	0.1–0.4	0.4–1.0	1–5
Successful preventive strategies	No specific measures	LDUH (q12h), LMWH, IPC, and ES	LDUH (q8h), LMWH, and IPC	LMWH, oral anticoagulants, IPC (+ LDUH or LMWH), and ADH

ADH, adjusted-dose heparin; LDUH, low-dose unfractionated heparin; LMWH, low-molecular-weight heparin; IPC, intermittent pneumatic compression stockings; ES, elastic stockings.
Modified from Clagett GP, Anderson FA Jr, Geerts W, et al. Prevention of venous thromboembolism. Chest 1998;114 (suppl):531S–560S, with permission.

prolonged VTE prophylaxis in patients who do not fit neatly into the standard risk categories.

Methods of Prophylaxis

Methods of thromboprophylaxis are generally divided into two categories, pharmacologic and mechanical. In the setting of an acutely ill patient, the former generally relies on a heparin preparation (with the exception of elective hip replacement) and the latter on intermittent pneumatic compression (IPC) boots with or without elastic compression stockings, which are viewed as minimizing venous stasis and dilation as well as stimulating local fibrinolysis. In patients perceived to be at highest risk of VTE, the heparin regimens most frequently recommended use unfractionated heparin (UH) given in doses adjusted sufficiently high to prolong the partial thromboplastin time (aPTT) or a low-molecular-weight heparin (LMWH) in a fixed dose. Because of the need for laboratory monitoring, the lack of widely available standards for determining the institution-specific therapeutic range for the aPTT, and the rare case of heparin-induced thrombocytopenia with thrombosis, the use of adjusted-dose UH is rapidly falling into disuse in favor of fixed-dose LMWH, especially with the highest-risk patients. The heparin-based regimens of prophylaxis are widely held to pose a risk of bleeding, though most controlled studies show at most an increased incidence of superficial, minor bleeding when compared to placebo. Mechanical methods of prophylaxis pose no known risk of bleeding. IPC is as effective as fixed-dose UH in postoperative patients,[26] though its efficacy compared to adjusted-dose UH or LMWH has not been evaluated. Because their presumed mechanisms of action are different, it is widely assumed that the efficacies and toxicities as mechanical and pharmacologic thromboprophylactic maneuvers are additive. Since there are no predictable toxicities of IPC, the general belief is that combined IPC and LMWH therapy will provide a degree of prophylaxis greater than either agent alone yet with no more toxicity than LMWH itself. That belief has been substantiated in at least one clinical trial of

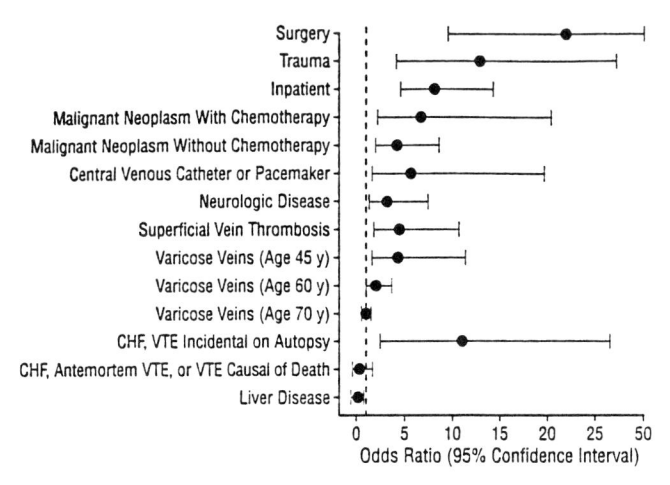

Figure 14-1 Odds Ratio and 95% confidence intervals of risk factors for first episode of VTE. CHF, congestive heart failure. (From Heit JA, Silverstein MD, Mohr DN, et al. Risk factors for deep vein thrombosis and pulmonary embolism: A population-based case-control study. Arch Intern Med 2000;160:809–815, with permission. Copyrighted 2000, American Medical Association.)

patients after cardiac surgery.[31] Such combined therapy is suggested for the highest-risk patients[26] and is a reasonable recommendation for the consultant to use in patients with a multiplicity of risk factors thought to be at high risk of failure with a single modality. It must be remembered, however, that IPC must be properly applied and monitored to be effective—something that is not always to be assumed can be accomplished in the hospital[32] let alone in an outpatient setting. In these highest-risk patients for whom the frequency of failure of prophylaxis is unknown and the consequences of failure can be catastrophic, monitoring for the development of asymptomatic DVT theoretically would be helpful; if found, aggressive therapy with anticoagulants, or possibly IVC filters, could be instituted. While this concept has proven valid, it has only been found to be helpful in situations where radiofibrinogen scanning for surveillance followed by venography confirmation of positive results was used. Radiofibrinogen scanning is no longer clinically available in the United States, and the only noninvasive method of detection of DVT that is available—duplex ultrasound—is not sensitive to asymptomatic DVT.[33] However, since many of these asymptomatic DVTs are short and/or nonocclusive[34] and (presumably) fatal PEs might come from larger thrombi more readily visualized with ultrasonography, ultrasound monitoring might be a reasonable suggestion for a patient perceived to be at high risk for failure of primary thromboprophylaxis.[35]

In addition to using combined mechanical/pharmacologic means to intensify prophylaxis, extending the duration of prophylaxis may also be helpful in the highest-risk patients. For years, studies of the efficacy of thromboprophylaxis in acutely ill patients was limited to the period of time the patient was hospitalized, basically because it was not easy to obtain study endpoints (venography or radiofibrinogen monitoring) as an outpatient, a time the patient's clinical care was generally not in the control of an investigating physician. Most practitioners, however, have seen patients return with symptomatic VTE several weeks postoperatively, underscoring the fact that the prothrombotic stimuli did not resolve once the patient left the confines of the hospital for home. An increasing body of literature, generally examining hip replacement patients as a risk model, demonstrates a significant frequency of VTE that develops in the 4 or so weeks posthospitalization[36–39] with an incidence in the 20% range. However, most of these are asymptomatic DVTs (the incidence of symptomatic VTE is lower, about 2%)[40] prompting some investigators to question their significance.[26] They still mark the presence of a disorder with life-threatening potential and are, consequently, clinically significant—all the more so if they are preventable. Results of four randomized, prospective, venogram endpoint trials show that LMWH, and possibly UH, given for 3 to 4 weeks postoperatively lowers the rate of DVT by about half.[36–38,41] While posthospital warfarin therapy is often used in these situations and is recommended based on the belief that it is safe and effective,[26] there are no direct data to substantiate either the belief or the practice. Indeed, results of a recent study evaluating hip replacement patients with ultrasound exams for a month postoperatively while being treated with warfarin shows that this therapy has a failure rate of at least 15%,[42] almost as high as the 19% to 25% incidence of DVT seen in patients not given any posthospital prophylaxis.[39,41] For patients at high risk of development of posthospital VTE, protracted prophylaxis seems a reasonable recommendation for the consultant to consider. Since there is some evidence that weight-bearing exercise lowers the rate of VTE following hip replacement,[41] a reasonable duration to consider is an open-ended one, namely until the patient is back to full weight-bearing activity.

Hospitalized General Medical Patients

While patients with acute medical illness have long been recognized as having a greater than normal risk of VTE, the use of thromboprophylaxis has not been as well studied as it has in surgical patients. Until recently, the largest trials of thromboprophylaxis in general medical patients used fixed-dose UH and used mortality as a primary endpoint, not VTE. Meta-analyses of these trials have suggested that the use of heparin might lower mortality by as much as 20%.[43,43a] This reduction in mortality was apparent beginning with the first day of therapy. In both timing and magnitude, it is doubtful that the improved mortality attributable to heparin prophylaxis is due to prevention of fatal PE because of differing methods used to detect VTE.[43a] Consequently, while UH might affect overall mortality among patients with acute medical illness, there were few data on the actual prevalence of VTE in this population or the effect of UH on it until recently. A pair of prospective, randomized, controlled trials have shed some light on these issues.[44,45] In the larger trial, two doses of LMWH (20 and 40 mg of enoxaparin daily) were compared to placebo with predismissal venography and 110-day symptomatic VTE as endpoints.[45] To facilitate the consultant in determining which medical patients were studied, so that one might duplicate these patients in their clinical practice, the inclusion and exclusion criteria are listed in Table 14–3. This study showed that patients randomized to placebo have a 14.9% incidence of VTE prior to dismissal (virtually all asymptomatic) and an additional 2.2% incidence of symptomatic VTE over the subsequent 100 days. The patients randomized to 20 mg of enoxaparin had outcomes indistinguishable from those of the placebo group, but the patients randomized to 40 mg had a significant reduction to a 5.5% incidence of in-hospital events and an additional 1.5% incidence of posthospital symptomatic VTE—for the first time demonstrating a therapy that affects the natural history of VTE in a well-defined group of medically ill patients with a moderate VTE risk. Another study in a similar number of patients with medical illness showed no difference in the frequency of radiofibrinogen scan positivity with 20 mg of enoxaparin once daily and 5000 units UH twice daily. The combination of the two studies suggests that 5000 units UH twice daily and 20 mg enoxaparin daily are equivalent and no more efficacious than

Table 14–3 • ENROLLMENT CRITERIA FOR A STUDY OF THE EFFICACY OF LMWH IN PREVENTING VTE IN PATIENTS WITH ACUTE MEDICAL ILLNESS

Inclusion Criteria
- \>40 years old, not immobilized for more than 3 days prior to hospitalization
- Congestive heart failure (NYHA class III or IV), *or*
- Acute respiratory failure (not intubated), *or*
- At least one of the following from A plus at least one from B:
  A. Acute infection, without shock
     Acute rheumatic disorders
     Acute inflammatory bowel disease
  B. \>75 years old
     Previous venous thromboembolism
     Obesity (body mass index > 30 for men, 28.6 for women)
     Varicose veins
     Cancer
     Hormone therapy (except for postmenopausal replacement)
     Chronic heart or respiratory failure

Exclusion Criteria
- Creatinine >1.7
- Stroke or major surgery in past 3 months
- Human immunodeficiency virus infection
- Uncontrolled hypertension (>200 mm Hg systolic or >120 mm Hg diastolic)
- Active peptic ulcer
- Required anticoagulant therapy for other reasons

These data can be used to help determine if any given patient might benefit from use of enoxaparin.

From Samama MM, Cohen AT, Darmon J-Y, et al. A comparison of enoxaparin with placebo for the prevention of venous thromboembolism in acutely ill medical patients. N Engl J Med 1999;341:793–800, with permission.

placebo, while 40 mg enoxaparin daily is effective in preventing VTE in patients with common acute medical illnesses. As with joint replacement patients, there is no reason to believe that the risk of VTE ends with hospital dismissal in medical patients. Indeed, there is a baseline frequency of symptomatic VTE of about 2% after dismissal in this population and it does not appear to be affected by in-hospital therapy.[45] Consequently, in medical patients perceived to be at highest risk of VTE, prolonged posthospital prophylaxis is reasonable to consider until lack of efficacy or undue toxicity is proven in clinical trials. As with surgical patients, the duration should be open-ended—until the patient returns to his pre-hospital functional status. Since LMWH (40 mg of enoxaparin daily) is safe and efficacious during the acute portion of their illness and is effective in preventing postdismissal VTE in hip replacement patients, it seems reasonable to suggest its use in the convalescent period of their illness until something is proven to work as well, or better.

Travel

Much is often made of the risk of VTE complicating travel, particularly airline travel, where the term *economy class syndrome* has been coined to describe it.[46] While patients who have been traveling do indeed develop VTE, the assumption has been made that they have an unusually high incidence of VTE is based on the premise that they have venous stasis due to their cramped position and prolonged immobility. However, as previously pointed out, stasis alone has never been shown to predispose to VTE.[8] Consequently, the basis for the assumption that travel alone predisposes to VTE is erroneous. When looked at objectively, a history of travel (even prolonged air travel) is found as often in patients suspected, but found not to have, VTE as it is in patients who actually have VTE[47] or is recalled by patients as often preceding a 4-year follow-up visit as it was at presentation.[48] While travel in excess of 5 hours is more common in patients with VTE than in unmatched controls,[49] those with VTE related to travel often have other accepted risk factors for thrombosis.[46,50,50a] Consequently, the decision to use VTE prophylaxis in patients planning a trip should be based as much on patient-specific variables as on the type and duration of the travel. It seems reasonable to use effective prophylaxis, including pharmacologic methods, in patients with known risk factors for VTE if they are planning a trip requiring several hours of relative immobility or an airline flight in excess of 3000 miles.[50b] The most effective type and duration of prophylaxis, or whether intermittent bursts of aerobic activity during the trip would suffice in the absence of medication, is not known. Until more is known about travel as an additive risk for VTE, it seems reasonable to assume that the more risk factors that are present, the longer and/or more intense the prophylaxis should be.

Prophylaxis with Inferior Vena Cava Filters

Placement of an inferior vena cava (IVC) filter is occasionally recommended to prevent fatal PE in high-risk patients, often to the exclusion of other means of thromboprophylaxis. However, despite their generalized use in clinical practice for almost 30 years, there has never been a controlled study that demonstrates that, in the absence of anticoagulant therapy, they prevent any PE (let alone fatal PE) in any patient population. In the only prospective, randomized trial of IVC filters (in active DVT, not as primary prophylaxis), patients randomized to receive a filter had a similar rate of PE and mortality but a higher incidence of symptomatic DVT in the 1.5 years of follow-up after anticoagulation was discontinued compared to patients initially treated with anticoagulants alone.[51] This landmark study (which will be discussed in more detail in the Therapy section) suggested that filters may not do what they were designed to do: prevent fatal PE and eliminate the need for (and risk of) anticoagulant therapy. Consequently, IVC filters should be considered as primary thromboprophylaxis only in patients with a predictably high incidence of failure of proven forms of prophylaxis or a predictably high likelihood of complications of these maneuvers. Unfortunately, data do not exist that would allow this author to provide guidelines more specific than this. Such patients will be very rare in clinical practice. (See Chapters 37 and 38.)

DIAGNOSIS

Background and Significance

Whereas the risk of VTE to life and limb is considerable, therapy of VTE involves very real risks to the patient: the risks of death or disability from anticoagulant or fibrinolytic therapy. In addition to the obvious risks of prolonged use of anticoagulants, the diagnosis of idiopathic VTE colors virtually all the medical decisions that will be made for the remainder of the patients' life (contraception, pregnancy, postmenopausal hormone replacement, aggressiveness of evaluating new cardiopulmonary symptoms, intensity of postoperative thromboprophylaxis, etc.), especially if the thrombosis is recurrent. Consequently, the diagnosis of VTE, both the initial and recurrent events, has profound and long-reaching implications for patient care and should be approached accordingly. Even though it has been recognized for a generation that the clinical diagnosis of DVT and PE is unreliable and that objective means of diagnosis are mandatory, as recently as 1997, treatment for PE was often prescribed without definitive imaging diagnosis.[52] An encyclopedic evaluation of all of the objective means for making or excluding a diagnosis of VTE is beyond the scope of this chapter. Even if it were the goal, such a chapter would be doomed to failure because of the rapid advance of the technology of vascular imaging. Instead, this chapter will provide information on diagnostic problems frequently encountered by the hematology consultant.

Recurrent DVT of the Leg: A Major, Common Problem

Since the advent of duplex ultrasonography, the diagnosis of the initial episode of DVT in the veins proximal to the knee has almost ceased to be a major quandary. This readily available procedure is quite sensitive and specific and has virtually replaced all other diagnostic tools in both clinical practice and in clinical research. Now the major area of concern to the consultant is the diagnosis of recurrent DVT of the leg. Recurrent DVT generally results in potentially more toxic forms of therapy than the index case. If the DVT recurs while on anticoagulant therapy, more aggressive degrees of anticoagulation or addition of an IVC filter is often recommended. If it recurs after cessation of anticoagulant therapy, a more protracted course of anticoagulation is generally prescribed. Consequently, the diagnosis of recurrent DVT should not be made lightly. In the case of alleged recurrence while on anticoagulation, the consultant can often be helpful by simply knowing the response to standard therapy. It is widely assumed that once anticoagulant therapy has begun, all thrombus formation ceases and the endogenous fibrinolytic system rapidly begins to "dissolve" the clot, eliminating all traces of the thrombus prior to cessation of the standard course of anticoagulation and preventing long-term sequelae of the DVT. This is not necessarily true. In their seminal 1977 study comparing fibrinolytic and anticoagulant therapy of DVT, Marder and coworkers found a 33% incidence of thrombus extension (as determined by pre- and post-therapy venograms) after 5 days of what was assumed to be "adequate" heparin therapy.[53] The doses of heparin and the PTTs achieved were similar in patients with and without thrombus extension. Since then, using repeat venograms or ultrasound exams, studies have shown that standard anticoagulant therapy is associated with a remarkably consistent 26% to 44% incidence of thrombus extension over the initial 5 to 30 days of therapy.[54-59] Indeed, surveillance ultrasound studies have shown that while on anticoagulant therapy, 6% of patients are found to develop new DVT in the leg contralateral to the one with the initial DVT.[59] Thrombus propagation generally occurs in the first 5 or 6 weeks after initiation of therapy, but is often seen in the first week, and is generally asymptomatic. Where studied, neither the degree of anticoagulation nor classical risk factors for VTE generally correlated with asymptomatic extension of or development of new DVT. One study demonstrated that the fraction of the time that anticoagulation was considered adequate by laboratory parameters (INR above 2.0 or heparin concentration above 0.2 units/mL) was inversely proportional to the risk of extension,[58] while another reported that extension was more common in patients with extensive venous thrombosis at presentation.[59] Studies focusing only on symptomatic recurrences (DVT extension, new DVT, or PE) show a lower incidence of recurrence, generally in the 5% to 8% range.[60-63] Symptomatic recurrences (seen after the patient has been on warfarin for some time) can generally be divided into two definable categories: those associated with predictably inadequate degrees of anticoagulation and those with underlying malignancy.[64,65] The long-term clinical outcome of the patients observed to have thrombus extension relative to those without extension generally is not reported in these studies, but one has shown that propagation is more likely to be associated with development of venous valvular insufficiency.[59] None of the studies suggest that there is a greater mortality rate associated with extension while on therapy (with the exception of those patients whose recurrence was associated with malignancy, whose deaths were attributed to the cancer rather than the thrombus extension).

How can this knowledge be helpful to the hematology consultant and the patients he or she is called to see? Often, repeat ultrasound studies are done after beginning therapy to "see how the clot is doing" or to investigate complaints of recurrent swelling or discomfort that the patient experiences after leaving the enforced bed rest of hospitalization for the unrestricted, upright activity of daily life. When these studies show that the thrombus is affecting a segment of vein that was not involved at presentation, "therapeutic failure" is declared and consultation is sought. In these instances, the consultant should examine the data to determine the precise anatomic degree of extension and try to determine the prognosis of the extension relative to adverse long-term events (greater likelihood of subsequent venous insufficiency or death from PE) as well as any reversible risk factors for subsequent extension (degree of anticoagulation predictably associated with recurrence by laboratory parameters, underlying malignancy). The consultant should examine the laboratory data defining the intensity of the patient's anticoagulant response to therapy. Frequently, it was the referring physician's intent to achieve adequate degrees of anticoagulation rather than the actuality. If the anatomic degree of thrombus extension is limited and the additive clot burden is thought to be of little additional threat to the patient's life or lifestyle, then continuation of medical therapy without intensification is reasonable given the recognition that this is a common occurrence in patients given standard therapy, especially in the first few weeks of treatment, and poses no as yet well-defined risk to the patient. A temporary increase in the intensity of anticoagulation is not unreasonable as long as it is not so intense or given for such a protracted period as to pose an additional significant risk of toxicity. The temptation to label these patients failures of medical therapy, stop anticoagulants, and rely on an IVC filter alone must be avoided. Also, if these small extensions occur while on warfarin therapy, especially in the first few weeks after cessation of heparin, the patients should not be labeled as "refractory to warfarin" and consigned to long-term heparin therapy. If the extension while on warfarin is highly symptomatic or anatomically large, a detailed search for an underlying malignancy should be considered. If the large or symptomatic recurrence occurs while on heparin therapy (or shortly after its discontinuance), a diagnosis of heparin-induced thrombosis with thrombocytopenia (or with a major drop in the platelet count) should be strongly considered—so strongly that heparin therapy should be withheld until this diagnosis can be ruled out reasonably. The diagnostic and therapeutic considerations when evaluating the possibility of warfarin failure are outlined in Table 14–4.

Thrombi that enlarge asymptomatically while on standard anticoagulant therapy are often encountered in clinical practice because they are easily found by surveillance ultrasonography. The fact that these asymptomatic thrombi occur frequently and without obvious immediate adverse outcomes makes it difficult to know how to intervene when it occurs—a syndrome easily diagnosed but with uncertain therapeutic implications. At the other end of the clinical spectrum is the patient with recurrent symptoms suggesting a new DVT but who does not have recurrence. Therapy of these patients (at least in reference to their anticoagulant therapy) is straightforward, but the lack of recurrence is difficult to diagnose. To understand this syndrome, the consultant has to be familiar with the long-term course of treated DVT. Anatomically, resolution of DVT detectable by ultrasound occurs in only 40% to 70% of patients treated with standard anticoagulant therapy.[66–70] Persistent abnormalities, including noncompressibility of the vein (the hallmark finding of acute DVT), are present in a majority to significant minority of patients after their first episode of DVT. It is assumed that the initially fibrin/platelet thrombus gradually becomes replaced with collagenous cicatrix at an unknown rate after anticoagulant therapy is begun and that these persistent imaging abnormalities represent scar tissue that will remain as an occlusion of the vein indefinitely. While much is often made in clinical practice about the ultrasonographic appearance of the persistent imaging abnormalities relative to its age (new versus old), none of the ultrasound characteristics often reported have been validated as being either sensitive or specific for recurrent thrombosis.[71] Consequently, persistent incompressibility of the vein in a patient with recurrent symptoms of DVT is not specific for recurrent thrombosis—it may be the original thrombus having undergone the process of organization. These findings would be only academic save for the fact that most patients have recurrent symptoms (pain and/or swelling) after their first episode of DVT that are clinically indistinguishable from recur-

Table 14–4 • CONSIDERATIONS WHEN EVALUATING POSSIBLE WARFARIN FAILURE

Diagnosis	Explanation	Therapeutic Options
Clot has extended, degree of extension is small	Occurs in up to 45% of patients in first month of therapy; no known adverse outcomes	Resist labeling a "warfarin failure" Resist IVC filter Continue therapy
Clot has extended, degree of extension is large	Trousseau syndrome Lower than target INR Unstable INR with disparate prothrombin and protein C levels Heparin-induced thrombocytopenia with thrombosis	Focused cancer search, switch to heparin if found Consider adding heparin until INR is stable in 2.0–3.0 range if cancer is not found Check platelet count and assay for heparin-dependent antiplatelet antibodies, start alternative anticoagulant if positive
No clot extension	Postphlebitic syndrome: worsens after cessation of bed rest	Resist labeling a "warfarin failure" Resist IVC filter Add support stockings Continue therapy
No clot found	Alternative diagnoses Baker's cyst hematoma, cellulitis, etc.	Diagnose and treat new disease

rence, but are caused by venous hypertension (the postphlebitic syndrome). Such symptoms occur in between 30% and 70% of DVT patients.[72–74] The hematology consultant is frequently called in to adjudicate whether the new patients symptoms associated with venous incompressibility on ultrasonography reflect a new DVT or are due to venous insufficiency. Patients with symptoms suggestive of recurrent DVT were referred to by Hull and colleagues as "a diagnostic challenge" in 1983[75] and remain inhabitants of "a problematic area" of diagnostic medicine in 1999.[71] Unfortunately, the diagnostic armamentarium of the modern imaging services has limited value to the consultant in these cases. For anything resembling a logical way to deal with these patients, we have to go back to diagnostic modalities in common use 20 years ago but not readily available today. At that time, contrast venography, impedance plethysmography, and radiolabeled fibrinogen scanning were readily available tools for diagnosis of DVT. A large cohort of patients (270 in total) who were not on anticoagulant therapy presenting with symptoms of recurrent DVT were evaluated initially with plethysmography followed by venography if the plethysmogram was abnormal and radiolabeled fibrinogen scanning if normal.[75] Anticoagulation was withheld unless the plethysmogram was abnormal and the patient had an intraluminal filling defect on venography or if the radiofibrinogen scan was positive. In this study, 181 patients (67%) had normal studies, had anticoagulation withheld, and were followed a mean of 20 months. This group had a 1.7% incidence of objectively verified recurrent VTE during the follow-up period, suggesting that two thirds of patients with symptoms of recurrent DVT after cessation of anticoagulant therapy do not have recurrence, and that this could be determined accurately with these two noninvasive diagnostic techniques. Seventy of the patients (26%) had abnormal plethysmograms and 45 of them had intraluminal filling defects on subsequent venography, suggesting that an abnormal plethysmogram at the time of recurrent symptoms was a reasonable indicator of recurrent DVT. The plethysmogram had reverted to normal after the initial episode of DVT in 12 of the patients presenting with recurrent DVT. At time of recurrence the plethysmogram had reverted from normal to abnormal in all 12, suggesting that serial plethysmography could be helpful in evaluating patients with symptoms of recurrent DVT. In all, 64 patients were found to have recurrent DVT by venography or radiofibrinogen scanning; plethysmography detected 45 (70%) and scanning found the other 18 patients. Observations of the utility of serial plethysmography after the initial DVT were extended in 1988 when it was demonstrated that 95% of patients had plethysmography that returned to normal by 1 year after the initial DVT.[76] Of this initial cohort, 31 patients presented with symptoms suggesting recurrent DVT after cessation of anticoagulation; 18 had persistently normal studies and anticoagulation was withheld with no adverse consequences. Of the 13 whose plethysmograms had converted from normal to abnormal, venography showed intraluminal filling defects in all cases. This study confirmed that (1) most patients with symptoms and signs suggesting recurrent DVT do not have recurrence; by inference, their symptoms were probably due to venous insufficiency caused by the initial DVT, and (2) if patients had undergone plethysmography as part of the follow-up of their initial DVT, plethysmography alone could dictate therapy in almost 85% of patients presenting with symptoms of recurrence. Unfortunately, the epidemic of blood-borne viral disease in the mid-1980s eliminated the feasibility of radiofibrinogen scanning and the advent of ultrasonography for diagnosis of first DVT in the early 1990s caused most vascular laboratories to relegate plethysmographs to the closet or the scrap pile.

So how do modern ultrasound imaging techniques help in the diagnosis of recurrent DVT? In short, they have not been well studied. The strength of ultrasonography in the diagnosis of first DVT—its specificity derived from its ability to image the veins in which thrombi are most likely to develop—may be its weakness in diagnosing recurrent DVT. In the group of patients in whom the thrombus never resolves, the collaterals that develop which allow venous return in the face of persistent obstruction of the major veins could thrombose. Since the precise anatomic location of these collaterals is unpredictable and, presumably, varies from patient to patient, the ultrasonographer has no idea where to look for them. If they cannot be found reliably, they cannot be imaged. Consequently, it is not unreasonable to infer that ultrasonography may miss those recurrent thromboses that develop in collateral veins, limiting the overall sensitivity of ultrasonography in the detection of recurrent DVT. The lack of anatomic specificity of plethysmography (it detects the rate of outflow of venous blood from the leg, independent of the vein through which the outflow occurs) may be the reason for its fairly high degree of sensitivity in cases of recurrent DVT. In the only study of ultrasonography for the detection of recurrent DVT published to date, a cohort of 145 patients with a DVT initially underwent ultrasonography and venography. They were then followed with repeat ultrasound exams at 1, 3, 6 and 12 months, which showed regression of clot size in most patients.[77] A total of 29 patients presented with signs and symptoms suggesting recurrence during this follow-up period and underwent repeat ultrasonography and venography. Of these 29, 10 patients (34%) were found to have new intraluminal filling defects in proximal veins on venography (confirming that only a minority of patients with symptoms of recurrence actually have recurrence). Of these 10 with recurrent DVT, 3 had new segments of incompressible vein that were normal on their most recent follow-up exam (not necessarily compared to the exam performed at time of initial diagnosis) and 7 had a 2-mm or greater increase in the diameter of previously noncompressible segments. The ultrasonographic findings on the patients without recurrence on venography showed no change or even improvement from previous exams. In two recent reviews of the subject, ultrasound exam was thought to be potentially helpful in the diagnosis of recurrent DVT only if results from ultrasound exams from the recovery phase (not from time of initial diagnosis) of the initial DVT were available for comparison,[71,78] something not generally available in clinical practice. While much is often made of the ultrasonographic appearance of the thrombus relative to its age ("old thrombi are echogenic, new thrombi are not"), this does not withstand objective scrutiny[79] and should not be relied upon in practice.

This information can be very helpful to the hematology consultant called to evaluate a patient with symptoms or signs suggestive of recurrent DVT. First the consultant should establish a working relationship with a vascular laboratory that is willing to perform plethysmography. Second, the consultant can work with the physicians who frequently refer patients to have them get follow-up ultrasonography and plethysmography on their DVT patients, particularly at the time anticoagulation is stopped and/or at approximately 1 year following the initial diagnosis. These follow-up studies provide invaluable comparators for studies done at the time of possible recurrence. If the pleythysmogram and the venous diameter on ultrasonography have not changed and no major new segments are noncompressible, then recurrence reasonably can be ruled out. For those rare patients with persistently abnormal plethysmograms or no readily available old studies for comparison, the diagnosis of recurrence cannot be made with any degree of objectivity. When symptoms suggestive of recurrent DVT occur in these patients, anticoagulant therapy would be reasonable until old records or old ultrasound videotapes can be obtained or the patient can be followed for several months to determine the course of the imaging abnormality. The importance of obtaining data on prior studies performed at other institutions cannot be overemphasized in these situations. If old studies simply do not exist, then following the patient while on anticoagulant therapy can be helpful. If plethysmography improves or the venous diameter decreases, then it is reasonable to infer that the patient suffered a recurrence and that continued anticoagulation is appropriate. Of course, venography could be performed on these patients, looking for intraluminal filling defects. However, without old venograms for comparison, objective interpretation will be difficult. Perhaps newer studies indicative of active thrombus formation such as D-dimer or thrombus-directed radiopharmaceuticals will make the diagnosis of recurrent DVT easier in the future. This area warrants close monitoring by consultants dealing with patients suffering from VTE.

Calf Vein Thrombosis

The diagnosis of acute calf vein thrombosis is made difficult by the multiplicity, small diameter, and often unpredictable anatomic location of these veins. Some of these veins are not routinely evaluated by compression ultrasonography in many labs. Unfortunately, isolated thrombi in veins not routinely interrogated, such as the soleal and gastrocnemial veins, account for almost half of the calf vein thrombi in some series.[80] Unless all the named veins are routinely evaluated, ultrasonography has a limited sensitivity for calf vein thrombosis compared to venography—a sensitivity as low as 36%.[81] While venography is considered the "gold standard" for the diagnosis of calf vein thrombosis, it also has its practical limitations. In addition to the obvious invasiveness and expense, it is a procedure that is rapidly becoming a lost art. It requires an experienced operator using a well-studied standardized technique and a cooperative patient to perform it well. Venographic techniques differ in their ability to produce evaluable studies by as much as 50%.[82] Even in academic medical centers, the percentage of venograms that are deemed "inadequate" by a panel of independent reviewers is as high as 41% in some series.[83] When venograms done under strict clinical research protocols are reviewed by different radiologists, discordant readings occur in up to 15% of patients.[84] If the consultant is relying on a venogram for a diagnosis, he or she should review the films personally and be convinced of the accuracy of their interpretation before proceeding with therapy. Magnetic resonance imaging (MRI) is being evaluated in some centers and is a promising tool. However, it will take some time, if ever, for this tool to be readily available to many of patients in whom the diagnosis of calf vein thrombosis is being considered. Given the lack of a simple, reliable imaging study, how should the diagnosis be approached by the consultant? The answer is that it depends on whether the thrombus would be treated if it is found (see the Treatment section). For many patients, thrombosis will not be treated until it is sufficiently large as to pose a risk of clinically significant embolization, generally indicated by propagation into the popliteal and more proximal veins. In these instances, serial ultrasound exams can be used to detect such propagation. However, in cases where the presence of calf vein thrombosis would result in treatment, ultrasonography can be tried. Despite its low sensitivity it has a specificity that is fairly high and treatment can be reasonably given if a positive result is obtained. However, if the ultrasonography does not reveal a thrombus, venography should be considered.

Pulmonary Embolism

Despite an increasingly large arsenal of diagnostic tools, the diagnosis of PE is still a clinical problem. The difficulty occurs mainly in patients with acute and chronic illness rather than the relatively rare, otherwise healthy patient with idiopathic VTE. The reasons behind the difficulty with the diagnosis of PE in patients with acute and chronic illnesses are many, and not always openly stated. In these patients simple, cheap, readily available, and nontoxic diagnostic modalities often do not give definitive results and more definitive studies involve predictable medical, social, and financial risks. Lung scans rarely are read as either normal or high probability because of underlying lung disease. D-dimer assays are usually not normal because of concurrent acute inflammatory disease. Patients are too ill to cooperate for spiral computed tomography (CT), and their renal function is often too borderline to risk contrast medium toxicity for angiography or CT; they may have too much

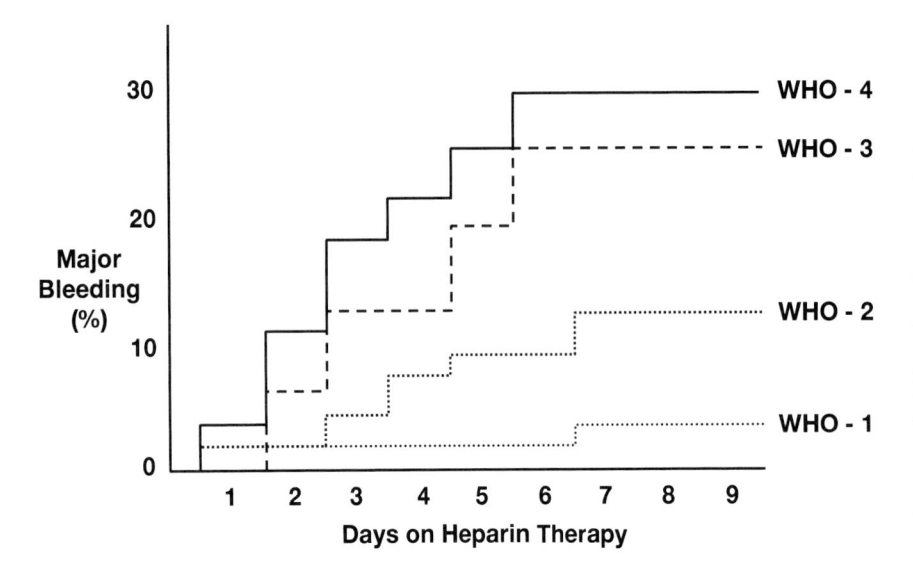

Figure 14-2 Cumulative incidence of major bleeding during the initial therapy of acute VTE with heparin or LMWH. WHO, World Health Organization functional status. WHO-1 is "restricted in physically strenuous activity, but ambulatory, and able to do light work"; WHO-2 is "ambulatory and capable of self-care, but unable to carry out any work"; WHO-3 is "capable of only limited self-care, confined to bed or chair 50% of waking hour"; WHO-4 is "completely disabled, unable to carry on any self-care." (Modified from Nieuwenhuis HK, Albada J, Banga JD, et al. Identification of risk factors for bleeding during treatment of acute venous thromboembolism with heparin or low molecular weight heparin. Blood 1991;78:2337–2343, with permission.)

implanted or attached hardware to undergo MRI, be reluctant to be transferred to institutions with selective angiography capability, or have already cost so much money that all involved in their care are not willing to spend more for an expensive imaging study with a less than 100% likelihood of being definitive. Despite all these problems of imaging, the major impediment to the diagnosis of PE in this population is the fact that it is not seriously considered in the differential diagnosis of the patient's syndrome. While it seems self-evident, studies confirm that if the diagnosis of PE is considered and attempts to pursue the diagnosis are made, PE is much more likely to be found.[85] It is less likely to be considered and pursued in elderly patients and those with acute lung disease.[85] The hematology consultant can be helpful here by continually trying to maintain awareness of the problem in the physicians who send referrals by advocating and aggressively recommending thromboprophylaxis and including PE in the differential diagnosis of appropriate patients.

The consultant is often called to help determine the presence or absence of PE in hospitalized patients with several risk factors for VTE, a clinical syndrome compatible with PE (but several other disease processes as well) and a non-high-probability lung scan. At this point, the consultant must start the evaluation by using his or her general medical background to determine what the patient's likelihood of having a PE is and what the patient's risk of bad outcome is if PE is present but not treated or treated but not present. In large part, the answers to these questions will determine how aggressively he or she will suggest pursuing the diagnosis. The likelihood of having a PE is directly proportional to the number and strength of the patient's risk factors and inversely proportional to the number of rational alternative explanations for the patient's syndrome. In patients with a high likelihood (greater than 80% to 90%) of having PE and a low likelihood of major bleeding complications from therapy (less than 5% to 7%), the consultant may be justified in accepting an imperfect imaging study and recommending anticoagulant therapy.[86] On the other hand, if the probability of PE is lower and/or

the risk of therapeutic toxicity is higher (as they both tend to be in many patients with acute and chronic disease) then the risk of more definitive imaging studies like angiography is justified. This is especially true in patients with a risk factor such as immobilization, leg trauma, and central venous instrumentation where lung scans read as "very low probability" have a prevalence of PE as high as 20%.[87] While the likelihood of PE is impossible to quantitate in any individual patient, recent studies have suggested that the risk of anticoagulant-related bleeding is reasonably predictable using readily available clinically definable parameters, and is as high as 23% over a 3-month period in many patients with serious underlying disease (Figs. 14–2 and 14–3).[88,89] Modern studies show that pulmonary angiography is a

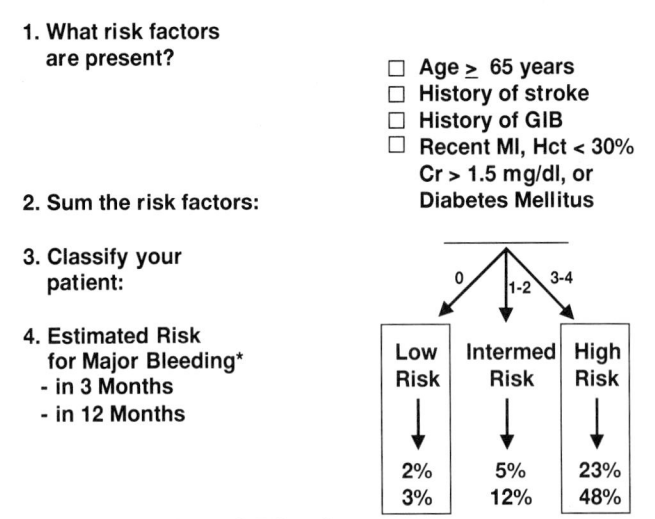

1. What risk factors are present?
   - ☐ Age ≥ 65 years
   - ☐ History of stroke
   - ☐ History of GIB
   - ☐ Recent MI, Hct < 30% Cr > 1.5 mg/dl, or Diabetes Mellitus

2. Sum the risk factors:

3. Classify your patient:

   0 → Low Risk
   1-2 → Intermed Risk
   3-4 → High Risk

4. Estimated Risk for Major Bleeding*
   - in 3 Months
   - in 12 Months

   Low Risk: 2% / 3%
   Intermed Risk: 5% / 12%
   High Risk: 23% / 48%

*based on 1 cohort of 556 patients

Figure 14-3 The "Outpatient Bleeding Risk Index," derived from a prospective evaluation of a cohort of 556 patients. The index can be used to estimate the risk of major bleeding during outpatient warfarin therapy. GIB, gastrointestinal bleeding; MI, myocardial infarction; Hct, hematocrit; Cr, serum creatinine concentration. (Modified from Beyth RJ, Quinn LM, Landefeld CS. Prospective evaluation of an index for predicting the risk of major bleeding in outpatients treatment with warfarin. Am J Med 1998;105:91–99, with permission from Excerpta Medica Inc.)

procedure with a sufficiently good risk : benefit ratio to use in these difficult cases, even in elderly individuals,[90-92] in whom the incidence of diagnostic lung scans decreases.[93] Consequently, in cases like these, the consultant should initially answer the question "Why should the patient *not* undergo angiography?"

Most referring physicians are well aware of the fact that pulmonary angiography is as close to being the definitive diagnostic technique for PE as is possible short of an autopsy, but are asking the consulting hematologist to recommend another objective diagnostic technique that is less invasive. In this regard, the consultant has an ever-enlarging spectrum of options from which to choose. Unfortunately, the information available to date is insufficient to objectively support the creation and use of an algorithm that is appropriate for even a majority of patients, clinical situations, and geographic locations. Using techniques for diagnosing DVT (from ultrasonography to MRI) and, if found, inferring that the patient's cardiopulmonary syndrome is due to PE is an approach that is often used and reasonable. Unfortunately, this method of diagnosing PE has a fairly low specificity,[94] assumes the luxury of withholding therapy to allow serial imaging studies to be performed,[95] generally has no proven clinical validity (depending of the imaging technique), and is subject to the previously discussed limitations in patients with prior DVT (often a reason PE is clinically suspected in the first place). While simple techniques such as leg vein ultrasonography are reasonable to suggest in these situations, the consultant should not expect them to resolve the question with any degree of frequency. Newer CT and MRI techniques for directly imaging PE are being actively investigated.[96-98] In studies that are generally small and/or do not report results on consecutive patients, these techniques appear to have a specificity sufficient for clinical practice (85% to 95%) but have insufficient sensitivity to rule out the diagnosis.[99] The reported reasons for false positive, false negative, and uninterpretable CT scans are listed in Table 14-5. These imaging modalities are not universally available, do not (in the case of CT) obviate the need for iodinated contrast material, require an often ill patient (and all life-support equipment) be transported to an imaging suite, are expensive, have an accuracy that is thought to be in part dependent on local expertise,[100] and all too often do not yield a definitive answer for the consultant, especially when PE is not seen or the study is technically suboptimal. Consequently, what these imaging techniques have to gain over angiography in an individual patient must be considered before they are recommended in difficult clinical situations. Further experience with these and other new imaging modalities will doubtless be forthcoming and may allow the consultant more definitive options in the future. Until then, the diagnostic approach must be individualized based on the patient's perceived likelihood of PE, toxicity of the diagnostic tools available, and toxicity of therapy (recognizing the therapy includes the several months of anticoagulant treatment after resolution of the acute illness). Often, the patient's clinical status is sufficiently tenuous to allow only one trip to the imaging suite and one bolus of radiographic contrast material. In these situations, the tool that can provide the most definitive information—whether or not a PE is documented—should be suggested. Where available, pulmonary angiography most often fits this description. The consultant should not be hesitant to make this recommendation.

Another reason the hematology consultant is often called to help with management is that the PE patient's condition is not improving despite anticoagulant therapy or is postulated to have recurrent PE while on anticoagulation. In these cases the consultant should initially question the diagnosis of PE. Some diagnoses mimic PE both clinically and on indirect imaging studies such as the classic ventilation/perfusion lung scan. Cocaine, when smoked, can be such a mimic, presumably by causing intense pulmonary arteriolar vasoconstriction.[101] In this situation the symptoms and scan abnormalities generally resolve within a few days. Fat embolism, occasionally due to causes other than trauma, and tumor embolism,[102] including marrow embolism in patients with myeloproliferative diseases,[103] should also be considered in these patients. The presence of a patent foramen ovale can predispose PE patients to refractory hypoxia, systemic embolization (including stroke), and death.[104,105] This concurrent diagnosis should be sought

Table 14-5 • REPORTED REASONS FOR UNSATISFACTORY RESULTS OF SPIRAL VOLUMETRIC COMPUTED TOMOGRAPHY[a]

Causes of false positive results
- Volume averaging of enhancing vessels with adjacent lymphadenopathy or atelectatic lung (2)
- Hilar areas of hypoattenuation caused by hilar lymph nodes (1)
- Breathing artifact (1)
- Asymmetry in pulmonary vascular opacification secondary to trauma with effusion and consolidation (1)
- Partial volume effects in obliquely oriented vessels, such as the lingula and right middle lobe arteries, suboptimal contrast, and/or intersegmental lymph nodes (3-6)

Causes of false negative results
- Subsegmental clot (10)
- Patient's large size (1)
- Right middle lobectomy (1)
- Embolus in the anterior segmental artery of the right lower lobe (1)

Causes of indeterminate scans or technical failures
- Inadequate depiction of right middle lobe and/or lingular segmental arteries (4)
- Breathing at the end of scanning (2)
- Interruption of contrast injection before the end of data acquisition (1)
- Limitation of breathing caused by pleuritic chest pain (1)
- Severe dyspnea (2)
- Patent foramen ovale (2)
- Technical difficulty with intravenous contrast connections (1)
- Poor enhancement, poor signal-to-noise ratio, and/or excessive patient motion (4)
- Moderate vascular opacifiation of the right lower lobe arteries (1)

[a] Number of patients in the literature on which this observation is based is given in parentheses.
Modified from Mullins MD, Becker DM, Hagspiel KD, et al. The role of spinal volumetric computed tomography in the diagnosis of pulmonary embolism. Arch Intern Med 2000;160:293-298, with permission. Copyrighted 2000, American Medical Association.

in patients not responding well to anticoagulant therapy as their situation may improve when the pulmonary artery pressure (PAP) is lowered with fibrinolytic therapy.

TREATMENT

General Considerations

Over the past 40 years, the treatment of VTE has been fairly straightforward: hospitalize the patient, start a heparin infusion, monitor the aPTT, and then start warfarin therapy. While this is a time-honored approach that most current practitioners are comfortable with, the hematology consultant increasingly will be required to choose from an ever-enlarging number of therapeutic options. Unfortunately, it is unlikely that the consultant will have definitive clinical trials directly comparing the various therapeutic modalities to use in making the choice. Because of the lack of definitive data, firm consensus among the full medical community on the best therapeutic approach will probably not be forthcoming. Consequently, as with the difficult diagnostic decisions, the consultant will have to rely in large part on his or her background as a generalist in performing the risk:benefit analysis for an individual patient—considering the known data on responses to various therapies and the unquantifiable data from the patient estimating his risk of therapeutic toxicity as well as the value of the therapeutic outcomes that are offered by various treatments. As newer treatments become available, the consultant must continually evaluate what potential (or proven) advantages they may offer over standard therapy and which patient populations might most benefit from these advantages. For instance, therapy designed to prevent the 10-year sequelae of DVT (such as catheter-directed fibrinolysis) might be inappropriate for a patient with a 90% likelihood of death from lung cancer within 1 year, but might prevent occupational disability in a construction worker with no limitation of life span. Many of these decisions often require intense discussion with the patient, his or her family, and the referring physician, often considering topics (such as prognosis of underlying disease, financial resources, lifestyle choices, etc.) that have not been previously discussed in depth. The consultant should not shy away from bringing these points out in the open, for without their consideration development of a logical therapeutic plan is not possible.

Pulmonary Embolism

As with diagnostic modalities, a definitive discussion of all therapeutic options is beyond the scope of this chapter. This chapter will consider questions most often posed to the hematology consultant and will consider therapy in the acute and chronic phases of the illness separately. In the acute phase of VTE, the consultant should first consider whether the patient might benefit from fibrinolytic therapy. Only after this question has been answered to his satisfaction should the consultant consider recommending other forms of therapy—such as anticoagulation or IVC interruption.

There is a moderately large body of data on the outcomes of fibrinolytic therapy of PE that goes back over 30 years. This information has conclusively shown that, compared to standard anticoagulant therapy, fibrinolytic therapy can improve most of the anatomic and physiologic sequelae of PE more rapidly—macroscopic clot size as quantitated by angiography, microvascular perfusion as estimated by perfusion lung scanning, pulmonary artery and right atrial pressures measured by catheterization,[106,107] and right ventricular size and contractility as seen on transthoracic echocardiography.[108] However, despite 30 years of evaluation, no study has been powered to determine the effect of fibrinolytic therapy on mortality from PE and very few studies have examined its effect on morbidity. Additionally, fibrinolytic therapy has generally been thought to pose a higher risk of major bleeding complications, though no modern study has tested this hypothesis. Because there is no direct evidence that fibrinolytic therapy reduces mortality or long-term morbidity compared to anticoagulant therapy (which is associated with an overall mortality rate that may be as low as 1.5%[109]) and it is perceived to be more toxic, fibrinolytic therapy classically has been reserved for those patients in need of rapid improvement of their cardiac status—those thought to be hemodynamically unstable or in shock (both terms otherwise undefined in most reviews). While this conservative approach is reasonable for most patients, it must be understood that it is based on lack of direct data to contradict it rather than on hard data demonstrating its superiority, and that there is another modest body of indirect data that the hematology consultant should consider when making recommendations for an individual patient. First is the recent demonstration that mortality after diagnosis of PE may not be as acceptable as previously reported. It may be as high as 40% at 1 week and 45% at 1 month,[27] suggesting standard anticoagulation may not be as helpful as we have thought in patients with this manifestation of VTE. Next is the demonstration that a pulmonary artery pressure (PAP) of over 50 mm Hg at time of PE diagnosis is associated with persistent pulmonary hypertension (relative risk 3.3 compared to patients with a PAP of less than 50 mm Hg) and the persistent pulmonary hypertension (over 35 mm Hg) was independently associated with 5-year mortality (odds ratio 9.2) and need for pulmonary thromboendarterectomy, suggesting that marked pulmonary hypertension at presentation is a bad prognostic indicator, even in the absence of hemodynamic instability or shock.[110] Since fibrinolytic therapy has been shown to lower PAP to a greater extent than anticoagulant therapy (at least in the early phase of treatment), it is conceivable that it might improve the long-term outcome of PE patients with marked pulmonary hypertension at presentation. In a randomized trial comparing fibrinolytic and anticoagulant therapy of PE, anticoagulant therapy was associated with recurrent PE and death only in patients with right ventricular hypokinesis at presentation (suggestive of pulmonary hypertension), indirectly supporting this concept.[108] Right ventricular dysfunction with or without pulmonary hypertension (as judged by echocardiography) in normotensive patients has also been associated with a 10% incidence of subsequent progression to shock, which itself has a 50% mortality rate.[111] A nonrandomized registry of over 700 consecutive hemodynamically stable PE patients observed that the only independent predictor of 30-day mortality was the receipt of fibrinolytic therapy at presentation (odds ratio 0.46 compared to anticoagulant therapy).[112] This study also associated fibrinolytic therapy with a lower incidence of recurrent symptomatic PE and a higher risk of nonfatal major bleeding complications (21.9% versus 7.8%). Follow-up studies of subgroups of patients randomized to fibrinolytic or anticoagulant therapy in the UPET/USPET studies of the late 1960s and early 1970s show that patients randomized to fibrinolytic therapy are more likely to have normal diffusing capacity of the lung for carbon dioxide and pulmonary capillary blood volume measurements,[113] less likely to have resting- and exercise-induced pulmonary hypertension and less likely to have clinically severe congestive heart failure.[114] While these indirect data suggest a potential clinical benefit of fibrinolytic therapy in hemodynamically stable patients with PE, several points must be considered in its interpretation:

1. Studies of PAP after PE do not include measurements of the pressure before the PE. Persistent pulmonary hypertension after PE may reflect the patients' baseline PAP, with the pulmonary hypertension being a marker of severe underlying lung disease. The high 5-year mortality rate seen in these patients may reflect the prognosis of their underlying lung disease rather than the outcome of their PE.
2. While fibrinolytic therapy improves the extent of pulmonary hypertension after 24 hours of treatment in randomized trials, its effect on long-term cardiopulmonary hemodynamics has been poorly studied. Indeed, while not a prospective evaluation, fibrinolytic therapy had no effect on 30-day post-therapy PAP as judged by echocardiography.[110]
3. Patients given fibrinolytic therapy in the nonrandomized registry might well have had a better overall prognosis (fewer comorbidities) than patients who were given anticoagulant therapy alone. The lower mortality in the fibrinolytic therapy group may simply reflect that they were intrinsically less sick than those who received less aggressive therapy.
4. The higher major bleeding rate seen in with fibrinolytic therapy in the registry of PE patients suggests that conventional wisdom may be correct—that fibrinolytic therapy of PE is more toxic than anticoagulant therapy (though the toxicity may not be fatal).

Given this information, can fibrinolytic therapy be reasonably considered in any patient judged to be hemodynamically stable? This is an area where reasonable practitioners have reasonable differences in opinion, but this author believes that it can—based in large part on the degree of pulmonary hypertension in a given patient and the extent to which PE is thought to be responsible for the hypertension, tempered by the perceived risk of major bleeding complications posed by fibrinolytic versus anticoagulant therapy in that patient. Past history, previous echocardiograms, extent of apical wall motion abnormalities (greater in acute than chronic cor-pulmonale[115]), and extent of thrombotic occlusion on CT/angiography can all reasonably be used to infer the contribution of the PE to the PAP. Another factor that reasonably can be considered is the patient's response to standard anticoagulant therapy. Pulmonary emboli treated with anticoagulant therapy resolve over a period of weeks, not days, particularly in patients with extensive PE.[116] Fibrinolytic therapy can be effective when given as much as 2 weeks after presentation.[117] For patients in whom the risk of bleeding complications of fibrinolytic therapy is thought to be unacceptable, a trial of anticoagulant therapy can be given and the patient's condition (including PAP, as monitored by serial echocardiography) monitored. If the rate of improvement is clinically acceptable, nothing further would be indicated. However, lack of improvement or resolution of the bleeding risk (healing of surgical wound, improvement of gastritis, etc.) could prompt reconsideration of the risk : benefit analysis of fibrinolytic therapy at a later time. Patients for whom clinical improvement is not seen but are still believed to be at high risk of bleeding could also be considered for mechanical thrombectomy. While this has classically been done via thoracotomy, modern percutaneous catheter-directed techniques are now possible,[118] making it a less heroic, more practical consideration where the expertise is available.

Superficial and Calf Vein Thrombosis

Treatment of thrombosis of deep veins of the calf or of superficial veins of the legs is dictated by the likelihood of these thrombi to result in either pulmonary embolization or venous insufficiency. In the absence of these complications, superficial or calf vein thrombi pose few, if any, major medical risks beyond their associated pain and discomfort. The discomfort caused by these thrombi generally responds well to elevation of the leg and analgesic and anti-inflammatory medications. Determining the likelihood of embolization or subsequent venous insufficiency, therefore, is crucial in determining whether more aggressive therapy with anticoagulants is warranted. Studies done through the 1970s suggested that calf vein thrombi resolved rapidly and rarely were associated with symptomatic or asymptomatic pulmonary embolization, in contradistinction to thrombi in the popliteal and more proximal veins, where as many as half of the patients were found to have PE (albeit frequently asymptomatic).[119] Whether calf vein thrombi really embolize less frequently than more proximal thrombi or whether, by virtue of being smaller cloths in smaller veins, they generate smaller emboli that are less likely to be symptomatic or seen on perfusion lung scan is not known. The risk of subsequent, clinically significant venous insufficiency is debated but valvular reflux often is found.[81] Similar outcomes have been reported with thrombi in the superficial veins of the legs. Because thrombi in these locations generally are not routinely associated with symptomatic embolization or venous insufficiency, the dogmatic position that they never need anticoagulant therapy is often taken with very little thought—occasionally to the patient's detriment.

There are several points about thrombi in these locations that the consultant should consider before withholding anticoagulant therapy. One is that not all series report a negligible incidence of embolization with calf vein thrombosis. As many as 25% to 35% of patients will be found to have PE on surveillance scans (reviewed by Giannoukas and coworkers.)[81] Consequently, patients at high risk for adverse outcome of embolization (those with significant cardiopulmonary disease) should be considered for anticoagulation. The next is that 15% to 30% of calf vein thrombi will extend to involve the popliteal and more proximal veins,[81,120–122] where there is a greater likelihood of embolization, and there is no method for predicting which patients' thrombi will extend. Consequently, if anticoagulation is withheld, serial imaging studies over the subsequent few weeks is warranted to detect this progression. Finally, patients with calf vein thrombosis have a high likelihood of recurrent thrombosis, up to 29% in 3 months, and these recurrences can be prevented with anticoagulant therapy.[123] Consequently close monitoring of patients clinically, and possibly with imaging studies, is indicated, especially if the patient's condition suggests that their definable risks for thrombosis will not quickly resolve (cancer, inflammatory bowel disease, hereditary prothrombotic states, etc.). For patients with superficial venous thrombosis, the consultant should be sure that the thrombus is truly in only a superficial vein. It must be remembered that the superficial femoral vein is actually part of the deep venous system of the thigh[124] and that thrombi in this vein have a high embolic potential and should be treated accordingly. Superficial venous thrombosis can coexist with[125,126] or progress to[127] thrombosis of the deep veins. Such progression should be anticipated and monitored for. Also, not all superficial veins are small veins. The superficial veins of the thigh, particularly the proximal greater saphenous vein, are large veins that can harbor large thrombi. Thrombosis of these large superficial veins is more likely to be associated with detectable PE than thrombosis of smaller superficial veins[128] and anticoagulant therapy should be considered, especially in those patients at risk for adverse outcomes of PE. Finally, neither calf vein nor superficial vein thrombosis are thought to occur in "normal" individuals. Many patients will be found to have underlying prothrombotic states, both acquired and congenital,[129–131]—states that require specific treatment (such as cancer) or predispose to more severe thrombosis, complications of pregnancy, paradoxical embolization, and so forth. These underlying problems should not be overlooked by the consultant. Points to be considered in the treatment of superficial and calf vein thrombosis are listed in Table 14–6.

Deep Vein Thrombosis

The case for fibrinolytic therapy of DVT is more difficult to make than it is for PE. Until recently, all the data that existed from which to make clinical decisions were derived from studies performed in the 1970s when streptokinase was given via a peripheral arm vein, generally for protracted periods of time—often several days—and the venographic results compared to that seen with the standard heparin therapy of the time. These studies were often not randomized, and generally did not provide results of long-term clinical follow-up. When pooled, the results of these trials suggested that there was a greater degree of thrombolysis achieved acutely (within several days to a week) but with a higher frequency of major bleeding complications.[132] The two studies providing long-term follow-up of patients treated with either anticoagulant or systemic fibrinolytic therapy provided data from 78 patients and suggested that patients who had severe postphlebitic symptoms were more likely to have received heparin and those free of such symptoms were more likely to have been treated with streptokinase.[133] When these studies were reviewed, diametrically opposed feelings were expressed at the turn of the last decade of the millennium, ranging from "SK is clearly beneficial in the treatment of DVT..."[134] to questioning "Can lytic therapy be

Table 14–6 • CONSIDERATIONS IN TREATMENT OF SUPERFICIAL OR CALF VEIN THROMBOSIS

Problem	Solution
Be sure there is no concurrent thrombosis of the deep veins of the thigh	Ultrasound the deep veins of the thigh Remember: the superficial femoral vein *is* a deep vein of the thigh
Be sure that patient can tolerate hemodynamically small pulmonary emboli	If the patient has significant cardiopulmonary disease, consider anticoagulation
Be sure that you will detect thrombus extension to the deep veins of the thigh if it occurs	Use surveillance ultrasonography for the duration of the patient's risk of thrombus extension If the patient has many risk factors for thrombus, consider anticoagulation until they resolve
Be sure the thrombus is not large enough to cause symptoms if it embolizes	Consider anticoagulation for large thrombi in the proximal saphenous vein
Recognize that calf and superficial vein thrombosis are indicative of an underlying prothrombotic state	Monitor patient for subsequent thrombi Use intense thromboprophylaxis in future high-risk situations Consider a focused search for cancer

Table 14-7 • LYSIS GRADE ACCORDING TO DURATION OF SYMPTOMS OF DVT

Type of Symptoms	Grade I (<50%)	Grade II (50% to 99%)	Grade III (100%)
Acute (n = 202)	27 (13%)	106 (52%)	69 (34%)
Chronic (n = 53)	17 (32%)	26 (49%)	10 (19%)
Acute and Chronic (n = 57)	10 (17%)	30 (53%)	17 (31%)
Total (n = 312)	54 (17%)	162 (52%)	96 (31%)

The cut-off between acute and chronic symptoms was 10 days. The number in parentheses is the percentage.
Modified from Mewissen MW, Seabrook GR, Meissner MH, et al. Catheter-directed thrombolysis for lower extremity deep venous thrombosis: Report of a national multicenter registry. Radiology 1999;211:39–49, with permission.

justified?"[135] The 1990s brought new fibrinolytic technology to the clinical arena in the form of new medications (tissue plasminogen activator) and new tools to allow the medications to be infused directly into the thrombus rather than into an arm vein distant from the clot. The use of these techniques brought very favorable reports from physicians and centers with interest in the technique and the technology to provide it.[103] High rates of acute thrombus resolution and rapid relief of acute symptoms were described, with particular attention to patients with extensive thrombosis of the iliac and femoral veins. Medical toxicity was acceptable, but questions were raised regarding the acceptability of the financial toxicity—over $20,000 when urokinase (the drug most extensively studied in that decade) was used.[136] These issues have not been worked out to everyone's satisfaction to date. However, there are now more data to help with the medical risk:benefit analyses, if not the financial ones. The data come not in the form of randomized, prospective trials but from a large registry of DVT patients treated with catheter-directed fibrinolysis.[137] This technique resulted in complete clot lysis in 31% of patients and more than 50% lysis in another 52% (Table 14–7). Complete lysis was achieved more often in patients with acute rather than chronic symptoms. Patency at 12 months was significantly more frequent in cases of iliofemoral thrombi compared to femoral-popliteal thrombi, and was more frequent if greater degrees of lysis were achieved (Figs. 14–4 and 14–5). Major bleeding, generally at the venipuncture site, occurred in 11% of cases. Clinical follow-up on a cohort of these patients has shown that they have less severe symptoms of postphlebitic syndrome than a contemporary cohort of patients treated with anticoagulation alone.[138] The major points that the consultant must keep in mind when considering fibrinolytic therapy of DVT are as follows:

1. That catheter-directed fibrinolytic therapy is used to maximize efficacy, not minimize toxicity. It is probably more effective than peripherally infused fibrinolytic therapy, and has a higher frequency of bleeding than does anticoagulant therapy.
2. The goal of therapy is to minimize physical disability from the postphlebitic syndrome. This goal has *not* been proven to be accomplished by the current standard of proof of efficacy—the prospective, randomized (and, preferably, double-blinded) clinical trial.
3. Catheter-directed fibrinolytic therapy is far more expensive and requires a greater degree of expertise than anticoagulant therapy. Not every patient is willing to pay for the possible benefits (nor does every patients stand to gain much from the theoretical benefits) and not every health care facility is equipped to perform the procedures.

The decision to use catheter-directed fibrinolytic therapy in any given patient will depend on the perceived likelihood of development of the postphlebitic syndrome (possibly, but not necessarily, related to size and location of the thrombus), the possible detriment that postphlebitic symptoms will have on the patient's occupational and avocational lifestyle, the likelihood of clot dissolution (related to the location of the clot and duration of symptoms), the patient's willingness to pay the

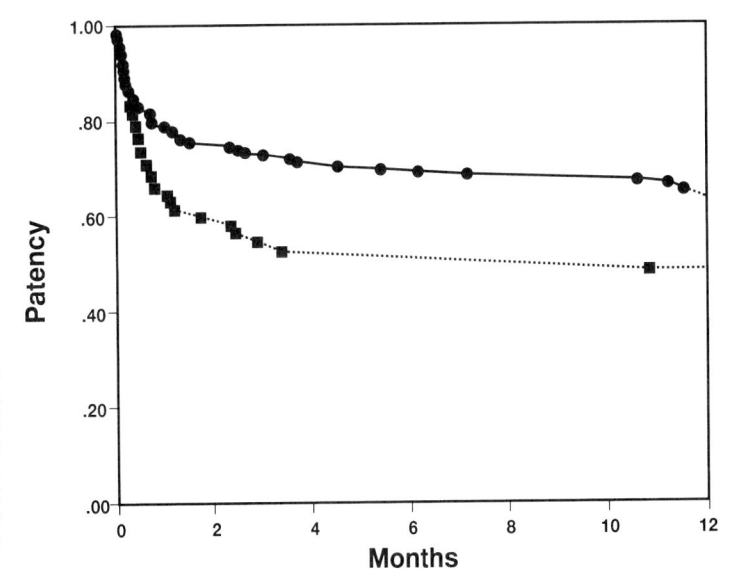

Figure 14–4 Cumulative primary patency curves for 221 patients with iliofemoral DVT (*solid line*) and 79 patients with femoral-popliteal DVT (*dashed line*). Patients with iliofemoral DVT were more likely to have maintained patency at 1 year than were patients with femoral-popliteal DVT (63.7% vs. 46.8%, $p < 0.01$). (From Mewissen MW, Seabrook Gr, Meissner MH, et al. Catheter-directed thrombolysis for lower extremity deep venous thrombosis: Report of a national mulicenter registry. Radiology 1999;211:39–49, with permission.)

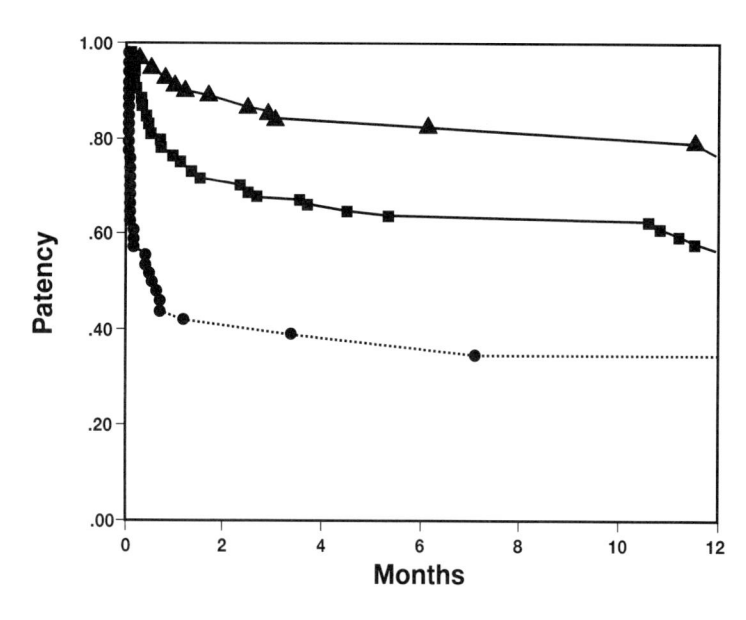

Figure 14–5 Cumulative primary patency curves after thrombolysis according to grade of lysis. The 1-year patency rate in limbs with complete lysis (triangles) was 78.9%, whereas the rate with 50% lysis (circles) was 32.3% ($p < 0.001$). Intermediate degrees of lysis are represented by squares. (From Mewissen MW, Seabrook GR, Meissner MH, et al. Catheter-directed thrombolysis for lower extremity deep venous thrombosis: Report of a national multicenter registry. Radiology 1999;211:39–49, with permission.)

price (both in terms of the bleeding risk and the financial cost), and the availability of the personnel and equipment to perform the procedure. The hematology consultant should establish a working relationship with a vascular interventionist and his team before these cases present to learn the extent of their experience with catheter-directed fibrinolysis and their degree of enthusiasm for getting involved in these cases. An ideal patient and enthusiastic hematologist with an inexperienced or uninterested interventional team is not the best combination with which to work.

Once the decision for or against fibrinolytic therapy has been made, anticoagulant therapy to prevent thrombus extension or recurrence is required. Currently, this is accomplished with a heparin derivative, but the future holds promise of other agents that might work as well or better. This is yet another area that bears close attention on the part of the consultative hematologist. Classically, unfractionated heparin has been given as an intravenous infusion whose dose was adjusted based on the aPTT result. While qualitatively there is no question that this approach works (nonuse of heparin results in an unacceptable rate of recurrence[139]), the use of the aPTT to quantitate heparin dose is a concept that is based on weak data. While some studies have shown that patients in whom the requisite degree of prolongation of the aPTT was not achieved have an inordinately high incidence of recurrence (almost 25% of patients!),[62] subsequent studies of similar patients reported from the same group of investigators using the same techniques failed to show such an unusually high rate of therapeutic failure.[63] Even if a good correlation between the aPTT results and the rate of recurrence existed, the admonition not to mistake correlation for causation must be kept in mind. No study has ever tried to demonstrate that changing the aPTT in a prospective manner alters patients outcomes. Indeed, many of the investigators whose work formed the basis for the wide clinical acceptance of the aPTT as a means to quantitate heparin dose have recently stated that whatever correlation between the aPTT and clinical outcomes there might be, they

disappear in patients given a threshold dose (above 35,000 units/day) of heparin acutely.[140] All the discussion of heparin monitoring in the usual patient with VTE is now moot, however, because of the introduction of low-molecular-weight heparins (LMWH) into clinical practice. They are at least as effective as unfractionated heparin when given as a fixed, unmonitored dose.[141] The hematology consultant should be familiar with the increasing number of commercially available LMWH preparations and their use in treating acute VTE, for they will probably replace unfractionated heparin for this indication in the majority of patients. On their downside, however, LMWH has a significantly longer half life than unfractionated heparin, cannot be readily quantitated by plasma measurement and is not reliably reversed by protamine. This makes treatment of major bleeding in patients on LMWH difficult save for standard supportive care measures. LMWH is also excreted renally, probably more from tubular secretion than by glomerular filtration, making its dose/response unpredictable in patients with renal disease. At this point, LMWH should probably be avoided in patients whose anticoagulation must be controllable from minute-to-minute because their high risk of bleeding from underlying disease and in patients with renal disease. In these patients, use of unfractionated heparin is probably the better part of valor.

The final decision regarding the acute therapy of VTE often faced by the hematology consultant is whether or not to suggest use of an IVC filter. Unfortunately, these devices became part of standard therapy at a time that threshold for clinical acceptance was much lower than modern standards. While reports of the use of these devices are legion, they are virtually all confined to case reports, registries with incomplete and/or nonobjective follow-up exams, or uncontrolled case series. Their use is based on three as yet unproven premises:

1. That there exist a number of clinical situations where toxicity of anticoagulation is predictably and unacceptably high.

2. That the devices lower the incidence of PE (by trapping emboli before they reach the pulmonary circulation without causing local thrombi that can embolize) in the absence of anticoagulation.
3. That the devices cause few clinically unacceptable complications.

Since these devices are often used in patients with active VTE and do nothing to treat concurrent DVT, their use is often based on the premise that the outcome of toxicity of anticoagulation is less clinically acceptable than the outcome of subsequent DVT or DVT extension without anticoagulation. The only study of these devices using anything close to acceptable modern techniques of clinical research prospectively randomized a large group of patients with DVT to anticoagulant therapy alone or anticoagulation combined with an IVC filter.[51] No attempt at standardization of filter type or of length of outpatient anticoagulation was made. After the first week or so of anticoagulant therapy with heparin, the patients randomized to receive filters indeed had fewer PE, suggesting that when combined with anticoagulant therapy filters probably do lower the incidence of acute PE. However, at the end of 2 years of follow-up, during which time most patients had been off anticoagulant therapy for 12 to 18 months, the incidence of PE was not different between the groups with and without filters and the group in whom filters were placed had a higher incidence of symptomatic DVT! These follow-up data from the only prospective, randomized trial of IVC filters calls into question the last two of the three premises on which their use in based! Until further information is available on the safety and efficacy of their use in patients with active VTE, the consultant should be hesitant to recommend the use of IVC filters to the exclusion of other forms of therapy with proven efficacy (such as anticoagulation). If the consultant believes that a given patient's risk of unacceptable toxicity with anticoagulant therapy is predictably high (higher than the risk of unacceptable outcomes of extension of old or development of new DVT) then IVC filter placement is reasonable clinical practice. However, patients with small emboli[142] or patients who have no detectable DVT on serial ultrasound exams[143] are probably better off with no specific therapy than with a filter. If the patient's perceived risk of anticoagulant toxicity changes (healed wounds, gastritis, etc.) during follow-up, strong consideration should be given to institution of anticoagulant therapy.

In the context of acute VTE, conventional wisdom has held that bed rest is one of the cornerstones of treatment, presumably preventing embolization of the thrombus present in the leg veins by preventing it from being fractured by the trauma inherent in movement of the leg. While experimental thrombi 2 hours old in dogs can be induced to embolize by "massaging. . . along the course of the femoral vein and by gently exercising the legs,"[3] there are no data attempting to determine objectively if this actually happens in clinically apparent venous thrombi (which are probably much older than 2 hours) in humans. In fact, the necessity of enforced bed rest to prevent embolization was based on such shaky evidence that two recent international clinical trials were allowed to randomize prospectively patients with DVT to home therapy with LMWH without enforced bed rest or in-hospital bed rest and infusional unfractionated heparin.[144,145] In both of these studies the incidence of clinically apparent embolization was similar in the patients treated at home and in the hospital, suggesting that enforced bed rest is not protective against embolization. However, neither of these studies used the same treatment regimen for both groups, and neither looked for asymptomatic embolization. A subsequent study gave all patients subcutaneous LMWH and randomized them to unrestricted activity at home (while wearing compression stockings) and enforced bed rest in the hospital and performed perfusion lung scans pre-therapy and 10 days later.[146] They showed a similar number of new perfusion defects in both groups. Other investigators have randomized DVT patients to bed rest without support stockings and ambulation with support stocking and formal walking exercises while receiving treatment with LMWH and found faster reduction in the pain and swelling with less propagation of the venous thrombus[147] and no increase in the rate of asymptomatic embolization in the ambulatory patient.[147,147a] Taken together, these observations refute the time-honored hypothesis that bed rest is protective against embolization of DVT and form the basis of the recommendation that patients with VTE be allowed a degree of physical activity commensurate with their symptoms, both of the thrombosis and any of coexistent disease, as long as the ambulation is carried out with the use of support stockings.

Phlegmasia Cerulea Dolens and Venous Gangrene

In daily clinical use the terms *phlegmasia cerulea dolens* and *venous gangrene* tend to be used interchangeably to define the situation of a patient with venous thrombosis extensive enough to occlude all venous circulation and with subsequent swelling sufficient to prevent arterial inflow into the leg, predisposing to infarction and necrosis of tissue. The term *phlegmasia cerulea dolens* was coined by French investigations in the late 1930s to distinguish DVT cases with tissue ischemia from the more common cases of DVT without ischemia, which were termed *phlegmasia alba dolens*.[148] Strictly speaking, however, the term *phlegmasia cerulea dolens* defines the presence of a painful leg with a bluish hue due to venous obstruction caused by thrombosis. The term quantitates neither the pain nor the intensity of bluish discoloration. Consequently, in clinical practice the term is applied to patients with a wide spectrum of disease severity, ranging from the common iliofemoral DVT (with the risk of PE and venous insufficiency) to the rare cases of occlusion of virtually all named and many unnamed veins leading to necrosis of tissue often requiring amputation. All cases progressing to venous gangrene can be classified as phlegmasia cerulea dolens, but not all cases of termed phlegmasia cerulea dolens will progress to tissue necrosis. Not only does this distinction pose a problem in determining the prognosis for a specific patient, it makes interpretation of reports of therapy difficult. For this discussion, only DVT cases with actual or impending necrosis of tissue will be given the term *phlegmasia cerulea dolens,* or PCD.

The pathophysiology of PCD involves the virtually complete occlusion of venous outflow from a significant portion of the leg, often caused by thrombotic occlusion to many of the large named veins and smaller tributary veins and vessels to small they are simply referred to as "microvasculature" in the areas of greatest tissue ischemia.[148] This causes profound venous engorgement and hypertension in the capillary bed, resulting in potentially massive third-space losses of intravascular volume. The resulting intravascular volume depletion and arteriolar hypotension coupled with the venous hypertension results in impaired capillary perfusion and tissue ischemia. The degree of hypovolemia in these patients can be profound, up to and including shock. This component of the pathophysiology of venous gangrene is often overlooked in practice because of the attention given to attempts at relief of the venous obstruction.

Classically, PCD is thought to be a consequence of the hypercoagulable state accompanying a malignancy, often an undiagnosed malignancy. However, there are enough reports in the literature linking PCD to the use of vena cava filters to think these devices may play a significant pathophysiologic role in some cases.[149-153] Recently, treatment of thrombosis complicating heparin-induced thrombocytopenia with high doses of warfarin has been thought to predispose to PCD.[154] In Many cases, however, the underlying cause is impossible to determine.

Treatment of this PCD is controversial because of the rarity of the disorder, the highly variable prognoses of patient comorbidities, and the lack of a standardized definition of the syndrome. The goal of therapy is to restore capillary perfusion, preventing or reversing tissue ischemia. Aggressive fluid resuscitation is a cornerstone of treatment. Intercompartmental pressures due to third spacing are often so high as to warrant fasciotomy to improve arterial inflow. Some investigators reasonably suggest using anticoagulant therapy with these measures initially, especially in patients with potentially fatal comorbidities such as cancer, and reserve attempts at clot removal for those patients whose condition deteriorates.[155] In patients for whom aggressive therapy is appropriate, catheter-directed thrombolysis should be attempted initially.[148,156,157] Venous thrombectomy, with[152] or without[158,159] local thrombolytic therapy, is also a reasonable consideration if the facilities are available. However, despite aggressive treatment the prognosis is poor, with many patients requiring amputation or progressing to death.

Chronic Secondary Prophylaxis

Once a decision has been made on the type of acute VTE therapy to use and the patient has stabilized, a decision on how to prevent subsequent thrombus formation must be made. Typically, this is done with warfarin. The hematology consultant should be aware, however, that other options are available from which to choose. Heparin derivatives are also an increasingly acceptable alternative. When used for 3 months on an outpatient basis, adjusted-dose heparin was found to be as effective as warfarin, but significantly less toxic, in a prospective randomized trial almost 20 years ago.[160] More recent trials have shown similar results with LMWH.[161-166] In the subgroup of patients with VTE who have concurrent malignancy, warfarin therapy may be more toxic and less efficacious than when used to treat VTE in patients without cancer.[65] This study demonstrated complication rates of 15% to 20% in this population (Figs. 14–6 and 14–7). Combining these data with the observation from a meta-analysis suggesting a survival advantage in cancer patients whose VTE was treated with LMWH acutely[141] provides a basis to recommend use of LMWH for long-term therapy in this population or any other patient perceived to be at high risk for hemorrhage with warfarin therapy. To date, such an approach has not been validated by clinical experimentation, but such trials are ongoing. This is another area for the hematology consultant to watch closely.

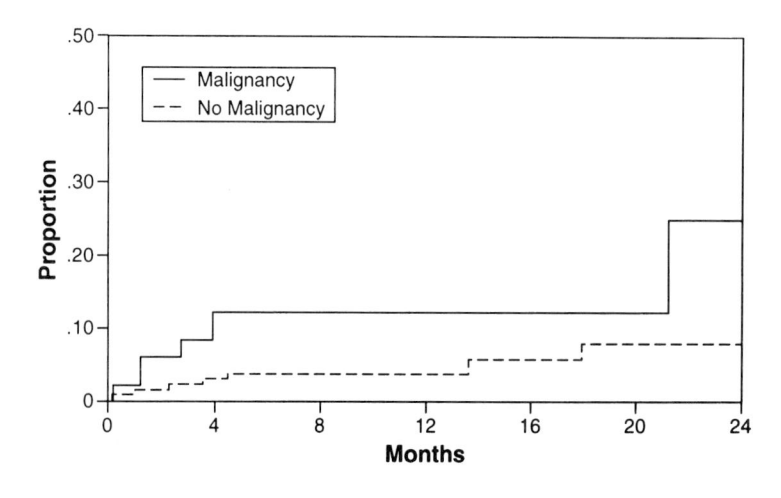

Figure 14–6 Cumulative incidence of first major hemorrhage in 53 patients with and 208 patients without malignancy at the initiation of warfarin therapy (for any indication, not just VTE). (From Gitter MJ, Jaeger TM, Petterson TM, et al. Bleeding and thromboembolism during anticoagulant therapy: A population-based study in Rochester, Minnesota, Mayo Clin Proc 1995;70:725–733, with permission.)

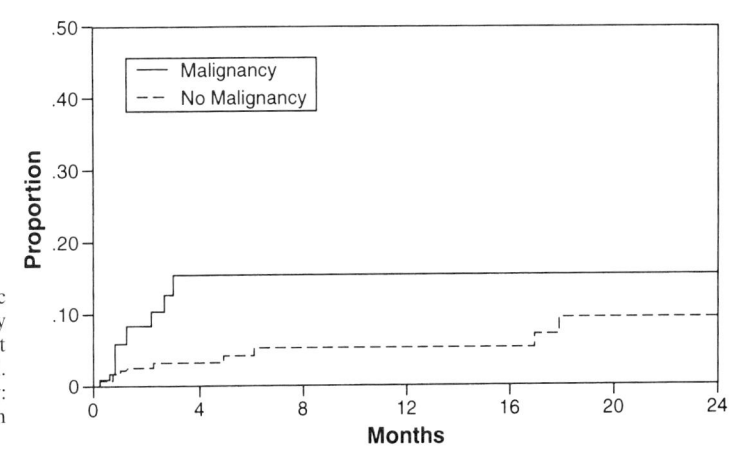

Figure 14-7 Cumulative incidence of first thromboembolic event in 53 patients with and 208 patients without malignancy at the initiation of warfarin therapy (for any indication, not just VTE). (From Gitter MJ, Jaeger TM, Petterson TM, et al. Bleeding and thromboembolism during anticoagulant therapy: A population-based study in Rochester, Minnesota. Mayo Clin Proc 1995;70:725–733, with permission.)

The duration of anticoagulant therapy after VTE is another question frequently posed to the consultant. Since most episodes of VTE occur as a complication of another disease process that is self-limited (infection, surgery, pregnancy, etc.), provision of anticoagulant therapy for a relatively short, fixed duration of time (3 to 6 months) has been the traditional answer to this question. Unfortunately, this approach results in recurrent VTE after cessation of anticoagulant therapy in an unknown percentage of patients, often over a protracted period of time.[167] Predicting which patients are likely to do well after a short course of anticoagulation and which patients are likely to have a recurrence is the subject of much ongoing debate and clinical research. Currently there are two approaches to the question proposed in the literature. The first is to subject the patient to a series of tests looking for a laboratory-defined abnormality that associated with a high incidence of VTE and, if found, providing a longer (but unspecified) period of anticoagulation.[168,168a] This approach ignores two facts: (1) that many patients with these laboratory-defined abnormalities have thromboses only when combined with obvious additive but temporary prothrombotic stimuli (such as surgery, pregnancy, etc.), and (2) in 40% to 50% of families with clear-cut tendencies to VTE we cannot define an abnormality. The former suggests some patients with laboratory-defined abnormalities may not benefit from protracted anticoagulant therapy while the latter implies that others who have no laboratory-defined abnormality might. The second suggested approach is to define clinical events leading to the patient developing VTE and determine if those circumstances are likely to recur: if the circumstances surrounding the episode of VTE are predictably unusual, of limited duration, and unlikely to recur, then provide a short course of anticoagulation; if there are no clinical circumstances that suggest the patient is VTE was provoked by reversible physiologic stimuli causing thrombosis, then provide a more protracted duration of anticoagulation.[19] By this second approach, patients with VTE complicating pregnancy, surgery, major trauma, severe medical illness, or (in some studies) estrogen therapies are thought to have VTE secondary to the physiologic changes caused by these self-limited events and have what is termed "secondary" VTE. Patients not fitting this category (either no or minor abnormalities such as prolonged air or auto travel) are thought to have "primary" or "idiopathic" VTE, probably as a consequence of an endogenous prothrombotic abnormality (congenital or acquired) that is unlikely to be reversible. Patients with secondary VTE have a much lower rate of recurrent VTE after a short (3- to 6-month) course of anticoagulant therapy than do patients with idiopathic VTE, consequently the latter group are often subjected to a longer duration of therapy. Indeed, even in patients with congenital prothrombotic states, those whose episode of VTE is "idiopathic" have a higher frequency of recurrence that those in whom it was "secondary."[169] To date neither approach to determine duration of anticoagulant therapy has been subjected to rigorous clinical investigation. In an attempt to determine if one approach is dramatically better in predicting rate of recurrent VTE after cessation of anticoagulation given to treat the initial thrombosis, the literature has been reviewed for publications describing rates of recurrence in idiopathic versus secondary VTE and in groups with and without specific laboratory-defined defects.[17–19,170–176] The results from each publication were converted to graphic form with a standard format, with time "0" being the time that anticoagulant therapy was discontinued in all groups. The results are illustrated in Figs. 14–8 and 14–9. These figures suggest that the rates of recurrence are similar in patients with idiopathic VTE and in patients with VTE associated with a definable laboratory abnormality—approximately 10% per year. The rate of recurrence in patients with secondary VTE might be a bit lower than the rate in patients with VTE who do not have the one laboratory abnormality sought in each individual study—generally in the 2% per year area. While these data do not lend themselves to formal statistical analysis, it suggests that the positive predictive value of "idiopathic" VTE is similar to that provided by laboratory testing and that the negative predictive value for

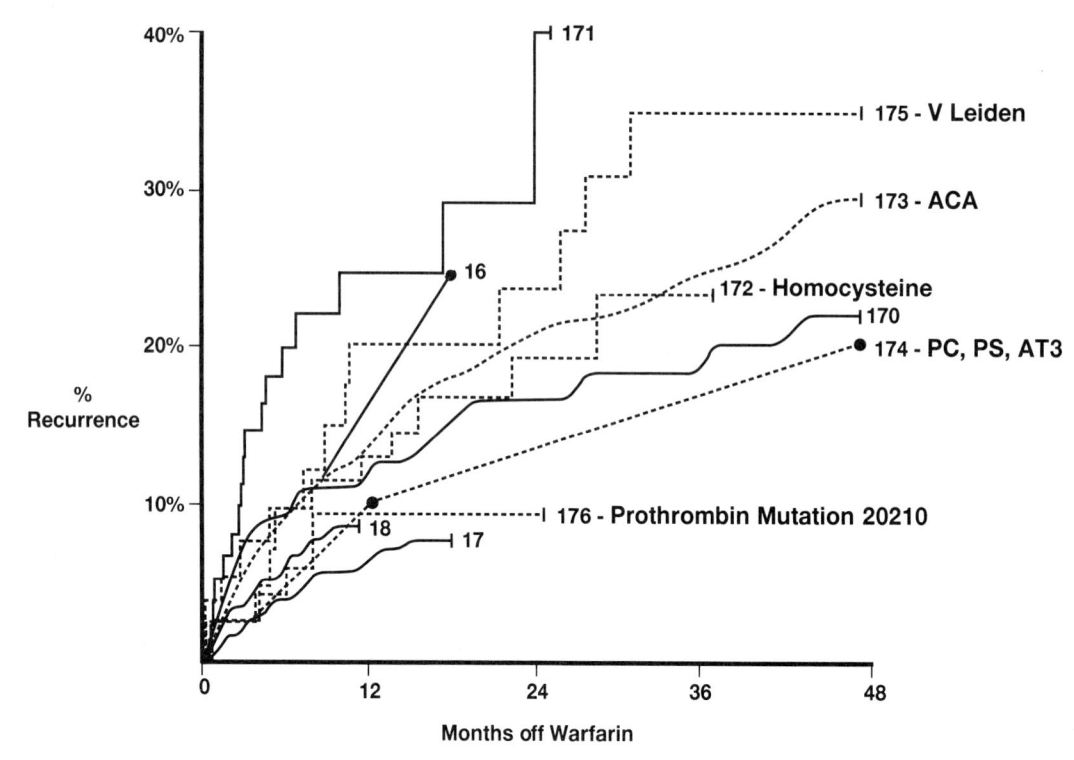

Figure 14-8 This figure represents rates of recurrent VTE after cessation of 6 months of warfarin therapy given for treatment of the initial episode of VTE. This figure was prepared by taking the rates of recurrence data from published series and converting them to graphic form when they were not presented graphically.[17, 174] With publications presenting recurrence rates graphically, the graphs were resized to standardize the axes. Time "0" in this figure is the time that warfarin therapy was discontinued. The solid lines represent rates of recurrent VTE in patients whose initial episode of VTE was defined as "idiopathic" (generally, in the absence of preceding surgery, trauma, major medical illness, or pregnancy). The dashed lines represent rates of recurrence in patients with a laboratory-defined prothrombotic abnormality. The number beside each line represents the reference from which the graph was derived. One can see that the rate of recurrent VTE after cessation of warfarin therapy is not detectably different in patients with a laboratory-defined prothrombotic defect and those whose thrombosis was idiopathic. Consequently, the consultant can predict the rate of recurrent thrombosis after cessation of standard therapy as well by simply taking a history (did the VTE occur in association with pregnancy, surgery, major trauma, or medical illness, or, possibly, estrogen therapy?) as he or she can be doing laboratory studies and finding a prothrombotic defect. Therapy for longer than the standard 6 months of warfarin treatment should be considered in both groups of patients.

"idiopathic" (i.e., "secondary") is no worse and may be a bit better than that provided by testing. Both of these methods of determining prognosis show that there is a group of patients with a high risk of recurrent VTE after completion of a short course of anticoagulation. The studies published to date do not give much information regarding recurrence rates beyond a year or two after cessation of anticoagulant therapy, so the precise duration of risk is currently unknown. However, the data available strongly suggest that the risk is high for up to 2 years after the first event. Most of these episodes of recurrence can be prevented with a more protracted course of warfarin.[177] Consequently, patients who are thought to be at high risk for recurrence, either by virtue of having idiopathic VTE or thrombosis in the face of a laboratory-defined abnormality, should strongly consider at least 1 to 2 years of anticoagulant therapy. The patient's clinical situation should be re-evaluated clinically to determine if the risk:benefit analysis of continued therapy has changed, based on new medical knowledge, intercurrent adverse effects of anticoagulant therapy, the patient's medical condition, or the patient's perception of the acceptability of the risks involved. This periodic reassessment of the individual patient's risk:benefit analysis is a service that is legitimately within the domain of the hematology consultant.

CONCLUSION

Accepting the role as consulting hematologist providing care to patients with hemostatic disorders is a demanding job. Just in the context of patients with DVT and PE it requires the skills of a generalist in being able to communicate with patients, families, and a wide spectrum of health care providers, including interventional radiologists, echocardiographers, obstetricians, surgeons of all specialties, pharmacists, and (most importantly) the referring physician. In the area of VTE, few clinical decisions are at all straightforward, particularly by the time the hematologist gets consulted. In this area, a detailed knowledge base is very helpful but the ability and willingness to communicate effectively the various risks and benefits to all involved is imperative. With the continual introduction of new techniques, med-

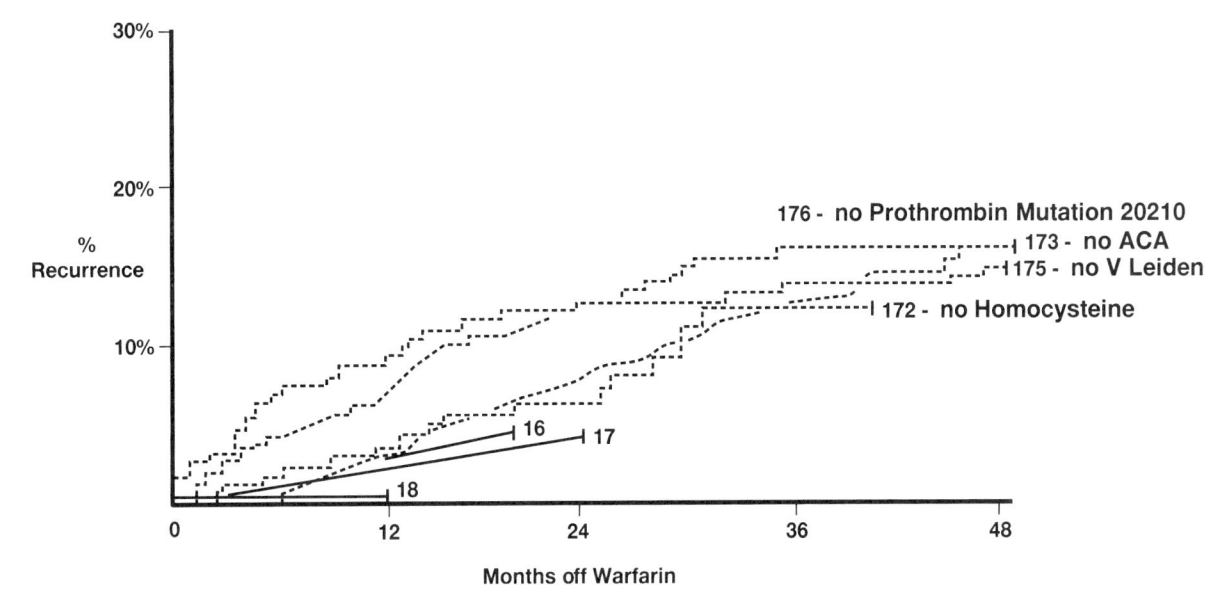

Figure 14–9 This figure represents rates of recurrent VTE after cessation of 6 months of warfarin therapy given for treatment of the initial episode of VTE. The figure was prepared as described for Figure 14–8. the solid lines represent rates of recurrence in patients whose initial episode of VTE was "secondary" (associated with antecedent surgery, trauma, major medical illness, or pregnancy). The dashed lines represent recurrence rate in patients testing negative for the single laboratory-defined prothrombotic abnormality investigated in the particular reference. The number beside each line represents the reference from which the graph was derived.

One can see that the rate of recurrent VTE after cessation of a standard 6 months of warfarin therapy is similar, if not slightly lower, in patients whose initial episode of VTE was secondary to reversible risk factors and in patients without laboratory-definable prothrombotic defects. Consequently, the consultant can estimate these patients' prognosis as well, if not slightly better, by simply taking a history as he or she can by performing a series of laboratory tests and finding no defect. Cessation of warfarin after 6 months or so of therapy should be considered in both groups.

ications, and concepts it is easy for the consultant to get caught up in the details involved in staying up-to-date. However, the most important part of their job is that of communication. Its requirements, though time consuming and occasionally frustrating, remain fairly constant.

REFERENCES

Chapter 14 References

1. Hull RD, Hirsh J, Carter CJ, et al. Pulmonary angiography, ventilation lung scanning, and venography for clinically suspected pulmonary embolism with abnormal perfusion lung scan. Ann Intern Med 1983;98:891–899.
2. Girard P, Musset D, Parent F, et al. High prevalence of detectable deep venous thrombosis in patients with acute pulmonary embolism. Chest 1999;116:903–908.
3. Moser KM, Cantor JP, Olman M, et al. Chronic pulmonary thromboembolism in dogs treated with tranexamic acid. Circulation 1991;83:1371–1379.
4. Nielsen HK, Husted SE, Krussel LR, et al. Silent pulmonary embolism in patients with deep vein thrombosis. Incidence and fate in a randomized, controlled trial of anticoagulation versus no anticoagulation. J Intern Med 1994;235:457–461.
5. Monreal M, Barroso CR, Manzano JR, et al. Asymptomatic pulmonary embolism in patients with deep vein thrombosis. Is it useful to take a lung scan to rule out this condition? J Cardiovasc Surg 1989;30:104–107.
6. Warlow C, Ogston D, Doublas AS. Deep venous thrombosis of the legs after strokes. Part I: Incidence and predisposing factors. Br Med J 1976;1:1178–1183.
7. Turpie AGG, Hirsh J, Jay RM, et al. Double-blind randomized trial of ORG 10172 low-molecular-weight heparinoid in prevention of deep-vein thrombosis in thrombotic stroke. Lancet 1987;1:523–526.
8. Comerota AJ, Stewart GJ, Alburger PD, et al. Operative venodilation: A previously unsuspected factor in the cause of postoperative deep vein thrombosis. Surgery 1989;106:301–309.
9. van der Poll T, Büller HR, ten Cate H, et al. Activation of coagulation after administration of tumor necrosis factor to normal subjects. N Engl J Med 1990;322:1622–1627.
10. Conkling PR, Greenberg CS, Weinberg JB. Tumor necrosis factor induces tissue factor-like activity in human leukemia cell line U937 and peripheral blood monocytes. Blood 1988;72:128–133.
11. van Hinsbergh VWM, Bauer KA, Kooistra T, et al. Progress of fibrinolysis during tumor necrosis factor infusions in humans. Concomitant increase in tissue-type plasminogen activator, plasminogen activator inhibitor type-1, and fibrin(ogen) degradation products. Blood 1990;76:2284–2289.
12. Binns M, Pho R. Femoral vein occlusion during hip arthroplasty. Clin Orthop Rel Res 1990;255:168–172.
13. Lentz Sr, Tsiang M, Sadler JE. Regulation of thrombomodulin by tumor necrosis factor-α: Comparison of transcriptional and posttranscriptional mechanisms. Blood 1991;77:542–550.
14. Nemerson Y. Tissue factor: Then and now. Thromb Haemost 1995;74:180–184.
15. Flynn PD, Byrne CD, Baglen TP, et al. Thrombin generation by apoptotic vascular smooth muscle cells. Blood 1997;89:4378–4384.
16. Prandoni P, Lensing AWA, Büller HR, et al. Deep-vein thrombosis and the incidence of subsequent symptomatic cancer. N Engl J Med 1992;327:1128–1133.
17. Schulman S, Rhedin A-S, Lindmarker P, et al. A comparison of six weeks with six months of oral anticoagulant therapy after a first episode of venous thromboembolism. N Engl J Med 1995;332:1661–1665.
18. Levine MN, Hirsh J, Gent M, et al. Optimal duration of oral anticoagulant therapy: A randomized trial comparing four weeks

with three months of warfarin in patients with proximal deep vein thrombosis. Thromb Haemost 1995;74:606–611.
19. Prandoni P, Lensing AWA, Cogo A, et al. The long-term clinical course of acute deep venous thrombosis. Ann Intern Med 1996;125:1–7.
20. Practice C. Thromboprophylaxis in elective orthopaedic surgery—what is the purpose? J Bone Joint Surg 1997;79B:889–890.
21. Fender D, Harper WM, Thompson JR, et al. Mortality and fatal pulmonary embolism after primary total hip replacement. J Bone Joint Surg 1997;79B:896–899.
22. Dahl OE. Commentary on thromboprophylaxis in hip replacement surgery. Acta Orthop Scand 1998;69:343–344.
23. Bratzler DW, Raskob GE, Murray CK, et al. Underuse of venous thromboembolism prophylaxis for general surgery patients. Arch Intern Med 1998;158:1909–1912.
24. Anderson FA, Wheeler HB, Goldberg RJ, et al. Changing clinical practice. Arch Intern Med 1994;154:669–677.
25. Comess KA, DeRook FA, Russell ML, et al. The incidence of pulmonary embolism in unexplained sudden cardiac arrest with pulseless electrical activity. Am J Med 2000;109:351–356.
26. Geerts WH, Heit JA, Clagett GP. Prevention of venous thromboembolism. Chest 2001;119:132S–175S.
27. Heit JA, Silverstein MD, Mohr DN, et al. Risk factors for deep vein thrombosis and pulmonary embolism: a population-based case-control study. Arch Intern Med 2000;160:809–815.
28. Kearon C, Salzman EW, Hirsh J. Epidemiology, pathogenesis, and natural history of venous thrombosis. In: Colman RW, Hirsh J, Marder VJ, Clowes AW, George JN (Eds.): Hemostasis and Thrombosis: Basic Principles and Clinical Practice, 4th ed. Philadelphia, Lippincott, Williams & Wilkins, 2001, pp. 1153–1177.
29. White RH, Zhou H, Romano PS. Incidence of idiopathic deep venous thrombosis and secondary embolism among ethnic groups in California. Ann Intern Med 1998;128:737–740.
30. Levine M, Hirsh J, Gent M, et al. Double-blind randomized trial of very-low-dose warfarin for prevention of thromboembolism in stage IV breast cancer. Lancet 1994;343:886–889.
31. Ramos R, Salem BI, De Pawlikowski MP, et al. The efficacy of pneumatic compression stockings in the prevention of pulmonary embolism after cardiac surgery. Chest 1996;109:82–85.
32. Comerota AJ, Katz ML, White JV. Why does prophylaxis with external pneumatic compression for deep vein thrombosis fail? Am J Surg 1992;164:265–268.
33. Wells PS, Lensing AWA, Davidson BL, et al. Accuracy of ultrasound for the diagnosis of deep venous thrombosis in asymptomatic patients after orthopedic surgery. Ann Intern Med 1995;122:47–53.
34. Ascani A, Radicchi S, Parise P, et al. Distribution and occlusiveness of thrombi in patients with surveillance detected deep vein thrombosis after hip surgery. Thromb Haemost 1996;75: 239–241.
35. Estrada CA, McElligott J, Dolezal JM, et al. Asymptomatic patients at high risk for deep venous thrombosis who receive inadequate prophylaxis should be screened. South Med J 1999;92:1145–1150.
36. Bergqvist D, Benoni G, Björgel O, et al. Extending enoxaparin 1 month after hospital discharge reduced thromboembolism after elective hip surgery. N Engl J Med 1996;335:696–700.
37. Planes A, Vochelle N, Darmon J-Y, et al. Risk of deep-venous thrombosis after hospital discharge in patients having undergone total hip replacement; double-blind randomised comparison of enoxaparin versus placebo. Lancet 1996;348:224–228.
38. Manganelli D, Pazzagli M, Mazzantini D, et al. Prolonged prophylaxis with unfractionated heparin is effective to reduce delayed deep vein thrombosis in total hip replacement. Respiration 1998;65:369–374.
39. Buehler KO, D'Lima DD, Petersilge WJ, et al. Late deep venous thrombosis and delayed weightbearing after total hip arthroplasty. Clin Orthop Rel Res 1999;361:123–130.
40. Leclerc JR, Gent M, Hirsh J, et al. The incidence of symptomatic venous thromboembolism during and after prophylaxis with enoxaparin. Arch Intern Med 1998;158:873–878.
41. Dahl OE, Andreassen G, Aspelin T, et al. Prolonged thromboprophylaxis following hip replacement surgery—results of a double-blind, prospective, randomised, placebo-controlled study with dalteparin (Fragmin®). Thromb Haemost 1997;77:26–31.
42. Caprini JA, Arcelus JI, Motykie G, et al. The influence of oral anticoagulation therapy on deep vein thrombosis rates four weeks after total hip replacement. J Vasc Surg 1999;30:813–820.
43. Lederle FA. Heparin prophylaxis for medical patients? Ann Intern Med 1998;128:768–770.
43a. Mismetti P, Laforte-Simitsidis S, Tardy B, et al. Prevention of venous thrombosis in internal medicine with unfractionated or low-molecular weight heparins: a meta-analysis of randomised clinical trials. Thromb Haemost 2000;83:14–19.
44. Bergmann J-F, Neuhart E. A multicenter randomized double-blind study of enoxaparin compared with unfractionated heparin in the prevention of venous thromboembolic disease in elderly in-patients bedridden for an acute medical illness. Thromb Haemost 1996;76:529–534.
45. Samama MM, Cohen AT, Darmon J-Y, et al. A comparison of enoxaparin with placebo for the prevention of venous thromboembolism in acutely ill medical patients. N Engl J Med 1999; 341:793–800.
46. Cruickshank JM, Gorlin R, Jennet B. Air travel and thrombotic episodes: the economy class syndrome. Lancet 1988;II:497–499.
47. Kraaijenhagen RA, Haverkamp D, Koopman MMW, et al. Travel and venous thrombosis. Lancet 2000;356:1492–1493.
48. Eekhoff EMW, Rosendaal FR, Vandenbroucke JP. Minor events and the risk of deep venous thrombosis. Thromb Haemost 2000;83:408–411.
49. Ferrari E. Chevalier T, Chapelier A, et al. Travel as a risk factor for venous thromboembolic disease: a case-control study. Chest 1999;115:440–444.
50. Arfvidsson B, Eklof B, Kistner RL, et al. Risk factors for venous thromboembolism following prolonged air travel: a "prospective" study. Vasc Surg 1999;33:537–544.
50a. Parsi KA, McGrath MA, Lord RSA. Traveller's venous thromboembolism. Cardiovasc Surg 2001;9:157–158.
50b. Lapostolle F, Surget V, Borron SW, et al. Severe pulmonary embolism associated with air travel. N Engl J Med 2001; 345:779–783.
51. Decousus H, Leizorovicz A, Parent F, et al. A clinical trial of vena caval filters in the prevention of pulmonary embolism in patients with proximal deep-vein thrombosis. N Engl J Med 1998;338:409–415.
52. Khorasani R, Gudas TF, Nikpoor N, et al. Treatment of patients with suspected pulmonary embolism and intermediate-probability lung scans: Is diagnostic imaging underused? Am J Radiol 1997;169:1355–1357.
53. Marder VJ, Soulen RL, Atichartakarn V, et al. Quantitative venographic assessment of deep vein thrombosis in the evaluation of streptokinase and heparin therapy. J Lab Clin Med 1977;89:1018–1028.
54. Krupski WC, Bass A, Dilley RB, et al. Propagation of deep venous thrombosis identified by duplex ultrasonography. J Vasc Surg 1990;12:467–475.
55. Arnesen H, Heilo A, Jakobsen E, et al. A prospective study of streptokinase and heparin in the treatment of deep vein thrombosis. Acta Med Scand 1978;203:457–463.
56. Nielsen HK, Husted SE, Krusell LR, et al. Anticoagulant therapy in deep venous thrombosis. A randomized controlled study. Thromb Res 1994;73:215–226.
57. van Ramshorst B, van Bemmelen PS, Hoeneveld H, et al. Thrombus regression in deep venous thrombosis. Quantification of spontaneous thrombolysis with duplex scanning. Circulation 1992;86:414–419.

58. Caps MT, Meissner MH, Tullis MJ, et al. Venous thrombus stability during acute phase of therapy. Vasc Med 1999;4:9–14.
59. Meissner MH, Caps MT, Bergelin RO, et al. Propagation, rethrombosis and new thrombus formation after acute deep venous thrombosis. J Vasc Surg 1995;22:558–567.
60. Basu D, Gallus A, Hirsh J, et al. A prospective study of the value of monitoring heparin treatement with the activated partial thromboplastin time. N Engl J Med 1972;287:324–327.
61. Hull RD, Raskob GE, Rosenbloom D, et al. Heparin for 5 days as compared with 10 days in the initial treatment of proximal venous thrombosis. N Engl J Med 1990;322:1260–1264.
62. Hull RD, Raskob GE, Hirsh J, et al. Continuous intravenous heparin compared with intermittent subcutaneous heparin in the initial treatment of proximal-vein thrombosis. N Engl J Med 1986;315:1109–1114.
63. Levine MN, Hirsh J, Gent M, et al. A randomized trial comparing activated thromboplastin time with heparin assay in patients with acute venous thromboembolism requiring large daily doses of heparin. Arch Intern Med 1994;154:49–56.
64. Schulman S, Lockner D. Relationship between thromboembolic complications and intensity of treatment during long-term prophylaxis with oral anticoagulants following DVT. Thromb Haemost 1985;53:137–140.
65. Gitter MJ, Jaeger TM, Petterson TM et al. Bleeding and thromboembolism during anticoagulant therapy: A population-based study in Rochester, Minnesota. Mayo Clin Proc 1995;70:725–733.
66. Cronan JJ, Leen V. Recurrent deep venous thrombosis: Limitations of US. Radiology 1989;170:739–742.
67. Killewich LA, Bedford GR, Beach KW, et al. Spontaneous lysis of deep venous thrombi: Rate and outcome. J Vasc Surg 1989;9:89–97.
68. Caprini JA, Arcelus JI, Hoffman KN, et al. Venous duplex imaging follow-up of acute symptomatic deep vein thrombosis of the leg. J Vasc Surg 1995;21:472–476.
69. Killewich LA, Macko RF, Cox K, et al. Regression of proximal deep venous thrombosis is associated with fibrinolytic enhancement. J Vasc Surg 1997;26:861–868.
70. Holmström M, Lindmarker P, Granqvist S, et al. A 6-month venographic follow-up in 164 patients with acute deep vein thrombosis. Thromb Haemost 1997;78:803–807.
71. Fraser JD, Anderson DR. Deep venous thrombosis: Recent advances and optimal investigation with US. Radiology 1999; 211:9–24.
72. Prandoni P, Lensing AWA, Cogo A, et al. The long-term clinical course of acute deep venous thrombosis. Ann Intern Med 1996;125:1–7.
73. Strandness DE Jr, Langlois Y, Cramer M, et al. Long-term sequelae of acute venous thrombosis. JAMA 1983;250:1289–1292.
74. Beyth RJ, Cohen AM, Landefeld CS. Long-term outcomes of deep-vein thrombosis. Arch Intern Med 1995;155:1031–1037.
75. Hull RD, Carter CJ, Jay RM, et al. The diagnosis of acute, recurrent deep-vein thrombosis: A diagnostic challenge. Circulation 1983;67:901–906.
76. Huisman MV, Büller HR, ten Cate JW. Utility of impedance plethysmography in the diagnosis of recurrent deep-vein thrombosis. Arch Intern Med 1998;148:681–683.
77. Prandoni P, Cogo A, Bernardi E, et al. A simple ultrasound approach for detection of recurrent proximal-vein thrombosis. Circulation 1993; 88(part 1):1730–1735.
78. Kearon C, Julian JA, Newman TE, et al. Noninvasive diagnosis of deep venous thrombosis. Ann Intern Med 1998;128:663–677.
79. Murphy TP, Cronan JJ. Evolution of deep venous thrombosis: A prospective evaluation with US. Radiology 1990;177:543–548.
80. Labropoulos N, Webb KM, Kang SS, et al. Patterns and distribution of isolated calf deep vein thrombosis. J Vasc Surg 1999; 30:787–793.
81. Giannoukas AD, Labropoulos N, Burke P, et al. Calf deep venous thrombosis: a review of the literature. Eur J Endovasc Surg 1995;10:398–404.
82. Kalebo P, Anthmyr BA, Eriksson BI, et al. Optimization of ascending phlebography of the leg for screening of deep vein thrombosis in thromboprophylactic trials. Acta Radiol 1997; 38:320–326.
83. ENOXACAN Study Group. Efficacy and safety of enoxaparin versus unfractionated heparin for prevention of deep vein thrombosis in elective cancer surgery: a double-blind randomized multicentre trial with venographic assessment. Br J Surg 1997; 84:1099–1103.
84. Couson F, Bounameaux C, Didier D, et al. Influence of variability of interpretation of contrast venography for screening of postoperative deep venous thrombosis on the results of a thromboprophylactic study. Thromb Haemost 1993;70:573–575.
85. Goldhaber SZ, Hennekens CH, Evans DA, et al. Factors associated with correct antemorten diagnosis of major pulmonary embolism. Am J Med 1982;73:822–826.
86. Stein PD, Hull RD. Relative risks of anticoagulant treatment of acute pulmonary embolism based on an angiographic diagnosis vs a ventilation/perfusion scan diagnosis. Chest 1994;106: 727–730.
87. Worsley DF, Palevsky HI, Alavi A. A detailed evaluation of patients with acute pulmonary embolism and low or very low probability lung scans. Arch Intern Med 1994;154:2737–2741.
88. Beyth RJ, Quinn LM, Landefeld CS. Prospective evaluation of an index for predicting the risk of major bleeding in outpatients treatment with warfarin. Am J Med 1998;105:91–99.
89. Nieuwenhuis HK, Albada J, Banga JD, et al. Identification of risk factors for bleeding during treatment of acute venous thromboembolism with heparin or low molecular weight heparin. Blood 1991;78:2337–2343.
90. Nilsson T, Carlsson A, Måre K. Pulmonary angiography: a safe procedure with modern contrast media and technique. Eur Radiol 1998;8:86–89.
91. Stein PD, Athanasoulis C, Alavi A, et al. Complications and validity of pulmonary angiography in acute pulmonary embolism. Circulation 1992;85:462–468.
92. Stein PD, Gottschalk A, Saltzman HA, et al. Diagnosis of acute pulmonary embolism in the elderly. J Am Coll Cardiol 1991; 18:1452–1457.
93. Righini M, Goehring C, Bounameaux H, et al. Effects of age on the performance of common diagnostic tests for pulmonary embolism. Am J Med 2000;109:357–361.
94. Turkstra F, Kuijer PMM, van Beek EJR, et al. Diagnostic utility of ultrasonography of leg veins in patients suspected of having pulmonary embolism. Ann Intern Med 1997;126:775–781.
95. Stein PD, Hull RD, Pineo G. Strategy that includes serial noninvasive leg tests for diagnosis of thromboembolic disease in patients with suspected acute pulmonary embolism based on data from PIOPED. Arch Intern Med 1995;155:2101–2104.
96. Meaney JFM, Weg JG, Chenevert TL. Diagnosis of pulmonary embolism with magnetic resonance angiography. N Engl J Med 1997;336:1422–1427.
97. Mullins MD, Becker DM, Hagspiel KD, et al. The role of spiral volumetric computed tomography in the diagnosis of pulmonary embolism. Arch Intern Med 2000;160:293–298.
98. Rathbun SW, Raskob GE, Whitsett TL. Sensitivity and specificity of helical computed tomography in the diagnosis of pulmonary embolism: A systematic review. Ann Intern Med 2000;132: 227–232.
99. Tapson VF. Editorial: Pulmonary embolism—new diagnostic approaches. N Engl J Med 1997;336:1449–1451.
100. Bergin CJ. Imaging of pulmonary thromboembolic disease. Semin Resp Crit Care Med 1998;19:505–514.
101. Smith GT, McClaughry PL, Purkey J, et al. Crack cocaine mimicking pulmonary embolism on pulmonary ventilation/perfusion lung scan: A case report. Clin Nucl Med 1995;20:65–68.
102. King Mb, Harmon KR. Unusual forms of pulmonary embolism. Clin Chest Med 1994;15:561–580.

103. Gordon JJ, Austin M, Kurtides ES. Pseudothromboembolism in myeloid metaplasia. Ann Intern Med 1998;108:837–838.
104. Estagnasie P, Djedaïni K, Le Bourdellès G, et al. Atrial septal aneurysm plus a patent foramen ovale. Chest 1996;110:846–848.
105. Konstantinides S, Geibel A, Kasper W, et al. Patent foramen ovale is an important predictor of adverse outcome in patients with major pulmonary embolism. Circulation 1998;97:1946–1951.
106. Walsh PN, Stengle JM, Sherry S. The urokinase pulmonary embolism trial. Circulation 1969;39:153–156.
107. A Cooperative Study: Urokinase-Streptokinase Embolism Trial. JAMA 1974;229:1606–1613.
108. Goldhaber SZ, Haire WD, Feldstein ML, et al. Alteplase versus heparin in acute pulmonary embolism: randomised trial assessing right-ventricular function and pulmonary perfusion. Lancet 1993;341:507–511.
109. Douketis JD, Kearon C, Bates S, et al. Risk of fatal pulmonary embolism in patients with treated venous thromboembolism. JAMA 1998;279:458–462.
110. Ribeiro A, Lindmarker P, Johnsson H, et al. Pulmonary embolism: One-year follow-up with echocardiography doppler and five-year survival analysis. Circulation 1999;99:1325–1330.
111. Grifoni S, Olivotto I, Cecchini P, et al. Clinical outcome of patients with pulmonary embolism, normal blood pressure and echocardiographic right ventricular dysfunction. Circulation 2000;101:2817–2822.
112. Konstantinides S, Geibel A, Olschewski M, et al. Association between thrombolytic treatment and the prognosis of hemodynamically stable patients with major pulmonary embolism: Results of a multicenter registry. Circulation 1997;96:882–888.
113. Sharma GVRK, Burleson VA, Sasahara AA. Effect of thrombolytic therapy on pulmonary-capillary blood volume in patients with pulmonary embolism. N Engl J Med 1980;303:842–845.
114. Sharma GVRK, Folland Ed, McIntyre KM, et al. Long term benefit of thrombolytic therapy in pulmonary embolism. Vasc Med 2000;5:91–95.
115. McConnell MV, Solomon SD, Rayan ME, et al. Regional right ventricular dysfunction detected by echocardiography in acute pulmonary embolism. Am J Cardiol 1996;78:469–473.
116. Tow DE, Wagner HN Jr. Recovery of pulmonary arterial blood flow in patients with pulmonary embolism. N Engl J Med 1967;276:1053–1059.
117. Daniels LB, Parker A, Patel SR, et al. Relation of duration of symptoms with response to thrombolytic therapy in pulmonary embolism. Am J Cardiol 1997;80:184–188.
118. Goldhaber SZ. Integration of catheter thrombectomy into our armamentarium to treat acute pulmonary embolism. Chest 1998;114:1237–1238.
119. Moser KM, LeMoine JR. Is the embolic risk conditioned by the location of deep venous thrombosis? Ann Intern Med 1981; 94:494–444.
120. Philbrick JT, Becker DM. Calf vein thrombosis: a wolf in sheep's clothing? Arch Intern Med 1988;148:2131–2138.
121. Kazmers A, Geoehn H, Meeker C. Acute calf vein thrombosis: outcomes and implications. Am Surg 1999;65:1124–1127.
122. Lohr JM, Kerr TM, Lutter KS, et al. Lower extremity calf thrombosis: to treat or not to treat? J Vasc Surg 1991;14:618–623.
123. Lagerstedt CI, Olsson CG, Fagher BO, et al. Need for long-term anticoagulant treatment in symptomatic calf-vein thrombosis. Lancet 1985;II:515–518.
124. Bundens WP, Bergan JJ, Halasz NA, et al. The superficial femoral vein: a potentially lethal misnomer. JAMA 1995;274:1296–1298.
125. Jorgensen JO, Hanel KC, Morgan AM, et al. The incidence of deep venous thrombosis in patients with superficial thrombophlebitis of the lower limbs. J Vasc Surg 1993;18:70–73.
126. Bounameaux H, Reber-WasemMA. Superficial thrombophlebitis and deep vein thrombosis: a controversial association. Arch Intern Med 1997;157:1822–1824.
127. Chenglis DL, Bendick PJ, Glover JL, et al. Progression of superficial venous thrombosis to deep venous thrombosis. J Vasc Surg 1996;24:745–749.
128. Verlato F, Zucchetta P, Prandoni P, et al. An unexpectedly high rate of pulmonary embolism in patients with superficial thrombophlebitis of the thigh. J Vasc Surg 1999;30:1113–1115.
129. Hanson JN, Ascher E, DePippo P, et al. Saphenous vein thrombophlebitis: a deceptively benign disease. J Vasc Surg 1998; 27:677–680.
130. De Moerloose P, Wutschert R, Heinzman M, et al. Superficial vein thrombosis of the lower limbs:influence of factor V Leiden, factor II G20210A and overweight. Thromb Haemost 1998; 80:239–41.
131. Martinelli I, Cattaneo M, Taioli E, et al. Risk factors for superficial vein thrombosis: the role of thrombophilic states (abstract). Blood 1998;92(suppl 1):559a.
132. Goldhaber SZ, Buring JE, Lipnick RJ, et al. Pooled analyses of randomized trials of streptokinase and heparin in phlebographically documented acute deep venous thrombosis. Am J Med 1984;76:393–397.
133. Comerota AJ. Thrombolytic therapy for acute deep vein thrombosis. In: Comerota AJ (Ed.): Thrombolytic Therapy for Peripheral Vascular Disease, Philadelphia, JB Lippincott, 1995, pp. 175–195.
134. Rogers LQ, Lutcher CL. Streptokinase therapy for deep vein thrombosis: A comprehensive review of the English literature. Am J Med 1990;88:389–395.
135. Sidorov J. Streptokinase vs heparin for deep venous thrombosis. Can lytic therapy be justified? Arch Intern Med 1989;149:1841–1845.
136. Horne MK, Chang R. Thrombolytic therapy for deep venous thrombosis? JAMA 1999;282:2164–2166.
137. Mewissen MW, Seabrook GR, Meissner MH, et al. Catheter-directed thrombolysis for lower extremity deep venous thrombosis: Report of a national multicenter registry. Radiology 1999; 211:39–49.
138. Comerota AJ, Throm RC, Mathias S, et al. Catheter-directed thrombolysis for iliofemoral DVT improved health related quality-of-life. J Vasc Surg 2000;32:130–137.
139. Brandjes DPM, Heijboer H, Büller HR, et al. Acenocoumarol and heparin compared with acenocoumarol alone in the initial treatment of proximal-vein thrombosis. N Engl J Med 1992; 327:1485–1489.
140. Anand SS, Bates S, Ginsberg JS, et al. Recurrent venous thrombosis and heparin therapy. An evaluation of the importance of early activated partial thromboplastin times. Arch Intern Med 1999;159:2029–2032.
141. Gould MK, Dembitzer AD, Doyle RL, et al. Low-molecular-weight heparins compared with unfractionated heparin for treatment of acute deep venous thrombosis. A meta-analysis of randomized, controlled trials. Ann Intern Med 1999;130:800–809.
142. Stein PD, Henry JW, Relyea B. Untreated patients with pulmonary embolism: outcome, clinical and laboratory assessment. Chest 1995;107:931–935.
143. Stein PD, Hull RD, Raskob GE. Withholding treatment in patients with acute pulmonary embolism who have a high risk of bleeding and negative serial noninvasive leg tests. Am J Med 2000;109:301–306.
144. Koopman MMW, Prandoni P, Piovella F, et al. Treatment of venous thrombosis with intravenous unfractionated heparin administered in the hospital as compared with subcutaneous low molecular weight heparin administered at home. N Engl J Med 1996;334:682–687.
145. Levine M, Gent M, Hirsh J, et al. A comparison of low molecular weight heparin administered primarily at home with unfractionated heparin administered in the hospital for proximal deep-vein thrombosis. N Engl J Med 1996;334:677–681.
146. Schwarz T, Schellong SM, Schmidt B, et al. Bed rest in deep vein thrombosis and the incidence of pulmonary embolism (abstract). Thromb Haemost (suppl) 1999:837.

147. Partsch H, Blattler W. Compression and walking versus bed rest in the treatment of proximal deep venous thrombosis with low molecular weight heparin. J Vasc Surg 2000;32:861–869.
147a. Aschwanden M, Labs K-H, Engel H, et al. Acute deep vein thrombosis: early mobilization does not increase the frequency of pulmonary embolism. Thromb Haemost 2001;85:42–46.
148. Perkins JMT, Magee TR, Galland RB. Phlegmasia cerulea dolens and venous gangrene. Br J Surg 1996;83:19–23.
149. Aruny JE, Kandarpa K. Phlegmasia cerulea dolens, a complication after placement of a bird's nest vena cava filter. AJR 1990;154:1105–1106.
150. Ihnat DM, Mills JL, Hughes JD, et al. Treatment of patients with venous thromboembolism and malignant disease: should vena cava filter placement be routine? J Vasc Surg 1998; 28:800–807.
151. Feinman LJ, Meltzer AJ. Phlegmasia cerulea dolens as a complication of percutaneous insertion of a vena cava filter. J Am Osteopath Assoc 1989;89:63–68.
152. Sciolaro C, Hunter GC, McIntyre KE, et al. Thrombectomy and isolated limb perfusion with urokinase in the treatment of phlegmasia cerulea dolens. Cardiovasc Surg 1993;1:56–60.
153. Harris EJ, Kinney EV, Harris EJ, et al. Phlegmasia complicating prophylactic percutaneous inferior vena caval interruption. J Vasc Surg 1995;22:606–611.
154. Warkentin TE, Elavathil LJ, Hayward CPM, et al. The pathogenesis of venous limb gangrene associated with heparin-induced thrombocytopenia. Ann Intern Med 1997;127:804–812.
155. Hood DB, Weaver FA, Modrall JG, et al. Advances in the treatment of phlegmasia cerulea dolens. Am J Surg 1993; 166:206–210.
156. Patel KR, Paidas CN. Phlegmasia cerulea dolens: the role of non-operative therapy. Cardiovasc Surg 1993;1:518–523.
157. Patel NH, Plorde JJ, Meissner M. Catheter-directed thrombolysis in the treatment of phlegmasia cerulea dolens. Ann Vasc Surg 1998;12:471–475.
158. Roder OC, Lorentzen JE, Hansen HJB. Venous thrombectomy for iliofemoral thrombosis: early and long-term results in 46 consecutive cases. Acta Chir Scand 1984;150:31–34.
159. Eklof B, Arfvidsson B, Kistner RL, et al. Indications for surgical treatment of iliofemoral vein thrombosis. Hematol Oncol Clin North Am 2000;14:471–482.
160. Hull R, Delmore T, Carter C, et al. Adjusted subcutaneous heparin versus warfarin sodium in the long-term treatment of venous thrmbosis. N Engl J Med 1982;306:189–194.
161. Gonzalez-Fajardo JA, Arreba E, Castrodeza J, et al. Venographic comparison of subcutaneous low-molecular weight heparin with oral anticoagulant therapy in the long-term treatment of deep venous thrombosis. J Vasc Surg 1999;30:283–292.
162. Veiga F, Escriba A, Maluenda MP, et al. Low molecular weight heparin (enoxaparin) versus oral anticoagulant therapy (acenocoumarol) in the long-term treatment of deep venous thrombosis in the elderly: a randomized trial. Thromb Haemost 2000; 84:559–564.
163. Das SK, Cohen AT, Edmondson RA, et al. Low molecular weight heparin versus warfarin for prevention of recurrent venous thromboembolism: a randomized trial. World J Surg 1996; 20:521–527.
164. Lopaciuk S, Bielska-Falda H, Noszczyc W, et al. Low molecular weight heparin versus acenocoumarol in the secondary prophylaxis of deep vein thrombosis. Thromb Haemost 1998;81:26–31.
165. Pini M, Aiello S, Manotti C, et al. Low molecular weight heparin versus warfarin in the prevention of recurrences after deep vein thrombosis. Thromb Haemost 1994;72:191–197.
166. Hull R, Pineo G, Mah A, Brant R. Long term low molecular weight heparin treatment versus oral anticoagulant therapy for proximal deep vein thrombosis (abstract). Blood 2000; 96(suppl 1):449a.
167. Heit JA, Mohr DN, Silverstein MD, et al. Predictors of recurrence after deep vein thrombosis and pulmonary embolism: a population-based cohort study. Arch Intern Med 2000;160: 761–768.
168. Hyers TM, Agnelli G, Hull RD, et al. Antithrombotic therapy for venous thromboembolic disease. Chest 1998;114 Supplement:561S–578S.
168a. Hyers TM, Agnelli G, Hull RD, et al. Antithrombotic therapy for venous thromboembolic disease. Chest 2001;119 Supplement:176S–193S.
169. Baglin C, Brown K, Luddington R, et al. Risk of recurrent venous thromboembolism in patients with the factor V Leiden mutation: effect of warfarin and prediction by precipitating factors. Br J Haematol 1998;100:764–768.
170. Petitti DB, Strom BL, Melmon KL. Duration of warfarin anticoagulant therapy and the probabilities of recurrent thromboembolism and hemorrhage. Am J Med 1986;81:255–259.
171. Kearon C, Gent M, Hirsh J, et al. A comparison of three months of anticoagulation with extended anticoagulation for a first episode of idiopathic venous thromboembolism. N Engl J Med 1999;340:901–907.
172. Eichinger S, Stümpflen A, Hirschl M, et al. Hyperhomocysteinemia is a risk factor of recurrent venous thromboembolism. Thromb Haemost 1998;80:566–569.
173. Schulman S, Svenungsson E, Granqvist S, et al. Anticardiolipin antibodies predict early recurrence of thromboembolism and death among patients with venous thromboembolism following anticoagulant therapy. Am J Med 1998;104:332–338.
174. van den Belt AGM, Sanson B-J, Simioni P, et al. Recurrence of venous thromboembolism in patients with familial thrombophilia. Arch Intern Med 1997;157:2227–2232.
175. Simioni P, Prandoni P, Lensing AWA, et al. The risk of recurrent venous thromboembolism in patients with an $Arg^{506} \to Gln$ mutation in the gene for factor V (Factor V Leiden). N Engl J Med 1997;336:399–403.
176. Eichinger S, Minar E, Hirschl M, et al. The risk of early recurrent venous thromboembolism after oral anticoagulant therapy in patients with the G20210A transition in the prothrombin gene. Thromb Haemost 1999;81:14–17.
177. Schulman S, Granqvist S, Homström M, et al. The duration of oral anticoagulant after a second episode of venous thromboembolism. N Engl J Med 1997;336:393–398.

CHAPTER 15

Venous Thromboses at Unusual Sites

Craig S. Kitchens, M.D.

Deep venous thrombosis (DVT) and its associated condition pulmonary embolism (PE) represent the most commonly encountered examples of venous thromboembolism (VTE). DVT and PE have been discussed thoroughly in Chapter 14. In this chapter we will discuss VTEs at unusual sites. These events are associated with acquired and congenital hypercoagulable disorders and, although less frequently encountered than DVT, account for a disproportionate amount of morbidity and mortality. Modern radiographic imaging and improved clinical understanding have resulted in more timely diagnosis and institution of effective treatment. Whereas in the past these unusual VTEs were autopsy suite curiosities, we can now deal with them in life, thus avoiding excessive morbidity and mortality.

HISTORICAL ASPECTS

Many founders of what we now call internal medicine complemented their vast clinical practice by precise observations made at the autopsy table. Both William Osler[1] and Austin Flint[2] in their textbooks a century ago discussed unusual sites of VTE. They both recognized that these conditions were characterized by vague and often subacute symptoms and that diagnosis was exceedingly rarely made in life, being made more often than not at autopsy. These observations pertained to thromboses of the hepatic veins, cerebral veins and sinuses, portal vein, and renal vein. Although Virchow[3] speculated 30 years prior to the Osler and Flint textbooks that abnormalities would be found in blood to complement inflammation and impaired circulation (thus creating Virchow's triad), neither Osler nor Flint mentioned his theory. Rather, they resorted to pathophysiologic theories we now regard as somewhat unusual. For instance, the known association of cerebral venous and sinus thrombosis with the puerperium was explained by propagation of clots from pelvic veins up through venous complexes along the spinal column and into the brain. They also speculated that renal vein thrombosis was caused by DVTs of the legs embolizing to a renal vein. These pathogenic mechanisms are no longer embraced. We now hold that these clots are formed in situ yet may coexist with DVTs and PEs, an association that they did appreciate. These great observational clinicians believed that most of these events were idiopathic, although association was made with marantic conditions and chronic infections.

Progress in our knowledge in this area of medicine has been exciting and intellectually satisfying as we have witnessed the replacement of theory, dogma, and the unknown by scientific discovery. Idiopathic causes are dwindling, being replaced by more specific diagnoses.[4] The tempo of knowledge acquisition has been rapid if one recalls that antithrombin III (ATIII) deficiency, the first thrombophilic disease discovered (which vindicated Virchow) was described in 1965, followed by protein C deficiency in 1981 and protein S deficiency in 1984. The factor V Leiden mutation and the prothrombin 20210 mutation were described in 1994 and 1996, respectively. Other disorders will no doubt be found in ensuing years. Not only has the idiopathic category been eroded but also pathogenic mechanisms have given way to more reasonable concepts. Thrombotic events are still best explained by a "double hit" in which there is an underlying hypercoagulable condition that does require an additional provocation such as pregnancy, surgery, infection, travel, or some other condition to tip the hemostatic scales in favor of thrombosis. Contributing provocations can be revealed in approximately 50% of cases of thrombosis using a thorough history, with the remaing half of the cases remaining seemingly spontaneous.[5]

The role of diagnostic imaging in the 21st century is nowwhere better exemplified than by the use of modern radiology in the elucidation of thromboses at unusual sites. Computed tomography (CT) is limited in some aspects, particularly in detecting cerebral vein and sinus thromboses, but it is excellent for imaging visceral thromboses. Ultrasonography has been extremely useful in diagnosis of visceral thromboses. Overall, magnetic resonance imaging/angiography (MRI/MRA) is the most sensitive and specific way to diagnose thromboses at unusual sites.

IMPORTANCE TO THE PATIENT AND CLINICIAN

DVT and PE remain the *sine qua non* of hypercoagulability. Using ATIII deficiency as the prototypic hypercoagulable disease, data are available to show that 25% of all patients with ATIII deficiency will at some time manifest their thrombophilia by thrombosis at an unusual site[6-9] (Table 15–1). These thromboses may be the initial presentation of thrombophilia, may coexist with DVT/PE, or may arise later in the course once the diagnosis of hypercoagulability has been established in either the patient or his kindred. A clue to the correct diagnosis of a thrombosis at an unusual site often is found in a past personal or family history of thromboembolism. Data presented by DeStefano et al.[5] substantiate the role of a heightened index of suspicion in the thrombophilic patient in sorting out the differential diagnosis of vague subacute symptoms. Whereas such symptoms may be of uncertain meaning in normal patients, those same symptoms in a thrombophilic patient may very well be interpreted rapidly as a cerebral or visceral thrombosis.

One could charge that the hematology community has been somewhat passive in the diagnosis, management, and follow-up of these patients, instead yielding to organ-specific physicians such as the hepatologist for a patient with hepatic vein thrombosis, the nephrologist for the patient with renal thrombosis, and the neurologist for the patient with cerebral vein thrombosis. It is obvious that the pathophysiologic link among these three examples is hypercoagulability, with the affected organ primarily an "innocent bystander." Having one organ manifest a thrombosis in no way protects other organs from thrombosis in patients with hypercoagulability. By virtue of having a cadre of hypercoagulable patients, the hematologist is in position to make a prompt diagnosis (Table 15–2).

Table 15–1 • THROMBOSES AT UNUSUAL SITES AND THE ROLE OF HYPERCOAGULABILITY

Established
Cerebral venous thrombosis
Mesenteric vein thrombosis
Hepatic venous thrombosis
Purpura fulminans
Splenic vein thrombosis
Portal vein thrombosis
Renal vein thrombosis
Axillary vein thrombosis
Adrenal hemorrhage
Probable
Retinal vein thrombosis
Placental infarction
Pituitary hemorrhage
Pelvic vein thrombosis
Doubtful
Priapism

Table 15–2 • FACTS REGARDING PATIENTS WITH THROMBOSES AT UNUSUAL SITES

- Thrombophilia will account for 75% of these unusual and rare conditions.
- Twenty-five percent of thrombophilic patients will experience at least one of these conditions in their lifetime.
- These conditions cause a considerable degree of morbidity and mortality if not diagnosed and treated aggressively.
- Familiarity with hypercoagulable patients allows the hematologist to maintain a high index of suspicion for these rare conditions.

MESENTERIC VEIN THROMBOSIS

Mesenteric venous thrombosis is a much less common event than mesenteric arterial thrombosis.[10] Arterial thrombosis is usually seen in older, hypertensive, and often diabetic patients presenting with an acute abdominal catastrophic event that rapidly leads to ischemia and death of the abdominal organs supplied by the superior mesenteric artery. Thrombosis of the superior mesenteric vein or the inferior mesenteric vein is less common and is much less precipitous, being subacute in nature. It has been difficult to diagnose historically because reliance on the usual radiographic images, such as flat plates and upright views of the abdomen as well as various barium studies does not lead to the diagnosis, which is much more readily made, even if accidentally, by CT with vascular contrast. The thrombosed superior mesenteric vein is seen as a large distended vessel that does not fill appropriately with contrast (Fig. 15–1). The bowel wall may be thick and edematous. We have observed in several cases a "misty mesentery"[11] by abdominal CT due to inflammation and edema from mesenteric vein thrombosis (Fig. 15–2). This totally resolves with successful therapy of the thrombosis.

Two adjacent articles in *Annals of Surgery* in 1895 provided seminal insight into mesenteric vein thrombosis. Delatour[12] described a fatal case of mesenteric infarction following elective removal of an enlarged spleen for what seems most likely to have been a myeloproliferative disorder. He opined that the hematologic condition "so changed her blood that coagulation was easily induced." Elliot[13] was able to remove infarcted bowel in a living patient yet noted that the patient suffered concomitantly bilateral femoral DVTs complicated by portal vein thrombosis.

Causes of mesenteric vein thrombosis are multiple. One must cautiously read older reviews of mesenteric

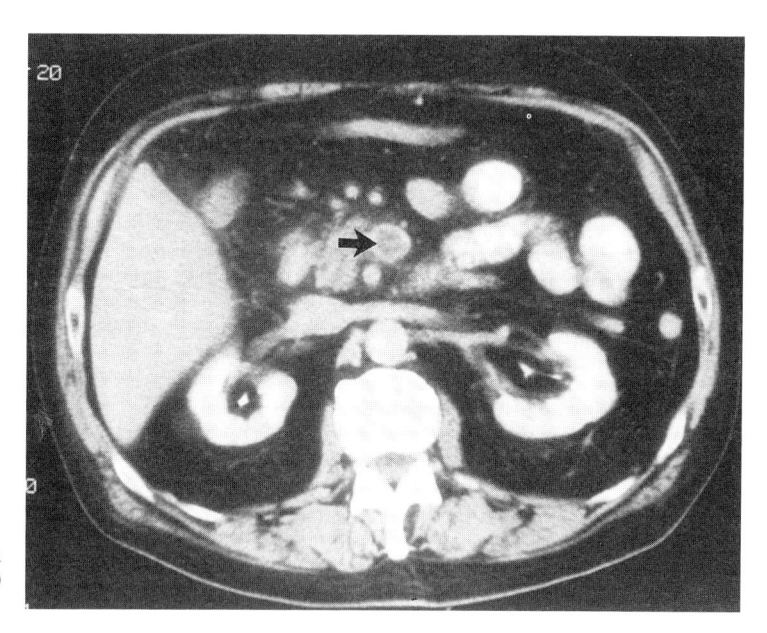

Figure 15–1 Mesenteric vein thrombosis. This CT scan with contrast shows an engorged superior mesenteric vein (*arrow*) that is distended with clot, outlined by a thin rim of dye.

vein thrombosis that garnered patients before the modern era of hypercoagulability as, by definition, causes cannot include thrombophilic diseases that had not yet been described. In one study, mesenteric vein thrombosis accounted for 0.01% of all surgical admissions and surgical autopsies[14] and, in another study, 0.06% of all surgical admission.[15] Clearly this is a rare disease. On the other hand, in cross-sectional studies, mesenteric vein thrombosis was found to have occurred in 3% of patients who were known to have deficiency of ATIII, protein C, or protein S,[5] whereas in another cross-sectional study, mesenteric vein thrombosis was found in 10% of patients with ATIII deficiency, in 6% of the patients with protein C deficiency, and in 4% of those with protein S deficiency. One can estimate that the incidence of mesenteric vein thrombosis is increased at least a hundred-fold in patients who have an identified thrombophilia. In one study, 80% of patients who had thrombophilia and mesenteric vein thrombosis had a history of a previous DVT or PE.[9] Estimates are not available for the more recently detected thrombophilias although Darnige and colleagues[16] described two patients with mesenteric vein thrombosis who harbored the prothrombin 20210 mutation. It is probable that these and yet-to-be-discovered thrombophilic conditions will continue to erode the "idiopathic" or "primary" category of mesenteric vein thrombosis.[4]

Whereas mesenteric vein thrombosis may appear to occur spontaneously in patients with thrombophilia, an additional provocation may be detected in about half the cases. This fact more likely than not accounts for older reviews that include such "causes" of mesenteric vein thrombosis as cirrhosis, heart failure, intra-abdominal malignancies, peritonitis, intra-abdominal abscesses, abdominal trauma, and abdominal surgery.[17] Whereas these provocations may well induce thrombosis in hypercoagulable patients, they could prove to be the sole cause in only the minority of cases. Synergy

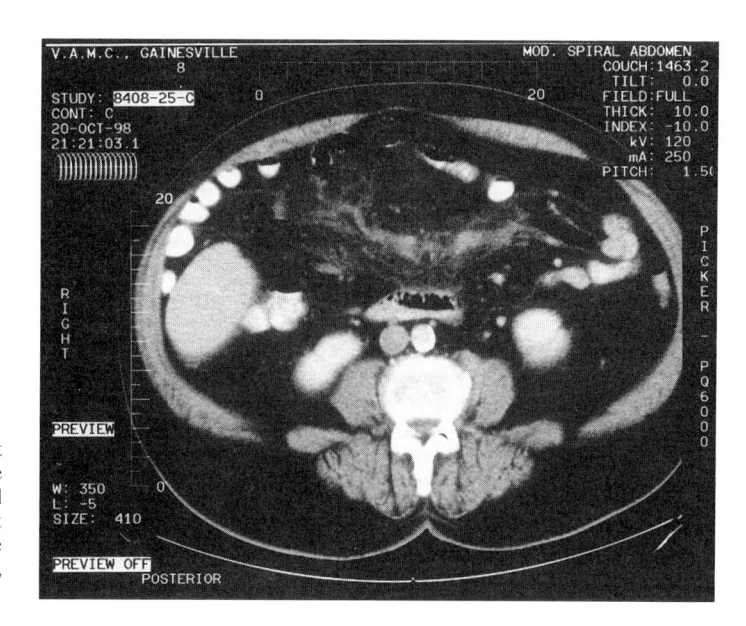

Figure 15–2 "Misty mesentery." This CT scan with contrast shows the mesentery as strands in a web-like configuration due to the edema and inflammation. This situation may have several causes but in this case of mesenteric vein thrombosis is most likely due to leakage of bacteria and bacterial products from the compromised ischemic small bowel. After successful treatment, follow-up images were normal.

between an underlying hypercoagulable disorder and a provocation is frequent. For example, we have seen several patients with antiphospholipid syndrome whose chronic oral anticoagulant therapy has been held in preparation for colonoscopy with polypectomy who develop abdominal pain several days later because of mesenteric vein thrombosis. The unopposed hypercoagulable disorder coupled with inflammation and bacterial showering from the biopsy site may have provoked this thrombosis in such high-risk patients.

Symptoms of mesenteric vein thrombosis are vague and nonspecific.[4,18] Abdominal pain is usually of insidious onset. The patient cannot find a position or maneuver that makes the pain disappear. In contrast with most abdominal catastrophes, bowel movements continue and frequently the patient continues to eat. Nausea is seen in less than half the cases. Typically the pain continues for days and may include even several evaluations from which no diagnosis is forthcoming. Routine abdominal roentgenograms are nearly always normal. Pain appears to be far worse than one can account for by physical examination. Rebound tenderness is not present unless the bowel is infarcted. Laboratory data show hemoconcentration and white cell count usually in the 15,000 to 30,000/μL range. The natural history of the process is such that if a diagnosis is not made after 10 to 20 days, the intestines will undergo ischemic infarction. At that time the symptoms evolve into those of a classical surgical abdomen, with rebound tenderness, rigidity, and increased morbidity and mortality due to venous infarction of the intestine.

Diagnosis is best made by CT scan at which time it may be haply discovered. We prospectively have made mesenteric vein thrombosis our initial diagnosis in hypercoagulable patients who presented with the above nondescript symptoms.

If the patient goes to surgery without the correct diagnosis, the surgeon usually finds a dusky but not frankly gangrenous intestinal wall (unless through-and-through infarction has taken place), and bounding mesenteric arterial pulses. If ischemia or infarction is present, it is not as clearly demarcated as in cases of acute arterial infarction. When the bowel wall is transected, tiny worm-like clots extrude from engorged veins in the edges of the resected bowel in a peculiar but pathognomonic way. Histologic examination shows extensive hyperemia and hemorrhage, with the degree of infarction determined by the duration of ischemia.

Surgery is to be avoided as the primary diagnostic method. Surgical exploration is now replaced by radiologic exploration. Once the thrombotic etiology of the disorder has been discovered it should be approached vigorously with aggressive anticoagulant therapy. Thrombolytic therapy has been used with success.[19] We have employed systemic thrombolysis with excellent results without excessive hemorrhage. We do not advocate catheter-directed thrombolytic therapy. Early surgical series before anticoagulant therapy or modern radiologic imaging described that about 65% of patients died, which was an improvement over the natural history without any therapy, for which mortality was estimated to be 95%. If the diagnosis is made at surgery and is followed promptly by anticoagulant therapy, observed mortality drops to approximately 35%. If the diagnosis is made radiographically and the patients are treated promptly with anticoagulants without any surgical intervention, mortality is currently about 10%.[4]

As the pathogenesis of this abdominal catastrophe is thrombosis it is appropriate that therapy be directed to reverse thrombotic potential. Such an approach is appropriate and additionally treats, even if inadvertently, other thromboses that the patient may harbor and of which the practitioner may be unaware. Modern reviews advocate early diagnosis and prompt aggressive anticoagulant or thrombolytic therapy.[17]

We favor chronic anticoagulant therapy with warfarin to maintain an INR in the range of 2.0 to 3.0 indefinitely because of the seriousness of this event as well as the fact the majority already have sustained a prior DVT/PE.

SPLENIC VEIN THROMBOSIS

Splenic vein thrombosis is subtle and rarely recognized at the time of initial thrombosis. However, vague acute abdominal pain and new-onset splenomegaly may lead to imaging studies that show acute splenic vein thrombosis. More often, splenic vein thrombosis is discovered during the evaluation of a patient with vague chronic abdominal pain or chronic splenomegaly, or serendipitously during the evaluation of pancreatitis and pancreatic carcinoma. Splenic vein thrombosis may complicate sclerotherapy for esophageal varices.[20]

Splenic vein thrombosis has been described in all manner of hypercoagulable disorders, whether congenital or acquired. In this disorder, intra-abdominal events, whether or not accompanied by hypercoagulable disorders, do directly cause a significant percentage of splenic vein thromboses. The chief offenders are pancreatitis and pancreatic carcinoma because of the intimate contact of the splenic vein with the pancreas. Splenic vein thrombosis has also been described in abdominal trauma and following abdominal surgery. It complicates 11% of all splenectomies but occurs at a much higher rate among patients having their spleens removed for hematologic indications.[21] Thus, the condition warranting splenectomy (such as a myeloproliferative disorder) probably is more "hypercoagulable" than the operation per se. Splenic vein thrombosis has also been related historically to splenectomy for immune thrombocytopenic purpura (ITP). That connection now is more likely than not due to the association of ITP with antiphospholipid syndrome (APLS), which explains both the ITP and splenic vein thromboses.

A common presentation for chronic splenic vein thrombosis is variceal bleeding, especially from the stomach and lower esophagus. When this occurs in the setting of normal serum liver function tests, without hepatomegaly but with isolated splenomegaly, the diagnosis of splenic vein thrombosis can be entertained strongly.[22] The syndrome has been called "left-sided portal hypertension." Splenectomy cures the portal hypertensive gastropathy and esophageal hemorrhage usually ceases at the time.[22,23]

The signs and symptoms (mentioned above) of splenic vein thrombosis are nonspecific. The diagnosis is most commonly made by ultrasonography, CT, or MRI.[21] Should the diagnosis of splenic vein thrombosis be made, acute anticoagulation is indicated not only to stop the process but also to limit potential propagation of thrombosis into the mesenteric and portal veins.[21] Long-term anticoagulant therapy is also indicated, particularly if the patient has an underlying hypercoagulable condition. Most practitioners would maintain an INR at 2.0 to 3.0 with continued use of warfarin. Continued follow-up by the hematologist is also appropriate as a significant number of these patients who do not currently have manifestations of a myeloproliferative disorder will develop them in time.[24]

PORTAL VEIN THROMBOSIS

Like splenic vein thrombosis, portal vein thrombosis is usually not recognized in its acute phase. It is characterized by relatively painless increasing splenomegaly and ascites without concomitant worsening of hepatic function. Portal vein thrombosis appears to have been described first by Belfour and Stewart in 1869.[25] Whereas portal vein thrombosis has been described in the recent literature as being associated with most of the acquired or congenital hypercoagulable disorders,[26] it is still seen in patients with common-variety portal hypertension, especially when due to hepatic cirrhosis. It remains to be seen if these two risk factors, namely hypercoagulability and portal hypertension, are synergistic in the genesis of portal vein thrombosis.[26a] Other causes include intra-abdominal neoplasia, especially carcinoma of the pancreas; infection, with particular reference to spontaneous bacterial peritonitis; and abdominal trauma, including surgery. Additionally, sclerotherapy for esophageal varices has been implicated in several cases. Portal vein thrombosis may complicate neonatal umbilical vein catheterization but this will not be further discussed here. Hypercoagulability should be considered strongly in patients who have no history of hepatic disease, intra-abdominal infections, or an inflammatory or neoplastic process. As with splenic vein thromboses, the myeloproliferative disorders (acquired causes of hypercoagulability) are notoriously common, particularly if patients are followed long enough to manifest their previously occult myeloproliferative disorder.[27] When splenectomy is performed in patients with myeloproliferative disorders, the incidence of portal vein and mesenteric vein thrombosis is approximately 30% for patients not receiving prophylactic anticoagulation.[28,29] Accordingly, when splenectomy is performed in patients with a known hypercoagulable or myeloproliferative disease, antithrombotic prophylaxis is indicated.

Diagnosis is usually made by nonivasive radiologic methods.[27] With color Doppler techniques, the direction of portal vein blood flow can be determined reliably. Contrast CT and MRI/MRA are equally powerful but somewhat more expensive (Fig. 15–3).

Management of this thrombosis depends on the manifestations of the process. If the process produces acute variceal hemorrhage, attention should be paid to that disorder. Discussion of the treatment of variceal esophageal hemorrhage is not within the scope of this chapter; however, patients with pure portal vein thrombosis who do not have liver disease generally survive acute upper gastrointestinal hemorrhage far better than those who have liver disease. If the portal vein thrombosis is thought to be secondary to an intra-abdominal process such as infection, neoplasia, or other inflammation, therapy should be directed toward those problems. Chronic portal hypertension due to chronic portal vein thrombosis is occasionally treated surgically by various decompressive mechanisms.[27]

The role of anticoagulant therapy has been somewhat controversial but as more patients have presented and more proof has accrued that this disorder is frequently a manifestation of hypercoagulability, anticoagulant therapy has become more attractive. This therapeutic option is particularly appealing in those patients who do not have prior portal hypertension on the basis of liver disease but who have experienced spontaneous thrombosis due to a hypercoagulable disorder. In these conditions, it is rational to initiate acute anticoagulant therapy in order not only to reverse the thrombotic process but also to minimize further progression of the thrombosis into the splenic or mesenteric veins. Anticoagulant therapy is also indicated strongly in patients who have undergone a shunt procedure for chronic portal hypertension due to chronic portal vein thrombosis. In that situation the patient's well-being is dependent upon the shunt remaining patent and therefore anticoagulant therapy, particularly for an identified underlying hypercoagulable disorder, is the treatment of choice. The concern of increased bleeding in patients with esophageal varices treated with concomitant anticoagulant therapy is always raised but may be more theoretical than actual experience; ironically, as anticoagulant therapy addresses the underlying pathophysiology, bleeding, over time, seems better controlled. We treat those patients with esophageal varices from portal hypertension due solely to hypercoagulable disorders with chronic warfarin therapy, maintaining in INR of 2.0 to 3.0. We have done this in 10 patients for a cumulative time period of about 100 patient-years. Not only have these patients not progressed, they have fared very well. We have only had four episodes of esophageal variceal hemorrhage in those 100 patient-years and these were easily treated in part because of their normal hepatic function (unpublished data). Patients treated with chronic oral anticoagulant therapy have been described who have recanalized their portal veins, thereby reversing portal hypertension.[27] Thrombolytic therapy has been tried in small number of the cases with encouraging results; use of thrombolytic therapy is most attractive if the thrombosis is fairly acute.

RENAL VEIN THROMBOSIS

The association of renal vein thrombosis and renal disease, with particular reference to the nephrotic syndrome, has been known since 1840.[30] Previously debate

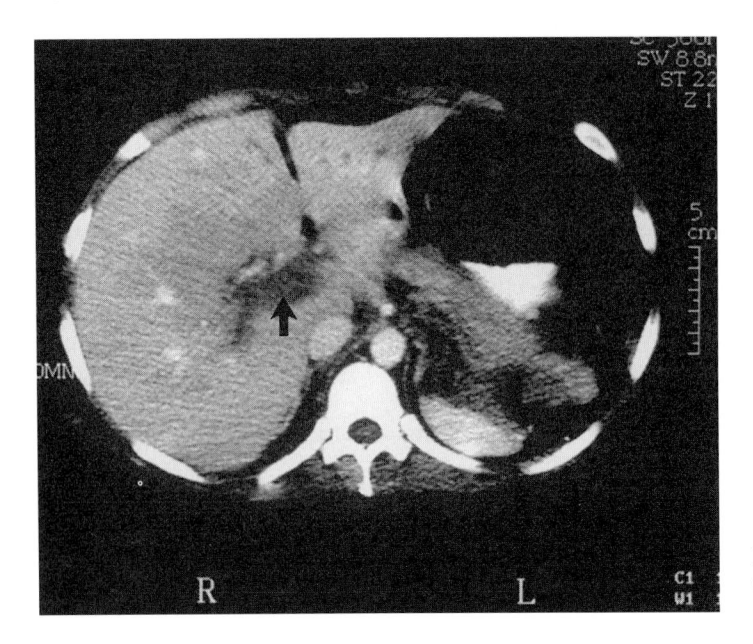

Figure 15–3 Portal vein thrombosis. This CT scan with contrast shows a distended portal vein that is devoid of contrast material (*arrow*) at the porta hepatis.

existed whether renal vein thrombosis caused the nephrotic syndrome or vice versa; it is now appreciated that the nephrotic syndrome is the pre-existent problem and the hypercoagulability of the nephrotic syndrome gives rise not only to thrombosis of renal veins but also to veins throughout the body and frequently to pulmonary embolism.[31,32] One putative mechanism for this hypercoagulability is that of decreased plasma levels of ATIII resulting from urinary loss of this small plasma protein paralleling the degree of albuminuria. Others have described a decrease in free protein S explained either by urinary loss or by excessive binding to increased levels of C4B binding protein characteristic of nephrotic syndrome.[33,34] The latter mechanism is especially attractive for the antiphospholipid syndrome, which is increasingly recognized as one of the common associations with the nephrotic syndrome.[35–37] Renal vein thrombosis also can occur in neonates during periods of acute dehydration. Whether these sporadic cases are associated with an underlying hypercoagulable disorder is not currently known.

The classic syndrome of acute renal vein thrombosis, namely acute flank pain, hematuria, and sudden deterioration of renal function, is only seen in about 10% to 20% of all adults with renal vein thrombosis. The remaining patients have a more chronic variety that is usually detected by subtle worsening of renal insufficiency, progressive proteinuria, and edema, usually without pain or hematuria. Nephrotic syndrome in adults appears to be more thrombogenic than in children and nephrotic syndrome due to membraneous nephropathy appears to be more thrombogenic than nephrotic syndrome secondary to diabetes.[38]

The chronic form of renal vein thrombosis occurs much more commonly than is appreciated and accordingly, if one waits for symptoms, the disorder will be underdiagnosed. Cross-sectional studies have shown that as many as 30% to 50% of all patients with chronic nephrotic syndrome studied will have evidence of renal vein thrombosis.[38,39]

Thrombosis from hypercoagulability with renal vein thrombosis may be self-perpetuating.[40] Concurrent PE is seen in 20% to 30% of patients diagnosed with renal vein thrombosis. Among these patients with PE only 5% are symptomatic.[38,41] Renal vein thrombosis is bilateral in half of all cases. Clots protrude from the renal vein into the inferior vena cava in 40% of cases. Anticoagulant therapy is the hallmark of successful therapy although increasingly systemic thrombolytic therapy is advocated; the few case reports available employing thrombolytic therapy describe gratifying results in acute situations.[41,42] The general systemic nature of such hypercoagulability potentially involving multiple sites clearly warrants systemic rather than catheter-directed therapy. Thrombolytic therapy should be considered especially in those patients with acute renal failure, bilateral renal vein thrombosis, or concomitant thrombosis at other sites.[37]

The diagnosis is aided by a high index of suspicion in the occasional patient with pre-existing acute or chronic renal insufficiency who then develops flank pain, hematuria, and sudden worsening of renal failure or more commonly an unexplained increase in renal insufficiency as well as in the azotemic patient who has an increase in proteinuria and peripheral edema. Renal vein thrombosis is also known to occur in patients without renal disease who have other hypercoagulable disorders. Regardless of presentation, the diagnosis is still best made by imaging using ultrasonography or MRI/MRA after discussion with the radiologist of one's suspicion of renal vein thrombosis[43] (Fig. 15–4).

The role of chronic anticoagulation with warfarin is debatable but such therapy appears to be efficacious in the prevention of rethrombosis either of the renal vein or elsewhere. Importantly, it is not known whether chronic oral anticoagulant therapy will help preserve renal function given the natural slow deterioration of renal function in patients with ongoing renal disease. However, rapid return of renal function to the patient's

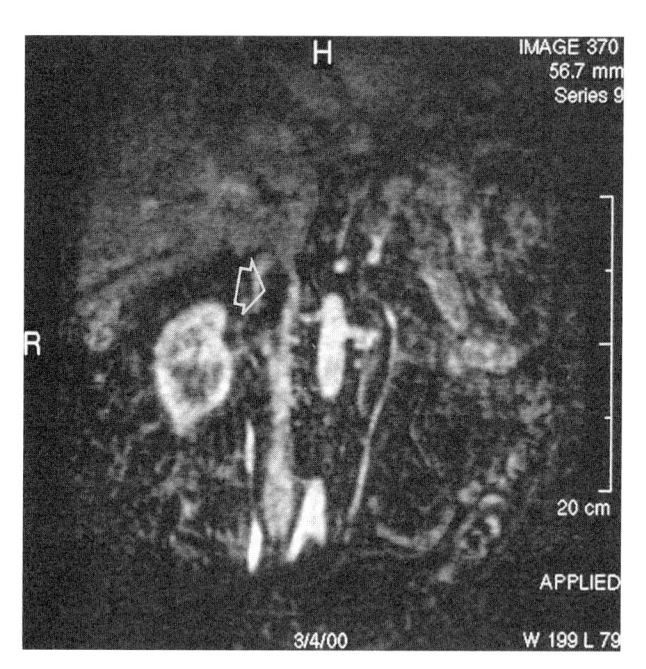

Figure 15-4 Renal vein thrombosis. This MRA scan demonstrates a large clot in the right renal vein that is extending (*arrow*) as a large mass into the suprarenal IVC.

chronic baseline level is expected with successful treatment of the acute syndrome.[41]

CEREBRAL VENOUS THROMBOSIS

Cerebral venous thrombosis refers to thrombosis of superficial and deep cerebral veins as well as the venous sinuses. This condition, like most conditions included in this chapter, is diagnosed increasingly because of increased knowledge of its existence and increased facility of diagnosis by modern imaging techniques.

Gates and Barnett have reviewed the history of cerebral venous thrombosis,[44] noting that Ribes first described cerebral venous thrombosis in 1825 in a man with disseminated carcinoma. Three years later Abercrombe described cerebral venous thrombosis in a woman in her puerperium. In 1873 Parrot described neonatal cerebral venous thrombosis. Gowers in 1888 associated cerebral venous thrombosis with both congestive heart failure and cachexia. In 1904 Nonne first used the term *pseudotumor cerebri*. In an important neurosurgical review in 1967, Krayenbuhl[45] clearly separated the infectious from the noninfectious etiologies of cerebral venous thrombosis. He was prescient in stating that neurosurgery had a limited and decreasing role in the treatment of this disease, stating anticoagulants were the treatment of choice. He further correctly pointed out that as opposed to other ischemic brain syndromes, central nervous system dysfunction due to cerebral venous thrombosis has an outstanding recovery rate, often with no permanent sequelae if treated aggressively and appropriately.

In the preantibiotic era the most common causes of thrombophlebitis in the skull and its contents were chronic suppurative infections due to inner-ear infections, skull osteomyelitis, and erysipelas. Infectious causes have been recently and thoroughly reviewed.[45a]

Whereas the puerperium represents a strong provocation for hypercoagulability and particularly thrombosis at unusual sites, this association is nowhere more apparent than in cerebral venous thrombosis. The reason for these repeated observations is not known. Cerebral venous thrombosis appears to be the only thrombosis at an unusual site that has a strong sex predilection, with a 3:1 ratio favoring women, the difference explained by the puerperium and/or the use of oral contraceptive agents.[46-49] Cerebral venous thrombosis has been associated with all the known hypercoagulable disorders, both congenital and acquired. Recent series have also documented a relative risk for cerebral venous thrombosis of 6 to 10 among patients having factor V Leiden mutation.[46-49] A recent paper estimates a relative risk of 10 due to the prothrombin 20210 mutation.[46] Data document that risk factors are not simply additive: a relative risk for cerebral venous thrombosis of 22 exists in patients using birth control pills and a relative risk of 10 exists with women having the prothrombin 20210 mutation, while the relative risk factor escalates to 150 among women with the prothrombin 20210 mutation who also use oral contraceptives.[46]

As dangerous as the disease is, it is difficult to diagnose because of its nonspecific and nonsensitive subacute presentation and fairly broad differential diagnosis. It is thought that symptoms are caused both by increased intracranial pressure due to venous congestion and by local inflammation due to phlebitis[50] (Table 15-3). Headaches are experienced in the vast majority of the cases. Papilledema occurs in approximately half the cases. When the headache and papilledema occur without focal neurologic signs, the term *pseudotumor cerebri* may be used.[51] Although pseudotumor cerebri has several causes besides cerebral venous thrombosis, this condition remains one of its more important causes. Typically the headache progresses over several days followed by confusion, stupor, and finally coma if the process is not interrupted. Conspicuously absent are sensory loss and motor weakness. Examination of the cerebrospinal fluid and electroencephalogram shows nonspecific findings, thus not supporting other entries within the differential diagnosis. CT has usually been performed by this time in the evaluation but is notoriously nonspecific if not even misleading. The classic "empty delta sign" is seen in only 21% of cases; therefore a normal CT scan should never be used to exclude

---

Table 15-3 • CLINICAL FEATURES OF CEREBRAL VENOUS THROMBOSIS

Headache 75%
Papilledema 49%
Fever 45%
Seizures 37%
Altered mental states 30%

Data from Ameri A and Bousser M-G. Cerebral venous thrombosis. Neuro Clin 1992;10:87-111.

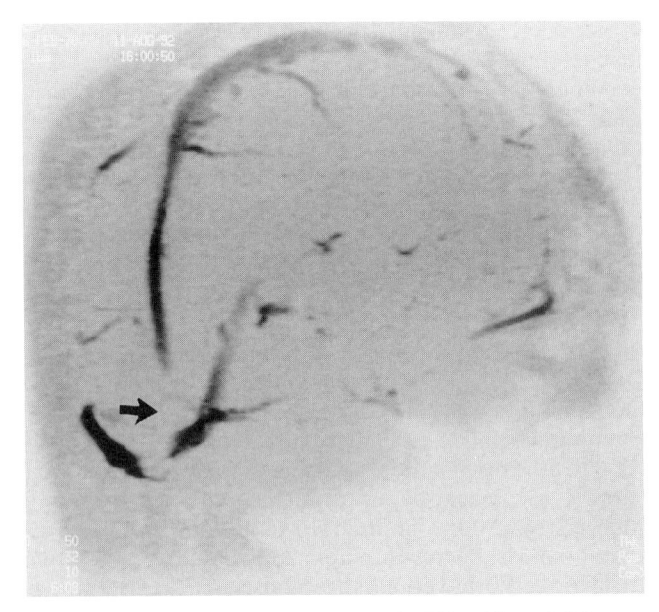

Figure 15–5 Cerebral venous thrombosis. This oblique MRI scan demonstrates a contrast-outlined superior sagittal sinus and both transverse sinuses. A large clot occupies the torcular Herophili, which is nonvisualized because of the absence of contrast medium (*arrow*).

this important diagnosis.[50] The diagnosis is best established by MRI/MRA[52–54] (Fig. 15–5), which is also sensitive for diagnosing the subtype known as deep cerebral venous thrombosis; this includes thrombosis of the internal cerebral veins and/or the great vein of Galen.[53,55] Once the diagnosis is made, prompt and aggressive therapy is indicated. The lingering fear of hemorrhage with anticoagulant therapy is probably based on older reports of the natural history of cerebral venous thrombosis that terminates in intracerebral hemorrhage due to infarctive ischemia. Both historical[56] and level 1[57] studies have shown that patients who are treated with heparin achieve approximately 80% full recovery, with only 15% to 20% having any sequelae. A very small number or none of the patients die when administered heparin. Conversely, as shown in Table 15–4, of patients who do not receive heparin, approximately 25% die and 50% survive but with sequelae, with only 25% having complete recovery. The efficacy of heparin therapy has been clearly noted, with improvement beginning as early as the second or third day of therapy,[57] even in patients who by imaging have evidence of some hemorrhage. Evidence for hemorrhage should no longer be viewed as an absolute contraindication to heparin therapy.[55,57] In a study involving small numbers of patients with the rarer subtype of deep cerebral venous thrombosis, none of 7 patients receiving heparin therapy died, while all 10 patients who did not receive heparin therapy died.[53] Most reviews of the subject agree that vigorous heparin therapy followed by warfarin is the treatment of choice.[48–53,55]

A small number of patients have been treated with thrombolytic agents successfully and without experiencing undue bleeding; however, that therapy cannot be recommended routinely at this time but should be given consideration because of such uniformly high efficacy. Safety of thrombolytic therapy compared to standard heparin therapy has not been evaluated thoroughly. Patients should be maintained on chronic warfarin in doses to keep the INR at 2.0 to 3.0 for at least a year and then for an uncertain period of time.

HEPATIC VENOUS THROMBOSIS

Hepatic venous thrombosis, previously known as Budd–Chiari syndrome, has been an area of semantic confusion since it was described. The history of this disorder has been detailed by Wang.[58] The English internist Budd described a case of thrombotic occlusion of the hepatic veins in 1845 and the Austrian pathologist Chiari described autopsies of 10 patients who had intrahepatic venous thrombosis. Osler[59] described a case of obliteration of the inferior vena cava by fibrotic stenosis at the orifices of the hepatic veins. It has become increasingly clear that there are two entities that initially appeared to be similar but are now being considered two disorders. Table 15–5 addresses the two types, which differ in locality, tempo, lethality, and other manifestations. It is interesting that most scholars believe that the obliterative hepatocavopathy (which is seen in Africa, India, and Asia) is the end result of thrombosis, resulting in formation of webs and intravascular diaphragms or scarring and obliteration of the vessels as described by Osler. Whether or not both the Eastern and Western types of this syndrome are due to thrombosis, and if so, why it would be manifest as an acute veno-occlusive disease in the Western world and a chronic fibrosing disease in Africa, India, and Asia, is not known.

Many clinicians advocate using the term *hepatic venous thrombosis* for the Western disease and the cumbersome term *obliterative hepatocavopathy* for the Eastern type.[60–63] The remainder of this discussion will center around the more acute thrombotic disease, for which we will use the term *hepatic venous thrombosis*.

Our understanding of this process has been changed by rapid dignosis owing to advances in roentgenographic imaging and changes in therapy (Figs. 15–6 and 15–7). It is thought that the disease has an excellent prognosis when it is detected early and is limited to only the

Table 15–4 • OUTCOME OF CEREBRAL VENOUS THROMBOSIS WITH AND WITHOUT HEPARIN THERAPY

	Historical Study[a]		Level 1 Study[b]	
	Heparin	No Heparin	Heparin	No Heparin
Complete recovery	85%	53%	80%	10%
Some sequelae	15%	20%	20%	60%
Died	0%	27%	0%	30%

[a] Data from Bousser M-G, Chiras J, Bories J, et al. Cerebral venous thrombosis: A review of 38 cases. Stroke 1985;16:199–210.
[b] Data from Einhaupl KM, Villringer A, Meister W. Heparin treatment in sinus venous thrombosis. Lancet 1991;338:597–600.

Table 15-5 • HEPATIC VENOUS THROMBOSIS[a]

	Hepatic Venous Thrombosis	Obliterative Hepatocavopathy
Locality	Western World	Africa, India, Asia
Pathogenesis	Acute thrombosis of hepatic veins and suprahepatic IVC	Webs and obliteration of intrahepatic IVC
Tempo	Acute (<3 months)	Chronic (>24–36 months)
Lethality	High	Low
Hepatic encephalopathy	30%	<10%
Splenomegaly	20%	55%
Ascites	95%	60%
Abdominal surface veins	<1%	65%
Pregnancy and hypercoagulability	High association	Low association
Hepatocellular cancer	Not associated	Associated
Idiopathic	Increasingly rare	Common
Surgical approach	Portocaval shunt	Cavoatrial shunt

[a] Hepatic venous thrombosis is now recognized as being two separate syndromes differing by locality, tempo, lethality, and other characteristics.[58,60,61]
IVC, inferior vena cava.
Data from Dilawari JB, Bambery P, Chawla Y, et al. Hepatic outflow obstruction (Budd-Chiari syndrome). Experience with 177 patients and a review of the literature. Medicine (Baltimore) 1994;73:21–36; Okuda K, Kage M, Shrestha SM. Proposal of a new nomenclature for Budd-Chiari syndrome: Hepatic vein thrombosis versus thrombosis of the inferior vena cava at its hepatic portion. Hepatology 1998; 28:1191–1198; and Wang ZG, Jones RS. Budd-Chiari syndrome. Curr Probl Surg. 1996;33:83–211.

peripheral smaller hepatic veins. If larger veins are occluded partially the morbidity is about 30%, and in cases with total obstruction of the major hepatic vessels and suprahepatic inferior vena cava the mortality is 67%.[64,65]

Hepatic venous thrombosis is due principally to hypercoagulable disorders yet is exacerbated frequently by provocations such as pregnancy, birth control pill usage, and infection. The syndrome is acute and is recognized clinically by the triad of acute painful abdomen, sudden enlargement of the liver, and ascites, with those symptoms present in 82%, 86%, and 100% of cases, respectively.[63] In acute cases of hepatic venous thrombosis there may be a lag of 1 or 2 days in elevation of standard liver function tests, which occasionally obscures the diagnosis.[66] Diagnosis can also be made by liver biopsy,[67] which may reveal the early phase of the disease when thrombosis is limited to the smaller hepatic veins.

Before the recent descriptions of the factor V Leiden mutation and the prothrombin 20210 mutation, Valla and colleagues[62] opined that approximately 30% of their cases were due to myeloproliferative disorders (notoriously polycythemia vera) and about 10% of the cases were due to paroxysmal nocturnal hemoglobinuria (PNH) alone. Given the rarity of PNH, the penetrance of hepatic venous thrombosis in that rare disease is exceptional. As these French investigators[62] have demonstrated, acute hepatic venous thrombosis may be the initial presentation of myeloproliferative disorders, and occasionally these hematologic disorders are not clinically apparent until after years of follow-up. More recent reviews indicate that the antiphospholipid syndrome is now the second most common cause of the disease,[68] accounting for approximately 30% of cases, while congenital hypercoagulable disorders account for up to another 30% of cases.[26,69]

With the advent of modern radiographic imaging the diagnosis is made increasingly early. Imaging now is very effective, with ultrasonography yielding the diagnosis in 75% of cases very rapidly. Using the combination of ultrasonography, MRI/MRA, and occasional angiography, Valla[62] and colleagues confirmed the diagnosis rapidly in over 90% of their cases. Experts favor anticoagulant therapy,[62,63,70] with many advocating an early, aggressive role of thrombolytic therapy whether systematically or by local infusion.[58,71] Early use of thrombolytic therapy coupled with anticoagulants has moved previously favored orthotopic liver transplantation to the therapy of last resort for those patients who have failed thrombolytic therapy or those who present late with fulminant hepatic failure and coma.[63,65,69] Long-term management should include chronic anticoagulant

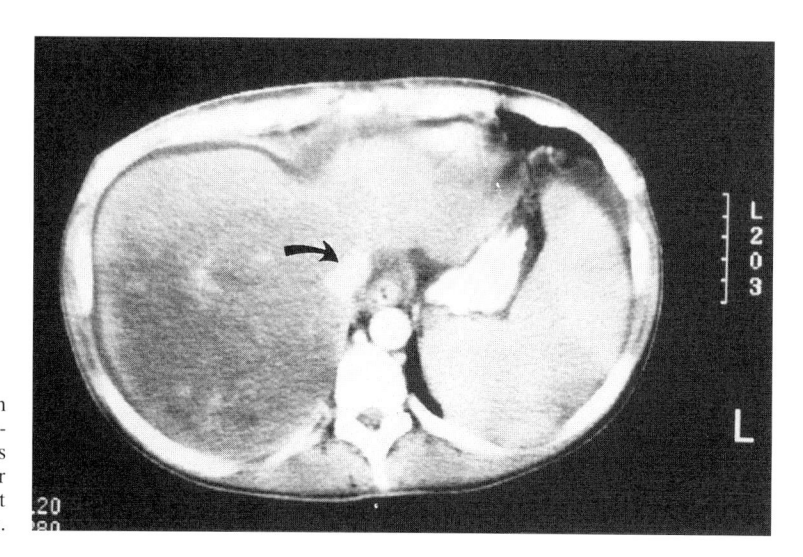

Figure 15-6 Hepatic venous thrombosis. This CT scan with contrast shows an enlarged, tense liver with a heterogeneous perfusion pattern. At this level, the hepatic veins should be clearly outlined by contrast media as they enter the contrast-filled inferior vena cava (arrow). They are not visualized because of total thrombosis of the hepatic veins.

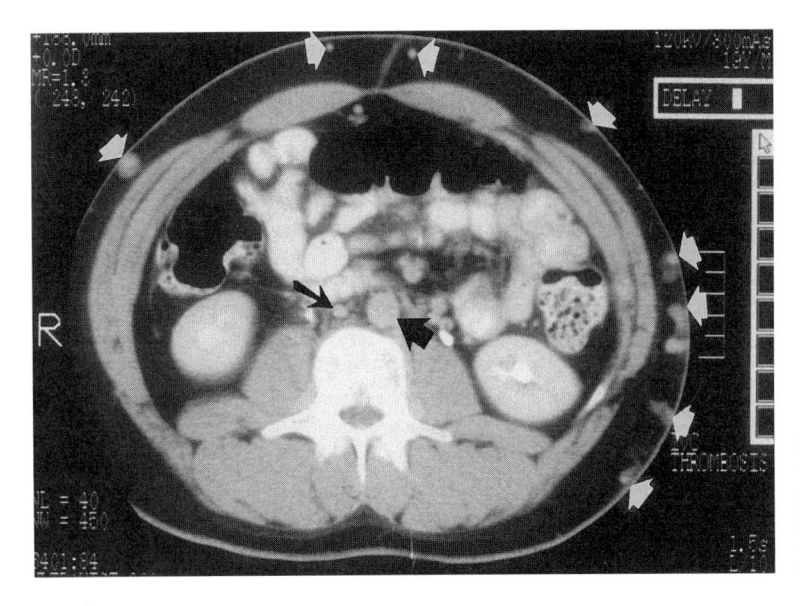

Figure 15–7 Obliteration of the inferior vena cava (IVC) with extensive collateral flow. In this case of chronic hepatic vein thrombosis the IVC is obliterated. The aorta (*large arrow*) and azygos vein (*small arrow*) are seen. Multiple large subcutaneous collaterals are seen in the abdominal wall (*white arrows*).

therapy in order to prevent recurrence of the disease locally and other manifestations of any underlying hypercoagulable disorder.[58,63,68,72]

If symptomatic portal hypertension persists and if vascular decompressive operations are indicated, various types of decompressive surgery are available and have been reviewed elsewhere.[58,61]

RETINAL VEIN THROMBOSIS

The history of our knowledge of retinal vein occlusion, which is often divided into branch retinal vein occlusion (BRVO) and central retinal vein occlusion (CRVO), has been reviewed by Williamson.[73]

Previous reviews, and indeed some very recent reviews in the ophthalmology literature, continue to focus on the time-honored observation of an apparent correlation between both BRVO and CRVO and increased plasma fibrinogen level, diabetes mellitus, hypertension, and hyperviscosity as well as decreased exercise.[73-77] Curiously, none of these recent reviews focus attention on the possibility of an association with hypercoagulable disorders and one[73] minimizes the role of anticoagulant therapy in afflicted patients.

A renaissance of investigation in retinal vein thrombosis has occurred in the 1990s.[78] Although reported results of several studies are seemingly mutually incompatible, several groups have noted an association between the presence of antiphospholipid antibodies and retinal vein occlusion and other retinal disorders.[79] Case reports include an association with antiphospholipid syndrome in a young woman who had depressed levels of free protein S.[80] Glueck et al.[81] noticed that 43% of their patients had laboratory evidence consistent with antiphospholipid syndrome, while only 3% in a control group had such laboratory evidence. In one study in Saudi Arabia,[82] 50% of their patients with retinal venous occlusion had laboratory evidence for antiphospholipid syndrome. There was a six-fold increase in patients harboring the factor V Leiden mutation in one study,[81] while another noticed a two-fold increase in factor V Leiden,[83] a third group[84] had reported an eight-fold increase, and a fourth group noted a three-fold increase.[85] A case of bilateral CRVO occurred in a patient heterozygous for factor V Leiden.[86] In one report, 8.3% of patients with retinal vein occlusion tested positive for the prothrombin 20210 mutation compared with 0% in a control group.[84] Four studies[87-90] failed to find an increased incidence of the factor V Leiden mutation but found evidence of resistance to activated protein C at a rate five times higher than that of controls. One group reported that resistance to activated protein C was the most common cause of retinal vein occlusion in the young,[88] while another[91] found it was the most common (25%) biochemically identified risk factor among patients with CRVO. Of interest, the same investigator[92] a year later was unable to duplicate those findings when he reported that among 55 patients with retinal vein occlusion, the incidence of resistance to activated protein C was precisely the same as his control group. Gottlieb and colleagues[93] were unable to find any evidence of increased resistance to activated protein C or factor V Leiden mutation in 21 of their patients, while Delahousse[94] determined that the incidence of prothrombin 20210 mutation was precisely the same (3.6%) in his patients with retinal vein occlusion as in his control group. One study found a 60% incidence of hyperhomocystinemia in patients with ocular venous occlusion.[95]

It is difficult to resolve these differing data but the preponderance of evidence published in the last several years suggests the possibility of an underlying disorder such as factor V Leiden mutation, prothrombin 20210 mutation, resistance to activated protein C, possibly hyperhomocystinemia, and particularly antiphospholipid syndrome in patients suffering from this eye disease. Some editorialists[82,96] urge an open mind and indicate that larger studies need to be done. They also note that much as with hypercoagulability and thrombosis in other sites, it may take a combination of a hypercoagulable disorder and a second provocation, in these cases such as age, diabetes, hypertension, and hyperfibrinogenemia, to cause the process to become manifest.

Other matters to consider include the unique anatomy of the optic sheath through which both the retinal vein and retinal artery travel. Accordingly, perturbations of the retinal artery due to hypertension, diabetes, or aging may encroach upon the adjacent retinal vein. Giorgi and colleagues recommended chronic warfarin therapy in patients with retinal vein occlusion thought to be due to a thrombotic process.[97] While oral anticoagulant therapy has been successfully used by others,[98] studies have yet to be done to establish the best therapy.

Two clinics[99,100] have administered systemic intravenous thrombolytic therapy in both acute and subacute retinal vein occlusion, reporting very good results. In fact, the vision in half the patients significantly improved even though therapy was given weeks after the occlusion.

Patients with this disorder should be investigated and strong consideration given to thrombolytic therapy in an acute or subacute phase and chronic oral anticoagulant therapy in doses to maintain an INR at 2.0 to 3.0 for the foreseeable future.

AXILLARY AND SUBCLAVIAN VEIN THROMBOSIS

Thrombosis of these vessels appears to be increasing, probably because of the combination of increased ease of diagnosis by modern imaging and increased use of intravascular devices such as indwelling catheters that are placed into these vessels. Although the incidence and causes of thrombosis of these vessels will vary according to the perspective of the physician and clinic reporting them, roughly one third will be found to be due to so-called primary or effort thrombosis, approximately one third due to the presence of indwelling catheters, and the remaining third will appear to be more or less idiopathic, including those due to hypercoagulable situations. Of course any of these causes could be additive, as Virchow predicted. Thrombophilic situations including ATIII deficiency, have been associated with axillary and subclavian vein thromboses. However, the inherited hypercoagulable disorders seem to play a lesser role in arm venous thrombosis than in deep[101] or superficial[102] vein thromboses of the leg. Antiphospholipid syndrome and Trousseau syndrome are common among the acquired causes of hypercoagulability.[103-105]

Thrombosis of the axillary and subclavian veins accounts for only about 2% of all DVTs. There is a male:female predilection of about 2:1, largely due to effort thrombosis, which is chiefly seen among males. It occurs bilaterally about 10% of the time, especially with effort thrombosis. Signs and symptoms of the disorder include swelling (100%), venous engorgement (82%), pain (73%), mild cyanosis of the involved arm (55%), and a palpable cord (26%).[106] The palpable cord often is appreciated only in the very dome of the axilla, where the enlarged, tender, inflamed subclavian vein may be palpated. Fortunately, upper-extremity venous gangrene occurs in only about 1% of all cases.[106] There has been debate whether PE can arise from axillary or subclavian vein thrombosis. Whereas this certainly can occur[106,107] such emboli are only infrequently of size sufficient to cause circulatory compromise that is characteristic of emboli originating from the legs.[104] Effort thrombosis may result from prolonged heavy use of the arms, particularly if the arms are maintained in somewhat less than usual positions. Examples include prolonged weightlifting, pole vaulting, playing of racquet sports, and rifle practice. A subset of patients with effort vein thrombosis will also be found to have as an extenuating circumstance some type of thoracic outlet obstruction, including anatomic abnormalities of these veins coursing under the first rib or the scalene muscle. This factor is often discovered by follow-up venography of a previously thrombosed vessel.

The use of various indwelling catheters into veins of the arm, the subclavian vein, and the internal jugular vein is a frequent trigger for upper-extremity vein thrombosis. In a prospective study of patients admitted to intensive care units, Timsit and colleagues[108] found that 33% of internal jugular vein catheter placements and 10% of subclavian vein catheter placements were associated with thromboses of those contiguous vessels when in place for 9 ± 5 days. There was a positive correlation between older patients and patients who were not receiving heparin. Catheter-related thrombosis also resulted in a 2.6-fold increase in risk for catheter-related sepsis. It is unknown if there is an association between catheter-related thrombosis and underlying thrombophilic conditions.

The subclavian and axillary veins may be associated with tumors either from resultant hypercoagulability associated with the tumor (including Trousseau syndrome) or from direct pressure of a tumor mass, most commonly lung cancer and lymphoma.

Thrombosis of these vessels is best documented by imaging techniques, typically starting with ultrasonography. These thromboses may be found serendipitously on imaging of the thorax for other reasons. The index of suspicion should be heightened in anyone with a swollen, tender arm with increased, engorged surface veins. A concern is cephalad propagation of thromboses up into the internal jugular and even into the cerebral venous drainage system; this is manifested by signs and symptoms of cerebral venous thrombosis, notably headache and papilledema.[109]

Once the diagnosis is made, most experts recommend anticoagulant therapy. Withholding anticoagulant therapy has not led to a good outcome, with the result often being a chronic swollen, heavy, and disfigured arm. Accordingly, treatment with anticoagulants and thrombolytic therapy are being proposed, whether systemically or, in the case of thrombolytics, site-directed.[106,110-115] Anticoagulation has acutely supplanted the indication for acute thrombectomy.[115] Thrombolytic therapy was shown by one group[106] to result in a 50% reduction in residual signs and symptoms of upper-extremity postphlebitic syndrome. Thrombolytic therapy should be considered seriously for the rare person presenting with upper-extremity venous gangrene.[113]

If a patient has received anticoagulation and subsequently is found to have thoracic outlet obstruction, surgery is indicated, with selected use of first-rib resection with or without scalenectomy, and appears to improve long-term follow-up. Otherwise, there is approximately a 50% relapse rate in these patients who do not undergo anatomic relief of their obstruction.[114,115] Others have recently recorded a more favorable long-term prognosis with conservative therapy alone.[116]

Studies have demonstrated that unmonitored low-dose (1 mg daily) warfarin[117] or low-dose low-molecular-weight heparin[118] decreases the risk of upper-extremity venous thrombosis in patients with long-term catheter or central venous line placement.

CUTANEOUS MICROVASCULAR THROMBOSIS (PURPURA FULMINANS)

Thrombosis of the dermal microvasculature results in discoloration and infarction of the skin and subcutaneous tissues. In its most dramatic and florid state this process is referred to as *purpura fulminans*.[119,120] Although not limited to disseminated intravascular coagulation (DIC), purpura fulminans is characteristically seen in this condition; the reader is referred to Chapter 12 for further details.

The leading category of causes of purpura fulminans is infectious diseases,[121] which can be viral, bacterial, rickettsial, or protozoan. Key in the pathophysiology of infectious purpura fulminans appear to be not only unchecked thrombin production but collapse of the fibrinolytic system, primarily through gross reductions of protein C and protein S, and concomitant increase in plasminogen activator inhibitor (PAI-1).[122] In at least one case transient severe depression of protein S was due to transient autoantibodies directed against protein S.[122]

Dermal necrosis secondary to capillary infarction is also the hallmark of warfarin skin necrosis, which is discussed in Chapter 11. Warfarin skin necrosis may occur in patients who have either congenital or acquired deficiency of protein C or protein S[123-127] and occasionally in patients with paroxysmal nocturnal hemoglobinuria.[128,129]

Skin necrosis occurs spontaneously in newborns who are homozygous for either protein S or protein C deficiency.[130,131] In these situations, consanguinity may be encountered. Neonatal purpura fulminans has also been described in patients doubly heterozygous for protein C deficiency[132] or protein S deficiency.[133]

Some investigators have questioned why only some patients with diseases such as meningococcemia develop purpura fulminans while other patients with the same illness do not.[120] They speculate that these patients also might harbor an underlying thrombophilia that may aid and abet microcirculatory thrombosis in that large increases in PAI-1 levels seen in patients with purpura fulminans are restricted to unique hyperreactors. There are five reports[134-138] involving 12 patients ranging in age from infancy through adolescence and full adulthood who have had infectious diseases associated with excessive purpura fulminans, all of whom were found to be heterozygous for the factor V Leiden mutation. In another report,[139] seven children who suffered purpura fulminans from varicella infection were all found to have strong lupus anticoagulants and transient severe deficiency of protein S. These findings have led some[138,140] to recommend routine screening for congenital thrombophilic disorders in patients who exhibit purpura fulminans. On the other hand, Westendorp and colleagues analyzed blood from patients who survived meningococcemia and from the parents of those patients who died, and although they found evidence for congenital thrombophilia in 7 of 50 consecutive patients, they determined that this incidence was the same as that in the general population.[141] This question is an interesting point not yet resolved.

Therapy depends on prompt diagnosis and, in the cases associated with DIC, therapy should be directed toward any treatable underlying cause. The treatment of warfarin skin necrosis is discussed in Chapter 11. Owing to the central role of depletion of protein C, many have advocated infusion with protein C concentrates[120] and limited case reports have shown a hint of efficacy. A therapeutic trial has been advocated.[142,143] Others[144] have advocated tissue plasminogen activator therapy. Because of extensive skin loss, these patients may best be treated in a burn unit.[145]

Chronic replacement therapy with protein C has been advocated for the rare unfortunate children with homozygous deficiency of protein C. This has been administered chronically intravenously[146] or, more recently, subcutaneously.[147]

OTHER SITES OF THROMBOSIS

It is now believed that **adrenal gland hemorrhage** is initiated by thrombosis of the adrenal veins. Thrombosis is followed by infarction and subsequent hemorrhage[148] into this very vascular organ. Adrenal vein hemorrhage occurs in stressful situations and increasingly is being recognized in association with antiphospholipid syndrome, heparin-induced thrombocytopenia with thrombosis,[149] and purpura fulminans. Whereas traditionally adrenal gland hemorrhage has been detected at autopsy, it has now been recognized in life in patients who are in stressful situations and develop abdominal pain of uncertain cause. Enlargement and hemorrhage of the gland subsequently is found when abdominal exploration is made by CT scanning[150] (Fig. 15-8).

Hemorrhagic infarction secondary to thrombosis of the **pituitary gland** has been described as a cause of hypopituitarism in patients with antiphospholipid syndrome.[151] This diagnosis may be entertained in the appropriate clinical setting in patients who exhibit evidence of hypopituitarism.

Priapism is caused by engorgement of the corpora cavernosa with blood, not by thrombosis. A minority of cases are called "high flow," characterized by increased inflow (hemorrhage) into the corpora cavernosa, which leads to engorgement. This may be caused by lacerated

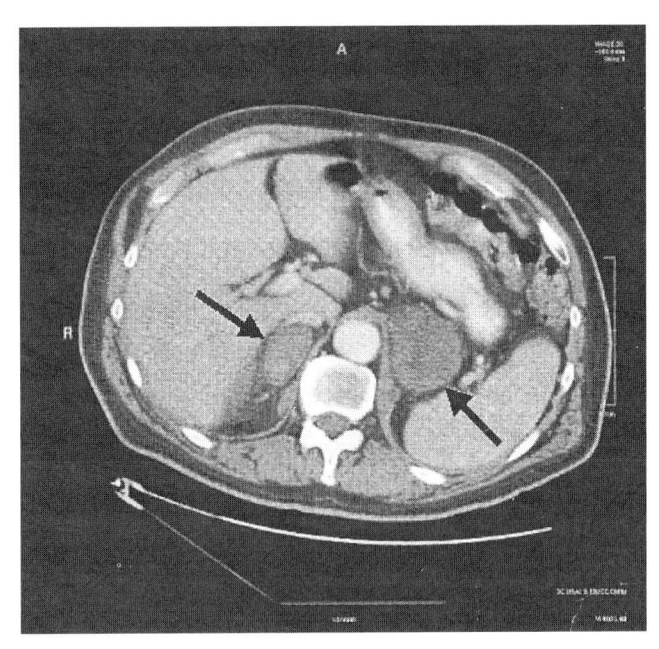

Figure 15–8 Adrenal gland hemorrhage. This CT scan with contrast shows bilateral adrenal hemorrhage (*arrows*) more advanced on the left.

cavernous arteries following blunt trauma. The more common cause, referred to as "low flow," is due to impairment of the vessels emptying the corpora cavernosum.[152] Causes include illicit drugs and psychotropic and anti-hypertensive drugs. It is a hallmark manifestation of sickle cell anemia.[153,154] Of interest, warfarin has been listed as a cause of priapism through unknown mechanisms.[153,154] Comprehensive reviews of hypercoagulable disorders fail to mention priapism, while reviews of priapism do not mention personal or family histories consistent with hypercoagulability. There has been a report of priapism in a patient who also had protein C deficiency[155] and another report of a patient who was homozygous for factor V Leiden defect[156] who had had no prior personal or family history of VTE. Treatment with anticoagulants was not mentioned in that case report.[156] These associations, of course, may be coincidental. Two cases of "high-flow" priapism due to lacerated cavernous arteries were actually treated with fresh clot embolization.[152] It is very unlikely that thrombosis plays an etiologic role in priapism.

Thrombosis of the **ovarian veins** occurs almost exclusively during the postpartum period.[157] It is rather rare, being seen in approximately 1 in every 2000 deliveries, although in one extensive prospective study, Witlin and colleagues[158] found only 11 cases out of 77,000 deliveries over a 10-year period, representing an incidence of less than 0.01%. Of interest, all of their cases were associated with vaginal deliveries. In their review they were unable to find features peculiar to or unusual about the nature of the pregnancy or the delivery predisposing to the thrombosis. The typical patient was admitted 7 to 13 days postpartum, usually for the combination of fever, right pelvic pain, and leukocytosis. The admitting diagnosis was endometritis in three quarters of the cases and in the other quarter was pyelonephritis; none were suspected to have postpartum ovarian vein thrombosis. These patients are considered clinically to be infected and are typically treated with antibiotics.

Because of the overwhelming predominance of this event occurring in the right pelvic vein as opposed to the left pelvic vein by virtue of the unique drainage of the right ovary, appendicitis is often included in the differential diagnosis. When patients' symptoms fail to respond to antibiotic therapy, deeper diagnostic thought is required. The correct diagnosis is almost always made by the combination of failure to respond to antibiotics followed by visualization of the abdominal and pelvic contents by modern imaging. One group found that MRI, CT, and ultrasonography had sensitivities and specificities as follows: 92% and 100%, 100% and 99%, and 50% and 99%, respectively. Imaging led to correct diagnosis in 76 consecutive cases of postpartum fevers that were refractory to antibiotic therapy.[159] The thrombosed postpartum ovarian vein can be surprisingly large. Therapeutic efforts are directed toward anticoagulation once the diagnosis is made. Whereas it is often cited in the obstetric literature that the defervescence of fever in response to heparin therapy occurs characteristically within 24 to 48 hours, Witlin and colleagues found in their study that the response usually requires 3 to 4 days. The disease is thought to be due to septic thrombophlebitis.[160,161] Because modern imaging yields the correct diagnosis, surgical exploration is no longer required. Taking advantage of cases found at surgery in premodern imaging days, however, Munsick and Gillanders[161] cultured the clots excised from thrombosed ovarian veins and found that in six of seven cases, they were able to culture bacteria, thereby solidifying the theory that this is in fact septic thrombophlebitis. Further evidence that this is not typically associated with congenital thrombophilia is the fact that pelvic thrombophlebitis has been described only rarely in patients with both processes. One case of protein C deficiency[155] and one case of protein S deficiency have been implicated.[162] A recent review, however, found 11 of 22 patients with ovarian vein thrombosis had a thrombophilic condition but had negative personal and family histories of prior VTE.[163,164] These experts suggested that warfarin be administered for several months following establishment of the diagnosis and initial heparin therapy. They were not certain about the role of antibiotics but noted that almost all of the patients had already completed a course of antibiotics prior to discharge. Although it is known that thrombi from the ovarian vein can protrude into either the inferior vena cava or veins of the legs, clinically significant PE is very rare. Excellent imaging studies of postpartum ovarian vein thrombosis have been published.[163] Ovarian vein thrombosis has also been found in nonpregnant women, usually incidentally when staging an oncologic disorder. These asymptomatic thromboses of the ovarian veins probably do not need to be treated with heparin but argument could be made to serially monitor the process.[164]

Antiphospholipid syndrome has been regarded as the chief cause of **infarctive placental dysfunction** but other hypercoagulable disorders are being found by systematic evaluation of women who have experienced late fetal loss and stillbirth. Kupferminc and colleagues found that among 110 women with complications of pregnancy that were associated with abnormal placenta vasculature, 71 (65%) had laboratory evidence for thrombophilia compared to 18% in controls ($p <0.001$).[165] Brenner and colleagues found that 49% of women who had undergone a spontaneous abortion had the factor V Leiden mutation, prothrombin 20210 mutation, or abnormalities in methylenetetrahydrofolate reductase (MTHFR) compared to 22% of controls ($p <0.0001$).[166] Gris and coworkers found similar defects in 21% of women with late fetal loss or stillbirth compared to 4% in controls.[167] Both these last two reports additionally confirmed that those harboring more than one hypercoagulable defect had a yet higher rate of fetal wastage (increasing from 7% with one abnormality to 23% with more than one) consistent with the synergism of risk factors described for thromboses at other sites.[168] Martinelli and colleagues calculated a relative risk of late fetal loss of 3.0 for women heterozygous for either the factor V Leiden or prothrombin 20210 mutation.[169] Among women known to have deficiency of either protein S, protein C, or ATIII, fetal loss was experienced in 22% of pregnancies when the women were not treated with anticoagulants; among control women without these deficiencies, 11% experienced fetal loss.[170] Although it is yet to be proven beneficial in most congenital hypercoagulable disorders as it has for pregnancy in women with antiphospholipid syndrome (see Chapter 29), it appears prudent to administer anticoagulant therapy throughout pregnancy and the puerperium for such women in order to increase chances for a live birth.

CONSULTATION CONSIDERATIONS

The consulting hematologist will be asked to see patients with thromboses at unusual sites through two pathways. First, the patient with an established hypercoagulable history may develop nonspecific yet serious signs and symptoms that defy a diagnosis. However, a knowledgeable physician is justified in elevating thrombosis at an usual site from a rarity buried in the differential diagnosis to very high on the list because the patient is thrombophilic. In the second instance, the question will arise whether a patient who develops an unusual thrombosis has an underlying hypercoagulable disorder.

As in all internal medicine, the history and physical examination are fundamental. One should search aggressively for clues in the past history for signs or symptoms of a previous thrombosis. Subtle signs include varicose veins, hemosiderin deposition in the skin of the legs, and chronic edema. Family history should be combed for evidence of members who have unexplained sudden death or a thrombophilic history, or who are on chronic warfarin therapy.

It is important to work closely with other specialists in order to plan for long-term management. Thrombosis is the unifying pathologic event in the genesis of syndromes with expressions as varied as abnormal liver function tests from hepatic vein thrombosis to altered mental status from cerebral venous thrombosis. Physicians who might not by training or interest be attuned to thromboembolism may need special guidance and assistance in therapeutic maneuvers, especially ophthalmologists and obstetricians/gynecologists. Radiologists participate in the diagnostic pursuit as special techniques, special contrasts, and special timing are in order when selecting modern expensive imaging studies.

LABORATORY EVALUATION

It is ironic that laboratory evaluation is best not carried out during the acute part of a VTE as thrombosis itself and treatment thereof may affect levels of protein C, protein S, and ATIII, and often detection of antiphospholipids/anticardiolipins. DNA-based testing using polymerase chain reaction (PCR) analyses such as detection of the factor V Leiden mutation or the prothrombin 20210 mutation will not be affected by these events. It is important to query family members who visit the patient as frequently a member may have a history of a previous thrombosis.

Analysis for protein C, protein S, ATIII, factor V Leiden mutation, prothrombin 20210 mutation, homocysteine, and antiphospholipids/anticardiolipins combined costs approximately $1000. As timing is not important and therapeutic decisions rarely rely on specific biochemical diagnoses, testing can wait.

COST CONTAINMENT

Frequently the consulting physician will have already ordered an expensive battery of tests for hypercoagulability in a patient who has had an acute VTE and is under therapy. These will be difficult to interpret and, if abnormal, the results may be altered by the acute condition or therapy as to any underlying disorder. Although these funds will have already been spent, it is important to clarify in the medical record for future reference the clinical condition and medications the patient was receiving at the time these tests were drawn. An incorrect diagnosis on a discharge summary is extremely difficult to undo. Frequently there is a significant delay or even discharge before results return and many parties will have forgotten these details. Cost containment is also favorably impacted by rapid diagnosis and rapid therapy even if it includes the expense of thrombolytic agents, as these will significantly decrease hospital stay, morbidity and mortality, and frequently extremely expensive procedures such as orthotopic liver transplantation in cases of hepatic vein thrombosis.

■ REFERENCES

Chapter 15 References

1. Osler W. The Principles and Practice of Medicine, 2nd ed. New York, Appleton and Co, 1896.

2. Flint A. A Treatise in the Principles and Practice of Medicine, 6th ed. Philadelphia, Lea Brothers and Co, 1886.
3. Virchow R. Gesammette abhandlungen zur wissenschaftlichen medicin. Frankfurt, Meidinger Sohn, 1856, p. 477.
4. Kitchens CS. Evolution of our understanding of the pathophysiology of primary mesenteric venous thrombosis. Am J Surg 1992;163:346–348.
5. DeStefano Y, Leone G, Mastrangelo S, et al. Clinical manifestations and management in inherited thrombophilia: Retrospective analysis and follow-up after diagnosis of 238 patients with congenital deficiency of antithrombin III, protein C, protein S. Thromb Haemost 1994;72:352–358.
6. Thaler F, Lechner K. Antithrombin III deficiency and thromboembolism. Clin Haematol 1981;10:369–390.
7. Cosgriff TM, Bishop DT, Hershgold EJ, et al. Familial antithrombin III deficiency: Its natural history, genetics, diagnosis, and treatment. Medicine 1983;62:209–220.
8. Winter JH, Fenech A. Familial antithrombin III deficiency. QJ Med 1982;51:373–395.
9. Pabinger I, Schneider B. Thrombotic risk in hereditary antithrombin III, protein C, or protein S deficiency. A cooperative, retrospective study. Gesellschaft fur Thrombose- und Hamostaseforschung (GTH) Study Group on Natural Inhibitors. Arterioscler Thromb Vasc Biol 1996;16:742–748.
10. Clavien PA, Durig M, Harder F. Venous mesenteric infarction: A particular entity. Br J Surg 1988;75:252–255.
11. Mindelzum RE, Jeffery RB Jr, Lane MJ, et al. The misty mesentery on CT: Differential diagnosis. Am J Radiol 1996;167:61–65.
12. Delatour HB. Thrombosis of mesenteric vein as a cause of death after splenectomy. Ann Surg 1895;21:24–28.
13. Elliot, JW. The operative relief of gangrene of the intestine due to occlusion of the mesenteric vessels. Ann Surg 1895;21:9–23.
14. Hansen HJB, Christofferson JK. Occlusive mesenteric infarction, a retrospective study of 83 cases. Acta Chir Scand 1976;472 (suppl):103–108.
15. Ottinger LW, Austen WG. A study of 136 patients with mesenteric infarction. Surg Gynecol Obstet 1967;124:251–261.
16. Darnige L, Jezequez P, Amoura Z, et al. Mesenteric venous thrombosis in two patients heterozygous for the 20210A allele of the prothrombin gene. Thromb Haemost 1998;80:703.
17. Chen MC, Brown MC, Willson RA, et al. Mesenteric vein thrombosis. Four cases and review of the literature. Digest Dis. 1996;14:382–389.
18. Abdu RA, Zakhour BJ, Dallis DJ. Mesenteric venous thrombosis, 1911 to 1984. Surgery 1987;101:383–388.
19. Robin R, Gruel Y, Lang M, et al. Complete thrombolysis of mesenteric vein occlusion with recombinant tissue-type plasminogen activator. Lancet 1988;1:1391.
20. Leach SD, Meier GH, Gusberg RJ. Endoscopic sclerotherapy: A risk factor for splanchnic venous thrombosis. J Vasc Surg 1989;10:9–13.
21. Petit P, Bret PM, Atri M. Splenic vein thrombosis after splenectomy: Frequency and role of imaging. Radiology 1994;190:65–68.
22. Han DC, Feliciano DV. The clinical complexity of splenic vein thrombosis. Am Surg 1998;64:558–561.
23. Elizalde JI, Castells A, Panes J, et al. Portal hypertensive gastropathy in splenic vein thrombosis. J Clin Gastroenterol 1994;19:310–312.
24. Teofili L, DeStefano V, Leone G, et al. Hematologic causes of venous thrombosis in young people: High incidence of myeloproliferative disorder as underlying disease in patients with splenic venous thrombosis. Thromb Haemost 1992;67:297–301.
25. Belfour GW, Stewart TG. Case of enlarged spleen complicated by ascites, both depending upon varicose dilation and thrombosis of the portal vein. Edinburgh Med J 1869;14:589–598.
26. Janssen HLA, Melmardi JR, Vleggaar FP, et al. Factor V Leiden mutation, prothrombin gene mutation, and deficiencies in coagulation inhibitors associated with Budd-Chiari syndrome and portal vein thrombosis: Results of a case-control study. Blood 2000;96:2364–3368.
26a. Amitrano L, Brancaccio V, Guardascione MA, et al. Inherited coagulation disorders in cirrhotic patients with portal vein thrombosis. Hepatology 2000;31:345–348.
27. Cohen J, Edelman RR, Chopra S. Portal vein thrombosis: A review. Am J Med 1997;92:173–182.
28. Broe PJ, Conley CL, Cameron JL. Thrombosis of the portal vein following splenectomy for myeloid metaplasia. Surg Gynecol Obstet 1981;152:488–492.
29. Valla D, Casadevall N, Huisse MG, et al. Etiology of portal vein thrombosis in adults. A prospective evaluation of primary myeloproliferative disorder. Gastroenterology 1988;94:1063–1069.
30. Rayer PFO. Traite des maladies des reins et des alteret lens de la secretions urinaire. Paris, France, Baillieve, 1840;2:550–559.
31. Llach F. Hypercoagulability, renal vein thrombosis, and other thrombotic complications of nephrotic syndrome. Kidney Int 1985;28:429–439.
32. Laville M, Aquilera D, Maillet J, et al. The prognosis of renal vein thrombosis: A re-evaluation of 27 cases. Nephrol Dial Transplant 1988;3:247–256.
33. Vigano-D'Angelo S, D'Angelo A, Kaufman DE Jr, et al. Protein S deficiency occurs in the nephrotic syndrome. Ann Intern Med 1987;107:42–47.
34. Gouault-Heilmann M, Gadelha-Parente T, Levent M, et al. Total and free protein S in nephrotic syndrome. Thromb Res 1988;49:37–42.
35. Ko WS, Lim PS, Sung YP. Renal vein thrombosis as a first clinical manifestation of the primary antiphospholipid syndrome. Nephrol Dial Transplant 1995;10:1929–1931.
36. Morgan RJ, Feneley RC. Renal vein thrombosis caused by primary antiphospholipid syndrome. Br J Urol 1994;74:807–808.
37. Asherson RA, Buchanan N, Baguley E. et al. Postpartum bilateral renal vein thrombosis in the primary antiphospholipid syndrome. J Rheumatol 1993;20:874–876.
38. Harris RC, Ismail N. Extrarenal complications of the nephrotic syndrome. Am J Kidney Dis 1994;23:477–497.
39. Velasquez FF, Garcia PN, Ruiz MN. Idiopathic nephrotic syndrome of the adult with asymptomatic thrombosis of the renal vein. Am J Nephrol 1988;8:457–462.
40. Kitchens CS. Thrombotic storm: When thrombosis begets thrombosis. Am J Med 1998;104:381–385.
41. Markowitz GS, Brignol F, Burns ER, et al. Renal vein thrombosis treated with thrombolytic therapy: Case report and brief review. Am J Kidney Dis 1995;25:801–806.
42. Lam KK, Lui CC. Successful treatment of acute inferior vena cava and unilateral renal vein thrombosis by local infusion of recombinant tissue plasminogen activator. Am J Kidney Dis 1998;32:1075–1079.
43. Kanagasundaram NS, Bandyopadhyay D, Brownjohn AM, et al. The diagnosis of renal vein thrombosis by magnetic resonance angiography. Nephrol Dial Transplant 1998;13:200–202.
44. Gates PC, Barnett, HJM. Venous disease: Cortical veins and sinuses. In Barnett HJM, Stein BM, Mohr JP, et al. (eds.): Stroke: Pathophysiology, Diagnosis, and Management. New York, Churchill Livingstone, 1986.
45. Krayenbuhl H. Cerebral venous and sinus thrombosis. Clin Neurosurg 1967;14:1–24.
45a. Southwick FS. Septic thrombophletis of major dural venous sinuses. In Remington JS, Swartz MN (eds.): Current Clinical Topics in Infectious Diseases. Boston, Blackwell Science, 1995, pp. 179–203.
46. Martinelli I, Sacchi E, Landi G, et al. High risk of cerebral vein thrombosis in carriers of a prothrombin-gene mutation and in users of oral contraceptives. N Engl J Med 1998;338:1793–1797.

47. Martinelli I, Landi G, Merati G, et al. Factor V gene mutation is a risk factor for cerebral venous thrombosis. Thromb Haemost 1996;75:393–394.
48. Zuber M, Toulon P, Marnet L, et al. Factor V Leiden mutation in cerebral venous thrombosis. Stroke 1996;27:1721–1723.
49. Reschiens MA. Coagulation studies, factor V Leiden, and anticardiolipin antibodies in 40 cases of cerebral venous thrombosis. Stroke 1996;27:1724–1730.
50. Ameri A, Bousser M-G. Cerebral venous thrombosis. Neurol Clin 1992;10:87–111.
51. Parnass SM, Goodwin JA, Patel DV, et al. Dural sinus thrombosis: A mechanism for pseudotumor cerebri in systemic lupus erythematosus. J Rheumatol 1987;14:152–155.
52. Uziel Y, Laxer RM, Blaser S, et al. Cerebral vein thrombosis in childhood systemic lupus erythematosus. J Pediatr 1995;126:722–727.
53. Crawford SC, Digre KB, Palmer CA. Thrombosis of the deep venous drainage of the brain in adults. Analysis of seven cases with review of the literature. Arch Neurol 1995;52:1101–1108.
54. Madan A, Sluzewski M, van Rooij WJ, et al. Thrombosis of the deep cerebral veins: CT and MRI findings with pathologic correlation. Neuroradiology 1997;39:777–780.
55. Erbguth F, Breener P, Schuierer G. Diagnosis and treatment of deep cerebral vein thrombosis. Neurosurg Rev 1991;14:145–148.
56. Bousser M-G, Chiras J, Bories J, et al. Cerebral venous thrombosis: A review of 38 cases. Stroke 1985;16:199–210.
57. Einhaupl KM, Villringer A, Meister W. Heparin treatment in sinus venous thrombosis. Lancet 1991;338:597–600.
58. Wang ZG, Jones RS. Budd-Chiari syndrome. Curr Probl Surg 1996;33:83–211.
59. Osler W. Case of obliteration of vena cava inferior, with great stenosis of orifices of hepatic veins. J Anat Physiol 1878;13:291–294.
60. Dilawari JB, Bambery P, Chawla Y, et al. Hepatic outflow obstruction (Budd-Chiari syndrome). Experience with 177 patients and a review of the literature. Medicine (Baltimore) 1994;73:21–36.
61. Okuda K, Kage M, Shrestha SM. Proposal of a new nomenclature for Budd-Chiari syndrome: Hepatic vein thrombosis versus thrombosis of the inferior vena cava at its hepatic portion. Hepatology 1998;28:1191–1198.
62. Valla D, Benhamou J-P. Obstruction of the hepatic veins or suprahepatic inferior vena cava. Dig Dis 1996;14:99–118.
63. Min AD, Atillasoy EO, Schwartz MG, et al. Reassessing the role of medical therapy in the management of hepatic vein thrombosis. Liver Transpl Surg 1997;3:423–429.
64. Maddrey WC. Hepatic vein thrombosis (Budd-Chiari syndrome). Hepatology 1984;4:44S–46S.
65. Valla D, Dhumeaux D, Babany G, et al. Hepatic vein thrombosis in paroxysmal nocturnal hemoglobinuria: A spectrum from asymptomatic occlusion of hepatic venules to fatal Budd-Chiari syndrome. Gastroenterology 1987;93:569–575.
66. Genti-Kocher S, Bernard O, Brunelle F, et al. Budd-Chiari syndrome in children: Report of 22 cases. J Pediatr 1988;113:30–38.
67. Nakamura H, Uehara H, Okada T, et al. Occlusion of small hepatic veins associated with systemic lupus erythematosus with the lupus anticoagulant and anti-cardiolipin antibody. Hepatogastroenterology 1989;36:393–397.
68. Pettetier S, Landi B, Piette J-C, et al. Antiphospholipid syndrome as the second cause of non-tumorous Budd-Chiari syndrome. J Hepatol 1994;21:76–80.
69. Mahmoud A, Elias E. New approaches to the Budd-Chiari syndrome. J Gastroenterol Hepatol 1996;11:1121–1123.
70. Langnas AN. Budd-Chiari syndrome: Decisions, decisions. Liver Transpl Surg 1997;3:443–445.
71. Raju GS, Felver M, Olin JW, et al. Thrombolysis for acute Budd-Chiari syndrome: Case report and literature review. Am J Gastroenterol 1996;91:1262–1263.
72. Campbell DA, Rolles K, Jamieson N, et al. Hepatic transplantation with peri-operative and long-term anticoagulation as treatment for Budd-Chiari syndrome. Surg Gynecol Obstet 1988;166:511–518.
73. Williamson TH. Central retinal vein occlusion: What's the story? Br J Ophthalmol 1997;81:698–704.
74. Sperduto RD, Hiller R, Chew E, et al. Risk factors for hemiretinal vein occlusion: Comparison with risk factors for central and branch retinal vein occlusion: The eye disease case-control study. Ophthalmology 1998;105:765–771.
75. Baumal CR, Brown GC. Treatment of central retinal vein occlusion. Ophthalmic Surg Lasers 1997;28:590–600.
76. The Eye Disease Case-Control Study Group. Risk factors for central retinal vein occlusion. Arch Ophthalmol 1996;114:545–554.
77. The Central Vein Occlusion Study Group. Natural history and clinical management of central retinal vein occlusion. Arch Ophthalmol 1997;115:486–491.
78. Hunt BJ. Activated protein C and retinal vein occlusion. Br J Ophthalmol 1996;80:194.
79. Dunn JP, Noorily SW, Petri M, et al. Antiphospholipid antibodies and retinal vascular disease. Lupus 1996;5:313–322.
80. Prince HM, Thurlow PJ, Buchanan RC, et al. Acquired protein S deficiency in a patient with systemic lupus erythematosus causing central retinal vein thrombosis. J Clin Pathol 1995;48:387–389.
81. Glueck CJ, Bell H, Vadlamani L. Heritable thrombophilia and hypofibrinolysis. Possible causes of retinal vein occlusion. Arch Ophthalmol 1999;117:43–49.
82. El-Asrav AMA, Al-Momen A-K, Al-Amro S, et al. Prothrombotic states associated with retinal venous occlusion in young adults. Int Ophthalmol 1996;20:197–204.
83. Linna T, Ylikorkala A, Kontula K, et al. Prevalence of factor V Leiden in young adults with retinal vein occlusion. Thromb Haemost 1997;77:214–216.
84. Albisinni R, Coppola A, Loffredo M, et al. Retinal vein occlusion and inherited conditions predisposing to thrombophilia. Thromb Haemost 1998;80:702–703.
85. Greiner K, Hafner G, Dick B, et al. Retinal vascular occlusion and deficiencies in the protein C pathway. Am J Ophthalmol 1999;128:69–74.
86. Spagnolo BV, Nasrallah FP. Bilateral retinal vein occlusion associated with factor V Leiden mutation. Retina 1998;18:377–378.
87. Williamson TH, Rumley A, Lowe GD. Blood viscosity, coagulation, and activated protein C resistance in central retinal vein occlusion: A population controlled study. Br J Ophthalmol 1996;80:203–208.
88. Larsson J, Olafsdottir E, Bauer B. Activated protein C resistance in young adults with central retinal vein occlusion. Br J Ophthalmol 1996;80:200–202.
89. Ciardella AP, Yannuzzi LA, Freund KB, et al. Factor V Leiden, activated protein C resistance, and retinal vein occlusion. Retina 1998;18:308–315.
90. Yesim F, Demirci FY, Guney DB, et al. Prevalence of factor V Leiden in patients with retinal vein occlusion. Acta Ophthalmol Scand 1999;77:631–633.
91. Guven D, Sayinalp N, Kalayei D, et al. Risk factors in central retinal vein occlusion and activated protein C resistance. Eur J Ophthalmol 1999;9:43–49.
92. Larsson J, Sellman A, Bauer B. Activated protein C resistance in patients with central retinal vein occlusion. Br J Ophthalmol 1997;81:832–834.
93. Gottlieb JL, Blice JP, Mestichelli B, et al. Activated protein C resistance, factor V Leiden, and central retinal vein occlusion in young adults. Arch Ophthalmol 1998;116:557–579.
94. Delahousse B, Arsene S, Piquemal R, et al. The 20210A allele of the prothrombin gene is not a risk factor for retinal vein occlusion. Blood Coagul Fibrinolysis 1998;9:447–448.

95. De Bruijne ELE, Keulen-de Vos GHJC, Ouwendijk RJT. Ocular venous occlusion and hyperhomocystinemia. Ann Intern Med 1999;130:78.
96. Greaves M. Aging and the pathogenesis of retinal vein thrombosis. Br J Ophthalmol 1997;81:810–811.
97. Giorgi D, Gabrieli CB, Bonomo L. The clinico-ophthalmological spectrum of antiphospholipid syndrome. Ocul Immunol Inflamm 1998;6:269–273.
98. Wiechens B, Schroder JO, Potzsch B, et al. Primary antiphospholipid antibody syndrome and retinal occlusive vasculopathy. Am J Ophthalmol 1997;123:848–850.
99. Hattenbach LO, Steinkamp G, Scharrer I, et al. Fibrinolytic therapy with low-dose recombinant tissue plasminogen activator in retinal vein occlusion. Ophthalmologica 1998;212:394–398.
100. Elman MJ. Thrombolytic therapy for central retinal vein occlusion: Results of a pilot study. Trans Am Ophthalmol Soc 1996;94:A471–504.
101. Martinelli I, Cattaneo M, Pangeri D, et al. Risk factors for deep venous thrombosis of the upper extremities. Ann Intern Med 1997;126:707–711.
102. Martinelli I, Cattaneo M, Taioli E, et al. Generic risk factors for superficial vein thrombosis. Thromb Haemost 1999;82:1215–1217.
103. Painter TD, Karpf M. Deep venous thrombosis of the upper extremity: 5 years' experience at a university hospital. Angiology 1984;35:743–749.
104. Becker DM, Philbrick JR, Walker FB IV. Axillary and subclavian venous thrombosis, prognosis and treatment. Arch Intern Med 1991;151:1934–1943.
105. Lindblad B, Tengborn L, Bergqvist D. Deep vein thrombosis of the axillary-subclavian veins: Epidemiologic data, effects of different types of treatment and late sequelae. Eur J Vasc Surg 1988;2:161–165.
106. Hurlbert SN, Rutherford RB. Primary subclavian-axillary vein thrombosis. Ann Vasc Surg 1995;9:217–223.
107. Roy TM, Byrd RP Jr, Lukeman R, et al. Primary subclavian vein thrombosis and pulmonary embolism. South Med J 1007;90:748–751.
108. Timsit JF, Farkas JC, Boyer JM, et al. Central vein catheter-related thrombosis in intensive care patients: Incidence, risks factors, and relationship with catheter-related sepsis. Chest 1998;114:207–213.
109. Birdwell BG, Yeager B, Whitsett TL. Pseudotumor cerebri. A complication of catheter-induced subclavian vein thrombosis. Arch Intern Med 1994;154:808–811.
110. Ameli FM, Minas T, Weiss M, et al. Consequences of "conservative" conventional management of axillary vein thrombosis. Can J Surg. 1987;30:167–169.
111. Druy EM, Trout HH III, Giordano JM, et al. Lytic therapy in the treatment of axillary and subclavian vein thrombosis. J Vasc Surg 1985;2:821–827.
112. Wilson JJ, Zahn CA, Newman H. Fibrinolytic therapy for idiopathic subclavian-axillary vein thrombosis. Am J Surg 1990;159:208–211.
113. Hicken GJ, Ameli FM. Management of subclavian-axillary vein thrombosis: A review. Can J Surg 1998;41:13–25.
114. Malcynski J, O'Donnell TF Jr, Mackey WC, et al. Long-term results of treatment for axillary subclavian vein thrombosis. Can J Surg 1993;36:365–371.
115. Azakie A, McElhinney DB, Thompson RW, et al. Surgical management of subclavian-vein effort thrombosis as a result of thoracic outlet compression. J Vasc Surg 1998;28:777–786.
116. Heron E, Lozinguez O, Emmerich J, et al. Long-term sequelae of spontaneous axillary-subclavian venous thrombosis. Ann Intern Med 1999;131:510–513.
117. Bern M, Lokich JJ, Wallach SR, et al. Very low doses of warfarin can prevent thrombosis in central venous catheters: a randomized prospective trial. Ann Intern Med 1990;112:423–428.
118. Monreal M, Alastrue A, Rull M, et al. Upper extremity deep vein thrombosis in cancer patients with venous access devices: prophylaxis with a low molecular weight heparin (Fragmin). Thromb Haemost 1996;75:251–253.
119. Seagle MB, Bingham HG. Purpura fulminans. Ann Plast Surg 1988;20:576–581.
120. Smith OP, White B. Infectious purpura fulminans: Diagnosis and treatment. Br J Haematol 1999;104:202–207.
121. Darmstadt GL. Acute infectious purpura fulminans: Pathogenesis and medical management. Pediatr Dermatol 1008;15:169–183.
122. Bergmann F, Hoyer PF, D'Angelo SV, et al. Severe autoimmune protein S deficiency in a boy with idiopathic purpura fulminans. Br J Haematol 1995;89:610–614.
123. Moreb J, Kitchens CS. Acquired functional protein S deficiency, cerebral venous thrombosis, and coumarin skin necrosis in association with antiphospholipid syndrome: Report of two cases. Am J Med 1989;98:207–210.
124. DeFranzo AJ, Marasco P, Argenta LC. Warfarin-induced necrosis of the skin. Ann Plastic Surg 1995;34:203–208.
125. Goldberg SL, Orthner CL, Yalisove BL, et al. Skin necrosis following prolonged administration of coumarin in a patient with inherited protein S deficiency. Am J Hematol 1991; 38:64–66.
126. Dominey A, Kettler A, Yiannias J, et al. Purpura fulminans and transient protein C and S deficiency. Arch Dermatol 1988;124:1442–1443.
127. Madden RM, Gill JC, Marlar RA. Protein C and protein S levels in two patients with acquired purpura fulminans. Br J Haematol 1990;75:112–117.
128. Draelos ZK, Hansen RC. Hemorrhagic bullae in an anemic woman, paroxysmal nocturnal hemoglobinuria. Arch Dermatol 1986;122:1325–1330.
129. Rietschel RL, Lewis CW, Simmons RA, et al. Skin lesions in paroxysmal nocturnal hemoglobinuria. Arch Dermatol 1978; 114:560–563.
130. Marlar RA, Montgomery RR, Broekmans AW. Diagnosis and treatment of homozygous protein C deficiency: Report of the working party on homozygous protein C deficiency of the subcommittee on protein C and protein S, International Committee on Thrombosis and Haemostasis. J Pediatr 1989;114:528–534.
131. Alessi MC, Aillaud MF, Paut O, et al. Purpura fulminans in a patient homozygous for a mutation in the protein C gene—prenatal diagnosis in a subsequent pregnancy. Thromb Haemost 1996;75:525–526.
132. Soria JM, Morell M, Jiminez-Astorga C, et al. Severe type I protein C deficiency in a compound heterozygote for Y124C and Q132X mutations in exon 6 of the PROC gene. Thromb Haemost 1995;74:1215–1220.
133. Pung-amritt P, Poort SB, Vos HL, et al. Compound heterozygosity for one novel and one recurrent mutation in a Thai patient with severe protein S deficiency. Thromb Haemost 1999;81: 189–192.
134. Jackson RT, Luplow RE III. Adult purpura fulminans and digital necrosis associated with sepsis and the factor V Leiden mutation. JAMA 1998;280:1829–1830.
135. Woods CB, Johnson CA. Varicella purpura fulminans associated with heterozygosity for factor V Leiden and transient protein S deficiency. Pediatrics 1998;102:1208–1210.
136. Gurgey A. Clinical manifestations in thrombotic children with factor V Leiden mutation. Pediatr Hematol Oncol 1999;16: 233–237.
137. Pipe SW, Schmaier AH, Nichols WC, et al. Neonatal purpura fulminans in association with factor V R506Q mutation. J Pediatr 1996;128(5 Pt 1):706–709.
138. Inbal A, Kenet G, Zivelin A. Purpura fulminans induced by disseminated intravascular coagulation following infection in 2 unrelated children with double heterozygosity for factor V Leiden and protein S deficiency. Thromb Haemost 1997;77:1086–1089.

139. Manco-Johnson MJ, Nuss R, Key N, et al. Lupus anticoagulant and protein S deficiency in children with postvaricella purpura fulminans or thrombosis. J Pediatr 1996;128:319–323.
140. Sackesen C, Secmeer G, Gurgey A, et al. Homozygous factor V Leiden mutation in a child with meningococcal purpura fulminans. Pediatr Infect Dis J 1998;17:87.
141. Westendorp R, Reitsma PH, Bertina RM. Inherited prethrombotic disorders and infectious purpura. Thromb Haemost 1996;75:899–901.
142. Rintala E, Seppala OP, Kotilainen P, et al. Protein C in the treatment of coagulopathy of meningococcal disease. Crit Care Med 1998;26:965–968.
143. Smith OP, White B, Vaughan D, et al. Use of protein C concentrate, heparin, and haemodiafiltration in meningococcus-induced purpura fulminans. Lancet 1997;350:1590–1593.
144. Aiuto LT, Barone SR, Cohen PS, et al. Recombinant tissue plasminogen activator restores perfusion in meningococcal purpura fulminans. Crit Care Med 1997; 25:1079–1082.
145. Brown DL, Greenhalgh DG, Warden GD. Purpura fulminans: A disease best managed in a burn center. J Burn Care Rehabil 1998;19:119–123.
146. Muller FM, Ehrenthal W, Hafner G, et al. Purpura fulminans in severe congenital protein C deficiency: Monitoring of treatment with protein C concentrate. Eur J Pediatr 1996;155:20–25.
147. Sanz-Rodriguez C, Gil-Fernandez JJ, Zapater P, et al. Long-term management of homozygous protein C deficiency: Replacement therapy with subcutaneous purified protein C concentrate. Thromb Haemost 1999;81:887–890.
148. Asherson RA, Hughes GRV. Hypoadrenalism, Addison's disease and antiphospholipid antibodies. J Rheumatol 1991;18:1–3.
149. Warkentin TE. Clinical presentation of heparin-induced thrombocytopenia. Semin Hematol 1998;35(suppl 5):9–16.
150. Caron P, Chabannier MH, Cambus JP, et al. Definitive adrenal insufficiency due to bilateral adrenal hemorrhage and primary antiphospholipid syndrome. J Clin Endocrinol Metab 1998;83:1437–1439.
151. Pandolfi C, Gianini A, Fregoni V, et al. Hypopituitarism and antiphospholipid syndrome. Minerva Endocrinol 1997;22:103–105.
152. Kim SC, Park SH, Yang SH. Treatment of post-traumatic chronic high-flow priapisms by superselective embolization of cavernous artery with autologous clot. J Trauma 1996;40:462–465.
153. Macaluso JN Jr, Sullivan JW. Priapism: Review of 34 cases. Urology 1985;26:233–236.
154. Bertram RA, Webster GD, Carson CC III. Priapism: Etiology, treatment, and results in series of 35 presentations. Urology 1985;26:229–232.
155. Melissari E, Kakkar VV. Congenital severe protein C deficiency in adults. Br J Haematol 1989;72:222–228.
156. De Prost D, Delmas V, Lefebvre M, et al. Priapism revealing ARG 506 to GLN factor V mutation. J Urol 1996;155:1392.
157. Ballem P. Acquired thrombophilia in pregnancy. Semin Thromb Hemost 1998;24:41–46.
158. Witlin AG, Sibai BM. Postpartum ovarian vein thrombosis after vaginal delivery: A report of 11 cases. Obstet Gynecol 1995;85(5 Pt 1):775–780.
159. Twickler DM, Setiawan AT, Evans RS. Imaging of puerperal septic thrombophlebitis: Prospective comparison of MR imaging, CT, and sonography. Am J Roentgenol 1997;169:1039–1043.
160. Isada NB, Landy HJ, Larsen JW Jr. Postabortal septic pelvic thrombophlebitis diagnosed with CT, a case report. J Reprod Med 1987;32:866–868.
161. Munsick RA, Gillanders LA. A review of the syndrome of puerperal ovarian vein thrombophlebitis. Obstet Gynecol Surv 1981;36:57–66.
162. Giraud JR, Poulain P, Renaud-Giono A. Diagnosis of postpartum ovarian vein thrombophlebitis by color Doppler ultrasonography: About 10 cases. Acta Obstet Gynecol Scand 1997;76(8):773–778.
163. Salomon O, Apter S, Shaham D, et al. Risk factors associated with postpartum ovarian vein thrombosis. Thromb Haemost 1999;82:1015–1019.
164. Simons GR, Piwnica Worms DR, Goldhaber SZ. Ovarian vein thrombosis. Am Heart J 1993;126(3 Pt 1):641–647.
165. Kupferminc MJ, Eldor A, Steinman N, et al. Increased frequency of genetic thrombophilia in women with complications of pregnancy. N Engl J Med 1999;340:9–13.
166. Brenner B, Sarig G, Weiner G, et al. Thrombophilic polymorphisms are common in women with fetal loss without apparent cause. Thromb Haemost 1999;82:6–9.
167. Gris J-C, Quere I, Monpeyroux F, et al. Case-control study of the frequency of thrombophilic disorders in couples with late foetal loss and no thrombotic antecedent. Thromb Haemost 1999;81:891–899.
168. Rosendaal FR. Thrombosis in the young: epidemiology and risk factors. A focus on venous thrombosis. Thromb Haemost 1997;78:1–6.
169. Martinelli I, Taioli, E, Cetin I, et al. Mutations in coagulation factor in women with unexplained late fetal loss. N Engl J Med 2000;343:1015–1018.
170. Sanson B-J, Friederich PW, Simiani P, et al. The risk of abortion and stillbirth in antithrombin-, protein C- and protein S-deficient women. Thromb Haemost 1996;75:387–388.

CHAPTER 16

Prevention, Diagnosis, and Treatment of the Postphlebitic Syndrome

Patricio Rosa, M.D.
David L. Gillespie, M.D.
Sean D. O'Donnell, M.D.

INTRODUCTION/EPIDEMIOLOGY

Deep venous thrombosis (DVT) of the lower extremity occurs in 250,000, or 1 out of 1000, persons in the United States each year.[1] The postphlebitic syndrome, consisting of persistent pain, edema, hyperpigmentation, induration of the skin, and stasis ulceration,[2] is a well-recognized complication of acute DVT, estimated to affect up to 4% of the general population.[3] The most likely cause of the postphlebitic syndrome is venous hypertension, resulting from outflow obstruction and damage to venous valves. This venous hypertension is then transmitted to the skin microcirculation, leading to tissue hypoxia and lymphatic obstruction.[4] Two thirds of patients with postphlebitic symptoms have evidence of a clinically or phlebographically proven DVT.[5] As long as 5 to 10 years may be required for the postphlebitic syndrome to become evident, although in some studies, most cases were recognized within the first 2 years of the acute thrombotic event.[4] In one study of patients with acute DVT, 17% showed symptoms 1 week after the acute episode; this increased to 37% after the first month and 69% after the first year.[5] Approximately 25% to 33% of individuals with a history of DVT remain asymptomatic in the long term.[3,6] Studies have reported that 67% to 80% of patients will have both symptoms and abnormal venous hemodynamics[7,8] after DVT.

The presence of abnormal venous hemodynamics, with incompetent valves and reflux on a chronic basis, constitutes chronic venous insufficiency (CVI). Over time, CVI may lead to the symptom complex that we know as postphlebitic syndrome. The terms *chronic venous insufficiency* and *postphlebitic syndrome,* although strictly not the same, as one represents a pathophysiology and the other a complex of resultant symptoms, are often used interchangeably.

The postphlebitic syndrome varies from mild edema with little discomfort to incapacitating limb swelling with pain and ulceration. Mild postphlebitic skin changes and hyperpigmentation are observed in 15% to 30%,[3,9] and severe signs of postphlebitic syndrome and marked trophic skin changes progressing to ulceration are observed in 2% to 10% of patients from 5 to 10 years after their DVT[3,6,8,9] regardless of the initial site of thrombosis. Severe CVI can be highly debilitating and frustrating to patient and physician. Successful treatment is fraught with difficulty, patient noncompliance, and recurrence, despite sometimes the initial success of the treatment.[10] The incidence of severe CVI seems to increase with age.[11]

Retrospective studies report that in more than 80% of the affected limbs, cutaneous ulceration resulted 10 years after a DVT. Recent studies suggest a lower incidence of severe changes following an episode of DVT.[3] Some suggest that the aggressive use of heparin may have reduced the incidence of serious long-term changes of the postphlebitic syndrome, but other studies have reported that even with adequate laboratory control of heparin anticoagulation, up to 30% of patients will show extension of their DVT.[3]

Most studies have shown that patients who develop venous reflux after DVT have incompetence of the deep venous system, whereas about 15% have reflux of the superficial venous system alone.[5] Venous thrombosis results in the destruction of the delicate bicuspid venous valves that promote antegrade flow of blood from the leg. During the process of walking, with each step the soleus muscle compresses the lower-extremity veins and propels the column of blood toward the heart. With the destruction of the venous valves, however, blood is free to reflux into the distal extremity. This results in a constantly elevated ambulatory venous pressure (AVP).

The combination of a persistently elevated AVP and other factors yet to be fully elucidated results in the chronic skin changes of the lower extremity that we recognize as evidence of CVI or the postphlebitic syndrome. Although some data suggest this is most closely associated with the development of incompetent venous valves, the mechanism by which incompetence occurs, as well as its time course, is not completely understood.[2] For example, 15% of normal people have some degree of venous reflux, mostly in the superficial veins.[5]

PATHOPHYSIOLOGY

There are three anatomic components to the venous system of the lower extremity: the superficial, the perforator, and the deep venous systems. The postphlebitic syndrome may be the result of abnormalities in one or more of these systems. CVI may be primary or secondary. Primary CVI, in which no known cause can be identified, is usually due to primary valvular insufficiency. Secondary CVI is acquired, typically postphlebitic.[11,12] In primary valvular insufficiency, all the symptoms of typical CVI are identified, and yet the patients have no prior history or imaging evidence of previous thrombosis. Patients with secondary CVI suffer the consequences of the two major sequelae of DVT. These sequelae are obstruction to outflow due to the presence of residual thrombus, and reflux due to valvular damage.[3,5,13] Obstructive symptoms are most commonly associated with acute thrombosis and usually improve with recanalization of the vessel[11] and collateral formation around an area of occlusion.[2,14] Residual obstruction to outflow results from failure to recanalize the major deep veins of the leg. It is believed that reflux results from irreversible valve destruction. This results in valvular insufficiency preventing efficient function of the calf muscle pump. Distal venous hypertension develops equal to the hydraulic pressure of the vertical column of blood extending from the heart to the ankle in the standing position.[3,15] A common dilemma is whether valvular incompetence or venous outflow obstruction is the more important factor in the development of symptoms.[14] While it is likely a combination of both, reflux is usually thought to be the primary pathologic problem. As such, symptoms are more closely associated with valvular incompetence than residual obstruction.[2,7,11,12] However, many patients with severe reflux have only mild symptoms and additional factors must therefore contribute to the development of severe postphlebitic syndrome.[16] Chronic venous obstruction therefore plays at least a secondary role in the sequelae of postphlebitic syndrome.[7] It has been proposed that primary deep venous insufficiency in the thigh may play a role in the development of distal DVT, by allowing reflux, which induces stasis. Valve destruction by DVT then appears to increase reflux, although this has not been proven in any prospective studies.[12,17]

Following DVT, recanalization commences. In one study of patients treated with heparin, lysis of thrombi with recanalization was present in 44% of cases at 7 days, 94% at 30 days, and 100% at 90 days. This is not, however, a simple straightforward sequence, because many patients showed extension of thrombus despite therapeutic doses of anticoagulation. Some patients showed extension of thrombus as early as 7 days into their course, and some as late as between 30 and 180 days.[2] Incomplete recanalization or inadequate formation of collaterals may leave residual obstruction, resulting in venous hypertension. In the process of recanalization, however, some damage occurs to the venous valves, which ultimately results in valvular incompetence, reflux, and venous hypertension. Several mechanisms play a role in the recanalization of the thrombus; these include retraction of the thrombus, peripheral fragmentation, central softening of the thrombus, and spontaneous fibrinolysis.[2,7] Lytic clefts form around the valve cusps; this has been attributed to local fibrinolytic activity that may be higher on the valve cusps than in the surrounding endothelium. This fibrinolytic activity appears to be more efficient in small veins, suggesting a higher concentration of fibrinolytic activity at these sites. Such increased efficiency may contribute to valve preservation. It also appears that very large and very small thrombi are more likely to recanalize rapidly and that certain veins, such as the posterior tibial vein, which has a large number of valves, may have a decreased incidence of reflux. Analysis of lysis times of the thrombi in vivo suggests that early recanalization is important in preserving valve integrity.[2,7] It has been postulated that rapid resolution of the thrombus may preserve valvular function and decrease the incidence of the postphlebitic syndrome. In one study, early lysis using fibrinolytic agents resulted in a better clinical outcome after DVT than stabilization of the thrombus with heparin.[2] The theory that early and complete lysis reduces the incidence of the postphlebitic syndrome has been the basis for the use of early, aggressive thrombolysis in selected patients with acute DVT.

The factors contributing to the development of valvular incompetence are not completely understood. Following resolution of thrombosis, changes in the vein walls and valve degeneration occur within a few months, leading to postphlebitic reflux.[18] A strong association has long been established between severe postphlebitic syndrome and venous reflux, which is probably the major pathophysiologic component of ulceration.[16,17] The valve cusps rarely are involved by fibrocellular organization.[7] However, because of the surrounding inflammatory processes, loss of elasticity results in impairment of venous wall compliance.[17] The development of reflux, which coincides with or is preceded by complete clot lysis within a venous segment, has been reported as early as 7 days after onset of the DVT.[2] Some patients have transient reflux associated with recanalization. Because of incomplete clot lysis, valves are prevented from closing completely. With complete lysis, these valves eventually become functional again.[7] In other cases venous valvular incompetence develops much later than recanalization. Doppler data suggest that incompetence develops between the second and fifth months following DVT.[2] Van Bemmelen and coworkers proposed that the development of venous incompetence is a two-stage process. Initially the vein dilates in response to proximal venous obstruction. Valvular incompetence occurs because the cusps of the valves are not large enough to coapt with the increased venous diameter.[19] At this stage, which occurs between the first and second months, the incompetence is reversible. By approximately the sixth month, the valves are completely destroyed and thus permanently incompetent.[7] Thus, the presence of thrombus may not be the primary factor responsible for the development of valvular incompetence. These studies suggest that long-term permanent destruction may be related to the development of venous hypertension.[2] Investigators have attempted to document the chronologic changes of venous physiology following major thromboses. Akesson and coworkers[20] studied 20 patients for over 5 years after an acute iliofemoral thrombosis treated with conventional anticoagulation. Radionuclide angiography showed that 70% of the patients had obstructive lesions of the iliac vein, with only minor changes occurring from 6 months to 5 years. Despite this, plethysmographic evaluation demonstrated that the venous outflow improved over time. Venous reflux, however, worsened with time. The authors concluded that although venous outflow continuously improves following iliofemoral thromboses, valvular competence and muscle pump function continuously deteriorate.[20]

Obstruction to outflow, although not the primary cause of the postphlebitic syndrome, may be more common than has been realized, and may in fact be present in as many as one third of patients with severe symptoms.[3,14] It seems that collaterals may be sufficient sometimes to meet resting but not ambulatory flow.[2,14] Duplex abnormalities consistent with previous DVT often suggest the coexistence of reflux and chronic obstruction.[11] Venous obstruction, particularly of the proximal veins, is more often implicated in the cause of the uncommon symptom of venous claudication, defined as pain in the limb while walking. This symptom is due to venous hypertension resulting from occlusion of the proximal veins.[5]

Increasing severity of the postphlebitic syndrome seems to be related to the site and extent of the DVT.[5,11,21] Residual venous abnormalities in the popliteal and tibial veins are associated with an increased likelihood of developing the postphlebitic syndrome.[13,21] Isolated disease of the superficial system is most frequently responsible for the development of CVI, occurring in 18% to 30% of patients. Isolated perforator vein incompetence is uncommon, occurring in less than 5% of individuals. The majority of individuals with severe CVI will have combined abnormalities involving all three venous systems.[11] In another study correlating the incidence of symptoms to the site of disease, swelling was increased by distal or a combination of proximal and distal reflux regardless of which system was involved. Absence of superficial reflux was associated with a low incidence of ulceration even in the presence of deep venous insufficiency.[5]

It has been suggested that vena caval filters have an association with the postphlebitic syndrome by virtue of the associated incidence of inferior vena caval thrombosis. In a recent comprehensive review of all the literature related to venal filters, however, the incidence of postphlebitic syndrome following vena caval interruption varied from 14% to 41% depending on the type of filter used,[22] whereas the incidence of postphlebitic syndrome following DVT is recognized to be as high as 80%.[7,8] Further study would be required, therefore, before we can say that vena caval filters are associated with an increased incidence of postphlebitic syndrome. The relatively low incidence of postphlebitic syndrome associated with the filters is likely to be a reflection of relatively short follow-up.

At the microscopic level, cutaneous blood flow regulation is disturbed in severe CVI. The feedback system between the transmural pressure in the postcapillary venules and the precapillary resistance regulating arterioles is altered. Postural feedback remains disturbed and upregulated even after a venous ulcer has healed.[23] Skin biopsies from patients affected by CVI show marked structural derangements. These include collapsed, thickened, and reduplicated basement membranes of the blood vessels, numerous and complex interdigitations between contiguous endothelial cells, and a lack of open junctions, as well as extensive fibrosis in the connective tissue matrix. As a consequence, the capacity for fluid exchange is reduced in CVI.[24]

There are four major areas of basic science investigation into the development of lipodermatosclerosis (defined as thickening and induration of the skin) and ulceration associated with the postphlebitic syndrome. These areas of investigation include the role of cellular apoptosis, the regulation of tissue fibrosis by transforming growth factor (TGF)-β, leukocyte activation in the microcirculation of the skin, and the role of matrix metalloproteinases in tissue remodeling.

Mendez and coworkers[25] have shown that wound fibroblasts grown from biopsies of venous ulcers show an abnormally high rate of apoptosis as compared to fibroblasts from normal tissue. They also found that growth rates of wound fibroblasts were significantly lower in all patients than those of normal fibroblasts.

Pappas and coworkers[26] have shown increased levels of TGF-β in dermal biopsies of patients with advanced CVI as compared to normal tissue biopsies. In a recent study they demonstrated that pathologic dermal degeneration in patients with CVI seems to be associated with increased production of TGF-β in patients with skin induration, hyperpigmentation, and lipodermatosclerosis. In addition, they found significantly increased production of TGF-β in the skin of the patients with lipodermatosclerosis and active ulcers as compared to healthy skin. Finally, they were also able to show significantly increased production of TGF-β in lower-calf skin biopsies as compared to lower-thigh skin biopsies of the same patient.

Saharay and coworkers have shown that venous hypertension results in sequestration of activated neutrophils and monocytes in the microcirculation of the leg in patients with venous disease. They postulate that these cells bind to the endothelium and release L-selectin.[27] In a recent study Shoab and coworkers reported the efficacy of treating patients with CVI with oral micronized flavonoid fraction. In this study they demonstrated decreased surface expression of L-selectin by neutrophils and monocytes as well as reduction of endothelial activity of ICAM-1 and VCAM with the administration of oral flavonoid 500 mg twice daily for 60 days.[28] The clinical significance of their findings is yet to be determined.[29]

The increased proteolytic activity by proteases, particularly matrix metalloproteinases (MMPs), is a key feature in venous leg ulcer formation. It is believed that the proteolytic effect of MMPs initiates an elevated turnover of the extracellular matrix, with breakdown of the matrix resulting in venous ulceration.[30,31] Further research will be necessary before we understand the role of MMPs in venous stasis ulcer formation.

SYMPTOMS

Clinical features of the postphlebitic syndrome include pain, edema, pigment deposition resulting in hyperpigmentation, and ultimately ulceration.[5,15,32] In one fifth of the patients, however, there is no evidence of antecedent deep venous occlusion.[33] Typically there is unilateral lower leg swelling. In milder cases, the complaints are those of pain and edema. The early edema that follows a DVT is secondary to residual obstruction, while the late edema that forms part of the postphlebitic syndrome is secondary to valvular insufficiency.[2] The pain is more often described as an ache, throb, or heaviness, which worsens with prolonged standing and as the day progresses. Earlier in the course, the edema is pitting and may resolve with appropriate compression. It also worsens with prolonged standing and as the day progresses. As the disease progresses, the skin becomes chronically thickened and permanently indurated (lipodermatosclerosis) (Fig. 16–1), and is associated with subdermal scarring.[11] It is not uncommon to see evidence of previously healed ulcers. The areas of hyperpigmentation are usually located in the anteromedial lower leg and appear as clusters of multiple brownish spots. Over time, these may coalesce and appear as a single large area of hyperpigmentation involving the entire anteromedial mid to distal leg, or gaiter zone. Ulceration, when present, is classically in the medial aspect of the mid to distal leg. These ulcers are usually painless. Any significant pain or tenderness should raise the suspicion of infection. Ulcers are often moist and covered by exudate.

The CEAP (Clinical, Etiologic, Anatomic, and Pathophysiologic) classification is used to categorize the severity of CVI.[34] CEAP is therefore a clinical classification. A numeric value can be assigned to each of the four categories; in practice, the clinical, or "C," category is most frequently used. The higher the number, the worse is the process. A "C" value of 0 indicates no identified venous disease. C2 indicates the presence of varicose veins; C3 indicates edema; C4 indicates the presence of skin changes including brawny edema, venous eczema, thickening, pigmentation, and lipodermatosclerosis; C5 indicates a history of a previously healed ulcer; and C6 indicates the presence of an active ulceration[10,11] (Table 16–1). This classification is useful in providing a guide

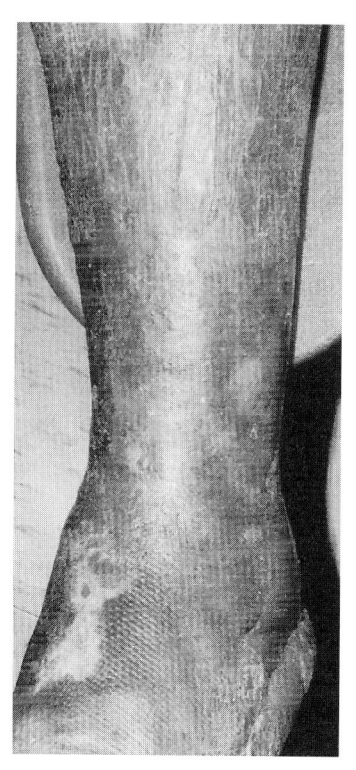

Figure 16–1 Postphlebitic syndrome. Notice areas of hyperpigmentation and healed and healing ulcers.

of how likely it is that a more complex form of therapy will be required in a particular patient. It will also facilitate interinstitutional studies.[34]

DIFFERENTIAL DIAGNOSIS

In considering the diagnosis of postphlebitic syndrome, as in any other condition, a differential diagnosis should be entertained. The conditions to be considered will vary depending on the stage and severity of the disease. In patients who have leg edema only, conditions causing peripheral edema should be considered. Most prominent in the differential are lymphedema (primary or secondary, or hereditary in cases of Milroy disease), congestive heart failure, cirrhosis, nephrotic syndrome and other conditions associated with hypoproteinemia, as well as possible hypo- and hyperthyroidism.

When the patient has an ulcer, the differential diagnosis includes arterial insufficiency, vasculitis, hypertensive (or Martorell) ulcer, pyoderma gangrenosum, squamous cell carcinoma, calciphylaxis, and other less common conditions.

A history of DVT and the presence of findings associated with venous insufficiency, such as hyperpigmentation and lipodermatosclerosis, assist in the diagnosis. Venous stasis ulcers are more often located in the medial malleolar area and, unless infected, are not painful. Most often, the correct diagnosis can be established based on the history and the physical examination alone.

Table 16-1 • CLINICAL, ETIOLOGICAL, ANATOMICAL, AND PATHOPHYSIOLOGICAL (CEAP) CLASSIFICATION OF VENOUS INSUFFICIENCY

CEAP Classification

Class	Clinical Characteristics	Clinical Significance
C0	No identified venous disease	Minimally symptomatic disease; not generally considered candidates for perforating vein surgery, although superficial venous ablation is appropriate for C2 or greater
C1	Telangiectasia	
C2	Varicose veins	
C3	Edema	
C4	Skin changes: brawny edema, venous eczema, thickening, pigmentation, and lipodermatosclerosis	C4–6 are considered candidates for perforating vein surgery
C5	Previously healed ulcer	
C6	Active ulceration	

RISK FACTORS

Multiple risk factors have been identified for the development of the postphlebitic syndrome. The triad of trauma to the venous wall, venous stasis, and hypercoagulability are the most common risk factors. Generally, we associate the development of postphlebitic syndrome with the previous occurrence of DVT, which is true in about 80% of patients.[33] The remaining 20% of patients, with no antecedent history of DVT, suffer from primary venous insufficiency, or equally possibly have had a DVT that was not appreciated by the patient. Some reports suggest that this number may be even higher. In a study in which ascending venography was performed on 51 limbs with postphlebitic syndrome, 32 had no radiologic evidence of recent or old thrombophlebitis. Instead, they had normal-appearing veins, suggesting primary incompetence of the deep and/or perforating venous valves rather than thrombophlebitis as the cause.[35] Older age, male sex, and obesity are also strongly associated with the development of CVI.[36] Somewhat less common associations are malignancy, superficial varicosities, family history of DVT, recent travel involving sitting for longer than 6 hours, cardiac failure, and pregnancy.[2] Some patients also essentially exist in a sitting position, eating, watching television, and even sleeping sitting in a chair or recliner with their legs dependent all night. This activity can and should be avoided.

Deficiencies of the fibrinolytic system have also been well documented in patients with the postphlebitic syndrome.[7] Patients with inherited or acquired hypercoagulable states are also at risk for postphlebitic syndrome.[37] For example, the prevalence of antithrombin III- (AT-III) deficient patients among those with the postphlebitic syndrome is reported at between 2% and 3%. Conversely, postphlebitic syndrome may be an initial presentation of antithrombin deficiency.[38] Diagnosis and treatment of the disorder with chronic warfarin therapy is indicated in order to reduce the incidence of recurrent venous thrombosis and the risk of pulmonary embolism.[39] Patients with DVT also may have lower levels of tissue plasminogen activator (tPA) or higher levels of plasminogen activator inhibitor (PAI-1).[2]

Other miscellaneous causes of lower extremity DVT include compression of the iliac vein, described by May and Thurner[40] and now known as May-Thurner syndrome. In these patients, the left common iliac vein is compressed against the vertebral column by the overlying right common iliac artery. This results in constant pulsation, which causes reactive changes in the vein and luminal narrowing with subsequent stasis and DVT.[41]

DIAGNOSIS

The postphlebitic syndrome is mostly a clinical diagnosis that is based on the typical signs and symptoms of pain, edema, hyperpigmentation and induration of the skin, and ulceration. More specific information is sometimes necessary in order to differentiate the syndrome from DVT or when surgical intervention is being considered. As many as two thirds of the patients who present with new symptoms after documented DVT actually have postphlebitic syndrome, which can often mimic or coexist with acute DVT. A skin biopsy, however, is neither necessary nor indicated in order to make the diagnosis of postphlebitic syndrome.

Duplex Scanning

When duplex scanning is used to diagnose a DVT, venous obstruction is indicated by the absence of spontaneous, augmentable, and phasic flow by pulsed-wave Doppler. Additional observations include the presence of thrombus visualized by B-mode ultrasonography and incompressibility of the vein in transverse section with probe pressure.[42] Absence of flow is considered the best method to determine total occlusion of a venous segment.[2,3,43] When assisting in the diagnosis of postphlebitic syndrome, duplex scanning can be used to diagnose chronic venous changes, indicated by the presence of incompetent valves and reflux, or to differentiate old from fresh clot based on the sonographic appearance of the thrombus.[42] Color flow duplex scanning is also the diagnostic test of choice to evaluate patients for the presence of reflux in the superficial, deep, and perforator systems. Competency of the saphenofemoral and saphenopopliteal junctions, the common femoral vein, and the origins of the deep and superficial femoral veins should be documented. Reflux should be evaluated with the patient in the standing position. Reflux of the lower leg is elicited either by manual compression of the calf with sudden release or by the use of a rapid cuff deflator.[19]

Incompetency of the tibioperoneal veins is best evaluated with the patient sitting with the foot resting supported off the floor. Duplex criteria for reflux in the deep system consist of retrograde flow persisting for longer than 0.5 seconds. Visualization of a venous lumen directly connecting a superficial and a deep vein is diagnostic of perforator vein incompetence.[2,5,11,32] Most surgically significant incompetent perforating veins are located on the medial calf. Medial calf perforating veins generally link the posterior tibial vein with tributaries of the saphenous system, most commonly the posterior arch vein. The two clusters corresponding to Cockett's II and III are the most commonly involved and are located between 7 and 9 cm and 10 and 12 cm proximal to the inferior border of the medial malleolus.

Air Plethysmography

Air plethysmography (APG) is a noninvasive test that provides reproducible information about the degree of venous outflow obstruction, and reflux and the efficiency of the calf pump.[44,45] An air-filled plastic bladder placed around the proximal calf is used to measure changes in the volume of the leg. These changes and the rates of these changes following certain maneuvers designed to fill or empty the venous system reflect the degree of venous obstruction. These maneuvers are done when the patient is supine, upright, or exercising. A series of measurements is obtained during the APG to assess the patient (Table 16–2). Immediately following a DVT, the venous outflow fraction (OF) is reduced because of obstruction. However, as recanalization and collateralization progress, OF gradually returns to normal and can become completely normal in a patient with evident postphlebitic syndrome. As the degree of reflux worsens, an increase in the venous filling index and residual volume fraction (RVF) is observed. These are characteristic of valvular incompetence.[5,11]

Venography

Venography may be used to demonstrate the level of reflux as well as the degree of venous obstruction. In ascending venography, a vein of the foot is cannulated and contrast administered in an antegrade fashion. As the contrast fills the veins from below, the venous anatomy and any obstruction to venous outflow will be evident (Fig. 16–2). Ascending venography may, however, fail to demonstrate the most proximal anatomy. Ascending venography may also be used to demonstrate perforator incompetence. With the use of tourniquets placed to obstruct the greater saphenous vein, contrast injected into a dorsal foot vein should demonstrate only the deep system. If perforator vein flow from deep to superficial system is demonstrated, those perforator veins are incompetent.

In descending venography, a more proximal vein is accessed, such as the contralateral common femoral vein, and contrast is injected in a retrograde fashion into the desired system. As the contrast fills and distends the veins from above, the venous valves and their ability or inability to prevent reflux will become evident. Descending venography cannot demonstrate distal disease in the presence of a competent proximal femoral valve because the valve will prevent the contrast from filling the most distal vein.[3]

Ambulatory Venous Pressure

An elevated AVP is the hallmark of chronic venous insufficiency and the postphlebitic syndrome. To measure the AVP, a catheter is inserted into a vein in the dorsum of the foot of the affected extremity and the venous pressure is transduced while the patient is ambulating on a treadmill. This is cumbersome and invasive and for these reasons not frequently done. Investigations have demonstrated that the RVF measurement during APG correlates directly with increased AVP.[46] However, since various operations have recently been

Table 16–2 • MEASUREMENTS USED TO ASSESS SEVERITY OF VENOUS OBSTRUCTION AND INSUFFICIENCY

Air Plethysmography (APG)

Ejection fraction	EF	Fraction of the blood volume expelled by the calf pump after a single tiptoe maneuver	Evaluates the calf pump function
Maximal venous volume	MVV	Maximum volume reached by the extremity, compared to baseline, when dependent and not weight bearing	Evaluates obstruction
Residual volume fraction	RVF	Fraction of the blood volume remaining after 10 tiptoe maneuvers, which are designed to completely empty the extremity	Evaluates the calf pump function
Venous filling index	VFI	Rate of filling of the venous system when going from a supine with the leg elevated to an upright position	Evaluates reflux
Venous outflow	VO	Volume of blood passively expelled from the elevated extremity by the action of gravity	Evaluates obstruction

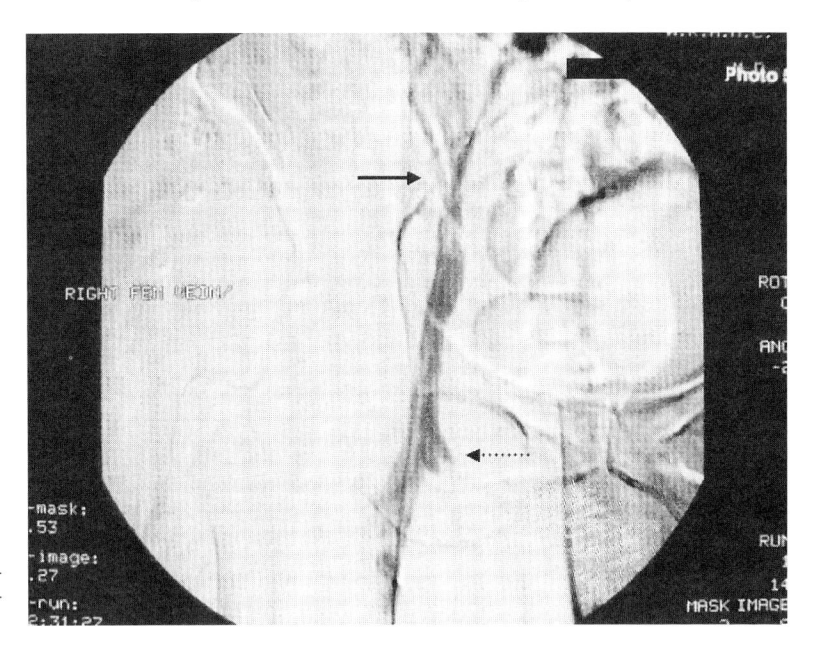

Figure 16–2 Ascending venography. Solid arrow demonstrates obstruction. Dashed arrow demonstrates valvular anatomy.

proposed to correct or bypass malfunctioning valves, precise demonstration of pathologic change is required to choose the appropriate procedure and to evaluate results.[35] Other tests, such as magnetic resonance imaging and radionuclide scintigraphy, may be useful in selected patients.[47]

PREVENTION

Prevention of the postphlebitic syndrome centers on prevention of venous valvular damage and reduction of AVP. For the vast majority of patients, this means prevention of DVT, or once a DVT has occurred, minimizing the damage to the venous valves with aggressive, adequate therapy. Health care professionals are responsible not only for recognizing and treating thromboembolic disorders, but also for taking all possible necessary measures to prevent recurrences. Individuals who have developed a venous thromboembolism remain at an elevated risk of having a recurrence; this is about 3% to 6% during the first 3 months, and although lower from then on, it remains elevated for years. This possibility is higher in patients with permanent risk factors such as inherited abnormalities of hemostasis than in those with post-traumatic or postoperative venous thrombosis.[6,48] Hospitalized individuals are at increased risk for DVT due to immobility, trauma, and underlying conditions that promote a hypercoagulable state, and these patients should be evaluated for the need for a prophylactic regimen such as compression devices that prevent stasis of blood in the extremities and/or the use of anticoagulants. Once a DVT has occurred, prompt resolution is probably the best measure that could be taken to minimize long-term impact. Clinically suspected DVT should be confirmed by objective tests since many patients with a clinically suspected DVT are shown to be negative on further evaluation.[42]

Although anticoagulation is critical to stabilize the thrombus and to reduce the incidence of pulmonary embolism following a DVT, anticoagulants may not prevent the sequelae of postphlebitic syndrome.[49] Unfortunately, no validated method exists to predict its occurrence.[50] The failure of anticoagulants to prevent the postphlebitic syndrome probably stems from their failure to clear the thrombus.[50]

The long-term clinical implications regarding the development of postphlebitic syndrome after isolated calf DVT, which has been estimated to occur in 5% to 33% of all DVT patients, are not clear. If not treated with anticoagulation, at least 8% of patients will have propagation of the thrombus proximally. The incidence of postphlebitic syndrome in this population has been reported to vary between 3% and 37%. The incidence of ulceration, however, is extremely low.[51] Based on this information, it would seem prudent that if the provider chooses not to use anticoagulation in DVT localized to the calf, follow-up studies should be obtained to monitor for propagation, which, if it occurs, requires anticoagulation therapy. The use of compression stockings, although perhaps not as critical, given the low incidence of ulceration, is probably still advisable in order to reduce the incidence of some of the less severe sequelae of the postphlebitic syndrome.

The use of thrombolytic agents to treat acute DVT is believed to reduce the sequelae of postphlebitic syndrome by affecting valve preservation. Although this has not been proved definitively, several studies suggest that this is true. Because of the large differences in the reported incidence of late postphlebitic syndrome after DVT, it has been suggested, however, that a minimal reopening rate is required to be of clinical value to the individual patient.[50] Thrombolytic therapy is most effective when initiated within 7 days of the onset of DVT. Thrombolytic therapy, however, has a higher incidence of hemorrhagic complications, of about 5% to 15%, and until conclusive evidence demonstrates its benefits, it should probably be reserved for those patients with massive DVT or DVT associated with relevant clinical signs, most often in patients with iliofemoral thrombosis.[1,52] The rationale of venous valve preservation is more attractive in young, healthy patients (e.g., postpartum patients) than in patients with short survival (e.g., cancer patients). It should also be considered in patients who have failed to respond to standard therapy, and in patients with a renal allograft on the same side of the DVT, in whom extension to the renal vein could result in loss of the transplant. The use of an inferior vena caval filter to prevent embolization during the thrombolytic treatment is not necessary.[1] The use of catheter-directed thrombolysis may reduce the incidence of systemic complications and provides more complete lysis,[53] although its use ignores the fact that 30% to 40% of such patients also have a coexisting pulmonary embolus or undetected DVT elsewhere. Although a large portion of the literature on thrombolysis has been written based on urokinase, with its disappearance from the market, the more frequent choice has been tPA over streptokinase. It is very likely that as providers become more familiar with the use of tPA, they will feel as comfortable as they once did with the use of urokinase. Reports of the use of thrombolytic agents during pregnancy are sparse. The successful use of urokinase in pregnancy has been reported in at least three patients[54] and of tPA, in at least one patient.[55] Anticoagulation therapy, instead of thrombolysis, will probably continue to be the mainstay of therapy because of factors such as limited extent of thrombosis, absence of tissue loss, complications associated with thrombolysis, and unfortunately, delay in referral for treatment beyond the 7 days or so when thrombolysis is most effective.[56]

The use of venous thrombectomy is rarely indicated and not frequently used in modern medicine. It should only be considered in instances of DVT involving the iliofemoral venous segment and when the age of the clot is thought to be less than 72 hours.[57,58] It is particularly indicated in the patient with phlegmasia cerulea dolens (see Chapter 14), in which the inherent delay associated with thrombolytic therapy would be unacceptable and rapid results are necessary to save the limb and possibly the patient's life. Even if the vascular patency is restored in a good percentage of cases, it is not particularly effective in preventing the postphlebitic syndrome.[49] Thrombectomy for venous thrombosis below the inguinal ligament has not been beneficial consistently. In the setting of widespread metastatic disease, rethrombosis rates are too high to justify thrombectomy in some patients[57]; rather, aggressive anticoagulant therapy is indicated.

Following management of acute DVT, compression is probably the most important form of management to prevent the more debilitating form of CVI, which is ulceration. It has been suggested that early application of external compression in patients with acute DVT may prevent the sequelae of the postphlebitic syndrome. A randomized trial comparing the use of stockings versus no stockings following a first episode of DVT showed reduction of development of postphlebitic syndrome by 50% at 2 years in patients wearing the stockings when compared to those not wearing the stockings.[4] Patients who have no symptoms will often not wear the stockings even though they have been prescribed.[3] Although the precise mechanism is not known, it is thought they stimulate the development of collaterals, reduce transcapillary filtration, increase fibrinolytic activity, and reduce overdistension of the venous system.[4,7] It is recommended that the use of appropriately sized graded compression stockings be initiated within 2 to 3 weeks from the time of initial diagnosis and used for at least 2[4] and perhaps up to 5 years.[9]

TREATMENT

Medical Therapy

The mainstay of treatment of the postphlebitic syndrome is compression. Graded compression stockings are used to reduce ambulatory venous pressure mechanically. Stockings are typically available in three degrees of compression; moderate compression provides 15 to 20 mmHg, firm compression, 20 to 30 mmHg, and extrafirm compression, 30 to 40 mmHg. For the patient with minimal symptoms, moderate compression and even leg elevation at the end of the day are reasonable alternatives. For the patient with mild to moderate symptoms of heaviness, ache, and edema, firm compression is a reasonable starting point. Compression stockings should be used continuously in the patient who has suffered a previous ulcer formation in order to prevent a recurrence, and in the compliant patient most limbs are adequately controlled with graded compression stockings.[3] It is recommended for the patient to put the stocking on in the morning, before ambulating, and wear it all day. Stockings can be removed at night when the patient sleeps in the supine position and venous pressure is reduced to 0 mmHg. Due to loss of their elasticity, stockings should be replaced approximately every 6 months. For patients who have previously had an ulcer, conservative treatment has an initial treatment failure and recurrence rate that ranges from 54% to 69% at 1 to 3 years. In a study comparing compliance versus noncompliance with the use of stockings, the compliant group had a recurrence rate of 29%, but the noncompliant group had a 100% recurrence rate at 3 years. If the data were recalculated, the recurrence rate would be closer to 30% in the first year.[10] Patients with advanced CVI (CEAP 6) require daily care of their venous ulcer in addition to compression therapy. The ulcer should be cleaned properly with saline and a gentle detergent solution followed by adequate débridement. Various wound dressing alternatives are commercially available. The Unna boot is probably the best known. The dressing contains zinc oxide as the active ingredient, combined with a semirigid compression dressing. The goal is to apply the dressing using the model of graded compression, where the highest degree of compression is present at the foot, beginning just proximal to the toes, and the least compression is proximally, immediately below the knee. Following application, "boots" are kept in place for 3 to 7 days, depending on the amount of wound drainage and dressing soilage. A sponge dressing may be added to the Unna boot to absorb wound exudate.

Duoderm® is an example of this type of dressing. The use of a sponge dressing by itself does not improve the healing rate, but in combination with compression has been shown to result in faster healing rates than with the Unna boot.[59] A second type of nonelastic stocking is the CircAid® legging. It consists of multiple, pliable, yet unyielding, adjustable layers that are attached by the use of Velcro. This device is considered by some providers to be easier to apply than stockings.[60] This inelastic device has been shown to maintain limb size and reduced venous volume better than stockings.[61] A trial of sequential compression pump therapy is worthwhile for patients with severe postphlebitic syndrome. A sustained beneficial response can be expected in 80% of patients; this is slightly decreased to 75% with long-term continued use.[62] Pump therapy increases the transcutaneous pressure of oxygen; this is associated with a rise in the skin temperature and a decrease in the edema.[63]

Surgical Treatment

Various surgical alternatives have been developed over the years in an attempt to deal with the late sequelae of the postphlebitic syndrome. Some procedures attempt to eliminate venous hypertension in the superficial system by eliminating the diseased portions of the superficial system and by ligating incompetent perforating veins. Other procedures are aimed at reducing reflux and venous hypertension by restoring or reconstructing the valvular system. In any particular patient, surgery should be directed at the affected component, as identified by the proper preoperative studies.

Ligation and Stripping and Flush Ligation

Surgical treatment of the postphlebitic syndrome should be guided by preoperative venous testing.[64] In an effort to preserve the great saphenous vein for potential later use for coronary artery bypass graft or lower extremity bypass, surgical ablation of varicose veins should be selective and guided by preoperative color-flow duplex and/or APG or continuous wave doppler.

Subfascial Endoscopic Perforator Surgery

The first report from the NASEPS (North American Subfascial Endoscopic Perforator Surgery) registry emphasized the importance of superficial reflux in the causation of venous ulceration.[65] Perforator interruption, however, has remained a controversial issue.[10] The superficial system is managed by removal of the incompetent branches after these have been identified and marked. The perforator system recently has been the object of renewed interest with the advent of subfacial endoscopic perforator surgery (SEPS). Patients are not generally considered candidates for this type of procedure unless their CVI is rated CEAP 4 or higher. This procedure recreates in a minimally invasive fashion what previous procedures such as the Linton operation did, namely, ligature and interruption of the communication between the superficial and deep venous systems of the lower extremity, the perforating veins. The recurrence rate of ulceration following a Linton flap operation of the lower extremities is 14.5% at 6 months to 10 years follow-up.[66] However, the Linton operation was associated with a high wound complication rate and required an extensive incision in the leg. The success rate of the SEPS procedure is very similar to that of the Linton operation, with about 84% of the ulcers healed in one study at a median time of 54 days. The recurrence rate, in the same study, was 28% at 2 years. The wound complication rate, however, was 6%, which is lower than for the open procedures. A very high failure rate was noted in patients with residual venous occlusion. In four of nine patients, the ulcer failed to heal, and the other five had recurrence. A clear association has also been found to exist between missed or recurrent perforators and ulcer recurrence.[10]

Valve Reconstruction

Various operations have been designed with the purpose of recreating a normal valvular system. Options include valve transposition, reconstruction, and transplantation.[67-69] In valve transposition a normal segment of vein is swung into position to replace the diseased segment. In valve reconstruction the wall of the vein may be folded and sutured in place to recreate valve function. In valve transplantation a normal segment of vein from a distant position is removed and interposed in the area of disease.

Surgical repair of an incompetent femoral vein as an adjunct to conventional stripping of varices and subfascial interruption of perforating veins is associated with a 90% success rate.[70] However, isolated disease of the more proximal (iliofemoral) valves does not seem to correlate with disease severity yet distal incompetence, or combined distal and proximal incompetence, does appear to correlate with disease severity. Thus the value of proximal vein reconstruction is uncertain.[39] Furthermore, venous pressure measurements do not always return to normal after surgery.[68] The failure of the venous pressure to normalize in the presence of an otherwise successful operation may sometimes be explained by the presence of residual obstruction in association with reflux.[3]

Surgical Treatment for Obstruction

Surgical alternatives are available for the rare patient who presents with symptoms associated with the presence of clinically significant chronic venous obstruction. These procedures should be delayed for 6 months to allow for the likely development of adequate collateral circulation.[71] The principal goal of these alternatives is to bypass the obstructed area. Various options have been described, which include the use of either autologous or prosthetic material. Described configurations include saphenofemoral venous crossover,[71] femorofemoral crossover using expanded polytetrafluoroethylene (ePTFE),[72] crosspubic bypass, and saphenopopliteal bypass.[73] In addition, percutaneous angioplasty and stenting has been used for the treatment of May-Thurner syndrome.[74]

Pharmacologic Treatment

The role of pharmacology in the treatment of the postphlebitic syndrome has been very limited. Although several products have been suggested to provide benefit, none has been established as routine clinical practice. Pentoxifylline is reported to improve the healing rate of venous leg ulcers. The mechanism of action of pentoxifylline is believed to be a downregulating effect in leukocyte activation. This in turn reduces leukocyte-derived free radicals, proteolytic enzymes, cytokines, and a number of other noxious mediators.[75] Another product is venostat. An herbal medicine commercially available as Venastat®, it is marketed for the treatment of varicose veins and venous stasis among other conditions. As is the case with many herbal medicines, minimal or no scientific literature is available regarding its effectiveness.

CONSULTATION CONSIDERATIONS

Actions to attempt to prevent the postphlebitic syndrome should be the goal of every practioner who manages DVT. Prevention should begin with prescribing compression stockings, which can be done by physicians of any practionary speciality. In cases of iliofemoral thrombosis, preventive measures might involve thrombolysis, and consultation with a vascular surgeon should be considered.

Patients with evidence of established postphlebitic syndrome with active ulcers, new or recurrent, who continue to show evidence of progression despite compression therapy or who have associated varicose veins should be evaluated by a vascular surgeon.

Surgeons and hematologists can work best together if they communicate with each other in their particular institution and obtain an understanding of each others' practices in the management of the postphlebitic syndrome.

CONCLUSION

The postphlebitic syndrome is a dermatologic destruction of the microscopic lymphatics resulting from persistent lower-extremity venous hypertension. It is usually caused by valvular destruction following DVT. The mainstay of therapy is prevention through DVT prevention. Early venous thrombolysis decreases the incidence. The goal of treating the postphlebitic syndrome is reduction of venous hypertension associated with ambulation. Reduction in venous hypertension helps to prevent advanced CVI with ulceration (CEAP 6). The majority of patients with CVI may be treated with skin emolients and compression stockings. Surgical therapy of the postphlebitic syndrome is aimed at eliminating venous reflux through ligation or stripping of varicose veins, or valve reconstruction.

Unfortunately, reduction in ambulatory venous hypertension does not restore skin affected by lipodermatosclerosis to its healthy state. Patients require lifelong compression therapy and skin care. Ultimately the understanding and prevention of the postphlebitic syndrome awaits further investigation into its cause.

■ REFERENCES

Chapter 16 References

1. Silverstein MD, Heit JA, Mohr DN, et al. Trends in the incidence of deep venous thrombosis and pulmonary embolism. A 25-year population-based study. Arch Intern Med 1998;158:585–593.
2. Killewich LA, Bedford GR, Beach KW, et al. Spontaneous lysis of deep venous thrombi: rate and outcome. J Vasc Surg 1989;9:89–97.
3. Johnson BF, Manzo RA, Bergelin RO, et al. Relationship between changes in the deep venous system and the development of the postthrombotic syndrome after an acute episode of lower limb deep vein thrombosis: a one to six year follow-up. J Vasc Surg 1995;21:307–313.
4. Brandjes DPM, Buller HR, Heijboer H, et al. Randomised trial of effect of compression stockings in patients with symptomatic proximal-vein thrombosis. Lancet 1997;349:759–762.
5. Labropoulos N, Leon M, Nicolaides AN, et al. Venous reflux in patients with previous deep venous thrombosis: correlation with ulceration and other symptoms. J Vasc Surg 1994;20:20–26.
6. Leizorovicz A. Long-term consequences of deep vein thrombosis. Haemostasis 1998;28:Suppl 3:1–7.
7. Meissner MH, Manzo RA, Bergelin RO, et al. Deep venous insufficiency: the relationship between lysis and subsequent reflux. J Vasc Surg 1993;18:596–608.
8. Lindner DJ, Edwards JM, Phinney ES, et al. Long-term hemodynamic and clinical sequelae of lower extremity deep vein thrombosis. J Vasc Surg 1986;4:436–42.
9. Franzeck UK, Schalch I, Bollinger A. On the relationship between changes in the deep veins evaluated by duplex sonography and the postthrombotic syndrome 12 years after deep vein thrombosis. Thromb Haemost 1997;77:1109–1112.
10. Gloviczki P, Bergan JJ, Rhodes JM, et al. Mid-term results of endoscopic perforator vein interruption for chronic venous insufficiency: lessons learned from the North American Subfascial Endoscopic Perforator Surgery registry. J Vasc Surg 1999;29: 489–502.
11. Padberg FT. Endoscopic subfascial perforating vein ligation: its complementary role in the surgical management of chronic venous insufficiency. Ann Vasc Surg 1999;13:343–354.
12. Masuda EM, Kistner RL. Long-term results of venous valve reconstruction: a four- to twenty-one-year follow-up. J Vasc Surg 1994;19:391–403.
13. Johnson BF, Manzo RA, Bergelin RO, et al. The site of residual abnormalities in the leg veins in long-term follow-up after deep vein thrombosis and their relationship to the development of the post-thrombotic syndrome. Int Angiol 1996;15:14–19.

14. Illig KA, Ouriel K, DeWeese JA, et al. Increasing the sensitivity of the diagnosis of chronic venous obstruction. J Vasc Surg 1996;24:176–178.
15. Cardon JM, Cardon A, Joyeux A, et al. Use of ipsilateral greater saphenous vein as a valved transplant in management of post-thrombotic deep venous insufficiency: long-term results. Ann Vasc Surg 1999;13:284–289.
16. Milne AA, Stonebridge PA, Bradbury AW, et al. Venous function and clinical outcome following deep vein thrombosis. Br J Surg 1994;81:847–849.
17. Perrin M, Hiltbrand B, Bayon JM. Results of valvuloplasty in patients presenting with deep venous insufficiency and recurring ulceration. Ann Vasc Surg 1999;13:524–532.
18. Plagnol P, Ciostek P, Grimaud JP, et al. Autogenous valve reconstruction technique for post-thrombotic reflux. Ann Vasc Surg 1999;13:339–342.
19. van Bemmelen PS, Bedford G, Beach K, et al. Quantitative segmental evaluation of venous valvular reflux with duplex ultrasound scanning. J Vasc Surg 1989;10:425–31.
20. Akesson H, Brudin L, Dahlstrom JA, et al. Venous function assessed during a 5 year period after acute ilio-femoral venous thrombosis treated with anticoagulation. Eur J Vasc Surg 1990;4:43–48.
21. Monreal M, Martorell A, Callejas JM, et al. Venographic assessment of deep vein thrombosis and risk of developing post-thrombotic syndrome: a prospective study. J Intern Med 1993;233:233–238.
22. Streiff MB. Vena caval filters: a comprehensive review. Blood 2000;95:3669–3677.
23. Junger M, Hahn M, Klyscz T, et al. Influence of healing on the disturbed blood flow regulation in venous ulcers. Vasa 1996;25:341–348.
24. Scelsi R, Scelsi L, Cortinovis R, et al. Morphological changes of dermal blood and lymphatic vessels in chronic venous insufficiency of the leg. Int Angiol 1994;13:308–311.
25. Mendez MV, Stanley A, Park HY, et al. Fibroblasts cultured from venous ulcers display cellular characteristics of senescence. J Vasc Surg 1998;28:876–883.
26. Pappas PJ, You R, Rameshwar P, et al. Dermal tissue fibrosis in patients with chronic venous insufficiency is associated with increased transforming growth factor-beta1 gene expression and protein production. J Vasc Surg 1999;30:1129–1145.
27. Saharay M, Shields DA, Porter JB, et al. Leukocyte activity in the microcirculation of the leg in patients with chronic venous disease. J Vasc Surg 1997;26:265–273.
28. Shoab SS, Porter J, Scurr JH, et al. Endothelial activation response to oral micronised flavonoid therapy in patients with chronic venous disease—a prospective study. Eur J Vasc Endovasc Surg 1999;17:313–318.
29. Shoab SS, Porter JB, Scurr JH, et al. Effect of oral micronized purified flavonoid fraction treatment on leukocyte adhesion molecule expression in patients with chronic venous disease: a pilot study. J Vasc Surg 2000;31:456–61.
30. Herouy Y, Nockowski P, Schopf E, et al. Lipodermatosclerosis and the significance of proteolytic remodeling in the pathogenesis of venous ulceration. Int J Mol Med 1999;3:511–515.
31. Herouy Y, May AE, Pornschlegel G, et al. Lipodermatosclerosis is characterized by elevated expression and activation of matrix metalloproteinases: implications for venous ulcer formation. J Invest Dermatol 1998;111:822–827.
32. Halliday P. Development of the postthrombotic syndrome: its management at different stages. World J Surg 1990;14:703–710.
33. Jacobs P. Pathogenesis of the postphlebitic syndrome. Annu Rev Med 1983;34:91–105.
34. Kistner RL, Eklof B, Matsuda EM. Diagnosis of chronic venous disease of the lower extremities: the "CEAP" classification. Mayo Clin Proc 1996;71:338–345.
35. Train JS, Schanzer H, Peirce ED, et al. Radiological evaluation of the chronic venous stasis syndrome. JAMA 1987;258:941–944.
36. Scott TE, LaMorte WW, Gorin DR, et al. Risk factors for chronic venous insufficiency: a dual case-control study. J Vasc Surg 1995;22:622–628.
37. Gillespie DL, Carrington L, Griffen J, et al. Resistance to activated protein C: A common, inherited cause of venous thrombosis. Ann Vasc Surg 1996;10:174–177.
38. Jackson MR, Olsen SB, Gomez ER, et al. Use of antithrombin III concentrates to correct antithrombin III deficiency during vascular surgery. J Vasc Surg 1995;22:804–807.
39. Phifer TJ, Mills GM. Occult antithrombin III deficiency: a potentially lethal complication of the postphlebitic limb. J Vasc Surg 1990;11:586–590.
40. Thurner J, May R. [Problems of phlebopathology with special reference to phlebosclerosis]. Zentralbl Phlebol 1967;6:404–482.
41. Blattler W, Blattler IK. Relief of obstructive pelvic venous symptoms with endoluminal stenting. J Vasc Surg 1999;29:484–488.
42. Salcuni M, Fiorentino P, Pedicelli A, et al. Diagnostic imaging in deep vein thrombosis of the limbs. Rays 1996;21:328–339.
43. Barloon TJ, Bergus GR, Seabold JE. Diagnostic imaging of lower limb deep venous thrombosis. Am Fam Phys 1997;56:791–801.
44. Christopoulos DG, Nicolaides AN, Szendro G, et al. Air-plethysmography and the effect of elastic compression on venous hemodynamics of the leg. J Vasc Surg 1987;5:148–159.
45. Gillespie DL, Cordts P, Hartono C, et al. The role of air plethysmography in monitoring the results of venous surgery. J Vasc Surg 1992;16:647–678.
46. Christopoulos D, Nicolaides AN, Cook A, et al. Pathogenesis of venous ulceration in relation to the calf muscle pump function. Surgery 1989;106:829–835.
47. Cronnan JJ. Venous thromboembolic disease: the role of US. Radiology 1993;186:619–630.
48. Prandoni P, Lensing AW, Prins MR. Long-term outcomes after deep venous thrombosis of the lower extremities. Vasc Med 1998;3:57–60.
49. Halstuk K, Mahler D, Baker WH. Late sequelae of deep venous thrombosis. Diagnostic and therapeutic considerations. Am J Surg 1984;147:216–220.
50. Breddin HK. Treatment of deep vein thrombosis: is thrombosis regression a desirable endpoint? Semin Thromb Hemost 1997;23:179–183.
51. Masuda EM, Kessler DM, Kistner RL, et al. The natural history of calf vein thrombosis: lysis of thrombi and development of reflux. J Vasc Surg 1998;28:67–74.
52. Cina G, Marra R, Cotroneo AR, et al. Treatment of deep vein thrombosis. Rays 1996;21:397–416.
53. Semba CP, Dake MD. Catheter-directed thrombolysis for iliofemoral venous thrombosis. Semin Vasc Surg 1996;9:26–33.
54. Krishnamurthy P, Martin CB, Kay HH, et al. Catheter-directed thrombolysis for thromboembolic disease during pregnancy: a viable option. J Matern Fetal Med 1999;8:24–27.
55. Fleyfel M, Bourzoufi K, Huin G, et al. Recombinant tissue type plasminogen activator treatment of thrombosed mitral valve prosthesis during pregnancy. Can J Anaesth 1997;44:735–738.
56. Rutherford RB. Pathogenesis and pathophysiology of the postthrombotic syndrome: clinical implications. Semin Vasc Surg 1996;9:21–25.
57. Solis MM, Ranval TJ, Thompson BW, et al. Results of venous thrombectomy in the treatment of deep vein thrombosis. Surg Gynecol Obstet 1993;177:633–639.
58. Ganger KH, Nachbur BH, Ris HB, et al. Surgical thrombectomy versus conservative treatment for deep venous thrombosis; functional comparison of long-term results. Eur J Vasc Surg 1989;3:438–439.
59. Cordts PR, Hanrahan LM, Rodriguez AA, et al. A prospective, randomized trial of Unna's boot versus Duoderm CGF hydroac-

tive dressing plus compression in the management of venous leg ulcers. J Vasc Surg 1992;15:480–486.
60. Vernick SH, Shapiro D, Shaw FD. Legging orthosis for venous and lymphatic insufficiency. Arch Phys Med Rehabil 1987;68:459–461.
61. Bergan JJ, Sparks SR. Non-elastic compression: an alternative in management of chronic venous insufficiency. J Wound Ostomy Continence Nurs 2000;27:83–89.
62. Ginsberg JS, Magier D, Mackinnon B, et al. Intermittent compression units for severe post-phlebitic syndrome: a randomized crossover study. CMAJ 1999;160:1303–1306.
63. Kolari PJ, Pekanmaki K, Pohjola RT. Transcutaneous oxygen tension in patients with post-thrombotic leg ulcers: treatment with intermittent pneumatic compression. Cardiovasc Res 1988;22:138–141.
64. Villavicencio JL, Gillespie DL, Pikoulis E, et al. Superficial varicose veins. In: Raju S, Villavicencio JL (eds.): Therapeutic Options in Venous Surgery. Baltimore, Williams & Wilkins, 1997, pp. 373–390.
65. Gloviczki P, Bergan JJ, Menawat SS, et al. Safety, feasibility, and early efficacy of subfascial endoscopic perforator surgery: a preliminary report from the North American registry. J Vasc Surg 1997;25:94–105.
66. Szostek M, Skorski M, Zajac S, et al. Recurrences after surgical treatment of patients with post-thrombotic syndrome of the lower extremities. Eur J Vasc Surg 1988;2:191–192.
67. Nash T. Long-term results of vein valve transplants placed in the popliteal vein for intractable post-phlebitic venous ulcers and pre-ulcer skin changes. J Cardiovasc Surg 1988;29:712–716.
68. Taheri SA, Lazar L, Elias S, et al. Surgical treatment of postphlebitic syndrome with vein valve transplant. Am J Surg 1982;144:221–224.
69. Goff JM, Gillespie DL, Rich NM. Long-term follow-up of a superficial femoral vein injury: A case report from the Vietnam Vascular Registry. J Trauma 1997;44:209–211.
70. Kistner RL. Surgical repair of the incompetent femoral vein valve. Arch Surg 1975;110:1336–1342.
71. Haas GE. Saphenofemoral veins crossover bypass grafting in iliofemoral vein obstruction. J Am Osteopath Assoc 1989;89:511–518.
72. Yamamoto N, Takaba T, Hori G, et al. Reconstruction with insertion of expanded polytetrafluoroethylene (EPTFE) for iliac obstruction. J Cardiovasc Surg 1986;27:697–702.
73. Bergan JJ, Yao JS, Flinn WR, et al. Surgical treatment of venous obstruction and insufficiency. J Vasc Surg 1986;3:174–181.
74. Telian SH, Tretter JF, Watabe JT, et al. May Thurner syndrome: report of five cases treated with catheter-directed thrombolysis and stent placement. Curr Surg 1999;56:428–436.
75. Dormandy JA. Pharmacologic treatment of venous leg ulcers. J Cardiovasc Pharmacol 1995;25 Suppl 2:S61–S65.

CHAPTER 17

Thrombocytosis

Prabhas Mittal, M.D.
Craig M. Kessler, M.D.

INTRODUCTION AND EPIDEMIOLOGY

Thrombocytosis is defined as a platelet count above 400,000/μL, which is the upper limit of the normal reference range. Thrombocytosis can be categorized as a primary or secondary process, a critical differentiation since the management is altogether different for each entity.[1]

Secondary or reactive thrombocytosis is due to increased megakaryocyte production of platelets mediated by a physiologically normal megakaryocyte response to elevated circulating levels of cytokines. Megakaryocyte development is stimulated by various cytokines, including interleukin (IL) 1, IL-3, IL-6, IL-11, granulocyte colony-stimulating factor, granulocyte-macrophage colony-stimulating factor, and stem cell factor. Elevated levels of IL-1, IL-6, IL-4, and C-reactive protein are found in patients with reactive thrombocytosis whereas normal levels are observed in individuals with primary thrombocytopenia.[2–4] Secondary thrombocytosis is a common epiphenomenon of inflammatory (such as rheumatoid arthritis and inflammatory bowel disease) and neoplastic disease states, iron deficiency, and acute blood loss (Table 17–1). Secondary thrombocytosis is much more commonly encountered in clinical practice than is the primary process.[5] It is typically asymptomatic and is not associated with the thrombohemorrhagic complications seen in essential or primary thrombocytosis. The management of secondary thrombocytosis basically involves the treatment of the underlying condition responsible for the elevated platelet count.

Primary thrombocytosis is either idiopathic (also called *essential thrombocytosis, thrombocythemia,* or *primary thrombocythemia*) or associated with chronic myeloproliferative disorders (*myeloproliferative thrombocythemia*), such as polycythemia vera, chronic myeloid leukemia, and agnogenic myeloid metaplasia/myelofibrosis. Essential thrombocythemia (ET) is considered a distinct entity by itself and its diagnosis is based on the exclusion of other reactive causes of elevated platelet counts. Myeloproliferative thrombocythemia and essential thrombocythemia are characterized by the autonomous proliferation of platelets by megakaryocytes residing in an abnormal marrow microenvironment and/or perhaps by megakaryocytes that are intrinsically hypersensitive to thrombopoietin stimulation.[6] Essential thrombocythemia was first described in 1934 by Epstein and Goedel in a patient with history of repeated hemorrhagic events.[7,8] Although ET is the most common of the myeloproliferative disorders, it is a relatively uncommon disease state with an undetermined true incidence. The Olmstead County study estimated the annual incidence of ET to be approximately 2.38 patients/100,000 population[9]; however, the increasing use of automated blood counters has led to the detection of a significant number of incidental, asymptomatic cases of ET. This is reflected in the rising annual incidence of ET diagnosed in Denmark, which was 0.31/100,000 population in 1977 and increased to 1.00/100,000 by 1998.[10]

PATHOGENESIS OF ESSENTIAL THROMBOCYTHEMIA

ET was initially recognized as a disease arising from clonal platelet expansion by pluripotent stem cells in 1981. Utilizing X-chromosome-linked gene probes, such as for glucose-6-phosphate dehydrogenase, phosphoglycerate kinase, hypoxanthine phosphoribosyl transferase, and later the human androgen receptor (HUMARA) and RT-PCR analysis of RNA transcripts from genes for iduronate-2-sulphatase (IDS), palmitoylated membrane protein p55 and G6PD, it was possible

Table 17-1 • CAUSES OF THROMBOCYTOSIS

- Pseudothrombocytosis
- Primary thrombocytosis
    - Chronic myeloproliferative disorders: essential thrombocythemia, polycythemia vera, chronic myelogenous leukemia, agnogenic myeloid metaplasia/myelofibrosis
    - Myelodysplastic syndromes: 5q- syndrome, idiopathic acquired sideroblastic anemia
    - Hereditary or familial thrombocytosis
- Reactive or secondary thrombocytosis
    - Bacterial infections and tuberculosis
    - Inflammatory diseases
    - Advanced malignancies
    - Acute blood loss and hemolytic anemias
    - Postsplenectomy or asplenia (congenital or functional)
    - Rebound after chemotherapy-induced thrombocytopenia
    - Iron deficiency

to study larger populations of ET patients. It is now appreciated that ET is pathogenetically heterogeneous and that clonal thrombopoiesis, while frequent (in up to about 50% of patients), is not universal; some ET patients appear to have polyclonal progenitors.[11-14] No consistent gene(s) or chromosomal defect or causal gene(s) association for ET has been identified to date.

The recent cloning of the megakaryocyte growth and development factor, thrombopoietin (TPO), has refocused efforts to determine the etiology of ET. TPO is the primary regulator of platelet production and stimulates both the growth and differentiation of megakaryocyte progenitor cells in vitro and in vivo. Thrombopoietin binds to the c-*Mpl* receptors (the product of the c-*mpl* proto-oncogene) on the platelet membrane surface and is subsequently internalized and degraded.[15] Serum TPO levels appear to be regulated normally by the total platelet and megakaryocyte mass; serum TPO levels are quite elevated in patients with aplastic anemia. Interestingly, serum TPO levels are normal or slightly elevated in ET despite an expanded megakaryocyte and platelet mass.[16] This suggests that there may be dysregulation of the TPO-c-*Mpl* system in ET. Interestingly, ET patients have markedly decreased expression of c-*Mpl* protein on their platelets (and decreased mRNA expression), resulting in reduced TPO-binding capacity, impaired uptake and catabolism of TPO, and decreased clearance of TPO from the circulation. These findings explain the normal or slightly increased serum thrombopoietin levels in ET.[17-19] These findings suggest that megakaryocytes in ET may be hypersensitive to the stimulatory effects of TPO on production of platelets in vivo.[6] It is yet to be determined how reliable the detection of reduced expression of c-*Mpl* would be as a diagnostic marker for ET and primary thrombocytosis versus secondary causes for elevated platelet counts. Because TPO levels may be elevated in both reactive and clonal thrombocytosis, TPO assays available to date cannot reliably be used to differentiate between the two conditions.[20-22]

Another category of thrombocytosis, which is quite rare, is designated as *hereditary* or *familial thrombocythemia*. A number of families have been described in which extreme thrombocytosis was confirmed in multiple individuals in successive generations, affecting both sexes, and transmitted in an autosomal dominant inheritance mode.[23-27] Recently, different mutations in the TPO gene have been defined in several families with hereditary thrombocythemia.[28-30] Each mutation was associated with the over expression of mRNA causing increased production of TPO and platelets. Nevertheless, there must be other mechanisms responsible for the development of hereditary thrombocythemia since additional other families have not had any mutation(s) detected in their genes coding for TPO or its receptor c-*Mpl*.[31-32] The clinical and laboratory features in familial thrombocythemia are similar to that seen in ET, in which no TPO gene mutation has yet been appreciated.

A variety of inconsistent morphologic, biochemical, and functional abnormalities have been described in the platelets of ET patients. These include prolonged bleeding times; reduced platelet aggregation responses to epinephrine, collagen, and adenosine diphosphate (ADP); spontaneous platelet aggregation; acquired storage pool disease with alpha-granule deficits; defects in the structure and function of surface membrane glycoproteins and receptors; and abnormal arachidonic acid metabolism.[33] The adsorption of the larger molecular weight multimers from circulating von Willebrand factor (vWF) protein onto the surface membrane glycoproteins of ET platelets may produce laboratory changes (reduced vWF antigen and ristocetin cofactor activities, and occasionally reduced factor VIII coagulant activity) and clinical features consistent with acquired type 2A von Willebrand disease. Reduction of the platelet count to <1,000,000/μL usually restores the multimeric integrity of the vWF protein with the reappearance in plasma of the high- and intermediate-molecular-weight vWF multimers. There is also a normalization of the deficient vWF activities and a resolution of hemorrhagic manifestations. Altered vWF structure and function and the development of clinical bleeding rarely if ever occur in reactive thrombocytosis.[34-36] The high risk of thromboembolic complications in ET is also attributable in part to platelet pathophysiology, although the mechanisms remain poorly defined.

Elevated plasma levels of plasma β-thromboglobulin, the increased generation of thromboxane β-2, and the enhanced expression of P-selectin (CD62p) and thrombospondin on platelet surface membranes have been observed in ET patients. These findings suggest an enhanced in-vivo platelet activation and possible predisposition toward hypercoagulability. These changes are not detected in patients with reactive thrombocytosis.[37,38] The immediate and complete resolution of erythromelalgia in ET (presumably due to platelet-mediated thrombosis in the microvasculature; see below) after administration of aspirin is an additional compelling indication of the critical role of platelet activation in vivo and the contribution of prostaglandin endoperoxides to thrombotic complications in this condition.[39]

Spontaneous megakaryocyte and/or erythroid colony formation in in-vitro cell cultures is seen in 80% of patients studied with ET. This type of abnormal growth is not observed in reactive or secondary thrombocytosis, and therefore, this test could provide a useful means of distinguishing between the benign and myeloproliferative causes of thrombocytosis.[40]

CLINICAL FEATURES AND THROMBOHEMORRHAGIC COMPLICATIONS

The clinical features of ET range from the absence of symptoms to the very dramatic complications attributed to thrombosis and hemorrhage. The age of diagnosis of ET is important in this regard since thrombohemorrhagic manifestations are rare before the age of 60 years; however, analysis of the overall patient population with ET indicates that the median age of presentation for all ET patients is approximately 60 years; 10% to 25% of patients are less than 40 years old. One third of ET diagnoses are established in asymptomatic individuals.[41-45] Below the age of 60 years, ET is more common in females but thereafter there does not appear to be any gender predilection. Physical examination is usually unremarkable in early ET; some patients may have moderate or progressive splenomegaly and/or hepatomegaly[43,45,46] particularly as the disease progresses to myelofibrosis with agnogenic myeloid metaplasia. However, the prevalence of splenomegaly is much less than the 70% incidence observed in polycythemia rubra vera.[47]

One large longitudinal study of 187 consecutive ET patients reported that those diagnosed before 55 years of age had a significantly shorter life expectancy than healthy age-matched controls.[42] Nevertheless, the bulk of the literature does not support this observation despite the fact that there is relatively high morbidity in ET.[43,45,48] Life expectancy in ET was noted to be normal in those diagnosed at less than 60 years and without a prior history of venous or arterial thromboembolic episodes.[49] Furthermore, life expectancy is not affected substantially by the rare progression of ET into acute leukemia or transformation into myelofibrosis with agnogenic myeloid metaplasia. This probably reflects the indolent chronicity of ET until later life. Progression of ET to acute leukemia or development of myelofibrosis has been observed in 3% to 5% of cases, with acute leukemia occurring predominantly in older patients and those who previously received treatment with radiophosphorus or alkylating agents.[43,45] Tefferi and coworkers followed 74 young women with ET for up to 26 years, documenting only one case of acute leukemia and three cases of transformation to myeloid metaplasia.[50]

ET was originally classified as a hemorrhagic disease associated with thrombocytosis,[7] which set the stage for the early literature to focus mainly on the bleeding complications of this disease.[45,51,52] More recent observations indicate that thromboembolic episodes are far more frequent in ET patients than hemorrhagic complications. The incidence of major thrombosis has been reported to occur in about 25% to 30% of individuals with ET[41,43-45,48,53]; approximately 15% of patients present with thrombotic episodes.[49] The annual incidence of thrombotic complications is significantly greater in those over 60 years old (15%) compared to those less than 40 years old (2%). The majority of the thrombotic events in ET occur in those with prior hypercoagulable histories and cardiovascular risk factors. The potential contribution of the hereditary hypercoagulable states (factor V Leiden; prothrombin gene mutation; antithrombin, protein S or C deficiencies) to the incidence of thrombotic complications in ET patients has never been examined.

Arterial thromboses occur more frequently in ET than venous events at a ratio of 3.1:1.[42] Thromboses involve both the microcirculation (erythromelalgia) and large arteries of the extremities and cerebral, coronary, and visceral circulation. ET is one of the rare causes of angina pectoris and myocardial infarction in adults without atherosclerosis. Venous thromboses may occur in anatomically unusual places; about 60% involve veins in the abdomen and cerebral venous sinuses.[42,43] Reactive thrombocytosis is not associated with significant risks of thromboembolism.

Hemorrhagic complications usually affect the gastrointestinal tract and are frequently associated with, precipitated by, and exacerbated by concurrent use of antiplatelet aggregating medications. Uncontrolled thrombocytosis is a definite risk factor for these bleeding events.[41] Bleeding is characteristic of that seen in qualitative or quantitative platelet disorders with mucosal manifestations, such as epistaxis, ecchymoses, and gingival bleeding. Rarely do major bleeding problems, such as large hematomas, hemarthroses, intraocular and gastrointestinal bleeding, and post-traumatic or postsurgical bleeding occur. A minority of patients present with both thrombotic and hemorrhagic complications.

Symptomatic manifestations related to the arterial microcirculation, especially in peripheral and cerebral regions, comprise the most frequent clinical complications in ET.[54,55] Patients may present with erythromelalgia, which is characterized by warm, markedly erythematous, and congested extremities and an intense painful burning sensation over the fingers, soles, and toes. It is precipitated by heat and relieved by cold and can lead to acrocyanosis, paresthesias, and/or gangrene of the fingers and toes.[42,43] Other associated complications may include intermittent claudication and peripheral arterial occlusive disease of the lower extremities. These symptoms are most likely due to platelet activation in the microcirculation with microthrombi formation. These symptoms are so promptly relieved by aspirin that the response serves as a diagnostic function. Pregnancy may be complicated by spontaneous abortion, premature delivery, or abruptio placentae due to placental infarcts (see below).

Neurologic symptoms related to ET include headache, paresthesias, transient ischemic attacks, paresis, visual disturbances, and epileptic seizures[56,57] (Table 17-2).

PROGNOSTIC INDICATORS FOR THROMBOSES AND HEMORRHAGE

The numerous risk factors which predispose ET patients to thrombotic and hemorrhagic complications have

Table 17–2 • NEUROLOGIC SYMPTOMS IN ESSENTIAL THROMBOCYTHEMIA

- Headaches, often occipital
- Transient monocular blindness
- Transient hemiparesis
- Peripheral paresthesias in feet
- Scintillating scotomata
- Vertigo
- Blurred vision
- Unstable gait
- Dysarthria
- Epileptic seizures

been identified and used to develop risk stratification paradigms for treatment planning. Age and prior history of cardiovascular disease and/or thromboembolic events have emerged as primary prognostic factors for future or recurrent thrombotic complications in ET. A prospective analysis of ET patients has indicated that age above 60 years is associated with an annual incidence of thrombosis of almost 15%, compared to less than 2% in those younger than 40 years old.[50] A retrospective study of 148 ET patients determined that age above 60 years was associated with 35.6% incidence of major thromboembolic events within 6 years of diagnosis compared to 21.4% incidence in patients younger than 60 years.[55] These risks increase substantially at age 70 and with prolonged duration of thrombocythemia. In those individuals with a past medical history of thrombosis, the incidence of recurrent hypercoagulable events was 42.6% within 6 years of diagnosis.[55] There is no apparent increased risk for thrombosis in males less than 60 years old with no history of thrombotic complications and platelet count of 1,500,000/μL[58]; however, the risk in young women may be increased. In a series of young women with ET, Tefferi reports recurrent thrombosis in 45% of those with and 13% of those without a history of prior thrombosis, respectively.[59] The contributions of obesity, oral estrogen contraceptive use, and smoking need to be clarified in this population. The role of hypercholesterolemia in the development of thrombosis in ET is also unclear. Although one study reported a 59.5% incidence of thrombosis for ET patients with hypercholesterolemia,[55] no increased risk has been noted by others.[42,53] Furthermore, no increased risks for thrombosis in ET were observed with other vascular risk factors, such as diabetes, essential hypertension[42,53,55,60] or gender.[42,44] Cigarette smoking was linked to increased incidence of ischemic complication in one[61] study but not in others.[42,53,55,60]

In general, the platelet count is not a reliable risk factor for development of thromboses in individual patients with ET.[41,44,45,55,61] While most of the thrombotic events are associated with platelet counts over 500,000 to 600,000/μL,[41,42] even while patients are on aspirin, it is not uncommon to diagnose thrombotic, neurologic, or peripheral vascular symptoms at lower platelet counts.[62] Extreme thrombocytosis (more than 1,000,000 to 1,500,000/μL) appears to increase the risks of spontaneous bleeding events, particularly from the gastrointestinal tract with concomitant use of aspirin or other antiplatelet aggregation agents.[41,45,48]

Analysis of risk factors is important in determining which patients need cytoreductive therapy and when treatment should begin. Stratification of patients into low-, intermediate-, and high-risk categories for thrombohemorrhagic complications is recommended to establish the risk–benefit relationship for treatment since some of the cytoreductive medications have significant side effects and potentially are leukemogenic.[50,59] Patients of any age with a prior history of thrombosis, extreme thrombocytosis, and/or thrombotic or hemorrhagic symptoms should be classified as high risk. Those over the age of 60 years and having platelet counts above 450,000/μL are also classified as high risk by most physicians. Individuals of any age with extreme thrombocytosis but without active thrombohemorrhagic symptoms are considered intermediate risk. It is unclear whether cardiovascular risk factors (diabetes mellitus, hypertension, hyperlipidemia, etc.) contribute to the mortality or morbidity of ET but clearly these risk factors should be treated. ET patients who are younger than 60 years old, asymptomatic, without previous history of thrombosis and cardiovascular risks but with an elevated platelet count of less than 1,500,000/μL have been designated as low risk for major thromboembolic or hemorrhagic events. However, it is still unclear whether to treat these low risk individuals with ET. Most authors advocate a "wait and watch" policy.[58] Recent literature questions this conservative approach. Bazzan and coworkers reported that their ET patients under 55 years old at diagnosis had a significantly shorter life expectancy than healthy age-matched controls. The authors concluded that ET significantly decreases both quality of life and life expectancy for younger patients.[42] There is also evidence that early reduction of platelet counts in young, asymptomatic ET patients may favorably affect their long-term survival. These observations suggest that more aggressive cytoreductive therapy with newer, nonleukemogenic agents, like anagrelide or interferon alpha, should be considered to maintain platelet counts less than 400,000/μL.

DIAGNOSIS OF ESSENTIAL THROMBOCYTOSIS

In 1986, the Polycythemia Vera Study group proposed six criteria for the diagnosis of essential thrombocytosis: (1) platelet count of more than 600,000/μL; (2) hemoglobin level 13 g/dL or less or normal red blood cell mass; (3) stainable iron stores in the bone marrow or failure of iron supplementation to normalize the elevated platelet count; (4) absence of the Philadelphia chromosome; (5) collagen fibrosis less than one third of the bone marrow biopsy area without marked splenomegaly and without evidence of leukoerythroblastosis in the marrow or on the peripheral blood smear; and (6) no known cause for reactive thrombocytosis.[46] These parameters were intended to exclude reactive thrombocytosis and other clonal etiologies of thrombocytosis (chronic myelogenous leukemia [CML], polycythemia vera, and myelofibrosis). Some investigators have advocated the measurement of acute phase reactants, such as plasma IL-6 and C-reactive protein levels, to discriminate reactive thrombocytosis from clonal thrombocytosis.[3] In

Table 17–3 • POLYCYTHEMIA VERA STUDY GROUP CRITERIA FOR DIAGNOSIS OF ESSENTIAL THROMBOCYTOSIS

- Platelet count >600,000/µL
- Hematocrit <40%, or normal red cell mass (males <36mL/kg, females <32mL/kg)
- No cause for reactive thrombocytosis
- Absence of iron deficiency documented by stainable iron in marrow or normal serum ferritin or normal RBC mean corpuscular volume
- Absence of Philadelphia chromosome and bcr/abl gene rearrangement
- Absence of collagen fibrosis of marrow or, if present, it should be less than one third biopsy area without marked splenomegaly and without leukoerythroblastic reaction
- No cytogenetic or morphologic evidence of myelodysplastic syndrome

1997, the diagnostic criteria were revised to endorse the presence of a normal serum ferritin level with normal red blood cell mean corpuscular volume as sufficient evidence to exclude both reactive thrombocytosis secondary to iron deficiency and polycythemia vera masked by iron deficiency as the cause of thrombocytosis (Table 17–3).[63] Exclusion of CML required the use of PCR assays to detect for bcr/abl gene rearrangements when the Philadelphia chromosome was absent. Furthermore, there should be no cytogenetic or morphologic evidence of an underlying myelodysplastic process. These criteria would exclude the so-called 5q-syndrome, which is associated with the myelodysplastic syndrome and other myeloproliferative disorders yet can present with significant thrombocytosis.[64] There is a high incidence of 17p chromosome deletions in ET patients treated with hydroxyurea as their disease transforms into acute myeloblastic leukemia.

LABORATORY FINDINGS OF ESSENTIAL THROMBOCYTHEMIA

The most prominent and consistent laboratory abnormality seen in essential thrombocythemia is an elevated platelet count over 600,000/µL. In most studies, the average platelet count at diagnosis is around 1,000,000/µL.[43,45] The hematocrit is usually normal unless the clinical course is complicated by bleeding or iron deficiency. Mild leukocytosis in the range of 10,000 to 20,000/µL is commonly seen and may be associated with myeloid immaturity and left shift in the differential count. Basophilia and/or eosinophilia may be present, as it is in other myeloproliferative disorders. Examination of the peripheral blood smear often reveals abnormal platelet morphology with many large and bizarre forms and platelet aggregates, not characteristic of the normal platelets seen in secondary thrombocytosis. The bone marrow biopsy typically contains megakaryocytic hyperplasia with large dysplastic megakaryocytes. Large clusters of platelets dissociated from megakaryocytes are found scattered among cells. Moderate erythroid and myeloid hyperplasia may be seen along with increased reticulin content.[46] Platelet aggregation responses in vitro are usually suboptimal after the addition of the agonists epinephrine and ADP but occasionally normal in response to collagen, ristocetin, and arachidonic acid. Spontaneous platelet aggregation or hyperaggregability is variably observed.[43,45] Platelet aggregation in reactive thrombocytosis is generally normal. Serum potassium levels may be spuriously elevated because of the very high platelet count (pseudohyperkalemia).[46,65] The measurement of plasma potassium provides a more accurate assessment. One fourth of patients may have elevated serum lactate dehydrogenase and uric acid levels. Leukocyte alkaline phosphatase is normal in most patients although abnormally increased or reduced levels are not uncommon.[43]

DIFFERENTIAL DIAGNOSIS

Essential thrombocythemia is a diagnosis of exclusion and should be entertained when other causes of elevated platelet counts have been ruled out. Table 17–1 lists the major causes of thrombocytosis.[1,5] Careful examination of peripheral blood smear should be pursued to exclude the presence of "pseudothrombocytosis," spuriously indicated by automated complete blood cell count analyzers, which will misidentify red or white cell fragments as platelets in such conditions as thrombotic thrombocytopenic purpura, chronic lymphocytic leukemia, and microspherocytosis.

Reactive thrombocytosis is a much more common cause of elevated platelet counts than is ET. In one study of 280 patients with extreme thrombocytosis (platelet count 1,000,000/µL or high), 82% were found to have secondary causes of thrombocytosis and only 14% had myeloproliferative disorders causing a rise in platelet count.[5] Therefore, a careful history and physical examination should be done and relevant laboratory data obtained to exclude the causes of reactive thrombocytosis. Elevated levels of C-reactive protein, IL-6, sedimentation rate, and plasma fibrinogen suggest reactive thrombocytosis.[3] Table 17–4 lists important clinical and laboratory features that may help to differentiate between essential and reactive thrombocytosis.

TREATMENT OF ESSENTIAL THROMBOCYTHEMIA

Traditionally, the decision to initiate treatment for ET has been based on clinical symptoms and signs and risk factor analysis and not merely on platelet number or function (Tables 17–5 and 17–6). It remains unclear whether young (less than 60 years old), asymptomatic (low risk) patients should receive treatment. In a prospective study of 65 untreated ET patients, younger than 60 years, with no history of thrombosis or hemorrhage, and platelet counts less than 1,500,000/µL, the incidence of thrombosis in ET patients was 1.91 cases per 100 patient-years versus 1.5 cases of thrombosis in a normal, age- and sex-matched, control population after a median

Table 17-4 • LABORATORY AND CLINICAL CHARACTERISTICS OF ESSENTIAL THROMBOCYTHEMIA VERSUS REACTIVE THROMBOCYTOSIS

Feature	Essential Thrombocythemia	Reactive Thrombocytosis
Thrombosis or hemorrhage	Present	Absent
Splenomegaly	Occasionally present	Typically absent
Abnormal platelet morphology and platelet aggregates on peripheral blood smear	Present	Absent
Bone marrow reticulum/fibrosis	Present	Absent
Clusters of dysplastic megakaryocytes in bone marrow	Present	Absent
Increased acute phase reactants (IL-6, C-reactive protein)	Absent	Present
Spontaneous colony formation in in-vitro cell cultures	Present	Absent
Abnormal cytogenetics	Occasionally present	Absent
Suboptimal platelet aggregation responses in in-vitro/spontaneous platelet aggregation	Present	Absent

follow-up of 4.1 years. This was not statistically significant. Pregnancy and surgery were not associated with an increased incidence of thrombosis in these ET patients.[58] In contrast, cytoreductive therapy is clearly indicated for those patients who have symptoms or who have risk factors for thrombosis or hemorrhage, including age over 60 years, prior history of thrombosis, or extreme thrombocytosis (platelet count greater than 1,000,000/μL). Patients should be advised to cease smoking and to obtain proper management of hypertension and diabetes, each of which is an independent risk factor for hypercoagulability. Treatment options to reduce platelet counts in ET are listed in Table 17-5.

Hydroxyurea

Hydroxyurea is a nonalkylating S-phase-specific myelosuppressive agents with a mechanism of action that is not platelet specific. It inhibits ribonucleotide diphosphate reductase, the enzyme that catalyzes the conversion of ribonucleotide diphosphates to the corresponding deoxyribose forms. Clinical experiments reveal that hydroxyurea treatment reduces hematopoietic progenitor growth and CD34 positive cells in polycythemia vera and ET.[66] It is administered orally and appears to have good bioavailability. Hydroxyurea is predominantly used to treat myeloproliferative disorders; in CML to control leukocytosis, in ET to reduce platelet counts, and in polycythemia rubra vera to reduce red cell mass and elevated platelet counts. The initial starting dose is 15 to 20 mg/kg/day orally, taken as a single dose. Subsequent dosing traditionally was titrated to maintain platelet counts below 600,000/μL without excessive lowering of neutrophil counts. Recent data suggest that ET patients may benefit further by reducing platelet counts to below 400,000/μL and maintaining that level. Dose modifications should be considered for patients with renal insufficiency. Continuous treatment with hydroxyurea has been shown to reduce platelet counts to below 500,000/μL within the first 8 weeks in 80% of patients.[67-69] The advantages of hydroxyurea include its convenience, its efficacy, and its low level of toxicity. Major short-term adverse effects include reversible myelosuppression manifested as neutropenia and macrocytic anemia. Other side effects include nausea, vomiting, diarrhea, skin changes and ulceration (including severe painful ankle ulceration), and rarely drug fever. Sudden withdrawal is associated with rebound elevations of the platelet count.[70-72]

In 1970s and 1980s, hydroxyurea was considered the drug of choice to reduce platelet counts in ET because of the significant risk of developing secondary acute leukemias associated with alkylating agents and radioactive phosphorus (^{32}P). Hydroxyurea is definitely effective in reducing the incidence of thrombotic complications in high-risk patients with ET.[73] A recent update of the data generated from the original prospective, randomized, controlled study continues to demonstrate a significantly better thrombosis-free survival in the hydroxyurea-treated ET cohort after a median follow-up 73 months. Thrombotic complications occurred in 45% of patients in the untreated high-risk ET group versus 9% of patients in the hydroxyurea treatment cohort.[74]

There is considerable concern that the cancer- (leukemia) free survival was significantly reduced in ET patients who had received treatment with hydroxyurea plus busulphan (some patients had received busulphan prior to randomization) versus the untreated control group; however, cancer-free survival was equivalent between the hydroxyurea-alone group and the untreated control group.[74]

Numerous other studies have challenged the relative leukemogenic safety of hydroxyurea.[67-69,75-78] All incidence data must be interpreted carefully since there appears to be a natural, albeit low, progression of untreated ET to acute leukemia. The rate of background transformation to acute leukemia has been difficult to

Table 17-5 • CYTOREDUCTIVE OPTIONS TO TREAT ESSENTIAL THROMBOCYTHEMIA

- Hydroxyurea
- Anagrelide
- Interferon-alpha
- Alkylating agents (busulphan, chlorambucil, pipobroman, thiotepa)
- Radioactive phosphorus
- Plateletpheresis

Table 17-6 • RISK STRATIFICATION AND MANAGEMENT GUIDELINES FOR ESSENTIAL THROMBOCYTOSIS

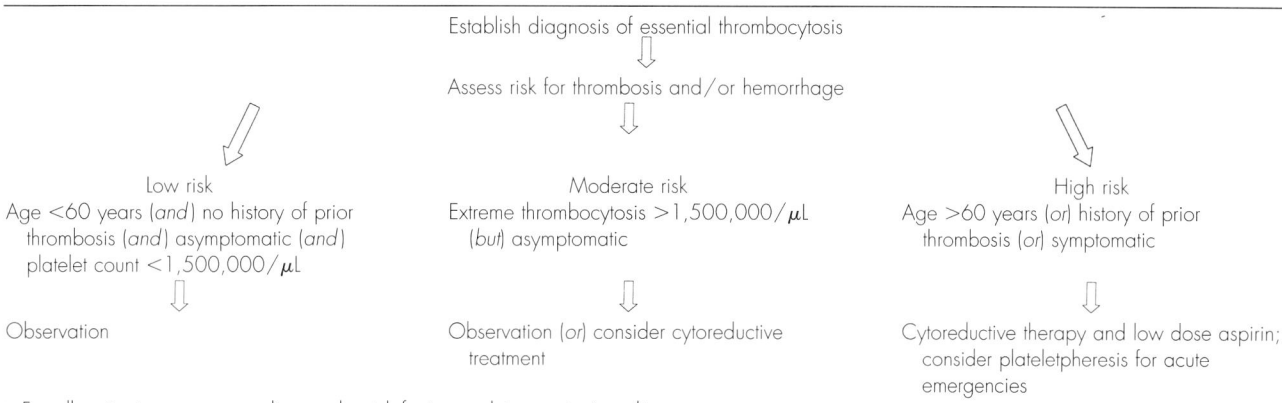

Establish diagnosis of essential thrombocytosis
⇩
Assess risk for thrombosis and/or hemorrhage

Low risk	Moderate risk	High risk
Age <60 years (and) no history of prior thrombosis (and) asymptomatic (and) platelet count <1,500,000/μL	Extreme thrombocytosis >1,500,000/μL (but) asymptomatic	Age >60 years (or) history of prior thrombosis (or) symptomatic
⇩	⇩	⇩
Observation	Observation (or) consider cytoreductive treatment	Cytoreductive therapy and low dose aspirin; consider plateletpheresis for acute emergencies

- For all patients, manage cardiovascular risk factors; advise against smoking.
- May consider low-dose aspirin in asymptomatic patients if there are no other contraindications and platelet count is less than 1,500,000/μL.
- Consider anagrelide or interferon-alpha as first line therapy in patients under 60 years.
- Consider hydroxyurea as a first-line therapy for patients 60 years and older.
- Consider low-dose aspirin and interferon-alpha, if indicated, in pregnancy.

quantitate since the majority of data was collected before PCR assays were available to exclude the presence of bcr/abl gene mutations, etc. Furthermore, the recently appreciated association of 17p chromosome deletions in ET, placing patients at higher risk of developing acute leukemia, suggests that there may be particularly susceptible cohorts of ET patients heretofore not stratified in clinical studies. The incidence of acute leukemia transformation is estimated to be approximately 3.5% at a median follow-up of 8.2 years when hydroxyurea is used alone. This risk increased to 14% when hydroxyurea was combined with other agents, in this study, pipobroman. A high proportion of cases (41%) were associated with deletions of the 17p chromosome, which is accompanied with dysgranulopoiesis and p53 mutations.[75] Thus, it appears that hydroxyurea administered as single-agent therapy carries an intrinsically small but definite genotoxic and mutagenic risk of inducing secondary malignancies. This risk increases significantly when hydroxyurea is administered in combination with other chemotherapy agents. Nevertheless, it is reasonable to continue to consider hydroxyurea the drug of choice for elderly patients (over 60 years) who have not received prior chemotherapy, since its cost–benefit ratio, tolerability, and safety profile are superior to those of anagrelide, interferon-alpha, and the alkylating agents. In younger patients at high risk of thrombosis or hemorrhage or in patients who had received prior chemotherapy, anagrelide or interferon-alpha should be considered as the initial choice. Administration of hydroxyurea may be a particularly effective and rapid means of shrinking spleen size over 2 to 3 months in those ET patients with massive splenomegaly.

Anagrelide

Anagrelide is an imidazo (2-1-b) quinazolin-2-1 compound that was originally developed as antithrombotic agent because of its powerful antiaggregating effect on platelets. It inhibits cyclic nucleotide phosphodiesterase and the release of arachidonic acid from phospholipase, possibly by inhibiting phospholipase A2. When anagrelide was first administered to humans, it had a potent thrombocytopenic effect, which had not been observed previously in any animal model system. Because anagrelide produces thrombocytopenia at doses significantly below those required to inhibit platelet aggregation, the potential risk of precipitating clinically important hemorrhagic complications is miniscule. Anagrelide has little or no immediate effect on myelopoiesis or erythropoiesis, but its long-term use has been associated with a 5% to 10% reduction in hemoglobin concentration in approximately one third of patients with ET.[79,80] This latter effect of anagrelide is probably mediated by an effect on erythropoietin levels since it can be readily reversed in vivo by the administration of therapeutic doses of recombinant erythropoietin.

The specific mechanism by which anagrelide induces thrombocytopenia remains unclear. The seminal clinical study published by Silverstein and coworkers demonstrated that anagrelide does not alter the cellularity of the bone marrow, the number of megakaryocytes in the bone marrow, or the circulating survival of platelets.[79] Anagrelide does not inhibit the proliferation of megakaryoctyic-committed progenitor cells (CFU-M) in vivo, although suprapharmacologic concentrations may inhibit megakaryocyte colony expansion in cell culture systems. Therefore, anagrelide-induced thrombocytopenia does not arise as the result of direct stem cell toxicity or from direct inhibition of megakaryocytopoiesis.[81] Anagrelide alters the maturation of megakaryocytes and thereby decreases their size and affects their morphology.[82] There is a left shift in the distribution of morphologic stages and decreased ploidy. The intracellular processes influenced by anagrelide have not been elucidated. In addition, it is not known whether anagrelide or a metabolite of the drug possesses the primary platelet-lowering property. Anagrelide in large concentrations can inhibit platelet aggregation in vitro; however, this mechanism is independent of its effects on thrombopoiesis and is rarely a significant issue from the clinical perspective.

The elimination half-life of anagrelide from the circulation is 76 hours. Seventy-five percent (75%) of the administered dose is excreted in the urine over 6 days and 10% is excreted in feces. The recommended initial dose of anagrelide is 0.5 mg two or four times daily. The dose should be increased by a maximum of 0.5 mg/day/week until the desired reduction in platelet count is achieved. The maximum dose of anagrelide ideally should not exceed 10 mg/day or 3 mg per dose.[83] Dose adjustments may be necessary in the presence of renal failure.

Anagrelide is licensed for use in the United States for the treatment of thrombocythemia associated with all myeloproliferative disorders. The broadest experience with anagrelide has been generated by the multicenter phase II clinical trial conducted by the Anagrelide Study Group. Of 577 patients with primary thrombocythemia (median platelet count of 990,000/μL), there was a 94% response rate (defined as reduction in the platelet count by 50% or maintained at less than 600,000/μL for at least 4 weeks) in individuals with ET treated with anagrelide. Patients initially received 1 mg anagrelide orally every 6 hours, which was later reduced to 0.5 mg four times a day, with increases of 0.5 mg/day every 5 to 7 days, depending on platelet count response. The median time to maximal response was 11 days and the dose needed to achieve a response ranged from 0.5 to 9.0 mg/day. However, 95% of patients responded to a dose of 4 mg/day or less.[80]

The rapid and effective control of thrombocythemia by anagrelide would be expected to substantially reduce the incidence and severity of thrombotic and hemorrhagic complications in ET. In fact, the number of adverse events appears to be reduced proportionally to the decrease in platelet counts, but as indicated in the original nonrandomized studies examining anagrelide use, the relationship was not linear. This suggests that other variables, such as total leukocyte counts, leukocyte properties, or intrinsic biochemical or physiologic characteristics of affected individuals with ET, may influence its clinical course (e.g., inherited hypercoagulability). Similar findings have been observed when hydroxyurea was used to control thrombocythemia. Unfortunately, there have been no randomized, controlled studies comparing the safety and efficacy of anagrelide, hydroxyurea, or interferon-alpha. It is possible that markedly decreasing the elevated platelet counts in ET, no matter by what means or medications, is more critical than how they are reduced.

One possible advantage that anagrelide has over hydroxyurea is that the "picket fence" or "peak–valley" pattern of platelet count reduction and rebound can be avoided. Fluctuating doses of hydroxyurea, necessitated by its effects on white blood cells, lead to a "peak–valley" effect on platelet counts compared to the stable, plateau of platelet count reduction produced by anagrelide. Consistent control of platelet counts may reduce thrombosis risk[53]; only randomized, controlled studies with both of these medications will determine if this is a real or theoretical advantage for anagrelide therapy in ET.

The major side effects noted with anagrelide administration are neurologic, gastrointestinal, and cardiac in nature (Table 17–7). These may be severe enough to cause patients to discontinue the medication. Petit and coworkers reported a 13% drop out rate in their anagrelide studies.[84] Most neurologic and gastrointestinal side effects develop during the first 2 weeks of therapy and resolve on average within 2 weeks. Postural hypotension may be produced at higher dosing level. In most cases, diuretics can control the fluid retention and peripheral edema induced by anagrelide use over time. Substantial normocytic and normochromic anemia is seen in about 25% of patients. There is no evidence of hemolysis. Originally believed to reflect hemodilution effects caused by intravascular fluid retention while on anagrelide, the anemia is more likely due to antierythropoietin properties of anagrelide. In fact, the administration of recombinant erythropoietin preparations can ameliorate the anemia. Cardiac adverse effects are observed in over one third of patients during anagrelide use and may be contraindicated in those with uncontrolled arrythmias.[80] Many individuals complain of frequent and anxiety-provoking palpitations, which are dose related. Restriction of caffeine intake and/or dose reduction often relieve or eliminate these symptomatic palpitations; occasionally β-blocker medications must be administered. The vasodilatory effects on the peripheral vasculature and the potent inotropic properties of anagrelide may induce cardiac symptoms. Rarely a cardiomyopathy may occur. This may be particularly problematic in elderly individuals, but may respond or be reversed by diuretics.[80] Severe headaches are reported in approxi-

---

Table 17–7 • MAJOR ADVERSE EFFECTS AND THEIR RELATIVE FREQUENCIES ASSOCIATED WITH ANAGRELIDE USE

Cardiovascular
Fluid retention or edema (24%)
Congestive heart failure (2.5%)
Palpitations and tachycardia (36%)
Irregular pulse (2.5%)
New or worsening angina (0.9%)

Neurologic
Headache (30%)
Dizziness (8%)

Gastrointestinal
Nausea (19%)
Diarrhea (15%)
Gas, eructation and bloating (8%)

Others (rare)
Rash and hyperpigmentation
Pulmonary fibrosis
Liver function abnormalities

mately one third of patients and are often described as "vascular" or "migraine-like." They are probably the result of the peripheral vasodilatory effects of anagrelide and may lead to intolerance of the medication in a substantial number of patients. Those with a pre-existing migraine history may be particularly susceptible to this side effect. Reduction of caffeine intake may be helpful. Finally, anagrelide is contraindicated in pregnancy as it crosses the placental barrier and may lead to fetal thrombocytopenia.[84]

Recombinant Interferon-Alpha

Recombinant interferon-alpha was first studied as alternative therapy for the treatment of polycythemia rubra vera, in which it was noted to reduce both the thrombocytosis and erythrocytosis in approximately two thirds of patients. Occasionally, massive splenomegaly disappeared and intense pruritis was ameliorated. Recombinant interferon-alpha administration significantly reduced the platelet count in approximately 85% of patients with ET and had beneficial effects on spleen size in about one third of recipients.[85] Numerous clinical trials have assessed the efficacy of interferon-alpha to reduce platelet counts in myeloproliferative disorders.[86–96] Interferon-alpha suppresses the proliferation of both pluripotent and lineage committed hematopoietic progenitors and inhibits the growth of megakaryocyte progenitors both in vivo and in vitro.[97–100] Interferon-alpha also reduces thrombopoiesis and causes modest shortening of platelet mean life span.[101] Interferon-alpha does not cross the placenta[102] and is not known to be teratogenic; it has been used safely in young pregnant women with CML and is the drug of choice for the treatment of ET in pregnancy. Interferon-alpha administration circumvents the theoretical concerns about the potential risks of teratogenicity with hydroxyurea and anagrelide. Interferon-alpha is nonleukemogenic and nongonadotoxic yet controls thrombocythemia very efficiently.

Recombinant interferon-alpha is administered usually at doses of 3 million units subcutaneously three times weekly. The response rate with respect to thrombocythemia approaches 90% and after initial cytoreduction is achieved, the interferon dose usually can be reduced. Discontinuation results in rapid relapse of thrombocythemia, which usually responds to the resumption of interferon therapy.[86–88,92–93] Sustained remissions have been documented in some patients after interferon-alpha therapy, suggesting that interferon-alpha has an antiproliferative effect on the neoplastic clone.[87,89,90,103] One clinical study has demonstrated decelerated proliferation of the neoplastic clone in five out of seven patients receiving interferon-alpha for their ET.[103] Interferon-alpha also antagonizes the action of platelet-derived growth factor (PDGF), a product of megakaryopoiesis, which initiates fibroblast proliferation. Interferon-alpha may reduce the inherent risks of progressive myelofibrosis and leukemogenesis in ET and the myeloproliferative disorders by its antiproliferative and immunomodulatory effects. There are no randomized studies comparing the safety, efficacy, leukemia-free survival, or thrombohemorrhagic event free survival of recombinant interferon-alpha with hydroxyurea or anagrelide in ET.

The major disadvantages of recombinant interferon-alpha in ET are its associated side-effects and its high cost.[104] Almost all patients experience an influenza-like syndrome during induction with fever, chills, myalgias, headache, and arthralgias. These symptoms are frequently controlled with acetaminophen. Long-term treatment can result in fatigue, anorexia, weight loss, alopecia, and autoimmune diseases, including autoimmune thyroiditis, autoimmune hemolytic anemia, autoimmune thrombocytopenia, and symmetric polyarthropathy. Patients can also develop clinically significant neuropsychiatric symptoms, including altered mentation, confusion, and deep depression.[85,92,104] The treating physician must be aware of suicide ideation in those with prior personal and/or family histories of depression. Neutralizing antibodies to recombinant interferon-alpha therapy may develop leading to rise in platelet count. Therapy with leukocyte interferon-alpha has been tried in such situation with excellent response.[105] In a review of 273 cases, interferon-alpha therapy was terminated in 25% patients. The most common reasons for withdrawal were interferon related side effects in 55% and patient refusal in 10%.[104] Many of these side effects dissipate over time with continued administration of the drug. Recombinant interferon-alpha is a very attractive therapeutic option for ET because it can (1) suppress the neoplastic clone; (2) efficiently lower platelet counts; (3) reduce and reverse massive splenomegaly and progression of myelofibrosis; and (4) circumvent potential teratogenicity of anagrelide, hydrea, and alkylating agents, and leukemogenicity of hydroxyurea and alkylating agents. Nevertheless, interferon-alpha remains underutilized in this disease, perhaps because of its price and spectrum of side effects. It has been reserved primarily for use in ET patients who are pregnant or who have massive splenomegaly.

Alkylating Agents and Radiophosphorous

The use of alkylating chemotherapeutic agents, such as busulphan, melphalan, and chlorambucil, was entertained for the treatment of ET after their success in reducing and controlling the thrombocythemia associated with polycythemia rubra vera in the Polycythemia Vera Study Group protocols. Similar good to excellent platelet responses also have been observed in ET; however, the 11.3% and 3.5% incidence of secondary acute leukemia associated with administration of chlorambucil and busulfan, respectively, has led to abandonment of their widespread use in both ET and polycythemia rubra vera. The risk of developing acute leukemias in patients given chlorambucil was 2.3 times that in patients given radioactive phosphorus and 13 times that in patients who were treated by phlebotomy alone.[106]

Radiophosphorous (^{32}P) yielded equally good success in controlling thrombocythemic states; however, this agent also has been generally avoided, except in very exceptional clinical situations, because of its inherent oncogenesis. The incidence of acute leukemia was 9.6% at 10 years postadministration in the Polycythemia Vera Study Group protocol and there was double the expected number of gastrointestinal tract and skin cancers, beginning 2 to 3 years after ^{32}P administration.[107]

At this time, the availability of relatively safer cytoreductive drugs, such as hydroxyurea, anagrelide, and interferon-alpha, has relegated the use of busulfan and ^{32}P only for high-risk ET patients who cannot tolerate the other medications and whose life expectancy is considered to be less than 10 years. Busulphan may be given 2 to 4 mg orally daily with careful monitoring of platelet and whole blood counts. After initial control of the platelet count, only intermittent courses of the drug are required. This limits the adverse effects experienced with the drug, including bone marrow aplasia, skin pigmentation, amenorrhea, and pulmonary fibrosis.[67,108]

^{32}P is a pure β-emitter with a half-life of 14.3 days and a maximum tissue range of 8 mm. Both oral and intravenous forms have been used to control thrombocythemia associated with essential thrombocytosis and polycythemia vera.[109-111] In one study, normalization of the full blood count was achieved in 50% of patients after a single administration of ^{32}P and in 73% after two treatments. Because oral ^{32}P may be more leukemogenic than the intravenous form, ^{32}P can be administered intravenously at 2.3 mCi/m^2 (capped at 5 mCi/m^2). Repeat dosing (may be escalated by 25% with a 7-mCi/m^2 cap) should be delayed for at least 3 months and administered only if adequate platelet control has not been achieved.

Pipobroman is a piperazine derivative that is structurally similar to alkylating agents but appears to act as a metabolic competitor of pyrimidine bases.[108,112] Most of the experience with this medication has been derived from its wide use in Europe for treatment of polycythemia rubra vera. It is not licensed for use in the United States. A randomized prospective study of hydroxyurea and pipobroman in 292 patients with polycythemia rubra vera revealed equal efficacy for either in disease control and an equal risk of leukemogenesis of approximately 10% at 13 years, with no significant difference between the two treatment arms.[113] In another study, the short-term incidence of acute myelogenous leukemia and myelodysplastic syndrome was 0% and 16%, respectively when pipobroman was used alone or with other agents (usually hydroxyurea).[75] Long-term use may be more problematic.[114] A high proportion of the cases of acute leukemia and myelodysplastic syndrome was associated with 17p-syndrome.[75]

Pipobroman has not been used widely in essential thrombocythemia. In two uncontrolled studies involving 21 and 24 patients, hematologic remission and platelet control were obtained in 86% and 92% of the cases respectively, with no observed secondary leukemia but the follow-up duration was relatively short in these studies.[115,116] Side effects include nausea, vomiting, abdominal cramps, diarrhea, and anemia. A rapid decline in hemoglobin associated with increase in serum bilirubin and reticulocyte count can occur. The initial dose is 1 mg/kg per day orally with dose titration according to the platelet counts and myelosuppressive effects.

Aspirin

The rationale for aspirin administration in low doses (81 mg/day) in ET is based on its irreversible inhibition of platelet cyclo-oxygenase activity and its excellent therapeutic and prophylactic profile in the control of platelet-mediated microcirculatory thrombotic disturbances. Similar benefits, although of briefer duration, may also be observed with indomethacin, but with more potential side effects. Aspirin is particularly useful in the treatment of erythromelalgia and acral cyanaosis as well as the prevention of thrombotic complications (transient ischemic attacks, amaurosis fugax, and unstable angina).[47] These benefits are observed even when the platelet counts remain elevated. Aspirin is very effective in prevention or reversal of potential platelet microthromboembolic complications associated with the in-vitro phenomenon of spontaneous platelet aggregation. High doses of aspirin (more than 325 mg/day) or aspirin used in combination with other medications with antiplatelet aggregation properties (such as dipyridamole or nonsteroidal anti-inflammatory drugs) should be avoided in ET since there is a significantly increased incidence of gastrointestinal bleeding. Fortunately, the incidence of serious bleeding, in general and specifically associated with the use of aspirin, is much less common in ET compared to polycythemia rubra vera. Care should be exercised when administering aspirin in the presence of qualitative platelet defects (as determined by platelet aggregation studies). Aspirin does not appear to exacerbate bleeding episodes in the acquired von Willebrand disease of ET, which may result from increased adsorption of the highest-molecular-weight multimers of circulating vWF protein onto receptors on the surface of platelets. Other medications with anticoagulant or antiplatelet activities, such as warfarin, sulfinpyrazone, dipyridamole, and ticlopidine, do not convey the same salutary effects in ET as aspirin.[47,52,117]

Plateletpheresis in Essential Thrombocythemia

The rapid reduction of extremely elevated platelet counts (usually over 1,000,000/μL) in ET is necessitated when emergent symptomatic or life-threatening thromboembolic and hemorrhagic complications occur. Cytoreductive agents may be initiated concurrently for long-term control; however, in certain clinical situations, such as pregnancy, the use of anagrelide and myelosuppressive medications may be contraindicated. Therefore, plateletpheresis, accomplished via the physical removal of platelets using an automated apheresis apparatus, can provide immediate and efficient benefits. Plateletpheresis is only a temporary measure and other cytoreductive strategies will be needed.[118-120] Reactive thrombocytosis is not symptomatic generally and should not require plateletpheresis.

Pregnancy and Essential Thrombocythemia

Pregnancy is a special clinical circumstance in ET since approximately 50% of such pregnancies are complicated by spontaneous miscarriage, intrauterine fetal death, abruptio placentae, intrauterine growth retardation, premature delivery, and pre-eclampsia. This is considerably higher than observed in the general population and may be due to placental vessel thrombosis and subsequent infarction. Spontaneous miscarriages occur most commonly during the first trimester and are unrelated to the degree of thrombocytosis or the type of treatment (including no treatment) received for the ET.[121] According to the observations of Beressi and coworkers, pregnancies which persist until term are not usually complicated by thrombohemorrhagic events or catastrophes at delivery.[122] Smoking should be avoided particularly in pregnancy since it may precipitate any potential hypercoagulability or platelet hyperaggregability. Hemorrhagic complications are quite uncommon in pregnancy. In some cases, a decrease in platelet count and even spontaneous remission of thrombocytosis has been noted to occur during pregnancy, perhaps due to hemodilution effects. Pregnancy is usually successful in such individuals.[123]

Management options during pregnancy should be tailored according to the perceived risk of developing thrombohemorrhagic complications. Low-risk (platelet count below 1,500,000/μL, asymptomatic, and no prior history of thrombosis) and intermediate-risk (platelet count above 1,500,000/μL, asymptomatic, and no history of thrombosis) pregnant women can usually be managed by careful observation alone with or without low-dose aspirin. Aspirin is the most frequently used medication during pregnancy in patients with ET. A successful pregnancy retention and delivery rate of 75% has been reported in association with aspirin administration compared to 43% in untreated women.[121] Moderate-dose aspirin (325 mg/day or less) is preferred to minimize bleeding risks and to avoid increased blood loss during delivery. Some have advocated that aspirin be stopped at least 1 week prior to delivery and then resumed postpartum.[121,124]

For high-risk pregnancies or women anticipated to be at high risk when pregnant (any high platelet count associated with prior miscarriage, neurovascular symptoms, prior thrombosis, hypertension, smoking, obesity, etc.) low-dose aspirin use should be combined with aggressive reduction of platelet counts. Cytoreduction can be achieved effectively with interferon-alpha, which does not cross the placenta and is unlikely to be teratogenic. There have been no reported birth defects associated with interferon-alpha use during pregnancies complicated by ET or CML.[121,124–127] Nevertheless, the manufacturers advise against using it in pregnancy. The side effects of interferon-alpha may be quite difficult to tolerate during pregnancy and the cost is considerable.

Hydroxyurea has been used successfully and safely in pregnancy in patients with ET, CML, and sickle cell disease despite its theoretical teratogenicity. Its initiation is often delayed until the second trimester. Currently, anagrelide is avoided in pregnancy because of its potential to cause fetal hemorrhage and teratogenicity.[84] More experience is needed to establish the safety of anagrelide during pregnancy. This may be gained by monitoring the administration of anagrelide in pregnant women intolerant of interferon-alpha or hydroxyurea. Alkylating chemotherapeutic drugs like busulfan should not be prescribed because of their increased risks of teratogenicity, although they have been used safely during pregnancies occurring in association with Hodgkin disease and non-Hodgkin lymphomas. With these other options, there is no reason to administer ^{32}P for platelet reduction in ET pregnancies. Plateletpheresis decreases platelet counts rapidly and safely but its benefits are temporizing until a more permanent solution to the thrombocythemia is implemented.

Summary: Treatment Strategies for Essential Thrombocythemia

The treatment of ET should be individualized and based on stratification of risk and modified according to extenuating clinical circumstances (e.g., pregnancy). The treatment of high-risk individuals is very straightforward. Advising treatment of low- and intermediate-risk patients with ET is considerably more difficult because of a dearth of properly performed, adequately sized, randomized, controlled, prospective studies. In the United States, treatment of these individuals generally has been more aggressive than the available literature would support; however, this is in response to the numerous medical-legal claims that arise when one of these individuals develops a life-threatening or fatal thrombohemorrhagic event. These complications are very infrequent in low- and intermediate-risk patients and the risk : benefit ratio of cytoreductive therapies remains to be established.

■ REFERENCES

Chapter 17 References

1. Pearson TC. Diagnosis and classification of erythrocytosis and thrombocytosis. Baillieres Clin Haematol 1998;11:695–720.
2. Hsu H-C, Tsai W-H, Jiang M-L, et al. Circulating levels of thrombopoietin and inflammatory cytokines in patients with clonal and reactive thrombocytosis. J Lab Clin Med 1999;134:392–397.
3. Tefferi A, Ho TC, Ahmann CJ, et al. Plasma interleukin-6 and C-reactive protein levels in reactive versus clonal thrombocytosis. Am J Med 1994;97:374–378.
4. Haznedaroglu IC, Ertenli I, Ozcebe OI, et al. Megakaryocyte-related interleukins in reactive thrombocytosis versus autonomous thrombocythemia. Acta Haematol 1996;95:107–111.
5. Buss DH, Cashell AW, O'Connor ML, et al. Occurrence, etiology and clinical significance of extreme thrombocytosis: A study of 280 cases. Am J Med 1994;96:247–253.
6. Axelrad AA, Eskinazi D, Amato D. Hypersensitivity of circulating progenitor cells to megakaryocyte growth and development of factor (PEG-rHu MGDF) in essential thrombocythemia. Blood 1998;92(suppl 1):488a.

7. Epstein E, Goedel A. Hamorrhagische thrombozythamie bei vascularer schrumpfmilz. Virchows Archiv A [Pathol Anat Histopathol] 1934;292:233–248.
8. Hoffman R. Primary Thrombocythemia. In Hoffman R et al. (Eds.): Hematology: Basic Principles & Practice, 3rd Ed. New York, Churchill Livingstone, 2000, pp. 1188–1204.
9. Mesa RA, Tefferi A, Jacobsen SJ, et al. The incidence and epidemiology of essential thrombocythemia and agnogenic myeloid metaplasia: An Olmstead County Study. Blood 1997; 90(suppl 1):347a.
10. Jensen MK, deNully BP, Nielsen DJ, et al. Incidence, clinical features and outcome of essential thrombocythaemia in a well defined geographical area. Eur J Haematol 2000;65:132–139.
11. Fialkow PJ, Faguet GB, Jacobson RJ, et al. Evidence that essential thrombocythemia is a clonal disorder with origin in a multipotent stem cell. Blood 1981;58:916–919.
12. Briere J, el-Kassar N. Clonality markers in polycythaemia and primary thrombocythaemia. Bailliere's Clin Haematol. 1998; 11:787–801.
13. el-Kassar N, Hetet G, Briere J, et al. Clonality analysis of hematopoiesis in essential thrombocythaemia, advantages of studying T-lymphocytes and platelets. Blood 1997;89:129–134.
14. Harrison CN, Gale RE, Machin SJ, et al. A large proportion of patients with a diagnosis of essential thrombocythemia do not have a clonal disorder and may be at lower risk of thrombotic complications. Blood 1999;93:417–424.
15. Kaushansky K. Thrombopoietin. N Engl J Med 1998;339: 746–753.
16. Wang JC, Chen C, Novetsky AD, et al. Blood thrombopoietin levels in clonal thrombocytosis and reactive thrombocytosis. Am J Med 1998;104:451–455.
17. Horikawa Y, Matsuma I, Hashimoto K, et al. Markedly reduced expression of platelet c-mpl receptor in essential thrombocythemia. Blood 1997;90:4031–4038.
18. Kiladjian J, el-Kassar N, Hetet G, et al. Study of the thrombopoietin receptor in essential thrombocythemia. Leukemia 1997; 11:1821–1826.
19. Matsumura I, Horikawa Y, Kanakura Y. Functional roles of thrombopoietin C-mpl-system in essential thrombocythemia. Leukemia Lymphoma 1999;32:351–358.
20. Harrison CN, Gale RE, Pezella F, et al. Platelet c-mpl expression is dysregulated in patients with essential thrombocythaemia but this is not of diagnostic value. Br J Haematol 1999;107:139–147.
21. Espanol I, Hernandez A, Cortes M, et al. Patients with thrombocytosis have normal or slightly elevated thrombopoietin levels. Haematologica 1999;84:312–316.
22. Verbeek W, Faulhaber M, Griesinger F, et al. Measurement of thrombopoietin levels: Clinical and biologic relationships. Curr Opin Haemotol 2000;7:143–149.
23. Fickers M, Speck B. Thrombocythemia, familial occurrence and transition into blastic crisis. Acta Haemat 1974;51:257–265.
24. Eyster ME, Saletan SL, Rabellino EM, et al. Familial essential thrombocythemia. Am J Med 1986;80:497–502.
25. Kikuchi M, Tayama T, Hayakawa H, et al. Familial thrombocytosis. Br J Haematol 1995;89:900–902.
26. Schlemper RJ, Mass APC van der, Eikenboom JCJ, et al. Familial essential thrombocythemia: Clinical characteristics of 11 cases in one family. Ann Hematol 1994;68:153–158.
27. Janssen JWG, Anger BR, Drexler HG, et al. Essential thrombocythemia in two sisters originating from different stem cell levels. Blood 1990;75:1633–1636.
28. Weistner A, Schlemper RJ., Mass APC, et al. An activating splice donor mutation in the thrombopoietin gene causes hereditary thrombocythaemia. Nat Gene 1998;18:49–52.
29. Kondo T, Okabe M, Sanada M, et al. Familial essential thrombocythemia associated with one-base deletion in the 5'-untranslated region of the thrombopoietin gene. Blood 1998;92:1091–1096.
30. Ghilardi N, Wiestner A, Kikuchi M, et al. Hereditary thrombocythaemia in a Japanese family is caused by a novel mutation in the thrombopoietin gene. Br J Haematol 1999;107:310–316.
31. Kunishima S, Mizuno S, Naoe T, et al. Genes for thrombopoietin and c-MPL are not responsible for familial thrombocythaemia: a case study. Br J Haematol 1998;100:383–386.
32. Wiester A, Padosch SA, Ghilardi N. Hereditary thrombocythaemia is a genetically heterogeneous disorder: exclusion of TPO and mpl in two families with hereditary thrombocythaemia. Br J Haematol 2000;110:104–109.
33. Schafer AI. Bleeding and thrombosis in the myeloproliferative disorders. Blood 1984;64:1–12.
34. Michiels JJ. Acquired von-Willebrand disease due to increasing platelet count can readily explain the paradox of thrombosis and bleeding in thrombocythemia. Clin Appl Thromb Hemost 1999;59:147–151.
35. van Genderen PJJ, Budde V, Michiels JJ, et al. The reduction of large von-Willebrand factor multimers in plasma in essential thrombocythemia is related to the platelet count. Br J Haematol 1996;93:962–965.
36. Budde V, Saharf RE, Franke P, et al. Elevated platelet count as a cause of abnormal von-Willebrand factor multimer distribution in plasma. Blood 1993;82:1749–1757.
37. Zahavi J, Zahavi M, Firsteter E, et al. An abnormal pattern of multiple platelet function abnormalities and increased thromboxane generation in patients with primary thrombocytosis and thrombotic complications. Eur J Haematol 1991;47:326–332.
38. Griesshammer M, Beneke H, Nussbaumer B, et al. Increased platelet surface expression of P-selectin and thrombospondin as markers of platelet activation in essential thrombocythaemia. Thromb Res 1999;96:191–196.
39. Michiels JJ, van Genderen PJJ, Lindemans J, et al. Erythromelalgic, thrombotic and hemorrhagic manifestations of 50 cases of thrombocythemia. Leukemia Lymphoma 1996;22(suppl): 147–156.
40. Juvonen E, Ikkala E, Oksanen K, et al. Megakaryocyte and erythroid colony formation in essential thrombocythaemia and reactive thrombocytosis: diagnostic value and correlation to complication. Br J Haematol 1993;83:192–197.
41. Fenaux P, Simon M, Caulier T, et al. Clinical course of essential thrombocythaemia in 147 cases. Cancer 1990;66:549–556.
42. Bazzan M, Tamponi G, Schinco P, et al. Thrombosis free survival and life expectancy in 187 consecutive patients with essential thrombocythemia. Ann Hematol 1999;78:539–543.
43. Hehlmann R, Jahn M, Baumann B, et al. Essential thrombocythemia: Clinical characteristics and course of 61 cases. Cancer 1988;61:2487–2496.
44. Colombi M, Radaelli F, Zocchi L, et al. Thrombotic and hemorrhagic complications in essential thrombocythemia: a retrospective study of 103 patients. Cancer 1991;67:2926–2930.
45. Bellucci S, Janvier M, Tobelem G, et al. Essential thrombocythaemia: clinical evolutionary and biological data. Cancer 1986; 56:2440–2447.
46. Murphy S, Iland H, Rosenthal D, et al. Essential thrombocythemia: An interim report from the Polycythemia Vera Study Group. Semin Hematol 1986;23:177–182.
47. Murphy S. Diagnostic criteria and prognosis in polycythemia vera and essential thrombocythemia. Semin Hematol 1999;36(suppl 2):9–13.
48. van Genderen PJJ, Mulder PGH, Waleboer M, et al. Prevention and treatment of thrombotic complications in essential thrombocythaemia: efficacy and safety of aspirin. Br J Haematol 1997;97:179–184.
49. Gugliotta L, Marchioli R, Fiacchini M, et al. Epidemiological, diagnostic, therapeutic and prognostic aspects of essential thrombocythemia in a retrospective study of the GIMMC group in two thousand patients. Blood 1997;90(suppl 1):348a.
50. Tefferi A, Solberg LA, Silverstein MN. A clinical update in polycythemia vera and essential thrombocythemia. Am J Med 2000;109:141–149.

51. Gunz FW. Hemorrhagic thrombocythemia: A critical review. Blood 1960;15:706–723.
52. Silverstein MN. Primary or hemorrhagic thrombocythemia. Arch Intern Med 1968;122:18–22.
53. Cortelazzo S, Viero P, Finazzi G. Incidence and risk factors for thrombotic complications in a historical cohort of 100 patients with essential thrombocythemia. J Clin Oncol 1990;8:556–562.
54. Griesshammer M, Bangerter M, Van Vliet HHDM, et al. Aspirin in essential thrombocythemia: Status quo and quo vadis. Semin Thromb Hemost 1997;23:371–377.
55. Besses C, Cervantes F, Pereira A, et al. Major vascular complications in essential thrombocythemia: a study of the predictive factors in a series of 148 patients. Leukemia 1999;13:150–154.
56. Jabaily J, Iland HJ, Laszlo J, et al. Neurologic manifestations of essential thrombocythemia. Ann Intern Med 1983;99:513–518.
57. Michiels JJ, Koudstaal PJ, Mulder AH. Transient neurologic and ocular manifestations in primary thrombocythemia. Neurology 1993;43:1107–1110.
58. Ruggeri M, Finazzi G, Tosetto A, et al. No treatment for low risk thrombocythaemia: results from a prospective study. Br J Haematol 1998;103:772–777.
59. Tefferi A. Risk based management in essential thrombocythemia. ASH Education Program Book, Hematology 1999;172.
60. Lengfelder E, Hochhaus A, Kronawitter U, et al. Should a platelet limit of 600×10^9/L be used as a diagnostic criterion in essential thrombocythemia? An analysis of the natural course including early stages. Br J Haematol 1998;100:15–23.
61. Watson KV, Key N. Vascular complications of essential thrombocythaemia. Br J Haematol 1993;83:198–203.
62. Regev A, Stark P, Blickstein D, et al. Thrombotic complications in essential thrombocythemia with relatively low platelet counts. Am J Hematol 1997;56:168–172.
63. Murphy S, Peterson P, Iland H, et al. Experience of the Polycythemia Vera Study Group with essential thrombocythemia: A final report on diagnostic criteria, survival, and leukemic transition by treatment. Semin Hematol 1997;34:29–39.
64. Swolin B, Weinfeld A, Ridell B, et al. On the 5q- deletion: Clinical and cytogenetic observation in ten patients and review of literature. Blood 1981;58:986–993.
65. Howard MR, Ashwell S, Bond LR, et al. Artefactual serum hyperkalemia and hypercalcemia in essential thrombocythemia. J Clin Pathol 2000;53:105–109.
66. Andreasson B, Swolin B, Kutti J. Hydroxyurea treatment reduces haematopoietic progenitor growth and CD34 positive cells in polycythemia vera and essential thrombocythemia. Eur J Haematol 2000;64:188–193.
67. Barbui T, Finazzi G. Management of essential thrombocythemia. Crit Rev Oncol Hematol 1999;29:257–266.
68. Finazzi G, Barbui T. Treatment of essential thrombocythemia with special emphasis on leukemogenic risk. Ann Hematol 1999;78:389–392.
69. Löfvenberg E, Wahlin A. Management of polycythemia vera, essential thrombocythaemia and myelofibrosis with hydroxyurea. Eur J Haematol 1988;41:375–381.
70. Daoud MS, Gibson LE, Pittelkow MR. Hydroxyurea dermopathy: a unique lichenoid eruption complicating long term therapy with hydroxyurea. J Am Acad Dermatol 1997;36:178–182.
71. Best P, Daoud MS, Pittelkow MR, et al. Hydroxyurea induced leg ulceration in 14 patients. Ann Intern Med 1998;128:29–32.
72. Starmans-Kool MSF, Fickers MMF, Pannebakker MAG. An unwanted side-effect of hydroxyurea in a patient with idiopathic myelofibrosis. Ann Hematol 1995;70:279–280.
73. Cortelazzo S, Finazzi G, Ruggeri M, et al. Hydroxyurea for patients with essential thrombocythaemia and a high risk of thrombosis. N Engl J Med 1995;332:1132–1136.
74. Finazzi G, Ruggeri M, Rodeghiero F, et al. Second malignancies in patients with essential thrombocythaemia treated with busulphan and hydroxyurea: Long term follow up of a randomized clinical trial. Br J Haematol 2000;110:577–583.
75. Sterkers Y, Preudhomme C, Laï J-L, et al. Acute myeloid leukemia and myelodysplastic syndromes following essential thrombocythemia treated with hydroxyurea: High proportion of cases with 17p deletion. Blood 1998;91:616–622.
76. Randi ML, Fabris F, Girolami A. Leukemia and myelodysplasia effect of multiple cytotoxic therapy in essential thrombocythemia. Leukemia Lymphoma 2000;37:379–385.
77. Nand S, Stock W, Godwin J, et al. Leukemogenic risk of hydroxyurea therapy in polycythemia vera, essential thrombocythemia and myeloid metaplasia with myelofibrosis. Am J Hematol 1996;52:42–46.
78. Liozon E, Brigaudeau C, Trimoreau F, et al. Is treatment with hydroxyurea leukemogenic in patients with essential thrombocythemia? An analysis of three new cases of leukaemia transformation and review of the literature. Hematol Cell Therapy 1997;39:11–18.
79. Silverstein MN, Petitt RM, Solberg LA, et al. Anagrelide: a new drug for treating thrombocytosis. N Engl J Med 1988;318:1292–1294.
80. Anagrelide Study Group. Anagrelide, a therapy for thrombocythemic states: experience in 577 patients. Am J Med 1992;92:69–76.
81. Mazur EM, Rosmarin AG, Sohl PA, et al. Analysis of the mechanism of anagrelide induced thrombocytopenia in humans. Blood 1992;79:1931–1937.
82. Solberg LA, Tefferi A, Oles KJ, et al. The effects of anagrelide on human megakaryocytopoiesis. Br J Haematol 1997;99:174–180.
83. Spencer CM, Brogden RN. Anagrelide: a review of its pharmacodynamic and pharmacokinetic properties and therapeutic potential in the treatment of thrombocythaemia. Drugs 1994;47:809–822.
84. Petitt RM, Silverstein MN, Petrone ME. Anagrelide for control of thrombocythemia in polycythemia and other myeloproliferative disorders. Semin Hematol 1997;34:51–54.
85. Elliott MA, Tefferi A. Interferon-α therapy in polycythemia vera and essential thrombocythemia. Semin Thromb Hemost 1997;23:463–472.
86. Sacchi S. The role of α-interferon in essential thrombocythaemia, polycythaemia vera and myelofibrosis with myeloid metaplasia (MMM): a concise update. Leukemia Lymphoma 1995;19:13–20.
87. Giles FJ. Maintenance therapy in the myeloproliferative disorders: the current options. Br J Haematol 1991;79(suppl 1):92–95.
88. Sacchi S, Tabilio A, Leoni P, et al. Interferon alpha-2b in the long-term treatment of essential thrombocythemia. Ann Hematol 1991;63:206–209.
89. Sacchi S, Tabilio A, Leoni P, et al. Sustained complete hematological remission in essential thrombocythemia after discontinuation of long-term α-IFN treatment. Ann Hematol 1993;66:245–246.
90. Kasparu H, Bernhart M, Krieger O, et al. Remission may continue after termination of rIFNα-2b treatment for essential thrombocythemia. Eur J Haemotol 1992;48:33–36.
91. Bentley M, Taylor K, Grigg A, et al. Long-term interferon-alpha 2A does not induce sustained hematologic remission in younger patients with essential thrombocythemia. Leukemia Lymphoma 1999;36:123–128.
92. Gisslinger H, Linkesch W, Fritz E, et al. Long-term interferon therapy for thrombocytosis in myeloproliferative diseases. Lancet 1989;634–637.
93. Middelhoff G, Boll I. A long-term clinical trial of interferon alpha therapy in essential thrombocythemia. Ann Hematol 1992;64:207–209.
94. Pogliani EM, Rossini F, Miccolis I, et al. Alpha interferon as initial treatment of essential thrombocythemia, An analysis after two years of follow up. Tumori 1995;81:245–248.

95. Rametta V, Ferrara F, Marottoli V, et al. Recombinant interferon alpha-2b as treatment of essential thrombocythemia. Acta Haematol 1994;91:126–129.
96. Gisslinger H, Chott A, Scheithauer W, et al. Interferon in essential thrombocythaemia. Br J Haematol 1991;79(suppl 1):42–47.
97. Gauser A, Carlo-Stella C, Greher J, et al. Effect of recombinant interferons alpha and gamma on human bone marrow derived megakaryocytic progenitor cells. Blood 1987;70:1173–1179.
98. Broxmeyer HE, Lu L, Platzer E, et al. Comparative analysis of the influences of human gamma, alpha and beta interferons on human multipotential (CFU-GEMM), erythroid (BFU-E) and granulocyte-macrophage (CFU-GM) progenitor cells. J Immunol 1983;131:1300–1305.
99. Carlo-Stella C, Cazzola M, Gasner A, et al. Effects of recombinant alpha and gamma interferons on the in-vitro growth of circulating hematopoietic progenitor cells (CFU-GEMM, CFU-MK, BFU-E and CFU-GM) from patients with myelofibrosis with myeloid metaplasia. Blood 1987;70:1014–1019.
100. Gugliotta L, Bagnara GP, Catani L, et al. In vivo and in vitro inhibitory effect of α-interferon on megakaryocyte colony growth in essential thrombocythemia. Br J Haematol 1989;71:177–181.
101. Wadenvik H, Kutti J, Ridell B, et al. The effect of α-interferon on bone marrow megakaryocytes and platelet production rate in essential thrombocythemia. Blood 1991;77:2103–2108.
102. Waysbort A, Giroux M, Mansat V, et al. Experimental study of transplacental passage of alpha interferon by two assay techniques. J Antimicro Chemother 1993;37:1232–1237.
103. Sacchi S, Gugliotta L, Papineschi F, et al. Alfa-interferon in the treatment of essential thrombocythemia: clinical results and evaluation of its biological effects on the hematopoietic neoplastic clone. Leukemia 1998;12:289–294.
104. Lengfelder E, Griesshammer M, Hehlmann R, et al. Interferon-alpha in the treatment of essential thrombocythemia. Leukemia Lymphoma 1996;22(suppl 1):135–142.
105. Törnebohm-Roche E, Merup M, Lockner D, et al. α-2a interferon therapy and antibody formation in patients with essential thrombocythemia and polycythemia vera with thrombocytosis. Am J Hematol 1994;48:163–167.
106. Berk PD, Goldberg JD, Silverstein MN. Increased incidence of acute leukemia in polycythemia vera associated with chlorambucil therapy. N Engl J Med 1981;304:441–447.
107. Najean Y, Rain J. The very long-term evolution of polycythemia vera: an analysis of 318 patients initially treated by phlebotomy or ^{32}P between 1969 and 1981. Semin Hematol 1997;34:6–16.
108. Van De Pette JEW, Prochazka AV, Pearson TC, et al. Primary thrombocythaemia treated with busulphan. Br J Haematol 1986;62:229–237.
109. "Leukemia and Hematosarcoma" Cooperative Group. European organization for research on treatment of cancer (E.O.R.T.C): Treatment of polycythemia vera by radiophosphorus or busulphan: A randomized trial. Br J Cancer 1981;44:75–80.
110. Brandt L, Anderson H. Survival and risk of leukaemia in polycythaemia vera and essential thrombocythaemia treated with oral radiophosphorus: Are safer drugs available? Eur J Haematol 1995;54:21–26.
111. Balan KK, Critchley M. Outcome of 259 patients with primary proliferative polycythaemia (PPP) and idiopathic thrombocythaemia (IT) treated in a regional nuclear medicine department with phosphorus-32, a 15 year review. Br J Radiology 1997;70:1169–1173.
112. Council on drugs. Evaluation of two antineoplastic agents: Pipobroman (Vercyte) and Thioguanine. JAMA 1967;200:139–140.
113. Najean Y, Rain Jean-Didier. Treatment of polycythemia vera: The use of hydroxyurea and pipobroman in 292 patients under the age of 65 years. Blood 1997;90:3370–3377.
114. Messora C, Bensi L, Vanzanelli P, et al. Myelodysplastic transformation in a case of essential thrombocythemia treated with pipobroman: Haematologica 1996;81:51–53.
115. Mazzucconi MG, Francesconi M, Chistolini A, et al. Pipobroman therapy of essential thrombocythemia. Scand J Haematol 1986;37:306–309.
116. Brusamolino E, Canevari A, Salvaneschi L. Efficacy trial of pipobroman in essential thrombocythemia: A study of 24 patients. Cancer Treatm Rep 1984;68:1339–1342.
117. Michiels JJ. Aspirin and platelet-lowering agents for the prevention of vascular complications in essential thrombocythemia. Clin Appl Thromb Hemost 1999;5:247–251.
118. Taft EG, Babcock RB, Scharfman WB, et al. Plateletpheresis in the management of thrombocytosis. Blood 1977;50:927–933.
119. Goldfinger D, Thompson R, Lowe C, et al. Long-term plateletpheresis in the management of primary thrombocytosis. Transfusion 1979;19:336–338.
120. Baron BW, Mick R, Baron JM. Combined plateletpheresis and cytotoxic chemotherapy for symptomatic thrombocytosis in myeloproliferative disorders. Cancer 1993;72:1209–1218.
121. Griesshammer M, Heimpel H, Pearson TC. Essential thrombocythemia and pregnancy. Leukemia Lymphoma 1996;22(Suppl 1):157–163.
122. Beressi AH, Tefferi A, Silverstein MN, et al. Outcome analysis of 34 pregnancies in women with essential thrombocythemia. Arch Intern Med 1995;155:1217–1222.
123. Samuelsson J, Swolin B. Spontaneous remission during two pregnancies in a patient with essential thrombocythaemia. Leukemia Lymphoma 1997;25:597–600.
124. Eliyahn S, Shalev E. Essential thrombocythemia during pregnancy. Obstet Gynecol Surv 1997;52:243–247.
125. Milano V, Gabrielli S, Rizzo N, et al. Successful treatment of essential thrombocythaemia in a pregnancy with recombinant interferon-α2a. J Maternal-Fetal Med 1996;5:74–78.
126. Pardini S, Careddu MF, Dore F, et al. Essential thrombocythemia and pregnancy. Haematologica 1995;80:392–393.
127. Delage R, Demers C, Cantine G. Treatment of essential thrombocythemia during pregnancy with interferon-α. Obstet Gynecol 1996;87:814–817.

CHAPTER 18

The Antiphospholipid Syndrome: Clinical Presentation, Diagnosis, and Patient Management

Barbara M. Alving, M.D.

INTRODUCTION AND HISTORICAL COMMENTS

Antibodies to phospholipid binding proteins, or antiphospholipid-protein antibodies (APA), were first described more than 50 years ago as "circulating anticoagulants" because of their interference in phospholipid-dependent assays.[1-3] Since they were often detected in patients with underlying systemic lupus erythematosus (SLE), they became known as *lupus anticoagulants* (LA), a misnomer that persists to the present time. Forty years ago Bowie and colleagues recognized their association with thrombotic events in patients with SLE.[4] In the decades following this report, the association of thrombosis, fetal loss, or thrombocytopenia with APA became known as the *antiphospholipid syndrome*.[5] During the past 20 years sensitive tests for antibody detection have become available,[6] and in the last 10 years the phospholipid-binding proteins that serve as antigens for these antibodies have been identified.[7-9]

The development of tests for APA has resulted in several different terms that are frequently used to define their activities (Table 18–1). Individuals may have IgG, IgM, or even IgA APA, although measurements for the latter isotype have not been well standardized. Approximately 90% of patients testing positive for LA also have anticardiolipin antibody (ACA) activity.[10] However, there is no direct correlation between the potency of the LA activity and the concentration of the ACA, which may reflect the heterogeneity of the APA.[5,10,11] Despite the difficulties in comparing studies in which only a test for LA or only an enzyme-linked immunosorbent assay (ELISA) has been utilized, associations between well-defined clinical problems and the presence of APA have emerged. This chapter will describe the clinical presentation of patients with the antiphospholipid syndrome, the appropriate laboratory testing, and patient management.

ANTIPHOSPHOLIPID SYNDROME: OVERVIEW OF CLINICAL MANIFESTATIONS

The antiphospholipid syndrome should be considered in patients, particularly those who are younger, presenting with one or more of the following clinical conditions: venous thrombosis, arterial thrombosis (stroke, myocardial infarction), or recurrent pregnancy loss.[12,13] Associated conditions include thrombocytopenia, vasculitic rashes, arthralgias, dermal necrosis of digits, livedo reticularis (see Color Plate 11-20), and pulmonary hypertension.[14] The diagnosis is confirmed if the patient also tests positive for autoantibodies that are detected in phospholipid-dependent clotting assays as LA or as ACA in ELISAs that contain cardiolipin along with β_2-glycoprotein I (β_2-GPI). Patients should be tested with both types of assay (immunologic and clot-based) and more than one test for LA is needed to rule out the diagnosis of antiphospholipid syndrome in a patient with a clinical presentation consistent with this disorder. The tests should be positive for LA or for moderate to high levels of ACA (IgG or IgM) on two occasions at least 6 weeks apart (Table 18–2).[13] The requirement for sustained positivity for APA is given because results may

Table 18-1 • COMMON TERMS FOR ANTIPHOSPHOLIPID ANTIBODIES

Antiphospholipid syndrome: Characterized by venous or arterial thrombosis, thrombocytopenia, and recurrent fetal loss in association with antiphospholipid-protein antibodies.
Antiphospholipid-protein antibodies (APA) or antiphospholipid antibodies: IgG, IgM, or IgA antibodies that are directed against proteins such as prothrombin or β_2-glycoprotein I (β_2-GPI) that bind to phospholipids. APA are described as lupus anticoagulants (LA) or anticardiolipin antibodies (ACA) according to the assay procedure used for their detection.
Lupus anticoagulant (LA): Antibody against a phospholipid-binding protein such as prothrombin or β_2-GPI that induces prolongation of a phospholipid-dependent clotting assay.
Anticardiolipin antibodies (ACA): Antibodies against β_2-GPI that have been detected in an ELISA containing cardiolipin as the phospholipid that binds β_2-GPI (which is present in the assay).

---

be positive only transiently and unrelated to clinical symptoms.[15]

In the absence of SLE or other autoimmune connective tissue disorders, the syndrome is considered as a *primary antiphospholipid syndrome* and is twice as common in women as in men. Many patients with primary antiphospholipid syndrome do not develop any signs of SLE with time.

The syndrome is known as a *secondary antiphospholipid syndrome* if it occurs in patients who have another autoimmune connective tissue disorder. In this patient group, the female:male ratio for development of the antiphospholipid syndrome is 9:1, which is the same gender ratio as that for SLE. An initial study in patients with SLE indicated that 61% had elevated levels of ACA antibodies of at least one isotype and 49% had detectable LA.[6] The overlap between LA and ACA was quite significant since ACA levels were increased in 91% of the patients who tested positive for LA. Subsequent prospective[16] and retrospective analyses have confirmed that LA and ACA antibodies are detectable in approximately 50% of patients with SLE. Patients with SLE who have a persistent elevation of ACA will have a significantly increased odds ratio (5.4) for a peripheral thromboembolic event compared to those who test positive for APA on only one occasion.[16]

NEUROLOGIC MANIFESTATIONS OF THE ANTIPHOSPHOLIPID SYNDROME

Neurologic manifestations of the antiphospholipid syndrome include single or recurrent cerebral infarcts, severe vascular headaches, transient ischemic attacks, and visual disturbances (Table 18-3).[17] Recurrent strokes are more likely in patients with the antiphospholipid syndrome who also have hypertension or other risk factors for cerebrovascular disease, such as cigarette smoking and hyperlipidemia.[17] As many as 80% of patients with the primary antiphospholipid syndrome have at least one of these additional risk factors. Cerebral angiography performed on such patients shows large-vessel occlusion or stenosis without evidence of vasculitis.

In one prospective study, 18% of young adults (ages 15 to 44 years) who had sustained ischemic stroke or transient ischemic attacks tested positive for ACA.[18] The patients with ACA had a higher probability of recurrent events than those who did not have the antibody.

In the older population, one large study shows no association between stroke and the presence of ACA. In a nested case-controlled study of men in the Physicians' Health Study, composed of men ages 40 to 84 years, the IgG ACA in 61 participants with ischemic stroke were not significantly different from those of controls ($p > 0.2$) and there was no evidence of increased risk for stroke in those with higher APA levels.[19] In a recent large prospective case-controlled study that included Caucasians, African Americans, and Hispanic patients, APA antibodies were found to be an independent stroke risk factor in all groups, causing a four-fold increase in the risk for ischemic stroke.[20] Although this area has not yet been clarified, the data suggest that for patients who have transient ischemic attacks at a young age or for those who have these events in association with other features of the antiphospholipid syndrome, testing for ACA and LA appears to be warranted. However, indis-

---

Table 18-2 • INDICATIONS FOR TESTING FOR THE ANTIPHOSPHOLIPID SYNDROME

Clinical
Venous thromboembolism (deep venous thrombosis, pulmonary embolism, and thrombosis in less common sites)
Peripheral arterial thrombosis
Myocardial infarction
Stroke or transient ischemic attacks (usually <55 years of age)
Recurrent fetal loss
Laboratory Confirmation[a]
Moderate to high positive anticardiolipin antibody titer (ACA IgG or IgM), or
Positive LA

[a] These tests must be positive on two occasions separated by at least 6 weeks.

Table 18-3 • NEUROLOGIC MANIFESTATIONS OF THE ANTIPHOSPHOLIPID SYNDROME

- One or more episodes of the following occurring in individuals at a relatively young age (<55 years):
  Vascular dementia
  Cerebral infarction
  Transient ischemic attack
  Amaurosis fugax
  Retinal infarction
  Myelopathy
  Acute ischemic encephalopathy
- Sneddon syndrome: progressive dementia and livedo reticularis

criminate testing of a general patient population with cerebrovascular events may not be indicated.

FETAL LOSS AND THE ANTIPHOSPHOLIPID SYNDROME

Many issues remain in the recognition and management of women with the antiphospholipid syndrome and fetal loss (see also Chapter 29). These include defining the criteria for the syndrome in pregnancy. Branch and Silver[21] have proposed that a pregnancy loss and fetal loss be accepted as criteria for APA if a woman who tests positive for LA or for IgG ACA (20 GPL units or more) has experienced: (a) one or more fetal deaths 10 weeks gestation or beyond with normal fetal morphology, (b) loss of one or more normal neonates due to complications of prematurity because of pre-eclampsia or severe placental insufficiency, or (c) three or more pre-embryonic or embryonic (less than 10 weeks gestation) losses with exclusion of other causes (genetic, anatomic, hormonal). With these definitions in mind, the clinician can more easily identify the possibility of the antiphospholipid syndrome in a woman who presents with a history of fetal loss.

Based on several small randomized studies, the treatment of choice for women with previous fetal loss and ACA is heparin at a dose of 5000 units subcutaneously twice daily[22] or a dose sufficient to prolong the aPTT to the upper range of normal (approximately 8000 units twice daily)[23,24] combined with aspirin (80 mg daily). The regimen of heparin combined with aspirin has resulted in a 70% to 80% fetal survival compared to 40% for women taking aspirin alone.[25] Prednisone is not indicated and is associated with maternal hypertension, weight gain, and diabetes.[25] The role of low-molecular-weight heparin (LMWH) in the treatment of the antiphospholipid syndrome has not been defined in any randomized clinical trials. A recent meta-analysis suggests that it may well be an acceptable substitute for unfractionated heparin in doses of 75 to 150 antifactor Xa units/kg/day.[26] Heparin use in pregnancy (both unfractionated and LMWH) is associated with loss of bone density that may or may not be symptomatic. Women receiving heparin for previous fetal loss due to APA should be supplemented with calcium, and heparin does not need to be initiated until the fifth to sixth week of pregnancy. A woman who has received anticoagulant therapy during pregnancy for the antiphospholipid syndrome should probably continue treatment for months postpartum. In the postpartum period, warfarin instead of heparin can be used, and the mother may nurse her infant since warfarin is not present in breast milk.

Pregnancy may cause changes in the pharmacokinetics of unfractionated and perhaps also LMWH and therefore monitoring antifactor Xa activity may be appropriate for some high-risk women.[27] Furthermore, larger trials are needed to define more clearly the optimum degree of anticoagulation with minimum side effects in pregnant women with APA. Until controlled studies can be done, clinical decisions will be made on the basis of outcomes derived from small clinical studies.[28]

The pathophysiology of fetal loss in the antiphospholipid syndrome is not completely understood. However, recent studies have focused on annexin V, a protein that is synthesized by placental trophoblasts and clusters on placental villous surfaces. Annexin V is postulated to prevent thrombosis by shielding the underlying phospholipids on the villi from contact with the flowing blood. Placentas from women with the antiphospholipid syndrome and pregnancy losses have reduced annexin V immunostaining on the villous surfaces, suggesting that these surfaces, with their exposed phospholipids, can promote thrombosis.[29] This is also suggested by the finding that in the presence of APA, endothelial cells and cultured primary trophoblasts have reduced annexin V and reduced anticoagulant activity.[30] The current hypothesis is that the binding of the APA to phospholipid–protein complexes may displace the annexin V on the placental surfaces, thus disrupting the antithrombotic "shield" and allowing exposed anionic phospholipids to serve as surfaces for promoting procoagulant activity.[31]

THROMBOCYTOPENIA AND THE ANTIPHOSPHOLIPID SYNDROME

A significant correlation between IgG ACA and thrombocytopenia has been reported in several studies. In one report of patients with thrombocytopenia and SLE (or related autoimmune disorders), 72% had increased levels of IgG ACA and in 44% levels of IgM ACA were increased.[32] In a similar patient group that did not have thrombocytopenia, increases in antibody levels were present in 38% (IgG ACA) and 20% (IgM ACA).[32] The association between either isotype and thrombocytopenia was significant.

In patients with idiopathic autoimmune thrombocytopenia (ITP) in the absence of other autoimmune disease, elevated levels of IgG and IgM ACA were present in 15% and 28%, respectively.[33] There was no correlation between levels of either isotype and levels of platelet-associated immunoglobulin. Others have found positivity for APA in as many as 46% of patients with ITP.[34] The presence of APA does not appear to affect outcome. In most patients with ITP and APA who have resolution of thrombocytopenia with prednisone, the titers of APA have remained elevated.

APA AND CARDIAC VALVE DYSFUNCTION

An increased incidence of cardiac valvular lesions and myocardial dysfunction occurs in patients with SLE and APA as well as in patients who have the primary antiphospholipid syndrome.[35–39] The valvular abnormalities include bland verrucous endocardial lesions composed of leukocytes, plasma cells, fibrous tissue, fibrin, and platelets. The lesions, which appear as small clusters, frequently affect the edges of the mitral valves and may produce no symptoms or cause valvular insufficiency or stenosis.[35-42]

Prospective studies utilizing two-dimensional echocardiography to detect cardiac abnormalities in patients with SLE have found a significant association between elevated APA and valvular lesions. The incidence of valvular disease was 40% in SLE patients with elevated APA compared to 12% to 14% in SLE patients without detectable antibodies.[36,37] At least half of the patients with cardiac lesions had other features of the antiphospholipid syndrome.[35] Serial studies in these patients indicated that hemodynamically significant cardiac valvular disease can develop with time[37] and that these patients may be at increased risk for cerebroembolic events.[43,44] Intramural cardiac thrombosis occurs rarely.[45] The studies suggest that all patients with SLE or patients with the antiphospholipid syndrome should undergo echocardiography.[39] Patients with asymptomatic vegetations should receive antibiotic prophylaxis before dental or surgical work; however, anticoagulation does not appear to be routinely indicated.[39]

APA have also been associated with myocardial vasculopathy that is sufficiently severe to induce myocardial infarction even in the presence of normal coronary arteries.[41] However, in a cohort study of the survivors of myocardial infarction divided into those younger or older than 51 years of age, ACA (measured as both the IgG and IgM isotypes) was not an independent risk factor for overall mortality, reinfarction, or thrombotic stroke.[43] The multivariate analysis was adjusted for age and HDL-cholesterol.

ASSOCIATION OF LA WITH PROTHROMBIN DEFICIENCY

Patients who have LA may have a slight prolongation of the prothrombin time (PT) depending on the sensitivity of the thromboplastin reagent. However, patients who have a significant prolongation of the PT (greater than 2 to 3 seconds above the upper limit of normal) should be evaluated for a true acquired deficiency of factor II (prothrombin). In one study of patients with LA and SLE or other autoimmune connective tissue disorders, the majority had IgG antibodies to prothrombin, although only 30% of patients with antibodies had a detectable prothrombin deficiency.[46] Prothrombin deficiency, when it does occur in patients with LA, appears to be due to the binding of the antibody to prothrombin in vivo, which results in increased clearance.

An acquired deficiency of prothrombin with clinical symptoms of bleeding may be the presenting feature in a patient who will later develop other manifestations of the antiphospholipid syndrome (and possibly SLE as well). Autoimmune-based prothrombin deficiency may also be suspected in a patient who is receiving warfarin as treatment for thrombotic complications of the antiphospholipid syndrome and who develops a gradually increasing international normalized ratio (INR) for no apparent reason. Evaluation includes measurement of the coagulation factor levels (II, V, VII, and X) of the extrinsic system.

The antibody production can usually be easily suppressed by administration of corticosteroids and azathioprine, as was demonstrated in one patient in whom the PT was normal 7 days after initiation of treatment.[47] In another study, the use of corticosteroids alone increased the prothrombin level even while the prothrombin–antibody complexes were still detectable.[48] If a patient is actively bleeding, treatment with fresh frozen plasma or prothrombin complex concentrates may be required.

Antibodies to prothrombin can also be detected in patients who have infections and LA. At least eight cases of LA and clinically significant hypoprothrombinemia have occurred in children under the age of 17 years in association with a viral illness.[49] In these cases, the diagnosis was established because of clinical symptoms that improved as the antibody spontaneously disappeared. Immunosuppression may be required in special circumstances. For example, in one report, a patient with severe hypoprothrombinemia and gastrointestinal hemorrhage was treated successfully with intravenous methylprednisolone followed by prednisone.[50]

LA AS A LABORATORY ABNORMALITY

LA are frequently found in patients hospitalized for a wide variety of disorders and are the most common cause of an unexplained prolongation of the aPTT in this population.[51] Patients who have LA or ACA in association with underlying infections or with use of medications are generally not at increased risk for thrombosis and do not require anticoagulation on the basis of this laboratory finding.[52-54] Conditions associated with LA include carcinoma, autoimmune disorders such as rheumatoid arthritis[55] and Sjögren syndrome, infection,[56-58] and use of drugs such as procainamide, hydralazine, chlorpromazine, quinidine, isoniazid, and methyldopa, which have also all been associated with the development of SLE.[52,53,59-62] Although thromboembolic events have been described in several patients who developed LA in association with procainamide,[54,63,64] the incidence of such events appears to be extremely low.[60,61,64] LA activity, which can be associated with the IgG or IgM isotype,[61] may be detected for months after the procainamide has been discontinued.[65]

APA (detected as LA or in ELISAs) develop in approximately 40% of patients who receive chlorpromazine[53,59] and may occur as early as 3 months after the initiation of treatment.[53] One group reported that phenothiazines other than chlorpromazine did not induce LA; however, LA that occurred in patients on chlorpromazine persisted when the patients were switched to other phenothiazines.[53] Other investigators have found APA in 27% of patients receiving phenothiazines other than chlorpromazine.[59]

Patients may have APA detected as LA only or as ACA, which is usually of the IgM isotype.[52,59] Additional frequent immunologic abnormalities include positive tests for antinuclear antibodies (ANA)[53,66] and antibodies to native DNA.[66] It is unlikely that LA positivity is a risk factor for thrombosis in these patients. Of 110 patients receiving phenothiazines who had either LA or ACA, only 3% had a history of thrombosis.[52,53,59]

LA are frequently associated with bacterial infections. Elevated levels of ACA have also been measured in patients with human immunodeficiency virus infections,[67] Lyme disease,[68] ornithosis, adenovirus, rubella, and chicken pox, as well as in those who have undergone vaccination against smallpox[69] or who have syphilis. The presence of LA does not increase the risk for thrombosis in these patients. In a recent study,[70] sera from 114 patients with infections (syphilis, tuberculosis, and *Klebsiella* infection) were tested for IgG antibodies against β_2-GPI and cardiolipin. All patients tested negative for antibodies to β_2-GPI; the incidence of ACA in these patients according to their underlying infections was as follows: tuberculosis, 6%: *Klebsiella* infection, 5%; and syphilis, 64%.

IMMUNOLOGY AND PATHOPHYSIOLOGY OF APA

Although APA are frequently directed against β_2-GPI and also prothrombin,[71,72] protein S and protein C may also be antigens. β_2-GPI is a 50-kDa proline-rich glycoprotein that can bind to negatively charged domains on lipoproteins, heparin, and platelets. β_2-GPI at concentrations as low as 1 μg/mL displays cofactor activity in an ELISA[7,8] and normal plasma values are 200 μg/mL. APA can recognize β_2-GPI in the absence of phospholipid if the protein is coated onto an oxygen-modified polystyrene surface.[73] Galli and coworkers have described APA as antibodies that recognize the human prothrombin–phospholipid complex and thus have LA activity only or as ACA that are directed against β_2-GPI on an anionic surface.[71,72]

Arnout has postulated that the pathogenesis of the antiphospholipid syndrome is very similar to that of heparin-induced thrombocytopenia since in both settings antibodies are directed against a protein complexed with either a polysaccharide or a phospholipid that is localized on a cell surface.[74] The Fc portion of the antibody can then activate platelets through the FcII receptors. In both syndromes, initial vascular damage appears to be an integral part of the thrombotic process, which results in venous and/or arterial thrombosis. In both settings, a double hit such as vascular injury and immune complex formation is needed. Greaves and coworkers have suggested that anti-endothelial cell antibodies, which are a common aspect of the antiphospholipid syndrome, may cause endothelial injury, thereby inducing tissue factor production and exposure of membrane phospholipid.[75] Circulating β_2-GPI could then bind to the phospholipid and the APA could in turn bind to the complex, inducing further damage.[75] Other investigators have shown that APA can also recognize heparin or heparin bound to β_2-GPI, thus inhibiting the interaction of heparin with antithrombin III.[76–78] None of these theories has gained broad acceptance. It is possible that APA are markers for other antibodies or processes that promote thrombosis. Several in-vitro studies have suggested that APA promote thrombosis by inhibiting the ability of protein C to inactivate factors Va and VIIIa.[79–81]

At least two groups have reported that APA can bind directly to circulating platelets without inducing platelet activation or aggregation.[82,83] Others have shown that APA can bind to activated platelets, although the binding does not affect the release reaction or aggregation.[84] Most human hybridoma LA do not bind to resting platelets in vitro.[85] Galli and coworkers reported that 40% of patients with the antiphospholipid syndrome and thrombocytopenia had antibodies against GPIIb/IIIa and/or GPIb/IX and that APA did not bind to resting platelets.[86]

ELISA FOR APA (CARDIOLIPIN ASSAY)

The assay is designed to measure the level of APA in patient sera in a quantitative fashion, utilizing microtiter plates coated with cardiolipin or another negatively charged phospholipid and containing β_2-GPI.[6,87–88] After an incubation period, the plates are washed and the antibodies are detected by labeled antihuman IgG or IgM. Test results are expressed in units of MPL or GPL (1 MPL is equal to 1 μg of IgM APA and 1 GPL is equal to 1 μg of IgG APA). The antibody concentrations are described qualitatively as high positive, moderately positive, low positive, or negative. For example, samples with less than 10 GPL or less than 10 MPL U/mL are considered negative.[89–91] The concordance among laboratories for high positive and negative IgG and IgM ACA is 90%; for medium and low positive results, the agreement is greater than 75%.[92] Although elevated IgA ACA levels have been reported in association with thrombosis, the quantitation is undergoing standardization and the clinical significance has yet to be defined.

TESTING FOR LA

LA is the designation given to APA that prolong the clotting time of phospholipid-dependent coagulation assays by blocking the binding of coagulation factors to the acidic phospholipid surfaces or by enhancing the binding of β_2-GPI to the procoagulant phospholipid surface (Table 18–4).[72,93] The assays involve dilution of the phospholipid to increase the ability to detect the antibody or increasing the concentration of the phospholipid to "normalize" the test result and to provide confirmation of LA.

LA are usually sufficiently potent to cause a prolongation of the activated partial thromboplastin time (aPTT). However, LA can be present even in plasmas that have a normal aPTT. Therefore, the presence or absence of LA is determined on the basis of performing specific tests that utilize phospholipid dilution to increase the sensitivity (Table 18–5).

An international standardization committee has recommended that more than one assay method be per-

Table 18-4 • INDICATIONS FOR TESTING FOR LUPUS ANTICOAGULANTS

- Patient suspected of having antiphospholipid syndrome:
  Perform at least two different assays for LA even if screening aPTT is normal.[a] (Also perform ELISA for ACA.)
- Evaluation of a prolonged aPTT, which is an incidental finding (no clinical suspicion for antiphospholipid syndrome)[b]:
  Confirm presence of LA if mixing studies suggest inhibitor and perform appropriate coagulation factor assays to establish factor levels. (No further evaluation if patient has no history suggestive of APA: that is, do not perform ELISA for ACA.)

[a] LA assays are based on phospholipid dilution and can therefore be positive in the presence of a normal aPTT.
[b] A positive test for LA is one of the most common reasons for a prolonged aPTT and is usually due to underlying infection or use of drugs such as phenothizines or procainamide.

formed to verify the presence of an LA.[94] In one study, the detection of LA increased from 73% with one test to 90% with two tests.[95] Phospholipid dilution assays are currently used for the detection of LA, especially in patients with an aPTT that is normal or only minimally prolonged. Perhaps the most sensitive test for LA is the kaolin clotting time, which relies only on the phospholipid in the plasma. Assays that are performed with dilution of phospholipid include the dilute Russell viper venom time (dRVVT)[96,97] and the dilute phospholipid aPTT,[98] both of which utilize only a single dilution of phospholipid. The dRVVT is a phospholipid dilution assay in which Russell viper venom, an activator of factor X, is used to initiate coagulation in the presence of phospholipid and calcium.[96] One laboratory reported a sensitivity and specificity of 97% and 100%, respectively, in detecting LA when two tests were utilized (the dRVVT and the dilute aPTT-LA [American Bioproducts, Parsippany, NJ]).[97]

The thromboplastin inhibition assay is simply a PT performed with a dilution of the thromboplastin reagent. It has been modified to provide increased sensitivity, although this has resulted in false-positive results in the presence of heparin. The dilute prothrombin time has gained increased sensitivity when a recombinant tissue thromboplastin has been used (Innovin, Baxter Diagnostics, Miami, FL).[99]

A newer assay based on a ratio of the clotting times of patient plasma obtained with the venom textarin to that of the venom ecarin has recently been developed.[100] Textarin activates prothrombin in a phospholipid-dependent fashion, whereas ecarin does not require phospholipid. Thus the ratio of the clotting times with textarin and ecarin will be increased in plasmas of patients with APA that have anticoagulant activity. The test can be falsely positive if the patient plasma contains heparin or antibodies against factor V.

For plasma with a prolonged aPTT, correction studies are performed by mixing normal and patient plasma and repeating the aPTT immediately and after 1 hour of incubation at 37°C. If an LA is present the results of the correction study will not change with the 1-hour incubation since the antibody is directed against the phospholipid that is added to the assay. In contrast, an abnormal correction study due to the presence of an antibody against a specific factor will be increasingly abnormal with incubation as the antibody gradually inhibits the normal factor in the normal plasma. Factor levels are measured in order to exclude a true factor deficiency or the presence of another inhibitor. If patient plasma has a prolonged aPTT and a normal PT, factors XII, XI, IX, and VIII are measured. Frequently LA are sufficiently potent to induce an apparent decrease in these coagulation factors. In this case, factor activity should increase toward the true value when measured in serial dilutions of the patient plasma. The dilution of the plasma also dilutes the inhibitory activity of the LA and allows for more accurate determination of the factor activity. If the patient has a real factor deficiency, such as deficiency of factor VIII, that is due to an antibody directed against the factor the determination of the factor level will not be influenced by the dilution at which the plasma is tested. If the PT is also prolonged, then measurement of factors VII, X, V, and II should be included. Occasionally in plasmas with LA, the PT can also be slightly prolonged in the absence of a true factor deficiency.[101,102] The most common true factor deficiency that is associated with the LA is prothrombin deficiency, as described above.

Table 18-5 • CHARACTERISTICS OF ASSAYS FOR LUPUS ANTICOAGULANT (LA)

	PNP	dRVVT	dPL-aPTT	KCT	TTI
Phospholipid[a]	Added	Diluted	Diluted	None	Diluted
False positive with heparin	Yes	Yes	Yes	Yes	No
False positive with factor deficiency	No	No[b]	No[b]	No[b]	No[b]
False positive with factor inhibitors	No	Yes	Yes	Yes	Yes

PNP, platelet neutralization procedure; dRVVT, dilute Russell viper venom time; dPL-aPTT, dilute phospholipid aPTT; KCT, kaolin clotting time; TTI, tissue thromboplastin inhibition test.
[a] All of these tests (with the exception of the PNP) can be performed with patient plasmas that have a normal aPTT.
[b] Test must be performed with a mixture of normal and patient plasma.

TREATMENT OF PATIENTS WHO HAVE THE ANTIPHOSPHOLIPID SYNDROME OR LABORATORY MANIFESTATIONS OF APA (LA OR ACA)

Major issues in the management of patients with the antiphospholipid syndrome and thrombosis are the intensity of anticoagulation that should be given, the duration of anticoagulation, and the appropriate monitoring (Table 18-6). One goal is to reduce other risk factors for thrombosis, such as uncontrolled hypertension,

Table 18–6 • TREATMENT ISSUES FOR PATIENTS WITH THE ANTIPHOSPHOLIPID SYNDROME MANIFESTED BY VENOUS OR ARTERIAL THROMBOSIS

Intensity of Anticoagulation
Anticoagulation with warfarin to maintain international normalized ratio (INR) of 2 to 3, with attempt to target the INR of 3 the best option (with or without aspirin daily at a dose of 75 to 325 mg daily). (Recurrent thrombotic events per year of follow-up ranging from 0.07 to 0.23.)

Duration of Anticoagulation
Anticoagulation to be on an indefinite basis after first thrombotic event. High rate of recurrence if anticoagulation is discontinued 3 months after initiation.

Issues with Respect to Monitoring
INR has been reported to be falsely increased in patients with LA and initial prolongation of PT. Test appears to be more reliable if recombinant tissue factor is not used in the PT reagent. The reliability of the test may also be increased by using plasmas with a calibrated INR as a standard for calculating the patient's INR instead of using the International Sensitivity Index (ISI) measured by the manufacturer.

smoking, and use of oral contraceptives.[103] Treatment of asymptomatic patients with LA or with moderate or high titers of ACA is controversial. Some physicians will prescribe low-dose aspirin (80 mg/day) and then use anticoagulation with warfarin or heparin at times of increased risk for thrombosis.[103]

Patients with the antiphospholipid syndrome and venous thromboembolism are at high risk for recurrence if anticoagulation is discontinued after a first episode of venous thrombosis.[104–106] In a retrospective study of 19 patients with secondary antiphospholipid syndrome who had 34 episodes of thromboembolism, the discontinuation of warfarin resulted in a 50% probability of recurrent episodes at 2 years, which increased to 78% at 8 years.[105] The rate of recurrence was highest (1.30 per patient-year) in the first 6 months after discontinuation of anticoagulation.[105] In contrast, continuation of warfarin (INR 2.5 to 4.0) resulted in 100% freedom from thrombosis at the 8-year follow-up.

The appropriate intensity of anticoagulation has not been studied carefully. However, one international trial that is in progress (Warfarin in the Antiphospholipid Syndrome study) randomizes patients to high-intensity treatment (INR 3 to 4.5) or to standard treatment.[107] In a prospective study comparing the clinical manifestations of patients with the primary and secondary antiphospholipid syndrome during a 2-year period, eight persons developed recurrent thrombosis, seven of whom had INR values below 3.[105] In a prospective study of the clinical relevance of APA in patients with venous thromboembolism but who did not have SLE, the authors found no recurrence in patients receiving warfarin at INR intensities of 2 to 2.9 and no difference in the rate of recurrence in patients with and without APA.[108] In a third prospective study, patients with an episode of venous thrombosis who had LA and were randomized to warfarin during a 4-year period had no recurrences when the INR was maintained between 2 and 3. The intensity of anticoagulation required may depend on whether or not the patient has underlying SLE; however, this issue has also not been resolved. In the meantime, for patients with antiphospholipid syndrome and thrombosis who are receiving warfarin, an INR of 2 to 3, with an attempt to maintain the INR nearer to 3, is recommended if there are no contraindications; furthermore, anticoagulation should be continued on an indefinite basis as long as the risks and consequences of bleeding are less than the risk of thrombosis. Low-dose aspirin may be added, depending on the whether or not thrombotic manifestations such as superficial thrombophlebitis persist.

One report has described variability in measuring the INR in patients with LA who also had an increased baseline PT as such a phenomenon could result in the underutilization of warfarin.[109] However, two other studies have shown that false prolongation of the INR in such patients appears not to be the case,[110,111] although in one study variability in the INR was greatly increased when a recombinant tissue factor was used as the PT reagent.[110] The authors also found increased reliability in measuring the INR when they calibrated patient plasmas against plasma standards that had three different levels of the INR. This was done instead of using the international sensitivity index (ISI) provided by the manufacturer to determine the INRs of the patient plasmas.

Patients with the antiphospholipid syndrome can present with an initial thrombosis followed by additional thromboses leading to severe morbidity or death if adequate anticoagulation is not promptly achieved.[112] Thus, before considering any other interventions in these patients such as placement of vena caval filters or plasmapheresis, consultants should be convinced that anticoagulation has been maximized. This may also include consideration of thrombolytic therapy for selected patients. The role of corticosteroids or plasmapheresis has not been documented for patients with the antiphospholipid syndrome. These treatments are reserved for patients with a "catastrophic antiphospholipid syndrome," defined as acute multiorgan failure in a patient with APA.[113] In this rare syndrome, mortality is 50%; plasmapheresis may be beneficial in patients who have not responded to heparin, corticosteroids, or immunosuppressive agents.[113]

COST CONTAINMENT AND MEDICOLEGAL ASPECTS OF TESTING FOR LA AND THE ANTIPHOSPHOLIPID SYNDROME

Two major reasons for ordering tests for LA are (1) for evaluation of an unexplained (and unexpected) prolongation of the aPTT and (2) to evaluate an individual who presents with clinical features suggesting the antiphospholipid syndrome. In the first case, in which testing is done for a prolonged aPTT, the finding of an LA does not mean that the test for ACAs with an ELISA needs to be performed. It is recommended that patients who have a prolonged aPTT and an LA also be tested for appropriate coagulation factor activities, especially if they are to undergo an invasive procedure. Patients may have apparent low factor VIII activity if a potent LA is present. However, in the test system the factor VIII activity will increase as the plasma is diluted, thus reducing the potency of the LA effect and allowing a more adequate assessment of the factor activity. For patients with a factor VIII antibody, the factor VIII activity is truly decreased and the same activity is achieved at all plasma dilutions in the test system. Testing the factor activities provides a safeguard against missing a possible factor deficiency; for example, factor VIII deficiency due to the presence of an antibody against factor VIII might be present in addition to the LA or the antibody against factor VIII might have been mistakenly described as an LA.

If testing is initiated because of the suspicion of the antiphospholipid syndrome, at least two different tests for LA should be performed as well as the ELISA for ACA in order to establish or exclude the diagnosis. If a test is positive, then the evaluation should again be performed in 6 weeks to confirm the persistence of the abnormality. Thus, the laboratory confirmation of the antiphospholipid syndrome is expensive and should be performed thoroughly once initiated. Such an evaluation should be based on strong clinical suspicion.

Patients with a history of thrombosis who are diagnosed as having the antiphospholipid syndrome are at high risk for recurrent thrombotic events, as described above. These patients may be prime candidates for using home monitoring devices to measure the INR, since continued and adequate anticoagulation is essential (see Chapter 35).

CONCLUSION

Although the pathophysiology of the antiphospholipid syndrome has not been well established, the specificity of the autoantibodies is now becoming more well defined and the diagnostic testing as well as the criteria for establishing the diagnosis has been greatly refined. A major issue is that of treatment[114]; the type, duration, and intensity of anticoagulation still have not been resolved but with the development of cooperative international clinical trials, some of these issues may soon be clarified. The antiphospholipid syndrome is a disorder that encompasses many specialties: hematology, neurology, obstetrics, and rheumatology. Thus, the approach to patients with this disorder must be truly interdisciplinary.

■ REFERENCES

Chapter 18 References

1. Conley CL, Rathbun HK, Morse WI II, Robinson JE Jr. Circulating anticoagulant as a cause of hemorrhagic diathesis in man. Bull Johns Hopkins Hospital 1948;83:288–296.
2. Mueller JF, Ratnoff O, Heinle RW. Observations on the characteristics of an unusual circulating anticoagulant. J Lab Clin Med 1951;38:254–261.
3. Margolius A Jr, Jackson DP, Ratnoff OD. Circulating anticoagulants: a study of 40 cases and a review of the literature. Medicine 1961;40:145–202.
4. Bowie EJW, Thompson JH Jr, Pascuzzi CA, Owen CA Jr. Thrombosis in systemic lupus erythematosus despite circulating anticoagulants. J Lab Clin Med 1963;62:416–430.
5. Hughes GRV. The antiphospholipid syndrome. Lupus 1996;5:345–346.
6. Harris EN, Gharavi EA, Boey ML, et al. Anticardiolipin antibodies: detection by radioimmunoassay and association with thrombosis in systemic lupus erythematosus. Lancet 1983;ii:1211–1214.
7. McNeil HP, Simpson RJ, Chesterman CN, Krilis SA. Anti-phospholipid antibodies are directed against a complex antigen that includes a lipid-binding inhibitor of coagulation: β_2-glycoprotein I (apolipoprotein H). Proc Natl Acad Sci 1990;87:4120–4124.
8. Galli M, Comfurius P, Maassen C, et al. Anticardiolipin antibodies (ACA) are directed not to cardiolipin but to a plasma protein cofactor. Lancet 1990;335:1544–1547.
9. Matsura E, Igarashi Y, Fujimoto M, et al. Anticardiolipin cofactor(s) and differential diagnosis of autoimmune disease. Lancet 1990;38:177–178.
10. Alving BM, Barr CF, Tang DB. Correlation between lupus anticoagulants and anticardiolipin antibodies in patients with prolonged activated partial thromboplastin times. Am J Med 1990;88:112–116.
11. McNeil HP, Chesterman CN, Krilis SA. Immunology and clinical importance of antiphospholipid antibodies. Adv Immunol 1991;49:193–280.
12. Greaves M. Antiphospholipid antibodies and thrombosis. Lancet 1999;353:1348–1353.
13. Wilson W, Gharavi AE, Koike T, et al. International consensus statement on preliminary classification criteria for definite antiphospholipid syndrome. Arthritis Rheum 1999;42:1309–1311.
14. Asherson RA. Anti-phospholipid antibodies. Clinical complications reported in medical literature. In: Harris EN, Exner T, Hughes GRV, Asherson RA (eds): Phospholipid-Binding Antibodies. Boston, CRC Press, Inc., 1991; pp. 388–402.
15. Vila P, Hernández MC, López-Hernández MF, Batlle J. Prevalence, follow-up and clinical significance of the anticardiolipin antibodies in normal subjects. Thromb Haemost 1994;72:209–213.
16. Long AA, Ginsberg JS, Brill-Edwards P, et al. The relationship of antiphospholipid antibodies to thromboembolic disease in systemic lupus erythematosus: a cross-sectional study. Thromb Haemost 1991;66:520–524.
17. Levine SR, Deegan MJ, Futrell N, Welch KMA. Cerebrovascular and neurologic disease associated with antiphospholipid antibodies: 48 cases. Neurology 1990;40:1181–1189.
18. Nencini P, Baruffi MC, Abbate R, et al. Lupus anticoagulant and anticardiolipin antibodies in young adults with cerebral ischemia. Stroke 1992;23:189–193.
19. Ginsburg KS, Liang MH, Newcomer L, et al. Anticardiolipin antibodies and the risk for ischemic stroke and venous thrombosis. Ann Intern Med 1992;117:997–1002.
20. Tuhrim S, Rand J, Wu X-X, et al. Elevated anticardiolipin antibody titer is a stroke risk factor in a multiethnic population independent of isotype or positivity. Stroke 1999;30:1561–1565.
21. Branch DW, Silver RM. Criteria for antiphospholipid syndrome: Early pregnancy loss, fetal loss, or recurrent pregnancy loss? Lupus 1996;5:409–413.
22. Rai R, Cohen H, Dave M, Regan L. Randomised controlled trial of aspirin and aspirin plus heparin in pregnant women with recurrent miscarriage associated with phospholipid antibodies (or antiphospholipid antibodies). Br Med J 1997;314:253–257.
23. Cowchock FS, Reece EA, Balaban D, et al. Repeated fetal losses associated with antiphospholipid antibodies: a collaborative randomized trial comparing prednisone with low-dose heparin treatment. Am J Obstet Gynecol 1992;166:1318–1323.
24. Kutteh WH, Ermel LD. A clinical trial for the treatment of antiphospholipid-antibody associated recurrent pregnancy loss with lower dose aspirin and heparin. Am J Reprod Immunol 1996;35:402–407.

25. Lockshin MD. Pregnancy loss in the antiphospholipid syndrome. Thromb Haemost 1999;82:641–648.
26. Sanson B-J, Lensing AWA, Prins MH, Ginsberg JS, et al. Safety of low-molecular-weight heparin in pregnancy: A systematic review. Thromb Haemost 1999;81:668–672.
27. Cowchock, S. Treatment of antiphospholipid syndrome in pregnancy. Lupus 1998;595–597.
28. Ginsberg J, Greer I, Hirsh J. Use of antithrombotic agents during pregnancy. Chest 2001;119:122S–131S.
29. Rand JH, Wu X-X, Guller S, et al. Reduction of annexin-V (placental anticoagulant protein-I) on placental villi of women with antiphospholipid antibodies and recurrent spontaneous abortion. Am J Obstet Gynecol 1994;171:1566–1572.
30. Rand JH, Wu X-X, Andree H, et al. Pregnancy loss in the antiphospholipid-antibody syndrome: a possible thrombogenic mechanism. N Engl J Med 1997;337:154–160.
31. Rand JH. Antiphospholipid antibody-mediated disruption of the annexin-V antithrombotic shield: a thrombogenic mechanism for the antiphospholipid syndrome. J Autoimmun 2000;15:107–111.
32. Harris EN, Asherson RA, Gharavi AE, et al. Thrombocytopenia in SLE and related autoimmune disorders: association with anticardiolipin antibody. Br J Haematol 1985;59:227–230.
33. Harris EN, Gharavi AE, Hegde U, et al. Anticardiolipin antibodies in autoimmune thrombocytopenic purpura. Br J Haematol 1985;59:231–234.
34. Stasi R, Stipa E, Masi M, et al. Prevalence and clinical significance of elevated antiphospholipid antibodies in patients with idiopathic thrombocytopenic purpura. Blood 1994;84:4203–4208.
35. Leung W-H, Wong K-L, Lau C-P, et al. Association between antiphospholipid antibodies and cardiac abnormalities in patients with systemic lupus erythematosus. Am J Med 1990; 89:411–419.
36. Nihoyannopoulos P, Gomez PM, Joshi J, et al. Cardiac abnormalities in systemic lupus erythematosus. Association with raised anticardiolipin antibodies. Circulation 1990;82:369–375.
37. Khamashta MA, Cervera R, Asherson RA, et al. Association of antibodies against phospholipids with heart valve disease in systemic lupus erythematosus. Lancet 1990;335:1541–1544.
38. Galve E, Ordi J, Barquinero J, et al. Valvular heart disease in the primary antiphospholipid syndrome. Ann Intern Med 1992;116:293–298.
39. Gleason CB, Stoddard MF, Wagner SG, et al. A comparison of cardiac valvular involvement in the primary antiphospholipid syndrome versus anticardiolipin-negative systemic lupus erythematosus. Am Heart J 1993;125:1123–1129.
40. Ford PM, Ford SE, Lillicrap DP. Association of lupus anticoagulant with severe valvular heart disease in systemic lupus erythematosus. J Rheumatol 1988;15:597–600.
41. Kattwinkel N, Villanueva AG, Labib SB, et al. Myocardial infarction caused by cardiac microvasculopathy in a patient with the primary antiphospholipid syndrome. Ann Intern Med 1992; 116:974–976.
42. Chartash EK, Lans DM, Paget SA, et al. Aortic insufficiency and mitral regurgitation in patients with systemic lupus erythematosus and the antiphospholipid syndrome. Am J Med 1989; 86:407–412.
43. Sletnes KE, Smith P, Abdelnoor M, et al. Antiphospholipid antibodies after myocardial infarction and their relation to mortality, reinfarction, and non-haemorrhagic stroke. Lancet 1992;339:451–453.
44. Pope JM, Canny CLB, Bell DA. Cerebral ischemic events associated with endocarditis, retinal vascular disease, and lupus anticoagulant. Am J Med 1991;90:299–309.
45. Leventhal LJ, Borofsky MA, Bergey PD, Schumacher HR, Jr. Antiphospholipid syndrome with right atrial thrombosis mimicking an atrial myxoma. Am J Med 1989;87:111–113.
46. Edson JR, Vogt JM, Hasegawa DK. Abnormal prothrombin crossed-immunoelectrophoresis in patients with lupus inhibitors. Blood 1984;64:807–816.

47. Bajaj SP, Rapaport SI, Fierer DS, et al. A mechanism for the hypoprothrombinemia of the acquired hypoprothrombinemia-lupus anticoagulant syndrome. Blood 1983;61:684–692.
48. Fleck RA, Rapaport SI, Rao VM. Anti-prothrombin antibodies and the lupus anticoagulant. Blood 1988;72:512–519.
49. Lee MT, Nardi MA, Hu G, et al. Transient hemorrhagic diathesis associated with an inhibitor of prothrombin with lupus anticoagulant in an 1 1/2-year-old girl: report of a case and review of the literature. Am J Hematol 1996;51:307–314.
50. Bernini JC, Buchanan GR, Ashcroft J. Hypoprothrombinemia and severe hemorrhage associated with a lupus anticoagulant. J Pediatr 1993;123:937–939.
51. Kitchens CS. Prolonged activated partial thromboplastin time of unknown etiology: A prospective study of 100 consecutive cases referred for consultation. Am J Hematol 1988;27:38–45.
52. Canoso RT, de Oliveira RM. Chlorpromazine-induced anticardiolipin antibodies and lupus anticoagulant: absence of thrombosis. Am J Hematol 1988;27:272–275.
53. Canoso RT, Sise HS. Chlorpromazine-induced lupus anticoagulant and associated immunologic abnormalities. Am J Hematol 1982;13:121–129.
54. List AF, Doll DC. Thrombosis associated with procainamide-induced lupus anticoagulant. Acta Haematol 1989;82:50–52.
55. Keane A, Woods R, Dowding V, et al. Anticardiolipin antibodies in rheumatoid arthritis. Br J Rheumatol 1987;26:346–350.
56. Boxer M, Ellman L, Carvalho A. The lupus anticoagulant. Arthritis Rheum 1976;19:1244–1248.
57. Schleider MA, Nachman RL, Jaffe EA, Coleman M. A clinical study of the lupus anticoagulant. Blood 1976;48:499–509.
58. Elias M, Eldor A. Thromboembolism in patients with the 'lupus'-type circulating anticoagulant. Arch Intern Med 1984; 144:510–515.
59. Lillicrap DP, Pinto M, Benford K, et al. Heterogeneity of laboratory test results for antiphospholipid antibodies in patients treated with chlorpromazine and other phenothiazines. Am J Clin Pathol 1990;93:771–775.
60. Bell WR, Boss GR, Wolfson JS. Circulating anticoagulant in the procainamide-induced lupus syndrome. Arch Intern Med 1977;137:1471–1473.
61. Edwards RL, Rick ME, Wakem CJ. Studies on a circulating anticoagulant in procainamide-induced lupus erythematosus. Arch Intern Med 1981;141:1688–1690.
62. Hess E. Drug-related lupus. N Engl J Med 1988; 318:1460–1462.
63. Li GC, Greenberg CS, Currie MS. Procainamide-induced lupus anticoagulants and thrombosis. South Med J 1988;81:262–264.
64. Asherson RA, Zulman J, Hughes GRV. Pulmonary thromboembolism associated with procainamide induced lupus syndrome and anticardiolipin antibodies. Ann Rheum Dis 1989;48:232–235.
65. Heyman MR, Flores RH, Edelman BB, Carliner NH. Procainamide-induced lupus anticoagulant. South Med J 1988;81:934–936.
66. Zarrabi MH, Zucker S, Miller F, et al. Immunology and coagulation disorders in chlorpromazine-treated patients. Ann Intern Med 1979;91:194–199.
67. Cohen AJ, Philips TM, Kessler CM. Circulating coagulation inhibitors in the acquired immunodeficiency syndrome. Ann Intern Med 1986;104:175–180.
68. Mackworth-Young CG, Harris EN, Steere AC, et al. Anticardiolipin antibodies in Lyme disease. Arthritis Rheum 1988;31:1052–1056.
69. Vaarala O, Palosuo T, Kleemola M, Aho K. Anticardiolipin response in acute infections. Clin Immunol Immunopathol 1986;41:8–15.
70. McNelly T, Purdy G, Mackie IJ, et al. The use of an anti-β_2-glycoprotein I assay for discrimination between cardiolipin antibodies associated with infection and increased risk of thrombosis. Br J Haematol 1995;91:471–473.

71. Galli M, Comfurius P, Barbui T, et al. Anticoagulant activity of β2-glycoprotein I is potentiated by a distinct subgroup of anticardiolipin antibodies. 1992;68:297–300.

72. Galli M, Finazzi G, Bevers EM, Barbui T. Kaolin clotting time and dilute Russell's venom time distinguish between prothrombin-dependent and β2-glycoprotein I-dependent antiphospholipid antibodies. Blood 1995;86:617–623.

73. Matsuura E, Igarashi Y, Yasuda T, et al. Anticardiolipin antibodies recognize β2-glycoprotein I structure altered by interacting with an oxygen modified solid phase surface. J Exp Med 1994; 179:457–462.;117:303–308.

74. Arnout J. The pathogenesis of the antiphospholipid syndrome: a hypothesis based on parallelisms with heparin-induced thrombocytopenia. Thromb Haemost 1996;75:536–541.

75. Greaves M, Hill MB, Phipps J, et al. The pathogenesis of the antiphospholipid syndrome. Thromb Haemost 1996;76:813–821.

76. Santoro SA. Antiphospholipid antibodies and thrombotic predisposition: underlying pathogenic mechanisms. Blood 1994; 83:2389–2391.

77. Pengo V, Biasiolo A, Fior MG. Binding of autoimmune cardiolipin-reactive antibodies to heparin: a mechanism of thrombosis? Thromb Res 1995;78:371–378.

78. Shibata S, Harpel PC, Gharavi A, et al. Autoantibodies to heparin from patients with antiphospholipid antibody syndrome inhibit formation of antithrombin III–thrombin complexes. Blood 1994;83:2532–2540.

79. Freyssinet J-M, Wiesel M-L, Gauchy J, et al. An IgM lupus anticoagulant that neutralizes the enhancing effect of phospholipid on purified endothelial thrombomodulin activity—a mechanism for thrombosis. Thromb Haemost 1986;55:309–313.

80. Cariou R, Tobelem G, Bellucci S, et al. Effect of lupus anticoagulant on antithrombogenic properties of endothelial cells—inhibition of thrombomodulin-dependent protein C activation. Thromb Haemost 1988;60:54–58.

81. Tsakiris DA, Settas L, Makris PE, Marbet GA. Lupus anticoagulant-antiphospholipid antibodies and thrombophilia. Relation to protein C-protein S-thrombomodulin. J Rheumatol 1990;17:785–789.

82. Out HJ, de Groot PG, van Vliet M, et al. Antibodies to platelets in patients with anti-phospholipid antibodies. Blood 1991;77:2655–2659.

83. Lin YL, Wang CT. Activation of human platelets by the rabbit anticardiolipin antibodies. Blood 1992;80:3135–3143.

84. Shi W, Chong BH, Chesterman CN. β2-Glycoprotein I is a requirement for anticardiolipin antibodies binding to activated platelets: differences with lupus anticoagulant. Blood 1993; 81:1255–1262.

85. Rauch J, Meng Q-H, Tannenbaum H. Lupus anticoagulant and antiplatelet properties of human hybridoma autoantibodies. J Immunol 1987;139:2598–2604.

86. Galli M, Daldossi M, Barbui T. Anti-glycoprotein Ib/Ix and IIb/IIIa antibodies. Thromb Haemost 1994;71:571–575.

87. Loizou S, McCrea JD, Rudge AC, et al. Measurement of anti-cardiolipin antibodies by an enzyme-linked immunosorbent assay (ELISA): standardization and quantitation of results. Clin Exp Immunol 1985;62:738–745.

88. Smolarsky M. A simple radioimmunoassay to determine binding of antibodies to lipid antigens. J Immunol Methods 1980; 38:85–93.

89. Harris EN. The second international anti-cardiolipin standardization workshop/the Kingston Anti-phospholipid Antibody Study (KAPS) Group. Am J Clin Pathol 1990;94:476–484.

90. Lockshin MD. Antiphospholipid antibody and antiphospholipid antibody syndrome. Curr Opin Rheumatol 1991;3:797–802.

91. Stewart MW, Etches WS, Russell AS, et al. Detection of antiphospholipid antibodies by flow cytometry: rapid detection of antibody isotype and phospholipid specificity. Thromb Haemost 1993;70:603–607.

92. Gharavi AE, Harris EN, Asherson RA, Hughes GRV. Anticardiolipin antibodies: isotype distribution and phospholipid specificity. Ann Rheum Dis 1987;46:1–6.

93. Pengo V, Thiagarajan P, Shapiro SS, Heine MJ. Immunological specificity and mechanism of action of IgG lupus anticoagulants. Blood 1987;70:69–76.

94. Brandt JT, Triplett DA, Alving B, Scharrer I. Criteria for the diagnosis of lupus anticoagulants: an update on behalf of the subcommittee on lupus anticoagulant/antiphospholipid antibody of the scientific and standardisation committee of the ISTH. Thromb Haemost 1995;74:1185–1190.

95. Societe Francaise de Biologie Clinique. Comparison of a standardized procedure with current laboratory practices for the detection of lupus anticoagulants in France. Thromb Haemost 1993;70:781–786.

96. Thiagarajan P, Pengo V, Shapiro SS. The use of the dilute Russell viper venom time for the diagnosis of lupus anticoagulants. Blood 1986;68:869–874.

97. Schjetlein R, Wisloff F. An evaluation of two commercial test procedures for the detection of lupus anticoagulant. Coag Transf Med 1995;103:108–111.

98. Alving BM, Barr CF, Johansen LE, Tang DB. Comparison between a one-point dilute phospholipid APTT and the dilute Russell viper venom time for verification of lupus anticoagulants. Thromb Haemost 1992;67:672–678.

99. Forastiero RR, Cerrato GS, Carreras LO. Evaluation of recently described tests for detection of the lupus anticoagulant. Thromb Haemost 1994;72:728–733.

100. Triplett DA, Stocker KF, Unger GA, Barna LK. The textarin/ecarin ratio: a confirmatory test for lupus anticoagulants. Thromb Haemost 1993;70:925–931.

101. Lazarchick J, Kizer J. The laboratory diagnosis of lupus anticoagulants. Arch Pathol Lab Med 1989;113:177–180.

102. Triplett DA, Brandt JT, Maas RL. The laboratory heterogeneity of lupus anticoagulants. Arch Pathol Lab Med 1985;109:946–951.

103. Khamashta MA. Management of thrombosis in the antiphospholipid syndrome. Lupus 1996;5:463–466.

104. Rosove MH, Brewer PMC. Antiphospholipid thrombosis: clinical course after the first thrombotic event in 70 patients. Ann Intern Med 1992;117:303–308.

105. Khamashta MA, Cuadrado MJ, Mujic F, et al. The management of thrombosis in the antiphospholipid-antibody syndrome. N Engl J Med 1995;332:993–997.

106. Kearon C, Gent M, Hirsh J, et al. A comparison of three months of anticoagulation with extended anticoagulation for a first episode of idiopathic venous thromboembolism. N Engl J Med 1999;340:901–907.

107. Galli M, Barbui T. Antiprothrombin antibodies: detection and clinical significance in the antiphospholipid syndrome. Blood 1999;93:2149–2157.

108. Ginsberg JS, Wells PS, Brill-Edwards P, et al. Antiphospholipid antibodies and venous thromboembolism. Blood 1995;86:3685–3691.

109. Moll S, Ortel TL. Monitoring warfarin therapy in patients with lupus anticoagulants. Ann Intern Med 1997;127:177–185.

110. Robert A, Le Querrec A, Delahousse B, et al. Control of oral anticoagulation in patients with the antiphospholipid syndrome-influence of the lupus anticoagulant on international normalized ratio. Thromb Haemost 1998;80:99–103.

111. Lawrie AS, Purdy G, Mackie IJ, Machin SJ. Monitoring of oral anticoagulant therapy in lupus anticoagulant positive patients with the anti-phospholipid syndrome. Br J Haematol 1997; 98:887–892.

112. Kitchens CS. Thrombotic storm: when thrombosis begets thrombosis. Am J Med 1998;104:381–385.

113. Asherson RA. The catastrophic antiphospholipid syndrome, 1998. A review of the clinical features, possible pathogenesis and treatment. Lupus 1998;7:S55–S62.

114. Schulman S, Svenungsson E, Granqvist S, and the Duration of Anticoagulation Study Group. Anticardiolipin antibodies predict early recurrence of thromboembolism and death among patients with venous thromboembolism following anticoagulant therapy. Am J Med 1998;104:332–338.

CHAPTER 19

Hemostatic Aspects of Cardiovascular Medicine

Richard C. Becker, M.D.
Scott D. Berkowitz, M.D.

The evolution of cardiovascular medicine has been based on an in-depth understanding of vascular biology, hemostasis, and thrombosis. Indeed, the development of pharmacologic therapies for preventing and treating coronary atherothrombosis is the result of collaborations between the cardiology, pathology, and hematology communities in response to several fundamental observations and key questions, which include (1) What are the anatomic and physiologic effects of atherosclerotic vascular disease?; (2) How does atherosclerosis influence the complex and delicate balance between thrombosis and "antithrombosis"?; (3) Can the thrombotic tendency in atherosclerotic vascular disease be tempered pharmacologically without compromising protective hemostasis?; and (4) Are there means to reproduce or mimic congenital hemostatic disorders in a "controlled fashion" for the purpose of attenuating thrombotic potential?

The following chapter will highlight cardiovascular medicine's rapid evolution with emphasis on the development of fibrinolytic and antithrombotic therapy, their clinical indications, and their potential impact on hemostatic capacity and hemorrhagic risk.

HISTORICAL PERSPECTIVES IN CARDIOVASCULAR MEDICINE

The rapid transformation of fluid blood to a gel-like substance (clot) has been a topic of great interest to scientists, physicians, and philosophers since the days of Plato and Aristotle.[1,2] However, it was not until the early 18th century that blood clotting was appreciated as a complex mechanism to stem blood following vascular injury.[3]

The microscope played a pivotal role in the understanding of coagulation. In the mid 17th century, Marcello Malpighi separated the individual components of a blood clot into fibers, cells, and serum.[4] The fibers were later found to be derived from a plasma precursor (fibrinogen) and given the name *fibrin*.[5] Further development in the mid 19th century included the recognition of an enzyme (later called *thrombin*) that was capable of coagulating fibrinogen (Table 19–1).[6]

The discovery of thrombin is particularly interesting because this enzyme plays such a prominent role in coagulation as we have come to understand it. In the latter half of the 19th century, the scientific community began to appreciate that thrombin could not be a constituent of normal plasma (otherwise clotting would occur continuously and at random).[7] This concept was vital to the understanding of the complex "checks and balances" system of coagulation, wherein inactive precursors are activated precisely where and when they are needed only to be deactivated soon thereafter in order to limit the thrombotic process. It also fostered the belief that blood contained many, if not all, of the necessary elements for intravascular coagulation (circulating predominantly in an inactive form). This hypothesis served as the basis for the theory of *intrinsic coagulation*.

Coagulation Cascades

Scientists were able to show that blood coagulated when it came into contact with a foreign surface and that some surfaces were more "thrombogenic" than others. This concept paved the way for an expanding knowledge of hereditary disorders of coagulation.[8,9] Developments in our understanding of extrinsic coagulation followed the pioneering work of several preeminent scientists,[10–13] all of whom described blood coagulation following the infusion of tissue suspensions (tissue factor, thromboplastin). A revised theory of *extrinsic coagulation* suggested that an exposed tissue surface (from a damaged blood vessel wall) was capable of stimulating blood clotting. Later discoveries included the direct contribution

Table 19–1 • A HISTORICAL TIMELINE FOR HEMOSTASIS

- Transformation of fluid blood to "gel-like" mass (Plato, Aristotle)
- Blood clots consist of fibers, cells, and serum (Malpighi, 1686)
- Blood clotting stems blood loss from wounds (Peitit, 1731)
- "Fibers," (later termed *fibrin*) are derived from fibrinogen (Babingon, 1830)
- Thrombin converts fibrinogen to fibrin (Buchanan, 1879)
- Blood contains "inactive" precursors that are "activated" by a foreign surface or exposed tissue (Schmidt, 1892)
- Platelets aggregate and represent the first step in hemostasis (Osler, 1874; Hayem, 1882)

of calcium, phospholipid, and other essential components of the prothrombinase complex (factors Va, Xa) to blood coagulation.

Platelets

The important contribution of platelets to the coagulation process can be traced to the original work of Alfred Donné, who discovered platelets with the assistance of a newly developed microscope lens (achromatic lens).[14] However, the clinical importance of platelets in normal hemostasis was not appreciated until the end of the 19th century, when Sir William Osler at age 25 described platelet aggregation[15] and Hayem cited the importance of platelet plugs in preventing blood loss after tissue injury.[16]

The development of electron microscopy subsequently made it clear that platelets adhered to damaged blood vessels and that platelets could become "activated" through a variety of pharmacologic (e.g., adenosine diphosphate, epinephrine, thrombin) or mechanical (e.g., shear stress) stimuli.

Fibrinolysis

The inability of blood to fully coagulate following death was observed centuries ago, possibly as early as the days of Hippocrates.[17] Pioneering work near the end of the 18th century described the process of fibrinolysis and a mechanism whereby a circulating precursor (plasminogen) generated (with the appropriate stimulus) an active enzyme (plasmin) capable of degrading clotted blood.[18,19]

The potential clinical ramifications of fibrinolysis and its application in treating thrombotic disorders theoretically began in 1921 with the work of Gratia, who observed that clots could be dissolved by staphylococcal extracts.[20] Tillet and Garner[21] later reported that bacteria-free filtrates of β-hemolytic streptococci contained a substance (streptokinase) capable of dissolving blood clots. Soon thereafter, the groundbreaking work of Sol Sherry[22] highlighted the potential use of fibrinolytics in treating humans thrombotic disorders.

Aspirin

The potential role of aspirin in the prevention and treatment of cardiovascular disease had been recognized by clinicians for decades; however, the landmark observations made in the ISIS-2 (Second International Study of Infarct Survival) study[23] firmly placed antithrombotic therapy with aspirin at the forefront of current management strategies for acute myocardial infarction (MI) (Fig. 19–1).

Myocardial Reperfusion

The recognition that sudden, complete coronary arterial occlusion was the proximate cause of acute ST-segment elevation MI, coupled with the work of Reimer and Jennings highlighting the "wavefront phenomenon" of myocardial necrosis and the "time-dependent" effect

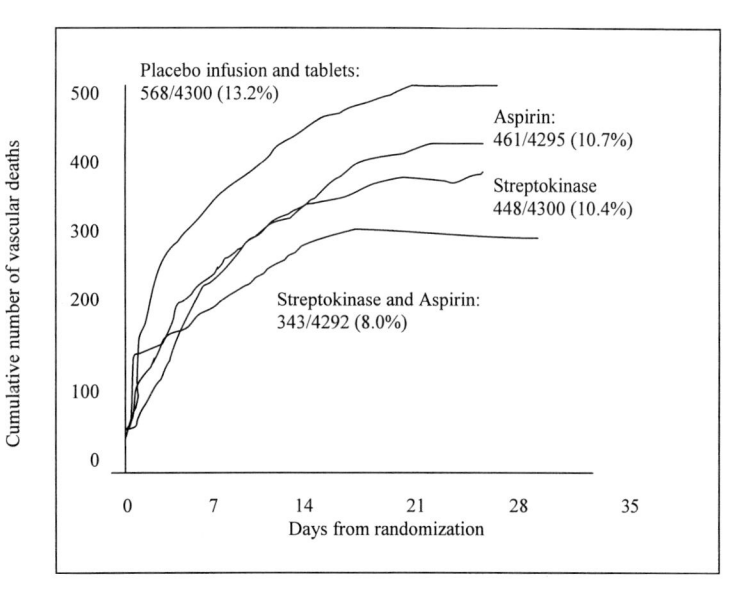

Figure 19–1 Cumulative vascular mortality rate (days 0–35) in the ISIS-2 study. (From ISIS-2 (Second International Study of Infarct Survival) Collaborative Group. Randomized trial of intravenous streptokinase, oral aspirin, both, or neither among 17,187 cases of suspected acute myocardial infarction: ISIS-2. Lancet 2:349, 1998, with permission.)

Hemostatic Aspects of Cardiovascular Medicine 281

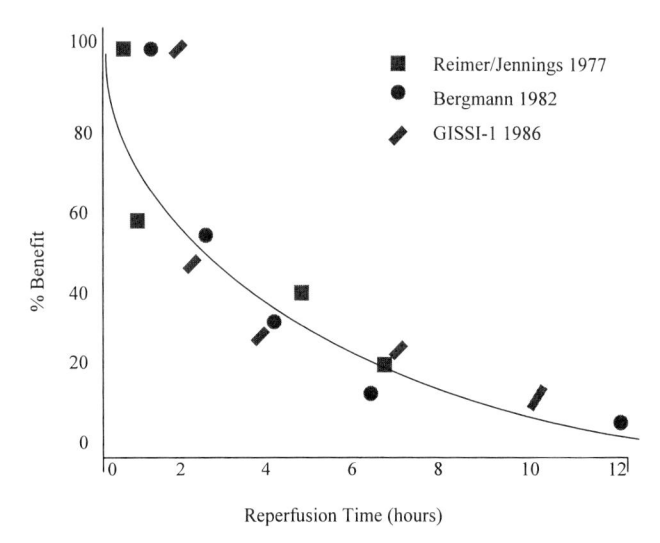

Figure 19-2 The time to reperfusion determines overall benefit following fibrinolytic therapy for acute MI (Adapted from Jaucherm JR, Lopez M, Sprague EA, et al. Mononuclear cell chemoattractant activity from cultured arterial smooth muscle cells. Exp Mol Pathol 1982;37:166–174.)

of coronary perfusion in limiting myocardial damage, paved the way for pharmacologic (fibrinolysis) and mechanical (coronary angioplasty, bypass grafting) reperfusion strategies that currently represent the standard of care[24-26] (Fig. 19-2). Efforts at the national level designed to reduce MI-related mortality have focused on education, early recognition, and prompt intervention (Fig. 19-3).

Low-Molecular-Weight Heparin

The contribution of coagulation proteins, including factor Xa and thrombin, to cardiovascular thrombosis stimulated interest in safe and effective antagonists. In acute coronary syndromes, as well as in acute venous thromboembolism, low-molecular-weight heparin (LMWH) has shown great promise and is rapidly becoming accepted therapy (Fig. 19-4).[27-31]

Platelet Glycoprotein IIb/IIIa Receptor Antagonists

Recognizing that the platelet is a pivotal component of arterial thrombosis and building on the knowledge of a congenital disorder characterized by the absence of a platelet surface receptor and a bleeding tendency (Glanzmann's thrombasthenia), the platelet glycoprotein (GP) IIb/IIIa receptor antagonists have, through intense investigation, become a mainstay in the treatment of high-risk patients with acute coronary syndromes and those undergoing percutaneous coronary intervention (Fig. 19-5).[32]

Combination Pharmacotherapy

Astute observations made over the past two decades regarding thrombosis, fibrinolysis, anticoagulants, and platelet antagonists will undoubtedly lead to their combined administration in clinical practice.[33] The challenge will be centered at establishing doses that will attenuate thrombosis while maintaining vascular and hemostatic integrity.

CORONARY ATHEROGENESIS

After monocytes attach to the morphologically intact but dysfunctional vascular endothelium, there is a net directed migration of cells through the endothelium to the subendothelial space, where they undergo differentiation. The phenomenon of "monocyte activation and differentiation" plays an important role in atherosclerosis, particularly with regard to plaque remodeling and lesion progression. This complex process proceeds by means of at least two mechanisms: (1) the generation of reactive oxygen species (free radicals); and (2) the phenotypic modulation and expression of a scavenger receptor or family of receptors. The chemical modification of low-density lipoprotein (LDL) results in its avid uptake by monocytes (now considered macrophages) and the subsequent transformation to foam cells. The

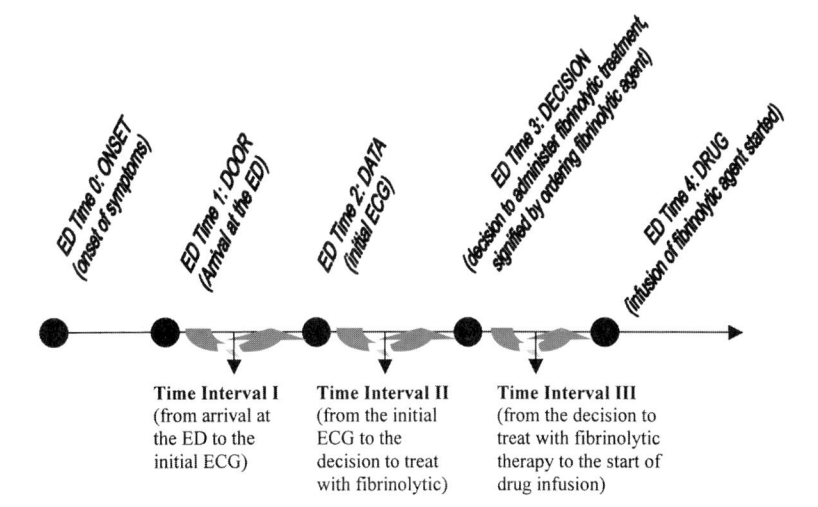

Figure 19-3 The four-D paradigm has been promoted by the National Heart Alert Program to hasten treatment for acute myocardial infarction. (Adapted from Hand M, Brown C, Horan M, et al. The National Heart Attack Alert Program: Progress at 5 years in educating providers, patients and the public: Future directions. J Thromb Thrombol 1998;6:9–17.)

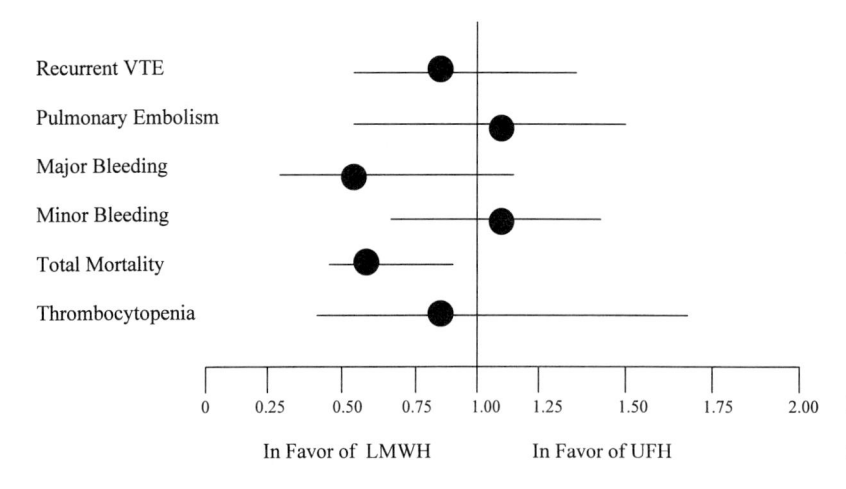

Figure 19-4 Low-molecular-weight heparin (LMWH) compares favorably to unfractionated heparin in patients with deep venous thrombosis.

specific receptor responsible for the uptake of modified LDL fails to effectively downregulate; as a result, a substantial amount of intracellular LDL cholesterol accumulates. When the influx of LDL particles exceeds the capacity of the macrophage scavenger receptors to remove them from the intracellular space, oxidized LDL particles accumulate within the arterial intima. These particles are cytotoxic, causing irreversible injury to endothelial cells, smooth muscle cells, and macrophages. The net result is disruption of the relatively fragile macrophage-derived foam cells, leading to release of their intracellular lipid into the extracellular compartment of the intima; this sequence of events gives rise to the origin of the pultaceous cholesteryl ester-rich core of the atherosclerotic plaque.[34-36]

CORONARY THROMBOGENESIS

The clinical expression of atherosclerotic disease activity is determined by pathologic events leading to coronary thrombosis. In this regard, there are two key factors: (1) the propensity of plaques to rupture, and (2) the thrombogenicity of exposed plaque components.

The morphologic characteristics of plaques that determine their propensity to rupture have been determined from analysis of lesions exhibiting disruption. Observational studies conducted by pathologists using necropsy and atherectomy tissue samples have shown convincingly that plaques causing intraluminal thrombosis are rich in extracellular lipid and that the lipid core of these "vulnerable or rupture-prone" plaques occupies a large proportion of the overall plaque volume. The degree of cross-sectional stenosis involving the vessel lumen is typically less than 50%.[37] In addition to the predominant lipid core, vulnerable plaques are characterized by a thin fibrous cap and high macrophage density.[38] Whereas most individuals with atherosclerotic coronary artery disease exhibit a diversity of plaque types, most have a preponderance of one specific type (vulnerable or nonvulnerable) (Fig. 19-6). The genetic and acquired determinants of plaque type are subjects of intense investigation.

VASCULAR THROMBOSIS

Under normal physiologic conditions, cellular blood components do not interact with an intact vascular endo-

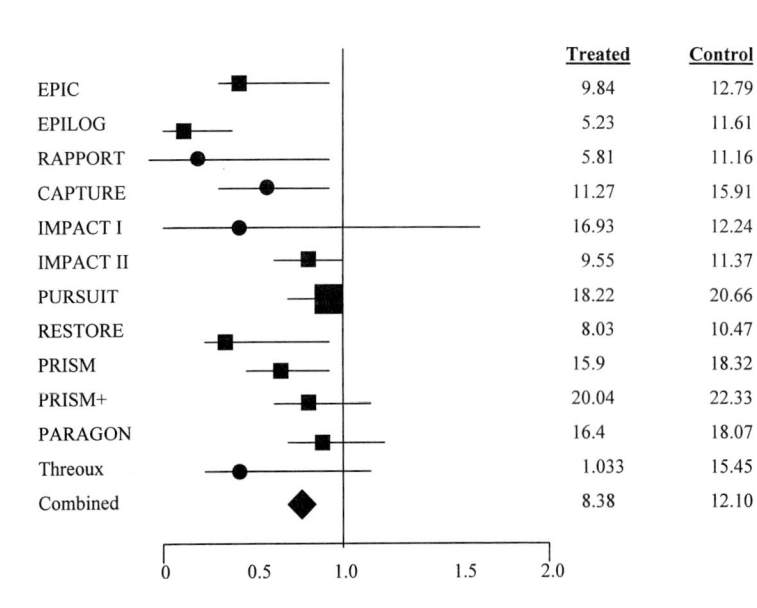

	Treated	Control
EPIC	9.84	12.79
EPILOG	5.23	11.61
RAPPORT	5.81	11.16
CAPTURE	11.27	15.91
IMPACT I	16.93	12.24
IMPACT II	9.55	11.37
PURSUIT	18.22	20.66
RESTORE	8.03	10.47
PRISM	15.9	18.32
PRISM+	20.04	22.33
PARAGON	16.4	18.07
Threoux	1.033	15.45
Combined	8.38	12.10

Figure 19-5 Risk of death, MI, or revascularization (odds ratio, 95% CI) at 30 days in large-scale clinical trials of GPIIb/IIIa receptor antagonists. (From Kong DF, Califf RM, Miller DP, et al. Clinical outcomes of therapeutic agents that block the platelet glycoprotein IIb/IIIa integrin in ischemic heart disease. Circulation 1998;98:2829-2835 with permission.)

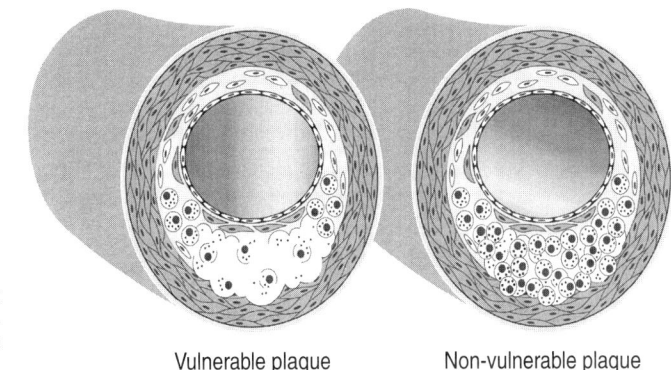

Figure 19-6 Vulnerable plaques are characterized by a prominent lipid core, a thin fibrous cap, and an active state of inflammation. In contrast, nonvulnerable plaques are fibrotic and less likely to disrupt (provoking thrombosis).

thelium. The exposure of circulating blood to disrupted or dysfunctional surfaces initiates a series of complex, yet orderly steps that give rise to the rapid deposition of platelets, erythrocytes, leukocytes, and insoluble fibrin, producing a mechanical barrier to blood flow.

In most instances, thrombosis occurring within the arterial circulatory system is composed of platelets and fibrin in a tightly packed network (white thrombus). By contrast, venous thrombi consist of a more loosely woven network of erythrocytes, leukocytes, and fibrin (red thrombus).

The process of vascular thrombosis, particularly in the coronary arterial system, is dynamic, with clot formation and dissolution occurring almost simultaneously. The overall extent of thrombosis and ensuing circulatory compromise is therefore determined by the predominant force that "shifts" the delicate balance in one direction or another. If local thrombotic stimuli exceed the vessel's own thromboresistant capacity, thrombosis will occur. If, on the other hand, the stimulus is not particularly strong and the intrinsic defenses are intact, clot formation of clinical importance is unlikely. In some circumstances, systemic factors contribute to or "magnify" local prothrombotic factors, shifting the balance toward thrombosis.

Overall, the site, size, and composition of thrombi forming within the arterial circulatory system are determined by the following:

1. alterations in blood flow;
2. thrombogenicity of endocardial and vascular surfaces;
3. concentration and reactivity of plasma cellular components; and
4. preservation and functional capability of physiologic protective mechanisms.

DEFINING STEPS IN ARTERIAL THROMBUS FORMATION

Platelet Deposition

Platelets attaching to nonendothelialized or disrupted surfaces undergo adherence, activation, and distribution along the involved area and subsequent recruitment to form a rapidly enlarging platelet mass. Under physiologic conditions this represents the primary step in hemostasis. In pathologic thrombosis, however, platelet adherence initiates a process that can escalate to an extent that causes circulatory compromise (Fig. 19–7).

The process of platelet deposition involves several processes:

1. platelet attachment to collagen or exposed surface adhesive proteins;
2. platelet activation and intracellular signaling;

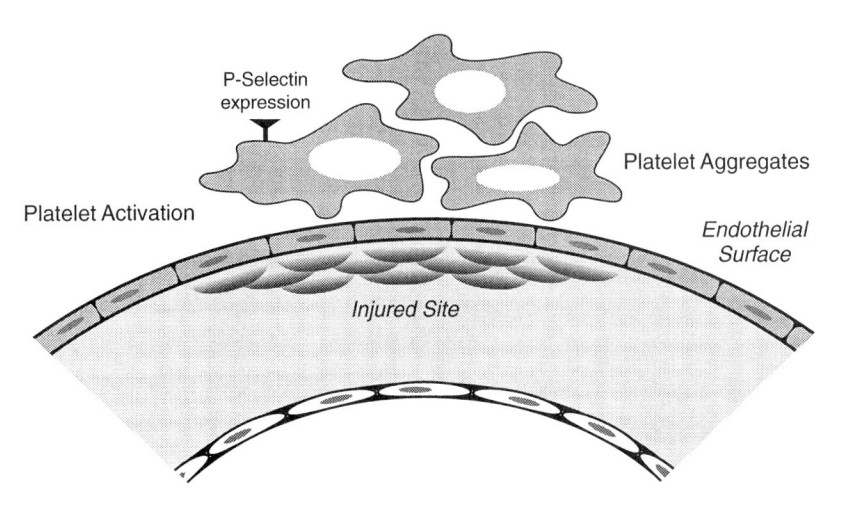

Figure 19-7 The initiating step in arterial thrombosis is *platelet dependent*.

3. the expression of platelet receptors for adhesive proteins;
4. platelet aggregation; and
5. platelet recruitment mediated by thrombin, thromboxane A$_2$, and adenosine diphosphate.

Activation of Coagulation Factors

Thrombin is generated rapidly in response to vascular injury. It also plays a central role in platelet recruitment and formation of an insoluble fibrin network. The thrombotic process is localized, amplified, and modulated by a series of biochemical reactions driven by the reversible binding of circulating proteins (coagulation factors) to damaged vascular cells, elements of exposed subendothelial connective tissue (especially collagen), platelets (which also express receptor sites for coagulation factors), and macrophages. These events lead to an assembly of enzyme complexes that increases local concentrations of procoagulant material; in this way, a relatively minor initiating stimulus can be greatly amplified to yield a thrombus (Fig. 19–8).

Fibrin Formation

The final phase in arterial thrombus formation involves the generation of a stable fibrin network, providing the structural support for circulating cellular elements and the scaffolding for vascular remodeling. In this pivotal process, thrombin cleaves two small peptides, fibrinopeptide A and fibrinopeptide B, to form fibrin monomers, which in turn polymerize to form soluble fibrin strands. An orderly assembly, branching, and lateral association of fibrillar strands follows, terminating with factor XIII-mediated covalent cross-linking to form a cohesive fibrin network (mature thrombus).

CURRENT MANAGEMENT OF ACUTE CORONARY SYNDROMES: PHARMACOLOGIC THERAPIES

The management of advanced atherosclerotic coronary artery disease causing unstable angina, non-ST-segment elevation MI, and ST-segment elevation/bundle branch block MI includes an increasingly vast array of fibrinolytic and antithrombotic agents. It is important for the hematology consultant to be familiar with these commonly used agents, their mechanism of action, and their impact on hemostasis (Table 19–2). Each will be discussed in greater detail in subsequent sections. The American Heart Association/American College of Cardiology has developed comprehensive management guidelines that provide a structured basis for pharmacologic and nonpharmacologic treatment and consistency in patient care (Figs. 19–9 and 19–10).[39,40]

Fibrinolytic Therapy

Mechanisms

In essence, fibrinolytic therapy makes use of the vascular system's native thromboresistant properties by accelerating and amplifying the conversion of an inactive precursor, plasminogen, to the active enzyme plasmin. In turn, plasmin hydrolyzes several key bonds in the fibrin (clot) matrix, causing dissolution (lysis). In the setting of MI or ischemic stroke, blood flow is restored, and with it perfusion of viable tissue is achieved.

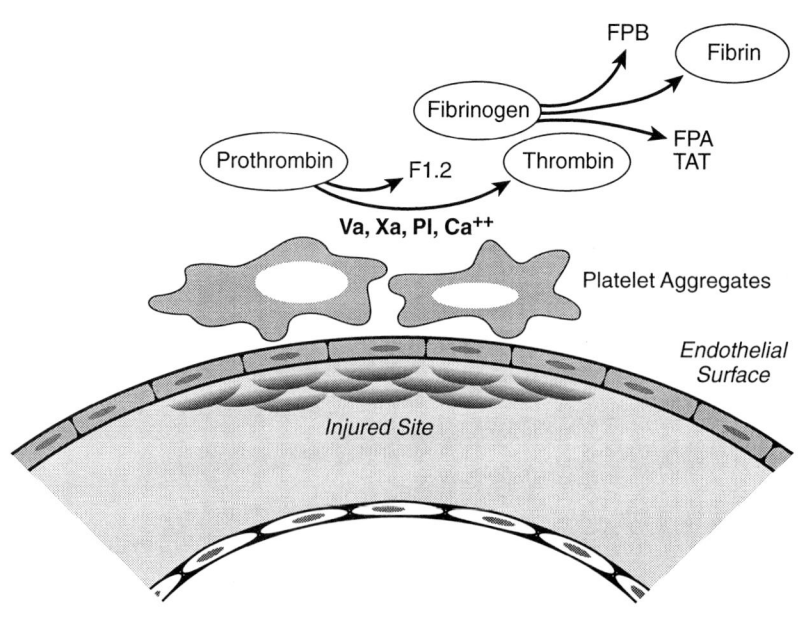

Figure 19–8 The growth phase of arterial thrombosis is *coagulation protein dependent*.

Table 19–2 • CLINICAL USE OF ANTITHROMBOTIC THERAPY IN ACUTE CORONARY SYNDROMES

Oral Antiplatelet Therapy

Aspirin	Initial dose of 162–325 mg nonenteric formulation followed by 75–160 mg/day of an enteric formulation
Clopidogrel (Plavix)	75 mg/day; a loading dose of 4 tablets (300 mg) can be used when rapid onset of action is desired
Ticlopidine (Ticlid)	250 mg twice daily; a loading dose of 500 mg can be used when rapid onset of inhibition is desired; assessment of platelet and white cell counts during treatment is required

Heparins

Dalteparin (Fragmin)	120 IU/kg subcutaneously every 12 h (maximum 10,000 IU twice daily)
Enoxaparin (Lovenox)	1 mg/kg subcutaneously every 12 h; the first dose may be preceded by a 30-mg IV bolus
Heparin (UFH)	Bolus 60–70 U/kg (maximum 5000 U) IV followed by infusion of 12–15 U/kg/h (maximum 1000 U/h) titrated to aPTT 1.5–2.5 times control

Intravenous Antiplatelet Therapy

Abciximab (ReoPro)	0.25-mg/kg bolus followed by infusion of 0.125 μg/kg/min (maximum 10 μg/min) for up to 24 h
Eptifibatide (Integrilin)	180-μg/kg bolus followed by infusion of 2.0 μg/kg/min for 72 to 96 h[a]
Tirofiban (Aggrastat)	0.4 μg/kg for 30 min, followed by infusion of 0.1 μg/kg/min for 48 to 96 h[a]

[a] Different dose regimens were tested in recent clinical trials before percutaneous interventions. UFH, unfractionated heparin.

First-Generation Agents

Streptokinase

Streptokinase is a nonenzymatic protein produced by β-hemolytic streptococci. It activates the fibrinolytic system indirectly by forming a 1:1 stoichiometric complex with plasminogen, which then activates plasminogen, converting it to the active enzyme plasmin.

Urokinase. Urokinase is a trypsin-like serine protease composed of two polypeptide chains connected by a disulfide bridge. It activates plasminogen directly, converting it to the active enzyme plasmin.

Second-Generation Agents

APSAC

Streptokinase and the plasminogen streptokinase activator complex are cleared rapidly from the circulation, with half-lives of 15 minutes and 3 minutes, respectively. By temporarily blocking the active center of plasminogen, the plasma half-life can be prolonged substantially.

Therefore, acylation of plasminogen (APSAC) protects the molecule from autodigestion and also prevents its inactivation by circulating inhibitors, resulting in a half-life of approximately 100 minutes. These features permit bolus dosing. APSAC is not a commonly used fibrinolytic agent.

Scu-PA

Scu-PA (single-chain urokinase-like plasminogen activator) is a single-chain glycoprotein containing 411 amino acids that can be converted to urokinase by hydrolysis of the Lys 148-149 peptide bond. Its fibrin specificity is not completely understood; however, the presence of intravascular fibrin, in and of itself, may neutralize a naturally occurring or inducible circulating scu-PA inhibitor.

Tissue-Type Plasminogen Activator

Native tissue-type plasminogen activator (t-PA) is a serine protease composed of one polypeptide chain containing 527 amino acids. The molecule is converted to a two-chain activator linked by one disulfide bond. This occurs by cleavage of the Arg 275-Ile 276 peptide bond yielding a heavy chain (M_r 31,000) derived from the amino-terminal part of the molecule and a light chain (M_r 28,000) comprising the carboxy-terminal region.

t-PA is a relatively weak enzyme in the absence of fibrin, but in its presence, plasminogen activation (and subsequent conversion to plasmin) is markedly enhanced. This unique property has been explained by an increased affinity of fibrin-bound t-PA for plasminogen without significant influence on the catalytic efficiency of the enzyme. Fibrin essentially increases the local plasminogen concentration by creating an additional interaction between t-PA and its substrate. The high affinity of t-PA for plasminogen in the presence of fibrin thus allows efficient activation on the fibrin surface (fibrin specificity), with little plasminogen activation in plasma.

Third-Generation Agents

A molecular based approach to constructing superior fibrinolytic agents uses site-directed mutagenesis with an end-product that either lacks specific structural or functional domains or duplicates specific domains. In this way, the most favorable properties of a given molecule can be used to their fullest potential, such as increasing fibrin specificity and the circulating half-life. Several mutants, hybrids, and variants of existing fibrinolytic agents have been developed and are currently undergoing evaluation.

The wild-type t-PA molecule (Table 19–3) has served as a template for several third-generation fibrinolytics with the following distinct goals in mind: (1) more rapid restoration of TIMI grade 3 (normal) coronary arterial blood flow; (2) restoration of TIMI grade 3 flow in a

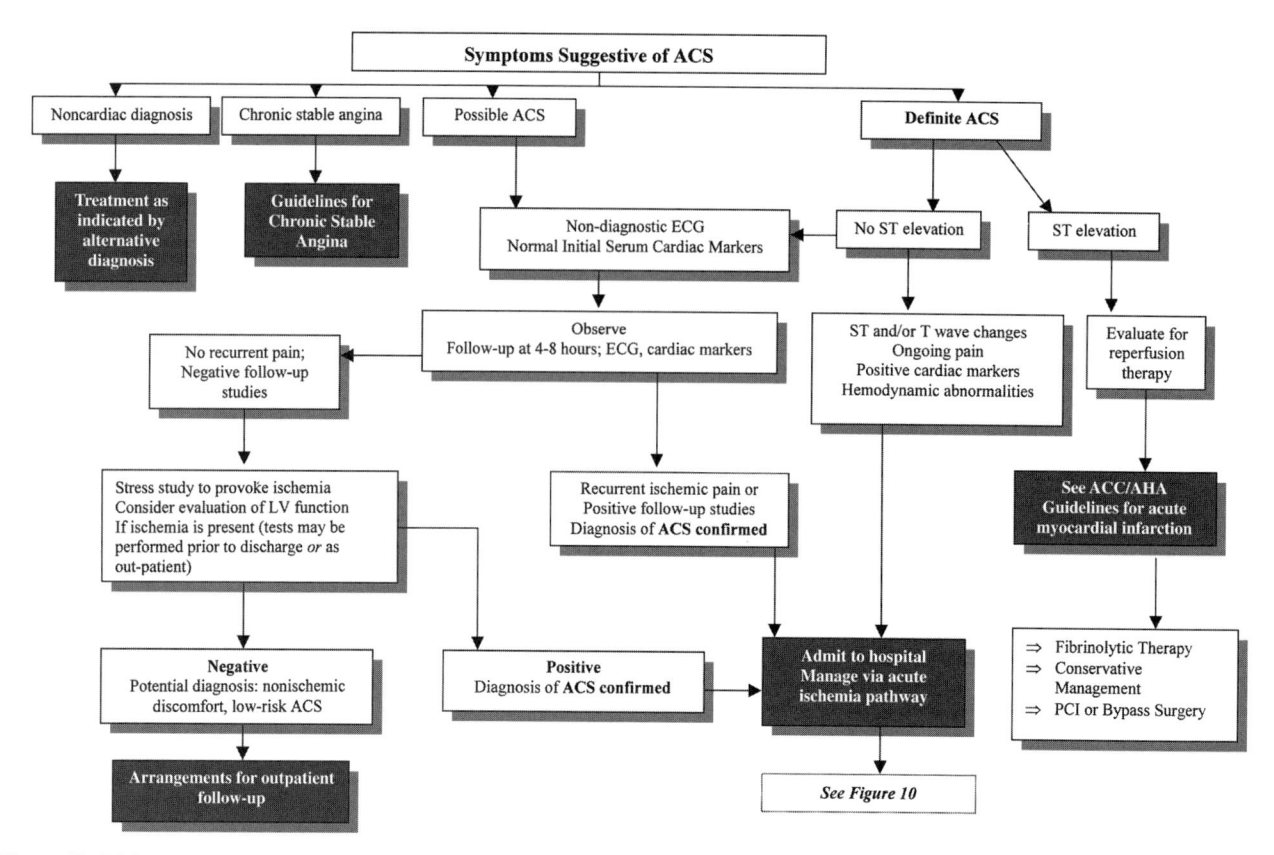

Figure 19–9 Management algorithm for patients with acute coronary syndromes (ACS). (From Braunwald E, Antman EM, Beasley JW, et al. ACC/AHA guidelines for the management of patients with unstable angina and non-ST-segment elevation myocardial infarction: a report of the American College of Cardiology/American Heart Association Task Force on Practice Guidelines (Committee on the Management of Patients with Unstable Angina). J Am Coll Cardiol 2000;36:970–1062 with permission.) PCI = percutaneous coronary intervention.

larger proportion of patients; (3) a longer circulating half-life, permitting bolus administration; (4) a lower risk of intracranial hemorrhage; and (5) an acceptable cost (promoting wide-scale use in daily clinical practice).

Reteplase (Retevase)

Recombinant plasminogen activator (r-PA) is a deletion mutant that contains the kringle-2 and protease domains of the parent t-PA molecule. It has a prolonged half-life (18 minutes) and is given in two abbreviated intravenous infusions (2 minutes) 30 minutes apart. Reteplase is a U.S. Food and Drug Administration (FDA)-approved fibrinolytic for the treatment of acute MI.[41]

TNK-t-PA (Tenecteplase)

TNK-t-PA is a multiple-point mutation of the parent t-PA molecule. In its mutant form T103N, N117Q, KHRR (296-299) AAAA, threonine 103 has been changed to asparagine 103, creating a new glycosylation site (and a longer half-life) (Table 19–4). The change in Asp117 (to glutamine) also contributes to the molecule's prolonged half-life (18 minutes), while the protease sequence change renders TNK more resistant to plasminogen activator inhibitor-1 (PAI-1).[42,43]

n-PA (Lanoteplase)

n-PA is a deletion and point mutant of wild-type t-PA. The finger and epidermal growth factor domains have been deleted, and a point mutation within the kringle-1 domain (Asp^{117}→Glu^{117}) contributes to the molecule's long circulation half-life (30 to 45 minutes).

Other Plasminogen Activators

Staphylokinase is a single-chain polypeptide (136 amino acids) derived from *Staphylococcus aureus*. Like streptokinase, it is not an active enzyme, but forms a 1:1 stoichiometric complex with plasminogen that activates other plasminogen molecules. In animal models, staphylokinase has fibrinolytic potency similar to streptokinase.

Clinical Indications

Fibrinolytic therapy is used predominantly for the early treatment of acute ST-segment elevation MI diagnosed

Hemostatic Aspects of Cardiovascular Medicine 287

Acute Ischemia Pathway

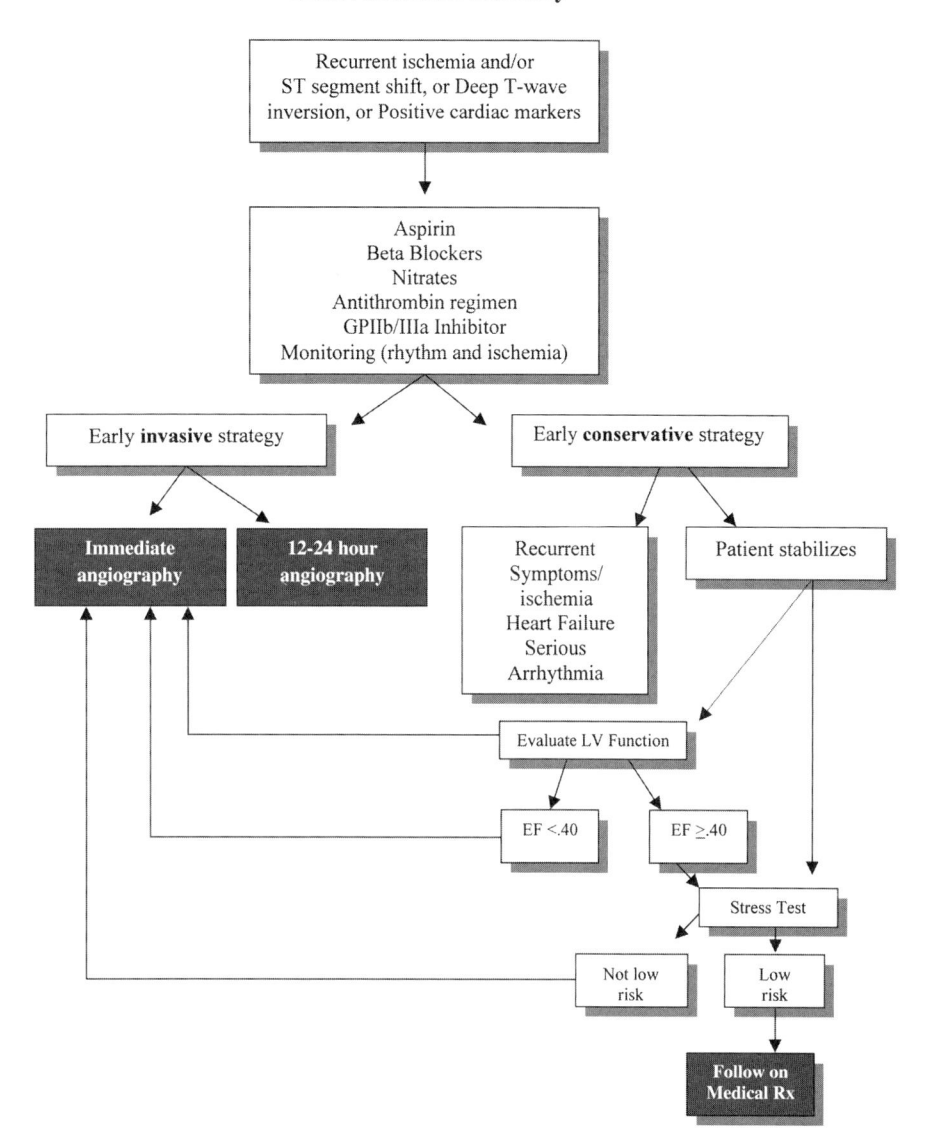

Figure 19–10 Management pathway for patients at high risk for MI and cardiovascular death. An early aggressive approach is recommended for most patients. (From Braunwald E, Antman EM, Beasley JW, et al. ACC/AHA guidelines for the management of patients with unstable angina and non-ST-segment elevation myocardial infarction: a report of the American College of Cardiology/American Heart Association Task Force on Practice Guidelines (Committee on the Management of Patients with Unstable Angina). J Am Coll Cardiol 2000;36:970–1062 with permission.)

within 12 hours of symptom onset. In the United States, t-PA is the most commonly used fibrinolytic agent, with practice patterns evolving toward third-generation drugs (TNK-t-PA, r-PA) that are given as either a "push" bolus or abbreviated infusion. Unfractionated heparin (UFH) (to a target aPTT of 50 to 70 seconds) is recommended as adjunctive therapy for the initial 24 to 48 hours. A transition to LMWH is likely in the near future as are innovative combined pharmacotherapies that include a third-generation fibrinolytic (half-dose), an anticoagulant (LMWH or very-low-molecular-weight heparin), and a platelet GPIIb/IIIa receptor antagonist.

Fibrinolytic therapy can also be used in the treatment of acute pulmonary embolism, particularly events that cause hemodynamic compromise and acute ischemic stroke, when administration is possible within 3 hours of symptom onset.

Complications

The most common complication of fibrinolytic therapy is hemorrhage, occurring in 3% to 5% of patients. Risk factors for major hemorrhage include advanced age, female gender, hypertension, low body weight (less than 70 kg), and high-intensity heparin anticoagulation (aPTT above 70 seconds).

Table 19–3 • STRUCTURE–FUNCTION RELATIONSHIP OF THE PARENT tPA MOLECULE

Domain/Region	Functional Property
Kringle-1	Receptor binding
Kringle-2	Fibrin binding (low affinity)
Fibronectin finger	Fibrin binding (high affinity)
Epidermal growth factor	Hepatic clearance
Protease	Catalytic activity; PAI-1 binding

PAI-1, plasminogen activator inhibitor-1.

Table 19-4 • ALTERATIONS IN THE STRUCTURE OF tPA THAT RESULT IN TNK-tPA

Designation	Substitution	Description
T	T103N	Adds glycosylation site resulting in decreased plasma clearance
N	N117Q	Removes glycosylation site resulting in decreased plasma clearance and increased fibrin binding
K	KHRR (296-299) AAAA	Increased fibrin specificity and increased resistance to PAI-1

Anticoagulants

Heparin Preparations

Heparin compounds consist of a heterogeneous mixture of polysaccharide chains varying in molecular weight and biologic activity. The chain lengths can vary from 5 to 100 or more saccharide units.

The pentasaccharide responsible for heparin–antithrombin binding is a critical part of its biologic activity. All heparins catalyze antithrombin-dependent factor Xa inactivation, but only those containing 18 or more saccharide units are capable of catalyzing thrombin inactivation.

Low-Molecular-Weight Heparin (LMWH). LMWH can vary in molecular weight from 2000 to 10,000 daltons. In both UFH and LMWH preparations, less than 40% of the constituent polypeptide chains contain the pentasaccharide sequence required for high-affinity interactions with antithrombin.

Bioavailability and Pharmacokinetics. The bioavailability of LMWH is essentially complete at a broad range of subcutaneous doses, and its plasma half-life is dose independent, with 90% bioavailability at all doses. This represents a favorable property compared to the inconsistent absorption of UFH, which is particularly poor at low doses. The half-life of intravenously administered LMWH is 5 to 8 hours. After subcutaneous administration, maximum anti-factor Xa activity persists for up to 12 hours. Because the elimination of LMWH depends mostly on renal excretion, its biologic half-life is increased in the setting of renal failure (creatinine clearance less than 40 mL/min). The persistence of anti-Xa activity appears vital its overall clinical efficacy. In addition, LMWH preparations have lower affinity for plasma proteins compared with UFH, especially acute phase reactants, resulting in more predictable circulating levels (and anticoagulation effects).

Indications. LMWH preparations are used clinically in a wide variety of settings that include venous thromboembolism (prophylaxis, treatment) and unstable angina/non-ST-segment elevation MI. The combined administration of LMWH and GPIIb/IIIa receptor antagonists is particularly attractive in acute coronary syndromes and percutaneous coronary interventions. Experience is growing rapidly with LMWH in the setting of atrial fibrillation, following mechanical heart valve surgery, and as "bridging therapies" that can be employed in the outpatient setting.[27-31]

Complications. The most common complication of anticoagulant therapy, including LMWH, is bleeding. Other reported but less frequent complications include anaphylactoid reactions, anaphylaxis (with shock), and heparin-induced thrombocytopenia.

Heparinoids

Derivatives of heparin, knows as heparinoids, have been under investigation for more than a decade. Heparan sulfate, a glycosaminoglycan, inactivates both thrombin and factor Xa. A subfraction of heparan sulfate contains the pentasaccharide sequence common to UFH and LMWH, which has significant affinity for antithrombin. It has been suggested that heparan sulfate also increases fibrinolytic activity. Dermatan sulfate has no affinity for antithrombin; however, it accelerates thrombin inhibition by interacting with heparin cofactor II, a natural inhibitor present in plasma. Interestingly, dermatan sulfate has no effect on calcium release from fetal rat calvaria, which theoretically could translate to an absence of osteoporosis with long-term administration.

Most of the experimental and clinical studies involving heparinoids have used danaparoid sodium (Orgaran, Lomoparan, Org 10172), a mixture of heparan sulfate (84%), dermatan sulfate (12%), and chondroitin sulfate (4%). Danaparoid is a more selective factor Xa inhibitor than either UFH or LMWH, with a 28:1 anti-Xa to anti-IIa ratio, and nearly 100% bioavailability following subcutaneous administration. Elimination occurs by both renal and nonrenal routes with a long elimination half-life (24.5±9.6h) of anti-Xa activity.

Indications. Danaparoid sodium has been used for the prevention and treatment of venous thromboembolism; however, its major indication is sustainment of anticoagulation in patients with heparin-induced thrombocytopenia (HIT).[44]

Complications. Bleeding is the most common complications associated with danaparoid administration. Cross-reactivity (in vivo) with heparin-related antibodies should be considered among patients with HIT who experience progressive thrombocytopenia and thrombotic events while receiving danaparoid.

Hirudin and Its Derivatives

Hirudin is extracted from the parapharyngeal gland of the medicinal leech *Hirudo medicinalis*. A number of derivatives and recombinant preparations have been developed, including hirugen, a synthetic C-terminal peptide fragment of hirudin; bivalirudin, a derivative of hirugen; and the following recombinant agents: desirudin (CGP 39393); lepirudin (HBW 023, Refludan); PEG-hirudin, a chemically defined conjugate of recombinant hirudin (r-hirudin) and two molecules of polyethylene glycol to prolong circulating half-life; and albumin r-hirudin fused molecules, also with prolonged half-lives.

Pharmacokinetics. Hirudin is this most potent direct thrombin antagonist known. It is capable of neutralizing thrombin faster than the physiologic reaction that takes place between thrombin and fibrinogen based on its rapid binding to thrombin's catalytic and fibrinogen-binding sites (hirugen and hirulog bind only to the fibrinogen-binding site). Hirudin also displaces thrombin from fibrinogen and its cellular receptors, and inhibits the activation of factors V, VIII, and XIII. It is an antithrombin-independent anticoagulant that is devoid of anti-factor Xa activity. It does not inhibit other activated clotting factors, but does inhibit thrombin's activation of platelets (but not their activation by other agonists). Hirudin's ability to inactivate clot-bound thrombin, contrary to heparin preparations, may confer a pathobiologic advantage in the treatment of thromboembolism.

Hirudin can be administered by either the intravenous or subcutaneous routes. The bioavailability of hirudin after subcutaneous injection is 85% to 90%, with peak concentrations reached after 1 to 2 hours and a terminal half-life of 2 to 3 hours. After subcutaneous injection (0.1 mg/kg), the aPTT increases by approximately twofold (from baseline). In subjects given hirudin by intravenous bolus, intravenous infusion, or subcutaneous injection, maximum aPTT prolongation is achieved at 10 minutes, 3 to 6 hours, and 2 to 3 hours, respectively. With multiple daily injection, the aPTT returns to normal 16 hours from the time of last injection, suggesting that the drug's pharmacodynamic and pharmacokinetic effects are not cumulative. Hirudin is cleared via the kidneys, a feature with an impact on dosing considerations among patients with renal insufficiency.

Indications. Although hirudin has been studied in the setting of acute coronary syndromes and venous thromboembolism (prophylaxis and treatment), its primary use is in the treatment of HIT. Management strategies for bypass grafting and percutaneous coronary interventions (PCI) are available (Table 19–5). Bivalirudin (Angiomax) is available for high-risk PCI.[47]

Argatroban (Argidipin)

Argatroban is a novel antithrombotic drug, belonging to a class of peptidomimetics that also includes inogatran, efegatran, and nasagatran. Argatroban, like hirudin, does not bind appreciably to plasma proteins, does not cause immune-mediated thrombocytopenia, and does not require antithrombin for production of an anticoagulant effect. Argatroban binds clot-bound thrombin and prevents thrombin-mediated platelet activation. It prolongs the PT, aPTT, and thrombin time in a dose-dependent manner following intravenous administration.

Indications. Argatroban is approved for the management of HIT.

Complications. As with other direct thrombin antagonists and anticoagulants, bleeding is the most common complication of argatroban administration.

Warfarin

The coumarin-derivative oral anticoagulants have been in use since the early 1940s and are well-established treatments in the management of patients with thrombotic disorders.

Mechanism. Warfarin produces its anticoagulant effect by interfering with the cyclic interconversion of vitamin K and its 2,3 epoxide through inhibition of vita-

Table 19–5 • PROCEDURAL MANAGEMENT STRATEGIES FOR HIRUDIN ADMINISTRATION

Procedure	Hirudin Dosing	Coagulation Assay	Target Level of Anticoagulation	Comments
Diagnostic coronary angiography	20 mg IV bolus[a]	Not required	Not required	30 mg IV for patients ≥ 100 kg
PCI	30 mg IV bolus 0.2 mg/kg/h infusion 5 mg IV bolus as needed	ACT	200–250 sec	Sheath removal > 6 h or ACT < 150 sec
Cardiopulmonary bypass (CPB)	0.2 mg/kg added to prime fluid 0.25 mg/kg IV bolus	ACT	> 400 sec	If infusion used, stop approx. 30 min before anticipated
	5–10 mg IV bolus as needed 0.5 mg/min infusion as needed	ECT	250–400 sec	CPB termination

[a] For patients determined to be at increased risk for thrombosis; ACT, activated clotting time; ECT, ecarin clotting time; PCI, percutaneous coronary intervention.

min K epoxide reductase. Vitamin K is an essential cofactor in the post-translational γ-carboxylation of several glutamic acid residues in the vitamin K-dependent coagulation factors II, VII, IX, and X. In the absence of γ-carboxylation, these proteins are unable to bind calcium and phospholipid and depending on the level of carboxylation, they manifest a reduced coagulant (i.e., enzymatic) potential.

Pharmacokinetics. Because of its excellent bioavailability and favorable pharmacokinetics, warfarin is the most commonly used oral anticoagulant in North America. It is highly water soluble and rapidly absorbed from the proximal portion of the gastrointestinal tract after oral ingestion. Peak absorption occurs within 60 to 90 minutes. Food can delay the absorption rate, but rarely reduces the extent of absorption.

Warfarin is a racemic mixture of stereoisomers, each with distinctive metabolic characteristics, half-lives, and anticoagulant potency. Overall, racemic warfarin has an average circulating half-life of 36 to 42 hours and a range of 15 to 60 hours. Variability in warfarin half-life as a result of intrinsic hepatic metabolism, disease states, and/or drug-induced alterations in drug catabolism accounts for the marked individual variation in initial response and daily requirements. Warfarin's effect also varies inversely with the amount of vitamin K absorbed (from the diet and metabolic by-products of gastrointestinal bacteria) and varies directly with the amount of warfarin absorbed or available (unbound to plasma proteins) to exert its anticoagulant effect.

Indications. Warfarin is a widely available and time-tested mainstay in the prevention and treatment of venous and arterial thrombotic disorders (Table 19–6).[46–48] The most common indications in cardiovascular medicine include prophylaxis against thrombosis in patients with atrial fibrillation, following mechanical heart valve replacement, and following acute MI, particularly large infarctions involving the anterior wall and ventricular apex.

Procedures in Patients Receiving Warfarin Anticoagulation Therapy. For patients on long-term anticoagulation requiring invasive procedures, physicians must assess the risk of thromboembolism if anticoagulation is stopped versus the risk of bleeding if anticoagulation is continued at the same or lower intensity. Based on this paradigm, there are several general strategies, including (1) discontinuing warfarin several days before the procedure to allow the INR to return to normal, then restarting therapy shortly after the procedure; (2) lowering the warfarin dose to maintain a lower or subtherapeutic range during the procedure; (3) discontinuing warfarin, admitting the patient to the hospital before surgery, and instituting heparin therapy that is discontinued after surgery when it is considered safe, followed by oral anticoagulation; and (4) administering LMWH on an outpatient basis. The last two options provide the shortest period of subtherapeutic anticoagulation if surgery cannot be done on the patient while anticoagulated.

An approach to anticoagulant therapy for patients undergoing procedures and elective surgery is outlined in Table 19–7.[49]

Platelet Inhibitors

The development of pharmacologic agents that selectively attenuate platelet function for use in the primary and secondary prevention of clinical events in patients with atherosclerotic cardiovascular disease stems from a growing appreciation of their contributory role in arterial thrombosis.

Aspirin

Aspirin, considered the prototypic platelet antagonist, has been available for over a century and currently represents not only a mainstay in the prevention and treatment of vascular events but also its use accounts for the single largest decrease in mortality from acute myocardial infarction over the past 25 years.[49a]

Mechanism. Aspirin irreversibly acetylates cyclooxygenase (COX), impairing prostaglandin metabolism and thromboxane A_2 (TXA_2) synthesis. As a result, platelet aggregation in response to collagen, adenosine diphosphate (ADP), thrombin (in low concentrations), and TXA_2 is inhibited.

Because aspirin more selectively inhibits COX-1 activity (found predominantly in platelets) than COX-2 activity (expressed in tissues following an inflammatory stimuli), its ability to prevent platelet aggregation is seen at relatively low doses, compared with the drug's potential anti-inflammatory effects, which require much higher doses.

Pharmacokinetics. Following oral ingestion, aspirin is absorbed rapidly in the proximal gastrointestinal tract

Table 19–6 • WARFARIN ANTICOAGULATION

Indication	Target INR (Range)
Prophylaxis of venous thrombosis (high-risk patients)	2.5 (2.0–3.0)
Treatment of venous thrombosis	2.5 (2.0–3.0)
Treatment of pulmonary embolism	2.5 (2.0–3.0)
Prevention of systemic embolism[a]	
Tissue heart valves	2.5 (2.0–3.0)
Atrial fibrillation (AF)	2.5 (2.0–3.0)
AF with recurrent systemic embolism	3.0 (2.5–3.5)
Mechanical prosthetic heart valves[b]	3.0 (2.5–3.5)
Postmyocardial infarction	3.0 (2.5–3.0)
Antiphospholipid syndrome with thrombosis	3.5 (3.0–4.0)
Long-term indwelling central vein catheters	Warfarin 1 mg daily

[a] In cases in which the risk of thromboembolism is great, a higher INR may be required.
[b] An INR of 2.5 may be adequate for mechanical valves in the aortic position if there are no other risk factors for thromboembolism.

Table 19-7 • RECOMMENDATIONS FOR PREOPERATIVE AND POSTOPERATIVE ANTICOAGULATION IN PATIENTS TAKING ORAL ANTICOAGULATION[a]

Indication	Before Surgery	After Surgery
Acute venous thromboembolism		
Month 1	IV heparin[b]	IV heparin[b]
Months 2 and 3	No change[c]	IV heparin
Recurrent venous thromboembolism[d]	No change	SC heparin
Month 1	IV heparin	IV heparin[e]
Mechanical heart valve	No change[c]	SC heparin
Nonvalvular atrial fibrillation	No change[c]	SC heparin

[a] IV heparin denotes intravenous heparin at therapeutic doses, and SC heparin denotes subcutaneous UFH or LMWH in doses recommended for prophylaxis against venous thromboembolism in high-risk patients.
[b] A vena caval filter should be considered if acute venous thromboembolism has occurred within 2 wk or if the risk of bleeding during intravenous heparin therapy is high.
[c] If patients are hospitalized, subcutaneous heparin may be administered, but hospitalization is not recommended solely for this purpose.
[d] The term refers to patients whose last episode of venous thromboembolism occurred more than 3 months before evaluation but who require long-term anticoagulation because of high risk of recurrence.
[e] Intravenous heparin should be used after surgery only if the risk of bleeding is low.
From Kearon C, Hirsh J. Management of anticoagulation before and after elective surgery. N Engl J Med 1997; 336:1500–1511, with permission. Copyright © 1997 Massachusetts Medical Society. All rights reserved.

(stomach, duodenum), achieving peak serum levels within 15 to 20 minutes and platelet inhibition within 40 to 60 minutes. As would be expected, enteric-coated preparations are less well absorbed, causing a delay in peak serum levels and platelet inhibition to 60 and 90 minutes, respectively.

The plasma concentration of aspirin decays rapidly, with a circulating half-life of approximately 20 minutes. Despite the drug's rapid clearance from plasma, platelet inhibition persists for the platelet's life span (7 ± 2 days), due to aspirin's irreversible inactivation of COX-1. Because 10% of circulating platelets are replaced every 24 hours, platelet activity (bleeding time, primary hemostasis) returns toward normal (50% activity or higher) by 5 to 6 days after the last aspirin dose.

Indications. Aspirin, perhaps more than any compound used in daily clinical practice, has withstood the test of time as a means to effectively prevent thrombotic events in patients with vascular disease.

Aspirin's beneficial effect is determined largely by the absolute risk of vascular events. Patients at low risk (healthy individuals without predisposing risk factors for vascular disease) derive minimal benefit, while those at high risk (those with unstable angina, prior MI) derive considerable benefit (Fig. 19–11). A risk-based approach to aspirin administration is recommended to avoid subjecting individuals who are unlikely to benefit from its potential adverse effects.

Enteric coating has not been shown to reduce the likelihood of major gastrointestinal adverse effects from either low- or high-dose aspirin. Patients with gastric erosions or ulcers who require treatment with aspirin should receive concomitantly a proton pump inhibitor (e.g., omeprazole) to minimize the risk of hemorrhage.

The impact of aspirin use on the hemodynamic effects of angiotensin-converting enzyme (ACE) inhibitors is a subject of considerable interest and clinical importance. Because COX-1 is believed to produce prostaglandins that regulate physiologic processes, including vascular homeostasis and renal perfusion, drugs with preferential COX-1 activity would be expected to interact with ACE inhibitors to a greater extent than COX-2 antagonists. The available evidence, derived from retrospective analyses, suggests that the antihypertensive and hemodynamic benefits are indeed attenuated when doses of aspirin in excess of 100 mg are administered daily. This effect may be particularly important in patients with poor ventricular performance and clinical heart failure. In these settings, alternative vascular/hemodynamic (e.g., angiotension II receptor antagonist) and antithrombotic (e.g., clopidogrel) therapies should be considered.

Complications. The adverse-effect profile of aspirin, considered predominantly from the perspective of hemorrhage, is determined largely by:

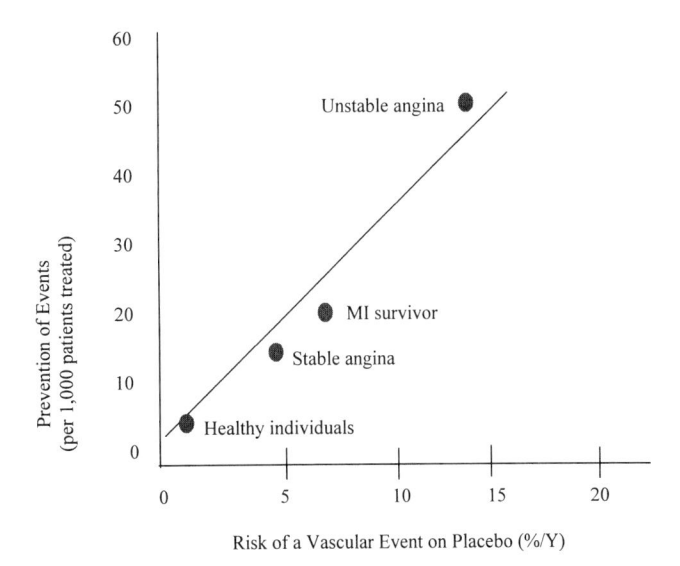

Figure 19–11 The benefit derived from aspirin is greatest for patients at high risk (for a vascular event).

- dose;
- duration of administration; and
- associated structural (peptic ulcer disease, *Helicobacter pylori* infection) and hemostatic (inherited, acquired) abnormalities.

Primary Prevention. Aspirin has been evaluated in three primary prevention trials involving over 30,000 healthy individuals. A fourth trial, designed to evaluate the benefit of low-dose aspirin in patients with hypertension, was recently completed. The Women's Health Initiative is currently evaluating the effects of low-dose aspirin prophylaxis (100 mg every other day) in 40,000 healthy women.[50–53]

Considered collectively, the data show convincingly that aspirin reduces the likelihood of MI, but at a cost of increased risk for hemorrhagic complications, including stroke. With increasing patient risk, additional benefit is gained, improving the net clinical benefit relationship.

Secondary Prevention. The Antiplatelet Trialists' Collaboration provides firm evidence in support of aspirin's ability to prevent vascular events, including nonfatal MI, nonfatal stroke, and vascular death in a wide range of high-risk patient groups. In high-risk patients as a whole, antiplatelet therapy (predominantly with aspirin) reduced nonfatal MI by approximately one third, nonfatal stroke by one third, and vascular death by nearly one quarter (Fig. 19–12). Although a majority of patients were treated for at least for 1 year, the favorable effect persisted beyond this time point, and those treated for longer periods (up to 3 years) derived increasing benefit.[54]

Although cardiac events that occur during aspirin administration are often considered a "failure of therapy," the nature of the event and clinical outcome must be considered carefully. For example, patients with acute coronary syndromes are less likely to experience an ST-segment elevation MI if they have taken aspirin in the days to weeks before a cardiac event.[55]

Dosing. Aspirin dose varied widely in the Antiplatelet Trialists' Collaboration overview, ranging from 75 to 1500 mg daily; however, indirect comparisons failed to identify differences that favored higher over lower doses. Accordingly, a maintenance dose of 75 to 100 mg daily may be adequate in a majority of high-risk patients. A somewhat higher dose (160 to 325 mg) is recommended when treatment is first being initiated.

Coronary Artery Bypass Grafting. Patients undergoing coronary artery bypass surgery are unique for several reasons. First, a majority of patients have advanced coronary atherosclerosis. Second, many individuals have concomitant peripheral vascular and cerebrovascular disease. Last, new vascular conduits (bypass grafts) provide an additional nidus for atherothrombosis. Over the years, upward of 24 clinical trials have been performed to determine the effectiveness of antiplatelet therapy in preventing early (up to 10 days following surgery) and late (6 to 12 months) saphenous vein graft occlusion. Ten of the trials investigated aspirin in doses ranging from 100 to 975 mg daily. Several also evaluated patients receiving internal mammary coronary bypass grafts.[56]

Considered collectively, and aided by the overview provided by the Antiplatelet Trialists' Collaboration, the data reveal improved saphenous vein graft patency with aspirin administration. Although a direct benefit on internal mammary bypass grafts has not been established, treatment is recommended given the common coexistence of vascular disease and the overall risk of thrombotic events.

Transient Ischemic Attacks/Stroke. The International Stroke Trial[57] and the Chinese Acute Stroke Trial[58] evaluated the efficacy and safety of aspirin given in a daily dose of 300 and 160 mg, respectively, in nearly 40,000 patients with acute ischemic stroke. Treatment was initiated within 48 hours of symptom onset and continued for 2 to 4 weeks. The combined results suggest an absolute benefit of 10 fewer deaths or nonfatal strokes per 1000 patients in the first month of treatment. The risk of hemorrhagic stroke was also increased (two excess events per 1000 patients).

Long-term aspirin administration reduces the likelihood of stroke (and other vascular events) in patients with transient ischemic attacks and completed minor strokes. Although there is an ongoing debate within the neurology community concerning the optimal daily dose, 50 to 325 mg is considered an acceptable range.

Percutaneous Coronary Interventions. Percutaneous coronary interventions (PCI), including standard balloon angioplasty, rotational atherectomy, and laser angioplasty, are associated with vascular injury, atheromatous plaque disruption, platelet activation, and at times, thrombotic occlusion. Based on data derived over the past two decades, antiplatelet therapy (predominantly

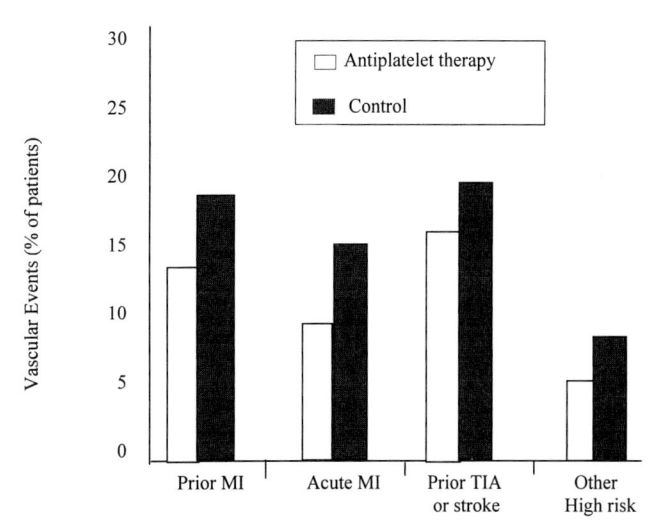

Figure 19–12 Antiplatelet therapy significantly reduces vascular event rates in high-risk patients. (From International Stroke Trial Collaborative Group. The International Stroke Trial (IST): a randomized trial of aspirin, subcutaneous heparin, both, or neither among 19,435 patients with acute ischaemic stroke. Lancet 1997;349:1569–1581 with permission.)

with aspirin) represents a standard of care for PCI, reducing periprocedural event rates by 50% to 60%.[59]

Ticlopidine

Ticlopidine (Ticlid) is a thienopyridine derivative that is structurally and functionally distinct from all other platelet antagonists.

In-Vitro Effects. In vitro, ticlopidine is a weak inhibitor of platelet aggregation. Against low concentrations of collagen, arachidonic acid, or ADP, ticlopidine exhibits much less antiaggregative activity than aspirin. In addition, the concentrations of ticlopidine required to achieve inhibition are in excess of those clinically achievable in clinical practice.

In addition to its modest in-vitro platelet-inhibiting properties, ticlopidine:

- attenuates endothelial cell growth;
- induces morphologic cellular changes; and
- increases endothelial cell-associated release of von Willebrand factor into plasma.

Ex-Vivo Effect on Platelet Function. After in-vivo administration (oral ingestion), ticlopidine becomes a concentration-dependent, potent inhibitor of ADP-mediated platelet aggregation. With standard dosing, platelet inhibition is evident within 24 to 48 hours; however, peak effects are not achieved for 3 to 6 days. The platelet-inhibiting effects of ticlopidine persist for 72 hours after the drug's discontinuation and progressively decline over the next 4 to 8 days.[60,61]

Pharmacokinetics. Following oral administration, 80% to 90% of a ticlopidine dose is absorbed, with peak plasma concentration occurring within 1 to 3 hours. Peak levels after a 250-mg dose are approximately 0.9 mg/L. Ticlopidine is rapidly and extensively metabolized in the liver to one or more metabolites that are responsible for the drug's platelet-inhibiting properties.[62]

Clinical Experience and Indications. The ability of ticlopidine to inhibit platelet aggregation in a dose-dependent manner, coupled with the synergistic effects observed when it is combined with aspirin, has led to a relatively large clinical experience in a variety of cardiovascular setting (Table 19–8).[63–74]

Complications. Approximately 10% to 15% of patients receiving ticlopidine at the recommended dosage of 250 mg twice daily (taken with food) experience side effects, the most common of which are gastrointestinal complaints and skin rashes. Bleeding is an uncommon side effect but is possible, particularly in individuals at increased risk and in those undergoing invasive/surgical procedures. Cholestatic jaundice and hepatitis have also been reported.

Table 19–8 • RANDOMIZED CLINICAL TRIALS OF TICLOPIDINE

Trial/Investigator	Study Population	Patients (n)	Treatment
Stroke and TIA			
CATS	Recent stroke	1072	Ticlopidine 250 mg bid or placebo
TASS	Recent TIA or minor stroke	3069	Ticlopidine 250 mg bid or ASA, 625 mg bid
TISS	Recent TIA amaurosis fugax or minor stroke	1632	Ticlopidine or indobufen (median doses 250 mg bid and 200 mg/d)
PAOD			
Swedish Ticlopidine Multicentre Study	Intermittent claudication	687	Ticlopidine 250 mg bid or placebo
Arcan et al.	Chronic intermittent claudication	169	Ticlopidine 250 mg bid or placebo
EMATAP	Intermittent claudication	615	Ticlopidine 250 mg bid or placebo for 24 weeks
Unstable Angina			
Balsano et al.[64]	Unstable angina	652	Conventional therapy with or without ticlopidine 250 mg bid
SVG Patency			
Chevigne et al.	Coronary bypass surgery	77	Ticlopidine 250 mg bid (started 3 days before surgery) or placebo
Limet et al.[66]	Coronary bypass surgery	173	Ticlopidine 250 mg bid (first dose on day 2) or placebo
Becquemin et al.	Femoropopliteal or femorofemoral bypass surgery	243	Ticlopidine 250 mg bid or placebo
Diabetic Retinopathy			
TMD	Nonproliferative diabetic retinopathy	435	Ticlopidine 250 mg bid or placebo

Abbreviations: ASA, aspirin; MI, myocardial infarction; PTCA, percutaneous transluminal coronary angioplasty; TIA, transient ischemic attack; CATS, Canadian American Ticlopidine Study; TASS, Ticlopidine Aspirin Stroke Study; TISS, Ticlopidine Indobufen Stroke Study; PAOD, peripheral arterial occlusive disease, EMATAP, Estudio Multicentrco de la Ticlopidine en las Arteriopatias perifericas; SVG, saphenous vein graft; TMD, Ticlopidine Microangiopathy of Diabetes.

The side effects of ticlopidine that cause the most concern are hematologic in origin and include agranulocytosis, neutropenia, erythroleukemia, thrombocytopenia, and thrombotic thrombocytopenic purpura (TTP). The occurrence of TTP, although rare, is perhaps more frequent than previously believed and high mortality rates have been reported, particularly in the absence of aggressive intervention (plasmapheresis).

In an overview of 60 cases of TTP associated with ticlopidine administration, the drug had been taken for less than 1 month by 80% of the patients and a normal platelet count was documented within 2 weeks of the disorder's onset.[75] A retrospective analysis of 43,322 patients undergoing coronary stenting at study sites participating in the Evaluation of Platelet GPIIb/IIIa Inhibitor for Stenting (EPISTENT) Study uncovered an incidence of 1 case per 4814 patients treated.[76] Although an infrequent occurrence, the 0.02% incidence is noteworthy (and clinically relevant) when the estimated 0.0004% incidence in the general population is considered. Thus close monitoring of platelet counts is recommended, particularly if therapy is continued for longer than 2 weeks.

Clopidogrel

Clopidogrel (Plavix) is a novel platelet antagonist that is several times more potent than ticlopidine yet is associated with fewer adverse effects.

In-Vitro and Ex-Vivo Effects on Platelets. Even at high concentrations (500 μM) clopidogrel does not inhibit ADP-mediated platelet aggregation in vitro.

At high doses (e.g., 375 mg or higher), clopidogrel reduces ADP-mediated platelet aggregation within 4 hours of administration (Fig. 19-13). Full inhibition of ADP-mediated platelet activation is produced within 2 hours by single loading doses of 525 mg or higher. At doses used in patients with vascular disease (75 mg daily), a modest degree of inhibition (25%) is seen within 48 hours, followed by a more substantial response (40% to 50% inhibition) after 3 to 4 days of daily administration. As with ticlopidine, the antiplatelet effects derived from clopidogrel are the result of an active metabolite (a carboxylic acid derivative generated by hepatic metabolism) that appears in the circulation. The plasma elimination half-life is 7.7 ± 2.3 hours.

Based on ADP-induced platelet aggregation studies, clopidogrel is approximately 100-fold more potent than ticlopidine. There are no known cumulative antiplatelet effects with prolonged oral administration.

Mechanism. The site(s) of action responsible for clopidogrel's platelet-inhibiting effects has not been fully elucidated. Clopidogrel has no direct effect on cyclooxygenase, thromboxane synthesis, phosphodiesterase, or adenosine uptake. In contrast, in-vitro experiments have shown that it does impair calcium mobilization and fibrinogen binding to the platelet GPIIb/IIIa receptor.[77,78] Although there is still some debate, several investigators have reported that clopidogrel derives its antiplatelet properties from inhibiting either a population of ADP-receptor sites or a region of the platelet between the ADP-binding site and the adentylate cyclase catalytic subunit.

Absorption and Metabolism. Clopidogrel is absorbed rapidly after oral administration and undergoes extensive metabolism in the liver. Less than 5% of the drug is excreted unchanged in the urine. As previously described, clopidogrel must undergo hepatic metabolism to be an active platelet antagonist.

Clinical Experience and Indications. The well-documented benefit derived from platelet inhibition in patients with vascular disease, coupled with a less than pristine adverse-effect profile witnessed with aspirin and ticlopidine, fostered the rapid development of clopidogrel as a potential alternative to existing therapies. The Clopidogrel versus Aspirin in Patients at Risk for Ischemic Events (CAPRIE) study[79] was designed to test the hypothesis that clopidogrel (75 mg daily) administered without aspirin would reduce vascular events in high-risk patients by approximately 15% compared with aspirin (325 mg daily). The study population consisted of patients with atherosclerotic vascular disease manifested as recent ischemic stroke, recent MI, or symptom-

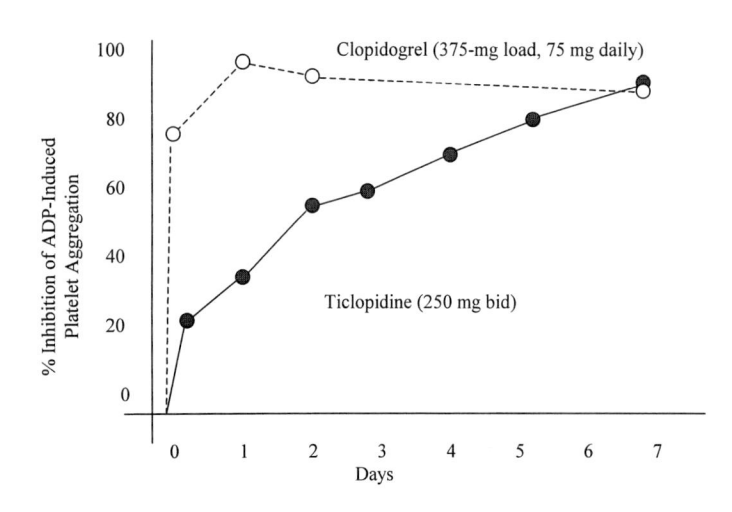

Figure 19-13 An "oral loading" strategy for clopidogrel administration provides rapid platelet inhibition.

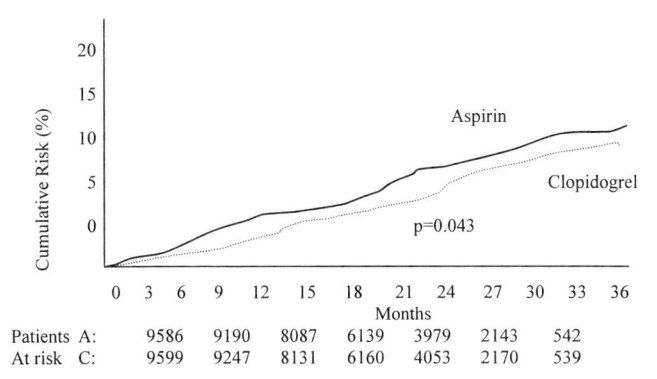

Figure 19–14 Cumulative risk of ischemic stroke, MI, or vascular death in the CAPRIE study. (From CAPRIE Steering Committee. A randomized, blind trial of Clopidogrel Versus Aspirin in Patients at Risk for Ischemic Events (CAPRIE). Lancet 1996;348:1329–1339 with permission.)

atic peripheral arterial disease. A total of 19,185 patients were enrolled in the international trial, with more than 6300 individuals in each of the prespecified subgroups. The mean follow-up was 1.91 years. Patients treated with clopidogrel (by intention-to-treat analysis) had a 5.32% annual risk of ischemic stroke, MI, or vascular death compared with 5.83% among aspirin-treated patients (Fig. 19–14) (relative-risk reduction 8.7%; 95% confidence interval 0.3 to 16.5; $p = 0.043$). A corresponding on-treatment analysis yielded a relative risk reduction of 9.4%.

For patients experiencing a stroke, the average event rate per year in the clopidogrel group was 7.15% compared with 7.71% in the aspirin group (relative-risk reduction 7.3%, $p = 0.26$). For patients with MI, the average event rate per year was 5.03% in the clopidogrel group compared with 4.84% in the aspirin group (relative-risk increase 3.7%; $p = 0.66$). In contrast, patients with peripheral vascular disease experienced a 3.71% annual event rate with clopidogrel and a 4.86% rate with aspirin (relative-risk reduction 23.8%; $p = 0.002$) (Fig. 19–15).

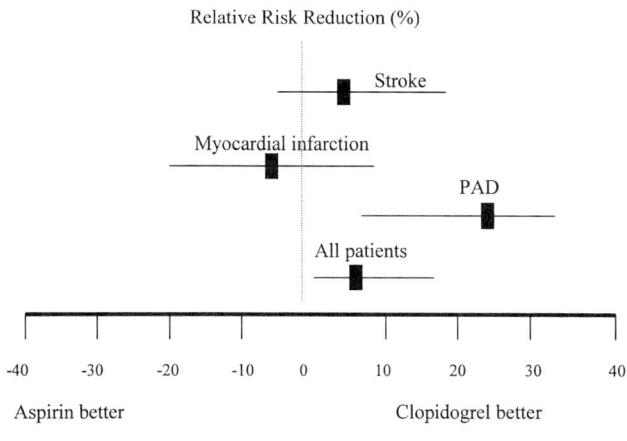

Figure 19–15 The relative risk of vascular events was lower in patients treated with clopidogrel, particularly those with peripheral vascular disease. (From CAPRIE Steering Committee. A randomized, blind trial of Clopidogrel Versus Aspirin in Patients at Risk for Ischemic Events (CAPRIE). Lancet 1996;348:1329–1339 with permission.)

Although there were no major differences in safety between treatment groups, a greater proportion of patients receiving aspirin had the study drug permanently discontinued because of gastrointestinal hemorrhage, indigestion, nausea, or vomiting. Approximately one out of the every 1000 patients treated with clopidogrel experienced significant neutropenia (less than 1.2×10^9/L); however, no cases of TTP were reported.

The combination of aspirin (325 mg) and clopidogrel (300 mg oral bolus, 75 mg daily) is considered optimal care for patients receiving coronary arterial stents. Although most experienced centers recommend 2 to 4 weeks of clopidogrel therapy, treatment for up to 6 months may offer extended benefit in high-risk patients subjects, including those who have experienced prior subacute stent thrombosis and patients undergoing intracoronary brachytherapy.

Complications. The occurrence of bone marrow suppression and other adverse effects is lower with clopidogrel than ticlopidine; however, TTP has been reported.[80]

Platelet Glycoprotein IIb/IIIa Receptor Antagonists

The GPIIb/IIIa (αIIb/β_3) receptor represents a final common pathway for platelet aggregation in response to a wide variety of biochemical and mechanical agonists. Accordingly, it represents an attractive target for therapies that can be applied to patients with acute coronary syndromes in whom platelet activation is heightened substantially and represents the predominant pathobiologic substrate.

The evolution of GPIIb/IIIa receptor antagonists represents a true "bench-to-bedside" metamorphosis that began with murine monoclonal antibodies and more recently has focused on small peptide or nonpeptide molecules that have structural similarities to fibrinogen and other circulating ligands. There are currently three intravenous GPIIb/IIIa receptor antagonists that have been approved by the U.S. FDA:

- Abciximab (ReoPro)
- Tirofiban (Aggrastat)
- Eptifibatide (Integrilin).

Abciximab

Abciximab (ReoPro) is the Fab fragment of the chimeric human-murine monoclonal antibody c7E3.

Pharmacokinetics. Following an intravenous bolus, free plasma concentrations of abciximab decrease rapidly, with an initial half-life of less than 10 minutes and a second-phase half-life of 30 minutes, representing rapid binding to the platelet GPIIb/IIIa receptor. Platelet function generally recovers over the next 48 hours; however, abciximab remains in the circulation for 10 or more days in the platelet-bound state.

Pharmacodynamics. Intravenous administration of abciximab in doses ranging from 0.15 to 0.3 mg/kg produces a rapid dose-dependent inhibition of platelet function as measured by ex-vivo platelet aggregation in response to ADP. At the highest dose, 80% of the platelet GPIIb/IIIa receptors are occupied within 2 hours and platelet aggregation, even with 20 μM ADP, is completely inhibited. Sustained inhibition is achieved with prolonged infusions (12 to 24 hours) and low-level receptor blockade is present for up to 10 days following cessation of the infusion. Platelet aggregation in response to 5 μM ADP returns to 50% or more of baseline within 24 hours in a majority of cases (Fig. 19–16).

Clinical Experience. In nearly 2100 patients undergoing either balloon coronary angioplasty or atherectomy who were judged to be at high risk for ischemic (thrombotic) complications, a bolus of abciximab (0.25 mg/kg) followed by a 12-hour continuous infusion (not to exceed 10 μg/min) was found to reduce the occurrence of death or MI and the need for an urgent intervention (repeat angioplasty, stent placement, balloon pump insertion, or bypass grafting) by 35%.[81]

The Evaluation in PTCA to Improve Long-term Outcome with Abciximab GPIIb/IIIa Blockade (EPILOG) study[80] included 2792 patients undergoing elective or urgent percutaneous coronary revascularization who received either abciximab with standard, weight-adjusted heparin (initial bolus 100 U/kg, target activated clotting time [ACT] 300 seconds or more); abciximab with low-dose, weight-adjusted heparin (initial bolus 70 U/kg, target ACT 200 seconds); or placebo with standard-dose, weight-adjusted heparin. At 30 days, the composite event rates were 5.4%, 5.2%, and 11.7%, respectively. The benefit was observed in both high-risk and low-risk patients, suggesting that GPIIb/IIIa receptor blockade:

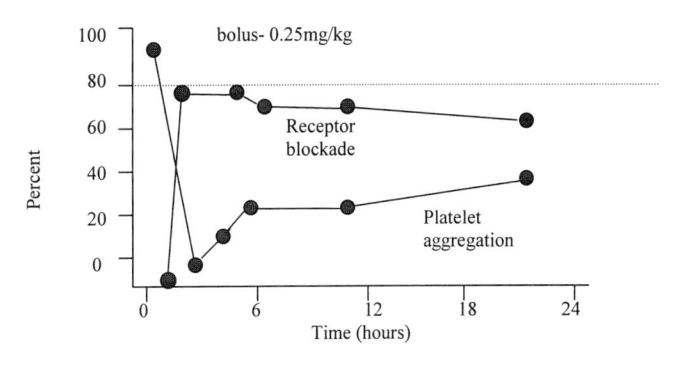

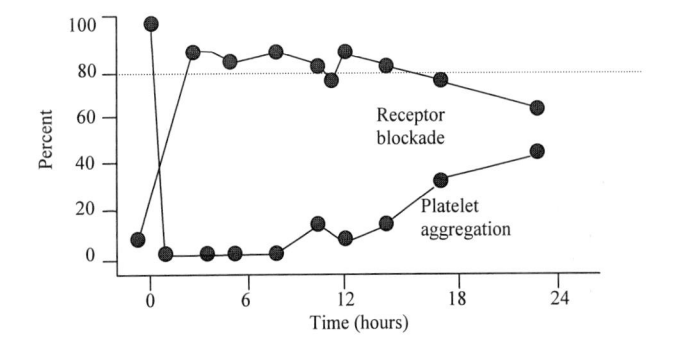

- has broad clinical use in reducing ischemic complications associated with coronary revascularization and
- can be used in combination with lower-intensity heparin anticoagulation.

The c7E3 Fab Antiplatelet Therapy in Unstable Refractory Angina (CAPTURE) study[85] was designed uniquely to assess whether abciximab, given during the 18 to 24 hours before coronary angioplasty, could improve outcome in patients with refractory (myocardial ischemia despite therapy with nitrates, heparin, and aspirin) unstable angina. A total of 1265 patients were randomly assigned to abciximab or placebo. By 30 days, the primary composite end point (death, MI, or urgent revascularization) occurred in 11.3% of abciximab-treated patients and in 15.9% of placebo-treated patients ($p = 0.012$). The rate of MI was lower before and during coronary interventions in those given abciximab.

Tirofiban

Tirofiban (Aggrastat), a tyrosine derivative with a molecular weight of 495 kd, is a nonpeptide inhibitor (peptidomimetic) of the platelet GPIIb/IIIa receptor.

Pharmacodynamics. Tirofiban, like other nonpeptides, mimics the geometric, stereotactic, and change characteristics of the RGD sequence, thus interfering with platelet aggregation.

Three doses of tirofiban were studied in a phase I study of patients undergoing coronary angioplasty who received one of three graduated regimens intravenously with a bolus dose of 5, 10, or 15 μg/kg and a continuous (16 to 24 hour) infusion of 0.05, 0.10, or 0.15 μg/kg/

Figure 19–16 Platelet inhibition in response to 5 μM ADP for abciximab (bolus) (**top panel**) and abciximab (bolus, infusion) (**bottom panel**). (Adapted from Uprichard AC. Handbook of Experimental Pharmacology. Berlin, Germany, Springer-Verlag, 1999.)

min.[84] A dose-dependent inhibition of ex-vivo platelet aggregation was observed within minutes of bolus administration and was sustained during the continuous infusion.

Clinical Trials and Experience. The Randomized Efficacy Study of Tirofiban Outcomes and Restenosis (RESTORE) trial[85] was a randomized, double-blind, placebo-controlled trial of tirofiban in patients undergoing coronary intervention within 72 hours of hospital presentation with an acute coronary syndrome.

Patients (n = 2139) received tirofiban as a 10-μg/kg intravenous bolus over a 30-minute period and a continuous infusion of 0.15 μg/kg/min over 36 hours. All patients received heparin and aspirin. The primary composite end point (death, MI, angioplasty failure requiring bypass surgery or unplanned stent placement, recurrent ischemia requiring repeat angioplasty) at 30 days was reduced from 12.2% in the placebo group to 10.3% in the tirofiban group (16% relative reduction).

The Platelet Receptor Inhibition in Ischemic Syndrome Management (PRISM) trial[86] included 3231 patients with unstable angina/non-ST-segment elevation MI. All patients received aspirin and were randomized to treatment with either unfractionated heparin or tirofiban, given as a loading dose of 0.6 μg/kg/min over 30 minutes followed by a maintenance infusion of 0.15 μg/kg/min for 48 hours (angiography/revascularization was discouraged during the infusion period). The primary composite end point (death, MI, refractory ischemia) at 48 hours was 3.8% in tirofiban-treated patients and 5.6% in placebo (aspirin/heparin)-treated patients (risk reduction 33%). Benefit was maintained but overall was less impressive at 7 and 30 days.

The PRISM in Patients Limited by Unstable Signs and Symptoms (PLUS) trial[87] included 1915 patients with unstable angina and non-ST-segment elevation MI who were treated with aspirin and heparin and randomized to either tirofiban (0.4 μg/kg/min for 30 minutes; then 0.1 μg/kg/min for a minimum of 48 hours and a maximum of 108 hours) or placebo (heparin). Angiography and revascularization were performed at the discretion of the treating physician. Tirofiban-treated patients had a lower composite event rate at 7 days than the placebo group, 12.9% versus 17.9%, risk reduction 34%. The benefit was due mainly to a reduced incidence of MI (47% risk reduction) and refractory ischemia (30% risk reduction). The benefit was maintained at 30 days (22% risk reduction in composite event rate) and at 6 months. The trial originally included a tirofiban-alone arm that was dropped because of excess mortality at 7 days. Although patients in this group did no worse at 48 or 30 days and the mechanism of potential detriment is unknown, concomitant treatment with heparin is recommended with tirofiban administration.

Eptifibatide

Eptifibatide (Integrilin) is a nonimmunogenic cyclic heptapeptide with an active pharmacophore that is derived from the structure of barbourin, a platelet GPIIb/IIIa inhibitor derived from the venom of the southeastern pigmy rattlesnake.[88]

Pharmacokinetics. The plasma half-life of eptifibatide is 10 to 15 minutes and clearance is predominantly renal (75%) and to a lesser degree hepatic (25%). The antiplatelet effect has a rapid onset of action and is rapidly reversible.

Pharmacodynamics. In a pilot study of patients undergoing PCI, patients were randomized to one of four eptifibatide dosing schedules:

- 180-μg/kg bolus, 1.0-μg/kg/min infusion;
- 135-μg/kg bolus, 0.5-μg/kg/min infusion;
- 90-μg/kg bolus, 0.75-μg/kg/min infusion; or
- 135-μg/kg bolus, 0.75-μg/kg/min infusion.

All patients received aspirin and unfractionated heparin and were continued on the study drug for 18 to 24 hours. The two highest bolus doses produced greater than 80% inhibition of ADP-mediated platelet aggregation within 15 minutes of administration in a majority of patients (greater than 75%). A constant infusion of 0.75 μg/kg/min maintained the antiplatelet effect, whereas an infusion of 0.5 μg/kg/min allowed gradual recovery of platelet function. In all dosing groups, platelet function returned to greater than 50% of baseline with 4 hours of terminating the infusion.[89]

Clinical Trials and Experience. The Integrilin to Minimize Platelet Aggregation and Coronary Thrombosis (IMPACT-II) trial[90] enrolled 4010 patients undergoing elective, urgent, or emergent coronary interventions. Patients were assigned to either placebo, a bolus of 135 μg/kg/min epitfibatide followed by an infusion of 0.5 μg/kg/min for 20 to 24 hours, or a 135-μg/kg bolus with a 0.75-μg/kg/min infusion. By 30 days, the composite end point (death, MI, unplanned revascularization, stent placement for abrupt closure) occurred in 11.4%, 9.2%, and 9.9% of patients, respectively. Although the benefit of treatment was maintained at 6 months, the differences between groups were not statistically significant. Review of the data derived from IMPACT II suggests that the greatest benefit from eptifibatide administration can be expected within the initial 24 to 72 hours of administration by reducing abrupt vessel closure and other ischemic complications.

The Enhanced Suspension of Platelet Receptor GPIIb/IIIa Using Integrilin Therapy (ESPRIT) trial designed to study eptifibatide as a 180-μg/kg bolus and a 2.0-μg/kg/min infusion followed by a second 180-μg/kg bolus 30 minutes later in patients undergoing either elective or urgent PCI was stopped prematurely because of benefit in eptifibatide-treated patients.

The Platelet Glycoprotein IIb/IIIa in Unstable Angina Receptor Suppression Using Integrilin Therapy (PURSUIT) trial[91] included patients with unstable angina or non-ST-segment elevation MI with symptoms within 24 hours and electrocardiographic changes within 12 hours (of ischemia). A total of 10,948 patients were randomized to eptifibatide: a 180-μg/kg bolus plus a 1.3-μg/kg/min infusion, or a 180-μg/kg bolus plus a 2.0-μg/

Table 19-9 • INDIVIDUAL CHARACTERISTICS OF THE GPIIb/IIIa RECEPTOR ANTAGONISTS

Characteristic	Abciximab	Eptifibatide	Tirofiban
Type	Antibody	Peptide	Nonpeptide
Molecular weight (daltons)	~50,000	~800	~500
Platelet-bound half-life	Long (h)	Short (s)	Short (s)
Plasma half-life	Short (min)	Extended (2 h)	Extended (2 h)
Drug-to-GPIIb/IIIa receptor ratio	1.5-2.0	250-2500	>250
50% return of platelet function (without transfusion)	12 h	~4 h	~4 h

Abbreviation: GP, glycoprotein; h = hour; s = seconds

kg/min infusion or placebo for up to 3 days (in addition to heparin [in most patients] and aspirin). The 30-day event rate of death or nonfatal MI was 14.2% with eptifibatide and 15.7% with placebo (1.5% absolute reduction). A reduction in MI or death (composite) with eptifibatide was observed at 96 hours, 7 days, and 30 days in medically or interventionally treated patients; however, the benefit was less impressive at later time points.

Similarities and Differences Between Intravenous GPIIb/IIIa Antagonists. Although considered collectively as GPIIIb/IIIa receptor antagonists, abciximab, tirofiban, and eptifibatide differ (Table 19-9) at several levels, including their

- molecular size
- receptor binding characteristics
- plasma concentration
- mechanism of clearance
- platelet-bound and biologic half-life
- potential reversibility

The duration of platelet inhibition following drug discontinuation and the potential for reversing the pharmacologic effect are particularly important properties in cases of emergent surgery and major hemorrhagic complications. In general, a return of platelet function toward a physiologic state (50% inhibition or less) occurs within 4 hours following the cessation of tirofiban and eptifibatide. In contrast, 12 hours are required for abciximab (Fig. 19-17). Some of the delayed return of physiologic platelet function following abciximab termination may be counterbalanced by its low free plasma concentration and drug-to-receptor ratio. These properties are responsible for the rapid return of hemostatic potential following platelet transfusions. In contrast, the high plasma concentrations observed with the small-molecule inhibitors limit the effectiveness of platelet transfusions. Fibrinogen supplementation (fresh frozen plasma, cryoprecipitate) is the more logical choice for restoration of hemostatic potential with tirofiban and eptifibatide, given the competitive nature of binding and relative availability of platelet GPIIb/IIIa receptors.[92]

Perhaps the most noteworthy distinguishing feature among GPIIb/IIIa receptor antagonists relates to their effect not on platelets but on other cells and proteins. In this regard, the nonspecific agent abciximab stands alone, with documented inhibitory effects on monocytes and the ubiquitous vascular protein vitronectin. Whether the non-platelet-related properties of abciximab have an important role in clinical outcome is currently under intense investigation (Fig. 19-18).

Major Clinical End Points. The intravenous GPIIb/IIIa receptor antagonists have been shown to reduce cardiac event rates in patients with acute coronary syndromes who are treated either by pharmacologic means alone or in the context of PCI. The available data suggest that the greatest overall benefit occurs in high-risk patients, many of whom require mechanical revascularization. Methodical differences between the major clinical trials make it difficult to compare the GPIIb/IIIa receptor antagonists, however, there is clear consistency among the agents with regard to efficacy and safety.[32] Meticulous attention to femoral arterial access, sheath care, and periprocedural heparin dosing has reduced vascular and major hemorrhagic complication substantially (Table 19-10).

Complications. The administration of GPIIb/IIIa receptor antagonists is associated with thrombocytopenia (platelet count less than 100,000/μL) in approximately 2% to 3% of patients.[93,94] A more marked reduction (less than 50,000/μL) is seen in less than 1% of patients and may be influenced by:

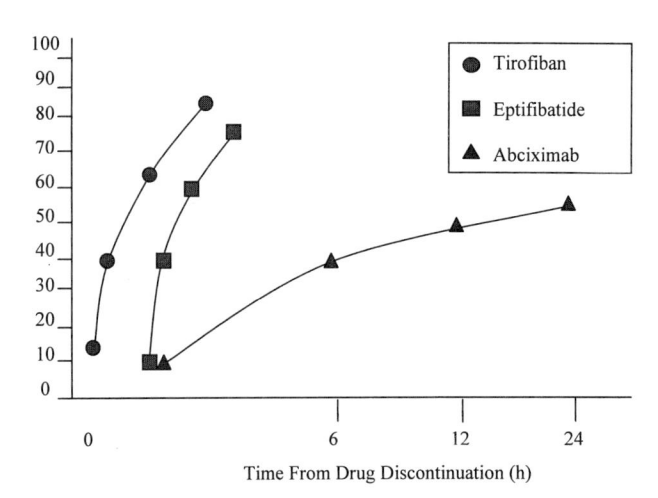

Figure 19-17 The biologic half-life for the small-molecule GPIIb/IIIa antagonists (eptifibatide, tirofiban) is relatively brief compared to abciximab.

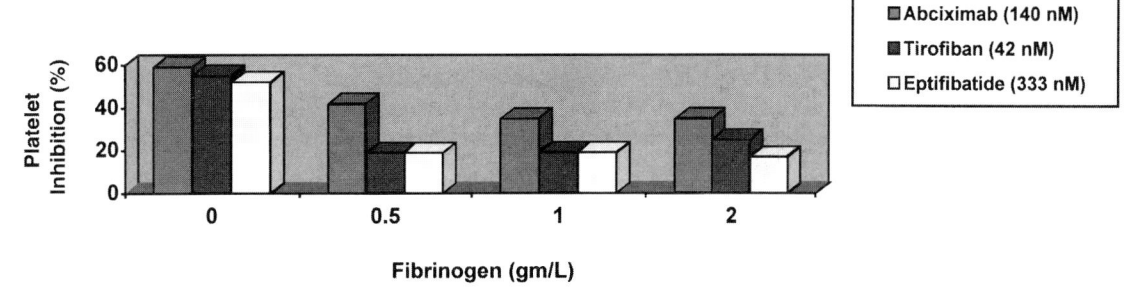

Figure 19-18 Fibrinogen supplementation can partially reverse the platelet-inhibitory effect of GPIIb/IIIa receptor antagonists. Reversibility is achieved more readily for small-molecule inhibitors.

- concomitant procedure (coronary interventions)
- medications (unfractionated heparin)
- age (older than 65 years)
- pretreatment platelet count
- duration of treatment
- repeat administration (even with a different agent)

Acute, profound thrombocytopenia (less than 2000/mm³) has been reported within 4 hours of abciximab treatment.

Although a majority of patients with thrombocytopenia do not experience major hemorrhagic events (in fact thrombosis during recovery is a greater concern), the risk is increased and careful observation is required.

Delayed thrombocytopenia (up to 10 days following treatment) has also been described in association with intravenous GPIIb/IIIa receptor antagonists. In this setting, a thorough evaluation of alternative causes of thrombocytopenia must be undertaken. Steroids and intravenous gamma immunoglobulin G, which have little role in the management of acute GPIIb/IIIa antagonist-induced thrombocytopenia, may be beneficial in the delayed form.

Oral GPIIb/IIIa Receptor Antagonists. The success enjoyed by intravenous GPIIb/IIIa receptor antagonists, coupled with the recognized risk for recurrent cardiac events incurred by patients with atherosclerotic coronary artery disease, stimulated interest in the development of oral agents that would provide continuous, low-level GPIIb/IIIa receptor inhibition. The experience to date in approximately 30,000 randomized patients has been disappointing. There are currently no FDA-approved oral GPIIb/IIIa antagonists.

CARDIOEMBOLISM

Embolic events involving the peripheral and cerebral vasculature frequently originate from left heart structures and the ascending aorta. Less commonly, thromboembolism originating within the venous circulatory system can migrate to the arterial system through a patent foramen ovale, atrial septal defect, or ventricular septal defect. This event is regarded as a "paradoxical embolism." Although a majority of cardioemboli have their origin within heart chambers (left atrium, left atrial appendage, left ventricle), native and prosthetic valves (aortic, mitral) and atherosclerotic plaques within the ascending aorta must always be considered during a comprehensive evaluation. Statistically, atrial fibrillation is the most common cause of cardioembolism.

Atrial Fibrillation

Epidemiology

Atrial fibrillation (AF) is one of the most common arrhythmias encountered in routine clinical practice and is an independent risk factor for stroke. More than 2 million adults in the United States have AF and the prevalence increases markedly with increasing age, affecting 4% of the population over age 60 and more than 10% of those over 80 (Fig. 19-19).

While nonvalvular AF was once considered a harmless disorder, it is now recognized as the second most common cardiovascular disorder leading to thrombotic events (following coronary atherosclerosis).

Patients with nonvalvular AF are at significant risk for stroke, but stroke rates rise even more dramatically for those with additional risk factors. Multivariate analyses of several randomized clinical trials demonstrate that independent risk factors for stroke in patients with AF include prior transient ischemic attacks (TIA) or stroke, history of hypertension, diabetes mellitus, congestive heart failure, angina, and increasing age.[95]

Antithrombotic Therapy

About two thirds of AF patients who are at risk for stroke are candidates for anticoagulant therapy, but too few actually receive it.

Five large randomized clinical trials performed in Denmark, the United States, and Canada show that oral anticoagulation therapy with warfarin in a highly statistically significant fashion reduces the risk of stroke, with very low risk of hemorrhage.[96-100]

Patient Selection

Risk stratification can be used to identify patients at greatest risk for stroke and those will benefit most from anticoagulant therapy (Table 19-11).

Table 19-10 • ADJUNCTIVE STRATEGIES AND CLINICAL OUTCOMES FOR THE MAJOR TRIALS OF GPIIb/IIIa RECEPTOR ANTAGONISTS

Trial	Patients	GPIIb/IIIa Receptor Antagonist	Heparin	Death (%)	Nonfatal MI (%)	Repeat PCI (%)	Unplanned Surgery (%)	Major Bleeding (%)	Time[c]
IMPACT II	1333	Eptifibatide bolus + infusion for 20–24 h (high)	100-U/kg bolus	0.8	6.9	2.9	2.0	5.2	30d
	1349	Eptifibatide bolus + infusion (low)	Target ACT 300–350 sec	0.5	6.6	2.6	1.6	5.1	
	1328	Placebo	No heparin after PCI	1.1	2.8	2.8	2.8	4.8	
PRISM	1616	Tirofiban bolus + infusion × 48 h	No heparin	0.2	0.9	3.5[a]	—	0.4	48 h
	1616	Heparin × 48 h		0.4	1.4	5.3[a]	—	0.4	
PRISM-Plus	773	Tirofiban bolus + infusion × 72 h	aPTT 2 × control	1.9	3.9	9.3[a]	—	4.0	7 d
	797	Heparin × 72 h	aPTT 2 × control	1.9	7.0	12.7[a]	—	3.0	
PURSUIT	4722	Eptifibatide	aPTT 50–70s[b]	3.5	10.7	—	—	10.8	30 d
	4739	Placebo	ACT 300–350[b] aPTT 50–70s[b] ACT 300–350s[b]	3.7	12.0	—	—	9.3	
EPIC	708	Abciximab bolus + infusion (12 h)	10–12 K bolus (additional bolus up to 20K)	1.7	5.2[a]	0.8[a]	2.4	14	30 d
	695	Abciximab bolus	ACT 300–350 sec	1.3	6.2	3.6	2.3	11	
	696	Placebo	Postprocedure to aPTT 1.5–2.5 × control for 12 h	1.7	8.6	4.5	3.6	7	
EPIC	708	Abciximab bolus + infusion (12 h)	10–12 K bolus (additional bolus up to 20K)	3.1	6.9	14.4[b]	9.4		1 yr
	695	Abciximab bolus	ACT 300–350 sec	2.6	8.0	19.9	9.9		
	696	Placebo	Postprocedure to aPTT 1.5–2.5 × control for 12 h	3.4	10.5	20.9	10.9		
EPIC	708	Abciximab bolus + infusion (12 h)	10–12 K bolus (additional bolus up to 20K)	6.8	10.7	—	34.8+	—	3 yrs
	698	Abciximab bolus	ACT 300–350 sec	8.0	12.2	—	38.6	—	
	696	Placebo	Postprocedure to aPTT 1.5–2.5 × control for 12 h	8.6	13.6	—	40.1	—	
CAPTURE	630	Abciximab bolus + infusion 18–24 h before PCI	Heparin to aPTT 2–2.5 × control before PCI, ACT 300 sec during PCI	1.0	4.1[b]	4.5	1.0	3.8	30 d
	635	Placebo		1.3	8.2	6.6	1.7	1.9	
EPILOG	918	Abciximab bolus + infusion (12 h)	100 U/kg target ACT 300 sec	0.4	3.8[a]	1.5[b]	0.9	3.5	30 d
	935	Abciximab bolus + infusion (12 h)	70 U/kg target ACT 200 sec	0.3	3.7[b]	1.2[b]	0.4	2.0	
	939	Placebo	100 U/kg target ACT 300 sec	0.8	8.7	3.8	1.7	3.1	

Abbreviations: MI, myocardial infarction; PCI, percutaneous coronary intervention; IMPACT II, Integrilin to Minimize Platelet Aggregation and Coronary Thrombosis; ACT, activated clotting time; PRISM, Platelet Receptor Inhibition in Ischemic Syndrome Management; PRISM-Plus, Platelet Receptor Inhibition in Ischemic Syndrome Management, Patients Limited by Unstable Signs and Symptoms; aPTT, activated partial thromboplastin time; PURSUIT, Platelet Glycoprotein IIb/IIIa Unstable Angina Receptor Supression Using Integrilin Therapy; EPIC, Evaluation of Platelet IIb/IIIa Inhibition for Prevention of Ischemic Complications; CAPTURE; Chimeric 7E3 Antiplatelet Therapy in Unstable Angina Refractory to Standard Treatment; EPILOG, Evaluation of PTCA to Improve Long-term Outcome by c7E3 GPIIb/IIIa Receptor.

[a] $P = 0.01$—refractory ischemia
[b] $P = 0.001$—heparin use at discretion of physician
[c] Time from randomization to determination of end point

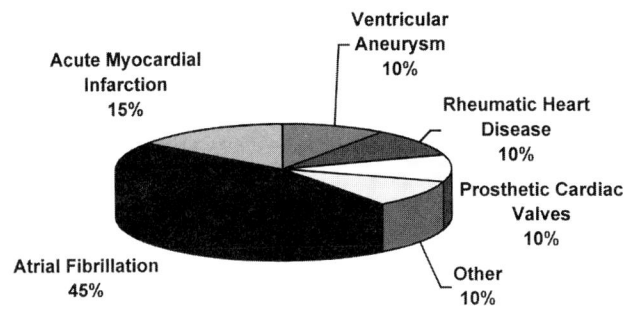

Figure 19–19 Atrial fibrillation is the most common cause of stroke among cardiac sources, accounting for nearly 50% of all events.

Native and Prosthetic Valvular Heart Disease

The most feared and devastating complication of native or prosthetic valvular heart disease is systemic embolism that can cause fatal or disabling stroke.

Mechanisms

Clinical, pathologic, and experimental evidence supports the view that there are two predominant mechanisms responsible for the initiation of thrombosis in patients with native or prosthetic valvular heart disease. The first involves disruption of the vascular endothelial surface and exposure of underlying prothrombotic substrate and/or the introduction of prothrombotic material into the circulation. The second is mediated by "triggering" of thrombosis in areas of stasis via activation of coagulation pathways. Early observations established that stasis alone requires prolonged periods of time to induce thrombosis; however, the combination of stasis and localized tissue abnormalities and/or a high concentration of coagulation factors is profoundly thrombogenic.[101,102] There is also evidence that prolonged periods of stasis impairs tissue perfusion, with resulting endovascular damage and compromised fibrinolytic activity (an important component of thromboresistance). Extension of thrombus into regions of relative stasis is common in both arterial and venous thromboembolism

and represents an important mechanism for thrombus growth following prosthetic heart valve surgery.

Prosthetic Heart Valve: Prothrombotic Conditions

The prerequisite conditions for prosthetic heart valve thrombosis can be defined conceptually in the context of Virchow's triad, with modifications for the introduction of a fourth component, an artificial surface. The traditional and widely cited components—abnormalities of the vascular/endothelial surface, stasis of blood flow, and abnormalities within the circulating blood—are all operational in the setting of prosthetic mechanical heart valve replacement, but vary according to the etiology, presence, duration, and extent of underlying valvular heart disease, prosthetic materials used, and the position of valvular insertion (aortic, mitral, or both).

The overall "thrombogenic surface" of prosthetic heart valves includes not only the artificial material itself but also the perivalvular excision tissue, sewing ring, and sutures as well. Each element is important, particularly in the early postoperative period when blood flow is reinitiated and the prothrombotic effects of surgery (platelet activation, circulating inflammatory mediators) are at their peak.

DETERMINING THROMBOEMBOLIC RISK

Native Valvular Heart Disease

The risk of thromboembolism in patients with native valvular heart disease is influenced strongly by the site of involvement, chamber dimension, ventricular performance, and the presence of concomitant risk factors such as paroxysmal or chronic AF. Prior thromboembolism is considered the strongest risk factor for recurrent events regardless of the valvular pathology.

Clinical Experience

The risk of thromboembolism in patients with prosthetic valvular heart disease is recognized and respected widely and has been the subject of clinical trials, case studies, and registries for over three decades. Despite methodologic limitations, the available information derived from relatively large studies and an ever-expanding clinical experience allows several general conclusions to be drawn:

- Thromboprophylaxis for mechanical prostheses is achieved most effectively with oral anticoagulants.
- Antiplatelet therapy alone does not offer adequate protection for patients with mechanical prostheses.
- The thrombogenicity of mechanical heart valves, from greatest to least, is as follows: caged ball> tilting disk >bileaflet.

Table 19–11 • ANTITHROMBOTIC THERAPY IN NONVALVULAR ATRIAL FIBRILLATION

Age (y)	Other Risk Factors[a]	Recommendation
<65	Absent	Aspirin
	Present	Warfarin (INR 2.5)
65–70	Absent	Aspirin or warfarin
	Present	Warfarin (INR 2.5)
>75	All patients	Warfarin (INR 2.5)

Abbreviations: INR, international normalized ratio
[a] Prior transient ischemic attack, systemic embolus or stroke, hypertension, poor left ventricular function, rheumatic mitral valve disease, prosthetic heart valve.
From Albers GW; Dalen JE, Laupacis A, et al. Antithrombotic therapy in atrial fibrillation. Chest 2001;119:194S–206S, with permission.

Table 19–12 • THROMBOEMBOLIC RISK SCALE FOR PROSTHETIC HEART VALVES

Low Risk
- Bioprosthetic heart valves (no other risk factors)
- Mechanical heart valve (St. Jude in aortic position) >3 months from surgery (no other risk factors)

Intermediate Risk
- Mechanical heart valve[a] (<3 months from surgery)
- Mechanical heart valve (aortic position)[a] plus AF
- Mechanical heart valve (aortic position)[a] plus LVEF <35%

High Risk
- Mechanical heart valve (mitral position; double valve, AF, LVEF <35%, prior thromboembolism, Starr-Edwards valve, Bjork-Shiley valve)

[a] Type of valve must be considered.
AF, atrial fibrillation; LVEF, left ventricular ejection fraction.

- High-risk patients benefit from combination (anticoagulant and platelet antagonist) antithrombotic prophylaxis.
- The risk of thromboembolism following bioprosthetic heart valve replacement is greatest during the first 3 postoperative months.

Risk Stratification

The management of patients with native and prosthetic valvular heart disease must be approached comprehensively, taking into consideration not only the valve itself but the "company that it keeps" as well. Risk stratification, although focused predominantly on the "thrombotic side" of the equation, must be balanced to include the potential risk of hemorrhage with systemic anticoagulant therapy, particularly in patients with valvular heart disease in whom surgical procedures are being considered (Tables 19–12 and 19–13).[103]

Table 19–13 • HEMORRHAGIC RISK SCALE FOR PATIENTS RECEIVING WARFARIN

Low Risk
- Dental procedures
- Cataract surgery
- Angiography
- Breast biopsy
- Arthroscopic surgery

Intermediate Risk
- Total hip or knee replacement
- Laparoscopic surgery
- Kidney or liver biopsy
- Hysterectomy
- Polypectomy
- Transurethral removal of the prostate (TURP)

High Risk
- Major abdominal surgery
- Major thoracic surgery
- Brain/central nervous system surgery
- Radical prostatectomy

Table 19–14 • SUMMARY OF RECOMMENDATIONS FOR PATIENTS WITH NATIVE VALVULAR HEART DISEASE

Native Valvular Heart Disease	Recommendations
Rheumatic Mitral Valvular Disease	
• Prior thromboembolism	Oral anticoagulants, INR 2.5
• Paroxysmal or chronic AF	Oral anticoagulants, INR 2.5
• LA diameter >5.5 cm	Oral anticoagulants, INR 2.5
• MVA <1.0 cm², LA enlargement	Strongly considered oral anticoagulants
• Recurrent embolism (despite oral anticoagulants)	Add aspirin (80 to 100 mg qd) or clopidogrel (75 mg qd)
Mitral Annular Calcification	
• Uncomplicated	No antithrombotic therapy
• AF or systemic embolism	Oral anticoagulants, INR 2.5
Mitral Valve Prolapse	
• Uncomplicated	No antithrombotic therapy
• TIA	Aspirin (325 mg qd)
• Recurrent TIA	Oral anticoagulants, INR 2.5
• Systemic embolism	Oral anticoagulants, INR 2.5
Aortic Valvular Disease	
• Sinus rhythm	No antithrombotic therapy
• Chronic AF or systemic embolism	Oral anticoagulants, INR 2.5

Abbreviations: INR, international normalized ratio; AF, atrial fibrillation; LA, left atrium; MVA, mitral valve area; TIA transient ischemic attack.

Anticoagulant Therapy: Recommendations and Management Guidelines

The recommended approach to patients with native and prosthetic valvular heart disease is based on a composite of clinical trial results and clinical experience[104]; the latter is particularly true of native valvular disease, for which few randomized clinical trials have been conducted (Tables 19–14 to 19–16).

Table 19–15 • SUMMARY OF RECOMMENDATIONS FOR PATIENTS WITH BIOPROSTHETIC HEART VALVES

Valve Type/Position	INR	Duration of Treatment
Mitral position	2.5	3 months
Aortic position	2.5	3 months
Atrial fibrillation	2.5	Long-term
LA thrombosis	2.5	3 to 6 months
Systemic embolism	2.5	3 to 12 months
Systemic embolism despite anticoagulant therapy	2.5[a]	Minimum 12 months

Abbreviations: INR, international normalized ratio; LA, left atrium (includes left atrial appendage).
[a] Add aspirin (80 to 100 mg qd) or clopidogrel (75 mg qd).

Table 19-16 • SUMMARY OF RECOMMENDATIONS FOR PATIENTS WITH MECHANICAL HEART VALVES

Valve Type/Position	INR
Bileaflet, aortic	2.5 (3.0 if AF, LA > 5.5 cm, or LVEF <35%)
Tilting disk, aortic	3.0
Bileaflet, mitral	3.0 or 2.5 plus ASA (80 to 100 mg qd)
Tilting disk, mitral	3.0 or 2.5 plus ASA (80 to 100 mg qd)
Caged ball/disk	3.0 plus aspirin (80 to 100 mg qd)
Systemic embolism despite anticoagulant therapy	3.0 plus aspirin (80 to 100 mg qd)

Abbreviations: INR, international normalized ratio; AF, atrial fibrillation; LA, left atrium; LVEF, left ventricular ejection fraction; ASA, aspirin.

MURAL THROMBOSIS AND EMBOLIC EVENTS

Left ventricular mural thrombus is observed either echocardiographically or at the time of autopsy among patients with MI,[105] particularly those with anterior infarction involving the apex.[106] In large clinical trials of anticoagulant therapy, researchers reported an incidence of cerebral embolism of 2% to 4% among the control patients, frequently causing either severe neurologic deficits or death. Of these trials, two showed a statistically significant reduction in stroke with early anticoagulation, whereas a third trial demonstrated a positive trend.

A meta-analysis performed by Vaitkus and coworkers supports the findings of prior studies. The odds ratio for increased risk of systemic embolism in the presence of echocardiographically demonstrated mural thrombus was 5.45 (95% confidence interval [CI] 3.02–9.83) and an event rate difference of 0.09 (95% CI 0.003–0.14). The odds ratio of anticoagulation versus no anticoagulation in preventing embolization was 0.14 (95% CI 0.04–0.52) with an event rate difference of −0.33 (95% CI −0.50 to −0.16). The odds ratio of anticoagulation versus control in preventing mural thrombus formation was 0.32 (95% CI 0.20–0.52) and the event rate difference was −0.19 (95% CI −0.09 to −0.28). The available data support the following conclusions: (1) mural thrombosis following acute MI increases the risk of systemic embolism; (2) anticoagulation can reduce mural thrombus formation; and (3) the risk of systemic embolism can be substantially reduced by anticoagulation.[107]

It is recommended that patients with acute MI at increased risk for systemic or pulmonary embolism because of severe left ventricular dysfunction (ejection fraction less than 35%), congestive heart failure, a history of venous or arterial embolism, echocardiographic evidence of mural thrombosis, or AF receive heparin in a dose sufficient to increase the aPTT 1.5 to 2.5 times control, followed by warfarin (INR target 2.5) for 1 to 3 months. LMWH may represent an acceptable alternative in the early post-MI setting. Continued treatment should be considered strongly in patients with recurrent embolic events, persistent left ventricular dysfunction, and chronic atrial fibrillation.

ATHEROMAS OF THE ASCENDING AORTA

The consistently high incidence of "cryptogenic stroke" in most stroke registries and databases led to further consideration of alternative etiologies beyond carotid artery disease, AF, and left heart cardioembolism. The development of transesophageal echocardiography and its use in the evaluation of patients experiencing acute ischemic stroke has provided much needed insight.[108,109] Atheromas of the ascending aorta are present in upward of 25% of patients with stroke and/or peripheral embolism. In this setting, the incidence of recurrent events is high, approaching 15% to 25% within 1 year of the original event. Features associated with an increased incidence of embolic events (atheroemboli, thromboemboli) include plaque thickness greater than 4 mm[110] and absence of calcification, ulceration, and superimposed thrombi (particularly with a mobile component).[111,112]

The treatment of atheromas of the ascending aorta has not been defined fully; however, a consensus is building. First, risk factor modification to include meticulous control of blood pressure, weight, and blood glucose as well as lipid-lowering with an HMG-CoA reductase inhibitor is recommended. Second, although atheroembolism may theoretically be precipitated by anticoagulant therapy, the risk is low and in patients with thromboembolism and mobile lesions imaged by transesophageal echocardiography warfarin therapy (target INR 2.5) has been associated with a 50% to 75% reduction in recurrent events.[26,80,81,113–115]

CARDIOVASCULAR HEMOSTASIS

The development of a wide range of potent antithrombotic agents for use in patients with coronary atherothrombosis, while providing considerable flexibility in management, also carries potential risk. A summary of antithrombotic agents, their mechanism of action, and recommended approach to hemorrhagic events appears in Table 19-17.

The platelet GPIIb/IIIa receptor antagonists warrant further discussion for several reasons. First, they are used widely in the treatment of patients with acute coronary syndromes, particularly those undergoing PCI. Second, as a class, they are among the most potent antithrombotic agents currently available for clinical use. Third, hemostatic abnormalities have been associated with hemorrhagic complications.[116] In a majority of cases, bleeding is of minor severity and attributable to the combined effects of platelet inhibition, concomitant heparin administration, and the performance of interventional procedures with resulting vascular trauma; however, major hemorrhage is seen in approximately 2% to 4% of treated patients. A large experience with GPIIb/IIIa antagonists derived from randomized clinical trials suggests that 50% to 80% of major hemorrhagic

Table 19–17 • AN AGENT-SPECIFIC APPROACH TO HEMORRHAGIC COMPLICATIONS

Agent	Aspirin	Clopidogrel	Ticlopidine	Abciximab	Tirofiban	Eptifibatide	UFH	LMWH	Lepirudin[a]	Argatroban	Danaparoid Sodium
Category Mechanism of action	Platelet antagonist Cyclooxygenase inhibition	Platelet antagonist ADP-Receptor inhibition	Platelet antagonist ADP-Receptor inhibition	Platelet antagonist GPIIb/IIIa receptor inhibition	Platelet antagonist GPIIb/IIIa receptor inhibition	Platelet antagonist GPIIb/IIIa receptor inhibition	Anticoagulant Thrombin inhibition (indirect)	Anticoagulant Thrombin inhibition (indirect)	Anticoagulant Thrombin inhibition (direct)	Anticoagulant Thrombin inhibition (direct)	Anticoagulant Thrombin inhibition (indirect)
Antidote	DDAVP	None	None	None	None	None	Protamine	Protamine (60%)	None	None	None
Available substrate for attenuating antithrombotic effects	Platelet transfusion	Platelet transfusion	Platelet transfusion	Platelet transfusion FFP, Cryoprecipitate	Cryoprecipitate FFP, Platelet Transfusion	Cryoprecipitate FFP, Platelet Transfusion			FFP, Plasmapheresis	FFP, Plasmapheresis	Plasmapheresis

UFH, Unfractionated heparin; LMWH, low-molecular-weight heparin; FFP, fresh frozen plasma.
[a] Similar approach for bivalirudin.

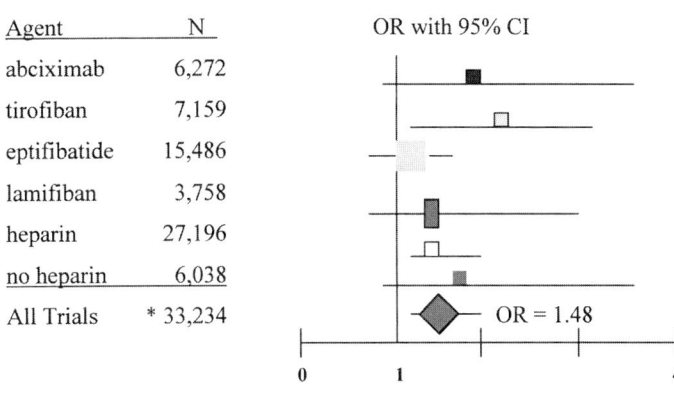

Agent	N	OR with 95% CI
abciximab	6,272	
tirofiban	7,159	
eptifibatide	15,486	
lamifiban	3,758	
heparin	27,196	
no heparin	6,038	
All Trials	* 33,234	OR = 1.48

* Total of all placebo and treated patients From published trials, including some agents not listed.

Abbreviations: OR = odds ratio

Figure 19–20 Thrombocytopenia occurs infrequently following GPIIb/IIIa receptor antagonist administration, but the incidence appears to differ among the available agents. (Adapted from Giugliano RP. Drug-induced thrombocytopenia—is it a serious concern for glycoprotein IIb/IIIa receptor inhibitors? J Thromb Thrombolysis 1998;5:191–202.)

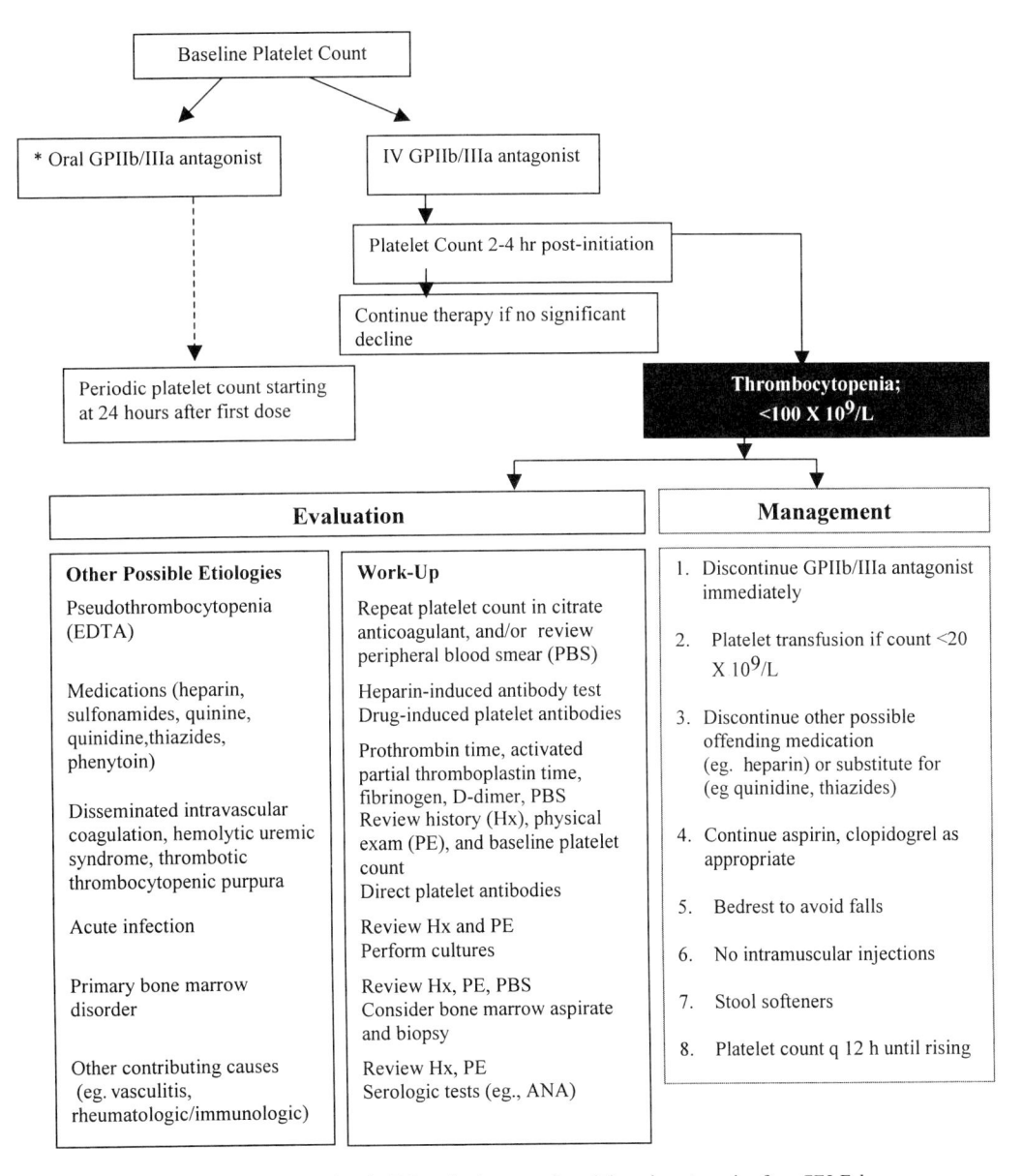

Baseline Platelet Count
→ * Oral GPIIb/IIIa antagonist
→ IV GPIIb/IIIa antagonist
→ Platelet Count 2-4 hr post-initiation
→ Continue therapy if no significant decline
→ Periodic platelet count starting at 24 hours after first dose
→ **Thrombocytopenia; <100 X 10⁹/L**

Evaluation

Other Possible Etiologies

Pseudothrombocytopenia (EDTA)

Medications (heparin, sulfonamides, quinine, quinidine, thiazides, phenytoin)

Disseminated intravascular coagulation, hemolytic uremic syndrome, thrombotic thrombocytopenic purpura

Acute infection

Primary bone marrow disorder

Other contributing causes (eg. vasculitis, rheumatologic/immunologic)

Work-Up

Repeat platelet count in citrate anticoagulant, and/or review peripheral blood smear (PBS)

Heparin-induced antibody test
Drug-induced platelet antibodies

Prothrombin time, activated partial thromboplastin time, fibrinogen, D-dimer, PBS
Review history (Hx), physical exam (PE), and baseline platelet count
Direct platelet antibodies

Review Hx and PE
Perform cultures

Review Hx, PE, PBS
Consider bone marrow aspirate and biopsy

Review Hx, PE
Serologic tests (eg., ANA)

Management

1. Discontinue GPIIb/IIIa antagonist immediately

2. Platelet transfusion if count <20 X 10⁹/L

3. Discontinue other possible offending medication (eg. heparin) or substitute for (eg quinidine, thiazides)

4. Continue aspirin, clopidogrel as appropriate

5. Bedrest to avoid falls

6. No intramuscular injections

7. Stool softeners

8. Platelet count q 12 h until rising

Reproduced with permission from Berkowitz DS et al. Acute profound thrombocytopenia after c7E3 Fab (abciximab) therapy. Circulation 1997;95:8091-813.

* Not currently available

Figure 19–21 The approach to thrombocytopenia following GPIIb/IIIa receptor antagonist administration requires a comprehensive evaluation of potential contributing causes and careful risk–benefit assessment.

events are related to the performance of coronary artery bypass surgery.[116]

Thrombocytopenia, which may at times be sudden (within several hours of drug administration) and profound (<20,000/μL) has been described in patients receiving GPIIb/IIIa antagonists.[117] The available evidence suggests that thrombocytopenia occurs more frequently with abciximab than the small-molecule antagonists tirofiban and eptifibatide (Fig. 19–20). This appears particularly true following readministration within several months of initial treatment.[118] A recommended approach to thrombocytopenia is outlined in Figure 19–21.

Management of Hemorrhagic Events

In the event of a hemorrhagic complication, aggressive efforts must be made to identify the source, assess the severity of bleeding and its hemodynamic consequences, and achieve hemostasis. The most common site of bleeding in patients undergoing cardiac procedures is the vascular access site. Prolonged manual or mechanical compression is recommended as the first step in management. If internal bleeding is suspected (e.g., retroperitoneal, gastrointestinal, or intracranial), or for external bleeding (e.g., from vascular access site) that is not easily controlled by external compression, the GPIIb/IIIa antagonist should be discontinued. A hemoglobin level, hematocrit, and platelet count should be obtained immediately, with serial measurements as needed.

Initially, crystalloid solutions are administered intravenously to support blood pressure, followed by red blood cell transfusions as needed. Clinicians are advised to transfuse on a unit-by-unit basis with a goal to relieve symptoms (e.g., hypotension, tachycardia, myocardial ischemia). Platelet transfusions are recommended for patients with thrombocytopenia (less than 50,000/μL with bleeding or less than 20,000/μL without bleeding). If profound thrombocytopenia (less than 2,000/μL) occurs, consideration should be given to discontinuing all concomitant antiplatelet therapy. Treatment may be re-

---

Table 19–18 • MANAGEMENT STRATEGIES TO LIMIT BLEEDING EVENTS IN PATIENTS TREATED WITH GLYCOPROTEIN IIb/IIIa INHIBITORS; FOCUS ON CORONARY INTERVENTIONS

Evaluate baseline risk factors:
- Screen for contraindication to GPIIb/IIIa inhibitor therapy
- Assess baseline risk for bleeding versus likelihood of benefit

Reduce procedural risk factors:
- Use GPIIb/IIIa inhibitors prophylactically rather than for "bailout" situations
- Obtain a baseline ACT
- Use "low-dose" weight-adjusted heparin (e.g., 70 U/kg initial bolus if baseline ACT <150)
- Achieve an ACT of >200 sec but <300 sec
- Obtain serial ACT measurements every 30 min throughout the procedure. Administer additional heparin (20 U/kg) as required to keep ACT 200–300 sec
- Avoid "through-and-through" arterial punctures or multiple arterial punctures
- Use a smaller arterial sheath size (<8F), if possible
- Avoid venous sheaths if possible
- Avoid intraprocedural fibrinolytics therapy; if thrombolytics are necessary, administer via intracoronary route and administer no more than 10% of systemic lytic dose (e.g., 10 mg IC tPA)
- Avoid treating patients receiving warfarin who have INR >2.0. In emergency cases involving such patients, if abciximab is considered necessary, administer heparin and IV fresh frozen plasma (2U), and consider vitamin K (5–10 mg IV)

Enhance postprocedural care:
- Discontinue heparin immediately following procedure
- Closely monitor patients postintervention. If hypotension should arise, rule out bleeding sources
- Establish routine nursing protocols for the care of PCI patients
- Remove sheaths at 4–6 hours or as soon as ACT <180 sec
- Assign sheath removal to trained, experienced, and dedicated individuals

- Monitor platelet count with 24 hours of starting GPIIb/IIIa inhibitor therapy to detect thrombocytopenia (Also, check platelet count at 2–4 hours after starting abciximab). If thrombocytopenia detected, consider discontinuation of infusion

Should bleeding occur:
- Rapidly identify the source
- Treat access site bleeding aggressively with manual compression, followed by mechanical compression for the duration of GPIIb/IIIa inhibitor, if necessary
- Discontinue GPIIb/IIIa inhibitor if internal bleeding suspected (e.g., retroperitoneal, gastrointestinal bleeding) or external bleeding (e.g., from vascular access site) that is not easily controlled by external compression
- Check hemoglobin, hematocrit, and platelet count immediately and obtain serial measurements. Initially use crystalloid to replace intravascular volume and follow protocol for erythrocyte transfusion
- Transfuse on a unit-by-unit basis to relieve symptoms (e.g., hypotension, tachycardia, ischemia)
- Transfuse platelets for thrombocytopenia if platelet count <50,000/uL with bleeding or <20,000/uL without bleeding

Emergency CABG:
- Discontinue heparin and GPIIb/IIIa inhibitor immediately
- If possible, delay surgery until antiplatelet effect of GPIIb/IIIa inhibitor no longer present (for abciximab: 12–24 hours; for eptifibatide or tirofiban; 4–6 hours)
- Consider "off-pump" CABG
- Do *not* administer standard heparin dosing (300 U/kg) for CPB
- Obtain ACT upon arrival in operating room
- Administer heparin as needed to achieve an ACT of 400–500 sec
- Administer platelet transfusion as patient is coming off CPB to facilitate perioperative hemostasis

ACT, activated clotting time; CP, cardiopulmonary; CB, cardiopulmonary bypass; CABG, coronary artery bypass graft surgery; GP, glycoprotein; IC, intracoronary; PCI, percutaneous coronary intervention; tPA, tissue-type plasminogen activator.
Data from EPILOG Investigators. Platelet glycoprotein IIb/IIIa receptor blockade and low-dose heparin during percutaneous coronary revascularization. N Engl J Med 1997;336:1689–1696.

instated once the platelet count recovers to greater than 20,000/μL.

Emergency Coronary Bypass Surgery

Although an infrequent occurrence, emergency coronary bypass surgery represents a major hemostatic challenge, and as a result, both heparin and the GPIIb/IIIa antagonist should be discontinued. When clinically acceptable, surgery should be delayed until the antiplatelet effects have significantly dissipated (approximately 12 to 24 hours for abciximab, and 4 to 6 hours for the small-molecule antagonists eptifibatide and tirofiban). Conventional heparin dosing for cardiopulmonary bypass (300 U/kg), when administered in the presence of GPIIb/IIIa receptor inhibition (particularly abciximab), will result in excess anticoagulation. An ACT should be obtained as soon as the patient arrives in the operating room, and heparin should be titrated to target ACT of 400 to 500 seconds (Table 19–18). Platelet transfusion during weaning from cardiopulmonary bypass may facilitate perioperative hemostasis.

■ REFERENCES

Chapter 19 References

1. Jewett B (Ed.). The Dialogues of Plato, 3rd ed. New York, Macmillan, 1892, pp. 3:339–543.
2. Lee HDP (translator). Aristotle: Meterologica. Loeb Classical Library. Cambridge, Harvard University Press, 1952.
3. Pettit JL. Dissertation sur la manie're d'arrester le sang dans les hemorrhagies. Mem Acad R Sci 1731;1:85–102.
4. Forester JM (translator). Milpighi M: De Polypo Cordis, 1686. Uppsala, Almquiest & Wiksels, 1956.
5. Babington BG. Some considerations with respect to the blood founded on one or two very simple experiments on that fluid. Med Chir Trans 1930;16:293–319.
6. Buchanan A. On the coagulation of the blood and other fibriniferous liquids. Lond Med Gaz 1845;1:617. Reprinted in J Physiol (Lond) 1879–1880;2:158–168.
7. Schmidt A. Zur Blutlehre. Leipzig, Bogel, 1892.
8. Otto JC. An account of an hemorrhagic disposition existing in certain families. Med Repository 1803;6:1–4.
9. Hay J. Account of a remarkable haemorrhagic disposition, existing in many individuals of the same family. N Engl J Med 1813;2:221–225.
10. Thackrah CT. An Inquiry into the Nature and Properties of the Blood. London, Cox and Sons, 1819.
11. De Blainville HMD. Injection de matiére cerebrale dans les veins. Gaz Med Paris 1834;2:524.
12. Howell WH. The nature and action of the thromboplastin (zymoplastic) substance of the tissues. Am J Physiol 1912;31:1–21.
13. Mills CA. Chemical nature of tissue coagulants. J Biol Chem 1921;46:135–165.
14. Donné A. De l'origine des globules du sang, de leur mode de formation et leur fin. CR Acad Sci (Paris) 1842;14:366–368.
15. Osler W. An account of certain organisms occurring in the liquor sanguinis. Proc Roy Soc Lond 1874;22:391–398.
16. Haycm G. Sur le méhanisme de l'arret des hemorrhages. CR Acad Sci 1885;95:18–21.
17. Konttinen YP. Fibrinolysis: Chemistry, Physiology, Pathology and Clinics. Tampere, Finland, Oy Star Ab, 1968.
18. Hedin SG. On the presence of a proteolytic enzyme in the normal serum of the ox. J Physioal (Lond) 1904;30:195–201.
19. Christensen LR, MacLeod CM. Proteolytic enzyme of serum: characterization, activation, and reaction with inhibitors. J Gen Physiol 1945;23:559–583.
20. Gratia A (quoted by Kontinnen YP). Fibrinolysis: Chemistry, Physiology, Pathology and Clinics. Tampere, Finland, Oy Star Ab, 1968.
21. Tillett WS, Garner RL. The fibrinolytic activity of hemolytic streptococci. J Exp Med 1933;58:485–502.
22. Sherry S, Fletcher A, Akljaersig N. Fibrinolysis and fibrinolytic activity in man. Physiol Rev 1959;39:343–381.
23. ISIS-2 (Second International Study of Infarct Survival) Collaborative Group. Randomized trial of intravenous streptokinase, oral aspirin, both, or neither among 17,187 cases of suspected acute myocardial infarction: ISIS-2. Lancet 1988;2(8607):349–360.
24. Lambrew CT. The National Heart Attack Alert Program: Overview and mission. J Thromb Thrombolysis 1996;3:247–248.
25. Hand M. Educational strategies to prevent prehospital delay in patients at high risk for acute myocardial infarction: A report by the National Heart Attack Alert Program. J Thromb Thrombolysis 1998;6:47–61.
26. Hand M, Brown C. Horan M, et al. The National Heart Attack Alert Program: Progress at 5 years in educating providers, patients and the public: Future directions. J Thromb Thrombolysis 1998;6:9–17.
27. Antman E for the TIMI 11B Investigators. Enoxaparin prevents death and cardiac ischemic events in unstable angina-non-Q-wave MI: Results of the TIMI 11b trial. Circulation 1999;100:1593–1601.
28. Cohen M, Demers C, Gurfinkel EP for the ESSENCE Investigators. A comparison of low-molecular-weight heparin with unfractionated heparin for unstable coronary artery disease. N Engl J Med 1997;337:447–452.
29. The FRISC Study Group. Low molecular weight heparin during unstability in coronary artery disease. Lancet 1996;347:561–568.
30. Klein W, Buchwald A, Hillis SE, et al. Comparison of low molecular weight heparin with unfractionated heparin acutely and with placebo for 6 weeks in the management of unstable coronary artery disease. Fragmin in Unstable Coronary Artery Disease Study (FRIC). Circulation 1997;96:61–68.
31. FRISC II Investigations. Long-term low-molecular mass heparin in unstable coronary artery disease: FRISC II prospective randomized multicentre study. Lancet 1999;354:701–707.
32. Kong DF, Califf RM, Miller DP, et al. Clinical outcomes of therapeutic agents that block the platelet glycoprotein IIb/IIIa integrin in ischemic heart disease. Circulation 1998;98:2829–2835.
33. Antman EM for the TIMI 14 Investigators. Abciximab facilitates the rate and extent of thrombolysis: Results of the TIMI 14 trial. Circulation 1999;99:2720–2732.
34. Jaucherm JR, Lopez M, Sprague EA, et al. Mononuclear cell chemoattractant activity from cultured arterial smooth muscle cells. Exp Mol Pathol 1982;37:166–174.
35. Schwartz CJ, Valente AJ, Sprague EA, et al. Atherosclerosis as an inflammatory process: the roles of monocyte-macrophage. Ann NY Acad Sci 1985;454:115–120.
36. Goldstein JL, Ho YK, Basu SK, et al. Binding site on macrophages that mediates uptake and degradation of acetylated low density lipoprotein, producing massive cholesterol deposition. Proc Natl Acad Sci USA 1979;76:333–337.
37. Little WC, Constantinescu M, Applegate RJ, et al. Can coronary angiography predict the site of a subsequent myocardial infarction in patients with mild-to-moderate coronary artery disease? Circulation 1988;78:1157–1166.

38. Davies MJ, Thomas AC. Plaque fissuring—the cause of acute myocardial infarction, sudden ischemic death and crescendo angina. Br Heart J 1985;53:363–373.
39. Braunwald E, Antman EM, Beasley JW, et al. ACC/AHA guidelines for the management of patients with unstable angina and non-ST-segment elevation myocardial infarction: a report of the American College of Cardiology/American Heart Association Task Force on Practice Guidelines (Committee on the Management of Patients with Unstable Angina). J Am Coll Cardiol 2000;36:970–1062.
40. Ryan TJ, Antman EM, Brooks NH, et al. 1999 Update: ACC/AHA guidelines for the management of patients with acute myocardial infarction. A report of the American College of Cardiology/American Heart Association Task Force on Practice Guidelines (Committee on Management of Acute Myocardial Infarction). J Am Coll Cardiol 1999;34:890–911.
41. The GUSTO III Investigators. A comparison of reteplase with alteplase for acute myocardial infarction. N Engl J Med 1997;337:1118–1123.
42. Van de Werf F, Cannon CP, Luyter A, et al. for the ASSENT-I Investigators. Safety assessment of single-bolus administration of TNK tissue plasminogen activator in acute myocardial infarction: The ASSENT-I trial. Am Heart J 1999;137:786–791.
43. Van de Werf F for the ASSENT II Investigators. Results of the ASSENT II trial. Circulation 1999;100:574 (abstr).
44. Magnani HN, Heparin-induced thrombocytopenia (HIT): An overview of 230 patients treated with Orgaran (Org 10172). Thromb Haemost 1993;70:554–561.
45. Bittl JA, Strony J, Brinker JA, et al. for the Hirulog Angioplasty Study Investigators. Treatment with Bivalirudin (Hirulog) as compared with heparin during coronary angioplasty for unstable or postinfarction angina. N Engl J Med 1995;333:764–769.
46. Gifford RH, Feinstein AR. A critique of methodology in studies of anticoagulation for acute myocardial infarction. N Engl J Med 1969;280:351–357.
47. Chalmers TC, Matta RJ, Smith H Jr, et al. Evidence favoring the use of anticoagulants in the hospital phase of acute myocardial infarction. N Engl J Med 1977;297:1091–1096.
48. Ansell J. Oral anticoagulant therapy—50 years later. Arch Intern Med 1993;153:586–596.
49. Kearon C, Hirsh J. Management of anticoagulation before and after elective surgery. N Engl J Med 1997;336:1506–1511.
49a. Heidenreich PA, McCellan M. Trend in treatment and outcomes for acute myocardial infarction: 1975–1995. Am J Med 2001;110:165–174.
50. The Steering Committee of the Physicians' Health Study research group. Final report on the aspirin component of the ongoing Physicians' Health Study. N Engl J Med 1989;321:129–135.
51. The Medical Research Council's General Practice Research Framework. Thrombosis prevention trial: randomized trial of low intensity oral anticoagulation with warfarin and low-dose aspirin in the primary prevention of ischaemic heart disease in men at increased risk. Lancet 1998;351:233–241.
52. Peto R, Gray R, Collins R, et al. Randomized trial of prophylactic daily aspirin in British male doctors. BMJ 1988;926:313–316.
53. Hansson L, Zanchetta A, Carruthers SG, et al. Effects of intensive blood-pressure lowering and low-dose aspirin in patients with hypertension: principal results of the Hypertension Optimal Treatment (HOT) randomized trial. HOT Study Group. Lancet 1998;351:1755–1762.
54. Antiplatelet Trialists' Collaboration. Collaborative overview of randomized trials of antiplatelet therapy: I. Prevention of death, myocardial infarction and stroke by prolonged antiplatelet therapy in various categories of patients (published correction appears in BMJ 1994;308:1540.) BMJ 1994;308:81–106.
55. Borzak S, Cannon CP, Kraft PL, et al. for the TIMI 7 Investigators. Effects of prior aspirin and anti-ischemic therapy on outcome of patients with unstable angina. Am J Cardiol 1998;81:678–681.
56. Goldman S, Copeland J, Moritz T, et al. Improvement in early saphenous vein graft patency after coronary artery bypass surgery with antiplatelet therapy: results of a Veterans Administration cooperative study. Circulation 1988;77:1324–1332.
57. International Stroke Trial Collaborative Group. The International Stroke Trial (IST): a randomized trial of aspirin, subcutaneous heparin, both, or neither among 19,435 patients with acute ischaemic stroke. Lancet 1997;349:1569–1581.
58. CAST (Chinese Acute Stroke Trial) Collaborative Group. CAST: randomized placebo-controlled trial of early aspirin use in 20,000 patients with acute ischaemic stroke. Lancet 1997;349:1641–1649.
59. Schwartz L, Bourassa MG, Lesperance J, et al. Aspirin and dipyridamole in the prevention of restenosis after percutaneous transluminal coronary angioplasty. N Engl J Med 1988;318:1714–1719.
60. O'Brien JR, Etherington MD, Shuttleworth RD. Ticlopidine antiplatelet drug: effects in human volunteers. Thromb Res 1978;13:245–254.
61. Ellis DJ, Roe RI, Bruno JJ, et al. The effects of ticlopidine hydrochloride on bleeding platelet function in man. Thromb Haemost 1981;46:176 (abstr).
62. DeMinno G, Cerbone AM, Mattioli PL, et al. Functionally thromboastenic state in normal platelets following the administration of ticlopidine. J Clin Invest 1985;75:328–338.
63. Berglund U, von Schenck H, Wallentin L. Effects of ticlopidine on platelet function in men with stable angina pectoris. Thromb Haemost 1985;54:808–812.
64. Balsano F, Rizzon P, Violi F, et al. Antiplatelet treatment with ticlopidine in unstable angina. A controlled multicenter clinical trial. Circulation 1990;82:17–26.
65. Knudsen JB, Kjoller E, Skagen K, et al. The effect of ticlopidine on platelet functions in acute myocardial infarction. A double blind controlled trial. Thromb Haemost 1985;53:332–336.
66. Limet R, David JL, Magotteaux P, et al. Prevention of aorta–coronary bypass graft occlusion. J Thorac Cardiovasc Surg 1987;94:773–783.
67. Sigwart U, Puel J, Mirkovitch V, et al. Intravascular stents to prevent occlusion and restenosis after transluminal angioplasty. N Engl J Med 1987;316:701–706.
68. Bertrand ME, Legrand V, Boland J, et al. Randomized multicenter comparison of conventional anticoagulation versus antiplatelet therapy in unplanned and elective coronary stenting. The Full Anticoagulation Versus Aspirin and Ticlopidine (FANTASTIC) Study. Circulation 1998;98:1597–1603.
69. Urban P, Macaya C, Rupprecht HJ, et al. for the MATTIS Investigators. Randomized evaluation of anticoagulation versus antiplatelet therapy after coronary stent implantation in high risk patients: the Multicenter Aspirin and Ticlopidine Trial After Intracoronary Stenting (MATTIS). Circulation 1998;98:2162–2132.
70. Leon MB, Baim DS, Gordon P, et al. Clinical and angiographic results from the stent anticoagulation regimen study (STARS). Circulation 1996;94 (suppl I): I–685 (abstract).
71. Arcan JC, Blanchard J, Boissel JP, et al. Multicenter double-blind study of ticlopidine in the treatment of intermittent claudication and the prevention of its complications. Angiology 1988;39:802–811.
72. Janzon L, Bergquist D, Boberg J, et al. Prevention of myocardial infarction and stroke in patients with intermittent claudication: effects of ticlopidine: results from STIMS, the Swedish Ticlopidine Multicenter Study (published correction appears in J Intern Med 1990;228:659). J Intern Med 1990;227:301–308.
73. Gent M, Blakely JA, Easton JD, et al. The Canadian-American Ticlopidine Study (CATS) in thromboembolic stroke. Lancet 1989;1:1215–1220.

74. Hass WK, Easton JD, Adams HP Jr, et al. A randomized trial comparing ticlopidine hydrochloride with aspirin for the prevention of stroke in high risk patients. Ticlopidine Aspirin Stroke Study Group. N Engl J Med 1989;321:501–507.
75. Bennett CL, Weinberg PD, Rozenberg-Ben-Dror K, et al. Thrombotic thrombocytopenic purpura associated with ticlopidine. A review of 60 cases. Ann Intern Med 1998;128:541–544.
76. Steinhubl SR, Tan WA, Foody JM, et al. for the EPISTENT Investigators. Incidence and clinical course of thrombotic thrombocytopenic purpura due to ticlopidine following coronary stenting. JAMA 1999;281:806–810.
77. Gachet C, Stierle A, Cazenave JP, et al. The thienopyridine PCR 4099 selectively inhibits ADP-induced platelet aggregation and fibrinogen binding without modifying the membrane glycoprotein IIb–IIIa complex in rat and in man. Biochem Pharmacol 1990;40:229–238.
78. Gachet C, Savi P, Ohlmann P, et al. ADP receptor induced activation of guanine nucleotide binding proteins in rat platelet membranes—an effect selectively blocked by the thienopyridine clopidogrel. Thromb Haemost 1992;68:79–83.
79. CAPRIE Steering Committee. A randomized, blind trial of Clopidogrel Versus Aspirin in Patients at Risk for Ischemic Events (CAPRIE). Lancet 1996;348:1329–1339.
80. Bennett CL, Connors JM, Carwile JM, et al. Thrombotic thrombocytopenic purpura associated with clopidogrel. N Engl J Med 2000;342:1773–1777.
81. Evaluation of Platelet IIb/IIIa Inhibition for Prevention of Ischemic Complications (EPIC) Investigators. Use of a monoclonal antibody directed against the platelet glycoprotein IIb/IIIa receptor in high-risk coronary angioplasty. N Engl J Med 1994;330:956–961.
82. EPILOG Investigators. Platelet glycoprotein IIb/IIIa receptor blockade and low-dose heparin during percutaneous coronary revascularization. N Engl J Med 1997;336:1689–1696.
83. CAPTURE Investigators. Randomized placebo-controlled trial of abciximab before and during coronary intervention in refractory unstable angina: the CAPTURE study (published correction appears in Lancet 1997;350:744). Lancet 1997;349:1429–1435.
84. Zkereiakes DJ, Kleiman NS, Ambrose J, et al. Randomized double-blind, placebo-controlled dose-ranging study of tirofiban (MK-383) platelet IIb/IIIa blockade in high risk patients undergoing coronary angioplasty. J Am Coll Cardiol 1996;27:236–542.
85. Randomized Efficacy Study of Tirofiban for Outcomes and Restenosis (RESTORE) Investigators. Effects of platelet glycoprotein IIb/IIIa blockade with tirofiban on adverse cardiac events in patients with unstable angina or acute myocardial infarction undergoing coronary angioplasty. Circulation 1997;96:1445–1453.
86. Platelet Receptor Inhibition in Ischemic Syndrome Management (PRISM) Study Investigators. A comparison of aspirin plus tirofiban with aspirin plus heparin for unstable angina. N Engl J Med 1998;338:1498–1505.
87. Platelet Receptor Inhibition in Ischemic Syndrome Management in Patients Limited by Unstable signs and Symptoms (PRISM PLUS) Study Investigators. Inhibition of the platelet glycoprotein IIb/IIIa receptor with unstable angina and non-Q wave MI. N Engl J Med 1998;338:1488–1497.
88. Phillips DR, Scarborough RM. Clinical pharmacology of eptifibatide. Am J Cardiol 1997;80:11B–20B.
89. Harrington RA, Kleiman NS, Kottke-Marchant K, et al. Immediate and reversible platelet inhibition after intravenous administration of a peptide glycoprotein IIb/IIIa inhibitor during percutaneous coronary intervention. Am J Cardiol 1995;76:1222–1227.
90. Integrilin to Minimize Platelet Aggregation and Coronary Thrombosis (IMPACT)-II Investigators. Randomized placebo-controlled trial of effects of eptifibatide on complications of percutaneous coronary intervention: IMPACT-II. Lancet 1997;349:1422–1428.
91. The Platelet Glycoprotein IIb/IIIa in Unstable Angina: Receptor Suppression Using Integrilin Therapy (PURSUIT) Trial Investigators. Inhibition of platelet glycoprotein IIb/IIIa with eptifibatide in patients with acute coronary syndromes. N Engl J Med 1998;339:436–443.
92. Becker RC, Spencer FA. Li T. Fibrinogen exerts varying effects on GPIIa/IIIa receptor-directed platelet inhibition in vitro. Circulation 1999;100(suppl):853 (abstr).
93. Berkowitz SD, Harrington RA, Rund MM, et al. Acute profound thrombocytopenia after c7E3 Fab (abciximab) therapy. Circulation 1997;95:809–813.
94. Giugliano RP. Drug-induced thrombocytopenia—is it a serious concern for glycoprotein IIb/IIIa receptor inhibitors? J Thromb Thrombolysis 1998;5:191–202.
95. Atrial Fibrillation Investigators. Risk factors for stroke and efficacy of antithrombotic therapy in atrial fibrillation. Analysis of pooled data from five randomized controlled trials (published correction appears in Arch Intern Med 1994;154:2254). Arch Intern Med 1994;154:1449–1457.
96. Peterson P, Boysen G, Godfredsen J, et al. Placebo controlled randomized trial of warfarin and aspirin for prevention of thromboembolic complications in chronic atrial fibrillation. The Copenhagen AFASAK Study. Lancet 1989;1:175–179.
97. Stroke Prevention in Atrial Fibrillation Investigators. Stroke Prevention in Atrial Fibrillation Study. Final Results. Circulation 1991;84:527–539.
98. Boston Area Anticoagulation Trial for Atrial Fibrillation Investigators. The effect of low-dose warfarin on the risk of stroke patients with nonrheumatic atrial fibrillation. N Engl J Med 1990;323:1505–1511.
99. Ezekowitz MD, Bridgers SL, James KE, et al. for the Veterans Affairs Stroke Prevention in Nonrheumatic Atrial Fibrillation Investigators. Warfarin in the prevention of stroke associated with nonrheumatic atrial fibrillation. N Engl Med 1992;327:1406–1412.
100. Connolly SJ, Laupacis A, Gent M, et al. Canadian Atrial Fibrillation Anticoagulation (CAFA) Study. J Am Coll Cardiol 1991;18:349–355.
101. Hewson W. Experimental inquiries. I. An inquiry into the properties of the blood, with some remarks on some of its morbid appearances; and an appendix relating to the discovery of the lymphatic system in birds, fish, and the animals called amphibians. London, T Cadell, 1771. Quoted by Wessler S. Thrombosis in the presence of vascular stasis. Am J Med 1962;33:648–666.
102. Wessler S. Thrombosis in the presence of vascular stasis. Am J Med 1962;33:648–666.
103. Hostkotte D, Piper C, Weimer M. Optimal frequency of patient monitoring and intensity of oral anticoagulation therapy in valvular heart disease. J Thromb Thrombolysis 1998;5:S19–S24.
104. Dalen JE, Hirsh J, Guyatt GH (eds.). Sixth ACCP Conference on Antithrombotic Therapy. 2001;119(suppl):1S–370S.
105. Visser CA, Kang, Meltzer RS, et al. Embolic potential of left ventricular thrombus after myocardial infarction. J Am Coll Cardiol 1985;5:1276–1280.
106. Keating EC, Gross SA, Schlamowitz RA, et al. Mural thrombi in myocardial infarction. Perspective evaluation by two dimensional echocardiography. Am J Med 1983;74:989–995.
107. Vaitkus PT, Barnathom ES. Embolic potential, prevention and management of mural thrombus complicating anterior myocardial infarction; A meta-analysis. J Am Coll Cardiol 1993;22:100–109.
108. Tunick PA, Kronzon I. Atheromas of the thoracic aorta: clinical and therapeutic update. J Am Coll Cardiol 2000;35:545–554.
109. Victor G, Da'vila-Roma'n MD, Murphy SF, et al. Atherosclerosis of the ascending aorta is an independent predictor of long-term neurologic events and mortality. J Am Coll Cardiol 1999;33:1308–1316.
110. Amarenco P, Cohen A, Tzouri C, et al. Atherosclerotic disease of the aortic arch and the risk of ischemic stroke. N Engl J Med 1994;331:1474–1479.

111. Maarenco P, Duyckaerts C, Tzourio C, et al. The prevalence of ulcerated plaques in the aortic arch in patients with stroke. N Engl J Med 1992;326:221–225.
112. Khatibzadeh M, Mitusch R, Stierle U, et al. Aortic atherosclerotic plaques as a source of systemic embolism. J Am Coll Cardiol 1996;27:664–669.
113. The Stroke Prevention in Atrial Fibrillation Investigators Committee on Echocardiography. Transesophageal echocardiography correlates of thromboembolism in high-risk patients with nonvalvular atrial fibrillation. Ann Intern Med 1998;128:639–647.
114. Dressler FA, Craig WR, Castello R, et al. Mobile aortic atheroma and systemic emboli: efficacy of anticoagulation and influence of plaque morphology on recurrent stroke. J Am Coll Cardiol 1998;31:134–138.
115. Ferrari E, Vidal R, Chevallier T, et al. Atherosclerosis of the thoracic aorta and aortic debris as a marker of poor prognosis. Benefit of oral anticoagulants. J Am Coll Cardiol 1999;33:1317–1322.
116. Madan M, Blankenship JC, Berkowitz SD, Bleeding complications with platelet glycoprotein IIb/IIIa receptor antagonists. Curr Opin Hematol 1999;6:334–341.
117. Turner NA, Monke JL, Kamat SG, et al. Comparative real-time effects on platelet adhesion and aggregation under flowing conditions of in vivo aspirin, heparin and monoclonal antibody fragment against glycoprotein IIb/IIIa. Circulation 1995;91:1384–1362.
118. Madan M, Berkowitz SD, Understanding thrombocytopenia and antigenicity with glycoprotein IIb/IIIa inhibitors. Am Heart J 1999;138:S317–S326.

CHAPTER 20

Novel Risk Factors for Arterial Thrombosis

Mary Cushman, M.D., M.Sc.
Paul M. Ridker, M.D., M.P.H.

Cardiovascular disease accounts for the largest portion of deaths annually in the United States, with nearly 1 million deaths a year. This is true despite improvements in acute coronary care, and resultant reduction in mortality attributable to acute myocardial infarction (MI) over the last 20 years. As reviewed elsewhere,[1] the known major risk factors, namely hyperlipidemia, hypertension, diabetes, smoking, and a positive family history, are not present in a large portion of individuals with MI. Thus, assessing new risk factors for improved identification of individuals at the highest risk for MI would be desirable. This chapter will outline the criteria that must be met for consideration of the clinical utility of newly discovered risk factors, and review data on the role of these risk factors in cardiovascular disease assessment.

Assessment of risk factors may be performed to direct primary prevention or secondary prevention efforts. Primary prevention concerns the use of preventive measures (i.e., lipid-lowering agents or smoking-cessation programs) to reduce the risk of new-onset disease in healthy patients. Secondary prevention refers to the use of similar measures among patients with established disease, with a goal of preventing recurrent events or death from the disease. The most problematic issue in primary and secondary prevention of any disease, including MI, is that most treated patients do not receive benefit from therapy, and some are even harmed. Even with basic risk factor knowledge, we currently have a finite ability to define the highest-risk individuals, who might benefit the most from preventive treatments. Apart from the effective application of known methods for risk factor reduction, improving current treatment requires not only the development and study of new drugs or new ways of administering old drugs, but also the improved ability to define the highest-risk subset of the population. Thus, drug development, clinical trials, and study of risk factors and their interrelationships with treatment are all important.

As we have recently reviewed elsewhere,[2] epidemiologic studies of new plasma and genetic markers for coronary risk have focused on three major domains: reduced fibrinolytic potential, increased thrombotic potential, and inflammation (Table 20–1). From an epidemiologic perspective, five biomarkers have been studied widely: fibrinogen, fibrinolytic capacity as assessed either by tissue-type plasminogen activator (tPA) or its primary inhibitor plasminogen activator inhibitor type-1 (PAI-1), lipoprotein(a), homocysteine, and inflammatory markers such as high-sensitivity C-reactive protein (hs-CRP). Genetic polymorphisms associated with these domains are being actively studied. Other emerging domains under study in relation to vascular risk include measures of subclinical atherosclerosis, hemostatic activation, lipid metabolism, plaque stability, and oxidative status.

From the perspective of a consulting hematologist, currently there is a limited direct role for the use of new cardiovascular disease risk markers in practice. In considering the clinical application of any potential new risk factor, several criteria must be met (Table 20–2). First, the plasma or genetic marker of interest must be measurable with an assay that is easy to apply to the population, and that has an appropriate sensitivity and specificity for screening. For analytes where assay characteristics are poor or where optimal methodology is controversial, no recommendation for clinical screening can be considered. For example, while lipoprotein(a) has been considered by many investigators to be an independent marker of risk for coronary events, standardization of lipoprotein(a) assays remains poor for commercially available tests.[3] Other analytes such as plasminogen activator inhibitor-1 (PAI-1) have found limited clinical use because of the difficulty of measuring this parameter in clinical settings and because of diurnal variation for fibrinolytic function.[4] On the other hand, in contrast to the laborious high-pressure liquid chroma-

Table 20–1 • NOVEL RISK MARKERS FOR MI

Impaired fibrinolysis
Plasminogen activator inhibitor (PAI-1)
Tissue-type plasminogen activator (tPA)
Lipoprotein(a)
Increased thrombotic potential
Fibrinogen
D-dimer
von Willebrand factor and factor VIII:C
Hyperhomocysteinemia
Inflammation
Fibrinogen
High-sensitivity C-reactive protein (hs-CRP)
Serum amyloid A
Interleukin-6
Intercellular adhesion molecule (ICAM-1)
Subclinical Atherosclerosis
Carotid intima–media thickness
Ankle–arm blood pressure index
Coronary calcium by electron–beam computed tomography

tography method, commercial enzyme-linked immunosorbent assays (ELISAs) for total plasma homocysteine are now widely available, allowing for the potential of population screening for high homocysteine.[5] Similarly, the availability of simple assays for markers of inflammation such as hs-CRP increases the potential for use of this analyte.[6] Regarding specificity, several new risk markers may also relate to the risk of total mortality.[7,8] Whether this is because of the high prevalence of atherosclerosis as a cause of mortality, or whether these markers detect risk of other chronic medical conditions is not clear at this time. For example, a few studies have reported that inflammatory biomarkers are associated with an increased risk for the future onset of diabetes mellitus.[9]

Second, prior to considering any new risk factor in the clinical setting, consistency of the association with the risk of MI must be established in studies representing the general population. In other words, application of risk factor assessment must be generalizable. For many of the biomarkers considered in this chapter, data are still lacking or minimal in significant populations, such as women and nonwhite ethnic groups. Because these factors may be important modifiers of the risk factor–disease relationship, this is an important consideration.

Third, even though epidemiologic studies cannot attribute causality, the optimal design of studies assessing new plasma-based biomarkers is the prospective design, where assessment of the exposure of interest is done *at baseline* in apparently healthy individuals at risk for future cardiovascular disease. Retrospective studies have a role in hypothesis generation, but the plasma concentrations of many novel risk markers, such as fibrinogen and the inflammatory markers, are altered as a consequence of disease occurrence,[10,11] so potential for clinical utility cannot be established with this study design. This study design element may be less important in studies of genetic risk factors, where the retrospective case-control design may be more efficient than the prospective study, and where issues of confounding of disease relationships are less important. In interpretation of retrospective study designs, one must consider the presence or absence of various types of bias, including ascertainment and recall bias, and the methods for selection of controls.

Fourth, because assessment of any new risk marker is not likely to replace traditional risk factor assessment, it is important to demonstrate that measurement of a new risk marker will add to our ability to predict risk beyond traditional risk factors.[12] Data demonstrating such additive effects with lipid parameters have been presented for inflammatory markers such as fibrinogen and hs-CRP.[13–16] Evidence that measurement of other new risk factors adds to risk prediction over and above lipid screening is less certain.

Fifth, any new screening method must be cost-effective. For screening methods that are expensive (such as the coronary artery calcium score), the impact on disease burden must be large to warrant general use.

Finally, assessment of a new risk factor should provide information on selection of a prevention strategy. Optimally, the risk factor assessed ought to be modifiable, or at least its assessment should indicate an appropriate treatment that might not otherwise be administered. An example of a modifiable new risk factor is plasma homocysteine. Pharmacologic B vitamin supplementation and population fortification are effective in lowering plasma homocysteine, however, it is not yet clear whether these interventions reduce the risk of vascular events, and if so, whether the mechanism for this is related directly to alterations in homocysteine.

Another important use of epidemiologic research related to new risk factors for vascular disease relates to the translation of hypotheses from epidemiologic studies to the laboratory for basic research. Over the last several years, increasing epidemiologic evidence supporting hs-CRP as a cardiovascular risk factor has been associated with renewed interest in determination of the biological roles of CRP in atherogenesis.[17–19]

In an update of a recent review of this topic,[2] this chapter provides an overview of six novel domains of assessing risk of MI: subclinical atherosclerosis, lipid metabolism measures, fibrinogen and inflammation, fi-

Table 20–2 • CRITERIA TO CONSIDER IN EVALUATING NEW BIOCHEMICAL RISK MARKERS

- Clinically applicable assay
- High sensitivity and specificity
- High within-person reproducibility
- Significant population variability
- Generalizable to diverse populations
- Data from valid epidemiologic study designs
- Additive predictive capacity to assessment of established risk factors
- Cost-effective
- Assessment defines a clinical approach that would not otherwise be used

brinolytic function, hemostatic activation, and total plasma homocysteine.

SUBCLINICAL ATHEROSCLEROSIS

In recent years, research tools for the noninvasive assessment of cardiovascular disease have been developed and studied in prospective epidemiologic studies.[20] Among apparently healthy individuals, subclinical atherosclerosis often is present.[21] Measurements such as ultrasonography-assessed intima–media thickness of the carotid artery and ankle–arm blood pressure index are associated with an increased risk for MI among apparently healthy individuals,[22,23] but the incremental value to assessment of cardiovascular risk factors has not been documented. Recently, a more direct measure of atherosclerosis in the coronary arteries has been developed. Electron-beam computed tomography assesses the presence of coronary calcium. Calcium occurs only in atherosclerotic vessels, so the noninvasive imaging provided by this modality may be useful in the recognition of individuals at risk of future coronary events. While early studies are promising in linking the presence of measurable coronary calcium in asymptomatic individuals with subsequent MI, long-term studies are lacking. As with other recently studied risk factors, the incremental value of coronary calcium score over traditional risk factors is not established, and this test cannot be justified at this time for identification of high-risk asymptomatic persons.[24]

LIPID METABOLISM MEASURES

Lipoprotein(a)

Lipoprotein(a) [Lp(a)] is composed of an apo B-containing lipoprotein structure virtually identical to low-density lipoprotein(LDL) cholesterol attached by a single disulfide bond to a long carbohydrate-rich protein designated apolipoprotein(a) (apo(a)). Apo(a) is highly homologous with plasminogen[25] and it has been hypothesized that Lp(a) competes for plasminogen binding to fibrin and endothelial cell surfaces, thus inhibiting fibrinolysis. Several lines of evidence support a biologic role for Lp(a) in atherothrombosis, including in-vitro inhibition of plasminogen binding to fibrin and inhibition of tPA catalyzed fibrinolysis.[26-28] A role in atherogenesis is suggested by other data: Lp(a) was more likely to accumulate in plaques from patients with unstable, compared to stable, angina, and it colocalized with macrophages in unstable plaques.[29] Lp(a) also induced monocyte chemoattractant activity in human vascular endothelial cells.[30]

Despite the basic laboratory evidence, the clinical role of Lp(a) as a marker of risk for future coronary events is controversial. Many retrospective studies indicate that patients with a prior history of MI or stroke have elevated levels of Lp(a). However, as levels of Lp(a) increase following acute ischemia, the relevance of these studies for risk prediction is limited. By contrast, prospective studies of Lp(a) avoid the potential for bias on this basis and are therefore more informative.

To date, over a dozen prospective studies of Lp(a) have been published, with many, but not all, reporting positive associations. For example, in three large studies there was no association between baseline plasma concentration of Lp(a) and subsequent vascular risk.[31-33] In contrast, four other studies reported positive graded associations between plasma Lp(a) level and risk of coronary heart disease.[34-37] Similarly, two large studies reported significant positive associations for electrophorectic detection of sinking pre-β lipoprotein, a surrogate for Lp(a).[38,39] A meta-analysis of prospective studies reported a relative risk of 1.7 (95% confidence interval 1.4 to 1.9) for Lp(a) in the top compared to the bottom third of the distribution (Fig. 20–1).[40]

Explanations offered for the lack of consistency in these prospective studies include use of different analytic methods, the effects of long-term sample storage on assay validity, genetic differences between populations, differences in the underlying extent of subclinical atherosclerosis between studies, and the potential role played by hyperlipidemia or aspirin therapy. On the other hand, careful analysis of the data also suggests that any true differences between "null" and "positive" studies of Lp(a) may be of little clinical consequence. Specifically, the 95% confidence intervals of virtually all major studies overlap each other and are consistent with a modest positive association.[40,41] Further, as the distribution of Lp(a) is skewed high and any potential increase in vascular risk may be limited to those with the very highest values, the vast majority of myocardial infarction events will occur among those with normal Lp(a) levels. Thus, from a clinical perspective, screening for Lp(a) may be of limited utility.

Other limitations exist for Lp(a) screening. First, recent data suggest that Lp(a) levels vary among different racial cohorts and at least one study has found no association between Lp(a) and vascular disease among African Americans.[42] Further, conflicting data in women suggest that findings in men cannot easily be generalized.[43] In addition, it is not apparent that the effects of Lp(a) are clearly additive to that of total or high-density lipoprotein (HDL) cholesterol. Rather, the predictive value of Lp(a) may be limited to those with underlying hyperlipidemia, a relationship attenuated by LDL reduction.[44] Finally, there is lack of uniformity in testing for Lp(a).[3] In part, the tandem-repeat structure of apo(a) has made commercial assays difficult to calibrate, an issue that can be overcome by developing assays that make use of apo(a) monoclonal antibodies specific for unique epitopes of the Lp(a) molecule. However, whether such specific antibodies will improve the predictive value of Lp(a) testing remains uncertain.

Because of these limitations most authorities do not recommend Lp(a) evaluation in general screening programs. In specific high-risk settings or in young patients without other apparent abnormalities, investigation of Lp(a) may nonetheless be warranted. Ongoing work evaluating specific genetic polymorphisms associated with Lp(a) isoforms may help to improve the predictive value of this lipoprotein. Typically used lipid-lowering

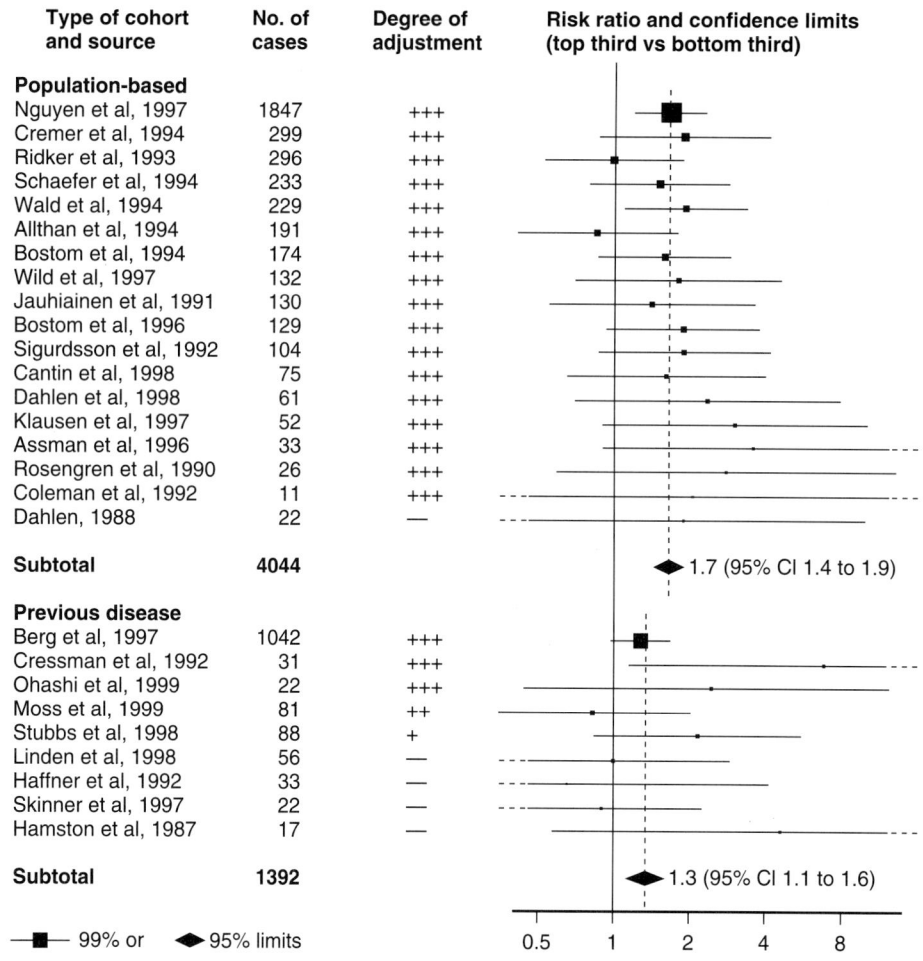

Type of cohort and source	No. of cases	Degree of adjustment
Population-based		
Nguyen et al, 1997	1847	+++
Cremer et al, 1994	299	+++
Ridker et al, 1993	296	+++
Schaefer et al, 1994	233	+++
Wald et al, 1994	229	+++
Allthan et al, 1994	191	+++
Bostom et al, 1994	174	+++
Wild et al, 1997	132	+++
Jauhiainen et al, 1991	130	+++
Bostom et al, 1996	129	+++
Sigurdsson et al, 1992	104	+++
Cantin et al, 1998	75	+++
Dahlen et al, 1998	61	+++
Klausen et al, 1997	52	+++
Assman et al, 1996	33	+++
Rosengren et al, 1990	26	+++
Coleman et al, 1992	11	+++
Dahlen, 1988	22	—
Subtotal	**4044**	
Previous disease		
Berg et al, 1997	1042	+++
Cressman et al, 1992	31	+++
Ohashi et al, 1999	22	+++
Moss et al, 1999	81	++
Stubbs et al, 1998	88	+
Linden et al, 1998	56	—
Haffner et al, 1992	33	—
Skinner et al, 1997	22	—
Hamston et al, 1987	17	—
Subtotal	**1392**	

Population-based subtotal: 1.7 (95% CI 1.4 to 1.9)
Previous disease subtotal: 1.3 (95% CI 1.1 to 1.6)

Figure 20-1 Prospective studies of Lp(a) and risk of coronary heart disease. (From Danesh J, Collins R, Peto R. Lipoprotein(a) and coronary heart disease: a meta-analysis of prospective studies. Circulation 2000;102:1082–1085, with permission.)

drugs, diet, and exercise do not lower Lp(a) levels, and few data are available on the potential clinical use of Lp(a) measurement. One recent study suggests a potential role. Despite an overall lack of benefit of randomized treatment with postmenopausal hormone replacement therapy,[45] the Heart and Estrogen/Progestin Interventions Trial reported that among women with established coronary disease, hormones lowered Lp(a) levels, and moreover, high Lp(a) predicted a modest beneficial effect of hormones on subsequent coronary events.[46] These intriguing data require confirmation given the current lack of certainty concerning the benefits of estrogen replacement on vascular disease health.[45]

Other measures of lipid-related risk are being studied actively. Proton nuclear magnetic resonance (NMR) spectroscopy, for determination of the concentrations of lipoprotein subclasses, is being extensively evaluated in population studies.[47] The clinical role of these tests remains to be determined. Studies are beginning to assess the role of genetic polymorphisms of lipid-related proteins. The ε4 allele of apolipoprotein E (APOE4) has been associated with coronary artery disease. This same allele is also prevalent among populations with Alzheimer disease. Variations of the cholesterol ester transfer protein have been related to HDL concentration and lipoprotein size.[48] In 1999, the cloning and identification of the ATP-binding cassette transporter 1 (ABC1) gene, as the basis for Tangier disease (severe HDL deficiency), led to new insights on the etiology of low HDL, an important lipid risk factor for MI.[49] Future studies relating ABC1 variants with MI and other vascular disorders will be of interest, as will efforts to develop interventions related to ABC1.

FIBRINOGEN

Plasma fibrinogen impacts directly on blood clotting, plasma rheology, platelet aggregation, and endothelial function. Further, fibrinogen plays a major role in monocyte adhesion, and both fibrinogen and fibrin degradation products have been shown to stimulate smooth muscle proliferation. Thus, through both hemostatic and inflammatory mechanisms, plasma fibrinogen level is closely related to thrombus formation.[50]

Of the major novel markers for coronary artery disease, fibrinogen was the earliest to undergo extensive epidemiologic evaluation. Prospective data from many studies[7,51–53] all confirm that higher fibrinogen is associated with the risk of future MI, stroke, or cardiovascular death, and in some cases noncardiovascular disease mortality. In pooled analyses, those with fibrinogen levels in the upper third of the distribution appear to have risks of future coronary heart disease 1.8 times that of individuals with levels in the lower third (95% confidence intervals 1.6 to 2.0).[51] In some studies[13,14] but not in others, evidence has been presented that assessment of fibrinogen adds to the predictive value of lipid screening.

Given the consistency of the prospective data and potential for additive value of fibrinogen over total and HDL cholesterol evaluation, many have suggested that fibrinogen be used as a clinical tool to determine coronary risk. However, this approach has not been widely adopted for several reasons. First, standardization of fibrinogen measurement remains poor and no single analytic technique has been adopted, leading to poor clinical acceptance. Second, fibrinogen levels are higher in the presence of other standard risk factors,[10] so the utility of fibrinogen screening among low-risk populations may be limited. Because there are differences in men compared to women, gender-specific definitions of elevated fibrinogen may be required. Overall, much fewer data are available on the role of fibrinogen in risk prediction among women, with at least two studies reporting no association of fibrinogen with future MI among older women.[7,54]

Apart from the above issues, fibrinogen screening may provide useful clinical information for risk prediction. However, there are no current therapies that specifically reduce fibrinogen without also lowering lipids, and the presence of high fibrinogen has not yet defined a specific intervention for risk reduction.

C-REACTIVE PROTEIN (hs-CRP) AND OTHER MARKERS OF INFLAMMATION

In addition to hyperlipidemia, vascular inflammation plays a major role in atherogenesis.[55] For example, atherosclerotic lesions are characterized by abundant monocyte and macrophage infiltration. In addition, unstable lesions may overexpress metalloproteinase activity, have increased levels of cytokine and adhesion molecule production, and preferentially express monocyte chemoattractant and growth factors.

Until recently, it had been assumed that inflammatory components associated with atherosclerosis were triggered by acute ischemia and that elevations of inflammatory markers were primarily a reflection of the acute phase response. However, a series of prospective epidemiologic studies indicate that plasma levels of several inflammatory markers are elevated years in advance of first-ever coronary events and that detection of inflammation in this way may provide a method of identifying high-risk individuals. Inflammatory markers evaluated to date include the hepatic proteins C-reactive protein, serum amyloid A, fibrinogen, and albumin, markers of cell surface adhesion such as soluble intercellular adhesion molecule (sICAM-1) and E selectin, and cytokines such as interleukin-6 and interleukin-1. The most compelling data available relate to C-reactive protein, particularly when measured with recently developed high-sensitivity assays (hs-CRP).

C-reactive protein is a nonspecific marker for systemic inflammation that rises several hundred-fold in response to acute injury. CRP production is dependent upon hepatic synthesis in response to circulating cytokines. In the absence of acute inflammation, hs-CRP levels tend to be stable within individuals over long periods of time and appear to provide an index of underlying low-grade inflammation.

Several biologic roles for CRP have been described in relation to atherosclerosis. Whether CRP has a direct role in thrombus formation is not clear, although the circulating level is directly correlated with some hemostasis factors,[56] and experimental evidence has shown that CRP can induce monocyte tissue factor expression.[57] CRP colocalizes with complement in atherosclerotic plaques,[58] can activate complement,[17] and may regulate of adhesion molecule expression by endothelial cells.[18] Further CRP is chemotactic for monocytes in plaques.[19]

A series of prospective epidemiologic studies links baseline levels of hs-CRP to future risks of MI, stroke, and coronary heart disease mortality among individuals free of known cardiovascular disease (Fig. 20–2).[59] The first report linking elevated hs-CRP with risk of future vascular events included patients with unstable angina.[60] Here, higher hs-CRP was associated with the development of recurrent acute coronary syndromes. In 1996 this finding was extended when a report from the Multiple Risk Factor Intervention Trial showed that baseline hs-CRP was associated with future fatal coronary heart disease among male smokers with other cardiac risk factors.[61] In this study hs-CRP was measured in blood samples drawn 5 to 17 years prior to the onset of clinical events, pointing out the potential for discriminating very long-term risk, and suggesting that hs-CRP measurement did not simply reflect generalized illness. In a larger study of apparently healthy middle-aged American men followed for 8 years, those with hs-CRP levels in the highest quartile at baseline had a twofold increase in the risk of future stroke, a threefold increase in the risk of MI, and a fourfold increase in the risk of undergoing surgery for peripheral vascular disease compared to study participants with lower levels of hs-CRP.[62,63] These effects were independent of other measured risk factors including fibrinogen, were present among nonsmokers, and were additive to total and HDL cholesterol in terms of risk prediction.[15] Similar data confirming these observations have been presented in studies of postmenopausal women (Fig. 20–3),[16] the elderly,[64] and middle-aged men.[65–67] A meta-analysis reported that hs-CRP concentrations in the top third of the population distribution were associated with a twofold increased risk of MI.[66] Among individuals with stable and unstable coronary syndromes, and in those who have a prior history of MI, hs-CRP also appears to have prognostic significance.[60,68–70]

The consistency of these studies supports a critical role for inflammation in plaque rupture, but associations with atherogenesis are less clear. Two studies did not find an association of hs-CRP with the presence of coro-

Type of cohort and source	No. of cases	Degree of adjustment	Risk ratio and confidence limits (top third vs bottom third)
Population based			
Present study	506	++++	
Ridker et al, 1997	246	++++	
Koenig et al, 1999	53	++++	
Kuller et al, 1996	246	+++	
Lowe et al, 1999	165	+++	
Tracy et al, 1997	150	+++	
Tracy et al, 1997	145	+++	
Witherell et al, 1999	100	+++	
Ridker et al, 1998	85	++++	
Agewall et al, 1998	16	+++	
Roivainen et al, 2000	241	++	
Subtotal	1953		2.0 (95% CI 1.6 to 2.5)
Pre-existing vascular disease			
Ridker et al, 1998	391	+++	
Toss et al, 1997	138	+++	
Haverkate et al, 1997	75	+++	
Subtotal	604		1.5 (95% CI 1.1 to 2.1)
Total	2557		1.9 (95% CI 1.5 to 2.3)

■— 99% or ◆— 95% limits

Figure 20–2 Prospective studies of hs-CRP as a risk factor for future cardiovascular disease in populations free of clinical disease. (From Danesh J, Whincup P, Walker M, et al. Low grade inflammation and coronary heart disease: prospective study and update meta-analysis. BMJ 2000;321:199–204, with permission.)

nary calcium assessed by electron-beam computed tomography,[71,72] although levels are associated with subclinical atherosclerosis in other vascular beds.[11] Like fibrinogen, hs-CRP tends to increase with age, body mass index, and smoking pattern.[11] However, most studies have found the predictive value of hs-CRP to be independent of these other risk factors, and one study suggested independence of the association from noninvasively assessed subclinical atherosclerosis.[64] In contrast to fibrinogen, hs-CRP increases with hormone replacement therapy,[73] data that further indicate that fibrinogen and hs-CRP reflect different pathophysiologic processes.

The inflammatory process associated with atherosclerosis may be a modifiable target for risk reduction. Two analyses derived from randomized controlled trials suggest that common preventive therapies may attenuate the inflammatory response. In the Physicians' Health Study, the male participants were randomly assigned at baseline to 325 mg of alternate-day aspirin and then followed for first occurrence MI. MI was reduced 44% with this intervention. However, the risk reduction associated with aspirin was greatest among those with the highest levels of baseline hs-CRP (55%) and smallest among those with the lowest levels of hs-CRP (13%).[62] These findings raise the possibility that, in addition to antiplatelet effects, low-dose aspirin may attenuate thrombosis through anti-inflammatory mechanisms. Subsequent studies have demonstrated this biochemical effect of low-dose aspirin on circulating cytokines.[74]

Interactions between hs-CRP and lipid reduction with HMG CoA reductase inhibitors ("statins") have also been demonstrated.[70,75] In the Cholesterol and Recurrent Events (CARE) trial of post-MI patients, randomized assignment to pravastatin was associated with a 24% reduction in risk of recurrent coronary events. However,

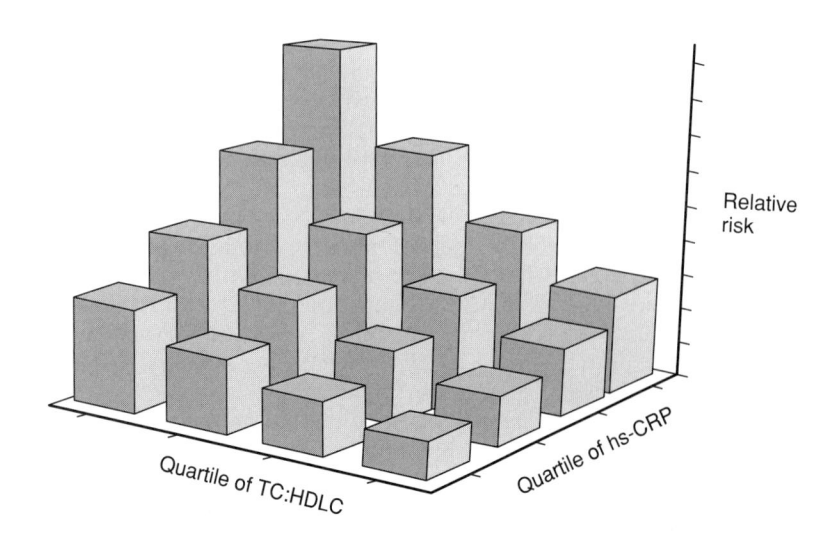

Figure 20–3 Relative risks of future myocardial infarction as predicted by the simultaneous assessment of hs-CRP and a standard lipid profile among men (left) and women (right). (From Ridker PM. High sensitivity C-reactive protein: Potential adjunct for global risk assessment in the primary prevention of cardiovascular disease. Circulation 2001;103:1813–1818, with permission.)

the risk reduction associated with pravastatin was almost twice as large among those with elevated levels of hs-CRP than among those with lower levels.[70] Moreover, the association between inflammation and risk of recurrent coronary events was present among those allocated to placebo, but markedly attenuated and no longer significant among those allocated to pravastatin. In additional data from the CARE trial, levels of hs-CRP were reduced over 5 years in the group treated with pravastatin, while no change was observed among those on placebo.[76] It has been hypothesized that the process of plaque stabilization associated with statin use may result in part from anti-inflammatory effects.[77]

At this time high-sensitivity assays for CRP are commercially available.[6,78] At least one new assay has been validated against data derived from a published research-based assay.[79] It is important to point out that, while they assess the same protein, standard clinical tests for CRP do not have adequate sensitivity to detect levels in the range that are relevant for coronary risk prediction.

IMPAIRED FIBRINOLYSIS

The balance between plasminogen activators, primarily tissue-type plasminogen activator (tPA), and its main inhibitor, plasminogen activator inhibitor type 1 (PAI-1), determine the activity of the fibrinolytic system. Synthesized and secreted by the vascular endothelium, adjacent smooth muscle, and, in the case of PAI-1, from adipocytes, these fibrinolytic proteins can be detected in plasma using sensitive assays for both antigen and activity levels. In general, an increased PAI-1 concentration is associated with impairment of fibrinolysis, which may lead to reduced plasmin formation, accumulation of fibrin, and activation of metalloproteinase activity.[80]

Based on these data, it has been hypothesized that, on a population basis, detection of impaired fibrinolytic function can be used to evaluate thrombotic risk. Support for this hypothesis is available from some, but not all available prospective studies that evaluated antigen levels of tPA or PAI-1, PAI-1 activity, or clot lysis time.[14,56,81–85] In some of these studies, important correlates of fibrinolytic function, such as components of the insulin resistance syndrome or obesity, have not been controlled for, or when adjustment was made for these, associations of fibrinolytic function were not independent predictors of MI.

It appears unlikely that assessment of fibrinolytic function using these biomarkers will prove to be clinically useful. In most studies, positive associations of fibrinolytic markers with MI were not independent of other risk factors for MI. Also, because of the circadian variation of fibrinolytic function and other preanalytical factors, the application of these techniques for screening appears limited.

Some of the difficulties in assessment of fibrinolysis might be overcome by assessing genetic markers of fibrinolytic function. Genetic variations associated with both PAI-1 and tPA production have been described. However, studies of an insertion–deletion polymorphism in the promotor of the PAI-1 gene and of an Alu-repeat insertion–deletion polymorphism in the tPA gene in relation to the risk of vascular disease have been inconsistent.

HEMOSTATIC ACTIVATION MARKERS

D-dimer is an activation marker that reflects the balance of procoagulant and fibrinolytic reactions. D-dimer is formed by the degradation of cross-linked fibrin by plasmin, therefore, its assessment reflects ongoing fibrin formation and breakdown. The association of D-dimer with future arterial thrombosis in healthy subjects has been addressed in only a few studies to date. Using sensitive assays, D-dimer above the 95th percentile predicted MI in apparently healthy middle-aged men, but the association was not independent of lipid levels.[86] This was not the case in the middle-aged Atherosclerosis Risk in Communities (ARIC) cohort, where baseline D-dimer in the highest compared to the lowest quintile of the population distribution was associated with a 4.2-fold higher risk of subsequent MI over 4.3 years of follow-up, independent of other factors.[87] Similarly, in a 2-year prospective study of 5201 men and women aged 65 and older, there was a 4.1-fold increased risk of MI for D-dimer in the top quartile of the population distribution.[56] This association also was independent of other risk factors, including hs-CRP and fibrinogen. D-dimer was a better predictor of events occurring within, rather than after, 12 months of follow-up. This suggests that D-dimer assessment might reflect plaque destabilization or hemostatic activation close to the time of occlusive events, and that serial assessment of D-dimer might have a clinical role in this age group. This time interaction was not observed in the younger participants of the ARIC study.

Other studies have assessed D-dimer among patients with pre-existing vascular disease and reported similar associations to those above.[88–90] Taken together, the epidemiologic studies suggest that D-dimer may have better predictive power for vascular events among those who have more underlying preclinical atherosclerosis. There are no data yet to suggest that D-dimer measurement adds to the predictive value of other risk factors, and the generalizability of this measurement remains uncertain.

From the laboratory perspective, D-dimer testing has acceptable within-person variability over time and the measurement is readily available using sensitive and reproducible ELISA or latex-agglutination assays. However, further research on D-dimer measurement is required to determine whether this biomarker fulfills the criteria necessary for clinical usefulness. If this can be demonstrated, like other analytes, laboratory standardization efforts would be required.

TOTAL PLASMA HOMOCYSTEINE

Homocysteine, a sulfhydryl amino acid, plays a major role in the metabolism of methionine. Patients with rare inherited deficiencies in the enzymes methionine synthase, methylenetetrahydrofolate reductase (MTHFR), and in particular cystathione β-synthase can have marked plasma elevations of homocysteine and often suffer from premature atherothrombosis or venous thrombosis. Several mechanisms may link severe hyperhomocysteinemia (plasma concentration above 100 μmol/L) to vascular damage, including direct endothelial toxicity, induction of vascular smooth muscle proliferation, impairment of endothelial derived relaxing factor, and accelerated oxidation of LDL cholesterol.[91] Some experimental data suggest that these processes may be reversible; homocysteine reduction may slow the rate of progression of carotid artery stenosis,[92] and acute hyperhomocysteinemia appears to induce reversible reduction of flow-mediated brachial artery reactivity.[93]

On a population basis, severe hyperhomocysteinemia is rare. However, mild to moderate hyperhomocysteinemia (plasma concentration above 15 μmol/L) is present in up to 10% of individuals. The principal cause of mild to moderate hyperhomocysteinemia is low dietary folate intake. Folic acid, cyanocobalamin (vitamin B$_{12}$) and pyridoxine (vitamin B$_6$) are all involved in the regulation of methionine metabolism, and several studies indicate inverse associations between homocysteine concentration and plasma levels of these vitamins. By contrast, folic acid supplementation in doses between 0.5 and 5.0 mg/day are known to reduce homocysteine levels.

A series of retrospective and cross-sectional studies provides support for a direct relationship between mild to moderate hyperhomocysteinemia and increased coronary risk. Overall these studies suggest that individuals with homocysteine levels above 15 μmol/L have an adjusted relative risk 1.4 times higher than those with levels below 10 μmol/L.[94] Based on this, it has been hypothesized that increased folate intake through supplementation might prevent as many as 30,000 premature deaths annually in the United States.[94]

Despite these provocative data, screening for hyperhomocysteinemia among asymptomatic individuals to determine risk is controversial and not currently recommended by either the American College of Cardiology or the American Heart Association.[94] This conservative approach reflects several issues. First, because homocysteine levels increase following acute MI and stroke, the observed association of homocysteine and atherothrombosis observed in cross-sectional and retrospective studies could be a consequence rather than a cause of vascular disease. Second, prospective studies of homocysteine as a marker of risk for future MI or stroke have been inconsistent (Fig. 20–4). In this regard, prospective studies from the United State[95] and Finland[96] report no evidence of association between moderate hyperhomocysteinemia and future vascular risk, while a second United States study of middle-aged male physicians found a positive association limited to those with the very highest baseline levels.[97] In this latter study no evidence of association was found on longer-term follow-up, a null finding similar to that observed among men and women enrolled in the prospective ARIC study,[98] in the Zutphen Elderly Study,[99] and the Caer-

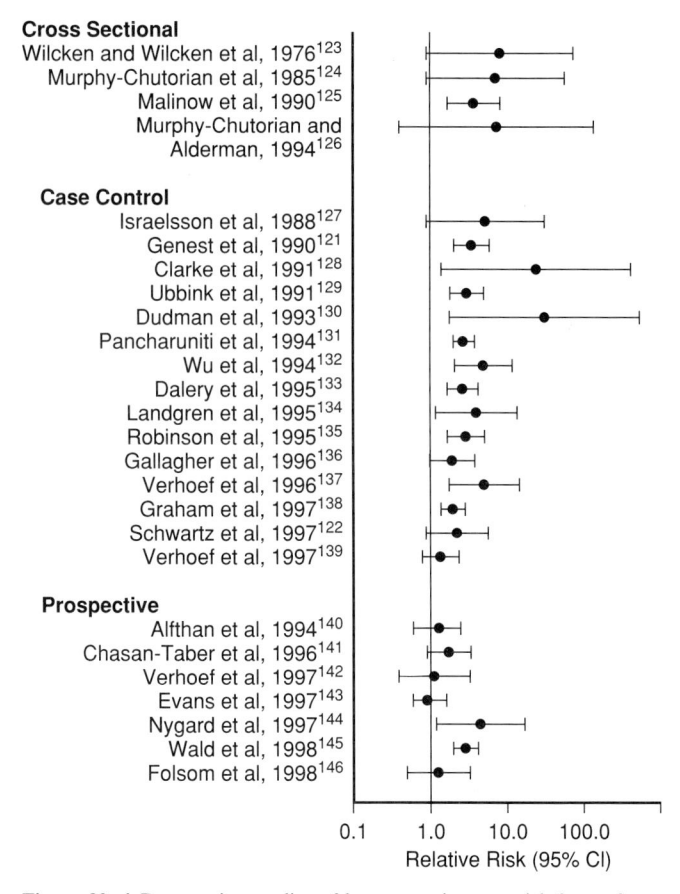

Figure 20–4 Prospective studies of homocysteine as a risk factor for future cardiovascular disease in populations free of clinical disease. (From Christen WG, Ajani VA, Glynn RJ, et al. Blood levels of homocysteine and increased risks of cardiovascular disease: causal or casual? Arch Intern Med 2000;160:422–434, with permission.)

philly cohort.[100] By contrast, other prospective studies of initially healthy individuals have reported a positive association between homocysteine and subsequent risk, in both middle-aged and older populations, with some studies confirming the threshold effect observed in the earlier study of male physicians.[101–104] In addition, among women, hyperhomocysteinemia has been related to all-cause mortality as well as vascular disease in two studies,[105,106] suggesting some nonspecificity.

Published reports on the relative risk of coronary heart disease with elevated homocysteine point out the differences between retrospective and prospective studies, and among the prospective studies.[107] There are several possible reasons for conflicting results among prospective studies. The studies may be too heterogeneous, either in methods or population source, to compare to one another. There appear to be larger associations in studies with shorter compared to longer follow-up. The use of adjustment for potential confounders, such as vitamin intake, has varied widely. The conflicting data suggest that the magnitude of any increased risk associated with hyperhomocysteinemia is likely to be modest and may be limited to those relatively few individuals with substantial elevations of total plasma homocysteine.

An important reason that homocysteine screening is not currently recommended for the general population is that it is not known whether homocysteine reduction reduces vascular risk. While folate supplementation is known to reduce homocysteine levels, randomized trials relating supplementation to clinical outcomes are not yet complete. It is important to note that the clinical relevance of homocysteine assessment may be limited because of fortification programs that were completed in the United States in 1997. In an effort to reduce the risk of neural tube defects during pregnancy, the Food and Drug Administration required that all enriched flour and grain products contain folic acid. The population impact of fortification on homocysteine levels has been considerable, with mean reductions of nearly 10%.[108] Whether supplementation will influence the effectiveness of B-vitamin therapy on vascular disease is uncertain. One study of women suggested that this will not be the case by reporting that homocysteine levels were associated with an increased risk of future coronary events, regardless of whether participants were taking folic acid-containing multivitamins.[106]

While current vascular disease prevention guidelines do not include homocysteine screening,[94] in certain high-risk conditions associated with high homocysteine levels, such as renal failure[109] or hypothyroidism,[110] screening and therapy may be beneficial. If screening were to be considered, accurate measurement of total plasma homocysteine concentration must be done fasting and must include assessment of the disulfide homocystine and cysteine-homocysteine. Standardization of assay methods, which include the gold standard high-performance liquid chromatography, the simpler enzyme or fluorescence polarization immunoassays, and capillary electrophoresis, is required.[111] Although methionine loading increases the sensitivity of homocysteine screening, this additional step is not needed for most patients.

In addition to diet, a common mutation in the thermolabile form of MTHFR has been associated with increased homocysteine levels. While some studies suggest that carriers of this polymorphism may be at increased coronary risk, most data have not confirmed this observation.[112]

THE HEMATOLOGIST'S PERSPECTIVE

Hematologists frequently are asked to provide consultation regarding the management of patients with arterial disease who have hemostatic risk factors that are more closely associated with the risk of venous thrombosis. These risk factors include deficiencies of the natural anticoagulant proteins, and heterozygous factor V Leiden or the prothrombin 20210A variant. Epidemiologic studies relating these disorders to arterial disease have been inconsistent and largely negative.[53,113-116] However, this does not necessarily mean that these disorders are not important in the pathogenesis of arterial occlusion in certain individuals. While there may be subgroups, such as young women, where associations of these factors with MI are present,[117,118] the optimal management of such patients and the role of anticoagulation, as compared to control of conventional risk factors, is not known. Because of this, evaluation must be individualized and no standard guidelines are available.

FUTURE DIRECTIONS IN CORONARY RISK PREDICTION

For clinicians attempting to better predict coronary risk, few screening guidelines are available that describe when to measure a novel marker. As stated throughout this chapter, the clinical application of these measures is not yet certain; there are insufficient data addressing sensitivity and specificity, and generalizability is not confirmed. Among all the markers discussed, hs-CRP assessment seems the most promising, but more study is required before general use in screening can be advocated.

Of equal importance to the future of cardiovascular risk reduction is the development of interventions that stabilize plaques and that incorporate evolving genetic approaches. With regard to novel therapeutic targets in atherothrombosis, agents in development include new anti-inflammatory and antimicrobial drugs, as well as antithrombotics and drugs that interfere with cytokine function, metalloproteinase activity, and nuclear receptor/transcription factors.[119]

Future directions in assessment of new risk factors are likely to involve studies of subclinical atherosclerosis, new ways to assess lipid metabolism, and inflammation. The clinical roles of coronary calcium measurement and other noninvasive tests of subclinical atherosclerosis in defining risk require clarification.

In the future, genetic screening is likely to represent a dramatic paradigm shift in coronary disease prevention. While it is clear that family history is a determinant of the risk of MI, the net impact of family history on risk is modest and in general, studies of single gene polymorphisms for atherothrombosis have been disappointing.[120] However, with the advent of high-throughput multilocus gene screening and the considerable promise of pharmacogenetics, such an approach to cardiovascular risk prediction will be a major research goal in the future.[120]

■ REFERENCES

Chapter 20 References

1. Jackson E, Skerrett PJ, Ridker PM. Epidemiology of arterial thrombosis. In: Colman RW, Hirsh J, Marder VJ, Clowes AW, George JN (Eds): Hemostasis and Thrombosis: Basic Principles and Clinical Practice. Philadelphia, Lippincott Williams & Wilkins, 2001, pp. 1179–1196.
2. Ridker PM. Novel risk factors and markers for coronary disease. Adv Intern Med 2000;45:391–418.
3. Tate JR, Rifai N, Berg K, et al. International Federation of Clinical Chemistry standardization project for measurement of lipoprotein(a). Phase 1. Evaluation of analytical performance of lipoprotein(a) assay systems and commercial calibrators. Clin Chem 1998;44:1629–1640.

4. Angleton P, Chandler WL, Schmer G. Diurnal variation of tissue-type plasminogen activator and its rapid inhibition. Circulation 1989;79:101–106.
5. Shiplander MT, Moore EG. Rapid, fully automated measurement of plasma homocyst(e)ine with the Abbott Imx Analyzer. Clin Chem 1995;41:991–995.
6. Ledue T, Weiner D, Sipe J, et al. Analytical evaluation of particle-enhanced immunonephelometric assays for C-reactive protein, serum amyloid A and mannose-binding protein in human serum. Ann Clin Biochem 1998;35:745–753.
7. Tracy RP, Arnold AM, Ettinger W, et al. The relationship of fibrinogen and factors VII and VIII to incident cardiovascular disease and death in the elderly: results from the Cardiovascular Health Study. Arterioscler Thromb Vasc Biol, 1999;19:1776–1783.
8. Harris TB, Ferruci L, Tracy RP, et al. Associations of elevated interleukin-6 and C-reactive protein levels with mortality in the elderly. Am J Med 1999;106:506–512.
9. Schmidt MI, Duncan BB, Sharrett AR, et al. Markers of inflammation and prediction of diabetes mellitus in adults (Atherosclerosis Risk in Communities study): a cohort study. Lancet 1999;353:1649–1652.
10. Cushman M, Yanez D, Psaty BM, et al. Correlates of fibrinogen and coagulation factors VII and VIII in the elderly: results from the Cardiovascular Health Study. Am J Epidemiol 1996;143:665–676.
11. Tracy RP, Psaty BM, Macy E, et al. Lifetime smoking exposure affects the association of C-reactive protein with cardiovascular disease risk factors and subclinical disease in healthy elderly subjects. Arterioscler Thromb Vasc Biol 1997;17:2167–2176.
12. Ridker PM. Evaluating novel cardiovascular risk factors: can we better predict heart attacks? Ann Intern Med 1999;130:933–937.
13. Heinrich J, Balleisen L, Schulte H, et al. Fibrinogen and factor VII in the prediction of coronary risk: Results from the PROCAM study in healthy men. Arterioscler Thromb 1994;14:54–59.
14. Thompson S, Kienast J, Pyke S, et al. Hemostatic factors and the risk of myocardial infarction or sudden death in patients with angina pectoris. N Engl J Med 1995;332:635–641.
15. Ridker PM, Glynn RJ, Hennekens CH. C-reactive protein adds to the predictive value of total and HDL cholesterol in determining risk of first myocardial infarction. Circulation 1998;97:2007–2011.
16. Ridker PM, Hennekens CH, Buring JE, et al. C-reactive protein and other markers of inflammation in the prediction of cardiovascular disease in women. N Engl J Med 2000;342:836–843.
17. Bhakdi S, Torzewski M, Klouche M, et al. Complement and atherogenesis: binding of CRP to degraded, nonoxidized LDL enhances complement activation. Arterioscler Thromb Vasc Biol 1999;19:2348–2354.
18. Pasceri V, Willerson JT, Yeh ETH. Direct proinflammatory effect of C-reactive protein on human endothelial cells. Circulation 2000;102:2165–2168.
19. Torzewski M, Rist C, Mortensen RF, et al. C-reactive protein in the arterial intima: role of C-reactive protein receptor-dependent monocyte recruitment in atherogenesis. Arterioscler Thromb Vasc Biol 2000;20:2094–2099.
20. Kuller LH, Shemanski L, Psaty BM, et al. Subclinical disease as an independent risk factor for cardiovascular disease. Circulation 1995;92:720–726.
21. Kuller L, Borhani N, Furberg K, et al. Prevalence of subclinical atherosclerosis and cardiovascular disease and association with risk factors in the Cardiovascular Health Study. Am J Epidemiol 1994;139:1164–1179.
22. O'Leary DH, Polak JF, Kronmal RA, et al. Carotid-artery intima and media thickness as a risk factor for myocardial infarction and stroke in older adults. Cardiovascular Health Study Collaborative Research Group. N Engl J Med 1999;340:14–22.
23. Newman AB, Shemanski L, Manolio TA, et al. Ankle-arm index as a predictor of cardiovascular disease in the Cardiovascular Health Study. Arterioscler Thromb Vasc Biol 1999;19:538–545.
24. O'Rourke RA, Brundage BH, Froelicher VF, et al. American College of Cardiology/American Heart Association expert consensus document on electron-beam computed tomography for the diagnosis and prognosis of coronary artery disease. Circulation 2000;102:126–140.
25. McLean JW, Tomlinson JE, Kuang WJ, et al. cDNA sequence of human apolipoprotein(a) is homologous to plasminogen. Nature 1987;330:132–137.
26. Hajar KA, Gavish D, Breslow JL, et al. Lipoprotein(a) modulation of endothelial cell surface fibrinolysis and its potential role in atherosclerosis. Nature 1989;339:303–305.
27. Harpel PC, Gordon BR, Parker TS. Plasmin catalyzes binding of lipoprotein(a) to immobilized fibrinogen and fibrin. Proc Natl Acad Sci USA 1989;86:3847–3851.
28. Loscalzo J, Weinfeld M, Fless G, et al. Lipoprotein(a), fibrin binding, and plasminogen activation. Arteriosclerosis 1990;10:240–245.
29. Dangas G, Mehran R, Harpel PC, et al. Lipoprotein(a) and inflammation in human coronary atheroma: association with severity of clinical presentation. J Am Coll Cardiol 1998;32:2035–2042.
30. Poon M, Zhang X, Dunsky KG, et al. Apolipoprotein(a) induces monocyte chemotactic activity in human vascular endothelial cells. Circulation 1997;96:2514–2519.
31. Jauhiainen M, Koskinen P, Ehnholm C, et al. Lipoprotein(a) and coronary heart disease risk: a nested case-control study of the Helskinki Heart Study participants. Atherosclerosis 1991;89:59–67.
32. Ridker PM, Hennekens CH, Stampfer MJ. A prospective study of lipoprotein(a) and the risk of myocardial infarction. JAMA 1993;270:2195–2199.
33. Cantin B, Gagnon F, Moorjani S, et al. Is lipoprotein(a) an independent risk factor for ischemic heart disease in men? The Quebec Cardiovascular Study. J Am Coll Cardiol 1998;31:519–525.
34. Schaefer EJ, Lamon-Fava S, Jenner JL, et al. Lipoprotein(a) levels and risk of coronary heart disease in men. The Lipid Research Clinics Coronary Primary Prevention Trial. JAMA 1994;271:999–1003.
35. Cremer P, Nagel D, Labrot B, et al. Lipoprotein(a) as a predictor of myocardial infarction in comparison to fibrinogen, LDL cholesterol and other risk factors: results from the prospective Gottingen Risk Incidence and Prevalence Study (GRIPS). Eur J Clin Invest 1994;24:444–453.
36. Wald NJ, Law M, Watt HC, et al. Apolipoproteins and ischaemic heart disease: implications for screening. Lancet 1994;343:75–79.
37. Wild SH, Fortmann SP, Marcovina SM. A prospective case control study of lipoprotein(a) levels and apo(a) size and risk of coronary heart disease in Stanford five-city project participants. Arterioscler Thromb Vasc Biol 1997;17:239–245.
38. Bostom AG, Gagnon DR, Cupples A, et al. A prospective investigation of elevated lipoprotein(a) detected by electrophoresis and cardiovascular disease in women: the Framingham Heart Study. Circulation 1994;90:1688–1695.
39. Nguyen TT, Ellefson RD, Hodge DO, et al. Predictive value of electrophoretically detected lipoprotein(a) for coronary heart disease and cerebrovascular disease in a community-based cohort of 9936 men and women. Circulation 1997;96:1390–1397.
40. Danesh J, Collins R, Peto R. Lipoprotein(a) and coronary heart disease: a meta-analysis of prospective studies. Circulation 2000;102:1082–1085.
41. Ridker PM. An epidemiologic reassessment of lipoprotein(a) and atherothrombotic risk. Trends Cardiovasc Med 1995;5:225–229.
42. Moliterno DJ, Jokinen EV, Miserez AR, et al. No association between plasma lipoprotein(a) concentrations and the presence or absence of coronary atherosclerosis in African-Americans. Arterioscler Thromb Vasc Biol 1995;15:850–855.

43. Sunayama S, Daida H, Mokuno H, et al. Lack of increased coronary atherosclerotic risk due to elevated lipoprotein(a) in women 55 years of age. Circulation 1996;94:1263–1268.
44. Maher VM, Brown BG, Marcovina SM, et al. Effects of lowering elevated LDL cholesterol on the cardiovascular risk of lipoprotein(a). JAMA 1995;274:1771–1774.
45. Hulley S, Grady D, Bush T, et al. Randomized trial of estrogen plus progestin for secondary prevention of coronary heart disease in postmenopausal women. JAMA 1998;280:605–613.
46. Shlipak MG, Simon JA, Vittinghoff E, et al. Estrogen and progestin, lipoprotein(a), and the risk of recurrent heart disease events after menopause. JAMA 2000;283:1845–1852.
47. Freedman DS, Otvos JD, Jeyarajah EJ, et al. Relation of lipoprotein subclasses as measured by proton nuclear magnetic resonance spectroscopy to coronary artery disease. Arterioscler Thromb Vasc Biol 1998;18:1046–1053.
48. Ordovas JM, Cupples LA, Corella D, et al. Association of cholesterol ester transfer protein—TaqIB polymorphism with variations in lipoprotein subclasses and coronary heart disease risk: the Framingham Study. Arterioscler Thromb Vasc Biol 2000; 20:1323–1329.
49. Remaley AT, Rust S, Rosier M, et al. Human ATP-binding cassette transport 1 (ABC1): genomic organization and identification of the genetic defect in the original Tangier disease kindred. Proc Nat Acad Sci USA 1999;96:12685–12690.
50. Ernst E, Resch KL. Fibrinogen as a cardiovascular risk factor: A meta-analysis and review of the literature. Ann Intern Med 1993;118:956–963.
51. Danesh J, Collins R, Appleby P, et al. Association of fibrinogen, C-reactive protein, albumin, or leukocyte count with coronary heart disease: meta-analyses of prospective studies. JAMA 1998;279:1477–1482.
52. Ma J, Hennekens CH, Ridker PM, et al. A prospective study of fibrinogen and risk of myocardial infarction in the Physician's Health Study. J Am Coll Cardiol 1999;33:1347–1352.
53. Folsom AR, Wu KK, Rosamond WD, et al. Prospective study of hemostatic factors and incidence of coronary heart disease: the Atherosclerosis Risk in Communities (ARIC) study. Circulation 1997;96:1102–1108.
54. Kannel WB, Wolf PA, Castelli WP, et al. Fibrinogen and risk of cardiovascular disease: the Framingham study. JAMA 1987; 258:1183–1186.
55. Ross R. Atherosclerosis—an inflammatory disease. N Engl J Med 1999;340:115–126.
56. Cushman M, Lemaitre RN, Kuller LH, et al. Fibrinolytic activation markers predict myocardial infarction in the elderly: the Cardiovascular Health Study. Arterioscler Thromb Vasc Biol 1999;19:493–498.
57. Cermak J, Key N, Bach R, et al. C-reactive protein induces human peripheral blood monocytes to synthesize tissue factor. Blood 1993;82:513–520.
58. Torzewski J, Torzewski M, Bowyer DE, et al. C-reactive protein frequently colocalizes with the terminal complement complex in the intima of early atherosclerotic lesions of human coronary arteries. Arterioscler Thromb Vasc Biol 1998;18:1386–1392.
59. Ridker PM, Haughie P. Prospective studies of C-reactive protein as a risk factor for cardiovascular disease. J Invest Med 1998; 46:391–395.
60. Liuzzo G, Biasucci LM, Gallimore R, et al. The prognostic value of C-reactive protein and serum amyloid A protein in severe unstable angina. N Engl J Med 1994;331:417–424.
61. Kuller LH, Tracy RP, Shaten J, et al. Relation of C-reactive protein and coronary heart disease in the MRFIT nested case-control study. Am J Epidemiol 1996;144:537–547.
62. Ridker PM, Cushman M, Stampfer MJ, et al. Inflammation, aspirin, and the risk of cardiovascular disease in apparently healthy men. N Engl J Med 1997;336:973–979.
63. Ridker PM, Cushman M, Stampfer MJ, et al. Plasma concentration of C-reactive protein and risk of developing peripheral vascular disease. Circulation 1998;97:425–428.
64. Tracy RP, Lemaitre RN, Psaty BM, et al. Relationship of C-reactive protein to risk of cardiovascular disease in the elderly: results from the Cardiovascular Health Study and the Rural Health Promotion Project. Arterioscler Thromb Vasc Biol 1997;17:1121–1127.
65. Koenig W, Sund M, Frolich M, et al. C-reactive protein, a sensitive marker of inflammation, predicts future risk of coronary heart disease in initially healthy middle-aged men: results from the MONICA (Monitoring Trends and Determinants in Cardiovascular Disease) Augsburg cohort study, 1984 to 1992. Circulation 1999;99:237–242.
66. Danesh J, Whincup P, Walker M, et al. Low grade inflammation and coronary heart disease: prospective study and updated meta-analysis. BMJ 2000;321:199–204.
67. Roivainen M, Viik-Kajander M, Palosuo T, et al. Infections, inflammation and the risk of coronary heart disease. Circulation 2000;101:252–257.
68. Haverkate F, Thompson SG, Pyke SDM, et al. Production of C-reactive protein and risk of coronary events in stable and unstable angina. Lancet 1997;349:462–466.
69. Morrow D, Rifai N, Antman E, et al. C-reactive protein as a potent predictor of mortality independently and in combination with troponin T in acute coronary syndromes. J Am Coll Cardiol 1998;31:1460–1465.
70. Ridker PM, Rifai N, Pfeffer MA, et al. Inflammation, pravastatin, and the risk of coronary events after myocardial infarction in patients with average cholesterol levels. Circulation 1998;98: 839–844.
71. Redberg RF, Rifai N, Gee L, et al. Lack of association of C-reactive protein and coronary calcium by electron beam computed tomography in postmenopausal women: implications for coronary artery disease screening. J Am Coll Cardiol 2000; 36:39–43.
72. Hunt ME, O'Malley PG, Vernalis MN, et al. C-reactive protein is not associated with the presence or extent of calcified subclinical atherosclerosis. Am Heart J 2001;141:206–210.
73. Cushman M, Legault C, Barrett-Connor E, et al. Effect of postmenopausal hormones on inflammation-sensitive proteins: the Postmenopausal Estrogen/Progestin Interventions (PEPI) study. Circulation 1999;100:717–722.
74. Ikonomidis I, Andreotti F, Economou E, et al. Increased proinflammatory cytokines in patients with chronic stable angina and their reduction by aspirin. Circulation 1999;100:793–798.
75. Horne BD, Muhlestein JB, Carlquist JF, et al. Statin therapy, lipid levels, C-reactive protein and the survival of patients with angiographically severe coronary artery disease. J Am Coll Cardiol 2000;36:1774–1780.
76. Ridker PM, Rifai N, Pfeffer MA, et al. Long-term effects of pravastatin on plasma concentration of C-reacrtive protein. Circulation 1999;100:230–235.
77. Crisby M, Nordin-Fredriksson G, Shah PK, et al. Pravastatin treatment increases collagen content and decreases lipid content, inflammation, metalloproteinases, and cell death in human carotid plaques: implications for plaque stabilization. Circulation 2001;103:926–933.
78. Wilkins J, Gallimore R, Moore E, et al. Rapid automated high sensitivity enzyme immunoassay of C-reactive protein. Clin Chem 1998;44:1358–1361.
79. Rifai N, Tracy RP, Ridker PM. Clinical efficacy of an automated high-sensitivity C-reactive protein assay. Clin Chem 1999;45: 2136–2141.
80. Collen D, Lijnen HR. Basic and clinical aspects of fibrinolysis and thrombolysis. Blood 1991;78:3114–3124.
81. Hamsten A, de Faire U, Walldius G, et al. Plasminogen activator inhibitor in plasma: risk factor for recurrent myocardial infarction. Lancet 1987;ii:3–9.
82. Jansson JH, Olofsson BO, Nilsson TK. Predictive value of tissue plasminogen activator mass concentration on long term mortality

in patients with coronary artery disease: a seven year follow-up. Circulation 1993;80:2030–2034.
83. Ridker PM, Vaughan DE, Stampfer MJ, et al. Endogenous tissue-type plasminogen activator and risk of myocardial infarction. Lancet 1993;341:1165–1168.
84. Meade TW, Ruddock V, Stirling Y, et al. Fibrinolytic activity, clotting factors, and long-term incidence of ischaemic heart disease in the Northwick Park Heart Study. Lancet 1993;342:1076–1079.
85. Thorgersen AM, Jansson JH, Boman K, et al. High plasminogen activator inhibitor and tissue plasminogen activator levels in plasma precede a first acute myocardial infarction in both men and women: evidence for the fibrinolytic system as an independent primary risk factor. Circulation 1998;98:2241–2247.
86. Ridker PM, Hennekens CH, Cerskus A, et al. Plasma concentration of cross-linked fibrin degradation product (D-dimer) and the risk of future myocardial infarction among apparently healthy men. Circulation 1994;90:2236–2240.
87. Folsom AR, Aleksic N, Park E, et al. A prospective study of fibrinolytic factors and incident coronary heart disease: the Atherosclerosis Risk in Communities (ARIC) Study. Arterioscler Thromb Vasc Biol 2001;21:611–617.
88. Fowkes FGR, Lowe GDO, Housely E, et al. Cross-linked fibrin degradation products, progression of peripheral arterial disease, and risk of coronary heart disease. Lancet 1993;342:84–86.
89. Lowe GDO, Yarnell JWG, Sweetnam PM, et al. Fibrin D-dimer, tissue plasminogen activator, plasminogen activator inhibitor, and the risk of major ischemic heart disease in the Caerphilly Study. Thromb Haemost 1998;79:129–133.
90. Moss AJ, Goldstein RE, Marder VJ, et al. Thrombogenic factors and recurrent coronary events. Circulation 1999;99:2517–2522.
91. Welch GN, Loscalzo J. Mechanisms of disease: homocysteine and atherothrombosis. N Engl J Med 1998;338:1042–1050.
92. Peterson JC, Spence JD. Vitamins and progression of atherosclerosis in hyperhomocysteinemia. Lancet 1998;351:263.
93. Chambers JC, McGregor A, Jean-Marie J, et al. Acute hyperhomocysteinemia and endothelial dysfunction. Lancet 1998;351:36–37.
94. Malinow MR, Bostom AG, Krauss RM. Homocyst(e)ine, diet, and cardiovascular disease. A statement for healthcare professionals from the Nutrition Committee, American Heart Association. Circulation 1999:178–182.
95. Evans RW, Shaten J, Hempel JD, et al. Homocysteine and risk of cardiovascular disease in the Multiple Risk Factor Intervention Trial. Arterioscler Thromb Vasc Biol 1997;17:1947–1953.
96. Alfthan G, Pekkanen J, Juahianen M, et al. Relation of serum homocysteine and lipoprotein(a) concentrations to atherosclerotic disease in a prospective Finnish population based study. Atherosclerosis 1994;106:9–19.
97. Stampfer MJ, Malinow MR, Willett WC, et al. A prospective study of plasma homocyst(e)ine and risk of myocardial infarction in US physicians. JAMA 1992;268:877–881.
98. Folsom AR, Nieto FJ, McGovern PG, et al. Prospective study of coronary heart disease incidence in relation to fasting total homocysteine, related genetic polymorphisms, and B vitamins. Circulation 1998;98:204–210.
99. Stehouwer CDA, Weijenberg MP, van den Berg M, et al. Serum homocysteine and risk of coronary heart disease and cerebrovascular disease in elderly men: a 10-year follow-up. Arterioscler Thromb Vasc Biol 1998;18:1895–1901.
100. Fallon UB, Ben-Shlomo Y, Elwood P, et al. Homocysteine and coronary heart disease in the Caerphilly cohort: a 10 year follow up. Heart 2001;85:153–158.
101. Arneson E, Refsum H, Bonaa KH, et al. Serum total homocysteine and coronary heart disease. Int J Epidemiol 1995;24:704–709.
102. Wald NJ, Watt HC, Law MR, et al. Homocysteine and ischemic heart disease—results of a prospective study with implications regarding prevention. Arch Intern Med 1998;158:862–867.
103. Bots ML, Launer LJ, Lindemans J, et al. Homocysteine and short-term risk of myocardial infarction among the elderly: the Rotterdam Study. Arch Intern Med 1999;159:38–44.
104. Whincup PH, Refsum H, Perry IJ, et al. Serum total homocysteine and coronary heart disease: prospective study in middle aged men. Heart 1999;82:448–454.
105. Bostom AG, Silbershatz H, Rosenberg IH, et al. Nonfasting plasma total homocysteine levels and all-cause mortality in elderly Framingham men and women. Arch Intern Med 1999;159:1077–1080.
106. Ridker PM, Manson JE, Buring JE, et al. Homocysteine and risk of cardiovascular disease among postmenopausal women. JAMA 1999;281:1817–1821.
107. Christen WG, Ajani UA, Glynn RJ, et al. Blood levels of homocysteine and increased risks of cardiovascular disease: causal or casual? Arch Intern Med 2000;160:422–434.
108. Jacques PF, Selhub J, Bostom AG, et al. The effect of folic acid fortification on plasma folate and total homocysteine concentrations. N Engl J Med 1999;340:1449–1454.
109. Bostom AG, Lathrop L. Hyperhomocysteinemia in end-stage renal disease: prevalence, etiology, and potential relationship to arteriosclerotic outcomes. Kidney Int 1997;52:10–20.
110. Nedrebo BG, Ericsson UB, Nygard O, et al. Plasma total homocysteine levels in hypothyroid and hyperthyroid patients. Metabolism 1998;47:89–93.
111. Tripodi A, Chantarangkul V, Lombardi R, et al. Multicenter study of homocysteine measurement—performance characteristics of different methods, influence of standards on interlaboratory agreement of results. Thromb Haemost 2001;85:291–295.
112. Brattstrom L, Wilcken DEL, Ohrvik J, et al. Common methylenetetrahydrofolate reductase gene mutation leads to hyperhomocysteinemia but not to vascular disease. The result of a meta-analysis. Circulation 1998;98:2520–2526.
113. Ridker PM, Hennekens CH, Lindpaintner K, et al. Mutation in the gene encoding for coagulation factor V and the risk of myocardial infarction, stroke, and venous thrombosis in apparently healthy men. N Engl J Med 1995;332:912–917.
114. Cushman M, Rosendaal F, Cook E, et al. Factor V Leiden does not increase cardiovascular risk in the elderly. Thromb Haemost 1998;79:912–915.
115. Ridker PM, Hennekens CH, Miletich JP. G20210A mutation in prothrombin gene and risk of myocardial infarction, stroke, and venous thrombosis in a large cohort of US men. Circulation 1999;99:999–1004.
116. Cushman M. Hemostatic risk factors for cardiovascular disease. In: Schechter GP, Hoffman R, Schrier SL, (Eds): Hematology 1999. Washington DC. The American Society of Hematology, 1999 pp; 236–242.
117. Rosendaal FR, Siscovick DS, Schwartz SM, et al. A common prothrombin variant (20210 G to A) increases the risk of myocardial infarction in young women. Blood 1997;90:1747–1750.
118. Doggen CJM, Manger Cats V, Bertina RM, et al. Interaction of coagulation defects and cardiovascular risk factors: increased risk of myocardial infarction associated with factor V Leiden or prothrombin 20210A. Circulation 1998;97:1037–1041.
119. Libby P. Molecular basis of acute coronary syndromes. Circulation 1995;91:2844–2850.
120. Ridker PM, Stampfer MJ. Assessment of genetic markers for coronary thrombosis: promise and precaution. Lancet 1999;353:687–688.
121. Genest JJ Jr, McNamara JR, Salem DN, et al. Plasma homocyst(e)ine levels in men with premature coronary artery disease. J Am Coll Cardiol 1990; 16:1114–1119.
122. Schwartz SM, Siscovick DS, Malinow MR, et al. Myocardial infarction in young women in relation to plasma total homocysteine, folate, and a common variant in the methylenetetrahydrofolate reductase gene. Circulation 1997;96:412–417.
123. Wilcken DEL, Wilcken B. The pathogenesis of coronary artery disease: a possible role for methionine metabolism. J Clin Invest 1976;57:1079–1082.

124. Murphy-Chutorian DR, Wexman MP, Grieco AJ, et al. Methionine intolerance: a possible risk factor for coronary artery disease. J Am Coll Cardiol 1985;6:725–730.

125. Malinow MR, Sexton G, Averbuch M, et al. Homocyst(e)inemia in daily practice: levels in coronary artery disease. Coron Art Dis 1990;1:215–220.

126. Murphy-Chutorian D, Alderman EL. The case that hyperhomocysteinemia is a risk factor for coronary artery disease. Am J Cardiol 1994;73:705–707.

127. Israelsson B, Brattstrom LE, Hultberg BL. Homocysteine and myocardial infarction. Atherosclerosis 1988;71:227–233.

128. Clarke R, Daly L, Robinson K, et al. Hyperhomocysteinemia: an independent risk factor for vascular disease. N Engl J Med 1991;324:1149–1155.

129. Ubbink JB, Vermaak WJH, Bennett JM, et al. The prevalence of homocysteinemia and hypercholesterolemia in angiographically defined coronary artery disease. Klin Wochenschr 1991;69:627–534.

130. Dudman NPB, Wilcken DEL, Wang J, et al. Disordered methionine/homocysteine metabolism in premature vascular disease. Arterioscler Thromb Vasc Biol 1993;13:1253–1260.

131. Pancharuniti N, Lewis CA, Sauberlich HE, et al. Plasma homocyst(e)ine, folate, and vitamine B12 concentrations and risk for early-onset coronary artery disease. Am J Clin Nurt 1994;59:940–948.

132. Wu LL, Wu J, Hunt SC, et al. Plasma homocyst(e)ine as a risk factor for early familial coronary artery disease. Clin Chem 1994;40:552–561.

133. Dalery K, Lussier-Cacan S, Selhub J, et al. Homocysteine and coronary artery disease in French Canadian subjects: relation with vitamins B_{12}, B_6, pyridoxal phosphate, and folate. Am J Cardiol 1995;75:1107–1111.

134. Landgren F, Israelsson B, Lindgren A, et al. Plasma homocysteine in acute myocardial infarction: homocysteine-lowering effect of folic acid. J Intern Med 1995;237:381–388.

135. Robinson K, Mayer EL, Miller DP, et al. Hyperhomocysteinemia and low pyridoxal phosphate: common and independent reversible risk factor for coronary artery disease. Circulation 1995;92:2825–2830.

136. Gallagher PM, Meleady R, Shields DC, et al. Homomcysteine and risk of premature coronary heart disease: evidence for a common gene mutation. Circulation 1996;94:2154–2158.

137. Verhoef P, Stampfer MJ, Buring JE, et al. Homocysteine metabolism and risk of myocardial infarction: relation with B_{12}, B_6, and folate. Am J Epidemiol 1996;143:845–859.

138. Graham IM, Daly LE, Refsum HM, et al. Plasma homocysteine as a risk factor for vascular disease: the European Concerted Action Project. JAMA 1997;277:1775–1781.

139. Verhoef P, Kok FJ, Kruyssen ACM, et al. Plasma total homocysteine, B vitamins, and risk of coronary atherosclerosis. Arterioscler Thromb Vasc Biol 1997;17:989–995.

140. Alfthan G, Pekkanen J, Jauhiainen M, et al. Relation of serum homocysteine and lipoprotein(a) concentrations to atherosclerotic disease in a prospective Finnish popluation-based study. Atherosclerosis 1994; 106:9–19.

141. Chasan-Taber L, Selhub J, Rosenberg IH, et al. A prospective study of folate and vitamin B6 and risk of myocardial infarction in US physicians. J Am Coll Nutr 1996;15:136–143.

142. Verhoef P, Hennekens CH, Allen RH, et al. Plasma total homocysteine and risk of angina pectoris with subsequent coronary artery bypass surgery. Am J Cardiol 1997;79:799–801.

143. Evans RW, Shaten BJ, Hempel JD, Cutler JA, Kuller LH, for the MRFIT Research Group. Homocyst(e)ine and risk of cardiovascular disease in the Multiple Risk Factor Intervention Trial. Arterioscler Thromb Vasc Biol 1997;17:1947–1953.

144. Nygard O, Nordrehaug JE, Refsum H, et al. Plasma homocysteine levels and mortality in patients with coronary artery diesaes. N Engl J Med 1997;337:230–236.

145. Wald NJ, Watt HC, Law MR, et al. Homocysteine and ischemic heart disease: results of a prospective study with implications regarding pervention. Arch Intern Med 1998;158:862–867.

146. Folsom AR, Nieto J, McGovern PG, et al. Prospective study of coronary heart disease incidence in relation to fasting total homocysteine, reltated genetic polymorphisms, and B vitamins. Circulation 1998;98:204–210.

CHAPTER 21

Hemostatic and Thrombotic Disorders of Malignancy

Frederick R. Rickles, M.D.
Mark N. Levine, M.D., M.Sc.

The propensity of cancer patients to develop venous thromboembolism (VTE) has been documented in the medical literature for over a century.[1,2] Virtually all patients with widespread malignant disease are thought to be at high risk for this complication, prompting the recommendation that such patients be routinely anticoagulated in preparation for surgery.[3–8] Hemorrhagic complications of cancer, with the exception of those due to thrombocytopenia secondary to chemotherapy (and/or radiation therapy-induced bone marrow failure) or the consumptive coagulopathy characteristic of acute promyelocytic leukemia (APL), are less common.[5] The most common bleeding complications of cancer for the most part either are prevented with the judicious use of growth factors or are reasonably well controlled with platelet transfusions. On the other hand, some investigators have even suggested that VTE remains the second most common cause of death in cancer patients,[9] supporting perhaps the major emphasis in this chapter on the understanding of the epidemiology, pathogenesis, and prevention of cancer-related VTE.

Clinical observers and experimentalists have recorded a variety of types of evidence linking tumor growth with robust activation of the clotting system. Histopathologic, clinical, laboratory, and pharmacologic evidence support the association of cancer with thrombosis (Table 21–1). When examining tumor growth in experimental animals and spontaneous human tumors, histopathologists have emphasized the geographic proximity of tumor cells, peritumor fibrin deposition, platelets, and inflammatory cells; more recently, unique patterns of fibrin deposition within the vascular endothelium of blood vessels supplying tumors have been described (Table 21–2).[2,3,6,11–19] These histologic observations are supported by experimental evidence that fibrin deposition enhances tumor growth.[6] The relationship between idiopathic VTE and certain types of tumors, including very small, occult cancers, has been well documented. The reverse is also true—patients with VTE are at increased risk for cancer (Table 21–3).[1,3–10,20,21] Laboratory studies of patients with cancer have generally revealed evidence of systemic activation of blood coagulation (Table 21–4),[6,22] and some evidence suggests the possibility of selecting for special intervention those cancer patients who are at particularly high risk for VTE.[22] Finally, a growing body of literature supports the interesting observation that anticoagulant drugs, in addition to their well-established utility for the prophylaxis and treatment of VTE in cancer, also inhibit tumor growth (Table 21–5).[6,23–27]

HISTORICAL OVERVIEW

The close relationship between tumor growth and the activation of blood coagulation has been known since 1865, when Professor Armand Trousseau described in a lecture to the New Sydenham Society the clinical association between idiopathic VTE and occult malignancy.[1] He noted that "I have always been struck by the frequency with which cancerous patients are affected with painful oedema of the superior or inferior extremities . . . in other cases, in which the absence of appreciable tumor made me hesitate as to the nature of a disease of the stomach, my doubts were removed, and I knew the disease to be cancerous when phlegmasia alba dolens appeared in one of the limbs." In describing the pathophysiology of this phenomenon, he wrote: "There appears in the cachexiae . . . a particular condition of the blood which predisposes it to spontaneous coagulation." To this day, one could hardly imagine a more perspicacious view of this syndrome, the full nature of

326   PART III   Thrombotic Processes

Table 21-1 • ASSOCIATION OF THROMBOSIS AND CANCER—TYPES OF EVIDENCE

- **Histopathologic**—fibrin deposition associated with tumor cells, platelets, inflammatory cells, and neoangiogenic blood vessels
- **Clinical**—venous thromboembolism (idiopathic or primary vs. secondary)
- **Laboratory**—hypercoagulability
- **Pharmacologic**—antitumor effects of anticoagulant, antiplatelet, and profibrinolytic drugs

Table 21-3 • CLINICAL EVIDENCE LINKING THROMBOSIS AND CANCER

- Idiopathic (primary) venous thromboembolism predicts occult cancer (Trousseau, 1865[1]; Prandoni et al., 1992[20]; Rickles and Levine, 2001[21])
- Increased risk of symptomatic venous thromboembolism in cancer patients (Rickles et al., 1992[3]; Prandoni, 1997[8]; Rickles and Levine, 2001[5])
- Increased risk of recurrent venous thromboembolism in cancer patients (Prandoni, 1997[8])

which is still unknown. Sadly, only 2 years later, in a letter to his student Peter, Trousseau wrote: "I am lost, the phlebitis that has just appeared tonight leaves me no doubt as to the nature of my illness."[28] Indeed, he succumbed to gastric cancer some 6 months later.

In 1878, the pathologist Billroth published his observations of fibrin clots in vessels draining malignant tumors at postmortem,[2] a finding confirmed 60 years later by Sproul and colleagues[11] and expanded in a large series by Saphir and colleagues,[12] in which 35% to 50% of autopsies of cancer patients revealed significant tumor-associated thrombosis. These observations from patients with cancer were defined further by: (1) relatively specific histochemical staining for fibrin[29]; (2) immunochemical identification of fibrin[30]; (3) electron microscopic confirmation of the characteristic periodicity of fibrin in apposition to tumors[31-35]; and (4) specific uptake of radiolabeled fibrinogen in experimental tumors[34,35] and human tumors.[36]

It might be fair to say that clinical thrombosis was not appreciated sufficiently as a significant complication of cancer until the era of widespread use of central venous access devices (CVADs) in the 1990s. The frequency of use in cancer patients and the prothrombotic character of the chemotherapy drugs infused through the catheters brought to light the increased propensity of these patients to develop clot in the catheters (an incidence rate of approximately 33%, as determined in two relatively small prospective studies).[37,38] It is now clear that cancer patients are at much higher risk for the development of VTE even without the use of CVADs—a realization that has stimulated the design of randomized, controlled intervention trials in this patient population to determine the best method for prevention of this very significant cause of morbidity and mortality.

PATHOGENESIS

Virchow's Triad

Patients with cancer have multiple reasons to develop VTE, which can be classified according to the same mechanisms first proposed by the famous German pathologist Rudolph Virchow in 1856[39] to explain the pathophysiology of all VTE. More recently, these mechanisms have been restated in the context of the cancer patient by Green and Silverstein[40] as follows: *stasis; vascular damage; hypercoagulability*. Cancer patients often suffer from *stasis* as a result of prolonged bed rest or obstruction of vascular flow from extrinsic compression or direct vascular invasion by tumor. *Vascular damage* may occur secondary to direct invasion by tumor, use of CVADs, and, most commonly, administration of cancer chemotherapy drugs. Indeed, virtually all of the commonly used intravenous cancer chemotherapy agents are capable of activating blood coagulation in vivo, presumably related to induction of vascular injury.[41] Finally, cancer patients have a primary *hypercoagulable state* the pathogenesis of which is exceedingly complex. The primary interactions between cancer cells and the vessel wall, which are thought to lead to thrombosis, are represented diagrammatically in Figure 21-1.[42] We will briefly review these mechanisms, which we believe reflect an aberrant host inflammatory response to a foreign invader—the tumor cell. The reader is referred to several recent reviews for a more detailed explanation of the proposed pathophysiologic mechanisms responsible for the hypercoagulability of cancer patients.[6,22,40,42]

Table 21-2 • HISTOPATHOLOGIC EVIDENCE LINKING THROMBOSIS AND CANCER

- Tumor thrombi (Billroth, 1878[2])
- Fibrin deposition surrounding tumors (Sproul, 1938[11]; Saphir, et al. 1947[12]; Dvorak et al., 1979[13]; Zacharski, et al., 1992[14]; Shoji, et al., 1998[15])
- Platelet adhesion to tumors (Gasic et al., 1973[16])
- Tumor-associated inflammatory cells and fibrin deposition (Dvorak et al., 1978[17], 1981[17,18]; Shoji et al., 1998[15])
- Tumor-associated endothelial cells and fibrin deposition (Contrino et al., 1996[19]; Shoji et al., 1998[15])

Table 21-4 • LABORATORY EVIDENCE FOR ACTIVATION OF CLOTTING IN BLOOD SAMPLES FROM CANCER PATIENTS

- Elevated levels of fibrinopeptide A and prothrombin F_{1+2}
- Elevated levels of thrombin–antithrombin complexes, fibrin monomers and fibrin D-dimers
- Increased plasma levels of tissue factor, factor VIIa, and tissue factor pathway inhibitor (TFPI)
- Reduced levels of antithrombin III, protein C, and free protein S
- Activated protein C resistance (in the absence of the factor V Leiden mutation)

Table 21-5 • HEMOSTATIC AGENTS CAPABLE OF ALTERING TUMOR GROWTH IN VIVO

- Warfarin sodium (Coumadin)
- Unfractionated heparin
- Low-molecular-weight heparin
- Antiplatelet agents (e.g., dipyridamole)
- Urokinase

Direct-Acting Tumor Procoagulants

Tumor cells themselves possess a variety of procoagulant properties, including the constitutive, cellular expression of the potent procoagulant tissue factor (TF), the secretion of the cysteine protease cancer procoagulant (CP), and the secretion of indirect procoagulant cytokines such as interleukins IL-1 and IL-8, tumor necrosis factor (TNF), and vascular endothelial growth factor (VEGF). The latter cytokines induce procoagulant properties in adjacent and distant host cells (Fig. 21-1). For example, tumor cell VEGF is chemotactic for both macrophages and endothelial cells, activating TF in both cell types. Tumor cells also activate platelets and, via integrin expression, form adhesive interactions with platelets and the endothelium of blood vessels.

Indirect-Acting Tumor Procoagulants–Tumor–Host Cell Interactions

Tumor cell interaction with the vessel wall reduces endothelial cell secretion of tissue plasminogen activator (tPA) and expression of thrombomodulin (TM), and increases endothelial cell synthesis of plasminogen activator inhibitor (PAI-1). Finally, substantial experimental evidence supports the presence of increased numbers of activated monocytes/macrophages in the circulation of cancer patients and in proximity to growing tumors.[6] These antigen-processing cells express TF on their surface, presumably as part of the host immune response to the tumor and/or in response to secretion of tumor products. Tumor-associated macrophages have been shown to assemble the entire coagulation cascade and form cross-linked fibrin on their surface in apposition to growing tumor.[6] The activation of coagulation in the tumor microenvironment, which routinely spills into the circulation of cancer patients (vide infra), may be a primitive effort on the part of the host to limit the spread of tumor cells. Of interest, macrophage TF expression in cancer patients (measured in cultured peripheral blood monocytes) correlates significantly with plasma levels of fibrinopeptide A (FPA), the first cleavage product of thrombin's action on fibrinogen.[6] Although correlation never proves causation, it is notable that cross-linked fibrin can be colocalized with TF in both tumor-

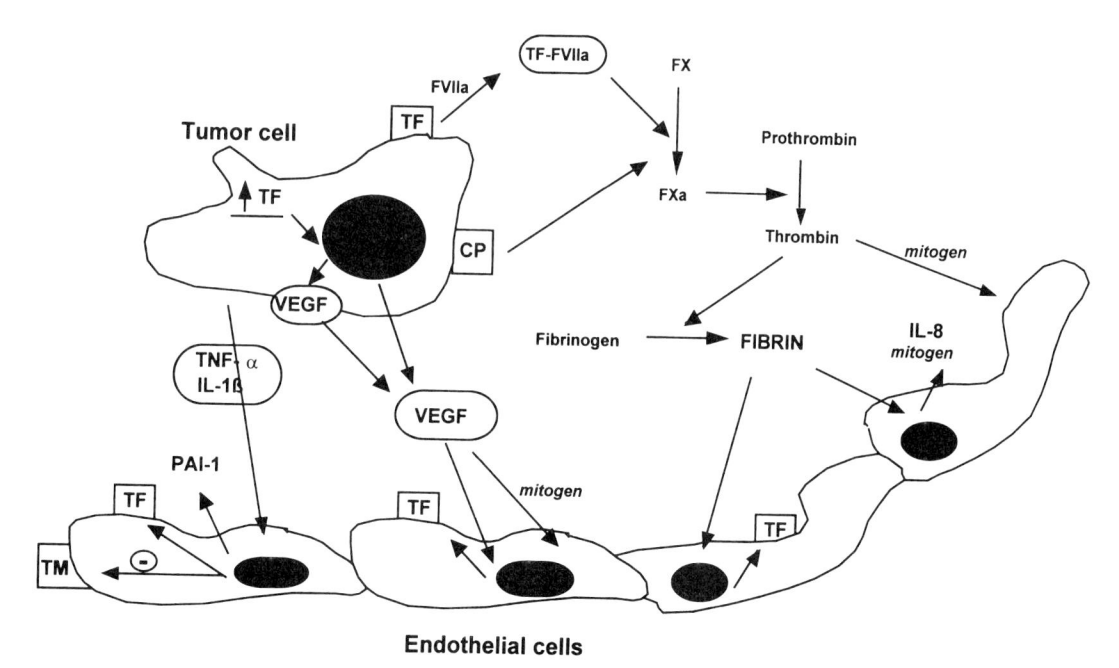

Figure 21-1 Regulation of tumor cell and endothelial cell procoagulant functions in the pathogenesis of thrombosis in cancer. Tissue factor (TF) and cancer procoagulant (CP) expression are synthesized and expressed on the surface of tumor cells. The effects of these tumor cell procoagulants are enhanced by the local production of the important proangiogenic cytokines interleukin-8 (IL-8 from the endothelial cell) and vascular endothelial growth factor (VEGF) and the inflammatory cytokines tumor necrosis factor-α (TNF-α) and interleukin-1β (IL-1β) from tumor cells. These cytokines convert the normal anticoagulant endothelium to a procoagulant endothelium as follows: (1) downregulation of thrombomodulin (TM) expression; (2) increased synthesis of TF and plasminogen activator inhibitor-1 (PAI-1). Fibrin, produced in response to activation of clotting by TF and CP, increases both TF and IL-8 production by the endothelium, further enhancing thrombogenesis and angiogenesis. TF also increases angiogenesis by the tumor cell by increasing the synthesis of VEGF. (From Rickels FR, Falanga A. Molecular basis for the relationship between thrombosis and cancer. Thromb Res (Vessels) 2001;102:V215–V224.

associated macrophages and within the endothelium of tumor-associated blood vessels in human breast and lung cancer.[15,19] The latter finding (i.e., TF expression in endothelial cells only in proximity to or within a growing tumor) lends further support to the concept that the new vessels, formed as a result of angiogenic signals generated by tumors, may be more susceptible to thrombogenesis.[19] Further, this observation has stimulated further exploration of a possible role for TF in the development of tumor angiogenesis[43,44] and as a marker of the so-called angiogenic switch,[45] the mechanism(s) by which otherwise normal endothelial cells become neoangiogenic.

HEMOSTATIC DISORDERS

Thrombocytopenia or Thrombocytosis

Quantitative platelet abnormalities are common in cancer patients, particularly in patients with solid tumors such as carcinomas of the lung and liver, as a complication of Hodgkin and non-Hodgkin lymphomas, and in chronic myelocytic leukemia.[46-49] Thrombocytopenia is the principal cause of bleeding in untreated cancer patients,[50] reflecting *reduced production, increased destruction,* or *sequestration* within an enlarged spleen.[47] Reduced production in cancer is usually secondary to replacement of bone marrow by tumor cells, sepsis, vitamin B_{12} or folate deficiency, or ineffective thrombopoiesis, and may result from the elaboration by tumor cells of mediators that inhibit platelet production.[46,47,51-53] Modest thrombocytosis (above 400,000 to 800,000/μL) is common, occurring in up to 60% of untreated patients in some series[3,46,48,49,51,53-57] and may provide an early marker of occult cancer.[49]

Several studies have called attention to increased platelet turnover and to evidence of platelet activation and consumption in patients with malignancy, abnormalities that generally respond to successful treatment of the underlying neoplasm.[58-61] Patients with very short platelet survival times tend to have the worst prognoses.[59] Disseminated intravascular coagulation (DIC) is probably the most common cause of increased platelet consumption, and platelet counts, whether elevated or depressed, may reflect the overall degree of compensation in DIC. This chronic form of DIC, however, may not be overt and may not present with laboratory abnormalities (i.e., prolongation of the prothrombin time [PT], activated partial thromboplastin time [aPTT], and thrombin time [TT]—vide infra) typical of acute DIC (see Chapter 12).

A symptom complex resembling idiopathic thrombocytopenic purpura (ITP), with accelerated, apparently immune, destruction of platelets has been reported repeatedly in patients with a variety of tumors, including Hodgkin disease, acute and chronic lymphocytic leukemia, and carcinomas of many sites; in these patients, thrombocytopenia may precede clinical evidence of neoplasia.[47]

Thrombocytopathy

Qualitative abnormalities of platelet function are not uncommon abnormalities in cancer patients and include reduced adhesion; impaired, increased, or spontaneous aggregation; and poor clot retraction.[62] A thrombocytopathy often accompanies dysproteinemia, in which tumor-secreted paraproteins coat platelets and interfere with their function; thrombocytopenia and/or clotting factor deficiencies also occur in these patients.[46] One or more of these defects is observed in up to 15% of patients with IgG myeloma, 38% of patients with IgA myeloma, and 60% of patients with Waldenstrom macroglobulinemia exhibit such abnormalities. An acquired storage-pool defect and other selective biochemical defects in the platelets have been described in cancer patients.[63,64]

Disseminated Intravascular Coagulation with Consumptive Coagulopathy

Clinically overt DIC with a consumptive coagulopathy and hemorrhage occurs infrequently in patients with cancer, except occasionally as a complication of therapy and in association with the tumor lysis syndrome. However, in patients with acute promyelocytic leukemia (APL), prior to the introduction of all-*trans* retinoic acid (ATRA) as standard induction therapy, the incidence of this complication of the chemotherapy was as high as 50%.[65] Much more common in cancer patients are subclinical hemostatic abnormalities manifested only as the result of laboratory testing. Cooper and colleagues coined the term *compensated DIC* to distinguish this group of patients from those with a consumptive coagulopathy, who were termed to have *decompensated DIC*. Nevertheless, these patients have been proven to be highly susceptible to the development of overt DIC.[56]

Abnormalities of one or more of the routine tests of coagulation have been reported in approximately 50% of all cancer patients at the time of presentation (before therapy), increasing to 90% of those patients with metastases.[53,66-68] The results of a serial study of 215 cancer patients reported by Edwards and colleagues[57] revealed the most common abnormalities at the time of entry into the study to be: (1) an elevated platelet count; (2) elevated plasma fibrinogen; and (3) elevated plasma levels of FPA. Although these individual findings are not specific and may be part of an acute-phase response or, in the case of thrombocytosis, may occur as the result of hemorrhage or iron deficiency, nevertheless they are consistent with the definition of "compensated DIC." Blood coagulation laboratory values (in particular FPA levels) in this study became progressively more abnormal with disease progression.[57] Many other clotting abnormalities have also been reported in cancer patients, such as those noted in Table 21-4, and are described in greater detail in recent reviews.[40,69]

These seemingly variable and even contradictory laboratory findings are to be anticipated in a disease in which excessive, but generally low-grade, coagulation, fibrinolysis, and compensatory homeostatic mechanisms are proceeding at different and changing rates. Individual cancer patients may lie at any point along a spectrum that extends from a "prethrombotic" or "hypercoagulable" state to DIC of varying degrees of severity and compensation. Cancer patients exhibit widely varying levels of DIC, from milder, more chronic forms without bleeding sequelae to severe forms with catastrophic bleeding. The underlying principle in all of these patients is that the clotting system is activated systemically, clotting factors are consumed, and fibrinolysis is activated.

In some cancer patients, clotting abnormalities are detected only with more sophisticated tests. Thus, the reported incidence of hemostatic abnormalities is not only a function of the type of tumor, the extent of tumor burden, and treatment; it also may be highly dependent on the sensitivity and specificity of the laboratory tests used. The clinical significance of abnormal laboratory tests of hemostasis in cancer patients requires a brief comment. We must emphasize that none of the clotting tests currently available is specific for cancer and, with the exception of the small study published by Falanga and colleagues,[70] no pattern of abnormal clotting studies has been demonstrated capable of predicting with a reasonable degree of certainty either bleeding or thrombosis in cancer patients.[71]

THROMBOTIC DISORDERS

Thrombophilia in Cancer: Congenital Versus Acquired

Congenital Thrombophilia

Conflicting results have been generated in studies attempting to determine if patients with cancer who develop thrombosis have an underlying, hereditary predisposition due to one or more defects of the anticoagulation pathway proteins. For example, Green and colleagues[72] found evidence of what they believed was an acquired resistance to activated protein C (APC-R), due to nonspecific elevation of levels of factor VIII and fibrinogen in 5 of 39 patients (13%) with advanced cancer. Only one patient was found to have the factor V Leiden mutation in association with APC-R, which confers increased risk for thrombosis in noncancer patients. The study was much too small, however, to provide useful data on thrombotic risk in the patients. In a much larger, case-controlled study, Melnyk and colleagues demonstrated a fivefold increased risk for thrombosis among cancer patients who were positive for the factor V Leiden mutation,[73] but no evidence of an increased incidence of congenital thrombophilia among the cancer patients.

Acquired Thrombophilia

On the other hand, a number of studies have suggested that cancer patients may acquire defects in one or more of the anticoagulant pathway proteins (e.g., protein C, protein S, antithrombin) as a result of the following mechanisms: (1) hepatic involvement by tumor with reduced synthesis; (2) protein-losing syndromes (enteropathy or nephrotic syndrome); and, (3) as a complication of chemotherapy.[67,74–81] The relationship, if any, of these defects to subsequent thrombosis remains uncertain. What is needed to resolve these conflicting reports are large prospective trials to assess the value of tests of hypercoagulability for predicting thrombotic risk in cancer patients.[71]

Occult Cancer Presenting as Idiopathic Venous Thromboembolism

Trousseau syndrome, as defined by his original description,[1] is characterized by "phlegmasia alba dolens," which is severe, symptomatic thrombophlebitis with some degree of secondary arterial insufficiency, often migratory in nature and often involving unusual anatomic sites such as the upper extremities. While this is a dramatic presentation of idiopathic VTE that quickly alerts the clinician to the likelihood that the patient has an occult malignancy, it is a rather uncommon presenting manifestation of cancer. In contrast, however, several well-designed studies have demonstrated that patients with carefully defined *idiopathic* VTE are at significantly higher risk for the subsequent diagnosis of malignancy when compared to patients who present with *secondary* VTE (i.e., VTE due to recognized causes, including congenital thrombophilia, use of oral contraceptives, pregnancy, immobilization, etc.) (reviewed by Rickles and Levine[21]).

Three types of studies are available in the literature that shed light on this question, including, in order of increasing confidence in the data (1) retrospective analyses of large numbers of unselected patients; (2) population-based, retrospective cohort analyses from large registries; and, best of all, (3) prospective studies of all patients with VTE followed according to a specified protocol after the presentation of an episode of VTE. Five large retrospective studies were reported from 1997 to 1998, with data from over 1800 patients.[82–86] In all but one of these studies,[86] the incidence of cancer in patients with presumed idiopathic VTE was significantly higher (two- to threefold) than in patients with secondary VTE. Nordstrom and coworkers[87] and Cornuz and coworkers,[88] in two additional retrospective studies, examined the cancer risk in 3505 patients with VTE compared to the expected risk in a group of 3256 control subjects (those evaluated for but not found to have VTE). While Nordstrom in a population-based study found a significant increased risk for cancer in subjects with VTE (4.8%) versus those without VTE (1.5%, $p < 0.0001$), Cornuz, in a single institution cohort study, did not (2.5% vs. 2.7%, $p = 0.20$). In two retrospective, population-based studies, Sorensen and coworkers[89] and Baron and coworkers[90] utilized cancer and thromboembolism registries in Sweden and Denmark, respectively, to calculate standardized incidence ratios (SIRs) for cancer in patients with VTE (observed number of cases ÷ expected number of cases in the same age group in the normal population). The incidence of cancer was increased during the first year following the diagnosis of VTE, an effect that persisted for up to 10 years in both populations. The SIR was 1.3 for patients in the smaller Swedish study[89] and 4.4 for the larger Danish study.[90]

Of interest, Baron and colleagues recently reported a follow-up to their study,[91] in which they examined the prognosis of the cancers found in three cohorts: (1) patients in whom cancer was diagnosed at the time of hospitalization for primary VTE (668 patients); (2) patients in whom cancer was diagnosed within the first year after hospitalization for VTE (560 patients); and, (3) patients in whom cancer was diagnosed 1 to 17 years after hospitalization for VTE (1907 patients). For each patient with cancer and VTE, 10 control patients were matched according to the type of cancer, sex, age at the time of the diagnosis of cancer, and year of the diagnosis of cancer. The survival curves for the first two cohorts were significantly worse than controls (12% alive at the end of 1 year in cohort 1 vs. 36% in controls, $p < 0.001$; 38% alive in cohort 2 vs. 47% of the controls, $p < 0.001$). These results led the authors to suggest that cancer presenting as VTE or complicated by VTE has a worse prognosis.

Retrospective studies, however, are problematic.[92] In particular, it is difficult to determine from registry data or even from retrospective chart reviews how often objective criteria were utilized to establish the diagnosis of VTE. Indeed, using the same Swedish Inpatient Registry as had been utilized by Baron and coworkers,[89] Schulman and his colleagues reported recently that "the diagnoses 'deep-vein thrombosis' and 'pulmonary embolism' were coded incorrectly in 10 to 20 percent of the registry cases."[93] Furthermore, in retrospective studies it is rare to find the data supporting the distinction between primary (or idiopathic) VTE and secondary VTE. It is often difficult to document if other risk factors have been rigorously excluded, such as congenital thrombophilia, pregnancy, use of oral contraceptives, and obesity. Of critical importance, the presence of a concurrent cancer must have been carefully eliminated in both groups of patients by comparable search strategies. Selection bias may be present in one or both groups unless consecutive patients are admitted to the study. In addition, comparing retrospective studies may be difficult, since different criteria may have been used to assemble the study inception cohort and consistent criteria for excluding patients with known malignancy may not have been used. Finally, a high degree of follow-up data is needed for both patient groups, which is often missing in retrospective studies.[5,92]

Fortunately, data from prospective studies support the important conclusions just discussed. In particular, we refer to the study by Prandoni and colleagues,[20] which was published in 1992. The investigators studied 145 patients with well-documented idiopathic VTE and 105 patients with equally well-documented secondary VTE, all of whom were followed closely for at least 1 year following the establishment of the diagnosis of VTE. The same careful cancer search strategy was applied to both groups of patients at the time of their initial presentation with VTE. Of the 145 patients in the idiopathic VTE group, 11 (7.6%) developed cancer within 12 months (most within 6 months), as compared to 2 of 105 (1.9%) patients with secondary VTE ($p = 0.043$). Patients with recurrent, idiopathic VTE had an even higher risk of developing cancer (up to ninefold, compared with those with secondary VTE).[20] Similar results have been reported in other prospective studies, although the data may not have always been collected and analyzed in a strictly prospective fashion.[94–96] Recent corroboration of these findings has been provided in another prospective study, albeit with a very different study design.[93]

Schulman and Lindmarker[93] used data analyzed retrospectively from the Duration of Anticoagulation Trial, the so-called DURAC study, which was designed to compare prospectively the efficacy of 6 weeks and 6 months of oral anticoagulation therapy.[97] The data analysis in the DURAC study regarding incidence of cancer in the two groups suffers from some of the same limitations discussed above for retrospective studies (e.g., failure to screen both groups prospectively for cancer at the time of entry into the study; failure to screen adequately both groups for other causes of thrombophilia; incomplete cancer screening at frequent follow up visits). Nevertheless, these investigators were able to calculate age- and sex-matched SIRs, both of which were significantly increased (3.4-fold) in the first year. The cumulative probability of cancer over 6 years of follow-up in those subjects categorized as having idiopathic VTE was nearly three times that of the group classified as having "nonidiopathic" VTE (17% vs. 5.8%).[93]

In spite of the data reviewed above, the question remains as to how aggressive the clinician should be in searching for an occult malignancy in the patient with true idiopathic VTE? What is the likelihood of discovering a treatable, let alone curable, tumor, particularly in view of the retrospective study of Sorensen and coworkers,[91] in which 44% of the VTE patients in cohort 1 (those in whom the diagnosis of cancer was established during the hospitalization for VTE) already had distant metastasis at the time of the cancer diagnosis? A prospective, randomized, controlled trial entitled "Screening for Occult Malignancy in Patients with Symptomatic Idiopathic Venous Thromboembolism," or SOMIT, designed to answer this critical question, is ongoing in Italy. Regrettably the SOMIT trial has had great difficulty in accruing adequate patient numbers and is not likely to provide a definitive answer as to the cost-effectiveness of aggressive screening of patients with idiopathic VTE for an underlying cancer. In view of the number of patients needed to answer this important question about the cost-effectiveness of screening (estimated to be approximately 1000 in each arm of the two-armed SOMIT study—aggressive screening vs. standard noninvasive screening), and the cost for underwriting such an invasive screening trial, it is unlikely that any prospective study of this magnitude will be funded in the near term. We can be hopeful that additional smaller, well-designed studies, like that of Prandoni and colleagues,[20] can be accomplished with sufficiently similar study designs to permit useful meta-analyses in the future. It will be imperative to include cost-effectiveness analysis in all such trials. Barosi and colleagues,[98] using a decision analysis model, reported possible gains in life expectancy with *targeted* screening for prostate, colon, and bladder cancer in men and for colon, breast, and endometrial cancer in women with idiopathic VTE. At this time, however, a strong recommendation cannot be made to screen broadly for occult malignancy in all patients with idiopathic VTE.

Venous Thromboembolism as a Complication of Cancer

Patients with a known diagnosis of cancer, particularly those with mucin-secreting adenocarcinomas of the gastrointestinal tract or ovary, are believed to represent a particularly high-risk group for the development of VTE.[4,7-10] Cancer patients have been stratified by the Consensus Conference of the American College of Chest Physicians into their highest risk category, compelling the routine use of anticoagulant therapy as prophylaxis against VTE short term during surgery, or long term in patients who have already experienced one episode of VTE.[9] The risk for recurrence of VTE in cancer patients with established VTE is approximately twice that of patients without cancer, even among those individuals who, when given oral anticoagulants, demonstrate appropriate prolongation of their prothrombin times (i.e., international normalized ratios [INRs] in the "therapeutic range")[8] (vide infra).

Use of Anticoagulants in Cancer Patients

Primary Prophylaxis

As indicated, cancer patients are clearly "hypercoagulable" and remain so as long as the cancer is active.[6,8] Cancer patients develop thromboembolism during different clinical situations, including the following: (1) surgery[8,101]; (2) during chemotherapy[99,100]; (3) as a result of placement of an indwelling central venous catheter[37,38]; and (4) following immobilization for any reason[102,103] (Table 21–6). Quantification of the additive risk for VTE in cancer patients is not always easy to determine, since many of the studies of risk factors contain only a subset of cancer patients.

Surgery. Patients with cancer undergoing surgery are at an approximate twofold increased risk of postoperative thrombosis compared to noncancer patients subjected to the same operations.[104-107] The risk of venous thrombosis in cancer patients undergoing specific types of surgery can be derived from the "no treatment" control arms of trials evaluating prophylactic measures in surgery.[108] The outcome measured typically in these studies was thrombosis, as detected by fibrinogen leg scanning, and the approximate rates were as follows: general surgery 29%; gynecologic surgery 20%; urologic surgery 41%; orthopedic surgery 50% to 60%; and, neurosurgery 28%. However, many of these thrombi were asymptomatic and some of the studies included patients without cancer.

Patients with cancer undergoing major surgery should receive antithrombotic prophylaxis. However, cancer patients are also at increased risk for perioperative bleeding.[109] Therefore, anticoagulant prophylaxis should be individualized to balance the competing risks of thrombosis and bleeding. A number of clinical trials have compared subcutaneous unfractionated heparin (UFH) with subcutaneous low-molecular-weight-heparin (LMWH) for the prevention of thromboembolism in patients undergoing major abdominal surgery and no difference was detected in postoperative VTE or bleeding between treatment groups. Many of these trials used leg scanning to detect postoperative leg vein thrombosis and some of the trials reported on the subgroup of cancer patients. In the Enoxacan trial, patients undergoing surgery for cancer of the abdomen or pelvis were randomized to LMWH (enoxaparin 40 mg daily) or UFH (5000 units three times a day).[110] All patients underwent mandatory venography prior to discharge from hospital. The rate of thrombosis in the LMWH group was 14.7% versus 18.2% in the UFH group, which was not statistically different. No difference was detected in the frequency of bleeding between the two groups. Thus, in general, cancer patients undergoing major abdominal or pelvic surgery should receive prophylaxis with either subcutaneous UFH or LMWH. In addition, graduated compression stockings should also be used in these patients. Patients undergoing orthopedic surgery are at very high risk of postoperative venous thromboembolism. Although many trials have evaluated prophylaxis in orthopedic patients, we are not aware of trials studying cancer patients undergoing orthopedic procedures. However, based on the results of studies in the general orthopedic population, LMWH or conventional intensity oral anticoagulant therapy is recommended for this high-risk population.[111]

In patients undergoing neurosurgery there is a general reluctance to use anticoagulant prophylaxis because of the concern for bleeding. Mechanical methods, graduated compression stockings, and external pneumatic compression, for example, are frequently used in such patients. Two randomized trials have compared LMWH plus graduated compression stockings to stockings alone in patients undergoing neurosurgery.[112,113] Many of the patients had brain tumors. In both trials, LMWH reduced the risk of thromboembolism over stockings alone without an increase in major bleeding. Finally, mechanical approaches remain the prophylactic methods of choice in any surgical patient with a high risk of

---

Table 21–6 • ADDITIONAL RISK FACTORS FOR VENOUS THROMBOEMBOLISM IN PATIENTS WITH CANCER

- Prolonged immobilization
- Surgical intervention
- Chemotherapy
- Indwelling central venous catheters
- Radiation therapy?

postoperative hemorrhage in whom anticoagulants may be contraindicated.

Medical Patients. The incidence of thrombosis in *ambulatory* cancer patients receiving anticancer agents can be determined from the randomized trials evaluating adjuvant systemic therapies. In the B20 trial of the National Surgical Adjuvant Breast Project (NSABP), for example, women with estrogen receptor-positive, node-negative (stage I) breast cancer received tamoxifen alone or tamoxifen plus chemotherapy.[114] The rates of VTE were 1.2% and 4.2%, respectively, supporting the hypothesis that chemotherapy increases the risk for VTE, even in this group of women with limited-stage disease. The rate of thrombosis in women with stage II breast cancer on chemotherapy varies in the literature between 5% and 13%,[115] with the highest rates of thrombosis observed in postmenopausal women.[101,116,117] Chemotherapy plus tamoxifen increases the risk for VTE over chemotherapy alone[116,117] and in one study the rate of thrombosis in patients with metastatic breast cancer receiving chemotherapy was 17.5%.[100] Other patients with advanced cancers receiving chemotherapy are likely to be at high risk for VTE, although reliable estimates of thrombotic rates in these groups of patients are not available, largely because many of the studies were small case series. Hence cancer patients receiving chemotherapy are at risk for VTE. The question is whether these patients should receive anticoagulant prophylaxis.

One randomized controlled trial provided some data on this question. Patients with metastatic breast cancer receiving chemotherapy were randomized to low-intensity warfarin (target INR 1.3 to 1.9), or placebo.[118] Prophylaxis with the oral anticoagulant was associated with an 85% relative reduction in the rate of thromboembolism without an increase in bleeding. Despite these results most oncologists do not use primary prophylaxis in patients with advanced cancer on chemotherapy. A suggested approach is to consider a patient's underlying baseline risk of VTE and then weigh the absolute reduction in the risk of VTE versus the risk of anticoagulant-induced hemorrhage. For example, a premenopausal woman with stage 2 breast cancer has a less than 5% risk of VTE. In this situation the magnitude of the benefit of anticoagulant prophylaxis in absolute terms is relatively small and for the individual patient might not outweigh the risk of hemorrhage. However, if this patient had a previous history of thromboembolism, her baseline risk of VTE is much higher and prophylaxis is likely to be worthwhile. A patient with metastatic cancer would be at a still higher baseline risk of VTE than a patient receiving adjuvant chemotherapy and thus the magnitude of the benefit in terms of the reduction in VTE with prophylaxis should outweigh any risks. However, patients with advanced cancer are at increased risk of anticoagulant-related hemorrhage. Hence the decision to use prophylaxis in such patients should be individualized. One situation that renders a patient with advanced cancer at particularly high risk of VTE is the presence of a large mass compressing a major vessel. In addition to chemotherapy, the use of hematopoietic growth factors may increase the risk of VTE, although no prospective data are available and the meta-analysis by Barbui and colleagues was inconclusive.[119]

Theoretically, radiation therapy should carry a risk similar to that of surgery for inducing VTE in patients with cancer. The rationale for primary prophylaxis in patients with large, bulky tumors, particularly mucin-secreting adenocarcinomas or tumors in patients with evidence of low-grade DIC (see Table 21–4) should be the same, therefore, as for surgery. However, no studies have been published to support this theory.

Prolonged *immobilization*, a particular risk factor for VTE in any patient admitted to an intensive care unit, is also a problem for cancer patients, who tend to be immobilized on a regular basis by pain, infection, cytopenias, or other complications of either chemotherapy or the primary disease. Shen and Pollak reported that in their series as many as 14% of hospitalized cancer patients died of pulmonary embolism (PE), as compared to a death rate from PE in noncancer patients of 8% ($p < 0.05$).[102] Samama and colleagues recently reported the results of the MEDENOX trial, in which hospitalized medical patients were randomized to LMWH (enoxaparin) or placebo.[103] The acutely ill medical patients had the following problems: (1) congestive heart failure (CHF); (2) acute respiratory failure not requiring ventilatory support; (3) acute infection without septic shock; (4) acute rheumatic disorders; (5) an acute episode of inflammatory bowel disease; (6) obesity; (7) age greater than 75 years; (8) varicose veins; (9) hormone therapy (antiandrogen or estrogen, except for postmenopausal hormone-replacement therapy); (10) chronic CHF; or (11) chronic respiratory failure. Fourteen percent of the patients in this series had cancer. All patients underwent routine venography between days 6 and 14, or earlier if thrombosis was clinically suspected. The rate of VTE was significantly reduced from 14.9% to 5.5% with LMWH. Therefore, extrapolating from the MEDENOX trial[103] and the data of Shen and Pollak,[102] it would seem reasonable that hospitalized cancer patients receive subcutaneous prophylactic doses of UFH or LMWH provided they are not at significant risk of bleeding.

Cancer patients with indwelling central venous catheters are at increased risk for thrombosis of the axillary/subclavian vein,[37,120] with the catheters themselves susceptible to thrombotic occlusion despite the use of routine heparin flushes. Ultra-low doses of warfarin (1 mg/day) that do not require monitoring[37] or prophylactic doses of LMWH[111] can prevent the occlusion of the catheters. A summary of the recommendations for primary prophylaxis against VTE in cancer patients is presented in Table 21–7.

Treatment of Established Venous Thromboembolism and Secondary Prophylaxis

The goals of treatment of patients with established VTE are important to the global management of patients with cancer and include (1) prevention of death from

Table 21-7 • PRIMARY PROPHYLAXIS IN CANCER

Indication	Recommendation
Prolonged immobilization	UH or LMWH (prophylactic doses)
Surgical intervention	UH or LMWH (in addition to standard noninvasive methods (e.g., intermittent pneumatic compression stockings); if low-grade DIC present, full therapeutic doses may be required)
Chemotherapy (high-risk tumors; e.g., mucin-secreting adenocarcinomas; high-risk patients, e.g., low-grade DIC present)	Further research UH, LMWH or warfarin in some situations (e.g., history of previous VTE)
Indwelling central venous catheters	Warfarin 1mg/day; or LMWH in prophylactic doses
Radiation therapy (high-risk tumors and patients, as for chemotherapy)?	No data available to support recommendation Further research

pulmonary embolism; (2) reduction of morbidity from the acute event; (3) reduction of risk for post-phlebitic syndrome; and (4) prevention of secondary pulmonary hypertension. A difficult question for the treating physician is whether VTE should be treated at all in a patient with a terminal illness, such as advanced cancer. However, treatment of VTE can be viewed as palliative if symptoms of acute VTE can be relieved (e.g., reduction of painful swelling of the leg from DVT and reversal of dyspnea and chest pain in PE) (Table 21–8). Nevertheless, the decision to treat with anticoagulants is particularly difficult in a patient with a very short life expectancy.

Initial Treatment. The traditional treatment for acute DVT or PE is an initial 5- to 7-day course of intravenous UFH followed by 3 months or more of oral anticoagulant therapy.[121] In many countries, LMWHs have replaced UFH for the initial treatment of acute DVT and PE. Oral anticoagulant therapy (e.g. warfarin) can be initiated simultaneously or anytime within the first 24 hours after beginning LMWH or UFH therapy. Patients with cancer should receive a minimum of 5 days of heparin therapy and care should be taken that the INR, used to monitor warfarin, has reached at least 2.0 to 2.5 prior to discontinuation of the heparin. The risk of

Table 21-8 • RATIONALE FOR TREATMENT OF VENOUS THROMBOEMBOLISM IN PATIENTS WITH ADVANCED CANCER

- Deep vein thrombosis
  Reduction of painful leg swelling
- Pulmonary embolism
  Reversal of dyspnea
  Reversal of pleuritic chest pain

clinically important bleeding in patients treated with LMWH or UFH is less than 5%.[111] However, published studies of bleeding risk in heparin-treated patients included predominantly patients without cancer, whose risk of bleeding may be less than cancer patients (vide infra).

In the situation where intravenous UFH is being used to treat acute VTE in a patient with malignant disease, some of these patients will require higher doses of UFH (i.e., more than 40,000 units per day) to achieve the therapeutic range of the aPTT test and are thus considered to be "heparin resistant."[122] In some of these patients, the circulating heparin level is dissociated from the corresponding aPTT. The resistance of the aPTT to prolongation is thought to be due to increased levels of factor VIII and fibrinogen as acute-phase reactants. Such patients should have their UFH levels confirmed by the antifactor Xa heparin assay using a target level of 0.3 to 0.9 U/mL.[122] This approach is safe and effective and results in less escalation of the heparin dose than occurs with monitoring of the aPTT alone.

LMWH has been demonstrated to be as safe and effective as UFH for the treatment of acute proximal DVT in hospitalized patients.[120,123,124] In three more recent clinical trials patients with acute proximal DVT were treated either with intravenous UFH in hospital or LMWH given as outpatient therapy.[125–127] In these trials there were a total of 405 cancer patients. Within this subgroup of patients no difference was detected in recurrent VTE between the treatment groups. The results demonstrated that LMWH can be used safely and effectively to treat patients with acute thrombosis in the home setting.

An issue to consider is whether results from such rigorous clinical trials can be generalized to the routine clinical situation. The results of recent cohort studies in patients with DVT[128,129] showed that nontrial patients can be treated safely at home; many of these patients had cancer. Treatment at home is particularly attractive for the cancer patient for whom quality of life is an important consideration. Clearly, not all cancer patients with acute thrombosis can be treated at home. Some require hospitalization because of symptoms from the cancer. If the patient is to be treated at home they must be reliable and compliant, and have a good support system. Fortunately, treatment of acute VTE with LMWH usually does not require laboratory monitoring, except if the patient has significant renal failure and/or is very obese. LMWH has been compared to intravenous UFH in two trials in hospitalized patients with PE[126,130] and, in a recent prospective cohort study, cancer patients with acute pulmonary embolism were treated at home with LMWH.[131]

Secondary Prevention (Prophylaxis) With Oral Anticoagulants. Patients with VTE who are treated with an initial course of heparin therapy require continuing oral anticoagulant therapy to prevent recurrence. Vitamin K antagonists (e.g., warfarin) have been shown to be effective in preventing recurrent thrombosis in patients with established VTE.[121] The target therapeutic range for patients with VTE (either DVT or PE) is an INR of 2.0 to 3.0. The risk of clinical bleeding with this intensity of oral anticoagulant therapy is relatively low (approximately 2% per year) in recent clinical trials.[122] However, it must be re-emphasized that this rate is based primarily on studies of patients without cancer. While it is generally agreed that cancer patients are at higher risk for hemorrhagic complications of warfarin,[132–134] the results of studies are conflicting. In studies by Prandoni and coworkers,[8,135] the rate of major bleeding was 3.4% in patients with cancer compared to 3.0% in patients without cancer. Similarly, in the study by Bona and coworkers,[134] no difference was detected in the rate of major bleeding between cancer patients and noncancer patients (0.004 events per patient months of treatment versus 0.003 events per patient months of treatment, respectively. However, other studies have reported increased rates of bleeding in cancer patients on warfarin compared to noncancer patients. Hutten and colleagues recently compared the rates of bleeding between cancer and noncancer patients in two randomized trials that compared LMWH with standard UFH for initial treatment of acute VTE.[136] There were 261 patients with malignancy and 1038 without malignancy in this study and the rates of bleeding were 13.3% per year versus 2.1% per year, respectively, $p = 0.002$. In a recent Italian population-based cohort study, the outcome of anticoagulation courses in 95 patients with malignancy was compared with the outcome in 733 patients without malignancy.[137] The investigators recorded a 21.6% rate of bleeding in cancer patients compared to 4.5% in noncancer patients, $P = 0.001$.

In the past it was the usual practice to continue warfarin therapy for 3 months following a first episode of proximal DVT or PE. The patient with active malignant disease who has had an episode of established thrombosis, however, is likely to be at continuing risk of recurrent VTE even after 3 months of warfarin,[8,118] due largely to the continued presence of the risk factors we have reviewed previously (see Fig. 21–1 and Table 21–6). The appropriate length of time to maintain warfarin therapy in patients with cancer is not known. However, three studies have considered this issue in patients with idiopathic DVT, a group considered to be at continuing risk of VTE.[11,97,138] In the first of these studies published by Schulman and the DURAC investigators, those patients with idiopathic proximal DVT who were randomized to receive 6 months of oral anticoagulant therapy after initial heparin therapy had a significant reduction in the rate of recurrent VTE, compared with those who received 6 weeks of therapy.[11] The DURAC investigators then randomized patients with a second episode of DVT to either 6 months or indefinite oral anticoagulant therapy, and patients who received the longer therapy had a significant reduction in recurrent VTE, with a small increase in incidence of bleeding.[97] More recently Kearon and coworkers reported a significant reduction in recurrence of VTE in favor of those patients with idiopathic DVT who received 2 years of warfarin over those who were treated with the conventional 3 months of therapy.[138] Based on the results of these trials, it would seem prudent to continue oral anticoagulant therapy in cancer patients beyond 3 months while these patients remain at high risk. In the patient at particularly high risk for bleeding, the dose of warfarin can be lowered to maintain an INR closer to 2.0.

Regardless of whether cancer patients are treated initially with UFH or LMWH, standard oral anticoagulant therapy for 3 months results in a twofold increased risk of recurrent VTE, compared to noncancer patients.[7,135,139] In the prospective cohort study of Prandoni and colleagues,[135] 355 consecutive patients with DVT were treated with UFH followed by oral anticoagulant therapy. The risk for recurrence of VTE in the 3-month follow-up period was increased in cancer patients (10.3%), as compared to noncancer patients (4.7%). This difference achieved statistical significance in the subgroup of patients with INRs of 2.0 to 3.0 (8.6% vs. 1.3%, $p < 0.01$), although the number of events on which this conclusion was based was quite small (5/58 vs. 4/297). Hutten and coworkers[136] performed a retrospective analysis of the rates of recurrent VTE and bleeding between cancer and noncancer patients in two previously conducted randomized trials. The two original studies had compared LMWH with standard UFH for initial treatment of acute VTE and included 261 patients with malignancy and 1038 without cancer. The rates of recurrent VTE were 27% per year versus 9% per year, respectively, $p = 0.003$.[136]

It is conceivable that longer-term LMWH therapy could prove more efficacious and safer than oral anticoagulant therapy in this group of patients. Two small randomized trials have compared long-term LMWH therapy with either UFH[140] or oral anticoagulant therapy,[141] although neither of these trials included a large number of cancer patients. Clinical trials have been initiated comparing long-term LMWH with long-term oral anticoagulant therapy in cancer patients with established VTE.

A cancer patient who develops recurrent thromboembolism with a subtherapeutic INR may be treated acutely with UFH or LMWH and restarted on oral anticoagulants, taking care to be certain that the INR is maintained between 2.0 and 3.0. Patients who develop a documented recurrent thrombosis while on therapeutic oral anticoagulant therapy represent a difficult therapeutic challenge. Several options exist after retreatment of the acute episode with UFH or LMWH, including (1) continued oral anticoagulant therapy at a higher targeted INR; (2) adjusted-dose subcutaneous UFH to maintain a therapeutic aPTT; or (3) LMWH. In patients at high risk for PE an inferior vena caval filter can be inserted in addition to the above measures. The use of an inferior vena caval filter without concomitant anticoagulant therapy should be limited to patients with active bleeding or those at very high risk of bleeding. In a randomized trial conducted in France, the use of a vena caval filter reduced the rate of recurrent pulmonary embolism over the short-term, but at the expense of recurrent DVT during longer follow-up.[142] Therefore, anticoagulation should be administered whenever possible. Without concomitant anticoagulation, thrombus may develop proximal to the filter and result in fatal pulmonary embolism.

Patients at Particular Risk of Hemorrhage

In patients with a "relative" contraindication to anticoagulation therapy (e.g., perhaps those with brain or pericardial tumors), it is reasonable to use LMWH as initial treatment for acute VTE and then to use either adjusted-dose heparin or LMWH to reduce the bleeding risk associated with long-term oral anticoagulant therapy and allow for the more rapid reversal of anticoagulation, if necessary. Alternatively, an inferior vena cava filter can be placed electively in such patients to avoid the need for long-term oral anticoagulation therapy (vide infra).

Inferior Vena Caval Filters

Placement of an inferior vena cava filter should be limited to patients who have active bleeding, those at high risk for bleeding, and those who develop recurrent VTE despite adequate anticoagulation therapy (as defined by appropriate doses of LMWH or appropriate laboratory test results when monitoring either UFH therapy or oral anticoagulant therapy). Clearly, more randomized controlled trials are needed to determine the optimal use of filters. This subject is covered in greater detail elsewhere in this text (see Chapters 37 and 38) and in a recent review.[143]

Catheter Thrombosis

Central vein access devices (CVADs) or catheters are used commonly in cancer patients, particularly for the administration of chemotherapy and long-term supportive care (e.g., antibiotics, blood products, growth factors). Thrombosis is a frequent complication of the use of such devices and can involve the tip of the catheter alone or the length of the catheter (forming a "fibrin sheath"), or may extend to involve the veins of the upper limbs, neck, and mediastinum.[144] The usual treatment for catheter tip thrombosis is low-dose thrombolytic therapy with either streptokinase, urokinase, or tPA,[144] while the treatment of symptomatic upper limb vein thrombosis related to a catheter is full-dose anticoagulant therapy with heparin (UFH or LMWH) followed by oral anticoagulant therapy. Insufficient data exist to allow recommendations as to whether thrombolytic therapy and/or catheter removal should be used (in addition to full-dose anticoagulant therapy) in the setting of upper-extremity VTE in association with a CVAD. Further research is needed on the optimal management of CVADs.

Anticoagulation Therapy and Cancer Mortality

Stimulated by a substantial literature documenting beneficial effects of anticoagulants, antifibrinolytic agents and antiplatelet agents in the treatment of cancer in experimental animals, investigators have attempted to repeat this experience in a variety of human cancers.[24,145–152] The animal studies provided a rationale for investigating the effects of each of these classes of drugs in the treatment of *human cancer*. Several early studies reported beneficial effects from the use of warfarin or antiplatelet drugs in human cancer patients, but these trials were methodologically weak.[26,153,154]

More recent, better-controlled studies have led to mixed results. In the Veterans Administration Cooperative Trial (CSP#75), patients with small cell carcinoma of the lung (SCCL) were randomized to receive either chemotherapy with standard doses of warfarin or chemotherapy with no anticoagulation therapy. Survival was twice as long in the warfarin group (50 weeks vs. 24 weeks, $p = 0.03$),[145] which could not be accounted for by protection against VTE or serious bleeding. A subsequent study of patients with SCCL with extensive disease published by Cancer and Leukemia Group B (CALGB) appeared to confirm these findings and also demonstrated significantly increased disease-free interval and incidence of tumor regression in warfarin-treated patients.[148] A more recent pilot study of warfarin treatment of SCCL patients with limited disease also appeared promising,[155] but a subsequent large randomized control trial with a similar group of SCCL patients failed to demonstrate significant improvement in outcome.[156]

In a second Veterans Administration Cooperative Trial (CSP#188), mopidamol (RA-233), a dipyridamole derivative and inhibitor of platelet function, favorably affected the survival of patients with defined limited burdens of non-SCCL[157] but neither mopidamol nor warfarin has been effective in patients with several other tumors, notably carcinomas of the colon, head and neck, or prostate.[25,157] Similar conflicting results can be found in the published studies of heparin treatment of cancer. Lebeau and colleagues demonstrated a significant increase in survival in patients with SCCL treated with unfractionated heparin in addition to chemotherapy.[158] However, von Templehoff and his colleagues found no significant survival benefit for patients with ovarian cancer treated with LMWH in a trial designed to test the efficacy of LMWH for prevention of postoperative thrombosis.[159] Two recent comprehensive reviews of UFH and LMWH and cancer treatment provide some insight into this difficult area.[26,27]

Nevertheless, these data, together with the results of subset analysis of recent, large, randomized clinical trials of LMWH versus UFH therapy in patients with acute proximal DVT,[160] have rekindled interest in the potential anticancer effect of antithrombotic agents—in particular, differences in potential survival benefits of cancer patients treated with LMWH. In the trial reported by Hull and colleagues,[161] the overall mortality rate was 9.6% in hospitalized patients receiving standard UFH compared to 4.7% in the patients treated with LMWH ($p = 0.05$). In the trial reported by Prandoni and colleagues,[162] the overall mortality rate in UFH-treated patients was 12% compared to 7% in the LMWH-treated patients (not statistically significant). In a meta-analysis of several large VTE trials, Lensing and coworkers[163] found an overall mortality rate of 3.9% for the patients treated with LMWH compared to 7.1% for those treated with standard UFH, a relative risk reduction of 47% ($p < 0.04$). In the 195 cancer patients in the studies subjected to meta-analysis, the mortality risk reduction was 64% in favor of LMWH ($p < 0.01$). A subsequent meta-analysis came to the same conclusion.[164]

Experimental evidence provides a theoretical basis for speculating that LMWH might exert an inhibitory effect on tumor growth superior to that observed with UFH, although it remains difficult to explain how short-term therapy (e.g., 7 days) with LMWH can impact on the natural history of a malignant tumor that has existed for months to years. Nevertheless, recent data published by Schulman and Lindmarker[93] has continued to provide "fuel for the fire"—provoking additional studies. These investigators were able to demonstrate in their retrospective analysis of data collected prospectively for the Swedish Tumor and Thrombosis Registries that patients in whom a subsequent diagnosis of cancer was established after being treated for 6 months with warfarin after an acute episode of VTE survived significantly longer than did a matched group of patients who had been treated for only 6 weeks with oral anticoagulant therapy. This survival difference persisted for several years into the study, again suggesting that anticoagulation therapy may alter the natural history of cancer. Clearly, additional prospective clinical trials evaluating long-term administration of anticoagulants, including warfarin and LMWH, are required to resolve this important issue.

CASE SCENARIOS

The following clinical scenarios illustrate some common management challenges in cancer patients with VTE.

CASE 1
A 62-year-old woman is recently diagnosed with early-stage breast cancer and tamoxifen therapy is recommended for adjuvant therapy. She has a history of DVT following major abdominal surgery 10 years ago. Does she require thromboprophylaxis?

Tamoxifen therapy is associated with an increased risk of VTE. The incidence of thrombosis in patients with early-stage breast cancer receiving tamoxifen is approximately 1% to 2%. The absolute risk in this patient may be higher because of her previous history of DVT. Because her DVT was secondary to a major transient risk factor (abdominal surgery) and had occurred many years ago, it is unlikely to alter her baseline risk at this time. Given that the risk of major hemorrhage in patients on standard intensity oral anticoagulant therapy (with a target INR of 2.0 to 3.0) is approximately 2% to 3% per year, the risk of bleeding would outweigh her risk of thrombosis. Therefore, *thromboprophylaxis using warfarin would not be recommended*.

In contrast, if her previous thrombotic event was idiopathic (i.e., not associated with a transient risk factor) or was in the very recent past (within the past year), thromboprophylaxis would be justifiable, since her risk of recurrent VTE would be higher. In the latter situation warfarin therapy with a targeted INR of 1.3 to 1.9 could be considered.

CASE 2
A 45-year-old man with metastatic pancreatic cancer presents with increasing swelling of his right leg while receiving warfarin therapy for atrial fibrillation. His INR has been therapeutic and is 2.6 on the day of presentation. Objective testing confirms acute DVT involving his right leg. What is the best treatment now? Is this an indication for insertion of an inferior vena caval filter?

This patient is "warfarin resistant" because he developed new thrombosis while on therapeutic oral anticoagulation, which is not unusual in cases of advanced malignancy, particularly adenocarcinomas. The best available treatment is full-dose LMWH, which can be self-administered safely on an outpatient basis. Inferior caval filter placement at this point is not indicated, since caval interruption does not treat the underlying thrombotic problem and may worsen his leg symptoms. A filter can also become thrombosed and filters have not been proven to be superior to anticoagulant therapy in reducing the risk of PE or decreasing mortality over the long term. If this patient develops recurrent thromboembolism while on therapeutic doses of LMWH, insertion of a filter should be considered.

CASE 3
A 66-year-old woman with lung cancer is on warfarin therapy following a PE. She now requires thoracentesis for drainage of a malignant pleural effusion and may require this on a repeated basis. How should her anticoagulation be managed?

Invasive procedures are commonly required in patients with cancer. Depending on the exact type of procedure, the associated hemorrhagic risk, and the time since the diagnosis of venous thrombosis, the management of anticoagulant therapy will vary. For patients with recently diagnosed thrombosis (within a few months), the risk of recurrence is high and therefore interruption of anticoagulant therapy should be avoided or minimized. This can be accomplished by switching the patient to LMWH injections 3 to 4 days before the procedure. This will allow the INR to normalize slowly. Alternatively, vitamin K can be given to hasten the normalization of the INR.[165,166] LMWH is stopped 24 hours before the procedure and is resumed after the procedure. LMWH and the oral anticoagulant can be restarted together once satisfactory hemostasis is achieved. The LMWH is discontinued when the INR is therapeutic again. For patients with a more remote history of thrombosis (greater than 6 months), stopping oral anticoagulant therapy 3 to 4 days before the procedure and restarting after the procedure is likely to provide adequate protection. For procedures associated with a minimal risk of bleeding (e.g., skin biopsy and percutaneous needle biopsy), interruption of anticoagulation may not be necessary at all as long as hemostasis can be achieved with local measures (e.g., prolonged pressure). Most procedures can be performed without causing excessive bleeding when the INR is less than 1.5.

CASE 4
A 29-year-old man has testicular cancer with metastases to his brain and lung. He is now diagnosed with left-leg DVT. Can he be safely treated with standard anticoagulant therapy?

At our centers, we routinely treat patients with standard anticoagulation (initial LMWH or UFH followed by warfarin) despite the presence of a primary brain tumor or brain metastases, as long as there is no history or evidence of intracranial hemorrhage. There is no evidence that the bleeding risk is increased as long as the anticoagulant therapy is closely monitored. The target INR should remain within the therapeutic range but we would aim for an INR below 2.5. The one exception to this practice is the patient with melanoma involving the central nervous system. These lesions are highly vascular and the bleeding risk is high. Therefore, we would consider inserting a caval filter in these patients rather than treating them with anticoagulant therapy. The final choice of therapy will depend on the overall status of the patient and the patient's informed decision.

These case studies are illustrative of only some of the unique challenges facing the clinician in the prevention and treatment of VTE in patients with cancer. In the near future more specific, targeted anticoagulants (e.g., heparin-like pentasaccharide, small-molecular-weight thrombin and/or factor Xa inhibitors, tissue factor pathway inhibitor, activated protein C) may provide improved risk/benefit ratios for patients with cancer. Similarly, the judicious use of thrombopoietin and/or other analogous megakaryocyte growth factors may reduce the risk of thrombocytopenic bleeding in cancer patients. Finally, a better understanding of the molecular pathogenesis of thrombosis and bleeding in cancer patients may provide opportunities for prevention and treatment of these complications hardly envisioned today. Nevertheless, the cancer patient will no doubt continue to be a challenge in terms of the prevention and treatment of bleeding and thrombosis.

ACKNOWLEDGMENTS

The authors acknowledge with gratitude the generous contributions to this chapter of Harold Dvorak, M.D., Mallinkrodt Professor of Pathology, Harvard Medical School, and Chairman, Department of Pathology, Beth Israel/Deaconness Medical Center, Boston. Dr. Dvorak provided many of the observations from the literature richly cited in his contributions to our chapter in *Hemostasis and Thrombosis,* 4th edition; from which several portions of the current chapter have their roots. We also acknowledge the contributions of Anna Falanga, M.D., Divisione di Ematologia, Ospedale Riuniti, Bergamo, Italy, in particular to the section on pathogenesis, and for the creation of the figure that appears both in this chapter and in our article in Thrombosis Research.[42]

■ REFERENCES

Chapter 21 References

1. Trousseau A. Phlegmasia alba dolens. In: Clinique medicale de l'Hotel-Dieu de Paris. Paris, JB Ballière et Fils, 1865; vol. 3; pp. 654–671.
2. Billroth T. Lectures on Surgical Pathology and Therapeutics: A Handbook for Students and Practitioners. Translated from the 8th edition. London, The New Sydenham Society, 1877–1878.
3. Rickles FR, Levine M, Edwards RL. Hemostatic alterations in cancer patients. Cancer Metastasis Rev 1992;11:237–248.
4. Edwards RL, Rickles FR. Thrombosis and Cancer. In: Pineo GF, Hull R (Eds): Disorders of Thrombosis. Philadelphia, WB Saunders, 1996; pp. 374–382.
5. Rickles FR, Levine MN. Venous thromboembolism in malignancy and malignancy in venous thromboembolism. Haemostasis 1998;28:43–49.
6. Rickles FR, Levine M, Dvorak HB. Abnormalities of hemostasis in malignancy. In: Hemostasis and Thrombosis, 4th ed. Colman RW, Hirsh J, Marder VJ, et al. (eds.) Philadelphia, Lippincott Williams & Wilkins, 2000; pp. 1131–1152.
7. Levine MN, Rickles FR. Treatment of venous thromboembolism in cancer patients. Haemostasis 1998;28:66–70.
8. Prandoni P. Antithrombotic strategies in patients with cancer. Thromb Haemost 1997;78:141–144.
9. Geerts WH, Heit JA, Claggett GP. Prevention of venous thromboembolism. Chest 2001;119:132S–175S.
10. Donati MB. Cancer and thrombosis: from phlegmasia alba dolens to transgenic mice. Thromb Haemost 1995;74:278–281.
11. Sproul EE. Carcinoma and venous thrombosis: The frequency of association of carcinoma in the body or tail of the pancreas with multiple venous thrombosis. Am J Med Sci 1938;34:566–585.
12. Saphir O. The fate of carcinoma emboli in the lung. Am J Pathol 1947;23:245–253.
13. Dvorak HF, Orenstein NS Carvalho AC, et al. Induction of a fibrin gel investment: An early event in line 10 hepatocarcinoma growth mediated by tumor-secreted products. J Immunol 1979; 122:166–174.
14. Zacharski LR, Costantini V, Ornstein DL, et al. Pathways of coagulation/fibrinolysis activation in malignancy. Thromb Haemost 1992;18:104–116.
15. Shoji M, Hancock WW, Abe K, et al. Activation of coagulation and angiogenesis in cancer. Immunohistochemical localization in situ of clotting proteins and vascular endothelial growth factor in human cancers. Am J Pathol 1998;152:399–411.
16. Gasic GJ, Gasic TB, Galanti N, et al. Platelet-tumor cell interactions in mice. The role of platelets in the spread of malignant disease. Int J Cancer 1973;11:704–718.
17. Dvorak AM, Connell AB, Proppe K, et al. Immunologic rejection of mammary adenocarcinoma (TA-3-St) in C57 BL/6 mice: participation of neutrophils and activated macrophages with fibrin formation. J Immunol 1978;120:1240–1248.
18. Dvorak HF, Dickersin GR, Dvorak AM, et al. Human breast carcinoma. Fibrin deposits and desmoplasia. Inflammatory cell type and distribution. Microvasculature and infarction. J Natl Cancer Inst 1981;67:335–345.
19. Contrino J, Hair GA, Kreutzer DL, et al. In situ detection of the expression of tissue factor in vascular endothelial cells: corre-

lation with the malignant phenotype of human breast disease. Nat Med 1996;2:209–215.
20. Prandoni P, Lensing AWA, Buller HR, et al. Deep-vein thrombosis and the incidence of subsequent symptomatic cancer. N Engl J Med 1992;327:1128–1133.
21. Rickles FR, Levine MN. Epidemiology of thrombosis in cancer. Acta Haemtol 2001;106:6–12.
22. Falanga A, Rickles FR. Pathophysiology of the thrombophilic state in the cancer patient. Semin Thromb Hemost 1999;25:173–182.
23. Zacharski LR, Donati MB, Rickles FR. Registry of clinical trials of antithrombotic drugs in cancer: second report. Thromb Haemost 1993;70:357–360.
24. Zacharski LR, Constantini V, Wojtukiewicz MZ, et al. Anticoagulants as cancer therapy. Semin Oncol 1990;17:217–227.
25. Zacharski LR, Rickles FR. Warfarin in the treatment of cancer In: Poller L, Hirsh J. (Eds.): Oral Anticoagulants. New York, Oxford University Press, 1996; pp. 229–238.
26. Zacharski LR, Ornstein D. Heparin and cancer. Thromb Haemost 1998;80:10–23.
27. Zacharski LR, Ornstein DL, Mamourian AC. Low-molecular weight heparin and cancer. Semin Thromb Hemost 2000;26 Suppl 1:69–77.
28. Solinsky CD. Trousseau's phenomenom. Blood 1983;62:1304.
29. O'Meara RAQ. Coagulative properties of cancers. Ir J Med Sci 1958;6:474.
30. Hiramoto R, Bernecky J, Jurandowski J, et al. Fibrin in human tumors. Cancer Res 1960;20:592–593.
31. Dvorak HF, Dvorak AM, Manseau EJ, et al. Fibrin gel investment associated with line 1 and line 10 solid tumor growth, angiogenesis, and fibroplasia in guinea pigs: Role of cellular immunity, myofibroblasts, microvascular damage, and infarction in line 1 tumor regression. J Natl Cancer Inst 1979;62:1459–1472.
32. Harris NL, Dvorak AM, Smith J, et al. Fibrin deposits in Hodgkin's disease. Am J Pathol 1982;108:119–129.
33. Dvorak HF. Tumors: Wounds that do not heal. Similarities between tumor stroma generation and wound healing. N Engl J Med 1986;315:1650–1659.
34. Dvorak HF, Harvey VS, McDonagh J. Quantitation of fibrinogen influx and fibrin deposition and turnover in line 1 and line 10 guinea pig carcinomas. Cancer Res 1984;44:33–48.
35. Brown LF, Van De Water L, Harvey VS, et al. Fibrinogen influx and accumulation of crosslinked fibrin in healing wounds and in tumor stroma. Am J Pathol 1988;130:455–465.
36. Spar IL, Bale WF, Marrack D, et al. ^{131}I-labelled antibodies to human fibrinogen. Diagnostic studies and therapeutic trials. Cancer 1967;20:865–870.
37. Bern MM, Lokich JJ, Wallach SR, et al. Very low doses of warfarin can prevent thrombosis in central venous catheters. A randomized prospective trial. Ann Intern Med 1990;112:423–428.
38. Monreal M, Alastrue A, Rull M, et al. Upper extremity deep vein thrombosis in cancer patients with venous access devices—prophylaxis with a low-molecular-weight heparin (Fragmin). Thromb Haemost 1996;75:251–253.
39. Virchow R. Gesammelte Abhaldungen zur Wissensdiafflichem Medicine. Frankfurt; Meidinger Sohn, 1856; p. 447.
40. Green KB, Silverstein RL. Hypercoagulability in cancer. Hematol Oncol Clin North Am 1996;10:499–530.
41. Edwards RL, Klaus M, Matthews E, et al. Heparin abolishes the chemotherapy-induced increase in plasma fibrinopeptide A levels. Am J Med 1990;89:25–28.
42. Rickles FR, Falanga A. Molecular basis for the relationship between thrombosis and cancer. Thromb Res 2001;102:V215–V224.
43. Shoji M, Abe K, Nawroth PP, et al. Molecular mechanisms linking thrombosis and angiogenesis in cancer. Trends Cardiovasc Med 1997;7:52–59.

44. Abe K, Shoji M, Chen J, et al. Regulation of vascular endothelial growth factor production and angiogenesis by the cytoplasmic tail of tissue factor. Proc Nat Acad Sci USA 1999;96:8663–8668.
45. Folkman J. Tumor angiogenesis and tissue factor. Nat Med 1996;2:167–168.
46. Steingart RH. Coagulation disorders associated with neoplastic disease. Recent Results Cancer Res 1988;108:37–43.
47. Ratnoff OD. Hemostatic emergencies in malignancy. Semin Oncol 1989;16:561–571.
48. Selroos O. Thrombocytosis. Acta Med Scand 1973;193:431–436.
49. Levin J, Conley CL. Thrombocytosis associated with malignant disease. Arch Intern Med. 1964;114:497–500.
50. Goldsmith GH Jr. Hemostatic disorders associated with neoplasia. In: Ratnoff OD, Forbes CD, (Eds.): Disorders of Hemostasis, 2nd ed. Philadelphia, Grune & Stratton, 1991, pp. 352–368.
51. Sun NC, McAffee WM, et al. Hemostatic abnormalities in malignancy, a prospective study of 108 patients. Am J Clin Pathol 1979;71:10–16.
52. Kies MS, Posch JJ, Giolma JP, et al. Hemostatic function in cancer patients. Cancer 1980;46:831–837.
53. Hagedorn AB, Bowie EJW, Elveback LR, et al. Coagulation abnormalities in patients with inoperable lung cancer. Mayo Clin Proc 1974;49:647–653.
54. Davis RB, Theologides A, Kennedy BJ. Comparative studies of blood coagulation and platelet aggregation in patients with cancer and nonmalignant disease. Ann Intern Med 1969;71:67–80.
55. Tranum BL, Haut A. Thrombocytosis: Platelet kinetics in neoplasia. J Lab Clin Med 1974;84:615–619.
56. Cooper HA, Bowie EJW, Owen CA Jr. Evaluation of patients with increased fibrinolytic split products in their serum. Mayo Clin Proc 1974;49:654–657.
57. Edwards RL, Rickles FR, Moritz TE, et al. Abnormalities of blood coagulation tests in patients with cancer. Am J Clin Pathol 1987;88:596–602.
58. Bidet JM, Ferriere JP, Besse G, et al. Evaluation of β-thromboglobulin levels in cancer patients: Effects of antitumor therapy. Thromb Res 1980;19:429–433.
59. Slichter SJ, Harker LA. Hemostasis in malignancy. Ann NY Acad Sci 1974;230:252–261.
60. Johannson S, Kutti J, Olsson LB. Rapid platelet consumption in a case of metastatic osteogenic sarcoma of the breast. Acta Pathol Microbiol Scand 1978;505:86A (abstr).
61. Schernthaner G, Ludwig H, Silberbauer K. Elevated plasma β-thromboglobulin levels in multiple myeloma and in polycythaemia vera. Acta Haematol (Basel) 1979;62:219–222.
62. Francis JL. Haemostasis and cancer. Med Lab Sci 1989;46:331–346.
63. Boneu B, Bugat R, Boneu A, et al. Exhausted platelets in patients with malignant solid tumors without evidence of active consumption coagulopathy. Eur J Cancer Clin Oncol 1984;20:899–903.
64. Sloand EM, Kenney DM, Chao FC, et al. Platelet antithrombin defect in malignancy: Platelet protein alterations. Blood 1987;69:479–485.
65. Barbui T, Finazzi G, Falanga A. The impact of all-trans-retinoic acid on the coagulopathy of acute promyelocytic leukemia. Blood 1998;91:3093–3102.
66. Luzzatto G, Schafer AI. The prethrombotic state in cancer. Semin Oncol 1990;17:147–159.
67. Nand S, Fisher SG, Salgia R, et al. Hemostatic abnormalities in untreated cancer: Incidence and correlation with thrombotic and hemorrhagic complication. J Clin Oncol 1987;5:1998–2003.
68. Rasche H, Dietrich M. Hemostatic abnormalities associated with malignant diseases. Eur J Cancer 1977;13:1053–1064.
69. Goad KE, Gralnick HR. Coagulation disorders in cancer. Hematol Oncol Clin North Am 1996;10:457–484.
70. Falanga A, Ofosu FA, Cortelazzo S, et al. Preliminary study to identify cancer patients at high risk of venous thrombosis following major surgery. Br J Haematol 1993; 85:745–750.

71. Falanga A, Barbui T, Rickles FR, et al. Guidelines for clotting studies in cancer patients. Thromb Haemost 1993;70:343–350.
72. Green D, Maliekel K, Sushko E, et al. Activated protein C resistance in cancer patients. Haemostasis 1997;27:112–118.
73. Melnyk A, Theriault R, Andreeff M, et al. Factor V Leiden (G1691A) and the risk of thrombosis in patients with solid tumors: a prospective case control study. Blood 1996; 88 Suppl: 176a (abstr).
74. Honegger H, Anderson N, Hewitt LA, et al. Antithrombin III profiles in malignancy, relationship to primary tumors and metastatic sites. Thromb Haemost 1981;46:500–503.
75. Rodeghiero F, Mannucci PA, Vigano S, et al. Liver dysfunction rather than intravascular coagulation as the main cause of low protein C and antithrombin III in acute leukemia. Blood 1984;63:965–969.
76. Rubin RN, Kies MS Posch JJ. Measurements of antithrombin III in solid tumor patients with and without hepatic metastases. Thromb Res 1980;18:353–360.
77. Wajima T. Fibrinolytic profiles in patients with small cell carcinoma of the lung. Semin Thromb Haemost 1991;17:280–285.
78. Troy K, Essex D, Rand J, et al. Protein C and S levels in acute leukemia. Am J Hematol 1991; 37, 159–162.
79. Feffer SE, Carmosino LS, Fox RL. Acquired protein C deficiency in patients with breast cancer receiving cyclophosphamide, methotrexate, and 5-fluorouracil. Cancer 1989;63:1303–1307.
80. Rogers JS, Murgo AJ, Fontana JA, et al. Chemotherpay for breast cancer decreases plasma protein C and protein S. J Clin Oncol 1988;6:276–281.
81. Rella C, Coviello M, Giotta F, et al. A prothrombotic state in breast cancer patients treated with adjuvant chemotherapy. Breast Ca Res Treat 1996;40:151–159.
82. Achkar A, Laaban JP, Horellou MH, et al. Prospective screening for occult cancer in patients with venous thromboembolism. Thromb Haemost 1997;78 Suppl:383(abst).
83. Monreal M, Fernandez-Llamazares, Perandreu J, et al. Occult cancer in patients with venous thromboembolism: which patients, which cancers? Thromb Haemost 1997;78:1316–1318.
84. Rance A, Emmerich J, Guedj C, et al. Occult cancer in patients with bilateral deep-vein thrombosis. Lancet 1997;350:1448–1449.
85. Hettiaranchchi RJ, Lok J, Prins MH, et al. Undiagnosed malignancy in patients with deep-vein thrombosis: incidence, risk indicators and diagnosis. Cancer 1998;83:180–185.
86. Rajan R, Levine M, Gent M, et al. The occurrence of subsequent malignancy in patients presenting with deep vein thrombosis. Results from a historical cohort study. Thromb Haemost 1998;79:19–22.
87. Nordstrom M, Lindbald B, Anderson H, et al. Deep vein thrombosis and occult malignancy: an epidemiological study. Br Med J 1994;308:891–894.
88. Cornuz J, Pearson SD, Creagor MA, et al. Importance of findings on the initial evaluation for cancer in patients with symptomatic idiopathic deep vein thrombosis. Ann Intern Med 1996;25: 785–793.
89. Baron JA, Gridley G, Weiderpass E, et al. Venous thromboembolism and cancer. Lancet 1998;351:1077–1080.
90. Sorensen HT, Mellemkjaer L, Steffensen FH, et al. The risk of a diagnosis of cancer after primary deep venous thrombosis or pulmonary embolism. N Engl J Med 1998;338:1169–1173.
91. Sorensen HT, Mellemkjaer L, Olsen JH, et al. Prognosis of cancers associated with venous thromboembolism. N Engl J Med 2000;343:1846–1850.
92. Prins MH, Lensing AWA, Hirsh J. Idiopathic deep vein thrombosis. Is a search for malignant disease justified? Arch Intern Med 1994;154:1310–1312.
93. Schulman S, Lindmarker P. Incidence of cancer after prophylaxis with warfarin against recurrent venous thromboembolism. N Engl J Med 2000;342:1953–1958.
94. Monreal M, Lafoz E, Casals A, et al. Occult cancer in patients with deep venous thrombosis: a systematic approach. Cancer 1991;67:541–545.
95. Monreal M, Casals A, Boix J, et al. Occult cancer in patients with acute pulmonary embolism. A prospective study. Chest 1993;103:816–819.
96. Bastounis EA, Karyiannakis AJ, Makri GG, et al. The incidence of occult cancer in patients with deep vein thrombosis: a prospective study. J Intern Med 1996;239:153–156.
97. Schulman S, Rhedin A-S, Lindmarker P, et al. for the Duration of Anticoagulation Trial Study Group. A comparison of six weeks and six months of oral anticoagulant therapy after a first episode of venous thromboembolism. N Engl J Med 1995; 332:1661–1665.
98. Barosi G, Marchetti M, Dazzi L, et al. Testing for occult cancer in patients with idiopathic deep vein thrombosis—a decision analysis. Thromb Haemost 1997;78:1319–1326.
99. Huber O, Bounameaux H, Borst F, et al. Postoperative pulmonary embolism after hospital discharge. An underestimated risk. Arch Surg 1992;127:310–313.
100. Goodnough LT, Saito H, Manni A, et al. Increased incidence of thromboembolism in stage IV breast cancer patients treated with a five-drug chemotherapy regimen: a study of 159 patients. Cancer 1984;54:1264–1268.
101. Levine MN, Gent M, Hirsh J, et al. The thrombogenic effect of anticancer drug therapy in women with stage II breast cancer. N Engl J Med 1988;318:404–407.
102. Shen VS, Pollak EW. Fatal pulmonary embolism in cancer patients: is heparin prophylaxis justified? South Med J 1980;73: 841–843.
103. Samama MM, Cohen AT, Darmon J-Y, et al. A comparison of enoxaparin with placebo for the prevention of venous thromboembolism in acutely ill medical patients. N Engl J Med 1999;341:793–800.
104. Kakkar VV, Howe CT, Nicolaides AN, et al. Deep vein thrombosis of the leg. Is there a high risk group? Am J Surg 1970; 120:527–531.
105. Claggett GP, Reisch JS. Prevention of venous thromboembolism in general surgical patients. Ann Surg 1988;208:227–240.
106. Ambrus JL, Ambrus CM, Mink JB, et al. Causes of death in cancer patients. J Med 1975;6:61–64.
107. Hills NH, Pflug JJ, Jeyasingh K, et al. Prevention of deep vein thrombosis by intermittent pneumatic compression of calf. Br Med J 1972;1:131–135.
108. Levine MN. Cancer patients. In: Goldhaber S (Ed.): Prevention of Venous Thromboembolism. New York; Marcel Dekker, 1993, pp. 463–483.
109. Cohen AT, Wagner MB, Mohamed RS. Risk factors for bleeding in major abdominal surgery using heparin prophylaxis. Am J Surg 1997;174:1–5.
110. Enoxacan Study Group. Efficacy and safety of enoxaparin versus unfractionated heparin for prevention of deep vein thrombosis in elective cancer surgery: a double-blind randomized multicentre trial with venographic assessment. Br J Surg 1997;84:1099–1103.
111. Levine M, Raskob G, Landefeld S, Kearon C. Hemorrhagic complications of anticoagulant treatment. Chest 2001;119:108S–121S.
112. Agnelli G, Piovella F, Buoncristiani P, et al. Enoxaparin plus compression stockings compared with compression stockings alone in the prevention of venous thromboembolism after elective neurosurgery. N Engl J Med 1998;339:80–85.
113. Nurmohamed MT, van Riel AM, Henkens CM; et al. Low molecular weight heparin and compression stockings in the prevention of venous thromboembolism in neurosurgery. Thromb Haemost 1996;75:233–238.
114. Fisher B, Dignam J, Wolmark N, et al. Tamoxifen and chemotherapy for lymph node negative, estrogen receptor positive breast cancer. J Natl Cancer Inst 1997;89:1673–1682.

115. Levine MN. Prevention of thrombotic disorders in cancer patients undergoing chemotherapy. Thromb Haemost 1997;78: 133–136.
116. Saphner T, Tormey DC, Gray R. Venous and arterial thrombosis in patients who received adjuvant chemotherapy for breast cancer. J Clin Oncol 1991;9:286–294.
117. Pritchard KI, Paterson AHG, Paul NA, et al., for the National Cancer Institute of Canada Clinical Trials Group. Increased thromboembolic complications with concurrent tamoxifen and chemotherapy in a randomized trial of adjuvant therapy for women with breast cancer. J Clin Oncol 1996;14:2731–2737.
118. Levine M, Hirsh J, Gent M, et al. Double-blind randomised trial of very-low-dose warfarin for prevention of thromboembolism in stage IV breast cancer. Lancet 1994;343:886–889.
119. Barbui T, Finazzi G, Grassi A, Marchioli R. Thrombosis in cancer patients treated with hematopoietic growth factors—a meta-analysis. Thromb Haemost 1996;75:368–371.
120. Monreal M, Alastrue A, Rull M, et al. Upper extremity deep vein thrombosis in cancer patients with venous access devices—prophylaxis with a low molecular weight heparin (Fragmin). Thromb Haemost 1996;75:251–253.
121. Ginsberg JS. Management of venous thromboembolism. N Engl J Med 1996;335:1816–1824.
122. Levine MN, Hirsh J, Gent M. A randomized trial comparing activated thromboplastin time with heparin assay in patients with acute venous thromboembolism requiring large daily doses of heparin. Arch Intern Med 1994;154:49–56.
123. Hirsh J, Levine MN. Low molecular weight heparin. Blood 1992;79:1–17.
124. Nurmohamed MT, Roendaal FR, Buller HR, et al. Low molecular weight heparin versus standard heparin in general and orthopedic surgery. A meta-analysis. Lancet 1992; 340:152–155.
125. Levine M, Gent M, Hirsh J, et al. A comparison of low molecular weight heparin administered primarily at home with unfractionated heparin administered in the hospital for proximal deep vein thrombosis. N Engl J Med 1996; 334:677–681.
126. The Columbus Investigators. Low molecular weight heparin in the treatment of patients with venous thromboembolism. N Engl J Med 1997;337:657–662.
127. Koopman MMW, Prandoni P, Piovella F, et al. Treatment of venous thrombosis with intravenous unfractionated heparin administered in the hospital as compared with subcutaneous low molecular weight heparin administered at home. N Engl J Med 1996;334:682–687.
128. Harrison L, McGinnis J, Crowther M, et al. Assessment of outpatient treatment of deep vein thrombosis with low molecular weight heparin. Arch Intern Med 1998;158:2001–2003.
129. Wells P, Kovacs MJ, Bormanis J, et al. Expanding eligibility for outpatient treatment of deep vein thrombosis and pulmonary embolism with low molecular weight heparin. Arch Intern Med 1998;158:1809–1812.
130. Simonneau G, Sors H, Charbonnier B, et al. A comparison of low-molecular-weight heparin with unfractionated heparin for acute pulmonary embolism. N Engl J Med 1997;337:663–669.
131. Kovacs MJ, Anderson D, Morrow B, et al. Outpatient treatment of pulmonary embolism with Dalteparin. Thromb Haemost 2000;83:209–211.
132. Gitter MJ, Jaeger TM, Peterson TM, et al. Bleeding and thromboembolism during anticoagulant therapy: a population-based study in Rochester, Minnesota. Mayo Clin Proc 1995;70:725–733.
133. Wester JPJ, deValk HW, Nieuwenhuis HK, et al. Risk factors for bleeding during treatment of acute venous thromboembolism. Thromb Haemost 1996;76:682–688.
134. Bona RD, Sivjee KY, Hickey AD, et al. The efficacy and safety of oral anticoagulation in patients with cancer. Thromb Haemost 1995;74:1055–1058.
135. Prandoni P, Lensing AWA, Cogo A, et al. The long-term clinical course of acute deep venous thrombosis. Ann Intern Med 1996;125:1–7.
136. Hutten BA, Prins MH, Gent M, et al. Incidence of recurrent thromboembolic and bleeding complications among patients with venous thromboembolism in relation to both malignancy and achieved International Normalized Ratio: a retrospective analysis. J Clin Oncol 2000;18:3078–3083.
137. Palareti G, Legnani C, Lee A, et al. A comparison of the safety and efficacy of oral anticoagulation for the treatment of venous thromboembolic disease in patients with or without malignancy. Thromb Haemost 2000;84:805–810.
138. Kearon C, Gent M, Hirsh J, et al. A comparison of three months of anticoagulation with extended anticoagulation for a first episode of idiopathic venous thromboembolism. N Engl J Med 1999;340:901–907.
139. Levine MN, Lee A. Treatment of venous thrombosis in cancer patients. Semin Thromb Hemost 1998;25:245–249.
140. Monreal M, Lafoz E, Olive A, et al. Comparison of subcutaneous unfractionated heparin with low molecular weight heparin (Fragmin) in patients with venous thromboembolism and contraindications to coumarin. Thromb Haemost 1994;71:7–11.
141. Pini M, Aiello S, Manotti C, et al. Low molecular weight heparin versus warfarin in the prevention of recurrences after deep vein thrombosis. Thromb Haemost 1994;72:191–197.
142. Decousus H, Leizorovicz A, Parent F, et al. A clinical trial of vena caval filters in the prevention of pulmonary embolism in patients with proximal deep-vein thrombosis. Prevention du Risque d'Emblie Pulmonaire par Interruption Cave Study Group. N Engl J Med 1998;338:409–415.
143. Streiff MB. Vena caval filters: a comprehensive review. Blood 2000;95:3669–3677.
144. Bona RD. Thrombotic complications of central venous catheters in cancer patients. Semin Thromb Hemost 1999;25:147–157.
145. Zacharski LR, Henderson WG, Rickles FR, et al. Effect of sodium warfarin on survival in small cell carcinoma of the lung: VA Cooperative Study #75. JAMA 1981;245:831–835.
146. Bastida E. The metastatic cascade: Potential approaches for the inhibition of metastasis. Semin Thromb Hemost 1988;14:66–72.
147. Zacharski LR, Henderson WG, Rickles FR, et al. Rationale and experimental design for the VA Cooperative Study of anticoagulation (warfarin) in the treatment of cancer. Cancer 1979; 44:732–741.
148. Chahinian AP, Propert KJ, Ware JH, et al. A randomized trial of anticoagulation with warfarin and alternating chemotherapy in extensive small cell lung cancer by the Cancer and Leukemia Group B. J Clin Oncol 1989;7:993–1002.
149. Torngren S, Rieger A. The influence of heparin and curable resection on the survival of colorectal cancer. Acta Chir Scand 1983;149:427–429.
150. Zacharski LR, Henderson WG, Rickles FR, et al. Platelets and malignancy: Rationale and experimental design for the VA Cooperative Study of RA233 in the treatment of cancer. Am J Clin Oncol 1982;5:593–609.
151. Frost P, Hart I, Kerbel R. The hemostatic system in malignancy. Cancer Metastasis Rev 1992;11:223–234.
152. Kramer B. Historical overview of clinical experience with anticoagulant therapy. In: Honn KV, Sloane BF (Eds.): Hemostatic Mechanisms and Metastasis. Boston; Martinus Nijhoff, 1984; pp. 355–368.
153. Gastpar H. Platelet–cancer cell interaction in metastasis formation. J Med 1977;8:103–114.
154. Thornes RD. Oral anticoagulant therapy of human cancer. J Med 1974;5:83–91.
155. Aisner J, Goutsou M, Maurer LH, et al. Intensive combination chemotherpay, concurrent chest irradiation, and warfarin for the treatment of limited disease small cell lung cancer: a Cancer and Leukemia Group B pilot study. J Clin Oncol 1992;10:1230–1236.
156. Maurer LH, Herndon JE II, Hollis DR, et al. Randomized trial of chemotherapy and radiation therapy with or without warfarin for limited stage small cell lung cancer: a Cancer and Leukemia Group B study. J Clin Oncol 1997;15:3378–3387.

157. Zacharski LR, Moritz TE, Baczek LA, et al. Effect of RA233 (Mopidamole) on survival in carcinoma of the lung and colon. J Natl Cancer Inst 1988;80:90-97.
158. Lebeau B, Chastang CL, Brechot JM, et al. Subcutaneous heparin treatment increases survival in small cell lung cancer. Cancer 1994;74:39–45.
159. von Tempelhoff GF, Dietrich M, Niemann F et al. Blood coagulation and thrombosis in patients with ovarian malignancy. Thromb Haemost 1997;77:456–461.
160. Green D, Hull RD, Brant R, Pineo GF. Lower mortality in cancer patients treated with low molecular weight versus standard heparin. Lancet 1992;339:1476 (letter).
161. Hull RD, Raskob GL, Pineo GF. Subcutaneous low molecular weight heparin compared with continuous intravenous heparin in the treatment of proximal vein thrombosis. N Engl J Med 1992;326:975–982.
162. Prandoni P, Lensing AWA, Buller HR. Comparison of subcutaneous low molecular weight heparin with intravenous standard heparin in proximal deep vein thrombosis. Lancet 1992;339:441–445.
163. Lensing AW, Prins MH, Davidson BL, et al. Treatment of deep venous thrombosis with low molecular weight heparins. A meta-analysis. Arch Intern Med 1995;155:601–607.
164. Siragussa S, Cosmi B, Piovella F, et al. Low molecular weight heparins and unfractionated heparin in the treatment of patients with acute venous thromboembolism: results of a meta-analysis. Am J Med 1996;100:269–277.
165. Wentzien TH, O'Reilly RA, Kearns PJ. Prospective evaluation of anticoagulant reversal with oral vitamin K1 while continuing warfarin therapy unchanged. Chest 1998;114:1546–1550.
166. Crowther MA, Julian J, McCarty D, et al. Treatment of warfarin-associated coagulopathy with oral vitamin K: a randomized controlled trial. Lancet 2000;356:1551–1553.

CHAPTER 22

Thrombotic Thrombocytopenic Purpura

Joel L. Moake, M.D.

Thrombotic thrombocytopenic purpura (TTP) is the most extensive and dangerous intravascular platelet clumping disorder. For about 55 years after the initial recognition of the disease, almost everyone with TTP died quickly. Physicians were both fascinated by the dramatic clinical presentations and horrified by the near-100% mortality rate. Many hematologists, even with their limited experience trying to manage the rarely encountered patient, believed intuitively that understanding the mechanism of systemic intravascular platelet aggregation in TTP would provide important insights into this enigmatic condition and also into the pathophysiology of common, localized forms of arterial platelet thrombosis (e.g., heart attack and stroke).

Until the 1970s and 1980s, most physicians had never seen a case of TTP. Hematologists after years in practice could recall one or two patients, at most. Then, for unknown reasons, the disease increased in prevalence. About 1000 to 2000 new cases of acute idiopathic TTP now occur annually in North America. At the Texas Medical Center, 30 to 40 new TTP patients are admitted each year (compared with 0 to 2 per year in the 1970s). This is a true increase in acute idiopathic TTP, and not simply improvement in recognition of a disorder with long-established clinical and laboratory characteristics. Furthermore, several drugs in common usage in the 1990s (e.g., ticlopidine) have been found to induce in a fraction of the many exposed patients TTP that is clinically indistinguishable from the acute idiopathic type. Therefore, the remark several years ago about paroxysmal nocturnal hemoglobinuria by Dr. Wendell Rosse of the Duke University Medical Center that "more people study the disease than have it" no longer applies to TTP.

HISTORICAL REVIEW

Eli Moschcowitz was born in Hungary in 1879 and was brought to the United States at the age of 2 years. He received his M.D. degree from the College of Physicians and Surgeons of Columbia University in 1900 and subsequently trained in surgery and histopathology in New York City and Berlin.[1]

On September 15, 1923, Moschcowitz admitted "Patient KZ," a 16-year-old girl, to the Beth Israel Hospital in New York City. She had the abrupt onset of petechiae, anemia, and pallor, and these were followed rapidly by paralysis, coma, and, on September 20, 1923, death. Moschcowitz believed that he had observed a new disease and reported his young patient in 1924 in the *Proceedings of the New York Pathological Society*.[2] Terminal arterioles and capillaries in the unlucky teenager were occluded by hyaline thrombi, later determined to be composed mostly of platelets, without perivascular inflammation or endothelial desquamation. Moschcowitz suspected a "powerful poison which had both agglutinative and hemolytic properties"[2] as the cause of this frightening new disease, now known as thrombotic thrombocytopenic purpura (TTP).

Before there was any inkling of the pathophysiology of TTP, Byrnes and Khurana[3] reported in 1977 that relapses in chronic TTP could be prevented or reversed by the infusion of only a few units of fresh frozen plasma (FFP) or its cryoprecipitate-poor fraction (cryosupernatant). It was also discovered by Byrnes and Khurana,[3] Bukowski,[4] and their colleagues (and subsequently confirmed by studies in several hundred patients[5,6]) that plasma infusion combined with plasmapheresis (plasma exchange) allows most patients to survive an episode of TTP. In the majority of these patients, the disorder neither recurs nor produces persistent organ damage.[6]

In 1982,[7] "unusually large" von Willebrand factor (vWF) multimers found in the plasma of patients with the rarest subtype of the disorder, chronic relapsing TTP, were proposed by Moake and coworkers as the agglutinative substance. Unusually large vWF multimers are: (1) more immense than even the largest vWF multimeric species normally in plasma; (2) similar to a subset of huge vWF forms secreted by human endothelial cells; (3) designed to entangle (after retrograde secretion by endothelial cells) with subendothelial fibrous components, in order to maximize vWF-mediated platelet adhesion onto subendothelium exposed by vascular damage; and (4) eliminated rapidly by a vigilant processing activity[7,8] in normal plasma that prevents the especially adhesive unusually large vWF multimers[7] from going far, or staying long, after their antegrade secretion into the bloodstream. The 1982 report concluded that "patients with chronic relapsing TTP have a defect in the processing of very large VIII:vWF multimers after synthesis and secretion by endothelial cells, and . . . this defect makes the patients susceptible to periodic relapses."[7]

CLINICAL MANIFESTATIONS OF TTP

Severe thrombocytopenia and hemolytic anemia with many fragmented red cells (schistocytes) on the blood smear, along with neurologic symptoms and signs, constitute the characteristic clinical triad. Neurologic disorders may range in severity from transient bizarre mentation and behavior to sensory-motor deficits, aphasia, seizures, or coma. The peripheral blood smear typically shows increased reticulocytes (polychromatic large erythrocytes) and often nucleated red blood cells, in response to the intense hemolysis. A minority of patients also have fever and some have renal dysfunction. The latter usually includes proteinuria and hematuria, as well as azotemia. Symptoms and signs of ischemia in the retinal (visual defects), coronary (conduction abnormalities), and abdominal circulation (abdominal pain) may be present. Abdominal presentations of TTP have become ever more commonly recognized during the past several years, so that perhaps 5% to 10% of TTP episodes may now begin with an abdominal presentation.

The early, evolving, and overt manifestations of an acute TTP episode, along with the therapeutic actions triggered, are summarized in Table 22–1. A patient can appear in the emergency department or physician's office in any stage of the disorder.

LABORATORY FINDINGS

In TTP, the degree of thrombocytopenia reflects the extent of intravascular platelet clumping. Platelet counts are often less than $20,000/\mu L$ during acute episodes of TTP. Erythrocyte fragmentation occurs as red cells attempt to bypass at high flow rates the microvascular platelet aggregates, producing the characteristic schistocytes on peripheral blood films (Fig. 22–1). Occasionally, schistocytes do not appear until a day or two following the initial clinical presentation. Hemolysis is predominantly intravascular and, along with tissue damage, contributes to the increased serum levels of lactate dehydrogenase (LDH). Most of the LDH is, however, derived from injured tissue cells.[9] Thrombocytopenia, hemolytic anemia, schistocytosis, and LDH elevations—as well as neurologic manifestations—are usually less extreme in hemolytic-uremic syndrome (HUS) than in TTP.

Coagulation studies are characteristically normal in the early stages of a TTP episode. If there is considerable tissue necrosis, however (as during an especially severe or protracted episode of TTP), secondary disseminated intravascular coagulation (DIC) may occur as a result of overactivation of the coagulation pathway. This overactivation follows the binding of factor VIIa to exposed tissue factor on injured tissue cells. The ominous development of secondary DIC can be detected by the appearance of elevated levels of D-dimers or fibrin degradation products, prolongation of the prothrombin or activated partial thromboplastin times, and a decreasing fibrinogen level.

TYPES OF TTP

Since the general application of plasma therapy, many patients have survived episodes of TTP. It has become apparent that there are several conditions associated with the disorder, and more than one etiology[10] (Table 22–2). The majority of adult patients with TTP (about two thirds) have a *single episode* that never recurs (presuming successful treatment). About one third of adult patients who recover from an initial TTP episode will have *recurrences* at irregular intervals. In the rarest type, *chronic relapsing TTP,* frequent episodes occur at regular (approximately 3 to 4 week) intervals. Children are

Table 22–1 • REAL-TIME CONSIDERATIONS IN TTP

	EARLY?	EVOLVING?	OVERT
Thrombocytopenia	75,000–100,000	30,000–75,000	<30,000 μL
Schistocytes	Occasional	Some	Many
Increased LDH	Slight	Several-fold	Extreme
CNS abnormalities	No	+/–	Usually
GI abnormalities	No	+/–	+/–
Renal abnormalities	No	+/–	+/–
ACTION	Observe	Glucocorticoids	Glucocorticoids
	Evaluate for other diagnosis	Plasma exchange	Plasma exchange

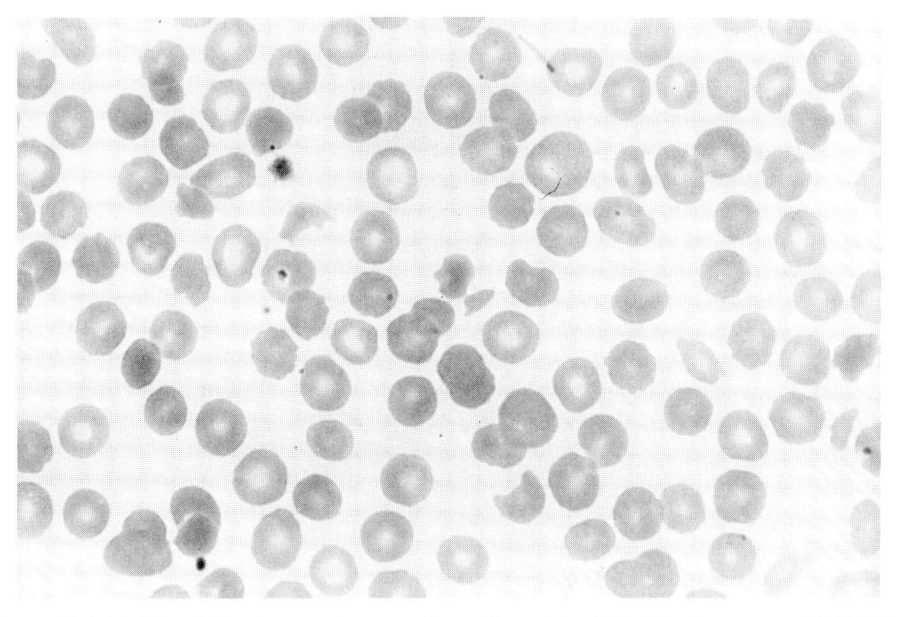

Figure 22–1 Peripheral blood smear from a patient with evolving TTP (platelet count = 54,000/μL).

more likely than adults to develop *chronic relapsing TTP*.[11,12]

During the past few years, the structurally similar platelet function inhibitors ticlopidine (Ticlid)[13,14] and clopidogrel (Plavix)[15] have been associated with the induction of TTP in a fraction of exposed patients. These two drugs, which differ from each other by a single carboxymethyl group, inhibit a platelet adenosine diphosphate (ADP) receptor site and are used to suppress arterial platelet thrombosis. A fraction of patients with human immunodeficiency virus-1 (HIV-1) infection also develop TTP (see Chapter 33).

HUS usually occurs as a single, nonrecurrent episode, occasionally during the postpartum period.[16] Rarely, however, does HUS occur *during* pregnancy. In contrast, TTP *does occur during pregnancy*, especially the last trimester.

Mitomycin C, cyclosporine FK506 (tacrolimus), *chemotherapeutic agents* in combination, and *total-body irradiation* have been associated with the subsequent development of thrombotic microangiopathy.[17–21] The syndrome often more closely resembles HUS than TTP, and usually develops weeks to months after exposure.[20,22] Patients who have been treated for various illnesses with bone marrow transplantation make up a relatively large subgroup.[22] Thrombotic microangiopathy has also been reported after kidney, liver, heart, and lung transplantation.[21]

PATHOPHYSIOLOGY

von Willebrand Factor

Early vascular lesions in TTP consist almost exclusively of platelet thrombi without evidence of perivascular inflammation or other overt vessel wall pathology.[23] Microvascular ("hyaline") occlusions are seen in most organs, including the lungs and eyes. Most frequently involved are the brain, heart, spleen, kidneys, pancreas, and adrenals.

TTP is likely to be the result of the abnormal presence in the circulation of a platelet-aggregating agent. In fact, the histiopathologic and clinical findings in human TTP suggest that organ ischemia and thrombocytopenia may be caused by direct, potentially reversible, platelet aggregation in the microcirculation of multiple organs concurrently. Any conclusions about the pathophysiology of platelet aggregation in TTP must be reconciled with the immunohistochemical studies of TTP thrombi by Asada and coworkers[24] that reveal an abundance of vWF with little fibrinogen/fibrin, implying that vWF is involved in microvascular platelet aggregation in TTP.

vWF monomers (280 kD) are linked by disulfide bonds into multimers of varying sizes that range into the millions of daltons. vWF multimers are produced within megakaryocytes and endothelial cells and are stored within the α-granules of platelets and the Weibel-Palade bodies of endothelial cells. The predominant sources of plasma vWF multimers are endothelial cells. The entire constellation of vWF multimers found in the normal circulation is produced within both megakaryocytes and endothelial cells. Additionally, both cell types construct vWF multimeric forms that are even larger in

---

Table 22–2 • CLINICAL TYPES OF TTP

Chronic relapsing
Acute idiopathic (± recurrence)
Drug-induced:
   Ticlopidine (Ticlid)
   Clopidogrel (Plavix)
   Mitomycin[a]
   Cyclosporin[a]
Bone marrow transplantation/chemotherapy[a]

[a] Clinical presentation often more similar to HUS than TTP.

size than those found in normal plasma (*unusually large [UL] vWF multimers*).[7] ULvWF forms may be more effective than the largest plasma vWF forms at binding under the influence of elevated fluid shear stresses to the glycoprotein (GP)Ib component of platelet GPIb-IX-V receptors, and to platelet GPIIb/IIIa complexes, resulting in aggregation.[25]

The laboratories of Tsai in New York[26] and Furlan and colleagues in Switzerland[27] described independently a metalloproteinase activity in normal plasma that is capable of degrading vWF multimers by cleaving the 842Tyr-843Met peptide bond of vWF monomeric subunits. This metalloproteinase can cleave vWF multimers in vitro if the vWF forms are partially unfolded mechanically (as by shear stress) or chemically (as by guanidine-HCl).[26,28] Alternatively, the metalloproteinase activity in vitro can be accentuated by low ionic strength or urea in the presence of divalent cations (especially Ba^{2+}).[27] Although these conditions for detecting activity of the vWF-cleaving metalloproteinase in vitro are artificial, one important finding suggests that the enzyme may have a role in normal physiology: cleavage in vitro of vWF and ULvWF multimers results in the generation of 176-kD and 140-kD vWF fragments identical to those found in normal plasma.[26]

Serial studies of plasma samples from patients during single episodes of TTP often have shown either the presence of ULvWF multimers or, alternatively, the absence of the largest plasma vWF forms.[7,29] The presence of ULvWF forms in TTP patient plasma may reflect the failure of TTP plasma to process adequately the ULvWF multimers released from endothelial cells. The disappearance of large plasma vWF forms in some TTP patient plasma samples during acute TTP episodes may be predominantly because these ULvWF forms, along with the largest plasma vWF multimers, bind to platelets causing aggregation and clearance of ULvWF from plasma.

Recently conducted serial flow cytometry studies of EDTA-whole blood samples from patients with initial episode, intermittent, or chronic relapsing TTP confirm that ULvWF and large vWF multimers are the likely aggregating agents in TTP.[30] The amount of vWF bound to single platelets is increased significantly during TTP relapses relative to remission periods in patients with acute idiopathic single-episode, intermittent, and chronic relapsing types of TTP. No concordance has been observed between vWF and P-selectin expression on most samples of TTP patient platelets. This latter finding suggests that the vWF bound to platelets in TTP is likely to be from plasma, rather than from platelet α-granules (platelet α-granules contain both vWF and P-selectin).

Several patients with chronic relapsing TTP reported in 1997 by Furlan and coworkers[12] were found to have decreased or absent vWF-cleaving metalloproteinase activity. This deficiency was not associated with an inhibitor and was, therefore, considered to be congenital. In 1998, Furlan[31,32] as well as Tsai and Lian,[33] independently reported data obtained on adult initial-episode and intermittent TTP patients. The two groups of investigators found that almost all TTP patient samples evaluated had deficient vWF-cleaving metalloproteinase activity during, but not after, TTP episodes. An inhibitor of the vWF-cleaving metalloproteinase activity was responsible for this deficiency in most of the patients with initial-episode and intermittent TTP studied further.[31–33] The inhibitor was an IgG antibody (presumably an autoantibody) in the patient samples analyzed for inhibitor type.

Chronic relapsing TTP patients almost always have unusually large vWF multimers in their plasma, especially between episodes when these gigantic multimeric forms may be less actively attaching to platelets.[7,29] Unusually large vWF forms are also often present in plasma samples from patients during, but not after, acute single TTP episodes.[29] The studies of Furlan and coworkers[12,31,32] and Tsai and Lian[33] imply that either chronic absence of the plasma vWF-cleaving metalloproteinase (in chronic relapsing TTP) or transient inhibition of the enzyme by autoantibodies (during acute idiopathic episodes) is the likely explanation for these findings. It has been determined recently that ticlopidine- or clopidogrel-associated TTP patients also have ticlopidine- or clopidogrel-induced antibodies against the vWF-cleaving metalloproteinase.[14,15]

What is the consequence of the failure to eliminate unusually large vWF multimers after their secretion from endothelial cells into the plasma? In children with chronic relapsing TTP, the unusually large vWF multimers are associated with periodic platelet aggregation that may be triggered by elevated shear stresses in the microcirculation.[11] Elevated fluid shearing forces induce platelet aggregation in vitro by stimulating the binding of large or unusually large vWF multimers to platelet GP Ib-IX-V and activated GP-IIb-IIIa receptors.[25,34,35] Fibrinogen cannot substitute for vWF in aggregation stimulated by high shear stresses.[25,34] It has been suggested by Moake and coworkers[11] that in chronic relapsing TTP, the accumulation of ULvWF forms in the bloodstream may periodically (about every 3 to 4 weeks) exceed a threshold level required for attachment to platelets (and intravascular aggregation) under the high-shear conditions of the microcirculation.

In summary, the plasma vWF multimeric patterns, platelet-bound vWF data, and studies of the vWF-cleaving metalloproteinase imply that adult TTP may often be an autoimmune disorder associated with the defective breakdown of a platelet-aggregating agent, i.e., ULvWF multimeric forms, after their release from systemic endothelial cells. The cause of this putative transient or intermittent defect of immune regulation is presently unknown, as is the reason the vWF-cleaving metalloproteinase is selectively targeted for autoantibody attack. The vWF-cleaving metalloproteinase autoantibodies may appear for only a brief period (single-episode TTP) or may recur at unpredictable intervals (intermittant TTP). If a TTP patient survives an initial episode and suffers no subsequent relapse, vWF multimeric forms in recovery samples are almost always normal. In contrast, ULvWF multimers found in adult-patient plasma samples after recovery may indicate persistent subclinical autoantibody-mediated interference with the vWF-cleaving metalloproteinase. In chronic relapsing TTP, which usually begins in childhood, there may be a congenital defect in the production or activity of the vWF-cleaving metalloproteinase. Occasional children or adolescents may produce autoantibodies against vWF metalloproteinase that are associated with single-episode or intermittently recurrent TTP (as in adults). The pathophysiology of platelet aggregation in bone marrow transplantation-associated microangiopathy, and in HUS, is not established. In neither condition is there a deficiency or inhibition of vWF-cleaving metalloproteinase activity.

Other Observations

In 1997, five patients from the rural midwestern United States with a TTP-like illness were reported to have rod-shaped, *Bartonella bacilliformis*-like organisms adherent to 0.1% to 2% of circulating erythrocytes during disease episodes.[36] Four of the five patients survived, and two of these four were treated with the tetracycline derivative, doxycycline, instead of plasma exchange! Previous claims of various causative microorganisms in TTP have not been verified. It will, therefore, be of intense interest to see if other clinical investigators confirm this provocative report.

Apoptosis is induced in cultured microvascular endothelial cells, but not in macrovascular human umbilical vein endothelial cells (HUVECs), by exposure to the serum of some TTP or HUS patients.[37] The mechanism of this in vitro phenomenon presently is unknown, but does not require endothelial cell GPIV or the presence of tumor necrosis factor-α (TNF-α) or other toxic cytokines.

Experimental findings from Canada and Italy support a relationship between TTP episodes and the presence in patient plasma of either a Ca^{2+}-dependent cysteine proteinase (calpain)[38] or a lysosomal-derived non-Ca^{2+}-dependent cathepsin-type cysteine proteinase.[39] It is possible that these cysteine proteinases may enter the bloodstream of some TTP or HUS patients from injured tissue sources or apoptic endothelial cells.

CAUSES OF TTP

About twice as many women as men develop acute idiopathic TTP. Most patients are in the 20- to 60-year age range, no racial or seasonal predisposition is obvious, and case clustering is rare. The majority of patients who develop acute idiopathic TTP have no identifiable associated risk factor, although TTP during pregnancy or the postpartum period accounts for a small percentage of cases. Neame[40] suggested that abnormal immune modulation might contribute to the etiology in these circumstances. Indeed, a specific defect in immune regulation is likely to be the basis for the "escape" of autoantibody production against the vWF-cleaving metalloproteinase in most acute idiopathic TTP patients. How ticlopidine or clopidogrel might promote this anti-vWF-cleaving metalloproteinase "escape" in occasional patients is not presently known.

The possibility that immunologic events are involved in acute idiopathic TTP is supported by studies that suggest macrophage/lymphocyte activation in some patients.[41,42] Elevated levels of interleukin (IL)-1, IL-6, the soluble IL-2 receptor, TNF-α, and transforming growth factor-β (TGF-β) have all been reported in the disorder. There is also preliminary evidence that patients lacking the class II HLA antigen, DR53, may be more susceptible to thrombotic microangiopathy.[43]

Acute, idiopathic TTP has been associated occasionally with diseases characterized by autoimmune or other types of abnormal immune responses, including systemic lupus erythromatosus (SLE),[44] autoimmune "idiopathic" thrombocytopenic purpura (ITP),[45,46] and the acquired immunodeficiency syndrome (AIDS)[46-48] (see Chapter 33).

Harkness and colleagues[23] found that early vascular lesions in the brain consist almost exclusively of platelet thrombi with little or no fibrin, and without evidence of perivascular inflammation or other vessel wall pathology. TTP may, therefore, be a disease of direct platelet aggregation in the microcirculation of the brain and other organs that is not preceded by endothelial desquamation and platelet adherence to exposed subendothelium. This putative direct platelet aggregation is potentially reversible by effective therapeutic intervention. Immunohistochemical study of early TTP lesions has revealed an abundance of vWF with little fibrinogen present.[24] The opposite findings are characteristic of thrombotic lesions in DIC[24] (see Chapter 12). vWF multimers within these thrombi may function as polymeric bridges promoting platelet–platelet cohesion (aggregation). The relative predominance of platelets (rather than fibrin) as the occlusive component in microvessels, as well as the paucity of laboratory coagulation abnormalities, also distinguish TTP from DIC.

REPRESENTATIVE CASES OF TTP

Case 1 • A 3-month-old girl became pale and jaundiced, and had several transient episodes of hemiparesis. Physical examination was normal. Hemoglobin was 8.4 g/dL, platelets were 11,000/μL, and there were reticulocytes (polychromatophilic red cells) and 3+/4+ schistocytes on her peripheral blood film. Serum LDH level was elevated five-fold and unconjugated bilirubin was increased. Computed tomography of the brain showed ischemic changes.

Platelet-bound vWF was abnormally elevated in an EDTA-whole blood sample obtained soon after admission using flow cytometry. Several days later it was determined that vWF-cleaving metalloproteinase activity was not detectable in a citrate-plasma sample obtained prior to any therapy, and that the sample did not contain any inhibitor directed against the vWF-cleaving metalloproteinase.

Packed red cells and FFP were administered, followed by rapid clinical and hematologic remission during the following 2 days. Neurologic recovery was complete.

A regimen of periodic FFP infusions was tentatively planned (10 mL/kg every 3 weeks) for her probable *chronic relapsing TTP*.

Case 2 • A 22-year-old man developed headache and confusion. He had been healthy previously and was taking no medicine. His hemoglobin was 6.7 g/dL and platelets were 5,000/μL. Schistocytes (4+/4+) and reticulocytes were prominent on his peripheral blood film. The serum LDH level was 10 times normal. Computed tomography did not show intracerebral hemorrhage.

Platelet-bound vWF was abnormally elevated in the admission EDTA-whole blood sample. The citrate-plasma sample obtained before treatment was later found to have no detectable vWF-cleaving metalloproteinase, along with a high titer inhibitor to the vWF-metalloproteinase in normal citrate-plasma.

The patient was given high dose methylprednisolone, packed red cells, immediate FFP infusion, and 3 days of plasma exchange (using FFP) commencing on the night of admission. On day 4 he became comatose, and cryosupernatant was substituted for FFP in the daily exchanges. He awakened on day 7, and neurologic symptoms disappeared by day 8. On day 10, platelets were 43,000/μL; by day 17, platelets were 203,000/μL and LDH levels were normal. Plasma exchange with cryosupernatant was continued for 5 additional days, and then stopped. Glucocorticoids were tapered over a period of weeks. The patient has not had a recurrence of the *acute idiopathic TTP* episode in the subsequent 2 years.

DIFFERENTIAL DIAGNOSIS OF TTP

The constellation of thrombocytopenia, hemolysis, and schistocytosis also occurs (to an extent that is usually less extreme than in TTP) in DIC, pre-eclampsia/eclampsia, the HELLP syndrome (pre-eclampsia-associated hemolytic anemia with elevated liver enzymes and low platelets), malignant hypertension, severe vasculitis, scleroderma with associated hypertension and renal failure, Evans syndrome (concurrent autoimmune thrombocytopenia and direct Coombs' test-positive autoimmune hemolysis), and in patients with a malfunctioning prosthetic cardiac valve (Table 22–3). Of these, the most frequently troublesome diagnostic dilemma is between TTP or HUS and DIC.

DISTINCTION BETWEEN TTP AND HUS

Platelet aggregates in the microcirculation in TTP produce fluctuating ischemia or infarction in various organs,

Table 22–3 • **DIFFERENTIAL DIAGNOSIS OF TTP**

Hemolytic uremic syndrome
Disseminated intravascular coagulation
Evans syndrome[a]
Malignant hypertension
Malfunctioning prosthetic cardiac valve
Severe vasculitis
Pregnancy ⎡ Pre-eclampsia/eclampsia
⎣   HELLP syndrome[b]

[a] Autoimmune thrombocytopenia/hemolysis.
[b] Hemolytic anemia, elevated liver enzymes, and low platelets.

Table 22–4 • **DISTINCTION OF TTP FROM HUS**

- Thrombocytopenia, schistocytosis, and LDH elevation usually more severe in TTP
- Renal ischemia/injury usually more severe in HUS
- Nonrenal organ ischemia usually more severe in TTP
- Plasma vWf-cleaving metalloproteinase activity low in TTP

including the brain in 50% to 71% of episodes.[5,6] In the closely related hemolytic-uremic syndrome (HUS), initially reported by Gasser and colleagues in 1955,[49] the ischemia is predominantly renal. Thrombocytopenia, erythrocyte fragmentation, and increased serum levels of LDH are usually less extreme in HUS (Table 22–4). However, the variability of organ dysfunction in TTP (including renal abnormalities in 50–75% of episodes)[5,6] and the occasional extrarenal manifestations in HUS can make the two syndromes difficult to distinguish.[5,6,16] If these clinical observations are combined with the fact that TTP and HUS are sometimes associated with similar inciting cofactors (e.g., pregnancy, chemotherapy/total-body irradiation), then it is no wonder that many hematologists suspect that TTP and HUS may be different clinical manifestations of some related intravascular platelet aggregation mechanism.

HUS is a triad of thrombocytopenia, acute renal failure, and intravascular hemolytic anemia with schistocytosis and elevated serum LDH. Renal dysfunction is severe in HUS, in contrast to most cases of TTP, and often requires dialysis. Oliguria, anuria, chronic renal failure, and hypertension sometimes complicate HUS, whereas this is uncommon in patients who recover from episodes of TTP. Although the microvascular platelet aggregation is usually predominantly renal, other organs may sometimes also be involved.[16,50] The occasional extrarenal manifestations in HUS can sometimes muddle the distinction between HUS and TTP.

Truly recurrent TTP (as opposed to a single protracted episode with brief intervening periods of incomplete remission[6]) occurs in at least 11% to 28% of TTP patients.[5,6] HUS usually occurs as a single episode, except in rare individuals who have a familial, recurrent type of the disease. In these latter patients (often children), the level of the plasma complement control protein, factor H, is abnormally low. The result is overactivation of complement component 3 (C3) whenever the alternative complement pathway is activated.[51] In adults, HUS may follow the administration of mitomycin, cyclosporin, quinine, total-body irradiation, or multiple chemotherapeutic agents.[10,16] In children, HUS is often associated with gastroenteritis caused by cytotoxin-producing serotypes of *Escherichia coli* (e.g., 0157:H7) or *Shigella* species.[52]

TTP and HUS are *clinical diagnoses*. Tissue obtained from the biopsy of bone marrow, gingiva, or kidney may be obtained at a time when there are only a few (or no) arterial thrombi in the microvessels of the area sampled. This may account for the finding of characteristic microvascular hyaline thrombi in only about 50% of gingival biopsies obtained from patients considered on the basis of clinical evidence to have TTP.[53] Biopsy samples are usually not necessary for diagnosis. In some circumstances, it is not even safe to do the procedure.

TTP and HUS may be manifestations of a similar mechanism of microvascular platelet aggregation. If the platelet aggregation is systemic and extensive, and especially if the central nervous system is involved, the disorder is called "TTP." If platelet aggregation is relatively less extensive, and predominantly involves the kidneys, the patient is considered to have "HUS." Severe renal involvement in a "TTP" patient, or extra-renal manifestations in a patient with "HUS," can hopelessly obfuscate clinical boundaries between the two syndromes. Furlan and colleagues[32] have provided evidence that a single laboratory test may enable physicians to untangle TTP from HUS. Patients diagnosed with TTP had little or no plasma vWF-cleaving metalloproteinase activity, whereas the plasma activity was normal (or nearly so) in patients considered to have familial or acquired HUS. These provocative findings may, at last, provide the basis for more precise differentiation of the two entities. The results probably also explain why plasma therapy, which is frequently so effective in TTP, is often disappointing in acquired HUS.

TREATMENT OF TTP

According to some series,[5,6] in nearly 90% of patients with acute TTP episodes the process can be treated successfully by intensive plasma manipulation. This is best done using daily *plasma exchanges,* i.e., the combination of plasmapheresis and plasma infusion with normal platelet-poor FFP (3 to 4 L) (Table 22–5). Skipping even 1 day prior to complete remission may lead to rapid relapse. More than one exchange per day has not been demonstrated to be beneficial. *Cryosupernatant* is at least as effective as FFP in plasma-exchange procedures.[54,55] Compared to FFP, cryosupernatant is relatively deficient in fibrinogen and fibronectin. Perhaps even more important, cryosupernatant does not contain the largest vWF forms that are present in normal FFP and in the cryoprecipitate fraction of FFP.[54] The process of treating plasma with a solvent and detergent to inactivate lipid-envelope viruses (HIV-1; hepatitis B and C) also removes large vWF multimers. Solvent/detergent-plasma is effective in treating TTP episodes.[11] Transfusions or exchange transfusions with fluids other than plasma, cryosupernatant, or solvent/detergent-treated plasma (e.g., albumin alone; concentrated immunoglobulin) are usually ineffective and cannot be recommended.

It is presumed that the infusion of normal plasma or cryosupernatant is providing supplemental quantities of the vWF-cleaving metalloproteinase that is inhibited by autoantibodies in single episode and intermittently recurrent TTP.[31–33] It is also presumed that harmful substances (ULvWF multimers[7] and autoantibodies against vWF-cleaving metalloproteinase) are being removed by plasmapheresis.

Relapses in children (or the rare adult) with true chronic relapsing TTP usually respond to, or are prevented by, the infusion of normal FFP alone, cryosupernatant alone, or solvent/detergent-plasma alone (in quantities varying from one to several units) without the need for concurrent plasmapheresis.[11] These observations are compatible with recent reports by Furlan and coworkers[12,56] that a deficiency of plasma vWF-cleaving metalloproteinase is the underlying cause of chronic relapsing TTP.

Older children with an initial episode of TTP may require plasma exchange, perhaps because TTP in this setting is due to autoantibody inhibition of vWF-cleaving metalloproteinase (as in adults), rather than a congenital deficiency of the vWF-cleaving metalloproteinase (as in infants and young children).

Infusion of normal FFP at the rate of about 30 mL/kg/day can be used initially in an adult TTP patient until plasma exchanges can be arranged. This should be within a few hours (but usually no more than 24 hours) in most circumstances. Plasma infusion alone is less effective than plasma exchange[5] and may result in volume overload. TTP patients with coma, cardiac failure, or severe renal dysfunction should receive plasma exchange commencing as soon as possible.

If a patient with a TTP episode is taking either ticlopidine or clopidogrel, or any other suspicious drug (e.g., mitomycin, cyclosporin, quinine), then this medicine should be stopped immediately.

Although some adult patients have recovered from TTP episodes without receiving glucocorticoids, in one large series a subset of TTP patients recovered in association with glucocorticoid therapy alone.[6] On the basis of this study by Bell and colleagues, it is probably prudent to institute glucocorticoid therapy—in association with plasma exchange—in all adult patients with initial or recurrent TTP episodes, unless there is a strong contraindication. The usefulness of glucocorticoids may reflect the proposed autoimmune pathogenesis in many adult patients (e.g., glucocorticoids may suppress the production of autoantibodies against vWF-cleaving metalloproteinase). Bell and coworkers[6] administered prednisolone intravenously immediately following diagnosis in a dosage of about 200 mg/day, and continued it until the patient recovered.

Depending on the hemoglobin level and intensity of hemolysis, red blood cell transfusions may be required. If the platelet count is very low and bleeding is a primary problem, or if intracranial bleeding is demonstrated by computed tomography or magnetic resonance imaging, then transfusion of platelets (at a slow rate) will be necessary. Otherwise, it is probably better to withhold

---

Table 22–5 • TREATMENT OF TTP

- Immediate infusion of FFP (30 mL/kg/day)
- Daily plasma exchange with FFP or cryosupernatant[a] (3–4 L/day)
- Glucocorticoids (e.g., intravenous prednisolone at 200 mg/day)
- Red cells as needed
- Platelets only for life-threatening, including intracerebral, hemorrhage

[a] Cryosupernatant = plasma minus vWf-rich cryoprecipitate

platelet transfusions because they have been temporally associated too frequently with exacerbation of the microcirculatory thrombotic process in the central nervous system.[23,57]

Plasma exchange should be continued for more than 3 days after patients attain complete remission (i.e., a normal neurologic status, a platelet count of 150,000 to 200,000/µL, a rising hemoglobin value, and a normal serum LDH level). Schistocytes in declining numbers often persist for many days on peripheral blood films, and so cannot be used as a reliable marker for remission. With only three additional postremission exchanges, incomplete response with rapid relapse is likely.[6] At least five additional postremission exchanges are currently used empirically in some centers. The procedure should then be stopped, and the glucocorticoid dosage tapered and discontinued over a period of several weeks. A decreasing frequency of plasma exchanges over days or weeks has not been demonstrated to provide any additional benefit in most patients. Platelet counts should be monitored regularly in order to detect incipient relapse. If TTP does recur (see Table 22–1), the same treatment program (i.e., glucocorticoids/plasma exchange) that has previously induced remission should be repeated.

In patients who achieve only a partial response, or worsen during therapy, plasma exchanges should be continued for a period of a few to many additional days in an effort to achieve a complete remission. In these patients, concomitant heparin-associated thrombocytopenia/thrombosis (HITT) should be suspected, especially if LDH values have decreased progressively toward normal during therapy. In the latter situation, all exposure of the patient to heparin should be eliminated (including via keep-open intravenous lines or indwelling catheters, during dialysis, or on the tips of Swan-Ganz catheters).

If a patient with TTP responds minimally within the first few days of therapy, or actually deteriorates, cryosupernatant should be substituted for FFP in the plasma exchange procedures.[54] Some adult TTP patients refractory to FFP exchanges will respond to exchange with cryosupernatant.[54]

Currently available treatment does not work in some patients with acute initial TTP episodes. It is not known if vWF-cleaving metalloproteinase autoantibodies are produced in higher titer, or for longer periods, in this refractory subset. Other forms of therapy can be added if plasma exchanges with FFP or cryosupernatant are incompletely successful—or unsuccessful (Table 22–6). These other options include: addition of vincristine,[58] which depolymerizes platelet microtubules and may alter the availability of GPIb-IX-V or GPIIb/IIIa receptors for vWF on platelet surfaces; splenectomy[59] (removal of immunologic cells involved in vWF-cleaving metalloproteinase autoantibody production?); and addition of other immunosuppressive agents to suppress production of these autoantibodies (e.g., azathioprine [Imuran]).[60] Additional possible newer immunosuppressive approaches are described in the following section.

In some adult patients who turn out to have intermittent TTP, the disorder may not recur for months to years after an initial episode. Recent study of a few patients of this type suggested that frequent relapses may be controlled by splenectomy.[61]

The use of aspirin during TTP episodes is controversial.[62,63] If shear stress-induced, vWF-mediated platelet aggregation in vivo is important in the pathogenesis of platelet aggregation, then aspirin would not be expected to be helpful. Blockade of cyclooxygenase-mediated platelet thromboxane A_2 generation by aspirin does not inhibit shear-induced aggregation in vitro.[64] Aspirin may actually exacerbate hemorrhagic complications in some patients,[62] especially those who are severely thrombocytopenic.

In *summary*, acute idiopathic single-episode (and intermittently relapsing) types of TTP, caused by autoantibody interference with vWF-cleaving metalloproteinase activity, require the infusion of large volumes of metalloproteinase-containing plasma products over days or weeks. Plasmapheresis is almost always also required probably to remove autoantibodies and unusually large vWF multimers (i.e., plasma exchange). Glucocorticoids may also reduce metalloproteinase autoantibody levels, and splenectomy may be required in some patients refractory to plasma exchange. Any drug suspected of inducing TTP should be stopped.

POSSIBLE FUTURE APPROACHES TO THERAPY

It is likely that new additives to blood products capable of destroying viruses without lipid envelopes (e.g., parvovirus B19) will be available soon to supplement, or supplant, the solvent/detergent combination that eliminates HIV, hepatitis B and C, and other lipid-envelope viruses from plasma.[11] It is also probable that the vWF-cleaving metalloproteinase will be purified and provided in concentrated form for therapeutic use.

The vWF-cleaving metalloproteinase has been purified[64a,64b] and determined to be a Zn^{2+}/Ca^{2+}-requiring enzyme of 190 kD encoded on chromosome 9 and produced predominantly by the liver.[64a-64c] The enzyme is now designated specifically as "ADAMTS 13" (A Disintegrin And Metalloproteinase with ThromboSpondin domains, number 13).[64c] Point mutations and deletions within the ADAMTS 13 gene result in severely reduced or absent vWF-cleaving metalloproteinase activity, and cause chronic relapsing TTP.[64d]

Table 22–6 • TREATMENT OF REFRACTORY TTP[a]

- Continued daily plasma exchange with cryosupernatant (3–4 L/day)
- Elimination of heparin from catheter lines and ports
- Vincristine (≤ 2 mg on day 1; then 1 mg on days 4, 7, 10)
- Splenectomy
- Azathioprine (Imuran; 50–150 mg/day)

[a] No remission with glucocorticoids/plasma exchange

If the explanation for TTP in many (or most) adult patients proves to be the production of vWF-cleaving metalloproteinase autoantibodies of IgG type, hope might be revived for protein-A column immunoadsorption as useful therapy. A recent retrospective study contended that column treatment was effective in 7 of 10 patients analyzed who had not responded optimally to plasma exchange.[65] Each daily column run removes only a small percentage of circulating IgG, however, and IgG has an extensive extravascular distribution. A convincing prospective demonstration of any consistent therapeutic effect of ex-vivo protein-A immunoadsorption in TTP using presently marketed columns is not available in the United States. Perhaps more efficient techniques for removing the autoantibodies, combined with infusion of concentrates of the purified enzyme (also not yet available) will increase survival in this desperate situation.

The binding of ULvWF or large vWF forms to platelet GPIb, followed by vWF binding to ADP-activated GPIIb/IIIa complexes, is required for platelet aggregation in fluid shear fields.[25,34,35,66–69] Substances that interfere with shear-induced aggregation may prove useful in the treatment of refractory TTP and, possibly, the prophylaxis of relapsing TTP. These compounds include: (1) recombinant fragments of the human vWF monomer (one is composed of amino acids 445-733) that contain the platelet GPIb binding site, bind to the GPIb component of platelet GPIb-IX-V in the absence of any modulator, and compete with large vWF multimers for binding to GPIb[70]; (2) 7E3Fab, or ReoPro, an intravenous chimeric mouse/human monoclonal antibody fragment directed against platelet GPIIb/IIIa that inhibits the attachment of large vWF multimers to GP IIb/IIIa under conditions of abnormally high shear stess (used to prevent coronary thrombosis or restenosis after angioplasty)[71]; (3) a cyclic heptapeptide, integrilin, containing the lysine-glycine-aspartate (KGD) sequence that is also capable of blocking the binding of vWF to platelet GPIIb/IIIa under high shear[72]; and (4) ADP purinoceptor blockers presently undergoing clinical trials (e.g., AR-C69931MX from AstraZeneca).[73] Each of these compounds could cause life-threatening hemorrhage in a severely thrombocytopenic patient, and so any initial trials will likely be confined to refractory TTP patients, or to other thrombotic microangiopathy patients whose lives are threatened because they are unresponsive to the usual therapeutic interventions.

Another approach suggested by the discovery of the autoantibody-induced blockade of the vWF-cleaving metalloproteinase in acute idiopathic TTP (as well as in ticlopidine/clopidogrel-associated TTP) is the use of new types of immunosuppressive agents, especially in refractory TTP patients. These might include: the chimeric mouse/human monoclonal antibody directed against CD20 antigens predominantly expressed on B lymphocytes (anti-CD20, or Rituximab)[74]; anti-CD40, which blocks the up-regulation of antigen-presenting cells by suppressing the attachment of CD40 ligand on activated T lymphocytes with CD40 on antigen-presenting cells[75]; a chimeric mouse/human monoclonal antibody (daclizumab, or Zenapax) against the interleukin-2-receptor α (anti-IL-2Rα), which prevents the T-lymphocyte growth factor, IL-2, from attaching to its receptor on T lymphocytes[76]; and the induction of apoptosis in type 1 helper T lymphocytes (Th1) by random copolymers of alanine, lysine, glutamic acid and tyrosine (glatiramer, or Copaxone).[77]

It remains to be determined if any of these emerging, relatively specific immunosuppressive agents will be safe and effective in TTP patients with anti-vWF-cleaving metalloproteinase autoantibodies who are refractory to conventional therapy.

COST CONTAINMENT

The treatment of acute types of TTP is labor intensive and prolonged, and usually requires the services of hematologists and transfusion medicine specialists. Large volumes of either FFP or the more expensive cryosupernatant are consumed. Cost reduction of consequence using presently effective therapy is unlikely. On the contrary, if solvent/detergent plasma or purified vWF-cleaving metalloproteinase is ultimately used in place of FFP and cryosupernant, then costs will increase further.

MEDICAL-LEGAL ISSUES

TTP is no longer a rare disorder, and so the diagnosis must be considered in every patient whose initial complete blood cell count shows thrombocytopenia and the presence of schistocytes. Until there is a heightened, almost reflex, wariness about the possibility of TTP among general and emergency physicians, the burgeoning cottage industry in TTP-related malpractice claims will continue to thrive.

Before any severely thrombocytopenic patient who is not exsanguinating is transfused with platelets, the treating physicians should specifically determine that neither schistocytosis nor an elevated serum LDH value is present.

If the constellation of severe thrombocytopenia, schistocytosis and an elevated LDH level indicates that the diagnosis of TTP is likely, or even possible, then the treating physician should make the presumptive diagnosis of TTP and proceed with therapy as an emergency. Procrastination is unwise and dangerous. FFP infusion as temporary therapy, accompanied by high-dose glucocorticoid administration, should commence as soon as possible. This should be followed by the insertion of a large-bore catheter and the initiation of plasma exchange. These latter procedures can be complicated by hemorrhage or volume overload, and will require a few to many hours (sometimes up to 24). The daunting logistical difficulties are compounded if the patient must be transferred from an admitting hospital lacking plasmapheresis equipment and personnel to another facility that has the capacity to perform plasma exchanges.

Even with rapid diagnosis and proper therapy, perhaps 10% to 20% of patients die during TTP episodes. Under these circumstances, it is essential to help family members understand how a previously healthy individual can succumb "out of the blue" to an unpronounceable, incomprehensible disorder. If this is not done thoughtfully, a frequent next step is to presume that the tragic outcome must be the fault of the treating physicians and hospital. The likelihood is near 100% that some malpractice attorney will agree.

CONSULTATIVE CONSIDERATIONS

Disorders characterized by thrombocytopenia, hemolysis, schistocytosis, and LDH elevation are summarized in Table 22–3. HITT, which often causes progressive thrombocytopenia and thrombosis, is not usually accompanied by schistocytes.

The consulting hematologist should review quickly and personally the peripheral blood smear, and then rapidly focus on the likely diagnosis using patient examination and the results of a few additional laboratory studies done as an emergency (prothrombin time, activated partial thromboplastin time, D-dimer, fibrinogen, direct Coombs' test, creatinine).

If the differential diagnosis in an adult patient is between TTP and HUS, then the patient should be presumed to have TTP and therapy should commence immediately.

■ REFERENCES

Chapter 22 References

1. Marcus AJ. Dr. Eli Moschcowitz. In Kaplan BS, Trompeter RS, Moake JL (Eds): Hemolytic Uremic Syndrome and Thrombotic Thrombocytopenic Purpura. New York, Marcel Dekker, 1992; pp. 19–27.
2. Moschcowitz E. Hyaline thrombosis of the terminal arterioles and capillaries: A hitherto undescribed disease Proc NY Pathol Soc 1924;24:21–24.
3. Byrnes JJ, Khurana M. Treatment of thrombotic thrombocytopenic purpura with plasma. N Engl J Med 1977;297:1386–1389.
4. Bukowski RM, Hewlett JS, Reime RR, et al. Therapy of thrombotic thrombocytopenic purpura: An overview. Semin Thromb Hemost 1981;7:1–8.
5. Rock G, Sumak K, BusKard N, et al. Comparison of plasma exchange with plasma infusion in the treatment of thrombotic thrombocytopenic purpura. N Engl J Med 1991;325:393–397.
6. Bell WR, Braine HG, Ness PM, Kickler TS. Improved survival in thrombotic thrombocytopenic purpura–hemolytic-uremic syndrome clinical experience in 108 patients. N Engl J Med 1991;325:398–403.
7. Moake JL, Rudy CK, Troll JH, et al. Unusually large plasma factor VIII: von Willebrand factor multimers in chronic relapsing thrombotic throbocytopenic purpura. N Engl J Med 1982; 307:1432–1435.
8. Moake JL, Byrnes JJ, Troll JH, et al. Effects of fresh-frozen plasma and its cryosupernatant fraction on von Willebrand factor multimeric forms in chronic relapsing thrombotic thrombocytopenic purpura. Blood 1985;65:1232–1236.
9. Cohen JA, Brecher ME, Bandarenko N. Cellular source of serum lactate dehydrogenase elevation in patients with thrombotic thrombocytopenic purpura. J Clin Apheresis 1998;13:16–19.
10. Byrnes JJ, Moake JL. Thrombotic thrombocytopenic purpura and the hemolytic-uremic syndrome: evolving concepts of pathogenesis and therapy. Clin Haematol 1986;15:413–442.
11. Moake J, Chintagumpala M, Turner N, et al. Solvent/detergent-treated plasma suppresses shear-induced platelet aggregation and prevents episodes of thrombotic thrombocytopenic purpura. Blood 1994;84:490–497.
12. Furlan M, Robles R, Solenthaler M, et al. Deficient activity of von Willebrand factor-cleaving protease in chronic relapsing thrombotic thrombocytopenic purpura. Blood 1997;89:3097–3103.
13. Bennett CL, Weinberg PD, Rozenberg B-DK, et al. Thrombotic thrombocytopenic purpura associated with ticlopidine: a review of 60 cases. Ann Intern Med 1998;128:541–544.
14. Tsai H-M, Rice L, Sarode R, et al. Antibody inhibitors to von Willebrand factor metalloproteinase and increased von Willebrand factor-platelet binding in ticlopidine-associated thrombotic thrombocytopenic purpura. Ann Intern Med 2000;132:794–799.
15. Bennett CL, Connors JM, Carwile JM, et al. Thrombotic thrombocytopenic purpura associated with clopidogrel. N Engl J Med 2000;342:1773–1777.
16. Moake JL. Haemolytic-uremic syndrome: basic science. Lancet 1994;343:393–397.
17. Rabadi SJ, Khandekar JD, Miller HJ. Mitomycin-induced hemolytic uremic syndrome: Case presentation and review of the literature. Cancer Treat Rep 1982;66:1244–1247.
18. Atkinson K, Biggs JC, Hayes J, et al. Cyclosporin A associated nephrotoxicity in the first 100 days after allogeneic bone marrow transplantation: Three distinct syndromes. Br J Haematol 1983; 54:59–67.
19. Mach-Pascual S, Samii K, Beris P. Microangiopathic hemolytic anemia complicating FK506 (tacrolimus) therapy. Am J Hematol 1996;52:310–312.
20. Charba D, Moake JL, Harris MA, Hester JP. Abnormalities of von Willebrand factor multimers in drug-associated thrombotic microangiopathies. Am J Hematol 1993;42:268–277.
21. Singh N, Gayowski T, Marino IR. Hemolytic uremic syndrome in solid-organ transplant recipients Transplant Internat 1996;9: 68–75.
22. Moake JL, Byrnes JJ. Thrombotic microangiopathies associated with drugs and bone marrow transplantation. Hematol/Oncol Clin North Am 1996;10:485–497.
23. Harkness D, Byrnes JJ, Lian EC-Y, et al. Hazard of platelet transfusion in thrombotic thrombocytopenic purpura. JAMA 1981;246:1931–1933.
24. Asada Y, Sumiyoshi A, Hayashi T, et al. Immunochemistry of vascular lesions in thrombotic thromocytopenic purpura, with special reference to factor VIII related antigen. Thromb Res 1985; 38:469–479.
25. Moake JL, Turner NA, Stathopoulos NA, et al. Involvement of large plasma von Willebrand factor (vWF) multimers and unusually large vWF forms derived from endothelial cells in shear stress-induced platelet aggregation. J Clin Invest 1986;78:1456–1461.
26. Tsai HM. Physiologic cleavage of von Willebrand factor by a plasma protease is dependent on its confirmation and requires calcium ion. Blood 1996;87:4235–4244.
27. Furlan M, Robles R, Lammle B. Partial purification and characterization of a protease from human plasma cleaving von Willebrand factor to fragments produced by in vivo proteolysis. Blood 1996;87:4223–4224.
28. Tsai HM, Sussman II, Nagel RL. Shear stress enhances the proteolysis of von Willebrand factor in normal plasma. Blood 1994; 83:2171–2179.
29. Moake JL, McPherson PD. Abnormalities of von Willebrand factor multimers in thrombotic thrombocytopenic purpura and hemolytic-uremic syndrome. Am J Med 1989;87:3N–9N.
30. Chow TW, Turner NA, Chintagumpala M, et al. Increased von Willebrand factor binding to platelets in single episode and recurrent types of thrombotic thrombocytopenic purpura. Am J Hematol 1998;57:293–302.
31. Furlan M, Robles R, Solenthaler M, Lammle B. Acquired deficiency of von Willebrand factor-cleaving protease in a patient with thrombotic thrombocytopenic purpura. Blood 1998;91:2839–2846.

32. Furlan M, Robles R, Galbusera M, et al. von Willebrand factor-cleaving protease in thrombotic thrombocytopenic purpura and hemolytic-uremic syndrome. N Engl J Med 1998;339:1578–1584.
33. Tsai HM, Lian EC-Y. Antibodies of von Willebrand factor cleaving protease in acute thrombotic thrombocytopenic purpura. N Engl J Med 1998;339:1585–1594.
34. Moake JL, Turner NA, Stathopoulos NA, et al. Shear-induced platelet aggregation can be mediated by vWF released from platelets, as well as by exogenous large or unusually large vWF multimers, requires adenosine diphosphate, and is resistant to aspirin. Blood 1988;71:1366–1374.
35. Peterson DM, Stathopoulos NA, Giorgio TD, et al. Shear-induced platelet aggregation requires von Willebrand factor and platelet membrane glycoproteins Ib and IIb-IIIa. Blood 1987;69:625–628.
36. Tarantolo SR, Landmark JD, Iwen PC. Bartonella-like erythrocyte inclusions in thrombotic thrombocytopenic purpura. Lancet 1997;350:1602.
37. Laurence J, Mitra D, Steiner M, et al. Plasma from patients with idiopathic and human immunodeficiency virus-associated thrombotic thrombocytopenic purpura induced apoptosis in microvascular endothelial cells. Blood 1996;87:3245–3254.
38. Moore JC, Murphy WG, Kelton JG. Calpain proteolysis of von Willebrand factor enhances its binding to platelet membrane glycoprotein IIb/IIIa: an explanation for platelet aggregation in thrombotic thrombocytopenic purpura. Br J Haematol 1990;74:457–464.
39. Consonni R, Falanga A, Barbui T. Further characterization of platelet-aggregating cysteine proteinase activity in thrombotic thrombocytopenic purpura. Br J Haematol 1994;87:321–324.
40. Neame PD. Immunologic and other factors in thrombotic thrombocytopenic purpura (TTP). Semin Thromb Hemost 1980;6:416–429.
41. Zauli G, Gugliotta L, Catani L, et al. Increased serum levels of transforming growth factor beta-1 in patients affected by thrombotic thrombocytopenic purpura (TTP): its implications on bone marrow haematopoiesis. Br J Haematol 1993;84:381–386.
42. Wada H, Kaneko T, Ohiwa M, et al. Plasma cytokine levels in thrombotic thrombocytopenic purpura. Am J Hematol 1992;40:167–170.
43. Joseph G, Smith KJ, Hadley TJ, et al. HLA-DR53 protects against thrombotic thrombocytopenic purpura/adult hemolytic uremic syndrome. Am J Hematol 1994;47:189–193.
44. Nesher G, Hanna VE, Moore TL, et al. Thrombotic microangiopathic hemolytic anemia in systemic lupus erythematosus. Semin Arthr Rheum 1994;24:165–172.
45. Zacharski LR, Lustad D, Glick JL. Thrombotic thrombocytopenic purpura in a previously splenectomized patient. Am J Med 1976;60:1061–1063.
46. Yospur LS, Sun NC, Figueroa P, Niihara Y. Concurrent thrombotic thrombocytopenic purpura and immune thrombocytopenic purpura in an HIV-positive patient: case report and review of the literature. Am J Hematol 1996;51:73–78.
47. Leaf AN, Laubenstein LJ, Raphael B, et al. Thrombotic thrombocytopenic purpura associated with immunodeficiency virus type I (HIV-1) infection. Ann Intern Med 1988;109:194–197.
48. Nair JM, Bellevue R, Bertoni M, Dosik H. Thrombotic thrombocytopenic purpura in patients with the acquired immunodeficiency syndrome (AIDS)-related complex: A report of two cases. Ann Intern Med 1988;109:209–212.
49. Gasser C, Gautier E, Steck A, et al. Hamolytisch-uramische syndrome: bilaterale nierenrindennekrosen bei akuten erworbenen hamolytischen anamien. Schweiz Med Wochenschr 1955;85:905–909.
50. Kaplan BS, Proesmans W. The hemolytic uremic syndrome of childhood and its variants. Semin Hematol 1987;24:1480–1488.
51. Warwicker P, Goodship THJ, Donne RL, et al. Genetic studies into inherited and sporadic hemolytic uremic syndrome. Kidney Int 1998;53:836–844.
52. Karmali MA, Petric M, Lim C, et al. The association between idiopathic hemolytic uremic syndrome and infection by verotoxin-producing Escherichia coli. J Infect Dis 1985;151:775–782.
53. Goodman A, Ramos R, Petrelli M, et al. Gingival biopsy in thrombotic thrombocytopenic purpura. Ann Intern Med 1978;89:501–504.
54. Byrnes JJ, Moake JL, Panpit K, Periman P. Effectiveness of the cryosupernatant fraction of plasma in the treatment of refractory thrombotic thrombocytopenic purpura. Am J Hematol 1990;34:169–174.
55. Rock G, Shumack KH, Sutton DM, et al. Cyrosupernatant as a replacement fluid for plasma exchange in thrombotic thrombocytopenic purpura. Br J Haematol 1996;94:383–386.
56. Furlan M, Robles R, Morselli B, et al. Recovery and half-life of von Willebrand factor-cleaving protease after plasma therapy in patients with thrombotic thrombocytopenic purpura. Thromb Haemost 1999;81:8–13.
57. Gordon LI, Kwaan HC, Rossi EC. Deleterious effects of platelet transfusions and recovery thrombocytosis in patients with thrombotic microangiopathy. Semin Hematol 1987;24:194–201.
58. Gutterman LA, Stevenson TD. Treatment of thrombotic thrombocytopenic purpura with vincristine. JAMA 1982;247:1433–1436.
59. Thompson CE, Damon LE, Ries CA, Linker CA. Thrombotic microangiopathies in the 1980s: clinical features, response to treatment, and the impact of the human immunodeficiency virus epidemic. Blood 1992;80:1890–1895.
60. Moake JL, Rudy CK, Troll JH, et al. Therapy of chronic relapsing thrombotic thrombocytopenic purpura with prednisone and azathioprine. Am J Hematol 1985;20:73–79.
61. Crowther MA, Heddle N, Hayward CPM, et al. Splenectomy done during hematologic remission to prevent relapse in patients with thrombotic thrombocytopenic purpura. Ann Intern Med 1996;125:294–296.
62. Rosove MH, Ho WG, Goldfinger D. Ineffectiveness of aspirin and dipyridamole in the treatment of thrombotic thrombocytopenic purpura. Ann Intern Med 1982;96:27–33.
63. del Zoppo GJ. Antiplatelet therapy in thrombotic thrombocytopenic purpura. Semin Hematol 1987;24:130–139.
64. Hardwick RA, Hellums JD, Moake JL, et al. Effects of antiplatelet agents on platelets exposed to shear stress. Trans Am Soc Artif Intern Organs 1980;26:179–184.
64a. Gerritsen HE, Robles R, Lammle B, Furlan M. Partial amino acid sequence of purified von Willebrand factor-cleaving protease. Blood 2001;98:1654–1661.
64b. Fujikawa K, Suzuki H, McMullen B, Chung D. Purification of human von Willebrand factor-cleaving protease and its identification as a new member of the metalloproteinase family. Blood 2001;98:1662–1666.
64c. Zheng X, Chung D, Takayama TK, et al. Structure of von Willebrand factor cleaving protease (ADAMTS 13), a metalloprotease involved in thrombotic thrombocytopenic purpura. J Biol Chem 2001;44:41059–41063.
64d. Levy GG, Nichols WC, Lian EC, et al. Mutations in a member of the ADAMTS gene family cause thrombotic thrombocytopenic purpura. Nature 2001;413:488–494.
65. Gaddis TG, Guthrie TH, Drew MJ. Treatment of plasma refractory thrombotic thrombocytopenic purpura with protein A immunoabsorption. Am J Hematol 1997;55:55–58.
66. Chow TW, Hellums JD, Moake JL, Kroll MH. Shear stress-induced von Willebrand factor binding to platelet glycoprotein Ib initiates calcium influx associated with aggregation. Blood 1992;80:113–120.
67. McCrary JK, Nolasco LH, Hellums JD, et al. Direct demonstration of radiolabeled von Willebrand factor binding to platelet glycoprotein Ib and IIb-IIIa in the presence of shear stress. Ann Biomed Eng 1995;23:787–793.
68. Goto S, Salomon DR, Ikeda Y, Ruggeri ZM. Characterization of the unique mechanism mediating the shear-dependent binding

of soluble von Willebrand factor to platelets. J Biol Chem 1995;270:23352–23361.
69. Konstantopoulos K, Chow TW, Turner NA, et al. Shear stress-induced binding of von Willebrand factor to platelets. Biorheology 1997;34:57–71.
70. Sugimoto M, Ricca G, Hrinda ME, et al. Functional modulation of the isolated glycoprotein Ib-binding domain of von Willebrand factor expressed in *Escherichia coli.* Biochemistry 1991;30:5202–5209.
71. Turner NA, Moake JL, Kamat SG, et al. Comparative real-time effects on platelet adhesion and aggregation under flowing conditions of in vivo aspirin, heparin, and monoclonal antibody fragment against glycoprotein IIb-IIIa. Circulation 1995;91:1354–1362.
72. Kamat SG, Turner NA, Konstantopoulos K, et al. Effects of Integrelin on platelet function in flow models of arterial thrombosis. J Cardiovasc Pharmacol 1997;29:156–163.
73. Turner NA, Moake JL, Turner JD, McIntire LV. Blockade of adenosine diphosphate receptors $P2Y_{12}$ and $P2Y_1$ is required to inhibit platelet aggregation in whole blood under flow. Blood 2001;98:3340–3345.
74. Reff M, Carner K, Chambers K, et al. Depletion of B cells in vivo by a chimeric mouse human monoclonal antibody to CD20. Blood 1994;83:435–445.
75. Aruffo A, Bajorath J, Buhlmann JE, et al. Immune regulation by CD40 and its ligand GP39. Annu Rev Immunol 1993;11:591–617.
76. Minami Y, Kono T, Miyazaki T, Taniguchi T. The IL-2 receptor complex: its structure, function, and target genes. Annu Rev Immunol 1993;11:245–267.
77. Duda PW, Schmied MC, Cook SL, et al. Glatiramer acetate (Copaxone) induces degenerate, Th2-polarized immune responses in patients with multiple sclerosis. J Clin Invest 2000;105:967–976.

CHAPTER 23

Heparin-Induced Thrombocytopenia

Theodore E. Warkentin, M.D.

HISTORICAL OVERVIEW

In 1958, a vascular surgeon, Rodger Weismann, and his resident, Richard Tobin, reported 10 patients from whom they had extracted unusual platelet-fibrin thrombi that formed during a 1- to 2-week treatment course with heparin [for review[1]]. These physicians suspected a causal relationship with heparin, perhaps via heparin-induced embolization of thrombus from the proximal aorta (the paucity of red cells in the thrombi argued against a cardiac origin). It was not until 1973, however, that another vascular surgeon, Donald Silver, and two residents, recognized the concurrence of thrombocytopenia in similar patients. They also observed that heparin rechallenge soon after platelet count recovery caused abrupt recurrence of thrombocytopenia. Moreover, patient plasma and heparin added to normal platelets in vitro caused platelet aggregation, suggesting that a patient-dependent factor such as immunoglobulin G (IgG) was responsible. In 1977, Silver and his colleagues described eight patients with apparent heparin-induced thrombocytopenia, noting thrombotic complications (usually affecting arteries) in seven of the patients. Drawing upon the similar clinical profile depicted by Weismann and Tobin almost two decades before, Silver proposed the existence of a heparin-induced, immunoglobulin-mediated prothrombotic disorder with a paradoxical association with thrombocytopenia and a predilection for causing arterial thromboembolism.

Over the next two decades, the clinical and pathologic features of this distinct syndrome—now known as heparin-induced thrombocytopenia (HIT)—gradually emerged.[1,2] The presence of heparin-dependent, platelet-activating, IgG antibodies became the laboratory hallmark of this syndrome, and sensitive and specific platelet *activation assays* to detect the antibodies were developed.[3] In 1992, Jean Amiral identified the target antigen of HIT—a multimolecular complex between platelet factor 4 and heparin[4]—a breakthrough that led to the development of a new class of *antigen assays* to detect the pathogenic HIT antibodies. Over time, it became apparent that the spectrum of thrombosis complicating HIT included venous thrombosis; indeed, deep venous thrombosis (DVT) and pulmonary embolism appeared to occur even more often than did arterial thrombosis.[5] The importance of venous thrombosis in HIT was underscored by the recognition in 1997 of an iatrogenic syndrome of limb loss in HIT—venous limb gangrene—in which warfarin treatment was implicated as a cause for progression of DVT to limb gangrene.[6] This study also found marked in-vivo thrombin generation in HIT, giving rise to the concept that activation of coagulation—rather than platelet activation alone—was central to the prothrombotic nature of HIT. This new concept coincided with the recognition that the most effective treatments of HIT are agents that reduce thrombin generation or inhibit thrombin directly.[2]

TERMINOLOGY

Most patients who develop thrombocytopenia during heparin treatment do not have HIT. Accordingly, various terms have been developed to distinguish HIT from other explanations for thrombocytopenia (Table 23–1).[2] The widely used term *heparin-induced thrombocytopenia* generally refers to the antibody-mediated syndrome, and will be used in this context in this chapter. Sometimes, however, *HIT type II* is used to indicate the immune-mediated syndrome. Although heparin may contribute to mild thrombocytopenia via nonimmune platelet-activating mechanisms (sometimes designated as *HIT type I*), from a practical standpoint, this phenomenon usually cannot be distinguished from other clinical explanations for the thrombocytopenia. Thus, the recommended term for these patients is *nonimmune heparin-associated thrombocytopenia*. Sometimes, such a patient's clinical picture so strongly resembles HIT that the term *pseudo-HIT* may be appropriate (vide infra).[7]

Table 23-1 • TERMINOLOGY OF THROMBOCYTOPENIA COMPLICATING HEPARIN TREATMENT

Terminology	Comment
Heparin-Induced Thrombocytopenia (HIT)	*Recommended term:* widely used and denotes role of heparin in inducing thrombocytopenia
HIT type II	Popular term first used by Chong[a]
Heparin-associated thrombocytopenia (HAT)	Confusing, as term used both for immune and nonimmune thrombocytopenia
Heparin-induced thrombocytopenia/ thrombosis syndrome (HITT or HITTS)	Sometimes used to specify that HIT patient has developed thrombosis
White clot syndrome	Sometimes used to indicate that patient has pale, platelet-rich thrombi in artery(ies)
Nonimmune Heparin-Associated Thrombocytopenia (Nonimmune HAT)	*Recommended term:* makes explicit the lack of immune etiology, as well as the uncertain relationship of platelet count fall to heparin
HIT type I	Popular term first used by Chong[a]
Heparin-associated thrombocytopenia (HAT)	Confusing, as term used both for immune and nonimmune thrombocytopenia
Pseudo-HIT	Clinical situation that strongly mimics HIT

[a] See ref. 1.

PATHOGENESIS

The main pathologic event in HIT is formation of heparin-dependent IgG antibodies that activate platelets via platelet FcγIIa receptors.[8] The antibodies recognize multimolecular complexes of heparin and a positively charged platelet α granule chemokine protein, platelet factor 4 (PF4).[4,9,10] The antigen appears to be one or more sites on PF4 that have been conformationally modified because of binding to heparin.[11,12] Certain negatively charged substances other than heparin also support antigenic modification of PF4: for example, the highly sulfated anticancer agent pentosan polysulfate can induce thrombocytopenia and thrombosis by antibodies indistinguishable from those generated in HIT. Also, PF4 bound to polyvinylsulfonate binds HIT antibodies, which is the basis for a commercial antigen assay for HIT. The nature of these PF4/heparin interactions could explain why low-molecular-weight heparin (LMWH) preparations are less likely to cause HIT[5]: heparin chains must be at least 12 to 14 saccharide units in length to form the HIT antigen together with PF4.

Figure 23-1 summarizes the pathogenesis of HIT and emphasizes the central role of thrombin generation.[2,13] Levels of thrombin-antithrombin complexes (a marker of in-vivo thrombin generation) are far greater in HIT patients than control subjects.[6,14] At least three factors contribute to increased thrombin generation. First, Fc receptor-mediated platelet activation by HIT-IgG antibodies causes formation of procoagulant, platelet-derived microparticles that accelerate coagulation reactions.[15–17] Second, the HIT antibodies cross-react with PF4 bound to endothelial surface glycosaminoglycans, which may lead to endothelial cell activation and generation of tissue factor.[10] And third, PF4 released from platelets neutralizes the anticoagulant effects of heparin.

No genetic predisposition to HIT has been identified.[18] Unlike certain other immune-mediated thrombocytopenic disorders, no HLA association with HIT has been identified. Although there is an ARG$_{131}$/HIS$_{131}$ FcγIIa receptor polymorphism known to affect antibody-induced platelet activation, there is conflicting evidence as to whether one of the genotypes is significantly more likely to be associated with HIT.[18] Finally, there is the surprising observation that repeated heparin exposure in patients with a previous history of HIT does not usually cause recurrence of HIT antibodies.[19] A related observation is that HIT antibodies are transient, and are usually not detectable 100 days following an episode of HIT.[19] Perhaps absence of long-lasting immunologic memory explains these unusual clinical features of HIT.

Only a few of the patients who form HIT antibodies during heparin treatment develop thrombocytopenia.[5,20] High-titer HIT antibodies of the IgG class[21] that are detectable using sensitive platelet activation assays[22] are most likely to cause thrombocytopenia. Although anecdotal reports suggest that IgM and/or IgA antibodies can cause HIT,[23] this remains to be confirmed in prospective studies.

Coexisting clinical factors strongly influence localization of thrombosis in HIT. For example, postoperative orthopedic patients who develop HIT are much more likely to develop venous thrombosis, including pulmonary embolism, than arterial thrombotic events. In contrast, medical patients are about as likely to develop arterial thrombosis as venous events.[20] Injury to blood vessels, such as by indwelling catheters, is strongly associated with thrombosis in the affected vein or artery.[24,25]

FREQUENCY

The type of heparin preparation, the duration of treatment, and the definition of thrombocytopenia used, as well as the patient population receiving the heparin, are among the factors that influence the frequency of HIT.[20]

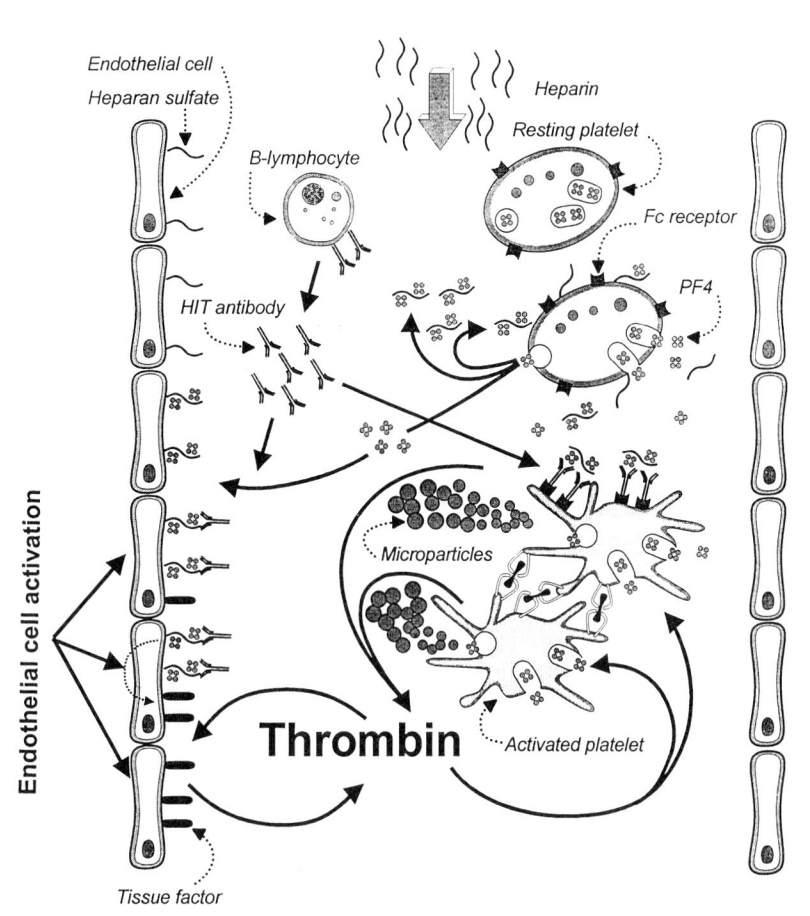

Figure 23-1 Pathogenesis of HIT: a central role for thrombin generation. (From Warkentin TE, Kelton JG. Thrombocytopenia due to platelet destruction and hypersplenism. In Hoffman R, Benz EJ Jr, Shattil SJ, et al. (Eds): Hematology. Basic Principles and Practice, 3rd ed. New York, Churchill Livingstone, 1999, pp. 2138–2154, with permission.)

Unfractionated heparin (UFH) causes HIT far more often than does LMWH (about eight-fold greater risk).[5,20] A meta-analysis found that heparin obtained from bovine lung is more likely to cause HIT than heparin derived from porcine gut.[20] This could be related to a greater chain length and higher degree of sulfation of bovine heparin.[20]

Since HIT typically begins after 5 or more days of heparin use, limiting heparin use to less than 5 days, when appropriate, should theoretically reduce the frequency of HIT. However, even this approach can fail, since even a brief exposure to heparin occasionally triggers formation of potent HIT antibodies that can cause thrombocytopenia and thrombosis beginning several days after the heparin has been discontinued, so-called "delayed-onset heparin-induced thrombocytopenia and thrombosis."[25,26]

Sometimes, the "standard" platelet count threshold indicating thrombocytopenia (150,000/μL) is inappropriate to define HIT. For example, transient thrombocytosis is common 1 to 2 weeks after major surgery. In such patients, an otherwise unexpected fall in the platelet count during heparin treatment that exceeds 50% from the postoperative peak strongly suggests HIT.[25] Using this definition of thrombocytopenia, the frequency of HIT is about 5% in postoperative orthopedic patients receiving UFH prophylaxis for 2 weeks.[25,26]

Some patient populations are at greater risk for HIT (Fig. 23–2).[22] For example, cardiac surgical patients are the most likely to form HIT antibodies (approximate 50% risk), but less than 5% of these antibody-positive patients develop HIT (overall, 1% to 2% frequency of HIT). In contrast, although only 15% of orthopedic patients form IgG antibodies detectable by antigen assay, as many as one third of these patients develop HIT (overall, 3%–5% frequency of HIT) (Fig. 23–2). The explanation for population-dependent differences in susceptibility to HIT is unknown.

CLINICAL FEATURES

Table 23–2 lists the typical clinical features of HIT.

Temporal Profile

The hallmark of HIT is a platelet count fall that begins between days 5 and 10 after starting heparin (first day of heparin use = day 0) (Fig. 23–3). Such a "typical" onset is observed in about 70% of patients with HIT. In the remaining patients, a "rapid" onset of HIT occurs. Generally speaking, this situation is characterized by a patient who has recently received heparin (within the past 100 days), and in whom resumption of heparin causes an abrupt fall in the platelet count (Fig. 23–4). This profile likely is caused by acute platelet activation in a patient with circulating, pre-existing HIT antibod-

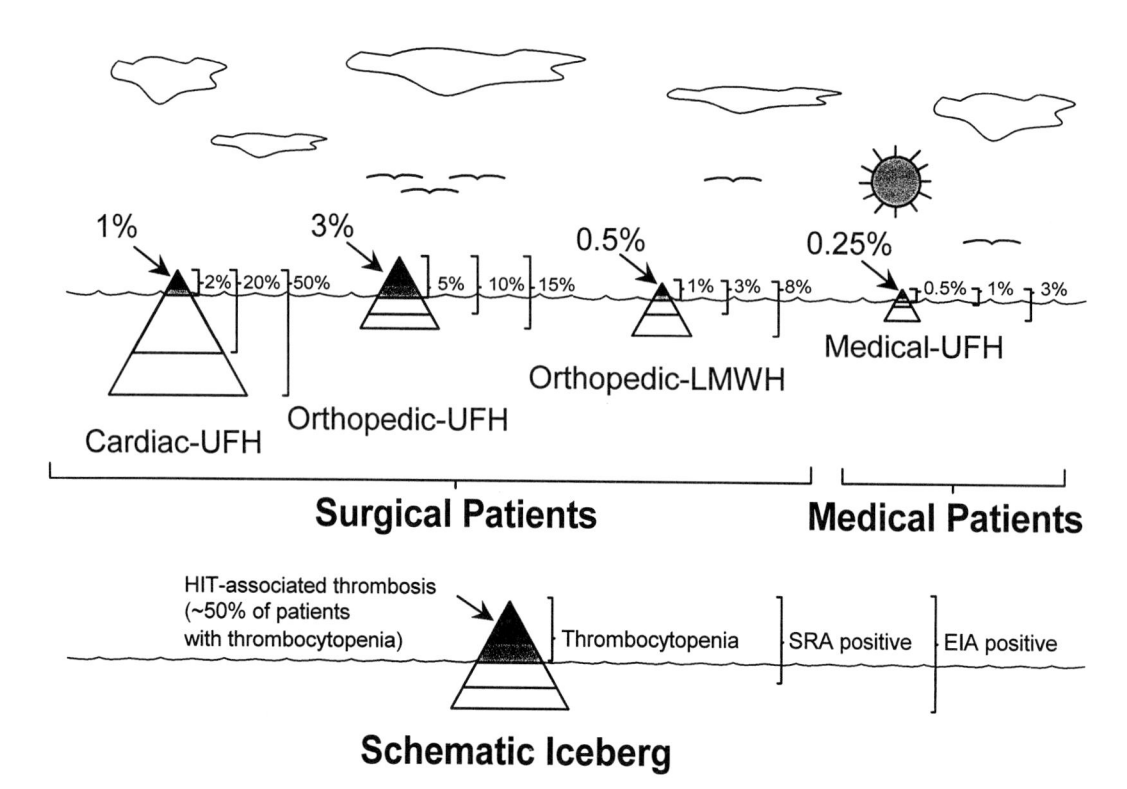

Figure 23–2 Multiple-iceberg model of HIT. A schematic "iceberg," shown on the lower "water line," illustrates the relations among HIT-associated thrombosis, thrombocytopenia, HIT antibodies detected by serotonin release assay (SRA), and HIT antibodies detected by PF4/heparin enzyme immunoassay (EIA). Above, the relative sizes of the various icebergs reflect the relative frequency of HIT antibody formation, thrombocytopenia, and HIT-associated thrombosis among several different patient populations. Note that unfractionated heparin (UFH) is more likely than low-molecular-weight heparin (LMWH) to cause HIT among orthopedic patients. However, patient population-dependent effects are also evident (e.g., although cardiac surgical patients are more likely to form HIT antibodies, among patients who form HIT antibodies, orthopedic patients are most likely to develop HIT). (From Lee DP, Warkentin TE. Frequency of heparin-induced thrombocytopenia. In Warkentin TE, Greinacher A (Eds): Heparin-induced Thrombocytopenia. New York, Marcel Dekker, 2000; pp. 81–112, with permission.)

Table 23–2 • CLINICAL FEATURES OF HIT

Timing of thrombocytopenia
  Typical onset: between days 5 and 10 after starting heparin
  Rapid onset: < 1 day following resumption of heparin (usually in a patient recently exposed to heparin, who therefore has residual circulating HIT antibodies)
Severity of thrombocytopenia
  Platelet count nadir: <20,000/μL in 10% of patients; <150,000/μL in 85% of patients
Thrombosis is common
  >50% develop new thrombosis
  Venous thrombosis: deep venous thrombosis > pulmonary embolism > warfarin-induced venous limb gangrene > adrenal hemorrhagic necrosis[a] > cerebral sinus thrombosis
  Arterial thrombosis: limb artery thrombosis > stroke syndrome > myocardial infarction > mesenteric artery thrombosis
Absence of petechiae (even when platelets <20,000/μL)
Skin lesions at heparin injection sites
  Severity ranges from erythematous plaques to skin necrosis
Acute systemic reactions following intravenous bolus heparin
  Acute inflammatory or cardiorespiratory signs and symptoms associated with abrupt platelet count fall

[a] There is evidence that adrenal hemorrhage complicating HIT is associated with adrenal infarction caused by thrombosis of the adrenal vein.

ies, formed in relation to the recent heparin exposure, rather than rapid regeneration of HIT antibodies because of an "anamnestic" (immune memory) response.[19]

Severity of Thrombocytopenia

Mild-to-moderate severity of thrombocytopenia is characteristic of HIT; the median platelet count nadir is about 60,000/μL,[27] and the platelet count falls below 20,000/μL in only 15% of patients (Fig. 23–5). Remarkably, even when a patient with HIT develops severe thrombocytopenia, petechiae usually are not seen. This clinical profile differs strikingly from that of patients with drug-induced immune thrombocytopenic purpura caused by quinine, quinidine, and sulfa antibiotics, in which the platelet count nadir is below 20,000/μL in most patients, and mucocutaneous hemorrhage is characteristic.

Venous Thrombosis

Venous thrombosis is the most common thrombotic complication. As many as 50% of HIT patients develop symptomatic DVT, and about half of these patients develop pulmonary embolism.[25,28] Some patients with

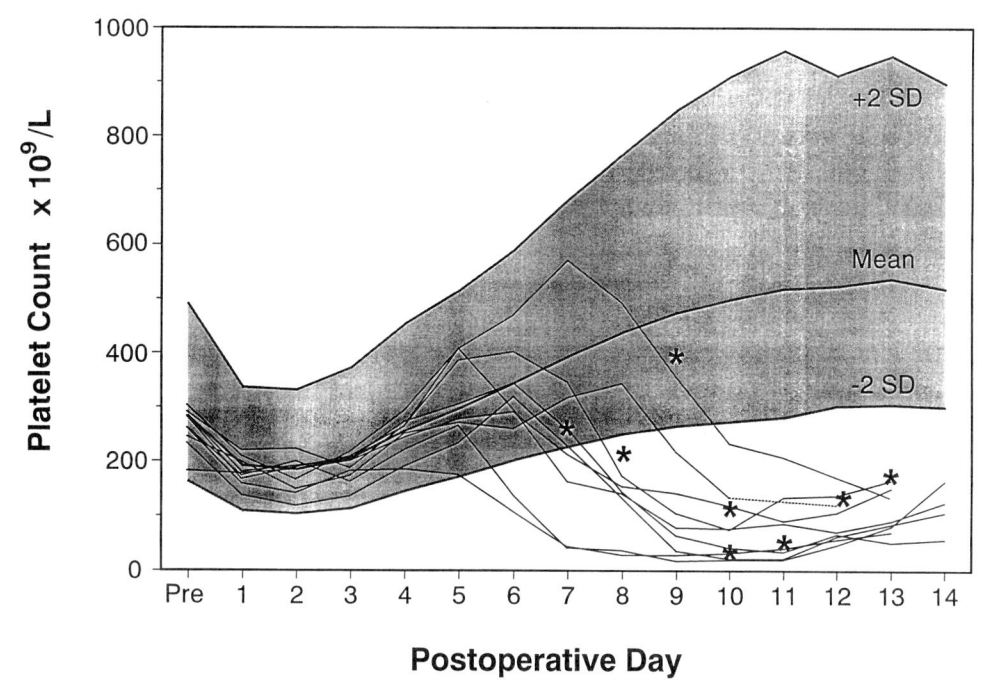

Figure 23–3 Platelet count profile of HIT in postoperative patients. The bold line and shaded area indicate the mean (± 2 SD) platelet count in normal postoperative orthopedic patients. Nine patients, shown by the thin lines, developed serologically confirmed HIT; eight of the nine patients developed HIT-associated thrombosis (time of thrombosis indicated by *). (From Warkentin TE, Levine MN, Hirsh J, et al. Heparin-induced thrombocytopenia in patients treated with low-molecular-weight heparin or unfractionated heparin. N Engl J Med 1995; 332:1330–1335, with permission.)

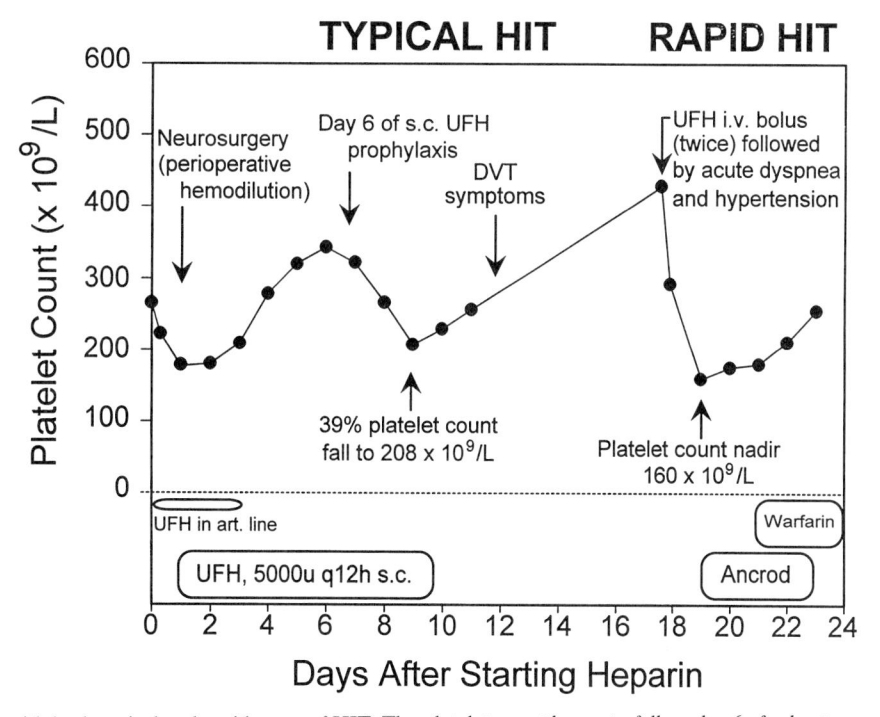

Figure 23–4 A patient with both typical and rapid onset of HIT. The platelet count began to fall on day 6 of subcutaneous (s.c.) unfractionated heparin (UFH) treatment (typical-onset HIT). However, following a subsequent intravenous (i.v.) UFH bolus given on day 18 for deep venous thrombosis (DVT), the platelet count fell abruptly (rapid-onset HIT). (From Warkentin TE. Clinical picture of heparin-induced thrombocytopenia. In Warkentin TE, Greinacher A (Eds): Heparin-induced Thrombocytopenia, 2nd ed. New York, Marcel Dekker, 2001, pp. 43–86, with permission.)

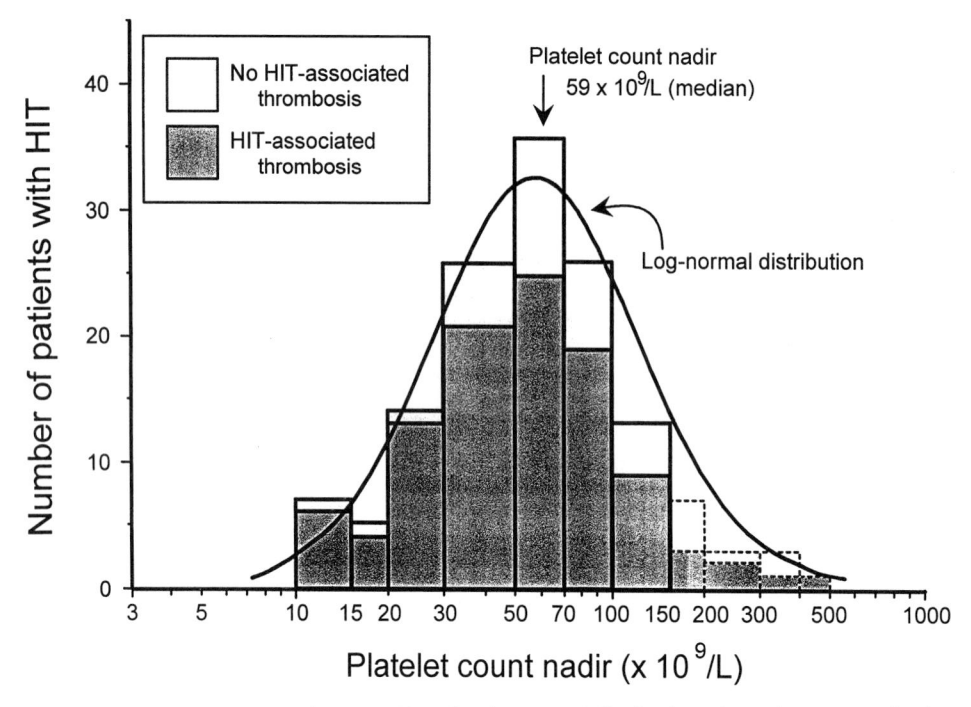

Figure 23–5 Platelet count nadirs of 142 patients with HIT. There is a log-normal distribution of platelet count nadirs (median platelet count naidr, 59,000/μL). HIT-associated thrombosis occurred in most patients with HIT, irrespective of the platelet count nadir. (From Warkentin TE. Clinical presentation of heparin-induced thrombocytopenia. Semin Hematol 1998;35 (Suppl 5):9–16, with permission.)

DVT develop severe limb ischemia, including phlegmasia cerulea dolens and venous limb gangrene (vide infra). Adrenal vein thrombosis is believed to be the explanation for adrenal hemorrhagic necrosis, which occurs in about 3% to 5% of patients with HIT.[25] Bilateral adrenal hemorrhage can cause acute or chronic adrenal failure, and prompt recognition of this complication, with institution of cortisol replacement can be life saving.[29] Cerebral sinus thrombosis is another unusual life-threatening venous thrombotic event that is associated with HIT.[30]

Arterial Thrombosis

Arterial thrombosis was the first complication identified as a feature of HIT.[1] The characteristic pale thrombi extracted by surgeons led to the term *white clot syndrome* that is still sometimes used to indicate HIT. The typical location of thrombi in HIT, namely lower limb artery occlusion > stroke syndrome > myocardial infarction, is reversed from that observed in the non-HIT population (myocardial infarction > stroke syndrome > lower limb artery occlusion).[25]

Limb Ischemic Syndromes

There are several explanations for limb-threatening ischemia in a given patient with HIT[25]: (1) occlusion of the distal aorta, iliofemoral, or other large limb arteries by occlusive platelet-rich thromboemboli; (2) microembolization to, or in-situ formation of small thrombi within, small arteries or arterioles (distal limb ischemia despite palpable or doppler-identifiable pulses); (3) severe DVT progressing to phlegmasia cerulea dolens; and (4) warfarin-induced venous limb gangrene. This last syndrome is discussed in the following section.

Prothrombotic Complications of Warfarin Treatment of HIT

Figure 23–6 illustrates two prothrombotic complications of warfarin therapy reported in patients with HIT[6,31,32]: "classic" warfarin-induced skin necrosis and warfarin-induced venous limb gangrene. In North America, warfarin is the most widely used coumarin agent, whereas in continental Europe, phenprocoumon has been implicated.[14] Table 23–3 summarizes the clinical features and pathogenesis of these syndromes, which are believed to result from a disturbance in procoagulant/anticoagulant imbalance, namely a failure of the protein C natural anticoagulant pathway to down-regulate thrombin in the microvasculature.[6,31,32]

Venous limb gangrene occurred in 8 of 66 (12%) patients with acute DVT complicating HIT in whom treatment included warfarin.[6] In some patients, concomitant use of a defibrinogenating snake venom, ancrod, may have contributed to this complication[6,33] by increasing thrombin generation.[34] Although the frequency of this syndrome may be less than 10% in patients receiving warfarin alone,[35] it is prudent to avoid warfarin anticoagulation in acute HIT until the patient is well anticoagulated with a parenteral agent that reduces thrombin generation and, preferably, the thrombocytopenia has largely recovered.

Heparin-Induced Thrombocytopenia 361

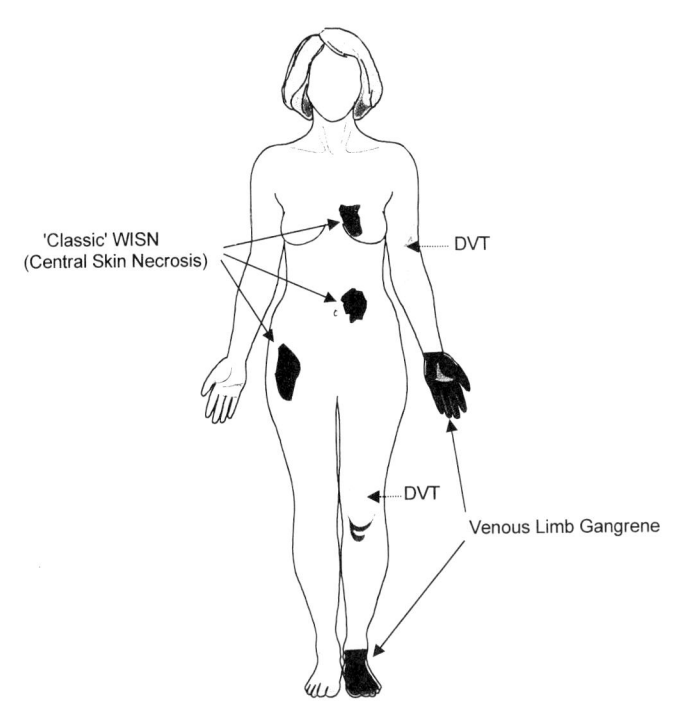

Warfarin-Induced Skin Necrosis (WISN)

Figure 23–6 Warfarin-induced complications of HIT. HIT is strongly associated with warfarin-induced venous limb gangrene, which is acral necrosis of a limb affected by deep venous thrombosis (DVT). Less commonly, HIT can be complicated by "classic" warfarin-induced skin necrosis (WISN), which typically affects central tissues. (From Warkentin TE. Heparin-induced thrombocytopenia: IgG-mediated platelet activation, platelet microparticle generation, and altered procoagulant/anticoagulant balance in the pathogenesis of thrombosis and venous limb gangrene complicating heparin-induced (HIT). Transfus Med Rev 1996;10:249–258, with permission.

Warfarin-induced venous limb gangrene has a distinct feature: a supratherapeutic international normalized ratio (INR) that coincides with the progression of DVT to distal limb necrosis. This characteristic elevation in INR is caused by a severe reduction in factor VII that parallels a severe reduction in protein C,[6] i.e., the high INR is a surrogate marker for a low protein C level.[36] Early recognition of this syndrome, and reversal of warfarin anticoagulation with vitamin K and fresh frozen plasma, may be limb saving.[6] Uncontrolled DIC associated with adenocarcinoma is another clinical situation that has been associated with limb gangrene during warfarin therapy.[7,36]

Heparin-induced Skin Lesions

Inflammatory, plaque-like or necrotic lesions that begin 6 or more days after commencing subcutaneous injections of UFH or LMWH is a manifestation of the HIT syndrome.[25,37,38] Most patients do not develop concomitant thrombocytopenia, even when HIT antibodies are detected by sensitive antigen or activation assays. Platelet counts should continue to be monitored for a few days in all patients with heparin-induced skin lesions, as thrombocytopenia and thrombosis sometimes occur after heparin therapy has been discontinued.[39]

Neurologic Syndromes

Stroke syndromes caused by arterial or even venous thrombosis are relatively common in HIT.[25] Cerebral sinus thrombosis[30,40] is suggested by headache, decreased level of consciousness, and focal neurologic defects. Transient global amnesia is a rare complication of HIT that can follow an intravenous bolus of heparin.[41] Lower-limb paralysis associated with infarction of the spinal cord or lumbosacral plexus can occur.

Cardiac Syndromes

Besides myocardial infarction, other complications of HIT that involve the heart include intraventricular and intra-atrial thrombus formation that can lead to peripheral or pulmonary embolism. Cardiopulmonary arrest occurring shortly after intravenous heparin bolus administration is another manifestation of HIT.[25,42]

Table 23–3 • WARFARIN-INDUCED SKIN NECROSIS VERSUS WARFARIN-INDUCED VENOUS LIMB GANGRENE

	Classic Warfarin-Induced Skin Necrosis (WISN)	**Warfarin-Induced Venous Limb Gangrene**
Clinical picture	Necrosis of skin and subdermal tissues, especially in central sites (e.g., breast, thigh, abdomen) that begins 3 to 7 days after starting warfarin therapy	Necrosis of acral (distal) tissues in limb(s) affected by deep venous thrombosis during warfarin therapy that results in a supratherapeutic INR (typically >4.0); this syndrome can follow a prodrome of phlegmasia cerulea dolens
Predisposing features	(1) congenital deficiency of natural anticoagulant: (protein C > protein S > antithrombin); (2) factor V Leiden (?); (3) acute HIT	(1) acute HIT; (2) adenocarcinoma-associated with DIC
Pathogenesis	Unknown; believed to be caused in some patients by acquired severe deficiency in protein C related to interaction of congenital deficiency and rapid further fall in protein C levels upon starting warfarin treatment (short half-life for protein C)	Acquired severe deficiency of protein C natural anticoagulant, usually during initiation of warfarin therapy; at the same time, warfarin fails to down-regulate increased thrombin generation associated with the underlying disorder (HIT or adenocarcinoma)

Outpatient Presentation of HIT

HIT is generally regarded as a diagnosis affecting hospital inpatients. However, some patients can develop potent platelet-activating antibodies after a brief course of heparin that results in thrombocytopenia and thrombosis beginning 5 or more days after cessation of heparin.[25,26] Figure 23–7 illustrates such a course in which the patient develops HIT-associated thrombosis as an outpatient 40 days after heparin exposure.

DIFFERENTIAL DIAGNOSIS

Thrombocytopenia occurs commonly in hospitalized patients, and most patients who develop thrombocytopenia during heparin therapy do not have HIT. When thrombocytopenia occurs early during heparin treatment (within the first 4 days), the explanation usually rests with the patient's reason for hospitalization (e.g., hemodilution/platelet consumption following surgery, septicemia, disseminated intravascular coagulation). However, HIT should be suspected in a patient with early-onset thrombocytopenia when the degree of thrombocytopenia is not in keeping with the patient's clinical situation, and the patient recently has been exposed to heparin (Fig. 23–4). Indeed, such a rapid onset of thrombocytopenia occurs in about one quarter of all patients recognized with HIT.[19]

Pseudo-HIT is a term used by the author to describe patients whose clinical profile appears to suggest HIT, but in whom HIT antibodies cannot be detected by sensitive assays (Table 23–4).[7] For example, Figure 23–8 illustrates the course of two patients with very similar platelet count profiles: one patient had HIT-associated pulmonary embolism, the other patient had pulmonary embolism-associated thrombocytopenia.[25] For the latter patient with pseudo-HIT, *increased* doses of heparin (to overcome heparin "resistance") resulted in improvement of the platelet count and clinical recovery (Fig. 23–8B).

In evaluating a patient for possible HIT, the physician should focus on four issues:

1. How unusual is the observed platelet count fall?
2. Did new, progressive, or recurrent thrombosis, or any other unexpected clinical event (e.g., skin lesions at heparin injection sites) accompany the thrombocytopenia?
3. To what extent can the thrombocytopenia or other clinical events be attributed to other suspected or established illnesses?
4. Are HIT antibodies detectable, and how "strong" are they?

Thus, HIT should be regarded as a clinicopathologic syndrome, i.e., the diagnosis is most reliably made when patients develop one or more clinical events (e.g., falling platelet count, progressive or new thrombosis) and the laboratory identifies the presence of the pathologic factor (i.e., HIT antibodies). Consequently, laboratory testing for HIT antibodies is crucial for confirming or refuting a diagnosis of HIT.

LABORATORY TESTING

Two major classes of assays detect HIT antibodies: activation (functional) and antigen assays. *Activation* assays, which include aggregation of platelets in citrate-anticoagulated platelet-rich plasma (developed in the 1970s) as well as assays utilizing washed platelets (devel-

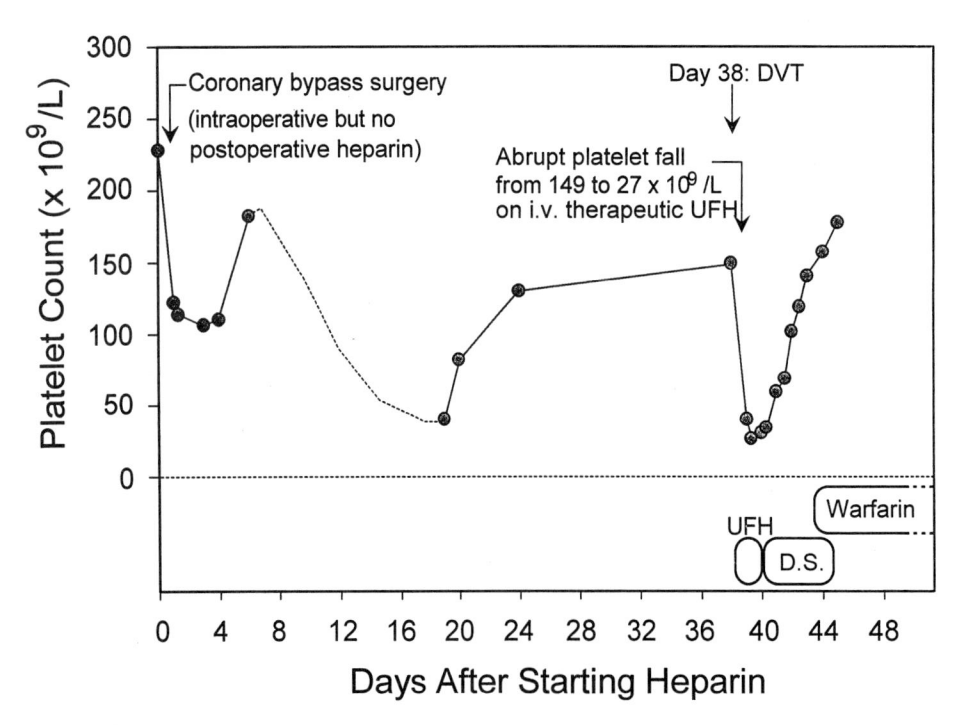

Figure 23–7 Outpatient presentation of HIT. A patient was found to have a platelet count of 40,000/μL 19 days following cardiac surgery. HIT was not diagnosed until an abrupt fall in the platelet count occurred following an intravenous (i.v.) unfractionated heparin (UFH) bolus given for deep venous thrombosis (DVT) on day 38. (From Warkentin TE. Clinical picture of heparin-induced thrombocytopenia. In Warkentin TE, Greinacher A (Eds): Heparin-induced Thrombocytopenia, 2nd ed. New York, Marcel Dekker, 2001, pp 43–80, with permission.)

Table 23-4 • PSEUDO-HIT DISORDERS: THROMBOCYTOPENIA AND THROMBOSIS

Pseudo-HIT Disorder	Pathogenesis of Thrombocytopenia and Thrombosis	Timing
Adenocarcinoma	DIC secondary to procoagulant material(s) produced by neoplastic cells	Late
Pulmonary embolism	Platelet activation via clot-bound thrombin	Early or late[a]
Diabetic ketoacidosis	Hyperaggregable platelets in ketoacidosis (?)	Early
Antiphospholipid syndrome	Multiple mechanisms described, including platelet activation by antiphospholipid antibodies (?)	Early
Thrombolytic therapy	Platelet activation by thrombin bound to fibrin degradation products	Early
Infective endocarditis	Infection-associated thrombocytopenia; ischemic events secondary to septic emboli	Early
Paroxysmal nocturnal hemoglobinuria	Platelets susceptible to complement-mediated damage; platelet hypoproduction	Early
Post-transfusion purpura (PTP)	"Pseudospecific" alloantibody-mediated platelet destruction (exception: bleeding, not thrombosis)	Late

These "pseudo-HIT" disorders can mimic HIT by causing thrombocytopenia and thrombosis in association with heparin treatment. An exception is post-transfusion purpura (PTP), which causes bleeding but not thrombosis; however, PTP can resemble HIT because both disorders usually occur about a week after major surgery requiring blood and postoperative heparin. The pseudo-HIT disorders can be categorized based on whether the onset of thrombocytopenia is typically "early" (less than 5 days) or "late" (more than 5 days) in relation to the heparin.
[a] See Figure 23-8A for an example of "late" thrombocytopenia associated with pulmonary embolism. (From Warkentin TE. Pseudo-heparin-induced thrombocytopenia. In Warkenton TE, Greinacher A (Eds): Heparin-induced Thrombocytopenia, 2nd ed. New York, Marcel Dekker, 2001, pp. 271-289, with permission.)

oped in the 1980s), imply the presence of HIT antibodies via their platelet-activating properties.[3] In contrast, *antigen* assays, which were developed in the 1990s,[4] detect HIT antibodies based upon their reactivity with PF4 complexed to heparin or other polyanions. Thus, laboratory testing for HIT parallels another hypercoagulable state, the antiphospholipid syndrome, in which both functional ("lupus anticoagulant" testing) and antigen (anticardiolipin antibody) assays are used for diagnosis (see Chapter 18).

Activation Assays

Activation assays detect HIT antibodies of the IgG class via their ability to cross-link platelet FcγIIa receptors

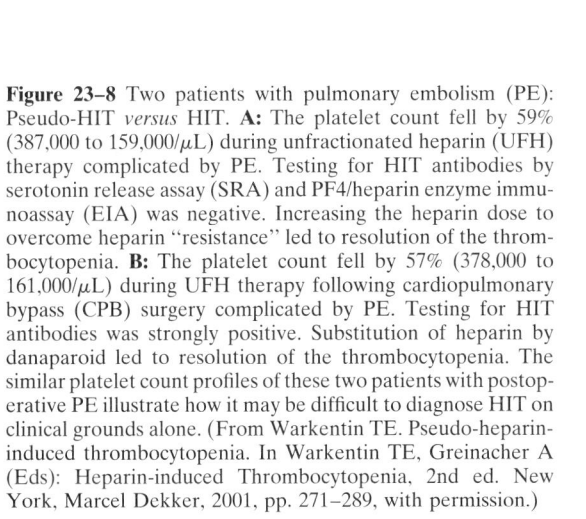

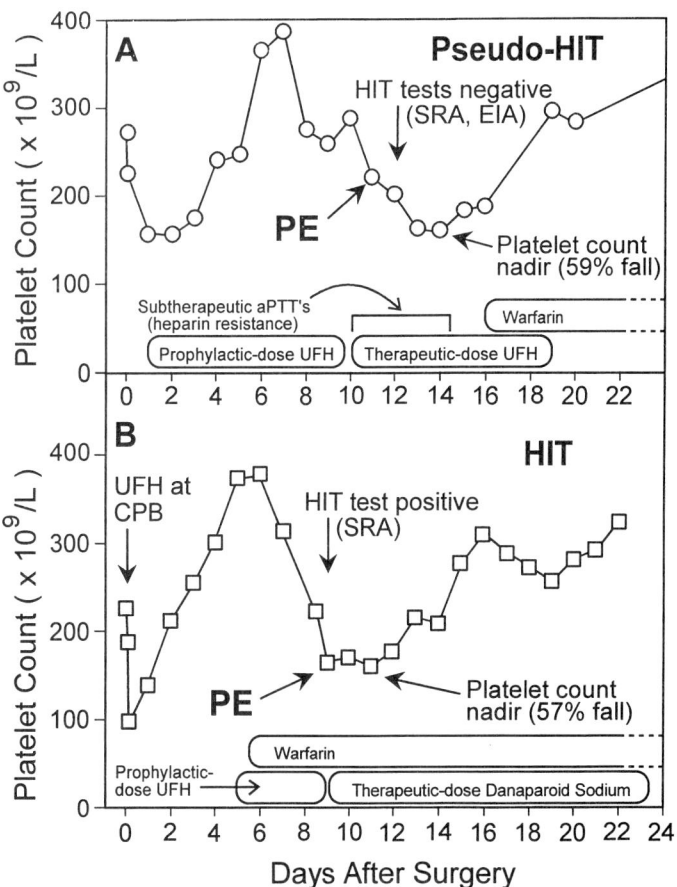

Figure 23-8 Two patients with pulmonary embolism (PE): Pseudo-HIT *versus* HIT. **A:** The platelet count fell by 59% (387,000 to 159,000/μL) during unfractionated heparin (UFH) therapy complicated by PE. Testing for HIT antibodies by serotonin release assay (SRA) and PF4/heparin enzyme immunoassay (EIA) was negative. Increasing the heparin dose to overcome heparin "resistance" led to resolution of the thrombocytopenia. **B:** The platelet count fell by 57% (378,000 to 161,000/μL) during UFH therapy following cardiopulmonary bypass (CPB) surgery complicated by PE. Testing for HIT antibodies was strongly positive. Substitution of heparin by danaparoid led to resolution of the thrombocytopenia. The similar platelet count profiles of these two patients with postoperative PE illustrate how it may be difficult to diagnose HIT on clinical grounds alone. (From Warkentin TE. Pseudo-heparin-induced thrombocytopenia. In Warkentin TE, Greinacher A (Eds): Heparin-induced Thrombocytopenia, 2nd ed. New York, Marcel Dekker, 2001, pp. 271-289, with permission.)

in the presence of heparin, causing platelet activation.[8] Since platelet activation is a nonspecific end point, care must be taken to distinguish HIT antibodies from thrombin, immune complexes, or other platelet activators.

Washed Platelet Activation Assays

Washed platelet activation assays, which use platelets resuspended in calcium-containing buffer, are reliable activation assays for HIT, provided that platelets are handled properly. For example, the use of apyrase (an enzyme that degrades adenine nucleotides) during platelet washing is important to maintain sensitivity of the platelets to subsequent stimulation by adenosine diphosphate (ADP), an important potentiating factor in HIT.[43]

The *platelet serotonin release assay* (SRA) quantitates the release of ^{14}C-labeled serotonin from platelets as a marker of platelet activation.[44,45] This assay's clinical usefulness has been validated: a positive test result was strongly associated with late-onset thrombocytopenia (beginning on or after 5 days of heparin therapy, thus indicating probable HIT) in a large study (odds ratio, approximately 80).[5] Use of a flow cytometer to detect platelet-derived microparticles employs similar platelet-handling methods but avoids a radioisotope.[46]

The *heparin-induced platelet activation* (HIPA) assay[47-49] assesses aggregation of washed platelets incubated with patient serum and heparin in U-bottomed polystyrene microtiter wells containing two stainless-steel spheres, under conditions of platelet stirring. At 5-minute intervals, the wells are examined against an indirect light source: a change in appearance of the reaction mixture from turbidity (nonaggregated platelets) to transparency (aggregated platelets) indicates platelet activation.

Advantages of washed platelet activation assays include: (1) their high sensitivity for detecting clinically significant HIT antibodies; (2) their (relative) low sensitivity for detecting clinically insignificant HIT antibodies, compared with antigen assays; and (3) their ability to permit batch evaluation of many patient samples under several reaction conditions, enhancing test specificity. Since washed platelets are activated by IgG, but not IgA and/or IgM HIT antibodies, washed platelet activation assays likely have greater specificity for clinical HIT, compared with antigen assays that detect antibodies of all three antibody classes.

Disadvantages include the technically demanding nature of these assays,[49] as well as the need for radiolabeling (SRA), expensive equipment (flow cytometer), or a subjective observer-dependent end point (HIPA). Further, the laboratory must maintain a panel of positive control sera. Test serum also must first undergo controlled heat treatment (to inactivate thrombin), which sometimes causes ex-vivo formation of IgG immune complexes, yielding an "indeterminate" test result (activation of platelets at all heparin concentrations).[3]

Quality control involves selecting blood donors whose platelets respond well to HIT sera, as well as testing various strong and weak positive control sera. Since HIT sera and washed platelets exhibit variable reactivity in a hierarchical manner,[45] a positive result using a "weak" positive HIT serum control ensures that the platelet handling was adequate to permit accurate interpretation of the test results.

Aggregation Assays that Utilize Platelet-Rich Plasma

Aggregation assays utilizing platelet-rich plasma are the most widely used activation assays to detect HIT antibodies, as they require the ubiquitous platelet aggregometer and involve relatively simple methods.[3,50,51] The aggregation response of platelets (prepared as citrated platelet-rich plasma from a normal donor) to citrate-anticoagulated platelet-poor plasma obtained from the patient, in the presence of therapeutic heparin levels (0.5 to 1.0 U/mL), is assessed, and compared with reactivity in the presence of buffer control and high heparin concentrations (100 U/mL). Unfortunately, these aggregation assays are relatively insensitive for diagnosing HIT: as few as 33% to 50% of samples that test positive in a washed platelet assay give a positive aggregation assay result.[48] Another problem is that nonspecific platelet activation may occur more commonly than with washed platelet methods, increasing the chance of a false-positive result.

Antigen Assays

Antigen assays use enzyme immunoassay (EIA) methodology to detect binding of HIT antibodies to their PF4-containing antigen target, usually immobilized to a solid-phase. Two antigen assay kits are available commercially. One assay (Asserachrom HPIA, Stago) utilizes PF4/heparin complexes, whereas the newer test (available from GTI, Brookfield, WI) uses PF4 bound to polyvinylsulfonate (PVS).[52] Both commercial tests detect HIT antibodies of the three major immunoglobulin classes (IgG, IgA, IgM). However, this might not be an advantage over antigen assays that detect only IgG HIT antibodies: our laboratory found that an "in-house" EIA that detected only IgG HIT antibodies[53] gave positive results in all 15 patients identified with HIT in prospective clinical trials (high sensitivity).[22]

A fluid-phase PF4/heparin EIA was developed by investigators in Australia.[54] In this method, patient serum or plasma reacts with biotin-PF4/heparin complexes in a fluid-phase, prior to capturing IgG antibodies—and any bound antigen—using staphylococcal protein A. The biotinylated antigen-antibody complexes, now bound to the protein G sepharose via the Fc moieties of HIT IgG, are separated from unbound antigen by centrifugation and washing. Streptavidin-conjugated peroxidase is used to quantitate the biotin-PF4/heparin/IgG complexes (streptavidin binds to biotin). This method may have a lower false-positive rate, because it avoids denaturation of the antigen caused by binding to a solid-phase, and also detects only IgG HIT antibodies. It also permits detection of in-vitro cross-reactivity of HIT antibodies against different heparins and heparinoids.[54]

Interpretation of HIT Antibody Test Results

Interpretation of HIT antibody test results is complicated by the fact that only a minority of patients who develop HIT antibodies develop thrombocytopenia.[5,55] A corollary is that a positive HIT test result may not therefore actually indicate HIT, particularly if a "weak" positive result is obtained, and if there is another convincing explanation for the thrombocytopenia.[3] Thus, it is important that tests for HIT be interpreted in the clinical context. Since antigen assays are more likely than activation assays to detect clinically insignificant HIT antibodies,[22,56] one algorithmic approach is to screen for HIT antibodies using a commercial antigen assay, but to perform further testing with a washed platelet activation assay if an unexpected positive result is obtained (Fig. 23–9). However, as existing antigen and washed platelet activation assays are very sensitive for detecting clinically significant HIT antibodies, negative results in one or (especially) both classes of assay is strong evidence against HIT, irrespective of the patient's clinical course. Occasionally, when an unexpected negative test result is obtained using an antigen assay, referral for further testing by activation assay may be needed,

as there is anecdotal evidence that a false-negative EIA result can rarely be caused by antibodies directed against "minor" antigens other than PF4/heparin (e.g., interleukin-8 or neutrophil-activating peptide-2); in such patients, sensitive activation assays give positive results.[57]

TREATMENT OF HIT-ASSOCIATED THROMBOSIS

Overall, about 50% to 75% of patients with serologically proven HIT develop new, progressive, or recurrent thrombosis during or soon after their episode of thrombocytopenia.[20,28] Thus, there is frequent need to use an alternative, rapidly acting, nonheparin anticoagulant for patients with HIT. Three major options are available in the United States: danaparoid, lepirudin, and argatroban. Oral anticoagulants are contraindicated as sole therapy for acute HIT, but are the main treatment for long-term management of thrombosis following an episode of HIT.

Danaparoid

Danaparoid sodium (Orgaran) is a mixture of anticoagulant glycosaminoglycans, predominantly heparan sulfate (84%), dermatan sulfate (12%), and chondroitin

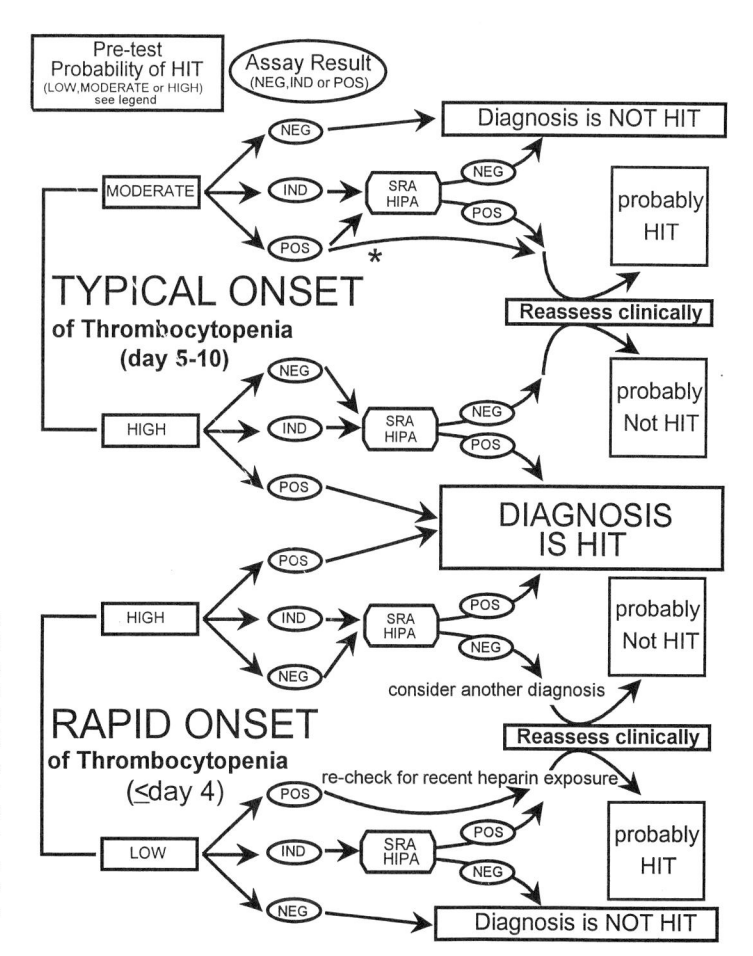

Figure 23–9 Diagnostic algorithm for HIT using an antigen assay (PF4/heparin enzyme immunoassay). The asterisk (*) indicates that a washed platelet activation assay, such as the SRA or HIPA, could be useful in a patient with a moderate pretest probability for HIT and a positive antigen assay, since a positive activation assay has a higher specificity for clinical HIT. Abbreviations: IND, indeterminate test result; NEG, negative test result; POS, positive test result; HIPA, heparin-induced platelet activation assay; SRA, serotonin release assay. (From Warkentin TE, Greinacher A. Laboratory testing for heparin-induced thrombocytopenia. In Warkentin TE, Greinacher A (Eds): Heparin-induced Thrombocytopenia, 2nd ed. New York, Marcel Dekker, 2001, pp. 231–269, with permission.)

sulfate (4%).[58,59] Heparan sulfate provides most of the anti-factor Xa activity of danaparoid, which is mediated via binding to antithrombin (formerly, antithrombin III). Dermatan sulfate, by binding to heparin cofactor II, provides some antithrombin (anti-IIa) activity. However, the anti-Xa/anti-IIa ratio of danaparoid is at least 22, which is much higher even than LMWH (usual ratio, approximately 2 to 4). Danaparoid has minimal nonspecific binding to plasma proteins, and thus "resistance" to its anticoagulant effect because of elevated acute phase reactants is usually not seen.

Danaparoid is well absorbed after subcutaneous administration, with peak levels reached 4 to 5 hours postinjection. The near-100% bioavailability makes it easy to determine the appropriate subcutaneous dosage for a stably anticoagulated patient receiving intravenous danaparoid: for example, 190 U/h by intravenous infusion is approximately equal to 2250 U given twice daily by subcutaneous injection (both provide about 4500 U/24 h). Despite the long half-life of its anti-factor Xa activity (about 25 hours), the drug should be given either intravenously or (at least) twice daily via the subcutaneous route, as the half-life for anti-thrombin activity is about 2 to 4 hours. Danaparoid is renally metabolized, and the dose should be reduced somewhat for patients with renal failure. There is no antidote for danaparoid.

Danaparoid prolongs neither the activated partial thromboplastin time (aPTT) nor the prothrombin time (PT) nor the INR, which facilitates assessment of overlapping warfarin therapy. Monitoring of danaparoid's anticoagulant effect, when needed, is by measuring plasma anti-factor Xa activity by chromogenic assay. This is similar to monitoring of LMWH, except that the standard calibration curve must be constructed using danaparoid (if a LMWH standard curve is used, danaparoid concentrations will be overestimated). Anti-factor Xa monitoring for danaparoid is not widely available, but since danaparoid gives predictable anticoagulant effects, monitoring is often not necessary if a standard dose is given (Table 23–5). However, patients in whom monitoring should be considered include those with substantial renal impairment, unusually low or high body weight, life- or limb-threatening thrombosis, or those in whom unexpected bleeding has occurred. The usual target therapeutic range for danaparoid is 0.5 to 0.8 anti-Xa U/mL, although a higher level (approximately 1 U/mL) in a patient with severe thrombosis seems appropriate.

Table 23–5 • DOSING SCHEDULE FOR DANAPAROID

For rapid intravenous therapeutic-dose anticoagulation:
Loading dose: 2250 U IV bolus,[a] followed by 400 U/h for 4 hours, 300 U/h for 4 hours;
Maintenance: 150–200 U/h for ≥5 days, aiming for anti-Xa level of 0.5–0.8 U/mL

[a] Adjust intravenous danaparoid bolus for body weight: less than 60 kg, 1500 U; 60–75 kg, 2250 U; 75–90 kg, 3000 U; more than 90 kg, 3750 U.

In the United States, danaparoid is approved for DVT prophylaxis following hip replacement surgery (750 U two or three times daily by subcutaneous injection). This low-dose regimen would be appropriate for a patient with previous HIT who requires postoperative antithrombotic prophylaxis. However, for patients with acute HIT, with or without thrombosis, a therapeutic regimen should be given (Table 23–5).[60,61] Although approved for DVT prophylaxis in the United States, Canada, and Europe, its high cost means that this agent is predominantly used as "off-label" treatment for HIT.[59]

A randomized clinical trial[62] found a higher thrombosis resolution rate in patients treated with danaparoid and warfarin, compared with dextran and warfarin, for patients either with mild thrombosis (92% versus 72%; $P = 0.04$) or serious thrombosis (92% versus 33%; $P < 0.001$). Retrospective case series also support the efficacy of danaparoid as a treatment for HIT-associated thrombosis.[60,63-65]

In-vitro cross-reactivity against danaparoid can be detected in some HIT sera.[54,65] However, the cross-reactivity is generally weak, and does not predict adverse clinical outcomes. In the author's opinion, treatment should not be delayed to perform in-vitro cross-reactivity studies, nor is detectable cross-reactivity a contraindication to use of danaparoid.

Lepirudin

Lepirudin (Refludan) is a derivative of hirudin—a direct thrombin inhibitor synthesized naturally by the salivary glands of the medicinal leech—and is manufactured by recombinant technology.[66] The 65-amino acid polypeptide differs minimally in structure from its natural counterpart. Hirudin and its synthetic derivatives form noncovalent but irreversible complexes with thrombin, binding to two sites on thrombin, its active site cleft, as well as its fibrinogen anion-binding site. Unlike heparin, hirudin acts independently of the plasma cofactors, antithrombin and heparin cofactor II. Hirudin also differs from heparin by its ability to inhibit clot-bound thrombin. Thus, dependable thrombin neutralization can occur even in the highly procoagulant milieu of HIT.

In normal subjects, the half-life of lepirudin is about 1.3 hours. However, this agent is renally excreted, and the half-life can rise to 48 hours in patients with renal failure, leading to substantial risk for drug accumulation and bleeding. Lepirudin is usually monitored using the aPTT, which gives a fair correlation with plasma drug levels. The target therapeutic range of 1.5 to 2.5 times the patient's baseline (if known), or the median of the laboratory normal range.[14] Although there are interpatient differences in lepirudin metabolism, most patients show stable anticoagulation during lepirudin treatment. However, the potential for developing antilepirudin antibodies—which paradoxically increases the anticoagulant response to lepirudin in a few patients—means that daily aPTT monitoring must be performed even in stably anticoagulated patients.[67] A high proportion of patients

Table 23-6 • DOSING SCHEDULE FOR LEPIRUDIN (RECOMBINANT HIRUDIN)

For rapid intravenous therapeutic-dose anticoagulation:
Loading dose: 0.4 mg/kg IV bolus
Maintenance: 0.15 mg/kg/h IV, with adjustments to maintain aPTT 1.5 to 2.5 times the median of the normal laboratory range

develop antihirudin antibodies.[67,68] No antidote for lepirudin exists.

Two prospective cohort studies (using historical controls for comparison)[69,70] of lepirudin for the treatment of HIT-associated thrombosis using a prespecified dosing schedule (Table 23-6) led to its approval for this indication both in the European Union (March 1997) and in the United States (March 1998). The first study[69] showed a significantly reduced frequency of a composite end point of mortality, limb amputation, and new thromboembolic complications, compared with the controls (10% versus 23% at day 7 follow-up, and 25% versus 52% at day 35 follow-up, respectively; $P = 0.014$). The second study[70] found a trend in favor of lepirudin (cumulative frequency of composite end point, 31% versus 52%; $P = 0.12$). A meta-analysis[14] of these two studies found that a subtherapeutic aPTT ratio (less than 1.5) was associated with an increased risk for thrombosis, whereas a therapeutic aPTT ratio above the therapeutic range (greater than 2.5) was associated with increased bleeding without any further reduction in antithrombotic efficacy. However, even for patients within the target therapeutic range, bleeding was increased significantly compared with historical controls (relative risk = 3.21 [95% confidence interval, 1.7 to 6.0]; $P<0.001$).

Argatroban

Argatroban is a small-molecule, direct thrombin inhibitor that was associated with a lower thrombotic event rate in a prospective treatment study that utilized historical controls.[71] In this study, patients received argatroban beginning at a dose of 2 μg/kg/min for an average of 6 days. Like lepirudin, the half-life of argatroban is short (less than 1 hour). In contrast to lepirudin, argatroban is excreted normally in patients with moderately severe renal failure; however, the dose of argatroban must be reduced in patients with hepatic failure. Table 23-7 provides a dosing schedule for argatroban

Table 23-7 • DOSING SCHEDULE FOR ARGATROBAN

For rapid intravenous therapeutic-dose anticoagulation:
Initial dose: 2 μg/kg/min IV
Maintenance: Above initial dose adjusted to maintain aPTT 1.5 to 3.0 times the initial baseline value (not to exceed 100 seconds)

in HIT. Argatroban was approved by the U.S. Food and Drug Administration (FDA) for the treatment of HIT-associated thrombosis as of June 30, 2000, and was launched for use in the United States in mid-November 2000. Since the clinical studies also included patients with isolated HIT, argatroban also received this second indication from the FDA (prevention of HIT-associated thrombosis). Identical (therapeutic) doses are recommended for patients either with isolated HIT or HIT-associated thrombosis.

Choice of Parenteral Anticoagulant

The choice of parenteral anticoagulant depends upon several factors, including patient renal and hepatic function, anticipated need to reverse anticoagulation quickly, monitoring methodologies, drug availability/cost, and physicians' experience with a given agent. Table 23-8 lists some of these features, including relative cost.[72,73]

Overlap of Parenteral and Oral Anticoagulation

Overlap of parenteral and oral anticoagulation is required to avoid paradoxical hypercoagulable complications of warfarin. Thus, warfarin should not be started until the patient is satisfactorily anticoagulated with a parenteral anticoagulant (danaparoid, lepirudin, or argatroban). Where possible, the author further recommends that oral anticoagulant therapy be delayed until the platelet count has risen to at least 100,000/μL, as this suggests HIT is responding to parenteral anticoagulant therapy. For patients in whom HIT is not diagnosed until treatment with warfarin has commenced, it may be necessary to reverse warfarin treatment, at least temporarily. The reason is that warfarin prolongs both the INR and the aPTT, and therefore suboptimal anticoagulation with lepirudin or argatroban could result using aPTT-based monitoring. Theoretically, such a reason to reverse warfarin would not be applicable to a patient treated with danaparoid, as there is no interference by danaparoid on the INR. Figure 23-8B shows an example of this situation, in which warfarin therapy was continued in a patient with HIT-associated thrombosis, although bridge therapy with therapeutic-dose danaparoid was given until platelet count recovery occurred.

Physicians should consult the product monographs[74,75] for detailed information regarding monitoring of anticoagulation during overlapping treatment with warfarin and either lepirudin or argatroban. For example, during initiation of warfarin in a patient receiving lepirudin for HIT-associated thrombosis, it is recommended[74] to reduce the dose of the parenteral anticoagulant until the aPTT is at the lower end of the therapeutic range before starting warfarin. In contrast, for a patient receiving argatroban in whom warfarin is commenced, it is recommended[75] to wait for the INR to rise above 4.0 prior to discontinuing argatroban: this is because this level of the INR corresponds to an INR between 2.0

Table 23-8 • FACTORS THAT CAN INFLUENCE THE CHOICE OF ANTICOAGULANT FOR TREATMENT OF ACUTE HIT

Clinical Situation	Relative Merit (i.e. More favored > Less favored)
HIT-associated venous thromboembolism requiring overlapping oral anticoagulation	Danaparoid > Lepirudin > Argatroban
Arterial thrombosis	Argatroban ≈ Lepirudin > Danaparoid[a]
Impending surgery or other invasive procedures (need to reverse anticoagulation)	Argatroban ≈ Lepirudin > Danaparoid
Isolated HIT	Argatroban ≈ Danaparoid > Lepirudin
Renal failure	Argatroban > Danaparoid ≫ Lepirudin
Hepatic failure	Danaparoid ≈ Lepirudin ≫ Argatroban
Ease of monitoring[b]	Lepirudin ≈ Argatroban > Danaparoid[b]
Cost (in the United States)[c]	Argatroban < Lepirudin ≈ Danaparoid

[a] The ability of lepirudin and argatroban to inhibit clot-bound thrombin, as well as the short half-lives of these agents, may be an advantage over danaparoid in patients with arterial thrombosis (potential for rapid reversal of anticoagulation if surgery is mandatory).
[b] Although monitoring of danaparoid's anticoagulant activity by anti-factor Xa chromogenic assay is not widely available, not all patients treated with danaparoid require monitoring (see text).
[c] Argatroban costs about $3000 for a 1-week treatment course for a 60-kg adult (assumes constant infusion of 2 μg/kg/min, and a wholesale acquisition cost of $600 for a 250-mg vial). Danaparoid costs about $4000 for a 1-week treatment course for a 60-kg adult[72] (assumes initial 2250 U bolus followed by accelerated infusion regimen and subsequent constant maintenance infusion rate of 150 U/h, as described in Table 23-5); the cost of lepirudin is also about $4000 for a 1-week therapeutic-dose treatment of a 60-kg adult.[73]

and 3.0, following discontinuation of the argatroban (provided that a sensitive thromboplastin with international sensitivity index [ISI] between 0.88 and 1.78 was used to measure the INR, and that argatroban dosing was no greater than 2 μg/kg/min). In contrast to the direct antithrombins, danaparoid has no effect on the INR and aPTT, and thus monitoring of overlapping warfarin therapy is unchanged. Since the half-life of danaparoid is relatively long, this drug usually can be stopped after 4 or 5 days of warfarin treatment, once the INR has reached the lower therapeutic range. For all these situations, it is prudent to start with expected maintenance doses of warfarin, rather than to give an initial loading dose.

Adjunctive Treatments

Adjunctive treatments may be useful in selected patients with HIT.[76] *Surgical thromboembolectomy* can be limb saving in patients with acute occlusion of large limb arteries by platelet-rich thromboemboli. Either danaparoid[59] or lepirudin[66] can be used for intraoperative anticoagulation of these patients undergoing vascular surgery. *Thrombolytic therapy* with streptokinase or tissue plasminogen activator can be tried in highly selected patients, but issues such as the optimal choice and dose of concomitant parenteral anticoagulant remain (thrombolytic agents increase thrombin availability, since thrombin bound to fibrin degradation products is relatively protected from inhibition by antithrombin[77]). *Plasmapheresis* has been used to treat HIT in uncontrolled reports.[78] Although the rationale has been to remove pathogenic HIT antibodies, this treatment could benefit by correcting acquired deficiencies in natural anticoagulant, such as AT or protein C. If so, it theoretically suggests that plasma, rather than albumin, should be used as replacement fluid for these patients. *High-dose intravenous gammaglobulin* can inhibit HIT antibody-mediated platelet activation,[79] and may therefore be a useful treatment adjunct to try in patients with severe thrombocytopenia, DIC, or microvascular ischemia.[80] *Antiplatelet agents*, such as aspirin, can be tried in patients at high risk for arterial thrombosis, but issues such as bleeding when combined with antithrombotic drugs are not yet resolved.

CAVEATS IN MANAGEMENT OF HIT

Physicians must be vigilant to ensure no inadvertent heparin is given to patients with acute HIT. Since heparin is often given routinely (e.g., via "flushes" to indwelling catheters, or as heparin bonded to pulmonary artery catheters), a simple order to "discontinue heparin" may not necessarily result in removal of all heparin sources. Also, it is now recognized that certain treatments that might have intuitive appeal can actually worsen treatment outcomes in HIT:

- *Warfarin-induced phlegmasia, venous limb gangrene, and skin necrosis syndromes.* As discussed earlier, oral anticoagulants can cause severe deficiency of protein C while at the same time not adequately reducing thrombin generation in acute HIT. Thus, during acute HIT, warfarin should be given only after adequate anticoagulation has been achieved with an agent such as danaparoid, lepirudin, or argatroban, and preferably only once the platelet count has recovered substantially. Occasionally, a patient may be recognized as having HIT once several days of warfarin have already been given. In these situations, it seems reasonable to continue warfarin therapy, provided that cautious dosing is used (to avoid a supratherapeutic INR) and the clinical signs of thrombosis are stable or improving. Particularly if such a patient had acute venous thromboembolism, the author would recommend adding "bridging" therapy with a rapidly effective anticoagulant (e.g., danaparoid) until the platelet count recovered, and it became clear that the thrombosis was under control (see Fig. 23–8B for an example of a patient recognized with HIT 5 days into warfarin therapy, treated with continued warfarin together with "bridge" therapy with danaparoid, until the platelet count recovered).

- *LMWH* is less likely than UFH to cause HIT antibody formation[5]; unfortunately, this does not mean that it is an acceptable treatment for HIT. Using sensitive activation assays, HIT antibodies are just as capable of activating platelets in the presence of LMWH as with UFH,[5,81] and clinical experience suggests that the risk for new, progressive, or recurrent thrombosis during treatment of HIT with LMWH approaches 50%.[82]
- *Platelet transfusions* are relatively contraindicated for prophylaxis of bleeding in patients with acute HIT.[76,83] This is because petechiae and other signs of bleeding are usually not clinical features of HIT, despite even severe thrombocytopenia.[25] Further, platelet transfusions have been associated with thrombotic events in anecdotal reports.[84,85] However, if bleeding caused by anatomic or other factors complicates HIT, therapeutic platelet transfusions in this clinical context may be appropriate.

TREATMENT OF ISOLATED HEPARIN-INDUCED THROMBOCYTOPENIA

Stopping heparin is an important step in managing proven or suspected HIT. However, several studies[14,28,69,70,85,86,87] indicate that cessation of heparin alone is inadequate therapy for HIT, including for patients in whom HIT was diagnosed on the basis of thrombocytopenia alone ("isolated HIT"). A large retrospective cohort study[28] estimated the risk for thrombosis to be 10% at 2 days, 40% at 7 days, and about 50% at 30 days follow-up. Other investigators reported[87] a 38% thrombotic event rate despite stopping heparin; surprisingly, the frequency of thrombosis was not lower in patients in whom the heparin had been stopped soon (less than 48 hours) after onset of HIT, compared with patients in whom the diagnosis was made late (45 versus 34%; $P = 0.26$). A high initial rate of thrombosis (10.4% over the mean 1.7-day period prior to starting lepirudin) was also found in prospective cohort studies performed in Germany.[14]

Tardy and colleagues[88] systematically performed either compression ultrasonography or contrast venography in patients with isolated HIT. They thereby identified subclinical DVT in 8 of 16 consecutive patients with isolated DVT. These eight patients were treated with therapeutic-dose danaparoid, and the remaining eight patients without thrombosis received danaparoid in prophylactic doses. One death from fatal thrombosis was observed using this treatment approach. The high frequency of subclinical DVT at first recognition of HIT may explain the high risk for developing clinically evident venous thrombosis (40% to 50%) when these patients are managed with heparin cessation alone.

Given this unfavorable natural history of isolated HIT, the Consensus Conference of the American College of Chest Physicians recommends that physicians consider giving a rapidly acting alternative anticoagulant for patients with isolated HIT[89,90] (Table 23–9). The author recommends giving *therapeutic* doses of an agent such as argatroban or danaparoid in this setting, as standard prophylactic doses may not suffice in a clinical setting such as acute HIT.[61] However, use of prophylactic doses may be a reasonable approach if subclinical DVT has been excluded by imaging studies, or the patient is judged to be at high risk for bleeding. Regardless of the dose of anticoagulants used, the author recommends that anticoagulation be continued until the platelet count has recovered to a stable plateau, and that duplex ultrasonography be performed prior to discontinuing the parenteral anticoagulant to be sure that ongoing warfarin anticoagulation is not needed.

RE-EXPOSURE TO HEPARIN OF A PATIENT WITH PREVIOUS HIT

Subsequent use of heparin is generally considered contraindicated in patients with a history of proven or suspected HIT.[2,76] However, there is evidence that it may be safe to use heparin again—at least for a brief period—in patients who have recovered from an episode of HIT.[19,76,91] This is because HIT antibodies are transient and are usually not detectable a few weeks or months after resolution of HIT.[19] Moreover, HIT antibodies may not recur quickly (or at all) upon re-exposure to heparin, requiring at least 5 days before clinically significant levels develop.[19]

From a practical point of view, however, such deliberate reuse of heparin in a patient with previous HIT is performed only in exceptional circumstances, for example, patients who require cardiac surgery,[19,91] for whom ideal alternative anticoagulants do not exist. Even in this situation, heparin would only be given for cardiopulmonary bypass itself. Heparin should be avoided completely in the preoperative and postoperative period, with alternative agents given for anticoagulation during heart catheterization or for postoperative anticoagulation.[59,66]

SPECIALIZED CLINICAL SITUATIONS

The management of acute HIT in patients requiring hemodialysis or cardiopulmonary bypass surgery can

Table 23–9 • RECOMMENDATIONS OF THE AMERICAN COLLEGE OF CHEST PHYSICIANS FOR TREATMENT OF HIT[a],[89]

1. We recommend the use of one of the following anticoagulant drugs to treat acute HIT complicated by thrombosis: danaparoid sodium (grade 1B), lepirudin (grade 1C), or argatroban (grade 1C).
2. We recommend that anticoagulation with one of these agents until the platelet count has recovered should also be considered for patients with acute HIT without thrombosis (isolated HIT), as there is a high risk for subsequent clinically evident thrombosis in these patients (all grade 2C in comparison to no treatment).
3. We recommend that clinicians do not use warfarin alone to treat acute HIT complicated by DVT because of the risk of causing venous limb gangrene (grade 1C).
4. Warfarin appears to be safe in acute HIT when it is given to a patient who is adequately anticoagulated with a drug that reduces thrombin generation in HIT, such as danaparoid, lepirudin, or argatroban, although it may be prudent to delay starting warfarin until the platelet count has risen above $100 \times 10^9/L$. We recommend that if warfarin is given to patients with acute HIT, it should be administered together with a drug that reduces thrombin generation in HIT until the platelet count has recovered. Then, warfarin can be continued alone (grade 1C).
5. LMWH is contraindicated in HIT. We recommend that clinicians do not administer LMWH for the treatment of acute HIT (grade 1C+).
6. We recommend that clinicians do not administer prophylactic platelet transfusions for the treatment of HIT (grade 2C).

[a] The implications of the Grades of Recommendations shown above are as follows:

Grade of Recommendation	Clarity of Risk/Benefit	Methodologic Strength of Supporting Data	Implications
1B	Clear	Randomized trials with important limitations	Strong recommendation; likely to apply to most patients
1C+	Clear	Overwhelming evidence from observation studies	Strong recommendation; can apply to most patients in most circumstances
1C	Clear	Observation studies	Intermediate-strength recommendation; may change when stronger evidence available
2C	Unclear	Observation studies	Very weak recommendation; other alternatives may be equally reasonable

Adapted from Hirsh J, Warkentin TE, Shaughnessy SG, et al. Heparin and low-molecular-weight heparin: mechanisms of action, pharmacokinetics, dosing, monitoring, efficacy, and safety. Chest 2001;119 (Suppl):64S–94S, and Guyatt G, Schünemann H, Cook D, et al. Grades of recommendation for antithrombotic agents. Chest 2001; 119(Suppl): 3S–7S.

pose special problems. A comprehensive discussion of these topics[92–94] is available elsewhere.

REFERENCES

Chapter 23 References

1. Warkentin TE. History of heparin-induced thrombocytopenia. In Warkentin TE, Greinacher A (Eds): Heparin-induced Thrombocytopenia, 2nd ed. New York, Marcel Dekker, 2001; pp. 1–18.
2. Warkentin TE, Chong BH, Greinacher A. Heparin-induced thrombocytopenia: towards consensus. Thromb Haemost 1998; 79:1–7.
3. Warkentin TE, Greinacher A. Laboratory testing for heparin-induced thrombocytopenia. In Warkentin TE, Greinacher A (Eds): Heparin-induced Thrombocytopenia, 2nd ed. New York, Marcel Dekker, 2001; pp. 231–269.
4. Amiral J, Bridey F, Dreyfus M, et al. Platelet factor 4 complexed to heparin is the target for antibodies generated in heparin-induced thrombocytopenia. Thromb Haemost 1992;68:95–96 (letter).
5. Warkentin TE, Levine MN, Hirsh J, et al. Heparin-induced thrombocytopenia in patients treated with low-molecular-weight heparin or unfractionated heparin. N Engl J Med 1995;332:1330–1335.
6. Warkentin TE, Elavathil LJ, Hayward CPM, et al. The pathogenesis of venous limb gangrene associated with heparin-induced thrombocytopenia. Ann Intern Med 1997;127:804–812.
7. Warkentin TE. Pseudo-heparin-induced thrombocytopenia. In Warkentin TE, Greinacher A (Eds): Heparin-induced Thrombocytopenia, 2nd ed. New York, Marcel Dekker, 2001; pp. 271–289.
8. Kelton JG, Sheridan D, Santos A, et al. Heparin-induced thrombocytopenia: laboratory studies. Blood 1988;72:925–930.
9. Greinacher A, Pötzsch B, Amiral J, et al. Heparin-associated thrombocytopenia: isolation of the antibody and characterization of a multimolecular PF4-heparin complex as the major antigen. Thromb Haemost 1994;71:247–251.
10. Visentin GP, Ford SE, Scott JP, Aster RH. Antibodies from patients with heparin-induced thrombocytopenia/thrombosis are specific for platelet factor 4 complexed with heparin or bound to endothelial cells. J Clin Invest 1994;93:81–88.
11. Newman PM, Chong BH. Further characterization of antibody and antigen in heparin-induced thrombocytopenia. Br J Haematol 1999;107:303–309.
12. Ziporen L, Li ZQ, Park KS, et al. Defining an antigenic epitope on platelet factor 4 associated with heparin-induced thrombocytopenia. Blood 1998;92:3250–3259.
13. Warkentin TE, Kelton JG. Thrombocytopenia due to platelet destruction and hypersplenism. In Hoffman R, Benz EJ Jr, Shattil SJ, et al. (Eds): Hematology. Basic Principles and Practice, 3rd ed. New York, Churchill Livingstone, 1999; pp 2138–2154.
14. Greinacher A, Eichler P, Lubenow N, et al. Heparin-induced thrombocytopenia with thromboembolic complications: meta-analysis of two prospective trials to assess the value of parenteral treatment with lepirudin and its therapeutic aPTT range. Blood 2000;96:846–851.
15. Warkentin TE, Hayward CPM, Boshkov LK, et al. Sera from patients with heparin-induced thrombocytopenia generate platelet-derived microparticles with procoagulant activity: An explanation for the thrombotic complications of heparin-induced thrombocytopenia. Blood 1994;84:3691–3699.
16. Warkentin TE, Sheppard JI. Generation of platelet-derived microparticles and procoagulant activity by heparin-induced thrombocytopenia IgG/serum and other IgG platelet agonists: a comparison with standard platelet agonists. Platelets 1999;10:319–326.
17. Hughes M, Hayward CPM, Warkentin TE, et al. Morphological analysis of microparticle generation in heparin-induced thrombocytopenia. Blood 2000;96:188–194.
18. Denomme GA. The platelet Fc receptor in heparin-induced thrombocytopenia. In Warkentin TE, Greinacher A (Eds):

Heparin-induced Thrombocytopenia, 2nd ed. New York, Marcel Dekker, 2001; pp. 189–214.

19. Warkentin TE, Kelton JG. Temporal aspects of heparin-induced thrombocytopenia. N Engl J Med 2001;344:1286–1292.

20. Lee DP, Warkentin TE. Frequency of heparin-induced thrombocytopenia. In Warkentin TE, Greinacher A (Eds): Heparin-induced Thrombocytopenia, 2nd ed. New York, Marcel Dekker, 2001; pp. 87–121.

21. Suh JS, Malik MI, Aster RH, Visentin GP. Characterization of the humoral immune response in heparin-induced thrombocytopenia. Am J Hematol 1997;54:196–201.

22. Warkentin TE, Sheppard JI, Horsewood P, et al. Impact of the patient population on the risk for heparin-induced thrombocytopenia. Blood 2000;96:1703–1708.

23. Amiral J, Wolf M, Fischer AM, et al. Pathogenicity of IgA and/or IgM antibodies to heparin-PF4 complexes in patients with heparin-induced thrombocytopenia. Br J Haematol 1996;92:954–959.

24. Warkentin TE, Hong AP. Frequency of upper limb deep venous thrombosis (UL-DVT) in relation to central venous catheter (CVC) use in patients with heparin-induced thrombocytopenia (HIT): evidence for interaction of systemic (HIT) and local (CVC) prothrombotic risk factors. Blood 1998;92 (Suppl 1):500a–501a (abstr).

25. Warkentin TE. Clinical picture of heparin-induced thrombocytopenia. In Warkentin TE, Greinacher A (Eds): Heparin-induced Thrombocytopenia, 2nd ed. New York; Marcel Dekker, 2001, pp 43–86.

26. Warkentin TE, Kelton JG. Delayed-onset heparin-induced thrombocytopenia and thrombosis. Ann Intern Med 2001;135:502–506.

27. Warkentin TE. Clinical presentation of heparin-induced thrombocytopenia. Semin Hematol 1998;35 (Suppl 5):9–16.

28. Warkentin TE, Kelton JG. A 14-year study of heparin-induced thrombocytopenia. Am J Med 1996;101:502–507.

29. Ernest D, Fisher MM. Heparin-induced thrombocytopaenia complicated by bilateral adrenal haemorrhage. Intensive Care Med 1991;17:238–240.

30. Meyer-Lindenberg A, Quenzel E-M, Bierhoff E, et al. Fatal cerebral venous sinus thrombosis in heparin-induced thrombotic thrombocytopenia. Eur Neurol 1997;37:191–192.

31. Warkentin TE, Sikov WM, Lillicrap DP. Multicentric warfarin-induced skin necrosis complicating heparin-induced thrombocytopenia. Am J Hematol 1999;62:44–48.

32. Warkentin TE. Heparin-induced thrombocytopenia: IgG-mediated platelet activation, platelet microparticle generation, and altered procoagulant/anticoagulant balance in the pathogenesis of thrombosis and venous limb gangrene complicating heparin-induced thrombocytopenia. Transfus Med Rev 1996;10:249–258.

33. Gupta AK, Kovacs MJ, Sauder DN. Heparin-induced thrombocytopenia. Ann Pharmacother 1998;32:55–59.

34. Warkentin TE. Limitations of conventional treatment options for heparin-induced thrombocytopenia. Semin Hematol 1998;35 (Suppl 5):17–25.

35. Wallis DE, Quintos R, Wehrmacher W, et al. Safety of warfarin anticoagulation in patients with heparin-induced thrombocytopenia. Chest 1999;116:1333–1338.

36. Warkentin TE. Venous limb gangrene during warfarin treatment of cancer-associated deep venous thrombosis. Ann Intern Med 2001;135:589–593.

37. Warkentin TE. Heparin-induced skin lesions. Br J Haematol 1996;92:494–497.

38. Wütschert R, Piletta P, Bounameaux H. Adverse skin reactions to low molecular weight heparins: frequency, management and prevention. Drug Saf 1999;20:515–525.

39. Warkentin TE. Heparin-induced thrombocytopenia, heparin-induced skin lesions, and arterial thrombosis. Thromb Haemost 1997;77 (Suppl):562 (abstr).

40. Pohl C, Klockgether T, Greinacher A, et al. Neurological complications in heparin-induced thrombocytopenia. Lancet 1999;353:1678–1679 (letter).

41. Warkentin TE, Hirte HW, Anderson DR, et al. Transient global amnesia associated with acute heparin-induced thrombocytopenia. Am J Med 1994;97:489–491.

42. Ansell JE, Clark WP Jr, Compton CC. Fatal reactions associated with intravenous heparin. Drug Intell Clin Pharm 1986;20:74–75 (letter).

43. Polgár J, Eichler P, Greinacher A, Clemetson KJ. Adenosine diphosphate (ADP) and ADP receptor play a major role in platelet activation/aggregation induced by sera from heparin-induced thrombocytopenia patients. Blood 1998;91:549–554.

44. Sheridan D, Carter C, Kelton JG. A diagnostic test for heparin-induced thrombocytopenia. Blood 1986;67:27–30.

45. Warkentin TE, Hayward CPM, Smith CA, et al. Determinants of platelet variability when testing for heparin-induced thrombocytopenia. J Lab Clin Med 1992;120:371–379.

46. Lee DP, Warkentin TE, Denomme GA, et al. A diagnostic test for heparin-induced thrombocytopenia: detection of platelet microparticles using flow cytometry. Br J Haematol 1996;95:724–731.

47. Greinacher A, Michels I, Kiefel V, Mueller-Eckhardt C. A rapid and sensitive test for diagnosing heparin-associated thrombocytopenia. Thromb Haemost 1991;66:734–736.

48. Greinacher A, Amiral J, Dummel V, et al. Laboratory diagnosis of heparin-associated thrombocytopenia and comparison of platelet aggregation test, heparin-induced platelet activation test, and platelet factor 4/heparin enzyme-linked immunosorbent assay. Transfusion 1994;34:381–385.

49. Eichler P, Budde U, Haas S, et al. First workshop for detection of heparin-induced antibodies: validation of the heparin-induced platelet activation (HIPA) test in comparison with a PF4/heparin ELISA. Thromb Haemost 1999;81:625–629.

50. Nguŷn P, Lecompte T, Groupe d'Etude sur l'Hémostase et la Thromboses (GEHT) de la Société Française d'Hématologie. Heparin-induced thrombocytopenia: a survey of tests employed and attitudes in haematology laboratories. Nouv Rev Fr Hematol 1994;36:353–357.

51. Chong BH, Burgess, J, Ismail F. The clinical usefulness of the platelet aggregation test for the diagnosis of heparin-induced thrombocytopenia. Thromb Haemost 1993;69:344–350.

52. Collins JL, Aster RH, Moghaddam M, et al. Diagnostic testing for heparin-induced thrombocytopenia (HIT): an enhanced platelet factor 4 complex enzyme linked immunosorbent assay (PF ELISA). Blood 1997;90 (Suppl 1):461a (abstr).

53. Horsewood P, Warkentin TE, Hayward CPM, Kelton JG. The epitope specificity of heparin-induced thrombocytopenia. Br J Haematol 1996;95:161–167.

54. Newman PM, Swanson RL, Chong BH. Heparin-induced thrombocytopenia: IgG binding to PF4-heparin complexes in the fluid phase and cross-reactivity with low molecular weight heparin and heparinoid. Thromb Haemost 1998;80:292–297.

55. Amiral J, Bridey F, Wolf M, et al. Antibodies to macromolecular platelet factor 4-heparin complexes in heparin-induced thrombocytopenia: a study of 44 cases. Thromb Haemost 1995;73:21–28.

56. Bauer TL, Arepally G, Konkle BA, et al. Prevalence of heparin-associated antibodies without thrombosis in patients undergoing cardiopulmonary bypass surgery. Circulation 1997;95:1242–1246.

57. Amiral J, Marfaing-Koka A, Wolf M, et al. Presence of autoantibodies to interleukin-8 or neutrophil-activating peptide-2 in patients with heparin-associated-thrombocytopenia. Blood 1996;88:410–416.

58. Meuleman DG, Hobbelen PMJ, Van Dedem G, Moelker HCT. A novel anti-thrombotic heparinoid (Org 10172) devoid of bleeding inducing capacity: a survey of its pharmacological properties in experimental animal models. Thromb Res 1982;27:353–363.

59. Chong BH. Danaparoid for the treatment of heparin-induced thrombocytopenia. In Warkentin TE, Greinacher A (Eds):

Heparin-induced Thrombocytopenia, 2nd ed. New York, Marcel Dekker, 2001; pp 323–347.

60. Farner B, Eichler P, Kroll H, Greinacher A. A comparison of danaparoid and lepirudin for heparin-induced thrombocytopenia. Thromb Haemost 2001;85:950–957.

61. Warkentin TE. Heparin-induced thrombocytopenia: yet another treatment paradox? Thromb Haemost 2001;85:947–949.

62. Chong BH. Low molecular weight heparinoid and heparin-induced thrombocytopenia. Aust NZ J Med 1996;26:331 (abstr).

63. Magnani HN. Heparin-induced thrombocytopenia (HIT): an overview of 230 patients treated with orgaran (Org 10172). Thromb Haemost 1993;70:554–561.

64. Tardy-Poncet B, Tardy B, Reynaud J, et al. Efficacy and safety of danaparoid sodium (ORG 10172) in critically ill patients with heparin-associated thrombocytopenia. Chest 1999;115:1616–1620.

65. Warkentin TE: Danaparoid (Orgaran®) for the treatment of heparin-induced thrombocytopenia (HIT) and thrombosis: effects on *in vivo* thrombin and cross-linked fibrin generation, and evaluation of the clinical significance of *in vitro* cross-reactivity (XR) of danaparoid for HIT-IgG. Blood 1996;88 (Suppl 1):626a (abstr).

66. Greinacher A. Recombinant hirudin for the treatment of heparin-induced thrombocytopenia. In Warkentin TE, Greinacher A (Eds): Heparin-induced Thrombocytopenia, 2nd ed. New York, Marcel Dekker, 2001; pp. 349–380.

67. Eichler P, Friesen H-J, Lubenow N, et al. Antihirudin antibodies in patients with heparin-induced thrombocytopenia treated with lepirudin: incidence, effects on aPTT, and clinical relevance. Blood 2000;96:2373–2378.

68. Song X, Huhle G, Wang L, et al. Generation of anti-hirudin antibodies in heparin-induced thrombocytopenic patients treated with r-hirudin. Circulation 1999;100:1528–1532.

69. Greinacher A, Völpel H, Janssens U, et al. for the HIT Investigators Group: Recombinant hirudin (lepirudin) provides safe and effective anticoagulation in patients with heparin-induced thrombocytopenia. A prospective study. Circulation 1999;99:73–80.

70. Greinacher A, Janssens U, Berg G, et al. for the Heparin-associated Thrombocytopenia Study (HAT) Investigators: Lepirudin (recombinant hirudin) for parenteral anticoagulation in patients with heparin-induced thrombocytopenia. Circulation 1999; 100:587–593.

71. Lewis BE, Wallis DE, Berkowitz SD, et al. for the ARG-911 Study Investigators: Argatroban anticoagulant therapy in patients with heparin-induced thrombocytopenia. Circulation 2001;103: 1838–1843.

72. Anonymous: Ardeparin and danaparoid for prevention of deep vein thrombosis. Med Lett 1997;39:94–95.

73. Anonymous: Lepirudin for heparin-induced thrombocytopenia. Med Lett 1998;40:94–95.

74. Hoechst Marion Roussel, prescribing information (as of March 1998) for Refludan™. HMR, The Pharmaceutical Company of Hoechst, Kansas City, MO.

75. SmithKline Beecham Pharmaceuticals, prescribing information (as of November 2000) for Argatroban, Philadelphia, PA.

76. Greinacher A, Warkentin TE. Treatment of heparin-induced thrombocytopenia: An Overview. In Warkentin TE, Greinacher A (Eds): Heparin-induced Thrombocytopenia, 2nd ed. New York, Marcel Dekker, 2001; pp. 291–322.

77. Weitz JI, Leslie B, Hudoba M. Thrombin binds to soluble fibrin degradation products where it is protected from inhibition by heparin-antithrombin but susceptible to inactivation by antithrombin-independent inhibitors. Circulation 1998;97:544–552.

78. Robinson JA, Lewis BE. Plasmapheresis in the management of heparin-induced thrombocytopenia. Semin Hematol 1999;36 (Suppl 1):29–32.

79. Greinacher A, Liebenhoff U, Kiefel V, et al. Heparin-associated thrombocytopenia: the effects of various intravenous IgG preparations on antibody mediated platelet activation—a possible new indication for high dose i.v. IgG. Thromb Haemost 1994;71: 641–645.

80. Frame JN, Mulvey KP, Phares JC, et al. Correction of severe heparin-associated thrombocytopenia with intravenous immunoglobulin. Ann Intern Med 1989;111:946–947.

81. Greinacher A, Michels I, Mueller-Eckhardt C. Heparin-associated thrombocytopenia: antibody is not heparin-specific. Thromb Haemost 1992;67:545–549.

82. Ranze O, Eichner A, Lubenow N, et al. The use of low-molecular-weight heparins in heparin-induced thrombocytopenia (HIT): a cohort study. Ann Hematol 2000;79 (Suppl. 1):P198 (abstr).

83. Contreras M. The appropriate use of platelets: an update from the Edinburgh Consensus Conference. Br J Haematol 1998;101 (Suppl 1):10–12.

84. Babcock RB, Dumper CW, Scharfman WB. Heparin-induced thrombocytopenia. N Engl J Med 1976;295:237–241.

85. Cimo PL, Moake JL, Weinger RS, et al. Heparin-induced thrombocytopenia: association with a platelet aggregation factor and arterial thromboses. Am J Hematol 1979;6:125–133.

86. Boon DMS, Michiels JJ, Stibbe J, et al. Heparin-induced thrombocytopenia and antithrombotic therapy. Lancet 1994;344:1296 (letter).

87. Wallis DE, Workman DL, Lewis BE, et al. Failure of early heparin cessation as treatment for heparin-induced thrombocytopenia. Am J Med 1999;106:629–635.

88. Tardy B, Tardy-Poncet B, Fournel P, et al. Lower limb veins should be systematically explored in patients with isolated heparin-induced thrombocytopenia. Thromb Haemost 1999; 82:1199–1200 (letter).

89. Hirsh J, Warkentin TE, Shaughnessy SG, et al. Heparin and low-molecular-weight heparin: mechanisms of action, pharmacokinetics, dosing, monitoring, efficacy, and safety. Chest 2001;119 (Suppl):64S–94S.

90. Guyatt G, Schunëmann H, Cook D, et al. Grades of recommendation for antithrombotic agents. Chest 2001;119 (Suppl):3S–7S.

91. Pötzsch B, Klovekorn WP, Madlener K. Use of heparin during cardiopulmonary bypass in patients with a history of heparin-induced thrombocytopenia. N Engl J Med 2000;343:515 (letter).

92. Fischer KG. Hemodialysis in heparin-induced thrombocytopenia. In Warkentin TE, Greinacher A (Eds): Heparin-induced Thrombocytopenia, 2nd ed. New York, Marcel Dekker, 2001; pp. 409–427.

93. Pötzsch B, Madlener K. Management of cardiopulmonary bypass anticoagulation in patients with heparin-induced thrombocytopenia. In Warkentin TE, Greinacher A (Eds): Heparin-induced Thrombocytopenia, 2nd ed. New York, Marcel Dekker, 2001; pp. 429–444.

94. Magnani HN, Beijering RJR, ten Cate JW, Chong BH. Orgaran anticoagulation for cardiopulmonary bypass in patients with heparin-induced thrombocytopenia. In Pifarré R (Ed): New Anticoagulants for the Cardiovascular Patients. Philadelphia, Hanley & Belfus, 1997; pp. 487–500.

PART IV

PHARMACOLOGIC AGENTS

CHAPTER 24

Antithrombotic and Thrombolytic Agents

Charles W. Francis, M.D.
Scott D. Berkowitz, M.D.

Antithrombotic and thrombolytic drugs are among the most frequently used in medicine. They include potent agents affecting hemostasis and are used to either prevent or treat thrombotic disease. Knowledge of their properties and skill in therapeutic application are necessary to achieve maximum benefit and limit the frequency of bleeding complications. This chapter will focus on practical issues in the use of commonly used antithrombotic and thrombolytic drugs and also consider several new agents that have been recently introduced into clinical practice.

ORAL ANTICOAGULANTS

Mechanism and Pharmacology

The oral anticoagulants include several coumarins that act as competitive inhibitors of vitamin K and thereby inhibit the carboxylation reactions required for synthesis of several coagulation proteins, including factors II, VII, IX, and X.[1] Proteins C and S, involved in inhibitory regulation of hemostasis, are also vitamin K dependent, and their levels also decrease during oral anticoagulation. The synthesis of all of these vitamin K-dependent proteins is inhibited to a similar extent, and steady-state levels during chronic therapy are reduced to the same degree. The initial rate of decrease, however, varies because of differences in plasma half-lives. Therefore, factor VII with a half-life of 6 hours declines rapidly, whereas prothrombin with a half-life of 72 hours decreases slowly after initiation of treatment.

In North America the commonly used coumarin is warfarin (Coumadin). Warfarin is nearly completely absorbed after oral administration, and treatment is administered orally, although an intravenous preparation is available for use in circumstances where oral intake is precluded. It does not work faster, however, than oral warfarin. Drug metabolism is complicated by binding to plasma proteins, including albumin, and also by hepatic metabolism, resulting in a variable plasma half-life. A number of drugs interact with warfarin by altering either protein binding or hepatic metabolism. Because warfarin is a competitive vitamin K antagonist, its biologic action is further complicated by variability in dietary vitamin K intake. Together, these effects result in wide biologic variability in response to warfarin so that close laboratory monitoring is required.

Administration and Monitoring

After starting therapy the onset of action is delayed as levels of vitamin K-dependent proteins decrease. Usually between 4 and 7 days of treatment are required to achieve comparably decreased levels of vitamin K-dependent factors. The anticoagulant effect is monitored by using the prothrombin time (PT) which is sensitive to decreases in vitamin K-dependent factors, and this is further standardized by conversion to the International Normalized Ratio (INR).[2] This reporting is now standard because different thromboplastins used to determine the PT vary in their sensitivity to the anticoagulant effect. Therefore, the degree of prolongation of the PT is variable using different thromboplastins, but the INR is independent of the thromboplastin used. Administration of a large initial dose ("loading") will result in rapid prolongation of the PT, an effect due largely to a rapid decrease in factor VII, which has a short half-life. This is, however, not an adequate reflection of true antithrombotic effectiveness, which depends on a balanced reduction of all vitamin K-dependent factors. Such treatment may result in excessive factor VII reduction, resulting in bleeding, or to a profound early decrease in the anticoagulant protein C, resulting in an unfavorable balance of antithrombotic and prothrom-

Table 24–1 • HINTS FOR THE SUCCESSFUL LONG-TERM USE OF WARFARIN

- Don't needlessly start and stop therapy (e.g., for biopsies or dental work). Low therapeutic INRs (2.0 to 2.2) will not result in excessive bleeding. Additionally, following this hint will minimize the risk of warfarin skin necrosis.
- It is helpful to think of a patient's warfarin dose in terms of a cumulative weekly quantity and then make adjustments in daily doses of warfarin small (i.e., only ±10% to 15%) in most cases. Skipping a day of therapy itself represents a 14% change in weekly dosage. Too frequently, changes are excessive, with undesirable results.
- When changing doses, do not expect reliable changes in the INR before 4 to 7 days. INR should not be drawn prior to 4 days into a dosage change. To do so more often results in misleading information and therapeutic overcompensation.
- Do not be frustrated by INRs such as 1.8 or 3.3 in patients who have a desired INR range of 2.0 to 3.0, which is actually a very narrow range achievable in only about 75% of the time under the best of circumstances.
- Significant variances (e.g., INRs less than 1.5 or greater than 6.0) nearly always have an explanation, such as missed or double doses, significant changes in diet, and especially the addition or substitution of some new drug or over-the-counter agent.
- Instruct patients not to take or discontinue any medications, over-the-counter drugs, drug samples, alternative medicines, or drugs from friends or family without your knowledge.
- If a new drug or therapy is added or diet significant changed, recheck the INR at day 4 to 5 to observe for effect. This is better than reliance on tables of drugs or one's memory.
- The most commonly encountered agents to greatly increase (i.e., at least double or triple) the INR include amiodarone, metronidazole, and cimetidine. Those greatly decreasing the INR include dietary supplements (e.g., Ensure and others) and multivitamin pills containing vitamin K.
- In reversing the anticoagulant effects of warfarin, recall that warfarin's action is through its antivitamin K action. Accordingly, vitamin K therapy is usually the most logical, cheapest, safest, fastest, and most enduring therapy. Even INRs greater than 20 are normalized within 6 to 8 hours following slow IV infusion of vitamin K. Fresh frozen plasma is slow, expensive, and cumbersome, and represents a major fluid challenge (6 to 8 units) in patients with very high INRs and its effects only last for the half-life of the replaced factors (i.e., on the order of only 6 to 8 hours).
- For long-term patient management, patients should become involved with their physicians in decisionmaking. Use of a "warfarin diary" maintained by the patient greatly helps with recording of drugs and INRs, and helps the patient realize that noticeable changes in INR can occur with changes in lifestyle and dietary alterations.
- The use of warfarin clinics, often run by a healthcare extender or a physician dedicated to running such a clinic, greatly facilitates and safens long-term warfarin therapy. This is accomplished, if by no other way, by INRs performed on site with notification of the patient within minutes. Accordingly the duration of over- or under-anticoagulation intensity is enormously minimized.
- Provide patients with a prescription for a small quantity of vitamin K tablets to take in case of an excessively elevated INR. This can save a trip to the Emergency Department.

botic effects.[3] Anticoagulation should be initiated with a dose close to the expected daily maintenance requirement, which is usually between 5 and 10 mg. Lower doses should be used for small, elderly, or poorly nourished patients or those with an increased bleeding risk and higher doses for patients at low risk of bleeding who are younger and larger. The effect should be monitored at least every other day during initiation of treatment and less frequently during chronic therapy depending on the stability of anticoagulation.

Problems with therapy include variability in the anticoagulant response, which is frequently due to drugs that can either increase or decrease the effect or to changes in the vitamin K content of the diet.[4] Patients should be advised to report any changes in medications to their physicians and to maintain a stable diet, particularly with respect to content of foods high in vitamin K, including green vegetables, and also dietary supplements containing vitamin K. Variability in anticoagulation can also result from changes in absorption due to gastrointestinal illness, poor compliance, excessive alcohol use, or over-the-counter alternative medications (Table 24–1).

Indications

Warfarin is used for prophylaxis of both venous and arterial thromboembolism. It is highly effective in primary prevention of venous thromboembolism in patients at high risk such as orthopaedic patients undergoing hip or knee replacement. Short-term administration for a period of 7 to 14 days postoperatively at an INR of 2 to 3 is effective in reducing the risk of venous thrombosis (Table 24–2). Oral anticoagulation is also highly effective as secondary prophylaxis to prevent recurrence after an initial episode of deep venous thrombosis or pulmonary embolism. Following initial acute treatment with heparin or low-molecular-weight heparin (LMWH), oral anticoagulation is continued chronically at an INR of 2 to 3 for variable periods depending on the risk of recurrence in the individual patient. Oral anticoagulation also is indicated for prophylaxis of arterial thromboembolism in patients with atrial fibrillation or with artificial heart valves who are at risk of systemic

Table 24–2 • RECOMMENDED INR VALUES DURING ORAL ANTICOAGULANT THERAPY

Condition	Target INR (Range)
Deep venous thrombosis treatment	2.5 (2.0–3.0)
Pulmonary embolism treatment	2.5 (2.0–3.0)
Deep venous thrombosis prophylaxis	2.5 (2.0–3.0)
Atrial fibrillation	2.5 (2.0–3.0)
Cardiac valve replacement	
Tissue valves	2.5 (2.0–3.0)
Mechanical valves	3.0 (2.5–3.5)
Acute myocardial infarction	2.5 (2.0–3.0)

Table 24-3 • REVERSAL OF WARFARIN THERAPY

Indication	Plan
Excessively long INR	
INR <6	Lower or hold dose
INR 6-10	Give vitamin K 1-2 mg PO or SQ; recheck INR 12-24 hours later
INR >10	Give vitamin K 2-4 mg PO or SQ; recheck INR 12-24 hours later
Serious bleeding or major overdose	Give vitamin K 5-10 mg IV, plus rarely fresh frozen plasma or prothrombin complex concentrate

embolization and stroke. In patients with mechanical heart valves, anticoagulation to a higher intensity of an INR of 2.5 to 3.5 is recommended. After an acute myocardial infarction (MI), oral anticoagulation is also indicated to prevent systemic embolization or recurrent MI.

Adverse Effects

The most serious and common complication of oral anticoagulation is bleeding, and its risk is related primarily to patient characteristics, the intensity of the anticoagulation and the length of therapy.[5-7] Older age has been related to bleeding risk in several studies. The risk of bleeding is increased with surgery or significant trauma during oral anticoagulation. Similarly, a history of gastrointestinal bleeding, particularly if recent, is a major risk; renal insufficiency, hypertension, and a history of cerebrovascular disease may also be related to bleeding risk. The intensity of anticoagulation as reflected by the INR is the most important predictor of bleeding risk, which is low in the usual therapeutic range but increases above 4.0. The cumulative risk of bleeding increases with a longer duration of treatment, whereas the absolute risk appears greatest early, possibly because of unmasking of asymptomatic pathologic lesions. Overall, the total risk of bleeding with a 3-month course of anticoagulation for venous thromboembolism is between 3% and 5%, and in patients anticoagulated for prosthetic heart valves or atrial fibrillation the yearly rate of major bleeding is also between 3% and 5%.

Warfarin skin necrosis is a rare complication of warfarin therapy that usually, but not always, occurs early in the course of anticoagulation. Initial complaints are typically burning and tingling at the affected site, such as the breast, buttock, or thigh, or at another location with significant underlying adipose tissue. Painful hemorrhagic full-thickness skin infarction develops which heals slowly and frequently requires skin grafting. Histopathology shows thrombosis in dermal and subdermal venules, and it is hypothesized that this is due to disproportionate rapid reduction of anticoagulant proteins C and S predisposing to thrombosis. The reason for its occurrence at anatomic sites with extensive subcutaneous fat is unknown.

Oral anticoagulation should be avoided in pregnancy because warfarin crosses the placenta and exposure during organogenesis in the first trimester can lead to fetal embryopathy with significant cranial bone malformations.[8] Anticoagulation later during pregnancy increases bleeding complications. Oral anticoagulants may be considered during the second trimester, but they are generally avoided because heparin or LMWH are reasonable alternatives.

Reversal of Oral Anticoagulation

Frequently, anticoagulation must be reversed because of bleeding, surgery, trauma, or, especially, overdose. For patients with excessively prolonged INRs (e.g., greater than 6) without bleeding, appropriate interventions are holding warfarin doses, administering low does of vitamin K, and increasing the frequency of monitoring (Table 24-3).[9,10] Serious bleeding or major warfarin overdose (e.g., INR greater than 10) require factor replacement and/or larger vitamin K doses that may need to be given intravenously. Anticoagulated patients who need invasive procedures represent a challenging management problem (Table 24-4).[11] Clinical decision should be based on balancing the risk of thromboembolism with that of bleeding (see Chapter 30).

The goal is to reduce anticoagulation and thereby bleeding risk during and immediately after surgery while avoiding thromboembolism. It is important to note that the risk of thromboembolism increases in the immediate postoperative period. In general, the bleeding risk is highest during surgery and decreases to baseline levels after approximately 1 week. Most surgery can be done with minimal bleeding risk in patients receiving warfarin with an INR near 1.5, although studies documenting an

Table 24-4 • REVERSING WARFARIN ANTICOAGULATION FOR SURGERY

Low risk of thrombotic recurrence: Hold warfarin 4 to 5 days preoperatively; Check the INR 1 day before surgery and perform surgery if it is less than 1.5. Warfarin can be started postoperatively.
Moderate risk of thrombotic recurrence: Hold warfarin 4 to 5 days preoperatively; Check INR 1 day before surgery to confirm it is below 1.5; start unfractionated heparin or LMWH in prophylactic doses preoperatively and continue until warfarin is in the therapeutic range after initiation postoperatively.
High risk of thrombotic recurrence: Effective anticoagulation must be maintained. Warfarin should be stopped 4 to 5 days preoperatively; when INR is below 2.0, heparin or LMWH begun in therapeutic doses either intravenously or subcutaneously, respectively. Heparin should be held 6 hours and subcutaneous LMWH 24 hours preoperatively. Start heparin or LMWH in therapeutic doses postoperatively as soon as the bleeding risk is decreased and acceptable. Restart warfarin. Stop heparin when a therapeutic INR is achieved.

ideal INR do not yet exist. Following acute thrombosis, the risk of recurrence is high initially and declines with time. For example, recurrent venous thromboembolism is high during the first 1 to 2 weeks after diagnosis but much less after 8 to 12 weeks. Elective surgery or other invasive procedures associated with a high bleeding risk should be postponed if possible during the first several months following thrombosis.

HEPARIN

Mechanism and Pharmacology

Heparin is a mixture of sulfated glycosaminoglycans and is the most commonly used rapidly acting parenteral anticoagulant.[12] It is extracted from lungs and intestinal tissue of cows and swine, and it is assayed biologically. Heparin has no direct anticoagulant effect, but it acts through antithrombin, a plasma serine protease inhibitor. Antithrombin inhibits thrombin, factor Xa, and other coagulation enzymes in a reaction that is relatively slow but accelerated approximately 1000-fold in the presence of heparin. Heparin is not absorbed after oral ingestion so it must be given either subcutaneously or intravenously. Heparin interacts with proteins and cells in the blood, resulting in complex pharmacokinetics characterized by rapid equilibration and slower clearance. Heparin causes release of endothelial cell-bound tissue factor pathway inhibitor, and this could contribute to its therapeutic actions. The plasma half-life increases with higher doses and is variable among individuals. After subcutaneous administration, bioavailability may be less than 50% and peak plasma levels occur after 30 to 60 minutes.

Administration and Monitoring

Heparin is usually given intravenously for full anticoagulation, and clinical studies have demonstrated a lower occurrence of bleeding complications with continuous intravenous rather than intermittent bolus therapy. The anticoagulant effect is immediate, but laboratory monitoring is needed because of variability in response among patients. This is most conveniently done with the aPTT. The appropriate aPTT range for heparin therapy is usually between 1.5 and 2.5 times the mean of the normal range, but varies depending on laboratory reagent and instrumentation, and each laboratory should establish a therapeutic range based on appropriate correlation with heparin levels. Clinically useful nomograms are available for adjusting heparin dose (Table 24–5).[13,14] Alternatively, heparin can be monitored using anti-Xa levels, and this approach is useful when the aPTT cannot be relied upon, such as in patients with baseline prolongation of the aPTT due to lupus anticoagulant. Other indications for using such heparin levels are listed in Table 24–6. The therapeutic range using a chromogenic anti-Xa assay is 0.3 to 0.7 U/mL. Maintenance of levels in the therapeutic range provides an adequate antithrombotic level and also limits bleed-

---

Table 24–5 • HEPARIN DOSING NOMOGRAMS

Fixed-Dose Nomogram[a]

aPTT (sec)[1]	Bolus Dose (units)	Stop Infusion (min)	Change Infusion Rate[2]	Time of Repeat aPTT
<50	5000	0	+3 mL/hr	6 hours
50–59	0	0	+3 mL/hr	6 hours
60–85	0	0	0	Next morning
86–95	0	0	−2 mL/hr	Next morning
96–120	0	30	−2 mL/hr	6 hours
>120	0	60	−4 mL/hr	6 hours

[a] From ref. 13. These are modifications following initial heparin loading and maintenance infusion.

Weight-Based Nomogram[b]

The initial dose is 80 U/kg as a bolus, then 18 U/kg per hour. The following dose adjustments are based on the aPTT values obtained every 6 hours.

aPTT (sec)[3]	Bolus (U/kg)	Infusion (U/kg/hr)
<35	80	increase rate by 4
35–45	40	increase rate by 2
46–70	0	no change
71–90	0	decrease rate by 2
>90	0	decrease rate by 3

Dose Adjustment column headers span Bolus (U/kg) and Infusion (U/kg/hr).

[b] From ref. 14.
[1] Reference range is 25 to 37 seconds. Therapeutic range is 60–85 seconds corresponding to a plasma heparin level of 0.3–0.7 U/mL by antifactor Xa activity.
[2] 1 mL/h equals 40 U/h.
[3] Reference range 20–30 seconds.

Table 24–6 • CLINICAL SITUATIONS IN WHICH IT IS APPROPRIATE TO MEASURE HEPARIN LEVELS

- Some clinical conditions are associated with a prolonged aPTT before heparin is administered. These include inherited factor deficiencies, severe liver deficiency, and antiphospholipid syndrome. Accordingly, monitoring heparin dosage by the aPTT is greatly obfuscated. Check a baseline aPTT and begin heparin therapy at a reasonable dose and confirm heparin levels to establish that the heparin level is in the therapeutic range.
- In some cases the clinical situation is such that one wishes to, on the one hand, treat a severe thrombotic episode with adequate heparin, but on the other hand, would not like to have excessive heparin levels. These would include situations where the patient is bleeding, has recently had surgery or a stroke, or severe thrombocytopenia.
- Treating massive thrombosis occasionally is complicated by what has been called heparin resistance. As more and more heparin is administered in an attempt to achieve a therapeutic aPTT, one becomes concerned. It is comforting to determine the heparin level when one is giving massive doses such as ≥40,000 units of standard heparin a day.
- In using LMWH or danaparoid, determination of an antifactor Xa activity is useful in all the above cases as well as where there is uncertainty regarding dosages in patients who are massively obese or in those who are renally insufficient. Should a patient have a bleeding episode while receiving what one had considered to be appropriate doses of these agents, it is of value to confirm the level at which the adverse effect took place.
- Obtaining heparin levels to rule out the presence of heparin when a patient theoretically had not been administered heparin is useful. One such clinical situation is postoperative bleeding with a very long aPTT, which strongly suggests the possibility of heparin. This can also be useful when an unexpectedly prolonged aPTT is obtained in a patient with an indwelling heparinized central line and the sample could be contaminated with heparin. Establishment that heparin was present or absent can narrow diagnostic considerations.

ing. Some patients appear to respond poorly to heparin, with inadequate prolongation of the aPTT despite apparently adequate or even high heparin dosage. This is often referred to as "heparin resistance," and is due rarely to antithrombin deficiency but more commonly to the acute phase response, which results in high levels of procoagulant proteins, particularly factor VIII. The antithrombotic effect of heparin correlates best with plasma heparin levels, which may be adequate in these circumstances despite an apparent subtherapeutic aPTT. Therefore, for patients requiring over 1500 U/h, monitoring with an anti-Xa assay is appropriate and provides a better indication of plasma heparin levels.[15] For prophylaxis of venous thromboembolic disease heparin is administered subcutaneously in doses of 5000 units every 8 to 12 hours, with the 8-hourly regimen more appropriate in patients at higher risk. Minor prolongation of the aPTT may occur, but monitoring is neither recommended nor required.

Indications

Heparin is commonly used in the prevention and treatment of venous thromboembolic disease. For treatment, therapy is initiated with a bolus followed by a constant infusion to maintain the desired anticoagulant effect for a minimum of 5 days and followed by a longer period of oral anticoagulation. Heparin is also used in the treatment of acute coronary syndromes and is effective in short-term treatment of unstable angina and MI, as an adjunct to thrombolytic therapy, and in preventing acute reocclusion after angioplasty or stenting. It is used to maintain vascular patency during vascular surgery and in high doses to permit extracorporeal circulation during hemodialysis or cardiopulmonary bypass. In patients with disseminated intravascular coagulation, heparin can be used attempting to reduce hemostatic activation, prevent microvascular occlusion, and improve overall hemostasis (see Chapter 12).

Heparin is often used for anticoagulation during pregnancy.[16] Acute short-term treatment is administered as in the nonpregnant patient, and long-term anticoagulation can be provided with subcutaneous administration. Heparin is often the anticoagulant of choice because warfarin cannot be used during pregnancy because of the risk of fetal effects. For full anticoagulation, subcutaneous doses of 17,000 units or more every 12 hours may be required with monitoring to maintain the aPTT in the therapeutic range 4 to 6 hours after administration. Heparin requirements may increase during pregnancy, particularly in the third trimester. Heparin does not cross the placenta and exerts no anticoagulant effect in the fetus. It can, however, increase bleeding during delivery, and heparin may be discontinued briefly at the beginning of labor or prior to planned operative delivery.

Adverse Effects

The most frequent complication of heparin administration is bleeding which is related to the dose and intensity of treatment and to patient characteristics. Considering the wide range of patients in whom heparin is used, it is difficult to provide an average bleeding risk. However, in large groups of patients receiving heparin for treatment of venous thromboembolic disease, approximately 3% may have a major bleeding complication. Lower doses, such as those used for prophylaxis, are rarely the sole or chief cause of hemorrhage.

Heparin-induced thrombocytopenia (HIT) (see Chapter 23) is an immune-mediated platelet consumption caused by an antibody directed against a complex of heparin and platelet factor 4.[12,17] Platelets can fall to low levels associated with bleeding yet HIT is more associated with severe arterial or venous thromboembolic complications. HIT occurs in about 3% of patients when defined as a 50% reduction in baseline platelet count or a platelet count of less than 150,000/μL during

Table 24-7 • APPROACH TO HEMORRHAGING PATIENTS RECEIVING HEPARIN

Questions	Considerations	Action
Is bleeding due to heparin?	Do not assume that hemorrhage is necessarily due to heparin. Consider and evaluate for structural defects such as tumor, ulcer, or nonligated vessel. Consider other inherited or acquired problems.	Apply local pressure if possible. Correct structural bleeding. Ligate vessels.
Are aggravating factors present?	Rule out contribution to hemorrhage by thrombocytopenia, antiplatelet agents such as aspirin or NSAIDs, thrombolytic agents, oral anticoagulants, or acquired vitamin K deficiency.	Administer DDAVP for antiplatelet agent reversal and vitamin K for that deficiency. Transfuse platelets for thrombocytopenia.
Is the concentration of heparin unacceptably high if actions thus far implicate heparin?	Identify time and dose (confirmed by discussion with pharmacy and nursing) of last heparin administration. Estimate half-life of remaining heparin. Check heparin level.	Cease heparin administration. Attempt protamine reversal in exceptional cases. Do not administer FFP.
Is the indication for continuing anticoagulation stronger than the contraindication?	Failure to treat thromboembolic indications with heparin is usually much more dangerous than the very rare hemorrhagic fatality using heparin.	Lower the dose of heparin and transfuse as necessary. Consider IVC devices in exceptional cases.

NSAIDs, Nonsteroidal anti-inflammatory drugs; DDAVP, desmopressin; FFP, fresh frozen plasma; IVC, inferior vena cava.

therapy. In patients receiving heparin for the first time, HIT usually occurs after 5 days but thrombocytopenia may develop earlier if there has been prior exposure. Platelet counts should be monitored during treatment and heparin discontinued if thrombocytopenia occurs. If a rapidly acting parenteral anticoagulant is needed, hirudin can be used as an alternative.

Long-term heparin therapy causes radiographic evidence of bone loss in over 15% of women receiving prolonged treatment during pregnancy. Symptomatic vertebral fractures occur in approximately 2%. The bone loss resolves after heparin is discontinued.[18,19] The risk with short-term use is not appreciable.

Reversal of Effect

A major advantage of heparin is its short half-life. Anticoagulant effect is eliminated within 2 to 3 hours after discontinuation of an intravenous infusion. Therefore, stopping the infusion and local measures are usually adequate to control bleeding (Table 24–7). In major or life-threatening bleeding, the anticoagulant effect of heparin can be neutralized with protamine sulfate, which is a basic polypeptide that binds tightly to the acidic heparin molecule. The usual dose of protamine is 1 mg to neutralize 100 units of heparin. The dose to be administered is based on an estimate of the amount of heparin remaining in the circulation. Protamine is routinely used to neutralize heparin after cardiopulmonary bypass using standard formulas and activated clotting time (ACT) monitoring. Fresh frozen plasma has no role in reversing heparin effect.

LOW-MOLECULAR-WEIGHT HEPARIN

Mechanism and Pharmacology

Significant clinical problems with heparin include unpredictable absorption and bioavailability after subcutaneous administration and variable binding to plasma proteins and cells. These together result in the need to monitor heparin therapy with coagulation tests and to adjust doses. Bleeding is a serious complication, osteoporosis can develop with prolonged use, and HIT develops in approximately 3% of patients. These limitations led to studies of structural and functional relationships with heparin and eventually to the development of low-molecular-weight heparins, which are now increasing in use. Low-molecular-weight heparin (LMWH) preparations are produced by treating heparin chemically or enzymatically to decrease the size of the polysaccharide chains, yielding a product with a restricted molecular weight distribution with a mean of approximately 4000 to 5000.[20] Like heparin, LMWH exerts its antithrombotic effect through interaction with antithrombin. In the presence of LMWH, antithrombin inactivates factor Xa as does unfractionated heparin but is less able to inactivate thrombin because of the shorter polysaccharide length. A comparison of important clinical properties of heparin and LMWH are shown in Table 24–8. Several LMWH preparations are available, and they share many clinical and pharmacologic properties. Also, effectiveness and safety have been similar in clinical trials. However, as each is produced by a different

Table 24-8 • DIFFERENCES BETWEEN HEPARIN AND LMWH

	Heparin	LMWH
Bioavailability after SQ injection	Dose dependent, low	High
Half-life	1–2 hours	3–5 hours
Need for monitoring	Routine	Occasional
Cost	Negligible	High
Prolongation of aPTT	Dose dependent	Minimal

SQ, subcutaneous.

method and has some unique properties, pharmacologic properties and clinical results may differ.

LMWH preparations can be administered intravenously, but they are usually given subcutaneously because of their nearly complete absorption and the obviously increased convenience. This is a clear benefit over unfractionated heparin, which exhibits variable and dose-dependent absorption after subcutaneous administration. Moreover, unlike heparin, LMWH shows much less binding to plasma proteins and cells. Consequently, blood levels and anticoagulant effects are more predictable after administration of LMWH. Also, LMWH preparations have a longer plasma half-life than unfractionated heparin, a desirable effect in the absence of bleeding. Together, these properties make possible once- or twice-daily subcutaneous LMWH regimens practical for prophylaxis and therapy. LMWH preparations have significant renal clearance, and high plasma levels can rapidly accumulate following repeated doses in patients with reduced renal function. Therefore, monitoring of anti-Xa levels and dose adjustments are needed in patients with renal impairment. Markedly obese patients also represent a difficult group, as dosing regimens have not been specifically tested in these patients and very high levels can result from weight-based dosing. Many experts "cap" the dose at the equivalent of approximately 12,500 units twice daily. Accordingly, in selected cases, heparin monitoring is very useful with LMWH therapy (see Table 24–6).

Clinical Use

The use of LMWH is expanding rapidly to encompass most applications for which heparin has been used traditionally. Extensive clinical studies are now available to guide prophylaxis and therapy of venous thromboembolic disease. The dosing regimens for LMWH preparations approved for use in North America and Europe are listed in Table 24–9. As of this date, enoxaparin (Lovenox), dalteparin (Fragmin), ardeparin (Normiflo), and tinzaparin (Innohep) are FDA approved for use in the United States. Each is marketed for specific indications, and labeling differs, with some assayed in anti-Xa units and some in milligrams. In general, 1 mg is approximately equivalent to 100 anti-Xa units. For details regarding indications and dosages, specific prescribing information should be reviewed.

For prophylaxis in surgery, regimens vary depending on the risk of thrombosis.[21] Lower doses are recommended for low-risk patients, with increased doses in higher-risk patients such as those undergoing surgery

Table 24–9 • TREATMENT REGIMENS WITH LMWH

	Drug[a]	Regimen
Prophylaxis		
General surgery		
Low risk	Dalteparin	2500 U, 1–2 hours preop and qd
	Enoxaparin	20 mg, 1–2 hours preop and qd
	Nadroparin	3100 U, 2 hours preop and qd
	Tinzaparin	3500 U, 2 hours preop and qd
High risk	Dalteparin	5000 U, 10–12 hours preop and qd
	Enoxaparin	40 mg 10–12 hours preop and qd
	Danaparoid[b]	750 U bid
Orthopedic surgery	Dalteparin	5000 U 8–12 hours preop and qd
	Enoxaparin	30 mg q12h starting 12–24 hours postop or 40 mg qd starting 12 hours preop
	Ardeparin	50 U/kg q12h starting 12–24 hours postop
	Nadroparin	40 U/kg 2 hours preop and qd for 3 d; then 60 U/kg qd
	Tinzaparin	50 U/kg 2 hours preop and qd; or, 75 U/kg qd starting 12–24 hours postop
	Danaparoid[b]	750 U 1–2 hours preop and bid
Spinal injury	Enoxaparin	30 mq q12h
Multiple trauma	Enoxaparin	30 mg q12h
Medical patients	Enoxaparin	20 mg qd (40 mg qd more effective in high-risk patients)
	Dalteparin	2500 U qd
	Danaparoid[b]	750 U bid
Treatment		
Venous thromboembolism	Enoxaparin	1 mg/kg q12h; or, 1.5 mg/kg qd
	Dalteparin	100 U/kg q12h; or 200 U/kg qd
	Nadroparin	90 U/kg q12h
	Tinzaparin	175 U/kg qd
Unstable angina	Enoxaparin	1 mg/kg q12h
	Dalteparin	100 U/kg q12h

[a] Brand names: dalteparin: Fragmin; enoxaparin: Lovenox; ardeparin: Normiflo; nadroparin: Fraxiparine; tinzaparin: Innohep; danaparoid: Orgaran.
[b] Danaparoid sodium is not a LMWH but a closely related glycosaminoglycan mixture composed of heparan sulfate, dermatan sulfate, and chondroitin sulfate.

for active malignancy. Orthopedic surgery patients are at particularly high risk, and increased daily or twice-daily doses are recommended. Generally, high doses are given either the night before or postoperatively rather than immediately preoperatively to decrease the risk of surgical bleeding. In patients receiving epidural anesthesia, the catheter should be placed either prior to administration of LMWH or at the time of anticipated trough level (see Chapter 39). Additional doses should be held for at least 2 hours after catheter insertion, withdrawal, or manipulation because of the risk of bleeding in the spinal canal.[22] LMWH is also effective in high-risk patients following spinal injury or multiple trauma. It can be used for prophylaxis in medical patients, and a recent large prospective study suggests that 40 mg of enoxaparin is more effective than 20 mg once daily in medical patients with acute illnesses.[23]

The pharmacokinetic properties of LMWH preparations make them suitable for treatment of acute deep venous thrombosis and pulmonary embolism using subcutaneous administration, and clinical studies have established the efficacy and safety of this approach.[24-26] High-dose regimens are used, and either once-or twice-daily administration has been effective. Similar doses are used for treatment of acute coronary syndromes, with evidence from clinical trials of improved outcomes in patients with unstable angina treated acutely with LMWH as compared to unfractionated heparin. LMWH does not cross the placenta and has been used successfully for prophylaxis and treatment of venous thromboembolic disease in pregnancy. Because of changing weight and renal function, occasional monitoring with anti-Xa levels is advisable.

Adverse Effects

The primary complication of LMWH is bleeding. Minor bruising at injection sites is common and annoying but of little clinical consequence. Major bleeding occurs with approximately the same frequency as with unfractionated heparin when used in similar patient groups for the same indication. HIT is much less common with LMWH, occurring only 10% to 15% as often as with heparin, suggesting that HIT could be reduced by 80% by the use of LMWH. However, cross-reactivity of the antibody occurs, and LMWH is not an acceptable choice for continued anticoagulation in patients with HIT. Animal studies suggest that osteoporosis may be less common with LMWH; few clinical data are available.

Choice of Heparin Versus LMWH

The factors governing choice of heparin or LMWH are effectiveness, safety, convenience, and cost. For prophylaxis in most surgical and medical patients, the evidence indicates that heparin and LMWH are equally effective, and the lower cost of heparin makes it an attractive choice. In orthopedic patients, LMWH is more effective than heparin and therefore preferable. For treatment of venous thromboembolic disease, the safety and effectiveness of heparin and LMWH are comparable and, therefore, choice of treatment rests on other factors. The subcutaneous regimens of LMWH offer better patient convenience, and outpatient home treatment is the preference of most patients. Outpatient therapy still requires intensive patient education, adequate medical supervision, and considerations of drug costs, insurance coverage, and adequate follow-up. The overall cost of outpatient therapy is much less than inpatient intravenous heparin treatment. There are some specific circumstances, however, in which unfractionated heparin may be preferable. In patients who may require an invasive procedure on an urgent basis, the short half-life of heparin administered intravenously is attractive. Also, patients with renal insufficiency have an increased bleeding risk and decreased LMWH clearance may lead to high levels; intravenous heparin offers some advantage. LMWH is incompletely reversed by protamine sulfate, making it difficult to use for bypass surgery. The use of LMWH for acute coronary syndromes is rapidly evolving and involves consideration of combination therapy, including potent antiplatelet agents and mechanical interventions. Some studies indicate greater effectiveness of LMWH for acute treatment of unstable angina.[27]

DANAPAROID SODIUM

Mechanism and Pharmacology

Danaparoid sodium is not a LMWH but is of the glycosaminoglycuronan class, composed of approximately 84% heparan sulfate, 12% dermatan sulfate, and 4% chondroitin sulfate (Table 24–10). Danaparoid sodium prevents fibrin formation in the coagulation pathway by its anti-Xa and anti-IIa (thrombin) effects. The anti-Xa:anti-IIa activity ratio is greater than 22. Because of this predominant anti-Xa activity, danaparoid sodium has little effect on the aPTT and PT. It has minimal effect on fibrinolytic activity and bleeding time, and only minor effect on platelet function and platelet aggregability. Danaparoid is eliminated mainly via the kidneys.

Indications and Clinical Use

Orgaran (danaparoid sodium) injection is indicated for the prophylaxis of postoperative DVT, which may lead to PE, in patients undergoing elective hip replacement surgery. Because danaparoid differs structurally from heparin, it has been used frequently in patients with HIT who require anticoagulation, although it does not as yet have U.S. Food and Drug Administration (FDA) labeling for this indication. Although there is some theoretical risk to this use as there is an in-vitro cross-reactivity rate of 10% to 20% of heparin antibodies with danaparoid,[28-30] actual in-vivo cross-reactivity appears to be extremely rare. Danaparoid has not been useful in treatment of arterial disease. To date only two papers describe its use in percutaneous coronary intervention, and this is in combination with abciximab in four HIT patients.[31,32] In the acute stroke study called the TOAST

Table 24–10 • COMPARISON OF PROPERIES OF ANTICOAGULANT AGENTS

	UFH	LMWH	Danaparoid	Lepirudin	Argatroban	Bivalirudin
Size	Very large	Large	Large	Small	V. small	Small
MW(dalton)	15,000	5000	6000	7000	527	2180
Thrombin inhibition	Indirect	Indirect	Indirect	Direct	Direct	Direct
Thrombin binding affinity	++	+	Minimal	+++	++	++
Route of administration	IV, SQ, (potentially PO)	IV, SQ, (potentially PO)	SQ	IV, SQ	IV	IV
Onset	Rapid	Rapid	Rapid	Rapid	Rapid	Rapid
Reversibility	Rapid	Slower	Slowest	Slow	Rapid	Rapid
Clearance	Hepatic	Renal	Renal	Renal	Hepatic	Renal; proteolysis
Inhibition of clot-bound thrombin	No	No	No	Yes	Yes	Yes
Tests for monitoring	aPTT	Anti-FXa	Anti-FXa	aPTT, ACT	aPTT, ACT	aPTT, ACT

trial,[33] despite an apparent positive response to treatment at 7 days, emergent administration of danaparoid was not associated with an improvement in favorable outcome at 3 months.

Administration and Monitoring

Danaparoid is intended for subcutaneous administration, and should not be administered by intramuscular injection. It has a very long half-life (anti-FXa activity 25 hours) and must be monitored with anti-Xa levels. The package insert should be reviewed before choosing a dose.

Adverse Effects

Hemorrhage injection site hematoma and skin rash are the main adverse effects reported.

Reversal of Effects

The effects of danaparoid on anti-Xa activity cannot be antagonized with any known agent. Protamine sulfate partially neutralizes the anti-Xa activity, but there is no evidence that protamine sulfate is capable of reducing severe nonsurgical bleeding during danaparoid therapy. In the event of serious bleeding, danaparoid should be stopped and blood or blood product transfusions should be administered as needed. Withdrawal of the medication is not associated with a rebound phenomenon.

HIRUDIN

Mechanism and Pharmacology

Hirudin, the anticoagulant present in the salivary glands of the medicinal leech, *Hirudo medicinalis,* is a highly specific direct inhibitor of thrombin (Table 24–10). The biosynthetic polypeptide molecule called lepirudin is composed of 65 amino acids and is identical to natural hirudin except for substitution of leucine for isoleucine at the *N*-terminal end of the molecule and the absence of a sulfate group on the tyrosine 63. Lepirudin (Refludan) binds tightly and nearly irreversibly to the catalytic site of thrombin, which imparts a prolonged duration of action. Lepirudin is renally excreted and so may accumulate in patients with renal impairment and potentially increase the risk of bleeding. The half-life appears to be 1 to 3 hours in normal volunteers but may be as long as 2 days in dialysis-dependent patients.

Administration and Monitoring

Lepirudin must be administered parenterally, and it results in dose-dependent prolongations of the aPTT, PT, and thrombin time. The usual dose is a bolus of 0.4 mg/kg intravenously followed by 0.15 mg/kg/hr as a continuous infusion. Therapy is monitored and the dose is adjusted based on the aPTT with a target range of 1.5 to 2.5 times the mean control. Because lepirudin is cleared by the kidneys, high plasma levels can result in patients with renal dysfunction and dose adjustments are required.

Indications and Clinical Use

Lepirudin is approved for anticoagulation in patients with HIT and associated thromboembolic disease in order to prevent further thromboembolic complications. It has been used successfully in clinical trials for the treatment of DVT and in patients with acute coronary syndromes. This direct thrombin inhibitor has no structural homology with heparin and thus no cross-reactivity with HIT antibodies. Two clinical trials of lepirudin use in patients with HIT have been completed.[34,35] In the HAT-1 trial, lepirudin was associated with rapid and sustained recovery of platelet counts and adequate anticoagulation as assessed by the aPTT.[34] In HAT-2, a follow-up study, investigators demonstrated that hirudin successfully prevented death, limb amputation, and new thromboembolic complications in HIT patients.[35] Several patients in the HAT trials were treated with lepirudin and underwent successful percutaneous coronary intervention.[34,35]

Adverse Effects

The primary adverse effects have been bleeding. Formation of antihirudin antibodies has been observed in about 40% of HIT patients treated with lepirudin, which may decrease drug clearance and thus *increase* the anticoagulant effect, possibly because of delayed renal elimination of lepirudin-antihirudin complexes, which retain anticoagulant properties.[36]

Reversal of Effect

There is no antidote to lepirudin. If overdosage or excess bleeding occurs, the infusion should be discontinued immediately, aPTT and other coagulation parameters obtained as appropriate, and assessment of the patient's hemoglobin concentration made with preparations for blood transfusion. Case reports suggested that hemofiltration or hemodialysis (using high-flux dialysis membranes with a cutoff point of 50,000 daltons) may be useful. Studies in pigs have shown reductions in bleeding with the infusion of von Willebrand factor.

ARGATROBAN

Mechanism and Pharmacology

Argatroban is a small-molecule (Mr 527) synthetic derivative of arginine that reversibly binds directly to the catalytic site of the thrombin molecule (Table 24–10).[37,38] It has no homology with heparin and thus no cross-reactivity. The primary route of metabolism is by the liver, with a terminal elimination half-life of 39 to 51 minutes.

Administration and Monitoring

The recommended initial dose of argatroban for adult patients without hepatic impairment is 2 μg/kg/min, administered as a continuous infusion. Therapy is monitored using the aPTT. Steady-state levels as determined by tests of anticoagulant effects (e.g., aPTT) typically occur within 1 to 3 hours after initiation of argatroban therapy. Dose adjustment may be required to maintain the target aPTT. Thus, the aPTT should be assessed 2 hours after initiation of therapy to confirm that the aPTT is within the desired therapeutic range. The dose is then adjusted as clinically indicated (not to exceed 10 μg/kg/min), until the steady-state aPTT is 1.5 to 3 times the initial baseline value (not to exceed 100 seconds). The package insert should be reviewed before dosing the patient.

Indications and Clinical Use

Argatroban recently received FDA approval labeling as an anticoagulant for prophylaxis or treatment of thrombosis in patients with HIT.[39] Argatroban has been evaluated in patients with HIT undergoing coronary angioplasty in two series.[40,41] Fifty patients were evaluated. Procedural success was achieved for 98% of patients and complications included one retroperitoneal hematoma and one abrupt vessel closure. The anticoagulant effect of the drug is often difficult to predict in the catheterization laboratory and there is no effective reversal agent.[40–42]

Adverse Effects

Hemorrhagic signs and symptoms and allergic reactions are the most common adverse effects reported.

Reversal of Effect

No specific antidote to argatroban is available. Excessive anticoagulation, with or without bleeding, may be controlled by decreasing the infusion rate or discontinuing argatroban. In clinical studies at therapeutic levels, anticoagulation parameters generally return to baseline within 2 to 4 hours after discontinuation of the drug. Reversal of anticoagulant effect may take longer in patients with hepatic impairment. If overdosage or excess bleeding occurs, the infusion should be discontinued immediately, aPTT and other coagulation parameters obtained as appropriate, and assessment of the patient's hemoglobin concentration made with preparations for blood transfusion.

BIVALIRUDIN

Mechanism and Pharmacology

Bivalirudin (Angiomaxx, The Medicines Company) (Table 24–10) is a 20-amino acid molecule that was engineered from naturally occurring hirudin to consist only of 2 amino acid sequences of hirudin that are important in binding to and inhibiting thrombin, connected by a bridge of 4 glycine residues. This bridge permits easy cleavage of the molecule, providing a more reversible interaction with the catalytic site of thrombin than hirudin, which may result in a significantly lower bleeding risk. The half-life is relatively short (24 to 45 minutes) and administration results in rapid, dose-dependent prolongation of the ACT. Elimination of bivalirudin is primarily by the liver. Approximately 20%

of standard doses are recovered in the urine. Bivalirudin has no structural similarity to heparin.

Administration and Monitoring

For reducing ischemic complications in unstable or post-infarction angina patients undergoing coronary angioplasty, bivalirudin has been given intravenously in a dose of 1 mg/kg as an initial bolus, followed by a continuous infusion of 2.5 mg/kg/h for 4 hours then 0.2 mg/kg/h for 14 to 20 hours. Bivalirudin was initiated immediately before angioplasty, and aspirin (300 to 325 mg) was also given to all patients.[43] The package insert should be reviewed before dosing the patient.

Indications and Clinical Use

In May 2000, The Medicines Company received an approval letter from the FDA for the use of bivalirudin (Angiomaxx) (formerly Hirulog) as an anticoagulant in patients with unstable angina undergoing percutaneous transluminal coronary angioplasty (PTCA). Bivalirudin has been shown to be a safe substitute for heparin in patients without HIT undergoing percutaneous coronary intervention in two clinical trials. In an open-label, dose-finding trial of 258 patients, bivalirudin was used as an alternative to heparin.[44] Bivalirudin was associated with lower bleeding complications, including retroperitoneal hemorrhage, need for transfusion, and major hemorrhage.

Adverse Effects

Bleeding is the most common adverse effect. Because of its small size and secondary structure, bivalirudin would not be expected to induce strong antibody responses upon readministration in contrast to larger molecules having more significant secondary structures (such as hirudin). Antibivalirudin antibodies have not been detected during or up to 4 weeks after intravenous bivalirudin therapy in several studies. No allergic phenomena have been reported to date.

Reversal of Effect

No specific antidote to bivalirudin is available. Excessive anticoagulation, with or without bleeding, may be controlled by decreasing or discontinuing the infusion of bivalirudin. If overdosage or excess bleeding occurs, the infusion should be discontinued immediately, aPTT and other coagulation parameters obtained as appropriate, and assessment of the patient's hemoglobin concentration made with preparations for blood transfusion.

FIBRINOLYTIC THERAPY

Fibrinolytic therapy is given to accelerate the slow physiologic process of fibrinolysis and induce rapid dissolution of occlusive thrombi and re-establishment of vascular patency. Fibrinolysis represents standard treatment for many patients presenting with acute MI as it accelerates reperfusion, decreases mortality, and reduces morbidity.[45,46] Fibrinolytic therapy has also become standard for many patients presenting with thrombosis of both native peripheral arteries and bypass grafts, and it may decrease mortality and improve functional outcome with the need for fewer surgical procedures.[47-50] It has been introduced recently for treatment of selected patients with thrombotic stroke, and its use may result in decreased disability. Fibrinolytic therapy results in less dramatic results in venous thromboembolic disease, but it is of value in selected patients to decrease long-term disability following DVT and to improve outcome in patients with PE associated with hemodynamic compromise.[51-53] Contraindications and cautions for thrombolytic use are listed in Table 24-11.

Fibrinolytic therapy is administered by infusing high doses of a plasminogen activator to accelerate the conversion of plasminogen to the active fibrinolytic enzyme, plasmin, the active agent regardless of the plasminogen activator employed. Specific biochemical and pharmacologic properties are important determinants of the administration regimen, the efficacy of clot lysis and the nature of adverse effects (Table 24-12).[54] For example, some plasminogen activators are active primarily at the fibrin surface and, therefore, have little effect on fibrinogen and other plasma proteins. Others, however, activate plasminogen less discriminately and convert circulating plasminogen to plasmin with profound fi-

Table 24-11 • CONTRAINDICATIONS AND CAUTIONS FOR THROMBOLYTIC USE

Absolute Contraindications
- Previous hemorrhagic stroke at any time
- Other strokes or cerebrovascular events within 1 year
- Active internal bleeding (does not include menses)
- Known intracranial neoplasm
- Suspected aortic dissection

Relative Contraindications
- History of prior cerebrovascular accident or known intracerebral pathology not covered in contraindications.
- Severe uncontrolled hypertension on presentation (blood pressure >180/110 mmHg) or chronic history of severe hypertension
- Current use of anticoagulants in therapeutic doses (warfarin INR 2.0-3.0)
- Known bleeding diathesis
- Noncompressible vascular punctures
- Recent (within 2 to 4 weeks) internal bleeding
- Recent trauma (within 2 to 4 weeks), including head trauma or traumatic or prolonged (>10 minutes) cardiopulmonary resuscitation or major surgery (less than 3 weeks)
- For streptokinase/antistreplase/staphylokinase: prior exposure (especially within 5 days to 2 years) or prior allergic reaction
- Active peptic ulcer or known gastrointestinal bleeding
- Pregnancy

Adapted from Ryan TJ, Anderson JL, Antman EM, et al. ACC/AHA guidelines for the management of patients with acute myocardial infarction. A report of the American College of Cardiology/American Heart Association Task Force on Practice Guidelines (Committee on Management of Acute Myocardial Infarction). J Am Coll Cardiol 1996 Nov 1;28:1328-1428.

Table 24-12 • PROPERTIES OF FIBRINOLYTIC AGENTS

Drug	Origin	Fibrin Specificity	Half-Life (min)	Antigenicity	Note
Streptokinase (Streptase)	Bacterial	No	20	Yes	Acts indirectly by forming 1:1 complex with plasminogen
Urokinase (Abbokinase)	Cell culture	Low	15	No	Normally present in urine. Currently not available because of manufacturing problems
Alteplase (Activase)	Recombinant	Moderate	5	No	Naturally occurring activator synthesized in endothelium
APSAC (Eminase)	SK-bacterial; plasminogen-plasma derived	Moderate	70	Yes	Complex of SK and plasmin-plasminogen with active site-blocked. Activates after administration.
Reteplase (Retavase)	Recombinant	Moderate	15	No	Modified form of t-PA with longer half-life
Tenecteplase (Metalyse)	Recombinant	Enhanced	30–120	No	Bioengineered variant of t-PA but with longer half-life, resistance to inactivation by PAI-1, and enhanced fibrin specificity

brinogenolysis. Over the course of the last 15 years, there has been great interest in developing new plasminogen activators with improved properties. Streptokinase and urokinase, the first generation of therapeutic plasminogen activators, are still available, but newer agents, including tissue plasminogen activator, acylated plasminogen streptokinase complex, and reteplase, have been introduced. Still newer plasminogen activators with uniquely favorable properties are undergoing clinical trial and offer promise for the future. Despite these advances, significant problems remain, including the inability of plasminogen activators to induce reperfusion in some patients, incomplete clot lysis in many, and, particularly, bleeding complications. Baseline patient predictors of bleeding complications determined from multivariable logistic regression models are listed in Table 24-13. Predictive models of noncerebral hemorrhage based on thrombolytic trial databases have been published.[55–57] A probability chart based on patients who did not undergo procedures in GUSTO I was developed to calculate the predicted value for their likelihood of experiencing a moderate or severe bleeding complication, and is provided in Table 24-14.

Streptokinase

Streptokinase is derived from β-hemolytic streptococci and was one of the first plasminogen activators to be identified and studied. It has a unique biochemical mechanism among plasminogen activators as it acts indirectly by combining with plasminogen to form an equimolar streptokinase-plasminogen complex that can then convert another plasminogen molecule to plasmin. When administered in therapeutic doses, streptokinase exhibits little fibrin specificity. Conversion of plasminogen to plasmin at the thrombus results in lysis of fibrin, whereas the same reaction in the blood causes systemic plasminemia and degradation of fibrinogen and other plasma proteins. The consumption of plasminogen in the blood can limit fibrinolysis, which requires an ongoing new supply of plasminogen at the site of thrombosis.[58] Proteolysis of platelet membrane proteins and platelet activation can also result from the systemic plasminemia. Streptokinase has a rapid plasma clearance of 20 minutes, necessitating continuous intravenous administration. The presence of pre-existing neutralizing antistreptococcal antibodies may further accelerate initial clearance and even lead to resistance.

Therapeutic Use

For treatment of venous thromboembolic disease, streptokinase usually is administered as an initial bolus of

Table 24-13 • BASELINE PATIENT PREDICTORS OF BLEEDING COMPLICATIONS WITH FIBRINOLYTIC THERAPY FROM MULTIVARIABLE LOGISTIC REGRESSION MODELS[a]

- Advanced age
- African ancestry
- Alteplase level 1500 ng/mL or higher
- Angiography or angioplasty
- Bypass surgery
- Cardiac decompensation
- Female sex
- Low fibrinogen
- History of hypertension
- Lower body weight
- Platelet count less than 100,000/μL

[a] Not in order of predictive power.
Data from Califf RM, Topol EJ, George BS, et al. Hemorrhagic complications associated with the use of intravenous tissue plasminogen activator in treatment of acute myocardial infarction. Am J Med 1988; 85:353–359; Bovill EG, Terrin ML, Stump DC, et al. Hemorrhagic events during therapy with recombinant tissue-type plasminogen activator, heparin, and aspirin for acute myocardial infarction. Results of the Thrombolysis in Myocardial Infarction (TIMI), Phase II Trial. Ann Intern Med 1991; 115:256–265; and Berkowitz SD, Granger CB, Pieper KS, et al. Incidence and predictors of bleeding after contemporary thrombolytic therapy for myocardial infarction. The Global Utilization of Streptokinase and Tissue Plasminogen Activator for Occluded Coronary Arteries (GUSTO) I Investigators. Circulation 1997; 95:2508–2516.

Table 24-14 • PREDICTION OF MODERATE OR SEVERE BLEEDING EVENTS FOR NONCATHETERIZED PATIENTS IN GUSTO-I

1. Find Points for each predictive factor:

Age		Weight		Pulse		Misc. RF		Risk Factor/Treatment Interaction				
									Treatment, Points			
Yr	Points	Kg	Points	BPM	Points	Factor	Points		t-PA	No t-PA	Combo	No Combo
40	0	120	0	40	91	Female sex	12	I. African ancestry				
50	6	100	0	60	91	SK-IV	13	No	0	0		
60	18	80	4	80	96			Yes	43	15		
70	29	60	20	100	100			II. Killip class				
80	41	40	37	120	98			I			15	3
90	53			140	91			II			25	0
100	64			160	77			III/IV			11	7
110	76			180	57							
				200	32							

2. Sum points for all predictive factors:

___ Age + ___ Weight + ___ Pulse + ___ Misc. RF + ___ Interaction I + ___ Interaction II = ___ Total points

3. Look up risk corresponding to total points:

Points	Predictive Value
142	5%
162	10%
175	15%
185	20%
192	25%
199	30%
206	35%
211	40%
217	45%
223	50%

BPM, beats per minute; Misc RF, miscellaneous risk factors; t-PA tissue plasminogen activator; SK + IV, streptokinase plus intravenous heparin treatment; Combo, combination (that is, t-PA and SK together) thrombolytic therapy; No combo, thrombolytic therapy with t-PA or SK only.
In Step 1, find the value most closely matching the patient's risk factors and circle the points. In Step 2, sum the points for all predictive factors. In Step 3, determine the risk corresponding to the total number of points.
Adapted from Berkowitz SD, Granger CB, Pieper KS, et al. Incidence and predictors of bleeding after contemporary thrombolytic therapy for myocardial infarction. The Global Utilization of Streptokinase and Tissue Plasminogen Activator for Occluded Coronary Arteries (GUSTO) I Investigators. Circulation 1997;95:2508-2516.

250,000 units followed by a constant infusion of 100,000 units/h for up to 3 days (Table 24-15). The purpose of the initial bolus is to overcome circulating neutralizing antibodies, which are common because of frequent previous streptococcal infections in the population. Occasional individuals will have particularly high-titer antibodies and neutralize this amount of streptokinase resulting in resistance. Therefore, it is useful to confirm evidence of the proteolytic effect of streptokinase after 1 to 2 hours of administration by measuring plasma fibrinogen concentration or thrombin clotting time. If these do not become abnormal, a second bolus infusion may be needed to overcome inhibition. Streptokinase is antigenic, and high-titer antibodies develop 1 to 2 weeks after use precluding retreatment until they decline. The antigenicity of streptokinase also accounts for occasional adverse febrile and hypotensive reactions during initial drug administration. The streptokinase regimen for treatment of acute MI differs from that recommended for venous thrombosis, using a higher dose over shorter time period to achieve maximum effect. For treatment of acute MI, streptokinase is usually administered in a dose of 1,500,000 units over 1 hour or as a single infusion.

Urokinase

Urokinase is a naturally occurring plasminogen activator synthesized by kidney cells and is present in the urine. A single-chain form of urokinase, scu-PA, is synthesized in endothelial cells and found in plasma and is converted to the two-chain form (urokinase) through proteolysis by plasmin or kallikrein. The two-chain form has been prepared for therapeutic use from embryonic kidney cell culture. Concern over possible viral contamination of urokinase has recently blocked commercial production and limited clinical use. Urokinase is a direct plasminogen activator that proteolytically converts plasminogen to plasmin. In usual doses it produces systemic

Table 24-15 • SYSTEMIC THROMBOLYTIC THERAPY REGIMENS

DVT AND PE

Drug	Dose	Duration
Streptokinase	250,000 loading dose IV followed by 100,000 U/h	PE—24 hours DVT—up to 3 days
Urokinase	2000 U/kg loading dose IV followed by 2000 U/kg/h	PE—12–24 hours DVT—up to 3 days
t-PA	100 mg	PE—2 hours DVT—not recommended

Thrombolytic Therapy for MI

Drug	Dose
Streptokinase	1,500,000 U over 1 hour IV
t-PA	15 mg bolus IV; then 0.75 mg/kg over 30 min (not to exceed 50 mg); then 0.75 mg/kg over 60 min (not to exceed 35 mg) or 100 mg total over 3 hours; 60 mg in first hour (6–10 mg as a bolus); 20 mg over the second hour and 20 mg over the third hour
APSAC	30 U over 5 min IV
Reteplase	10 U IV bolus; repeat ×1 after 30 min

Thrombolytic Therapy for Stroke

- t-PA 0.9 mg/kg (maximum 90 mg) IV, with 10% total dose as a bolus and the remainder over 60 min.
- Note: strict attention to criteria for patient selection required.

---

plasminemia with degradation of circulating fibrinogen, but this is generally less than occurs with streptokinase. Urokinase is cleared primarily by the liver and has a half-life of 15 minutes.

Urokinase has been used effectively in treatment of DVT, PE, MI, peripheral arterial occlusion, and stroke, but its primary use has been in venous thromboembolic disease and peripheral arterial occlusion. The same doses are used for treatment of DVT and PE; a shorter duration of treatment of 12 hours is typical for PE, whereas a longer duration of up to several days may be used for DVT. For peripheral arterial occlusion, urokinase is administered through a catheter placed within the thrombus. Several catheter techniques have been developed, including administering an initial bolus while withdrawing the catheter through the clot, or "lacing." Alternatively, a catheter with multiple side holes can be used in a "pulse spray" technique. Several doses and infusion rates can be used.[59] Thrombolysis results in a high rate of reperfusion, resulting in fewer amputations and a reduced need for surgical interventions but at the expense of increased bleeding complications.[47,48]

Tissue Plasminogen Activator

Tissue plasminogen activator (t-PA) is a naturally occurring plasminogen activator that is structurally and immunologically distinct from urokinase. It is elaborated by endothelial cells and other tissues. Originally produced from cell culture, t-PA is now synthesized for pharmacologic use by recombinant techniques. t-PA directly converts plasminogen to plasmin in a reaction that is strikingly accelerated in the presence of fibrin. This property accounts for the relative "fibrin specificity" of t-PA observed physiologically. In practice, t-PA is administered at a high dose, which often results in significant proteolysis of plasma fibrinogen, but this is less than occurs with treatment using either streptokinase or urokinase. Following intravenous administration, t-PA has a short half-life of 5 minutes, requiring a constant infusion to maintain therapeutic plasma levels.

t-PA has been evaluated in DVT, PE, MI, stroke, and peripheral arterial occlusion. Clinical trials using several regimens of t-PA in patients with DVT showed overall disappointing results, and t-PA is rarely used for this indication. However, t-PA has been evaluated in treatment of acute PE, and a regimen of 100 mg intravenously over 2 hours results in a high rate of clot lysis and hemodynamic improvement. t-PA has also been evaluated in numerous large studies for acute MI, demonstrating rapid reperfusion in the majority of patients with significant improvements in mortality and reduction in infarct-related morbidity. The drug is usually given in a "front-loaded" dosing schedule for maximum benefit (see Table 24–15).

Thrombolytic therapy is emerging as a useful modality in selected patients with stroke. Several studies using t-PA have shown overall beneficial effects.[60] In the National Institute of Neurologic Disorders and Stroke rt-PA Stroke Study,[61] patients were treated within 3 hours of onset of symptoms with placebo or rt-PA at 0.9 mg/kg. Patients treated with rt-PA showed reduced disability despite an increase in the incidence of intracerebral hemorrhage from 0.6% to 6.4%. Selective intra-arterial thrombolytic therapy is now being investigated with a catheter placed at the site of intracranial thrombosis. Initial studies show encouraging rates of recanalization.[62] Guidelines emphasize selection of patients presenting very early after onset of symptoms and avoidance of patients with an increased risk of intracranial bleeding.[63,64]

APSAC

A chemically modified streptokinase derivative with improved pharmacologic properties, anisoylated plasminogen streptokinase activator complex (APSAC), has been developed in which streptokinase is complexed with plasminogen that can mediate binding to fibrin in the thrombus. The active site is blocked with a p-anisoyl group so that it is enzymatically inactive until deacylation occurs either in the blood or after attachment to a thrombus. This strategy allows the enzymatically inert complex to be administered intravenously, and the fibrin-binding properties result in its attachment to fibrin, where deacylation results in conversion of plasminogen to plasmin. An important pharmacologic characteristic of APSAC is its relatively long half-life of approximately 40 minutes, allowing it to be administered for therapy in a bolus dose (see Table 24–12). The fibrin-binding properties of APSAC result in relatively greater activity at the site of fibrin deposition than systemically, and systemic plasminemia and fibrinogen depletion are less than with streptokinase or urokinase but more than with t-PA. The streptokinase moiety within APSAC is immunogenic, and resistance to therapy can occur in patients with pre-existing high-titer antistreptococcal antibodies. Also, high-titer neutralizing antibodies develop after administration, which may preclude re-treatment with this agent. Acute allergic reactions, including hypotension and bronchospasm, are less frequent than with streptokinase administration but can occur. APSAC has been evaluated clinically primarily in the setting of acute MI. A 30 unit intravenous bolus injection results in a high rate of coronary reperfusion.

Reteplase

Among the many attempts at engineering improvements over wild-type t-PA by recombinant technology, the most successful has been reteplase (Retavase). Reteplase lacks several domains of the t-PA molecule, and the structural modifications result in reduced fibrin binding but a significant longer half-life than t-PA (15 minutes versus 4 minutes) so that it can be administered as an intravenous bolus rather than a continuous infusion. Reteplase has been evaluated primarily as a treatment for acute MI, and has recently been approved for that indication. It is administered in two bolus injections of 10 units given 30 minutes apart.[65]

Tenecteplase

TNK-tissue plasminogen activator (TNK-t-PA) is a "third-generation" thrombolytic and the most recently FDA-approved thrombolytic agent. TNK-t-PA is a bioengineered variant of t-PA with a longer half-life, enhanced resistance to inactivation by plasminogen activator inhibitor-1, and improved fibrin specificity. Tenecteplase and alteplase have similar clinical efficacy for thrombolysis after MI, including similar rates of death and intracranial hemorrhage. Advantages include the longer half-life, greater fibrin specificity, ease and rapidity of administration, and lower noncerebral bleeding rates.[66,67]

Regional Therapy

Rheologic considerations indicate that adequate drug delivery into the thrombus is often the rate-limiting step in achieving effective thrombolysis.[68] Drug delivery through a catheter placed near or within the occlusive thrombus is attractive because a relatively high concentration of lytic agent can be delivered locally to maximize thrombolysis while potentially limiting systemic effects. For arterial thrombolysis, catheter-directed treatment has generally resulted in greater reperfusion, and it has been evaluated for coronary, cerebrovascular, and peripheral arterial occlusion.[59] This approach is rarely used for MI as systemic intravenous treatment is effective, widely available, less expensive, and can be administered rapidly. Also, primary angioplasty may be more effective in selected patients than thrombolysis if catheterization is acutely performed. For stroke, selective catheterization of the occluded middle cerebral artery may optimize treatment by maximizing thrombolysis and limiting bleeding, but this approach is limited to the few centers with sufficient experience and facilities to perform catheterization on an emergent basis. Studies of its effectiveness are evolving. The use of catheter-directed thrombolysis in peripheral arterial occlusion is routine as local therapy is much more effective than systemic administration, and clinical studies demonstrate that the ability to deliver drug into the thrombus is a critical determinant of thrombolytic success.

Catheter-directed thrombolysis is also effective in treatment of ileofemoral DVT in selected patients, but studies comparing its effectiveness to that of systemic thrombolysis are needed. Catheter-directed treatment is less successful in the goal of limiting systemic effects as the total dose of drug delivered exceeds the binding capacity of local fibrin deposits and bleeding complications result from systemic circulation. Additionally, the very rationale for catheter-directed therapy for DVT ignores the fact that 25% to 40% of all such patients may well harbor a concomitant PE or another venous thrombosis that may then go untreated.

Adjunctive Treatment

Administration of a thrombolytic agent represents only one aspect of the overall pharmacologic manipulation of hemostasis, which is designed to restore and maintain vascular patency. A comprehensive view of treatment includes consideration of antiplatelet, anticoagulant, vasodilator, and mechanical interventions to augment thrombolysis.[69] Additionally, thrombolysis may activate hemostasis directly and also releases fibrin-bound thrombin from the thrombus, which can have procoagulant properties. Appropriate selection of adjunctive therapy depends on the thrombus location, and it differs among venous thromboembolic disease, peripheral arterial occlusion, MI, and stroke. Generally, for DVT and PE, thrombolysis is given as an initial phase of treatment followed by standard anticoagulation with heparin or LMWH and long-term oral anticoagulants. Anticoagulation is not usually given concomitantly with the thrombolytic agent but is administered subsequently. For stroke, bleeding complications are a serious concern and treatment with anticoagulants or antiplatelet agents is avoided within 24 hours of administration of t-PA. This is in contrast to treatment of acute MI, which seeks to achieve maximum reperfusion and prevent reocclusion by combination therapy routinely, including antiplatelet agents and often heparin or LMWH concomitantly (see Chapter 19).

Bleeding Complications

The most frequent and serious complications related to thrombolytic therapy are due to bleeding caused by two problems. First, the accelerated fibrinolysis resulting from treatment is not limited to the symptomatic occlusive thrombus but acts on all fibrin deposits. Some of these may be physiologic intended to prevent bleeding at sites of vascular injury caused by catheters or pathologic lesions within the brain, gastrointestinal tract, or gentourinary tract. The second problem contributing to bleeding is the hypocoagulable state that results from the effects of fibrinolytic agents on platelets, fibrinogen, and other plasma proteins as well as pharmacologic effects of other anticoagulants and antiplatelet agents administered concurrently. The approach to this problem includes selection of patients to minimize complications, a high degree of suspicion, appropriate diagnostic tests, and finally an aggressive approach to managing bleeding complications when they occur.[70]

The most feared complication is intracranial hemorrhage, which occurs in less than 1% of individuals but has a high mortality and results in serious disability in most survivors. Some risk factors are intracranial vascular disease as indicated by a prior stroke, trauma, surgery, and tumor; fibrinolytic treatment typically should be avoided in patients known to have these risks.[71] Also, intracranial hemorrhage is more likely with advanced age, a higher dose of thrombolytic agent, and uncontrolled hypertension. Patients with stroke receiving thrombolytic therapy need to be selected carefully to minimize bleeding as the overall clinical benefit represents a balance between the deleterious effects of increased bleeding due to thrombolysis in comparison with the benefits of reperfusion. The second consideration is bleeding associated with invasive vascular procedures, including placement of arterial and venous lines. This problem can be reduced by limiting venous and arterial punctures to a minimum giving attention to arterial sites with local application of pressure and careful observation, recognizing that bleeding deep into tissues initially may appear only as pain and swelling. A separate problem is major bleeding resulting from pre-existing lesions in the gastrointestinal or gentourinary tract such as ulcers or unrecognized malignancies. These problems can be minimized by performance of a careful history and physical examination to avoid treating patients at high risk with a recurrent or recently identified bleeding lesion. Minor bleeding complications, including ecchymoses and microscopic hematuria, are frequent and troublesome but of little clinical consequence, especially considering the gravity of the illnesses for which fibrinolytic therapy is entertained.

The clinician should be fully prepared to deal with the challenge of bleeding complications that develop during fibrinolytic therapy (Table 24–16; Fig. 24–1). Accurate diagnosis is critical, and patients should be immediately evaluated if bleeding complications are suspected and the clinical course followed closely. Intracranial hemorrhage is the most serious and feared complication and may be suspected in patients who develop headache or neurologic dysfunction. Imaging will be required for accurate diagnosis. If intracranial hemorrhage is confirmed, neurosurgery should be consulted and all efforts undertaken to reverse abnormal hemostasis. Despite maximum efforts, the mortality and morbidity are high.

Major bleeding complications often involve deep tissue bleeding as well as gastrointestinal and genitourinary tract bleeding. Every effort should be made to identify the site of bleeding and determine if local therapy is needed. For example, a bleeding arterial puncture site from prior catheterization may require pressure or even surgical repair. Bleeding from sites in the gastrointestinal or genitourinary tract may require specific therapy. The systemic hemostatic abnormalities are related to direct effects of the fibrinolytic agent and the hypocoagulable state resulting from proteolysis of plasma pro-

---

Table 24–16 • TREATMENT OF FIBRINOLYTIC BLEEDING

If intracranial bleed is suspected, obtain imaging, consult neurosurgery and correct hemostasis as below.

For major bleeding:
- Send diagnostic test—aPTT, platelet count, fibrinogen.
- Attend to local hemostatic problems. Apply pressure if bleeding related to arterial puncture. Proceed with general supportive measures, including intravenous fluid hydration and transfusion of packed red cells if indicated. Proceed with diagnostic evaluation for gastrointestinal or genitourinary tract bleeding.
- Correct abnormal hemostasis
  —Prevent further fibrinolysis: stop fibrinolytic therapy; consider EACA or aprotinin.
  —Replacement therapy to repair hemostasis defect induced by fibrinolytic therapy: give cryoprecipitate 5–10 units and 2 U fresh frozen plasma; consider platelet transfusion
  —Correct other hemostatic defects: stop anticoagulant and antiplatelet agents; consider protamine to reverse heparin

```
                    ┌─────────────────────────────────────┐
                    │ Patient with serious bleeding within │
                    │     24 hours of thrombolytic therapy │
                    └─────────────────────────────────────┘
```

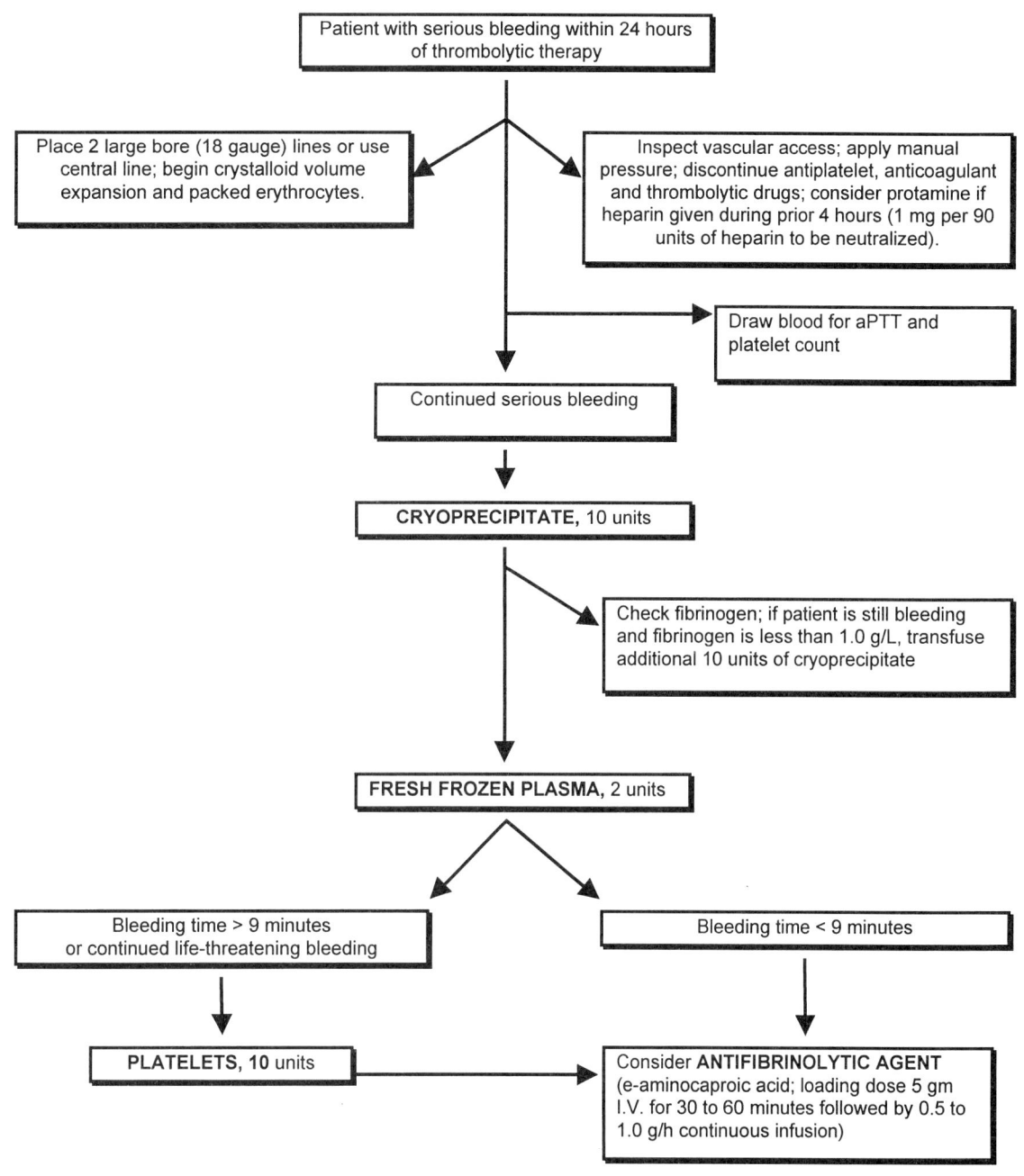

Figure 24–1. Algorithm for bleeding management in patients with serious bleeding after thrombolytic therapy. (Adapted from Sane DC, Califf RM, Topol EJ, et al. Bleeding during thrombolytic therapy for acute myocardial infarction: Mechanisms and management. Ann Intern Med 1989;111:1010–1022.)

Flowchart content:
- Patient with serious bleeding within 24 hours of thrombolytic therapy
  - Place 2 large bore (18 gauge) lines or use central line; begin crystalloid volume expansion and packed erythrocytes.
  - Inspect vascular access; apply manual pressure; discontinue antiplatelet, anticoagulant and thrombolytic drugs; consider protamine if heparin given during prior 4 hours (1 mg per 90 units of heparin to be neutralized).
  - Draw blood for aPTT and platelet count
- Continued serious bleeding
- CRYOPRECIPITATE, 10 units
  - Check fibrinogen; if patient is still bleeding and fibrinogen is less than 1.0 g/L, transfuse additional 10 units of cryoprecipitate
- FRESH FROZEN PLASMA, 2 units
  - Bleeding time > 9 minutes or continued life-threatening bleeding → PLATELETS, 10 units
  - Bleeding time < 9 minutes → Consider ANTIFIBRINOLYTIC AGENT (ε-aminocaproic acid; loading dose 5 gm I.V. for 30 to 60 minutes followed by 0.5 to 1.0 g/h continuous infusion)

teins and platelets, and also can be due to or abetted by adjunctive antiplatelet and anticoagulant therapy. Useful treatment can be directed at each of these problems. First, the fibrinolytic agent should be discontinued. This will result in rapid clearance of nearly all agents that have a circulating half-life as short as 5 minutes to as long as 70 minutes. For serious bleeding, the use of an antifibrinolytic agent such as ε-aminocaproic acid (EACA) should be considered to block fibrinolysis. In deciding whether to use an antifibrinolytic agent, the pharmacokinetics of the fibrinolytic agent administered should be considered. For example, 1 or 2 hours following discontinuation of t-PA, no drug will be left in the circulation, and EACA will be of no value. The second important consideration is to use replacement therapy to repair the hemostatic defect caused by systemic plasminemia. Fibrinogen replacement is important and can be accomplished by administration of 5 to 10 bags of cryoprecipitate, and fresh frozen plasma can be used to replace other hemostatic proteins. Replacement treatment should be monitored with repeat coagulation tests. Administration of platelet concentrates may be useful because fibrinolytic therapy results in platelet dysfunction. Finally, other antiplatelet or anticoagulant agents being used as adjuncts to thrombolysis should be discontinued. DDAVP administration may be effective. If high doses of heparin have been administered, its effect can be reversed with protamine.

REFERENCES

Chapter 24 References

1. Hirsh J, Dalen JE, Anderson DR, et al. Oral anticoagulants. Mechanism of action, clinical effectiveness, and optimal therapeutic range. Chest 2001;119(suppl):8S–21S.
2. Hirsh J, Fuster V. Guide to anticoagulant therapy. Part 2: Oral anticoagulants. AHA Medical/Scientific Statement Special Report. Circulation 1994;89:1469–1480.
3. Harrison L, Johnson M, Massicotte MP, et al. Comparison of 5-mg and 10-mg loading doses in initiation of warfarin therapy. Ann Intern Med 1997;126:133–136.
4. Wells PS, Holbrook AM, Crowther NR, et al. Interactions of warfarin with drugs and food. Ann Intern Med 1994;121:676–683.
5. Landefeld CS, McGuire E III, Rosenblatt MW. Risk for bleeding in patients starting anticoagulants. Am J Med 1990;89:569–578.
6. Fihn SD, Callahan CM, Martin DC, et al. The risk for and severity of bleeding complications in elderly patients treated with warfarin. Ann Intern Med 1996;124:970–979.
7. Levine MN, Raskob G, Landefeld CS, et al. Hemorrhagic complications of anticoagulant treatment. Chest 2001; 119(suppl):108S–121S.
8. Ginsberg, JS, Greer I, Hirsh J. Use of antithrombotic agents during pregnancy. Chest 2001;119(suppl):122S–131S.
9. Shetty HGM, Backhouse G, Bentley DP, et al. Effective reversal of warfarin-induced excessive anticoagulation with low dose vitamin K$_1$. Thromb Haemost 1992;67:13–15.
10. Crowther MA, Donovan D, Harrisons L, et al. Low-dose oral vitamin K reliably reverses over-anticoagulation due to warfarin. Thromb Haemost 1998;79:1116–1118.
11. Kearon C, Hirsh J. Management of anticoagulation before and after elective surgery. N Engl J Med 1997;336:1506–1511.
12. Hirsh J, Warkentin TE, Shaughnessy SG, et al. Heparin and low-molecular-weight heparin. Mechanisms of action, pharmacokinetics, dosing, monitoring, efficacy, and safety. Chest 2001; 119(suppl):64S–94S.
13. Cruickshank MK, Levine MN, Hirsh J, et al. A standard heparin nomogram for the management of heparin therapy. Arch Intern Med 1991;151:333–337.
14. Raschke RA, Reilly BM, Guidry JR, et al. The weight-based heparin dosing nomogram compared with a "standard care" nomogram. A randomized controlled trial. Ann Intern Med 1993; 119:874–881.
15. Levine M, Hirsh J, Gent M, et al. A randomized trial comparing activated thromboplastin time with heparin assay in patients with acute venous thromboembolism requiring large daily doses of heparin. Arch Intern Med 1994;154:49–56.
16. Ginsberg JS. Thromboembolism and pregnancy. Thromb Haemost 1999; 82:620–625.
17. Kaplan KL, Francis CW. Heparin-induced thrombocytopenia. Blood Rev 1999;13:1–7.
18. Dahlman T, Lindvall N, Helgren M. Osteopenia in pregnancy during long-term heparin treatment: a radiological study postpartum. Br J Obstet Gynaecol 1990;97:221–228.
19. Dahlman TC. Osteoporotic fractures and the recurrence of thromboembolism during pregnancy and the pueperium in 184 women undergoing thromboprophylaxis with heparin. Am J Obstet Gynecol 1993;168:1265–1270.
20. Weitz JI. Low-molecular-weight heparins. N Engl J Med 1997; 337:688–689.
21. Geerts WH, Heit JA, Clagett GP, et al. Prevention of venous thromboembolism. Chest 2001;119(suppl):132S–175S.
22. Horlocker TT, Heit JA. Low molecular weight heparin: biochemistry, pharmacology, perioperative prophylaxis regimens, and guidelines for regional anesthetic management. Anesth Analg 1997;85:874–885.
23. Samama MM, Cohen AT, Darmon J-Y, et al. A comparison of enoxaparin with placebo for the prevention of venous thromboembolism in acutely ill medical patients. N Engl J Med 1999; 341:793–800.
24. Koopman MMW, Prandoni P, Piovella F, et al. Treatment of venous thrombosis with intravenous unfractionated heparin administered in the hospital as compared with subcutaneous low-molecular-weight heparin administered at home. N Engl J Med 1996;334:682–687.
25. Levine M, Gent M, Hirsh J, et al. A comparison of low-molecular-weight heparin administered primarily at home with unfractionated heparin administered in the hospital for proximal deep-vein thrombosis. N Engl J Med 1996;334:677–681.
26. Gould MK, Dembitzer AD, Sanders GD, et al. Low-molecular-weight heparins compared with unfractionated heparin for treatment of acute deep venous thrombosis. A cost-effectiveness analysis. Ann Intern Med 1999;130:789–700.
27. Antman EM, Cohen M, Radley D, et al. Assessment of the treatment effect of enoxaparin for unstable angina/non-Q-wave myocardial infarction. TIMI 11B - ESSENCE Meta-Analysis. Circulation 1999;100:1602–1608.
28. Aster R. Drug-induced thrombocytopenia: An overview of pathogenesis. Semin Hematol 1999;36(Suppl 1):2–6.
29. Walenga JM, Jeske WP, Fasanella AR, et al. Laboratory tests for the diagnosis of heparin-induced thrombocytopenia. Semin Thromb Hemost 1999;25(Suppl 1):43–49.
30. Chong BH, Ismail F, Cade J, et al. Heparin induced thrombocytopenia: studies with new low molecular weight heparinoid Org 10172. Blood 1989;73:1592–1596.
31. Hale LP, Smith K, Braden GA, et al. Orgaran during rotational atherectomy in the setting of heparin-induced thrombocytopenia. Cathet Cardiovasc Diag 1998;45:318–322.
32. Cantor WJ, Leblanc K, Garvey B, et al. Combined use of Orgaran and ReoPro during coronary angioplasty in patients unable to receive heparin. Cathet Cardiovasc Interv 1999;46:232–244.
33. The TOAST Investigators. Low molecular weight heparinoid, ORG 10172 (danaparoid), and outcome after acute ischemic stroke: a randomized controlled trial. JAMA 1998;279:1265–1272.
34. Greinacher A, Volpel H, Janssen U, et al. Recombinant hirudin (lepirudin) provides safe and effective anticoagulation in patients with heparin-induced thrombocytopenia: a prospective study. Circulation 1999;99:73–80.
35. Greinacher A, Janssens U, Berg G, et al. Lepirudin (recombinant hirudin) for parenteral anticoagulation in patients with heparin-induced thrombocytopenia. Heparin-Associated Thrombocytopenia Study(HAT) Investigators. Circulation 1999;100:587–593.
36. Schiele G, Vuillemenot A, Kramarz P, et al. Use of recombinant hirudin as antithrombotic treatment in patients with heparin induced thrombocytopenia. Am J Hematol 1995;50:20–25.
37. Hursting MJ, Alford KL, Becker JP, et al. Novastan (brand of argatroban): A small molecule, direct thrombin inhibitor. Semin Thromb Hemost 1997;23:503–516.
38. Lewis BE, Walenga JM, Wallis DE. Anticoagulation with Novastan (argatroban) in patients with heparin induced thrombocytopenia and thrombosis syndrome. Semin Thromb Hemost 1997;23:197–202.
39. Lewis BE, Wallis DE, Berkowitz SD, et al. Study Investigators for the ARG-911 Study. Argatroban anticoagulant therapy in patients with heparin-induced thrombocytopenia: A prospective, historical controlled study. Circulation 2001;163:1838–1843.
40. Matthai WH. Use of argatroban during percutaneous coronary interventions in patients with heparin induced thrombocytopenia. Semin Thromb Hemost 1999;25(Suppl 1):57–60.

41. Lewis BE, Matthai W, Grassman ED, et al. Results of phase 2/3 trial of argatroban anticoagulation during PTCA of patients with heparin induced thrombocytopenia. Circulation 1997;96: I-217.
42. Lewis BE, Ferguson JS, Grassman ED, et al. Successful coronary interventions performed with argatroban in patients with heparin induced thrombocytopenia and thrombosis syndrome. J Invas Cardiol 1996;8:410–417.
43. Bittl JA, Strony J, Brinker JA, et al. for the Hirulog Angioplasty Study Investigators: Treatment with bivalirudin (hirulog) as compared with heparin during coronary angioplasty for unstable or post-infarction angina. N Engl J Med 1995;333:764–769.
44. Topol EJ, Bonan R, Jewitt D, et al. Use of a direct antithrombin, hirulog, in place of heparin during coronary angioplasty. Circulation 1993;87:1622–1629.
45. Anderson HV, Willerson JT. Thrombolysis in acute myocardial infarction. N Engl J Med 1993;329:703–709.
46. Fibrinolytic Therapy Trialists' (FTT) Collaborative Group. Indications for fibrinolytic therapy in suspected acute myocardial infarction: collaborative overview of early mortality and major morbidity results from all randomised trials of more than 1000 patients. Lancet 1994;343:311–322.
47. Ouriel K, Shortell CK, DeWeese JA, et al. A comparison of thrombolytic therapy with operative revascularization in the initial treatment of acute peripheral arterial ischemia. J Vasc Surg 1994;19:1021–1030.
48. The STILE Investigators. Results of a prospective randomized trial evaluating surgery versus thrombolysis for ischemia of the lower extremity. The STILE Trial. Ann Surg 1995;220:251–266.
49. Shortell CK, Francis CW. Thrombolytic therapy for arterial thrombosis. Curr Opin Hematol 1999;6:309–313.
50. Working Party on Thrombolysis in the Management of Limb Ischemia. Thrombolysis in the management of lower limb peripheral arterial occlusion—A consensus document. Am J Cardiol 1998;81:207–218.
51. Goldhaber SZ. Thrombolysis for pulmonary embolism. Prog Cardiovasc Dis 1991;34:113–134.
52. Goldhaber SZ, Kessler CM, Heit JA, et al. Recombinant tissue-type plasminogen activator versus a novel dosing regimen of urokinase in acute pulmonary embolism: A randomized controlled multicenter trial. J Am Coll Cardiol 1992;20:24–30.
53. Rogers LQ, Lutcher CL. Streptokinase therapy for deep vein thrombosis: A comprehensive review of the English literature. Am J Med 1990;88:389–395.
54. Weitz JI, Stewart RJ, Fredenburgh JC. Mechanism of action of plasminogen activators. Thromb Haemost 1999;82:974–982.
55. Califf RM, Topol EJ, George BS, et al. Hemorrhagic complications associated with the use of intravenous tissue plasminogen activator in treatment of acute myocardial infarction. Am J Med 1988;85:353–359.
56. Bovill EG, Terrin ML, Stump DC, et al. Hemorrhagic events during therapy with recombinant tissue-type plasminogen activator, heparin, and aspirin for acute myocardial infarction. Results of the Thrombolysis in Myocardial Infarction (TIMI), Phase II Trial. Ann Intern Med 1991;115:256–265.
57. Berkowitz SD, Granger CB, Piper KS, et al. Incidence and predictors of bleeding after contemporary thrombolytic therapy for myocardial infarction. The Global Utilization of Streptokinase and Tissue Plasminogen Activator for Occluded Coronary Arteries (GUSTO) I Investigators. Circulation 1997;95:2508–2516.
58. Önundarson PT, Haraldsson HM, Bergmann L, et al. Plasminogen depletion during streptokinase treatment or two-chain urokinase incubation correlates with decreased clot lysability ex vivo and in vitro. Thromb Haemost 1993;70:998–1004.
59. Kandarpa K. Catheter-directed thrombolysis of peripheral arterial occlusions and deep vein thrombosis. Thromb Haemost 1999; 82:987–996.
60. Hacke W, Ringleb P, Stingele R. Thrombolysis in acute cerebrovascular disease: indications and limitations. Thromb Haemost 1999;82:983–986.
61. The National Institute of Neurological Disorders; Stroke rt-PA Stroke Study Group. Tissue plasminogen activator for acute ischemic stroke. N Engl J Med 1995;333:1581–1587.
62. delZoppo GJ, Higashida RT, Furlan AJ, et al. PROACT: a phase II randomized trial of recombinant pro-urokinase by direct arterial delivery in acute middle cerebral artery stroke. Stroke 1998; 29:4–11.
63. Albers GW, Bates VE, Clark WM, et al. Intravenous tissue-type plasminogen activator for treatment of acute stroke. The standard treatment with alteplase to reverse stroke (STARS) study. JAMA 2000;283:1145–1150.
64. Katzan IL, Furlan AJ, Floyd LE. Use of tissue-type plasminogen activator for acute ischemic stroke. The Cleveland area experience. JAMA 2000;283:1151–1158.
65. The Global Use of Strategies to Open Occluded Coronary Arteries (GUSTO III) Investigators. A comparison of reteplase with alteplase for acute myocardial infarction. N Engl J Med 1997; 337:1118–1123.
66. Keyt BA, Paoni NF, Refino CJ, et al. A faster-acting and more potent form of tissue plasminogen activator. Proc Natl Acad Sci USA 1994;91:3670–3674.
67. Cannon CP, Gibson CM, McCabe CH, et al. TNK-tissue plasminogen activator compared with front-loaded alteplase in acute myocardial infarction: results of the TIMI 10B trial. Thrombolysis in Myocardial Infarction (TIMI) 10B Investigators. Circulation 1998;98:2805–2814.
68. Blinc A, Francis CW. Transport processes in fibrinolysis and fibrinolytic therapy. Thromb Haemost 1996;76:481–491.
69. Collins R, Peto R, Baigent C, et al. Aspirin, heparin, and fibrinolytic therapy in suspected acute myocardial infarction. N Engl J Med 1997;336:847–860.
70. Sane DC, Califf RM, Topol EJ, et al. Bleeding during thrombolytic therapy for acute myocardial infarction: Mechanisms and management. Ann Intern Med 1989;111:1010–1022.
71. Sobel BE. Intracranial bleeding, fibrinolysis, and anticoagulation. Causal connections and clinical implications. Circulation 1994; 90:2174–2182.

CHAPTER 25

Transfusion Medicine and Pharmacologic Aspects of Hemostasis

Charles D. Bolan, L.T.C., M.C., U.S.A.
Harvey G. Klein, M.D.

SYNOPSIS

Patients with disordered hemostasis present one of the greatest challenges to blood banks and transfusion practitioners. Early intervention with appropriate directed therapy can provide adequate hemostasis for a variety of bleeding conditions; however, the rapidly hemorrhaging patient can deplete the transfusion service's inventory and have a major impact on the hospital and the community. A variety of drugs and biologics are available to manage hemostatic disorders. This chapter will address various blood-derived biologics, non-blood-derived drugs, and strategies to prevent hemorrhage and manage hemostatic disorders.

INTRODUCTION AND HISTORICAL OVERVIEW

The evolution of the treatment of bleeding disorders with transfusions and pharmacologic therapy both parallels and differs from developments in traditional pharmacology. Early pharmaceutical preparations, such as digitalis, insulin, and vitamin B_{12}, were crude extracts that have been replaced by purer preparations or even by recombinant proteins. Similarly, the early use of whole-blood transfusion to treat conditions such as hemophilia, thrombotic thrombocytopenic purpura, and hemorrhagic disease of cattle after sweet clover ingestion has been supplanted by recombinantly derived clotting factors, specific blood component therapy, and USP standardized antidotes such as vitamin K to treat warfarin toxicity.[1,2] As progress in pharmacology has depended on an improved understanding of disease pathophysiology, so has progress in transfusion medicine depended on a detailed understanding of the mechanisms involved in hemostasis and the development of diagnostic laboratory assays to monitor management. To some extent, continued progress in rational transfusion management remains impeded by our lack of widely accessible assays to measure platelet function and to assess components of the fibrinolytic system.

Detection of past and emerging transfusion-transmitted infections, the effects of immunomodulation, and the role of long-lived cellular contaminants in transfusion recipients continue to challenge the transfusionist. The blood bank medical director has become a transfusion medicine consultant, heavily involved in the appropriate use of diverse therapies for patients with disordered hemostasis as well as in donor and inventory management and quality assurance.[3] While the primary responsibility is to assure optimal patient care, because newer blood components and plasma protein concentrates have become very costly, the transfusionist can also maximize cost-effectiveness and minimize waste of both funds and limited resources.

Several sentinel discoveries have played critical roles in adapting transfusion medicine and pharmacology for the care of the bleeding patient. Landsteiner's discovery of blood groups at the turn of the century allowed pretransfusion testing to be performed to avert reactions due to ABO-incompatible whole-blood transfusion. Blood group compatibility remains important for such hemostatic components as plasma and apheresis platelets, and blood group antibodies may still be found in some manufactured plasma fractions. With the development of citrate anticoagulant for blood storage, whole-blood transfusion was successfully adapted during the First World War, ultimately leading to the birth of the modern blood bank.

Edwin Cohn's investigations during the Second World War resulted in the cold ethanol plasma fractionation method, technology that still underlies the production of plasma with specific hemostatic activity. Pooling plasma on a large scale yielded standardized plasma fractions for patients with severe coagulation deficiencies and provided convenience and economy for the suppliers, which were blood centers. Unfortunately, military operations in the Korean War highlighted transfusion-transmitted hepatitis as a significant complication of pooled plasma, a problem that persisted until viral inactivation techniques were introduced in the mid 1980s.

The development of sterile interconnected plastic blood bags and of reliable blood cell separators in the 1960s ushered in the era of component therapy. This development provided the technology for large-scale production of fresh frozen plasma, cryoprecipitate, and platelet concentrates without which aggressive surgical, chemotherapeutic, and transplantation therapies could not have been undertaken. Cell separators permitted rapid therapeutic procedures, for example, "total plasma exchange" for patients with thrombotic thrombocytopenic purpura.

Blood banking aspects of the human immunoeficiency virus (HIV) epidemic of the 1980s remain indelibly imprinted in the philosophy of present-day transfusion medicine. However, the contamination of blood by HIV provided the stimulus to develop virus-inactivated plasma components and fractions, recombinant clotting factors, hemostatic drugs, and the more rational use of both blood components and pharmaceutical agents that affect hemostasis. To date, no such inactivation technologies have been licensed for cellular blood components.

Current challenges to the transfusion management of hemostasis have changed. With improved testing and screening, including polymerase chain reaction (PCR) techniques for hepatitis C and HIV contamination, the risk of known infection from a single donor exposure is once again extremely low. However, the risk of future unknown infections colors the use of single-donor and especially pooled-blood preparations. This fear has lead to increasingly stringent regulations designed to reduce the risk of disease and concomitant disruption of blood supplies and regional shortages at the same time that demand for blood is increasing. The cost of the new safer components and fractions has also risen dramatically. At the same time, the emergence of strategies for using pharmacologic agents to control bleeding associated with surgery may reduce the need for reoperation, improve overall mortality, reduce requirements for transfusion, and decrease exposure to allogeneic donors. Further, such agents may reduce the cost of therapy, and provide superior hemostasis when compared to traditional blood products. The treating physician now has a variety of choices and a variety of considerations when faced with a hemorrhaging patient or a patient being prepared for therapies or procedures that are likely to challenge the hemostatic system.[4]

TRADITIONAL BLOOD PRODUCTS

There is a wide range of blood components and plasma fractions, each with characteristic hemostatic properties and toxicities. Available products include those obtained by traditional single donation, either by centrifugal separation of whole blood or donor apheresis, as well as those obtained from fractions of pooled products processed from collections from thousands of donors. Recombinant blood proteins, although not blood derived, are often considered interchangeably with their plasma-derived relatives. Both the hemostatic properties and toxicities of these products are intimately related to the preparation processes. Increasingly, recombinant proteins have replaced virus-inactivated pooled plasma products for management of hemophilia A and B, while intermediate purity factor VIII preparations have replaced cryoprecipitate as treatment of von Willebrand disease (vWD). Cryoprecipitate remains the mainstay of treatment for fibrinogen and factor XIII deficiencies, while fresh frozen plasma (FFP) is the treatment of choice for other congenital factor deficiencies (factors XI, X, V, II, VII). Platelet concentrates and FFP are the blood components most frequently utilized for hemostasis; however, both red cells and granulocytes, as well as other preparations, may have important hemostatic effects related to either their plasma content or other properties.

Red Cells

Red blood cells (RBCs), commonly referred to as "packed cells" may be prepared either by whole-blood donation or by apheresis procedures. Although not typically considered a hemostatic component, RBCs may contribute to normal clot formation, or perhaps more accurately, a decrease in RBCs may contribute to a bleeding tendency. The template bleeding time prolongs as hematocrit falls, and RBC transfusions alone have been shown to improve hemostasis in patients with uremia[5] and chronic anemia.[6] The mechanism for this effect is not known, but may involve movement of platelets toward the vessel wall with increasing intravascular RBC mass,[7] or the action of RBC surface proteins that function as adhesion molecules.[8] RBC adhesion to endothelial cells plays a prominent pathologic role in malaria and sickle cell crisis, while the possible beneficial role of RBC adhesion during surgery or other conditions of compromised hemostasis is not known.

The adverse association of hematocrit with bleeding is greatest at low RBC concentrations (less than 6 g/dL),[6] and RBC transfusions may produce rapid hemostatic effects in addition to restoring oxygen-carrying capacity. RBC transfusions to maintain the hemoglobin above 9 g/dL produce no significant increment in hemostasis. Transfusions to patients to maintain a hemoglobin concentration above 9 g/dL may even be associated with decreased survival in intensive care units when compared to patients maintained at a hemoglobin concentration between 7 and 9 g/dL.[9]

Administration of the erythroid lineage cytokine erythropoietin (EPO) has been associated with a thrombopoietic effect. Although EPO administration may have effects on platelet reactivity,[10] the improvement in baseline hematocrit during EPO administration may account for the reduced incidence of bleeding in patients with uremia who are frequently treated with this agent.[11]

Exclusive reliance on RBC replacement in the rapidly bleeding patient may induce a hemostatic defect. Stored RBCs contain no functional platelets, and as little as 5% to 10% plasma depending on the preservative solution and method of collection. Serial testing for platelet count and screening coagulation assays such as the prothrombin time (PT) and activated partial thromboplastin time (aPTT) should be performed to guide component replacement when large numbers of RBC concentrates are transfused in trauma cases involving massive transfusion,[12] conventionally defined as transfusion exceeding one blood volume within 24 hours.

Platelets

Platelet concentrates can be prepared by pooling platelets obtained by centrifugation from individual units of whole blood. A "unit" of platelets has been defined as containing at least 5.5×10^{10} platelets—hence the term "six pack" describing a standardly prescribed dose of 3.3×10^{11}. Recent trends in blood center collection procedures have resulted in the majority of platelet products being obtained by single-donor apheresis, with the "dose" expressed by dividing the measured platelet content of the product by 3.0×10^{11}. These are arbitrary designations. Assessment of clinical response according to the dose of administered platelets and a post-transfusion platelet count measured within 1 hour of transfusion should be performed in all patients as a guide to future therapy (see below).

Apheresis or "single donor" collections result in fewer donor exposures for a given dose of platelets. Apheresis platelets may contain 200 to 250 mL of donor plasma, but heat-labile clotting factors decay rapidly at the storage temperature of 22°C. It has been surprisingly difficult to document an advantage of single-donor apheresis platelets over the pooled random-donor components, although one suspects that alloimmunization, bacterial contamination and virus transmission should all be reduced.

Platelets are transfused based on both prophylactic and therapeutic indications. Prophylactic transfusion triggers remain controversial. Previous recommendations for using $20,000/\mu L$ in stable patients were based on estimates of bleeding in children with leukemia, many of whom had received aspirin.[13] Subsequent studies indicate that even far lower numbers are safe.[14,15] Many clinicians now administer platelet transfusions to stable, nonbleeding patients with amegakaryocytic thrombocytopenia due to chemotherapy and/or leukemia prophylactically at platelet counts less than $5000/\mu L$.[16] A trigger of $20,000/\mu L$ may be more prudent for patients who are febrile, have rapidly falling counts, or have evidence of additional hemostatic defects. Platelet counts of $50,000/\mu L$ or so may be more reassuring when invasive procedures such as endoscopy, lumbar puncture, and bronchoscopy are anticipated although there is little evidence that such higher counts reduce morbidity or mortality. The clinical indications for therapeutic platelet transfusions are also controversial and should be based on the patient's clinical condition, the cause of bleeding, and the number and function of circulating platelets.[17]

Bleeding due to platelet defects acquired after cardiopulmonary bypass surgery or aspirin ingestion often responds to platelet transfusions; oozing related to uremia does not because the transfused platelets rapidly acquire the uremic defect.[17] Evolving algorithms for platelet transfusion in surgical settings based on point of care testing of platelet count and function have the potential to improve patient care as well as blood product utilization.[18]

Most platelet transfusions are administered to patients with defects in platelet production or function. However, some patients with immune-mediated thrombocytopenia may have satisfactory responses to platelet transfusions.[19] Platelet survival is generally no more than a few hours. Therefore these patients rarely benefit from prophylactic transfusions, while therapeutic transfusions may be life saving. Platelet transfusions are ordinarily considered to be contraindicated in patients with thrombotic platelet destruction such as those with thrombotic thrombocytopenic purpura (TTP), heparin-induced thrombocytopenia (HIT), and possibly disseminated intravascular coagulation (DIC).

Platelet transfusions should be monitored by baseline and post transfusion platelet counts. Some physicians prefer to standardize this evaluation by calculating a "corrected count increment" (CCI)[17]:

$$\text{CCI at 1 hour} = \frac{(\text{platelet count}_{post} - \text{platelet count}_{pre}) \times \text{body surface area (m}^2)}{\text{number of units transfused}}$$

A CCI above 4000 to $5000/\mu L$ suggests an adequate response to platelet transfusion, while two consecutive poor CCIs in the absence of fever, splenomegaly, active bleeding, consumption, ABO incompatibility, or other causes associated with increased platelet destruction suggest refractoriness. The development of platelet immune refractoriness presents a vexing clinical problem. Many patients can be managed well with platelets from human lymphocyte antigen (HLA)-compatible relatives or even unrelated matched donors. When such donors are unavailable, management of refractory patients, either by HLA "best-matching" or platelet cross matches, should be tried, but is cumbersome, expensive, and not uniformly efficacious. Repeated platelet transfusion in the absence of documented increments unnecessarily exposes patients to the potential risks of transfusion without evidence for any benefit and depletes an often scarce and costly blood resource.

Fresh Frozen Plasma

Fresh frozen plasma (FFP) is prepared by freezing the plasma component of a unit of whole blood within 6 to 8 hours of collection. The hemostatic activity of the coagulation factors is maintained even after storage for 1 year or longer, depending on the storage temperature. Once thawed, the plasma can be stored at refrigerated temperature for no more than 24 hours. On the average, 1 mL of FFP contains one unit of each coagulation factor. However, the volume of a "unit" of FFP, the concentration of coagulation factors, and the citrate anticoagulant concentration are variable, depending on the donor blood composition and anticoagulant solution. In one study of individual units collected from 51 regular plasma donors, the 5th and 95th percentiles for factor V concentrations ranged from 69 to 127 U/dL and for factor VII from 83 to 169 U/dL, while the fibrinogen concentration ranged from 180 to 370 mg/dL and antithrombin III from 92 to 129 U/dL.[20]

FFP remains the treatment of choice for deficiencies of factors XI, X, V, II, and VII.[21] FFP is commonly used to treat bleeding patients with acquired deficiency of multiple coagulation factors, such as patients with DIC, liver disease, dilutional coagulopathy, and TTP. FFP may also be used for rapid yet temporary reversal of the coagulopathy induced by oral anticoagulants (see below); these patients may require vitamin K therapy for long-term control, while those with cerebral hemorrhage may benefit from the higher concentration of vitamin K-dependent factors in prothrombin complex concentrates (PCCs).[22] FFP has also been employed for replacement of deficiencies of proteins C or S as well as other anticoagulant proteins in patients with thrombophilia. Prophylactic administration of FFP has not been found to improve patient outcome in the setting of massive transfusion unless bleeding is associated with documented coagulopathy; these patients should be followed with coagulation tests to guide replacement therapy.[23] Similarly, mild prolongations of the PT and aPTT (< 1.5 times midpoint of the normal range of the laboratory) do not call for FFP prophylaxis for trauma patients or for patients scheduled to undergo elective invasive procedures.[24,25] Indiscriminate transfusion of FFP for a mild, clinically insignificant prolonged PT is far too common, resulting in unnecessary allergic reactions and delays in diagnostic procedures as common consequences.[4] No clinical benefit has been documented.

Solvent detergent plasma is FFP that has been pooled and treated to inactivate lipid-encapsulated viruses such as HIV, hepatitis B virus (HBV), and hepatitis C virus (HCV). Solvent detergent treatment of pooled collections results in more uniform concentrations of these factors, and has reduced concentrations of high-molecular-weight vWF, a potential advantage for therapy of TTP, but a potential disadvantage in other hemostatic disorders.[26] Concentrations of protein S and α_2-antiplasmin are reduced as well.[26] The advantage of a product that is free of the major class of transfusion-transmitted viruses must be weighed against the potential disadvantage of trading a relatively safe single-donor component for one made from larger pools that may contain nonencapsulated viruses such as hepatitis A and parvovirus B19.

Cryoprecipitate

Cryoprecipitate is the cold insoluble material formed when FFP is thawed at 4°C. "Cryo" is rich in factor VIII, factor XIII, vWF, and fibrinogen.[21,27] The product can be stored frozen at −20°C for up to a year. When resuspended in a plasma volume of 10 to 20 mL after preparation from single-donor plasma, cryoprecipitate contains 80 to 100 units of factor VIII/vWF representing 40% to 70% of the original amount in the plasma, 100 to 250 mg fibrinogen, and approximately 30% of the original amount of factor XIII.[27] Because of its higher concentration of these factors compared to FFP, cryoprecipitate served for decades as the primary replacement therapy for patients with hemophilia A and vWD. Cryoprecipitate should no longer be used for these purposes, and has been replaced by DDAVP (below) for most mild cases of either disease, and by virus inactivated or recombinant preparations. Similarly, the use of cryoprecipitate to treat uremic bleeding (10 units per treatment) has largely been supplanted by DDAVP, estrogen therapy, or RBC transfusion and EPO therapy.[11] The use of cryoprecipitate as the source of fibrinogen for "home-brewed" "fibrin glue" preparations should disappear with the advent of standardized commercial products containing virus-inactivated human fibrinogen[28] (see Chapter 26).

Today, the main indication for cryoprecipitate is as replacement therapy in patients with hypofibrinogenemia that is congenital (rare) or acquired (i.e., following thrombolytic therapy, DIC, or massive transfusions).[12,21] When used for these indications, 10 to 20 units are normally pooled and infused, with repeat doses administered every 6 to 8 hours depending on the clinical status and measurements of laboratory tests of coagulation or fibrinogen concentration. Fibrinogen levels greater than 50 mg/dL are considered sufficient to support both physiologic hemostasis and result in a normal PT or aPTT. Cryoprecipitate may also be useful for treatment of factor XIII deficiency, a rare congenital deficiency, or an acquired disorder resulting from autoantibody formation.[21] Commercially prepared, virus-inactivated fibrinogen concentrates are not yet available in the United States.

Commercial Plasma Fractions

A variety of products prepared by special processing of plasma pools are used to treat hemostatic disorders. Among the earliest preparations are the so-called prothrombin complex concentrates (PCCs), which are impure mixtures of vitamin K-dependent proteins, isolated by ion-exchange chromatography from the cryoprecipitate supernatant of large plasma pools after removal of antithrombin III and factor XI.[29] Different processing techniques involving ion exchangers permit production of either four-factor concentrates, which include factor VII, or three-factor concentrates consisting mainly of factors II, IX, and X. The PCCs are standardized according to their factor IX content.[29] During production, activated clotting factors are produced which are then inactivated by a variety of processes including manipulation of pH and the addition of heparin and/or antithrombin III. These products may be further adjusted to produce activated PCCs used for treatment of patients with acquired factor VIII or IX inhibitors (see Chapters 4 and 6). PCCs are now treated to inactivate transfusion-transmitted viruses. Adverse events associated with PCCs include immediate allergic reactions, heparin-induced thrombocytopenia (for preparations containing heparin), and thromboembolic complications including DIC, arguably the most important side effect.[29] PCC administration is indicated only when the desired increase in factor activity cannot be achieved through other therapeutic measures (see treatment of cerebral bleeding in excessive oral anticoagulation with vitamin K, below). PCC should not be used for treatment of hemophilia B or congenital factor VII deficiency, with the exception of emergency situations when specific factor replacements are not available.[30]

Virus-inactivated, intermediate-purity factor VIII preparations with high vWF content have replaced cryoprecipitate as the primary therapy for vWD.[31-33] One of these products, Humate P, (Centeon L.L.C., Kanakee, Ill) has recently been approved by the Food and Drug Administration for treatment of vWD, and the product insert now provides the lot concentration of ristocetin cofactor activity to facilitate dosing.

Available treatments for hemophilia A and B have evolved to recombinant factor VIII and IX preparations, which are more expensive than virally inactivated pooled products, but provide physicians and patients a variety of products of high purity and safety (see Chapter 4). A recombinant factor VIIa preparation has been developed for treatment of those patients who develop inhibitors,[34] and has been recently applied to augment hemostasis in other bleeding conditions of diverse causes.[35,36] The costs of this therapy, along with other treatments for patients with inhibitors such as porcine factor VIII or high doses of human factor VIII, are formidable.

Adverse Effects

All single-donor components carry approximately equivalent risk for HIV, HBV, and HCV infection. The most widely quoted estimates of the risk of HIV transmission is 1 in 493,000 units transfused; of human T-cell leukemia virus (HTLV), 1 in 641,000; of HCV, 1 in 103,000; and of HBV, 1 in 63,000. The aggregate risk is 1 infection in 34,000 units, of which 88% is due to HBV and HCV.[37] The advent of nucleic acid testing for viral genome particles of HCV and HIV will likely reduce the risk of HIV transmission to 1 per million or less and the risk of HCV to about 1 in 350,000 units. However, residual infection due to HIV disease has been reported.[38] Thus, despite increasingly sophisticated testing and screening strategies, until activation procedures for cellular components are available, infections from current and emerging agents will prevent a zero-risk blood supply.[39]

Other adverse events are presently much more common than transfusion-transmitted viral infections. The most common associated with transfusion are febrile nonhemolytic transfusion reactions (FNHTR) from RBC or platelet transfusion, and urticarial reactions associated with FFP or plasma transfusions. These reactions are not life threatening, but may cause apprehension in the patient, and lead to significant delays in procedures or diagnostic studies until the cause is determined. FNHTRs typically occur in less than 1% of transfusions overall, but are more common with platelet transfusions and are observed in as many as 6% to 12% of adults with hematologic malignancies or pediatric patients.[40] Urticarial allergic reactions may occur in 1% to 3% of transfusions of RBCs, platelets, or FFP, while anaphylactic shock occurs once per 20,000 to 47,000 units of blood components transfused.[41] Severe hemolytic transfusion reactions are associated almost exclusively with incompatible RBCs, but hemolysis related to antibodies in plasma or platelet concentrates remains an important cause of morbidity and mortality.[42] Acute hemolytic transfusion reactions due to intravascular hemolysis may occur in one in 25,000 units, while delayed hemolytic transfusion reactions occur 5 to 10 times more frequently.[42] Both acute and delayed hemolytic reactions are associated with mortality, with an estimated risk of 1 in 630,000 and 1 in 1,150,000 units, respectively.[42]

The incidence of bacterial contamination and shock related to bacterial contamination is of particular concern in platelet transfusion. This component must be stored at room temperature and thus is particularly susceptible to bacterial growth. The true risk of contamination and frequency of reactions is unknown, but is probably underreported. Estimates from prospective studies indicate that bacterial contamination occurs in 0.3 of every 10,000 RBC units, 0.5 to 23 of every 10,000 apheresis platelet concentrates, and 5 to 30 of every 10,000 pooled random-donor platelet concentrates.[43] A wide variety of gram-positive and gram-negative organisms is associated with platelet contamination, while *Yersinia* sp. and other cryophilic organisms are most frequently implicated with RBC transfusions.[43] An estimated 25% of cases of transfusion-related bacterial sepsis are severe, resulting in septic shock or death.[43]

Less common, but dramatic reactions may occur in so-called transfusion-related acute lung injury (TRALI),[44] post-transfusion purpura (PTP),[45] and transfusion-associated graft-versus-host disease (TAGVHD).[46] The former two reactions are caused by plasma-containing components, while TAGVHD is associated with transfusion of cellular elements. The incidence of these reactions is likely underdiagnosed, but each may be associated with clinically significant reactions.

TRALI is a life-threatening complication, with severe acute pulmonary edema and hypoxemia associated with normal cardiac filling pressures and is indistinguishable from the adult respiratory distress syndrome, occurring within 1 to 6 hours (usually within 1 to 2 hours) of plasma-containing blood component transfusion.[44] The mechanism of TRALI is unknown, but is likely immunologically mediated by HLA-specific antibodies or leukagglutinins in donor plasma, particularly in plasma obtained from multiparous female donors. The incidence of TRALI is unknown, but may be as high as 0.001% to 0.34% of transfusions. TRALI has been implicated in 12% of all transfusion-related fatalities in one study. Treatment is supportive.

PTP is characterized by dramatic, precipitous thrombocytopenia occurring within 3 weeks of blood transfusion in a patient with a history of prior transfusion or pregnancy.[45] The sera of patients characteristically demonstrate potent antiplatelet reactivity induced by the transfusion, however, the mechanism responsible for the destruction of the patient's own platelets is unknown. The syndrome is most common after RBC transfusions, but may also occur after transfusion of single-donor plasma and platelet products. Patients are refractory to transfusion of either antigen-negative or -positive platelets, but may respond rapidly to intravenous immunoglobulin (IVIG) or plasmapheresis with albumin replacement.

TAGVHD is far less common than TRALI, although the precise incidence remains unknown.[46] The presentation mimics bone marrow transplant-related graft-versus-host disease, with the additional clinical finding of bone marrow aplasia, typically occurring 8 to 10 days (maximum of 4 weeks) after transfusion. TAGVHD occurs when immunocompetent donor T cells in the blood component engraft in the recipient. The most susceptible patients are closely matched family members of the donor or those who are immunocompromised, such as organ and bone marrow transplant recipients, premature infants, and patients with certain neoplasms. Once present, TAGVHD is almost always fatal. Leukocyte reduction is not effective prophylaxis. Blood product irradiation prevents TAGVHD and is indicated for susceptible patients.[47]

Hemostatic Effects of Transfusion Medicine Procedures

Apheresis procedures lower platelet counts in patients and in donors. The reduction in platelets is related to the volume of blood processed and number of procedures performed.[48] For example, donors of peripheral blood stem cells who undergo three consecutive daily large-volume apheresis procedures experienced a fall in platelet count, with a median nadir of 54,000/μL.[49]

Significant hemostatic effects also occur during plasmapheresis when plasma-free replacement fluid is used. Patients with normal hemostasis receiving plasmapheresis with 4L albumin replacement have sustained decreases of 50% in fibrinogen levels and activities of factors V and VIII and of vWF. These decreases have been associated with an 80% to 300% increase in the PT, aPTT, and thrombin time when measured immediately after the procedure.[48] The aPTT and thrombin time ordinarily return to pretreatment levels within 4 hours, while all hemostatic values normalize at 24 hours. Clinically significant bleeding episodes rarely occur. However, these changes should be considered when plasmapheresis is planned in patients with abnormal baseline screening tests (i.e., PT or aPTT) or when determining the timing of invasive procedures.

PHARMACEUTICAL AGENTS

Pharmaceutical agents occasionally replace but are more commonly used as adjunctive therapy to blood products in the treatment of patients with hemostatic disorders.[11,50] A broad spectrum of agents is available. For example, DDAVP, a synthetic analogue of L-vasopressin, can be used for most mild forms of hemophilia A and vWD, and is increasingly recognized to have multiple less well defined effects that have been applied in a variety of hemostatic defects. Lysine analogs that inhibit fibrinolysis, such as ε-aminocaproic acid (EACA) and tranexamic acid (AMCA), are used both systemically and locally for acquired and inherited defects in hemostasis and thrombocytopenia. Aprotinin, a bovine-derived serine protease inhibitor with potent antifibrinolytic activity, is widely employed to enhance surgical hemostasis after cardiopulmonary bypass. Vitamin preparations in the naphthoquinone family (vitamin K) are used to prevent neonatal bleeding syndromes as well as to reverse warfarin anticoagulation or to treat ingestion of superwarfarin-like rodenticides. Other agents may be utilized, such as estrogens to treat uremic bleeding, and protamine to reverse heparin-induced anticoagulation.

DDAVP

Background. The agent 1-deamino-8-D-arginine vasopressin, or desmopressin (DDAVP), is a synthetic analog of the antidiuretic hormone L-vasopressin[51] that has been used to control bleeding in patients with mild congenital or acquired hemorrhagic disorders for more than 25 years.[52,53]

The past decade has witnessed increasing use of at-home administration of DDAVP to prevent or treat bleeding episodes.[52] However, the past quarter of a century of clinical study and experience also refined the use of this drug even before the mechanisms of action were fully understood. For example, it is now recognized that DDAVP does not reduce blood loss in most surgical settings[54-56] except in patients with prior aspirin ingestion[57] or possibly with platelet dysfunction of other causes.[58] An overview of DDAVP is presented in Table 25-1. Current uses of DDAVP in adults and children have been summarized in several recent comprehensive reviews.[52,59]

Mechanisms of Action and Tachyphylaxis

The best-characterized hemostatic activity of DDAVP is to raise circulating factor VIII and vWF levels, which appears to be due to its chemical similarity to vasopressin.[51,52] Compared to vasopressin, DDAVP has increased affinity for V1 receptors, which cause renal free water retention and rapid release of factor VIII and vWF from preformed cellular stores, and markedly decreased affinity for V2 receptors, which mediate vasoconstriction.[51] In normal subjects, DDAVP increases

Table 25-1 • OVERVIEW OF DDAVP

Action
- Releases stored factor VIII and vWF within 30 to 60 minutes, peak effect at 2-4 hours, lasting 6-8 hours. Has other hemostatic effects on platelets and endothelium.

Administration
- Daily by intravenous, subcutaneous, and intranasal routes. Does not require concomitant use of antifibrinolytic agents. Tachyphylaxis may occur at more frequent dosing intervals, or after several daily administrations.

General Use
- Short-term control of various bleeding states. Initial efficacy should be established with a test infusion.
- Primary therapy for mild hemophilia A and vWD. More useful for type 1 than type 2 vWD, may be useful in some cases of type 3 vWD.
- Widely used to control bleeding in acquired and congenital platelet defects. Efficacy in this setting less well defined because of a lack of appropriate tests to assess platelet function.
- Use in surgical setting not consistently associated with improvement in hemostasis except after aspirin ingestion. Aprotinin and antifibrinolytics are superior in hemostatic control in cardiac bypass. Efficacy may be improved for selected patients identified by perioperative testing for platelet defects.

Possible Contraindications
- Worsens thrombocytopenia in some type IIB vWD patients.
- Use cautiously in elderly patients or those with coronary artery disease.

Toxicity
- Mild flushing, nausea are most common.
- Water retention, hyponatremia associated with seizures and headaches.
- Possibly associated with myocardial infarction in the cardiac bypass setting.

---

factor VIII and vWF levels within 30 minutes after infusion.[60] Levels peak at 300% to 400% of baseline in 1 to 2 hours, and persist for 6 to 12 hours.[52]

DDAVP induces a transient five- to sevenfold increase in tissue plasminogen activator (tPA) activity with resultant generation of plasmin, which is rapidly counteracted by endogenous levels of α_2-antiplasmin.[61] Recipients do not require antifibrinolytic agents in routine clinical practice.[11] In in-vitro studies, adhesion of both RBCs and platelets to endothelial cells has been found to be increased by DDAVP.[62,63] These effects might be produced by direct action on the vessel wall[63] or possibly by release of high-molecular-weight vWF at the endothelial cell surface.[64] In addition, shear stress at the vessel wall is decreased after infusion of DDAVP in patients with congenital platelet defects, possibly due to higher circulating levels of these high-molecular-weight multimers.[65–67] Other studies have shown that DDAVP may also (1) increase platelet microparticle formation,[68] (2) increase the expression of tissue factor on endothelial cells,[69] and (3) increase expression of P-selectin[70] and the adhesive glycoprotein 1b on platelet membranes.[71] One or more of these or other unidentified effects may explain the observations that DDAVP shortens the bleeding time in patients with severe vWD who have already received cryoprecipitate infusions,[72] and in qualitative platelet disorders such as uremia,[73] liver disease[74] and other acquired or congenital conditions,[74–76] in which levels of factor VIII and vWF are usually normal. In some of these studies, patients who had previously experienced severe bleeding during surgeries performed without the use of DDAVP experienced adequate surgical hemostasis after the use of DDAVP.[76]

The mechanisms of action of DDAVP explain some important clinical observations. First, infusion in hemophilia A and vWD produces short-term increases of circulating factor VIII and vWF, which decrease after their initial release from preformed intracellular stores.[52] Thus, DDAVP has been used alone in these conditions for minor surgical procedures or dental work, but is inadequate for procedures that require prolonged hemostasis. Second, repeat administration of DDAVP is associated with tachyphylaxis, with decreased laboratory and clinical response when administered at less than 24-hour intervals or repeatedly for several days.[77] The blunted response is presumably related to depletion of intracellular stores of factor VIII and vWF. The pattern of tachyphylaxis is not predictable, and is more marked in general for patients with hemophilia A compared to vWD. In one study of daily dosing, the responses after a second dose were 30% of the first-day response, but were not further reduced after the third and fourth dose.[77] In contrast to the diminished factor VIII and vWF responses after repeated doses, various fibrinolytic,[78] renal,[51] and platelet responses do not appear altered when doses are repeated frequently.[79] Although the hemostatic response to initial administration of DDAVP varies among patients, it is usually reproducible on each occasion for a given patient.[77] Ideally, all patients who may receive DDAVP should receive an initial test infusion to establish response at least several days prior to any planned invasive procedures.

Dosage and Administration

DDAVP may be administered by intravenous, subcutaneous, and intranasal routes (Table 25-2). The intravenous dose is 0.3 µg/kg, administered over 30 minutes in 50 mL of normal saline for adults (and in 10 mL for children weighing less than 10 kg). The maximum response occurs at intravenous doses of 0.3 µg/kg. The subcutaneous dose is 0.3 to 0.4 µg/kg, with peak responses approximately 230% above baseline at 60 minutes after administration, slightly lower and later than the peak dose after intravenous administration. The intranasal dose is an order of magnitude higher than the intravenous or subcutaneous dose, generally 300 µg in adults. Higher doses do not enhance efficacy, but may be associated with increased toxicity. A concentrated nasal spray formulation is available in both the United States and Europe. However, a concentrated preparation for subcutaneous use is not available in the United States, and the substantial volume (7 mL) required for subcutaneous treatment of a 70-kg individual may be uncomfortable. DDAVP is cleared by the liver and kidneys and has a plasma half life of 124 minutes. Because

Table 25–2 • HEMOSTATIC PREPARATIONS OF DDAVP

Route	Concentration	Dose[a]	Volume	Cost[b]	Peak Response[c]
Intravenous	4 μg/mL	21 μg (0.3 μg/kg)	5.25 mL (in 50 mL saline)	$116.00 per dose	30–60 min
Intranasal (Stimate)[d]	1500 μg/mL	300 μg total	0.1 mL per spray	$46.00 per dose	90–120 min
Subcutaneous	4 μg/mL	21 μg (0.3 μg/kg)	5.25 mL	$116.00	90–120 min
Subcutaneous[e]	40 μg/mL	21 μg (0.3 μg/kg)	0.52 mL	Not available in US	90–120 min

[a] For 70-kg adult.
[b] Average wholesale price.
[c] For factor VIII and vWF levels.
[d] One spray per nostril.
[e] This preparation is available only in Europe.

many of its known hemostatic effects are caused indirectly, blood DDAVP levels may be more relevant to renal effects and toxicity than to hemostasis.[80]

Indications

There are no controlled studies evaluating the use of DDAVP compared to placebo or factor concentrates in patients with hemophilia and vWD.[52] Since the bleeding tendency in hemophilia A, and to a lesser degree in vWD, correlates with measured blood levels of the deficient factor, the ability of DDAVP to transiently raise factor VIII and vWF has resulted in its approval for use in these disorders. Experience has confirmed its usefulness and DDAVP is now the treatment of choice for minor and even moderately invasive procedures in patients with these disorders who respond to a test infusion. However, the use of DDAVP in type 2B vWD remains controversial as these patients may develop mild thrombocytopenia related to the affinity of the vWF for platelets.[33] Infusion of DDAVP and release of endogenous vWF stores into circulation may worsen thrombocytopenia; nevertheless, several studies have reported improved hemostasis in type 2B vWD after infusion of DDAVP associated with little or only mild thrombocytopenia; therefore, it is reasonable to consider the use of DDAVP in carefully selected patients with type 2B vWD.[81,82] Although most patients with severe vWD do not respond to DDAVP, a minority of patients may achieve modest increases in factor VIII levels, providing sufficient hemostasis for minor procedures.[83] In patients with severe hemophilia A, factor VIII levels do not increase after DDAVP infusion; however, DDAVP may still provide potential benefit by increasing vWF levels, with an associated increased response in activity of infused factor VIII concentrates.[84] DDAVP may also further shorten the bleeding time in patients with severe vWD that was not fully corrected after infusion of cryoprecipitate infusions, possibly due to the nonspecific effects on hemostasis previously described.[72] Finally, DDAVP is useful in some mild cases of acquired vWD[85] but not when due to immune-mediated disease or in acquired vWD associated with monoclonal gammopathy of uncertain significance.[86]

DDAVP has also been found to augment hemostasis in a variety of acquired and congenital conditions with impaired hemostasis in which other treatment options are limited.[52] In one double-blind placebo-controlled study of patients with congenital platelet defects, DDAVP decreased the bleeding time most effectively in those with normal platelet dense granule stores.[87] In other studies, DDAVP has been shown to improve the bleeding time or be associated with adequate surgical hemostasis in patients with storage pool defect,[75,88] Bernard–Soulier disease,[89] aspirin ingestion,[79] and other defects in platelet hemostasis.[52,76] DDAVP has been utilized in patients without platelet disease, including limited studies in Ehlers-Danlos syndrome[90] and mild factor XI deficiency.[91] DDAVP shortens the bleeding time in some hemorrhagic diseases of multifactorial origin such as cirrhosis and uremia. Extrapolation of the utility of DDAVP in these conditions should be done with caution. Except in surgical studies of transfusion requirements after aspirin ingestion, most studies have determined the efficacy of DDAVP by observing a shortening of the bleeding time, or by assessing surgical hemostasis in uncontrolled studies of small numbers of patients. Since the bleeding time is a poor predictor of surgical bleeding, interpretation of these studies is problematic.[92] It may, however, be reasonable to consider the use of DDAVP in these conditions when other treatments are not available and after hemostasis has been maximized by local measures such as fibrin sealant or other methods.

Bleeding symptoms did not improve, and may have worsened, when DDAVP was combined with the vasoactive agent terlipressin for treatment of acute variceal hemorrhage in patients with cirrhosis, perhaps due to competitive inhibition of drug activity.[93] Similarly, its use in uremia seems to be diminishing as increasing use of erythropoietin and higher baseline hematocrits has decreased the frequency of uremic bleeding.[11] Other approaches may be useful in uremia, with long-term control achieved with the use of estrogens, while short-term bleeding may respond to RBC transfusions.[50]

Initial reports that DDAVP decreased blood loss and transfusion requirements after cardiac and spinal surgery have not been confirmed in follow-up studies.[52] A recent large meta-analysis revealed no reduction in bleeding after the use of DDAVP in cardiac surgery, in contrast to comparative studies with lysine analog antifibrinolytic agents and aprotinin.[94] Aprotinin was also associated with decreased mortality, while both aprotinin and antifibrinolytic agents were associated with a decreased need for repeat thoracotomy. Neither aprotinin nor antifibrinolytic agents increased the incidence of myocardial thrombosis. DDAVP had no effect on mortality or repeat thoracotomy, but was associated with a two- to fourfold increased risk of coronary thrombosis.[94] Although this study did not demonstrate a beneficial reduction in blood loss after the use of DDAVP, average surgical blood loss was relatively small. Earlier analyses have suggested a potential benefit for the use of DDAVP in cases having larger predicted blood loss.[95]

Methods to identify a subset of patients, prior to surgery, who might benefit from administration of DDAVP would be useful.[95] One such group appears to be patients with preoperative platelet defects, especially those who have been treated with aspirin. Blood loss was markedly reduced in patients with preoperative defects in platelet function identified by point-of-care testing who received DDAVP compared to those who received placebo.[58] Three randomized, double-blinded placebo-controlled trials have shown clinically significant reductions in blood loss and transfusion requirements after the use of DDAVP in patients who have ingested aspirin before cardiac surgery.[57,96,97] DDAVP also reduced bleeding in an unblinded comparison with placebo in patients who ingested aspirin before cholecystectomy.[98] In addition, DDAVP has been demonstrated to shorten the bleeding time in normal volunteers after aspirin ingestion,[74] perhaps due to direct effects on platelets or increases in vWF.[79] Aprotinin has also been demonstrated to reduce bleeding in aspirin-treated patients undergoing cardiac bypass, but has not been compared directly with DDAVP.[99]

DDAVP has been used without adverse effects to control hemorrhage during pregnancy in a patient with Ehlers-Danlos syndrome,[100] however, there is little additional information on the safety of DDAVP or other hemostatic agents in pregnant women with bleeding disorders.[101] A review of the use of intranasal DDAVP to treat 53 pregnant women with diabetes insipidus found no risk to mother or child. However, the average intranasal daily dose of DDAVP in these cases, 29 μg (range 7.5 to 100 μg), was significantly lower than that commonly used intranasally to augment hemostasis.[102]

While some studies have indicated that DDAVP is not effective in patients with afibrinogenemia,[103] thrombocytopenia,[74] or Glanzman disease,[74] other patients with Glanzman disease or thrombocytopenia have been reported to respond.[104,105]

Toxicity

Most side effects of DDAVP are minor. Facial flushing, often marked, and minimal elevation in pulse rate or blood pressure are observed more frequently with the intravenous than with the subcutaneous or intranasal routes.[106] The most common, clinically significant adverse event is hyponatremia, which results from the antidiuretic effect of this vasopressin analog. Hyponatremic seizures have been observed in children 1 month to 8 years of age, especially when hypotonic fluids and multiple doses of DDAVP are administered in the surgical setting.[59] Less severe but significant symptoms of headache, nausea, or lethargy have been reported in adults after intranasal[107] or repeated intravenous and subcutaneous administration.[108] Careful monitoring of intravenous fluids, urine output, and electrolytes is therefore important, especially for children who receive DDAVP perioperatively and in older patients when mild renal insufficiency decreases their ability to excrete free water. Patients should be instructed to restrict fluid intake for 24 hours.

Thrombosis is an obvious concern when drugs that enhance hemostasis are used. Isolated cases of thrombosis such as myocardial infarction, cerebral thrombosis, and unstable angina have been reported after use of DDAVP in patients at risk for thrombotic events.[109] In the surgical setting, one randomized, placebo-controlled study specifically designed to detect deep venous thrombosis in 50 patients undergoing hip surgery,[110] and an early meta-analysis[111] did not detect an increased incidence of thrombosis following DDAVP therapy. A recent meta-analysis reported a two- to fourfold (95% confidence intervals 1.02 to 5.60) increased risk of myocardial infarction in cardiac surgery patients who received DDAVP.[94] Some experienced hemophilia centers do not routinely administer DDAVP to elderly patients or those with risk factors for coronary artery disease.[112] It therefore seems prudent to carefully evaluate patients receiving DDAVP for possible occult coronary artery disease and to avoid the concurrent use of antifibrinolytic agents in these patients under most circumstances.

Lysine Analog Antifibrinolytic Agents

Background

Fibrinolysis occurs when plasmin, which has been generated from plasminogen by plasminogen activators, digests fibrin clots.[113] Both plasmin and plasminogen bind to fibrin through lysine binding sites.[114] The synthetic lysine analogs tranexamic acid (AMCA) and ε-aminocaproic acid (EACA) delay fibrinolysis by reducing the binding of plasminogen to fibrin.[114,115] These agents have been utilized for more than 30 years to inhibit fibrinolysis and ensure clot stability.[115,116]

AMCA was developed within a few years of EACA, and was noted to inhibit fibrinolysis more potently on a molar basis and to have a reduced incidence of gastrointestinal complaints at equivalent antifibrinolytic doses in healthy volunteers.[117] Much of the early use of antifibrinolytic agents in the United States involved EACA, while AMCA was used relatively more frequently in Europe.[115] Although AMCA and EACA have been considered as equivalent agents,[115] optimal dosing regimens have not been developed for either agent in most clinical settings, and reported toxicities vary.[118,119] Therefore, strict comparisons are difficult to make, and generalizations comparing studies should be performed cautiously.

Lysine analog antifibrinolytic drugs are effective and clearly indicated in rare inherited conditions associated with excessive fibrinolysis such as congenital α_2-antiplasmin deficiency.[120] However, much of the recent enthusiasm for these drugs has focused on their use in acquired disorders with evidence of excessive systemic fibrinolysis, especially cardiac bypass surgery, and to a lesser degree orthopedic surgery performed with the use of tourniquets. Importantly, both agents are useful when administered topically in areas with excessive local fibrinolysis such as the oral cavity and uterine cavity. In these instances, efficacy is well established, and side effects are reduced compared to systemic administration.[11,50,121] AMCA and EACA are also frequently administered to reduce bleeding in such conditions as amegakaryocytic and peripheral immune-mediated thrombocytopenia, where the indication is less obvious, and efficacy is presumably due to stabilization of fibrin clots.[122–125] As might be expected, there is less evidence of efficacy in these settings.[125] An overview of the use of these agents is given in Table 25-3.

Excessive thrombosis is a potentially devastating complication in clinical settings involving excessive procoagulant activity, such as DIC.[126,127] Thrombosis is not statistically increased with the use AMCA or EACA in most settings other than DIC. However, the risk of this complication may have limited the more widespread application of these drugs in conditions such as menorrhagia or upper gastrointestinal hemorrhage, despite randomized studies demonstrating benefit.[115,116]

Table 25-3 • OVERVIEW OF LYSINE ANALOG ANTIFIBRINOLYTIC AGENTS

Action
- Clot stabilization by rapid inhibition of fibrinolysis associated with competition at lysine binding sites of plasmin and plasminogen activators. AMCA is more potent on a molar basis than EACA.

Administration
- Every 4–8 hours by oral, intravenous, and topical routes. Dose should be reduced in patients with renal insufficiency, and has not been optimally determined in many conditions.

General Use
- Short- and long-term control of various bleeding states.
- Consistent benefit in blinded, randomized studies of upper gastrointestinal bleeding and menorrhagia.
- Effective topically, with decreased systemic effects, in oral and cardiac surgery, ophthalmologic conditions, and other conditions with excessive local fibrinolysis.
- Wide use in thrombocytopenic states, with less consistent benefit.
- Effective in rare acquired or congenital conditions characterized primarily by excessive fibrinolysis.
- Effective in cardiac bypass surgery; less expensive and possibly less effective overall than aprotinin at conventional doses.
- Anecdotal use in conditions that lack effective, specific therapy.

Contraindications
- Thrombotic disorders with compensatory fibrinolysis.
- Urologic bleeding conditions.

Toxicity
- Nausea, cramping, and diarrhea, more commonly with EACA.
- Myonecrosis after long-term oral use with EACA.
- Thrombosis in settings with compensatory fibrinolysis such as DIC.

Dosage and Administration

Both agents may be administered orally, intravenously, or topically. EACA and AMCA are well absorbed orally, and are cleared virtually unchanged by the kidneys.[114] The drugs are distributed widely throughout the body. AMCA crosses into cerebrospinal fluid, semen, synovial fluid, and cord blood, but is not secreted in saliva.[116] In the nonoperative setting, the half-life for both agents is approximately 1 to 2 hours in patients with normal renal function. The dose should be reduced in renal failure.[116,128] AMCA is approximately 6 to 10 times more potent than EACA on a molar basis,[114] however, few direct clinical pharmacokinetic and pharmacodynamic comparisons of the two agents have been performed.[116] A typical total daily oral dose for EACA is 10 to 24 g, administered as 2 to 4 g every 3 to 4 hours, and for AMCA 3 to 4 g, administered as 1 g every 6 to 8 hours. Dosage in individual studies varies widely.[115] Recent studies have attempted to optimize dosing for both agents in conditions such as cardiac surgery, where the clearance and distribution of these agents is altered.[128–130] Anecdotes and controlled studies have described improved control of bleeding using short-term, bolus,[131–133] and local or topical administration.[134–136] The optimum dose and route of administration may depend on the patient, the disease, or both.[116]

Indications

Data on the efficacy of AMCA and EACA to improve hemostasis in thrombocytopenic states are conflicting and difficult to interpret. Two retrospective uncontrolled studies of 31 patients with thrombocytopenia, including amegakaryocytic and immune-mediated etiologies, demonstrated a benefit with oral EACA.[122,123] A smaller study found that bleeding was controlled by EACA bolus infusion when platelet transfusions were unavailable or delayed.[132]

A randomized, double-blind, placebo-controlled study of AMCA administered to reduce bleeding in 38 patients with acute myeloid leukemia found a significant reduction in bleeding episodes and platelet transfusions during consolidation, but not during induction therapy.[124] However, a smaller study of eight patients with amegakaryocytic thrombocytopenia (seven with severe aplastic anemia and one with myelodysplasia) treated with AMCA in a placebo-controlled, double-blind, cross-over design, found no decrease in bleeding. Only three patients were able to complete all phases of the study. Bleeding increased in patients despite receiving AMCA.[125] Such studies are extremely difficult to perform,[137] yet antifibrinolytic agents continue to be widely utilized for this indication.[11]

Lysine analogs are often used in cardiac bypass surgery, where excessive bleeding and fibrinolysis are associated with extracorporeal devices. Although early studies did not reveal a uniformly beneficial effect, antifibrinolytic use has increased recently as a cost-effective alternative to aprotinin. In contrast to DDAVP, these agents are administered prior to bypass, and are associated with significant reductions in blood loss. A meta-analysis of placebo-controlled studies of antifibrinolytic agents in cardiac surgery that did not distinguish between AMCA and EACA demonstrated lower rates of re-exploration, improved mortality, and no significant increased risk of myocardial infarction in the treatment group.[94] The improvement in mortality and reoperation was less than that observed with aprotinin. In general, studies comparing these agents to each other, and to aprotinin, indicate that aprotinin is more effective than AMCA, which is more effective than EACA. However, these conclusions must interpreted cautiously, because the optimal dose of AMCA[129] or EACA[128] has yet to be determined.

Antifibrinolytic agents reduce bleeding in total knee arthroplasty where use of a tourniquet produces excessive fibrinolysis,[138] and reduce laboratory evidence of fibrinolysis in liver transplantation.[139] Transfusion requirements were not reduced in these settings. Studies that have attempted a cost-benefit analysis uniformly favor AMCA or EACA over aprotinin.[140–143] The issue of the optimal antifibrinolytic agent for bypass surgery continues to be actively debated.[144–146]

Other uses of lysine analogs include those based on well-designed studies as well as anecdote, with the strength of evidence often unrelated to clinical enthusiasm.[11,116] Although not widely used for control of gastrointestinal hemorrhage, AMCA was associated with a reduced incidence of rebleeding and a 30% to 40% reduction in mortality in a meta-analysis that included 1200 patients from double-blind, placebo-controlled trials.[147] A similar analysis found significant improvement in women with menorrhagia who received antifibrinolytic agents compared to hormonal methods and other modalities.[148] Concern for thromboembolism has tempered the widespread use of these agents for excessive menstrual bleeding; however, no studies have revealed an increased incidence of this complication.

AMCA reduced the incidence of rebleeding in patients with subarachnoid hemorrhage in two double-blind, placebo-controlled studies, however, its use in each study was not associated with improved neurologic outcome.[149,150] In the first study, there was an increased incidence of ischemic events in patients receiving AMCA.[149] In the second study, involving 462 patients who also received calcium channel blocking medications to prevent cerebral ischemia, poor outcome was associated with effects of the initial bleeding and delayed cerebral ischemia was not improved in patients who received AMCA (administered intravenously at 1 g every 4 hours for the first week, followed by 1 g orally every 4 hours for up to 2 additional weeks).[150] There were nonsignificant trends in this study toward a beneficial effect of AMCA in the patients with a normal level of consciousness on hospital admission, toward an adverse outcome for those with depressed consciousness on admission, and toward an increased incidence of pulmonary embolism in the AMCA group (four versus none in those receiving placebo).[150] Uncontrolled studies have proposed that shorter courses of high-dose EACA,[131] or lower-dose AMCA,[151] might reduce rebleeding and avoid the complications associated with long-term use in patients scheduled for early aneurysmal therapy to control subarachnoid hemorrhage.

Anecdotal reports indicate that antifibrinolytic agents may be successful in hereditary hemorrhagic telangiectasia (Osler-Weber-Rendu syndrome),[152] in disorders with excessive local fibrinolysis due to vascular malformations such as Klippel-Trenaunay[153] or Kasabach-Merritt syndrome,[154] and in rare disorders characterized by excessive fibrinolysis such as prostate cancer.[155] Use in the cases with excessive local coagulation due to vascular malformations was associated with thrombosis and obliteration of intravascular channels. Because of the potential for thrombosis in DIC, these drugs should be used with caution, if at all, in this setting.

Topical or local administration of these drugs has been successful in a variety of clinical settings. Topical AMCA dramatically reduced the incidence of rebleeding after traumatic hyphema, with decreased systemic symptoms compared to oral administration, and improved long-term outcomes compared to untreated controls.[136] Similarly, the utility of topical administration was illustrated in a double-blind study of cardiac surgery patients where a solution of tranexamic acid (1 g in 100 mL saline) was poured into the pericardial cavity and over the mediastinal tissues before closure. Chest tube drainage, but not the need for transfusion, was significantly reduced, without detectable AMCA blood levels.[156] In menorrhagia associated with the use of an intrauterine device, local administration of AMCA or aprotinin reduced the pain and symptoms of bleeding.[134]

The topical use of antifibrinolytic agents to control bleeding in dental surgery for patients with hemophilia and other conditions predisposing to excessive hemorrhage, including oral anticoagulation, deserves special mention. In this setting, antifibrinolytic agents are proposed to counteract excessive fibrinolysis in the oral cavity which exists because of the absence of salivary endogenous fibrinolytic inhibitors.[157] Blinded placebo-controlled studies 30 years ago demonstrated reduced bleeding and decreased requirements for clotting factor concentrates in patients with hemophilia A and B who received systemic oral administration of EACA, 6 g four times daily for 7 to 10 days.[158] More recently, AMCA mouthwash or placebo was administered to 20 patients as 10 mL of a 4.8% aqueous solution applied prior to sutures and as a 2-minute rinse four times a day for 7 days in a prospective, double-blind study. There were 10 bleeding episodes in 8 patients in the placebo group and only one bleeding episode in the treatment group. Only one patient had detectable blood levels of AMCA (2.5 μg per milliliter of plasma).[157] Since that time, topical administration of AMCA, along with the use of DDAVP and fibrin sealant, has become part of established multimodality therapy in hemophilia dental centers.[112]

With the increased use of oral anticoagulants to treat atrial fibrillation, local measures in oral surgery are preferred to temporary discontinuation of warfarin, which may result in thromboembolism and a hypercoagulable state.[159] Interestingly, in one placebo-controlled trial of patients receiving oral anticoagulants, the addition of AMCA mouthwash added no benefit to the use of local measures alone such as gelatin sponge and fibrin glue.[160] Since placebo rinses may interfere with the formation of stable clot in the oral cavity, these early placebo-controlled studies should be evaluated in the context of studies using improved local control measures. Similar results have been observed in treatment of epistaxis, where there was no difference in efficacy when using treatment with gel impregnated with AMCA or placebo.[161]

Toxicity

The most common side effects of lysine analog antifibrinolytic therapy are mild dose-dependent gastrointestinal symptoms such as nausea, cramping, and diarrhea. These symptoms are less frequently reported with AMCA than with EACA.[114–116] Myonecrosis, possibly due to inhibition of carnitine synthesis, has been described, although rarely, after long-term oral administration of EACA (therapy longer than 4 weeks).[118,119] Myonecrosis has not been reported after AMCA administration, and some patients who have developed this complication while on EACA therapy have been successfully treated for many months with AMCA.[116]

The drugs do not appear to differ in their potential to cause thrombosis at usual clinical doses. Widespread thrombosis has occurred in DIC, where increased fibrinolysis may protect against organ ischemia.[127] Some studies have attempted to utilize antifibrinolytic therapy in conjunction with heparin anticoagulation in DIC and "excessive" fibrinolysis characterized by low levels of α_2-antiplasmin. While bleeding decreased in most cases, some patients still developed generalized organ system failure attributed to thrombosis.[127] High-grade ureteral obstruction due to clot formation secondary to inhibition of urokinase may occur when antifibrinolytic agents are used to treat patients with hematuria. No increased risk of this complication was observed in nine patients with macroscopic hematuria of various causes using EACA at divided oral doses (150 mg/kg total daily dose administered every 6 hours for up to 21 days)[162]; in a contrasting report, thrombosis occurred in patients who had only microscopic hematuria who were treated with standard AMCA therapy (4 to 4.5 g total daily dose administered every 6 to 8 hours for 1 to 3 days).[163] Local therapy, administered by irrigation, has been successful for control of intractable urinary bleeding localized to the bladder.[135] Animal studies have indicated a possible teratogenic effect for EACA,[164] however, a recent review of AMCA in pregnancy found no significant increase in thrombosis or fetal injury.[165]

Aprotinin

Aprotinin is a bovine-derived protein with wide-ranging activity against multiple human proteases that has significant antifibrinolytic activity mediated predominantly by inhibition of plasmin.[166] Prior to its hemostatic applications, aprotinin had been widely used in Europe for treatment of pancreatitis and other inflammatory conditions.[146] During studies extended to trials designed to reduce neutrophil activation in cardiac bypass surgery,[167] investigators noted that the operative field was dry, and transfusion requirements markedly decreased in patients undergoing repeat open heart surgery.

The bleeding diathesis in cardiac bypass surgery is complex, and is characterized in part by abnormal platelet function, decreases in factor levels, and abnormalities associated with heparin and protamine sulfate in addition to activation of the fibrinolytic system (see below and Chapter 30).[50,168] The precise role(s) played by aprotinin in cardiac bypass surgery may be several.[146] A series of studies have clearly established aprotinin as effective in reduction of blood loss in open heart surgery.[94] Aprotinin may have similar activity in orthotopic liver transplantation, in which bleeding may also occur, in part due to excessive fibrinolysis.[169] Aprotinin is effective also in reducing blood loss in surgical patients treated with aspirin.[99] In a meta-analysis of pharmacologic strategies designed to reduce blood loss in cardiac surgery, aprotinin was the only agent associated with reduced mortality, while both aprotinin and lysine analog antifibrinolytic agents reduced overall transfusion requirements and the need for re-exploration.[94] However, aprotinin is significantly more expensive than lysine analog antifibrinolytics, and the cost-effectiveness and other merits of aprotinin compared to these agents continues to be debated.[141,143,144]

Interpretation of such studies remains complicated by methodology for assigning weight to endpoints such as mortality and re-exploration, as well as the effect of different dosing regimens.[142] While aprotinin-mediated inhibition of plasmin may be the primary mode of action for reduction of blood loss,[166] inhibition of other enzymes may be associated with its reported improvement in overall mortality.[94,146] The toxicity of most concern with aprotinin (a bovine protein) is anaphylaxis, which occurs in approximately 0.5% of initial exposures and up to 9% of repeat exposures, and may result in shock and death.[170]

Vitamin K

Background

The discovery of vitamin K, *koagulationvitamin*, was made in the 1930s by Henrik Dam, who demonstrated that chicks fed an ether-extracted diet developed a hemorrhagic diathesis that responded to a fat-soluble factor.[171] He demonstrated shortly thereafter that administration of vitamin K corrected the prolonged clotting tests of patients with obstructive jaundice, further noting that this correction occurred more rapidly after intramuscular compared to subcutaneous administration.[172] Vitamin K was soon demonstrated to correct bleeding in hemorrhagic disease of the newborn.[171] With recognition that the bleeding in "sweet clover disease of cattle" was due to a compound (identified later as bishydroxycoumarin, or Dicumarol) that interfered with vitamin K-dependent synthesis of active prothrombin, vitamin K subsequently acquired an established role in the management of excessive anticoagulation due to warfarin, super-rodenticides and other orally active anticoagulants with similar mechanisms of action. Vitamin K is also indicated in acquired vitamin K deficiency, which occurs frequently in intensive care settings,[173,174] and is effective in some cases of cirrhosis.[175]

Compounds with vitamin K activity exist in two forms in nature. Each possesses the 2-methyl 3-phytyl-1,4-naphthoquinone ring that is required for activity, but they differ in the 3 position side chain.[176] Vitamin K_1 (phylloquinone) is synthesized by plants, possessing the same phytyl side chain as chlorophyll, and is the major dietary source of vitamin K. The vitamin K_1 content varies widely between foods, and diet is a major potential source of variation in the response to oral anticoagulants. Absorption of dietary vitamin K occurs in the ileum and requires the formation of mixed micelles composed of bile salts and the products of pancreatic lipolysis.[176] Thus oral absorption is impaired in conditions of either biliary obstruction or pancreatic insufficiency. Vitamin K_2 (menadione) is synthesized by bacteria, and comprises a spectrum of molecular forms with side chains based on repeating unsaturated 5-carbon units. The physiologic importance of the large amounts of vitamin K_2 produced by bacterial flora of the large intestine is not clear.[176] Large amounts of vitamin K_2, which are stored in the liver, may have a reserve function to protect against dietary vitamin K deficiency, which is rare in healthy adults. Whether a slow chronic, inefficient absorption of high concentrations of colonic vitamin K_2 is physiologically relevant compared to the highly efficient absorption of lower concentrations of intermittent dietary vitamin K_1 in the ileum remains a matter of debate.[176,177]

Mechanism of Action

Vitamin K functions as an essential cofactor for the post-translational γ-carboxylation of glutamic acid moieties in the N-terminal region of a series of proteins.[178] Originally recognized as essential for the synthesis of functional prothrombin, vitamin K later was identified as necessary for coagulation factors (II, VII, IX, X), for naturally occurring anticoagulant proteins (protein C and S), and more recently for other proteins such as osteocalcin that are involved in bone metabolism.[177] γ-Carboxylation produces protein-constituent amino acids with stable divalent anionic charges which may interact with calcium ions by localizing clotting factors to appropriate areas of phospholipid membranes or by allowing formation of internal calcium channels.[178] Prior to participating in the carboxylation reaction, vitamin K must first be reduced to an active hydroquinone form. The carboxylation reaction produces a γ-carboxylic glutamic acid as the hydroquinone is converted to an inactive vitamin K epoxide. Vitamin K epoxide is reduced back to the active hydroquinone by vitamin K epoxide reductase, regenerating additional vitamin K to participate in carboxylation.[178] Thus, vitamin K is recycled in a process involving 100 to 1000 times more vitamin K daily than that absorbed from dietary or colonic sources.[176] Des-carboxylated, functionally inactive forms of vitamin K-dependent proteins (also called *proteins induced by vitamin K absence,* or PIVKA), may be detected in the circulation of patients on oral anticoagulant therapy or in those with vitamin K deficiency due to malabsorption, or with functional vitamin K deficiency induced by liver disease.[179]

The enzyme(s) that reduce and recycle vitamin K and vitamin K epoxide have different sensitivities to oral anticoagulant-induced inhibition.[178] This biochemical quirk explains why vitamin K functions as an antidote to excessive oral anticoagulation and why patients on warfarin therapy who receive higher doses of vitamin K may appear resistant to reinstitution of therapy. The primary site of inhibition by warfarin is vitamin K epoxide reductase, which under physiologic conditions is also the enzyme that reduces vitamin K to the active hydroquinone required for carboxylation.[178] However, a second reductase is present that is not inhibited by warfarin. This warfarin-insensitive reductase can reduce vitamin K to the active hydroquinone in the presence of high tissue concentrations of vitamin K. Thus, exogenous vitamin K can produce additional active vitamin K hydroquinone via this warfarin-insensitive step, bypassing the warfarin-induced inhibition of vitamin K epoxide reductase and reversing excessive anticoagulation.[178] If vitamin K levels accumulate, this same process may also lead to warfarin resistance upon resumption of anticoagulation.[180] Therefore only small doses of vitamin K should be administered to control excessive anticoagulation in patients who will require further antithrombotic therapy.

High doses of oral vitamin K do not affect the synthesis or raise the concentration of coagulation factors in normal, healthy subjects.[180] Lowered levels of vitamin K-dependent factors of patients on oral anticoagulant therapy recover at the same rate during the initial 8 hours following vitamin K administration; thereafter recovery depends on the rate of synthesis of new γ-carboxylated factors by the liver.[180] Levels of factor VII reconstitute most rapidly, followed by factors IX and X, and lastly by prothrombin.[180] The differential rate of circulating factor levels after vitamin K administration has practical importance in monitoring recovery from anticoagulant therapy. Oral anticoagulation is most frequently monitored using the International Normalized Ratio (INR), and the prothrombin time, on which the INR is based, is most sensitive to decreases in factor VII levels. Use of the INR attempts to account for the variable sensitivity of different thromboplastin reagents by adjusting the degree of prolongation of the prothrombin time according to the International Sensitivity Index (ISI) provided for the reagent used to perform the test.[181] During stable anticoagulant therapy, the INR is determined by decreases of several vitamin K-dependent coagulant and anticoagulant protein levels, which remain in relatively constant ratios to one another. However, the initial improvement of a markedly prolonged INR following administration of vitamin K for excessive anticoagulation may relate largely to a rapid increase in the factor VII level alone. In this setting, the slower recovery of factor IX may remain at clinically significant low levels. Thus the INR in this setting may be misleading and should not be interpreted as corresponding to levels obtained during stable anticoagulation. If available, measurement of factor levels may be useful to predict the bleeding risk before invasive procedures or to guide further therapy.

Dosage and Administration

Both vitamin K_1 and K_2 are active when administered orally or intravenously. However, the only preparation currently available in the United States is a vitamin K_1 preparation, phytonadione (AquaMEPHYTON, Merck & Co., West Point, Penn.). A similar product (Konakion, Roche Co., Nutley, NJ) for intravenous use is available in Europe and Australia. Both liquid preparations are prepared as a colloid solution, each milliliter containing 2 or 10 mg of phytonadione in a polyoxyethylated fatty acid derivative, which functions as a cremophor to solubilize the vitamin K. The AquaMEPHYTON preparation is effective when administered intravenously, subcutaneously, intramuscularly, or orally. Intramuscular administration may cause hemorrhage in anticoagulated patients and should be used only for prophylaxis against hemorrhagic disease of the newborn. The side effects reported with intravenous administration (see below) have limited its use, even though intravenous administration is more rapid and reliable than the subcutaneous or oral routes.[180,182,183] A colloidal system based on mixed micelles of lecithin and glycocholic acid to solubilize the lipophilic vitamin K was developed to reduce the toxicity attributed to the cremophor component of current preparations, however, significant symptoms have also been reported with this preparation and it is no longer under development.[184] Scored tablets are available, containing 5 mg phytonadione, permitting a dose as low as 2.5 mg. Although injectable and oral preparations have been available for nearly half a century, the appropriate dosage and route of administration remain controversial.[185] Despite careful pharmacodynamic studies, clinical guidelines have changed frequently[181,186,187] because of variability in patient responses and concerns regarding toxicity.[185]

Indications

Vitamin K is used most often to reverse excessive anticoagulation with warfarin. Indications include patients with serious bleeding as well as those requiring only temporary control of therapeutic anticoagulation in preparation for surgical procedures. The goals of therapy are prompt control of bleeding without toxicity, prevention of resistance to reinstitution of warfarin, and avoidance of subtherapeutic anticoagulation.[188] The response to vitamin K administration may depend on the direction, rate of change, and degree of prolongation of clotting times; the time, dose, and type of anticoagulant administered; and the presence of concurrent liver disease, antibiotics, or dietary factors.[189] The use of vitamin K and other effective therapies to reduce the INR in patients receiving warfarin are listed in Table 25–4.

Anticoagulant reversal is more prompt with intravenous than with subcutaneous administration of vitamin K[182,183] (Fig. 25–1). In a prospective, randomized, single-blind study of 22 patients, the INR decreased from a mean initial value of 8.0, to 4.6 and 3.1 after 8 and 24 hours, respectively, in patients who received 1 mg intravenously, compared to a mean initial value of 8.5, which decreased to 8.0 and 5.0 at the same times in patients who received 1 mg subcutaneously.[183] The response after oral ingestion of vitamin K is slower and less predictable than either subcutaneous or intravenous administration (Fig. 25–2), but is more rapid than that observed after simple discontinuation of warfarin,[185] which can be prolonged in elderly patients.[190] Oral doses as low as 0.5^{22} to $2.0^{22,187}$ mg have been recommended in patients at risk with mild to moderate prolongation of the INR who are not bleeding. An algorithm has been developed for determining the required oral dose based on the degree of prolongation of the INR.[191]

Simple discontinuation of warfarin for excessive anticoagulation may have unanticipated adverse thrombotic effects.[192] The use of large oral and subcutaneous doses of vitamin K has been associated with thrombosis and subsequent warfarin resistance requiring heparin therapy.[193] Thrombosis may be related to attaining subtherapeutic INR levels and more rapid recovery of factor VII and other coagulant enzymes compared to proteins C and S.[192] Smaller doses of 0.5 to 1 mg intravenously are frequently effective for reversal of excessive anticoagulation.[194-196] Similarly, in patients scheduled to have minor procedures while maintained on a stable dose of warfarin, 1 mg intravenous vitamin K transiently normalized the INR, with the effect vanishing within several days.[197] In another study of healthy volunteers receiving stable doses of oral anticoagulants, 1 mg of vitamin K intravenously lasted several days, while doses of 5 and 25 mg lasted up to 1 and 2 weeks, respectively.[180] Similar results have been obtained using low-dose oral vitamin K.[191] The subcutaneous route produces a more prolonged effect than the oral route and a higher frequency of subtherapeutic INR values,[185] with INR values below 2.0 observed in 5 of 22 (23%) subjects at 72 hours after intravenous treatment compared to 14 of 33 (42%) after subcutaneous therapy.[182]

In patients who require more rapid reversal of anticoagulation, plasma products produce results within minutes. If one discounts the 30 to 45 minutes generally required to thaw FFP plus the time for infusion, results with either FFP or PCCs are obtained more rapidly than with vitamin K, but are transient because of the 6- to 7-hour half-life of the infused factor VII. FFP possesses other side effects mentioned earlier in this chapter and the large volume load of FFP (10 to 15 mL/kg) required to provide adequate levels of vitamin K-dependent factors may be clinically difficult to administer, particularly in elderly patients. Additionally, the synthesis of new factors continues to be inhibited by warfarin following the use of FFP or PCCs. The use of either product should be monitored and supplemented with vitamin K as appropriate. Infusion of PCCs provides the most

Table 25-4 • VITAMIN K AND OTHER EFFECTIVE MEASURES TO REDUCE INR IN PATIENTS RECEIVING WARFARIN

Method	Mechanism	Clinical Situation	Advantages	Drawbacks
Reduce warfarin dosage	Decreases total warfarin dose	Outpatient INR 3-6 No bleeding	Safe, effective	Slow (days) Possibly confusing to patient
Hold warfarin dose 1-2 days, reduce dosage	Decreases total warfarin dose	Outpatient INR 5-8 No bleeding	Safe, effective	Slow (days) Often confusing to patient
Ingestion of spinach or salads	Increases vitamin K intake	Outpatient INR 5-8 No bleeding	Safe, probably effective	Slow (24 hours) Never systematically studied
Low dose ($\approx$ 1 mg) vitamin K PO	Increases vitamin K intake	Outpatient INR 6-12 No bleeding	Effective within 24 hours	Difficult to obtain small dose
Moderate dose (2-5 mg) vitamin K PO or SC	Increases vitamin K intake	Inpatient or outpatient INR 10-15 no bleeding OR INR 5-10 with bleeding	Effective within 24 hours	Takes $\approx$24 hours to work Often results in subtherapeutic INR
Low-dose (0.5 to 1 mg) vitamin K IV	Increases vitamin K intake	Inpatient or outpatient INR 6-12 with or without bleeding OR INR 2-5 prior to invasive procedure	Works within 6-8 hours, rarely results in subtherapeutic INR Useful for patients who should remain on warfarin	Rare anaphylaxis IV
High-dose (5-20 mg) vitamin K IV	Greatly increases vitamin K intake	Inpatient INR $\geq$ 8 with bleeding OR Accidental warfarin ingestion	Relatively safe Very rapid (6-8 hours) effect Inexpensive	Rare anaphylaxis IV Often results in subtherapeutic INR with warfarin resistance
Fresh frozen plasma (FFP)	Supplies missing coagulation factors	Inpatient INR $\geq$ 8 with bleeding	Effective in 2-4 hours in actual practice,[a] effective "immediately" in theory	Cumbersome, short half-life of factors, warfarin still active Risks of infusion include volume and infection
Prothrombin complex concentrates (PCCs)	Supplies missing coagulation factors	Inpatient INR $\geq$ 8 with bleeding CNS bleeding	Effective in 1-2 hours in actual practice	Not always available, expensive, risk of thrombosis and DIC,[b] short half-life of factors, warfarin still active

[a] Including time for ordering, thawing, procuring, and infusing.
[b] DIC, Disseminated intravascular coagulation.

rapid replacement of vitamin K-dependent factors, and may provide a superior clinical outcome compared to FFP for patients with intracranial hemorrhage.[198] As with FFP, the factor content of PCCs is variable, and a dose based on factor IX levels is often utilized. In such cases, the risk of thrombosis and DIC associated with PCCs must be balanced against the risk of the clinical condition and the risk of slower response to treatments with less toxicity. Infusion of vitamin K can surprisingly correct an astronomically high INR (estimated to be 288 in one case) rapidly in patients with good hepatic function.[199]

Vitamin K is established therapy for prevention of hemorrhagic disease of the newborn, due to transient vitamin K deficiency in the first week of life as well as vitamin K deficiency with onset weeks to months later.[200] The effectiveness in other uses is less well documented. Patients with cirrhosis[175] or liver cancer[201] may have circulating des-carboxylated coagulation factors similar to those seen in vitamin K deficiency, which may be due to an acquired deficiency of the vitamin K decarboxylase. Although the mechanism was not described, in one report, administration of 10 mg vitamin K subcutaneously for 3 days normalized prolonged PT values in 37% of patients with cirrhosis.[175] Vitamin K deficiency occurs commonly in malnourished patients in intensive care units, either with or without concomitant antibiotic use,[202] accounting for four or five cases yearly in one tertiary care referral center[173] and 20% of cases with prolongation of the PT (more than 1.5 times normal) in another.[174] Administration over 30 minutes of 5 to 25 mg intravenous vitamin K corrected the coagulopathy within 12 hours for these critically ill patients.[173,202] A much smaller dose of vitamin K, 1 mg intravenously, is effective within 24 hours when vitamin K deficiency is due to malabsorption in patients who are not critically ill, and the effect lasts 1 to 2 weeks.[180] Patients with the severe hemorrhagic diathesis due to

A

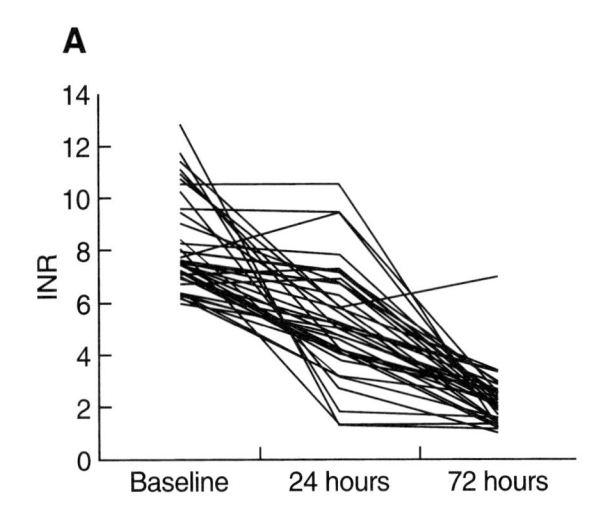

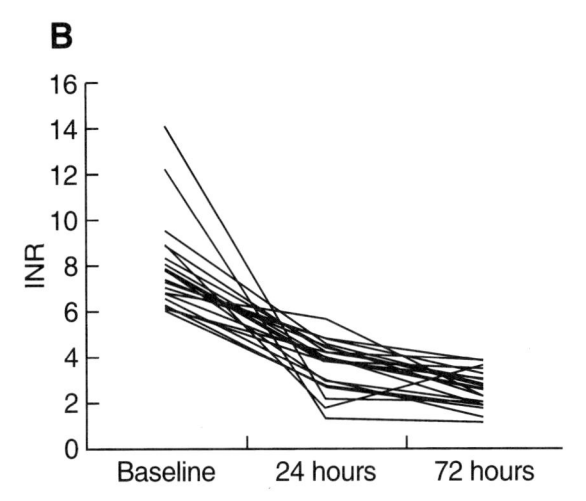

Figure 25-1 Individual values of the INR at baseline and at 24 and 72 hours after vitamin K therapy following subcutaneous administration in 33 patients (**A**) and intravenous administration in 22 patients (**B**). Subjects with an INR between 6 and 10 received 0.5 mg (25 subcutaneous and 20 intravenous), while those with an INR between 10 and 20 received 3.0 mg (8 subcutaneous and 2 intravenous). (Adapted from Nee R, Doppenschmidt D, Donovan DJ, Andrews TC. Intravenous versus subcutaneous vitamin K₁ in reversing oral anticoagulation. Am J Cardiol 1999;83:288, with permission from Excerpta Medica Inc.)

ingestion of the powerful rodenticide brodifacoum, may require initial oral administration of 100 mg daily of vitamin K for 2 months, then slow tapering over 300 days due to the extreme in vivo half-life of the poison.[203] In contrast, prolonged PT values associated with the relatively weaker anticoagulant activity of antibiotics with the N-methylthiotetrazole (NMTT) side chain (moxalactam, cefoperazone, cefamandole, cefotetan, and cefmetazole) respond rapidly to small doses in many cases.[204,205]

Toxicity

The major toxicity associated with administration of vitamin K is the rare, but dramatic occurrence of anaphylaxis, which has been associated with fatalities and is described only after intravenous administration.[206] Symptoms of flushing and chest pain after intravenous administration of phytonadione were described as early as 1952, and in the 1960s, cardiac irregularities were attributed to injections given more rapidly than 10 mg/min or to the propylene glycol content of an older preparation that has since been withdrawn from the market.[207] Although these reactions have been attributed to the cremophor excipient used in the preparation, severe anaphylaxis also occurred in a patient who received an intravenous injection of a mixed micelles vitamin K₁ preparation composed of glycocholic acid and lecithin designed to reduce anaphylaxis.[208] Intradermal skin testing with both preparations was positive; however, testing with individual components was negative. It is therefore not clear whether the vitamin, the excipient, formation of a hapten between the vitamin K and emulsifying agents, or nonimmunologic mechanisms led to these reactions.[208] What is known about reactions following vitamin K administration may be summarized as follows: (1) Anaphylactic reactions occur and are unpredictable. (2) Repeated administrations to the same patient do not necessarily carry the same risks. (3) Slow injection does not prevent these reactions, but permits interruption of the injection as soon as the onset of symptoms occurs[209]; although it is recommended that intravenous administration not exceed 1 mg/min, fatalities have occurred despite adherence to these guidelines.[206] (4) Severe reactions have been reported most frequently in elderly patients who have received doses greater than 5 mg, and after repeat dosing[206]; however, anaphylaxis has occurred in young patients even after the first administration. (5) Some patients have had no adverse events following subsequent administration after prior anaphylaxis.[210] (6) There is no obvious dose dependency in the frequency of reactions; however, reactions are rare when doses of 1 mg or less are used

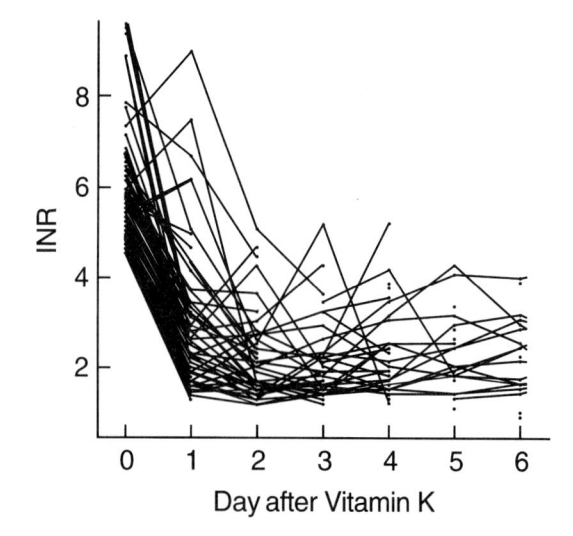

Figure 25-2 Individual values of the INR at baseline and at days 1 to 6 after oral administration of 1.0 mg vitamin K. Note the y axis scale difference between Figures 2-1 and 2-2. (Adapted from Crowther MA, Donavan D, Harrison L, et al. Low-dose oral vitamin K reliably reverses over-anticoagulation due to warfarin. Thromb Haemost 1998;79:1116-1118, with permission.)

and no fatalities have been reported at these doses.[180,182,183,194–197,211] (7) The cremophor excipients in various preparations used in the United States and overseas are not identical, but may have the same risks.[209] (8) Shock occurs in response to severe peripheral vasodilation, and treatment should be directed to counteract this effect.[210] One patient appeared to respond to an injection of high-dose steroids (100 mg dexamethasone).[212]

Caution should be exercised with intravenous vitamin K administration. However, when other routes are not feasible or when rapid, reliable dosing is required, it seems prudent to administer the preparation in 50–125 mL of isotonic solution and administer it carefully over at least 20 minutes. Small doses usually suffice, and the infusion should be halted if flushing or hypotension occurs.

OTHER AGENTS

Estrogens

Conjugated estrogens, which have been employed since the 1960s to augment hemostasis for a wide variety of conditions, also have hemostatic effects in uremia.[213–220] Livio and coworkers demonstrated in a double-blind, placebo-controlled study that conjugated estrogens at a dose of 0.6 mg/kg daily administered intravenously shortened the bleeding time in patients with uremia; the effect lasted 2 weeks and was first observed within 6 hours of the initial dose with the maximum effect achieved between 5 and 7 days.[216] Additional studies in patients with uremia have confirmed effectiveness in shortening the bleeding time with either single or repeated intravenous doses of 0.6 mg/kg, while administration of 0.3 mg/kg was ineffective.[221] A single dose of 25 mg of Premarin administered intravenously 2 hours prior to surgery produced no effect on hemostatic parameters and did not reduce blood loss.[222] Oral estrogens (50 mg daily of Premarin) also shorten the bleeding time and may control bleeding symptoms in uremic patients after 7.0 ± 4.2 days of therapy.[223] Similarly, transdermal estradiol administration of 50 or 100 μg/24 hours every 3.5 days has been reported to shorten the bleeding time in uremia and reduce transfusion requirements.[224]

Estrogens have also been used for patients with vWD. Three women who previously required blood product therapy for control of bleeding due to vWD were able to undergo successful surgical procedures after being treated with oral estrogens, given as replacement therapy or for contraception for 2 years prior to surgery and followed by 5 mg conjugated estrogens daily postoperatively. Each patient had previously exhibited a decrease in bleeding during pregnancies and subsequent normalization of coagulation tests during oral estrogen treatment; these same tests were abnormal when measured 8 weeks after discontinuation of treatment.[214]

The mechanism of action for estrogen therapy is not well characterized, and may involve effects on the mucopolysaccharide content of the vessel wall, increased synthesis of vWF by endothelial cells, or other less clearly defined effects on hemostasis.[213,225,226] These actions may explain the efficacy of oral estrogens in patients with gastrointestinal bleeding due to Osler-Weber-Rendu syndrome or angiodysplasia.[219] Significant hemostatic toxicity has not been reported. Mild gynecomastia, weight gain, and dyspepsia have been reported in men.[219] Similar side effects in men or gynecologic symptoms in women are frequently not specifically addressed.

Protamine

Protamine sulfate is a polycationic, highly positively charged protein derived from salmon sperm protein, of approximately 4500 daltons molecular weight.[227] Protamine has been used to neutralize anticoagulation due to unfractionated heparin (UFH) administration after cardiac bypass surgery in more than 2,000,000 patients yearly.[227] The mechanism of action involves binding to the negatively charged heparin molecules, forming a stable complex and displacing antithrombin III (ATIII) from the heparin-ATIII complex.[228] Protamine is the only effective available antidote to excessive anticoagulation produced by UFH; it is not nearly as effective against the anticoagulant activity of low-molecular-weight heparin and coagulation tests such as the aPTT are not useful in monitoring its action against these agents.[229] Protamine possesses additional intrinsic anticoagulant activities (including platelet clumping, thrombocytopenia, and interference with the formation of fibrin by thrombin)[230] so that doses in excess of those calculated to neutralize UFH should be avoided. Protamine administration may also be associated with other adverse effects during bypass surgery, including hypotension, increased pulmonary artery pressure, pulmonary neutrophil sequestration, and anaphylaxis, which are mediated by complement activation, histamine release, thromboxane and nitric oxide production, and antibody production.[227] The frequency of allergic reactions may be increased in patients with a history of prior insulin use, but probably not in those with a history of fish allergy or vasectomy.[227]

Protamine sulfate is administered by intravenous infusion. Its onset of action is immediate and its duration of action about 2 hours. Dosing strategies to neutralize excessive anticoagulation induced by UFH are often based on the use of 1 mg of protamine to neutralize 80 to 100 USP units of heparin.[230] Since the action of protamine is shorter that that of heparin, follow-up coagulation tests should be performed to reduce the risk of "heparin rebound" effect. Ordinarily, the dosage should not exceed 100 mg over 2 hours unless blood coagulation tests indicate a need for larger doses.

Protamine is administered after the completion of bypass surgery according to estimates of circulating heparin concentrations using dosing algorithms and measurement of the activated clotting time (ACT).[231] Monitoring protocols can markedly influence protamine doses used to neutralize UFH. Newer point-of-care hemostasis testing systems developed to replace traditional ACT-based empiric regimens have reduced both protamine dosage and postoperative bleeding in some,

Table 25-5 • COLLABORATIVE EDUCATIONAL AND TREATMENT ISSUES FOR HOSPITAL TRANSFUSION COMMITTEES

I. Transfusion of FFP
  A. Evaluation of PT triggers
  B. Disease indications and contraindications
II. Transfusion of platelets and RBCs
  A. Platelet thresholds in amegakaryocytic thrombocytopenia
  B. Platelet refractoriness
  C. RBC transfusion triggers
III. Transfusion of cryoprecipitate
IV. Plasma exchange therapy for TTP, other diseases
V. Determination of pharmaceutical agents to maintain in inventory and guidelines for use
  A. DDAVP for vWD, hemophilia A; use in uremia and other conditions
  B. Antifibrinolytics for surgery, thrombocytopenic states
  C. Guidelines for warfarin overdose, and administration of vitamin K
VI. Surgical support
  A. Massive transfusion guidelines
  B. Cell savers
  C. Autologous blood donation
  D. Point-of-care testing and collaborative treatment algorithms

but not all, prospective studies.[231] (See Chapter 35.) In addition to improved monitoring, UFH neutralization procedures may be improved in the future by the development of new agents such as low-molecular-weight protamine[228] and recombinant platelet factor 4, or heparinase.[231] The use of protamine in most outpatient settings has been greatly reduced by the use of low-molecular-weight heparin in place of UFH for most nonprocedural indications.

SUMMARY

Research and development of new blood products and pharmaceutical agents will continue to offer increasingly sophisticated approaches for the care and management of patients with disordered hemostasis.[3] Strategies for appropriate use may be best established in collaborative settings such as the Hospital Transfusion Committee (Table 25-5). For those patients with congenital hemostatic disorders, recombinant products and the advent of gene therapy promise additional safety and efficacy, but will also be associated with the potential for increased costs of development. Improved laboratory testing and rapid identification of appropriate therapy in surgical and other settings based on point-of-care testing and collaboratively developed guidelines promise additional benefits for those patients with acquired disorders.[58]

REFERENCES

Chapter 25 References

1. Ratnoff OD. Why do people bleed? In Wintrobe MM (Ed): Blood, Pure and Eloquent, New York, McGraw-Hill, 1980; pp. 601-658.
2. Diamond LK. A history of blood transfusion. In Wintrobe MM (Ed): Blood, Pure and Eloquent. New York, McGraw-Hill, 1980; pp. 659-690.
3. Klein HG. Transfusion medicine. The evolution of a new discipline. JAMA 1987;258:2108-2109.
4. Alving B, Alcorn K. How to improve transfusion medicine. A treating physician's perspective. Arch Pathol Lab Med 1999;123:492-495.
5. Livio M, Gotti E, Marchesi D, et al. Uraemic bleeding: role of anaemia and beneficial effect of red cell transfusions. Lancet 1982;2:1013-1015.
6. Ho CH. The hemostatic effect of packed red cell transfusion in patients with anemia. Transfusion 1998;38:1011-1014.
7. Turrito VT, Weiss HJ. Red blood cells: their dual role in thrombus formation. Science 1980;207:541-543.
8. Parsons SF, Spring FA, Chasis JA, et al. Erythroid cell adhesion molecules Lutheran and LW in health and disease. Baillieres Best Pract Res Clin Haematol 1999;12:729-745.
9. Hebert PC, Wells G, Blajchman MA, et al. A multicenter, randomized, controlled clinical trial of transfusion requirements in critical care. Transfusion Requirements in Critical Care Investigators, Canadian Critical Care Trials Group. N Engl J Med 1999;340:409-417.
10. Stohlawetz PJ, Dzirlo L, Hergovich N, et al. Effects of erythropoietin on platelet reactivity and thrombopoiesis in humans. Blood 2000;95:2983-2989.
11. Mannucci PM. Hemostatic drugs. N Engl J Med 1998;339:245-253.
12. Faringer PD, Mullins RJ, Johnson RL, et al. Blood component supplementation during massive transfusion of AS-1 red cells in trauma patients. J Trauma 1993;34:481-485.
13. Gaydos LA, Freireich EJ, Mantel N. The quantitative relation between platelet count and hemorrhage in patients with acute leukemia. N Engl J Med 1962;266:905-909.
14. Gmur J, Burger J, Schanz U, et al. Safety of stringent prophylactic platelet transfusion policy for patients with acute leukaemia. Lancet 1991;338:1223-1226.
15. Rebulla P, Finazzi G, Marangoni F, et al. The threshold for prophylactic platelet transfusions in adults with acute myeloid leukemia. Gruppo Italiano Malattie Ematologiche Maligne dell'Adulto. N Engl J Med 1997;337:1870-1875.
16. Beutler E. Platelet transfusions: the 20,000/μL trigger. Blood 1993;81:1411-1413.
17. Vengelen-Tyler V. Blood transfusion practice. In Vengelen-Tyler V (Ed): Technical Manual. 13th ed. Bethesda, Md, American Association of Blood Banks, 1999, pp. 451-481.
18. Despotis GJ, Skubas NJ, Goodnough LT. Optimal management of bleeding and transfusion in patients undergoing cardiac surgery. Semin Thorac Cardiovasc Surg 1999;11:84-104.
19. Carr JM, Kruskall MS, Kaye JA, et al. Efficacy of platelet transfusions in immune thrombocytopenia. Am J Med 1986;80:1051-1054.
20. Beeck H, Becker T, Kiessig ST, et al. The influence of citrate concentration on the quality of plasma obtained by automated plasmapheresis: a prospective study. Transfusion 1999;39:1266-1270.
21. Alving BM. Beyond hemophilia and von Willebrand disease: treatment of patients with other inherited coagulation factor and inhibitor deficiencies. In Alving BM (Ed): Blood Components and Pharmacologic Agents in the Treatment of Congenital and Acquired Bleeding Disorders. Bethesda, Md, AABB Press, 2000, pp. 341-356.
22. Guidelines on oral anticoagulation: 3rd edition. Br J Haematol 1998;101:374-387.
23. Ciavarella D, Reed RL, Counts RB, et al. Clotting factor levels and the risk of diffuse microvascular bleeding in the massively transfused patient. Br J Haematol 1987;67:365-368.

24. Counts RB, Haisch C, Simon TL, et al. Hemostasis in massively transfused trauma patients. Ann Surg 1979;190:91–99.
25. McVay PA, Toy PT. Lack of increased bleeding after liver biopsy in patients with mild hemostatic abnormalities. Am J Clin Pathol 1990;94:747–753.
26. Klein HG, Dodd RY, Dzik WH, et al. Current status of solvent/detergent-treated frozen plasma. Transfusion 1998;38:102–107.
27. Poon MC. Cryoprecipitate: uses and alternatives. Transfus Med Rev 1993;7:180–192.
28. Jackson MR, Alving BM. Fibrin sealant in preclinical and clinical studies. Curr Opin Hematol 1999;6:415–419.
29. Hellstern P. Production and composition of prothrombin complex concentrates: correlation between composition and therapeutic efficiency. Thromb Res 1999;95:S7–S12.
30. Hellstern P, Halbmayer WM, Kohler M, et al. Prothrombin complex concentrates: indications, contraindications, and risks: a task force summary. Thromb Res 1999;95:S3–S6.
31. Mannucci PM, Tenconi PM, Castaman G, et al. Comparison of four virus-inactivated plasma concentrates for treatment of severe von Willebrand disease: a cross-over randomized trial. Blood 1992;79:3130–3137.
32. Chang AC, Rick ME, Ross PL, et al. Summary of a workshop on potency and dosage of von Willebrand factor concentrates. Haemophilia 1998; 4(Suppl 3):1–6.
33. Montgomery RR. Structure and function of von Willebrand factor. In Colman RW, Hirsh J, Marder VJ, Clowes AW, George JN (Eds): Hemostasis and Thrombosis: Basic Principles and Clinical Practice, 4th ed. Philadelphia, Lippincott Williams & Wilkins, 2001, pp. 249–274.
34. Lusher J, Ingerslev J, Roberts H, et al. Clinical experience with recombinant factor VIIa. Blood Coagul Fibrinolysis 1998;9:119–128.
35. Kristensen J, Killander A, Hippe E, et al. Clinical experience with recombinant factor VIIa in patients with thrombocytopenia. Haemostasis 1996; 26(Suppl):159–164.
36. Kenet G, Walden R, Eldad A, et al. Treatment of traumatic bleeding with recombinant factor VIIa [letter]. Lancet 1999;354:1879.
37. Schreiber GB, Busch MP, Kleinman SH, et al. The risk of transfusion-transmitted viral infections. The Retrovirus Epidemiology Donor Study. N Engl J Med 1996;334:1685–1690.
38. Ling AE, Robbins KE, Brown TM, et al. Failure of routine HIV-1 tests in a case involving transmission with preseroconversion blood components during the infectious window period. JAMA 2000;284:210–214.
39. Klein HG. Will blood transfusion ever be safe enough? [editorial]. JAMA 2000;284:238–240.
40. Heddle NM, Kelton JG. Febrile nonhemolytic transfusion reactions. In Popovsky MA (Ed): Transfusion Reactions, 2nd ed. Bethesda, Md, AABB Press, 2001, pp. 45–82.
41. Vamvakas EC, Pineda AA. Allergic and anaphylactic reactions. In Popovsky MA (Ed): Transfusion Reactions, 2nd ed. Bethesda, Md, AABB Press, 2001, pp. 83–128.
42. Davenport RD. Hemolytic transfusion reactions. In Popovsky MA (Ed): Transfusion Reactions, 2nd ed. Bethesda, Md, AABB Press, 2001, pp. 1–44.
43. Goldman M, Blajchman MA. Bacterial contamination. In Popovsky MA (Ed): Transfusion Reactions, 2nd ed. Bethesda, Md, AABB Press, 2001, pp. 129–154.
44. Popovsky MA. Transfusion related acute lung injury (TRALI). In Popovsky MA (Ed): Transfusion Reactions, 2nd ed. Bethesda, Md, AABB Press, 2001, pp. 155–167.
45. McFarland JG. Posttransfusion pupura. In Popovsky MA (Ed): Transfusion Reactions, 2nd ed. Bethesda, Md, AABB Press, 2001, pp. 187–212.
46. Webb IJ, Anderson KC. Transfusion-associated-graft-verus-host disease. In Popovsky MA (Ed): Transfusion Reactions, 2nd ed. Bethesda, Md, AABB Press, 2001, pp. 171–186.
47. Leitman SF, Holland PV. Irradiation of blood products. Indications and guidelines. Transfusion 1985;25:293–303.
48. Flaum MA, Cuneo RA, Appelbaum FR, et al. The hemostatic imbalance of plasma-exchange transfusion. Blood 1979;54:694–702.
49. Anderlini P, Przepiorka D, Seong D, et al. Clinical toxicity and laboratory effects of granulocyte-colony-stimulating factor (filgrastim) mobilization and blood stem cell apheresis from normal donors, and analysis of charges for the procedures. Transfusion 1996;36:590–595.
50. Bolan CD, Alving BM. Pharmacologic agents in the management of bleeding disorders. Transfusion 1990;30:541–551.
51. Richardson DW, Robinson AG. Desmopressin. Ann Intern Med 1985;103:228–239.
52. Mannucci PM. Desmopressin (DDAVP) in the treatment of bleeding disorders: the first 20 years. Blood 1997;90:2515–2521.
53. Mannucci PM. Desmopressin: a nontransfusional form of treatment for congenital and acquired bleeding disorders. Blood 1988;72:1449–1455.
54. Laupacis A, Fergusson D. Drugs to minimize perioperative blood loss in cardiac surgery: meta-analyses using perioperative blood transfusion as the outcome. The International Study of Perioperative Transfusion (ISPOT) Investigators. Anesth Analg 1997;85:1258–1267.
55. Green D, Wong CA, Twardowski P. Efficacy of hemostatic agents in improving surgical hemostasis. Transfus Med Rev 1996;10:171–182.
56. Janssens M, Hartstein G, David JL. Reduction in requirements for allogeneic blood products: pharmacologic methods. Ann Thorac Surg 1996;62:1944–1950.
57. Dilthey G, Dietrich W, Spannagl M, et al. Influence of desmopressin acetate on homologous blood requirements in cardiac surgical patients pretreated with aspirin. J Cardiothorac Vasc Anesth 1993;7:425–430.
58. Despotis GJ, Levine V, Saleem R, et al. Use of point-of-care test in identification of patients who can benefit from desmopressin during cardiac surgery: a randomised controlled trial. Lancet 1999;354:106–110.
59. Sutor AH. DDAVP is not a panacea for children with bleeding disorders. Br J Haematol 2000;108:217–227.
60. Mannucci PM, Canciani MT, Rota L, et al. Response of factor VIII/von Willebrand factor to DDAVP in healthy subjects and patients with haemophilia A and von Willebrand's disease. Br J Haematol 1981;47:283–293.
61. Levi M, de Boer JP, Roem D, et al. Plasminogen activation in vivo upon intravenous infusion of DDAVP. Quantitative assessment of plasmin-alpha 2-antiplasmin complex with a novel monoclonal antibody based radioimmunoassay. Thromb Haemost 1992;67:111–116.
62. Tsai HM, Sussman II, Nagel RL, et al. Desmopressin induces adhesion of normal human erythrocytes to the endothelial surface of a perfused microvascular preparation. Blood 1990;75:261–265.
63. Barnhart MI, Chen S, Lusher JM. DDAVP: does the drug have a direct effect on the vessel wall? Thromb Res 1983;31:239–253.
64. Takeuchi M, Nagura H, Kaneda T. DDAVP and epinephrine-induced changes in the localization of von Willebrand factor antigen in endothelial cells of human oral mucosa. Blood 1988;72:850–854.
65. Ruggeri ZM, Mannucci PM, Lombardi R, et al. Multimeric composition of factor VIII/von Willebrand factor following administration of DDAVP: implications for pathophysiology and therapy of von Willebrand's disease subtypes. Blood 1982;59:1272–1278.
66. Sakariassen KS, Cattaneo M, Berg A, et al. DDAVP enhances platelet adherence and platelet aggregate growth on human artery subendothelium. Blood 1984;64:229–236.
67. Cattaneo M, Pareti FI, Zighetti M, et al. Platelet aggregation at high shear is impaired in patients with congenital defects of

platelet secretion and is corrected by DDAVP: correlation with the bleeding time. J Lab Clin Med 1995;125:540–547.
68. Horstman LL, Valle-Riestra BJ, Jy W, et al. Desmopressin (DDAVP) acts on platelets to generate platelet microparticles and enhanced procoagulant activity. Thromb Res 1995;79:163–174.
69. Galvez A, Gomez-Ortiz G, Diaz-Ricart M, et al. Desmopressin (DDAVP) enhances platelet adhesion to the extracellular matrix of cultured human endothelial cells through increased expression of tissue factor. Thromb Haemost 1997;77:975–980.
70. Wun T, Paglieroni TG, Lachant NA. Desmopressin stimulates the expression of P-selectin on human platelets in vitro. J Lab Clin Med 1995;126:401–409.
71. Sloand EM, Alyono D, Klein HG, et al. 1-Deamino-8-D-arginine vasopressin (DDAVP) increases platelet membrane expression of glycoprotein lb in patients with disorders of platelet function and after cardiopulmonary bypass. Am J Hematol 1994;46:199–207.
72. Cattaneo M, Moia M, Delle VP, et al. DDAVP shortens the prolonged bleeding times of patients with severe von Willebrand disease treated with cryoprecipitate. Evidence for a mechanism of action independent of released von Willebrand factor. Blood 1989;74:1972–1975.
73. Mannucci PM, Remuzzi G, Pusineri F, et al. Deamino-8-D-arginine vasopressin shortens the bleeding time in uremia. N Engl J Med 1983;308:8–12.
74. Mannucci PM, Vicente V, Vianello L, et al. Controlled trial of desmopressin in liver cirrhosis and other conditions associated with a prolonged bleeding time. Blood 1986;67:1148–1153.
75. Kobrinsky NL, Israels ED, Gerrard JM, et al. Shortening of bleeding time by 1-deamino-8-D-arginine vasopressin in various bleeding disorders. Lancet 1984;1:1145–1148.
76. Kentro TB, Lottenberg R, Kitchens CS. Clinical efficacy of desmopressin acetate for hemostatic control in patients with primary platelet disorders undergoing surgery. Am J Hematol 1987;24:215–219.
77. Mannucci PM, Bettega D, Cattaneo M. Patterns of development of tachyphylaxis in patients with haemophilia and von Willebrand disease after repeated doses of desmopressin (DDAVP). Br J Haematol 1992;82:87–93.
78. Vicente V, Estelles A, Laso J, et al. Repeated infusions of DDAVP induce low response of FVIII and vWF but not of plasminogen activators. Thromb Res 1993;70:117–122.
79. Lethagen S, Olofsson L, Frick K, et al. Effect kinetics of desmopressin-induced platelet retention in healthy volunteers treated with aspirin or placebo. Haemophilia 2000;6:15–20.
80. Pullan PT, Burger HG, Johnston CI. Pharmacokinetics of 1-desamino-8-D-arginine vasopressin (DDAVP) in patients with central diabetes insipidus. Clin Endocrinol (Oxf) 1978;9:273–278.
81. Fowler WE, Berkowitz LR, Roberts HR. DDAVP for type IIB von Willebrand disease [letter]. Blood 1989;74:1859–1860.
82. McKeown LP, Connaghan G, Wilson O, et al. 1-Desamino-8-arginine-vasopressin corrects the hemostatic defects in type 2B von Willebrand's disease. Am J Hematol 1996;51:158–163.
83. Castaman G, Lattuada A, Mannucci PM, et al. Factor VIII:C increases after desmopressin in a subgroup of patients with autosomal recessive severe von Willebrand disease. Br J Haematol 1995;89:147–151.
84. Deitcher SR, Tuller J, Johnson JA. Intranasal DDAVP induced increases in plasma von Willebrand factor alter the pharmacokinetics of high-purity factor VIII concentrates in severe haemophilia A patients. Haemophilia 1999;5:88–95.
85. Tefferi A, Nichols WL. Acquired von Willebrand disease: concise review of occurrence, diagnosis, pathogenesis, and treatment. Am J Med 1997;103:536–540.
86. Federici AB, Stabile F, Castaman G, et al. Treatment of acquired von Willebrand syndrome in patients with monoclonal gammopathy of uncertain significance: comparison of three different therapeutic approaches. Blood 1998;92:2707–2711.
87. Rao AK, Ghosh S, Sun L, et al. Mechanisms of platelet dysfunction and response to DDAVP in patients with congenital platelet function defects. A double-blind placebo-controlled trial. Thromb Haemost 1995;74:1071–1078.
88. Schulman S, Johnsson H, Egberg N, et al. DDAVP-induced correction of prolonged bleeding time in patients with congenital platelet function defects. Thromb Res 1987;45:165–174.
89. Noris P, Arbustini E, Spedini P, et al. A new variant of Bernard-Soulier syndrome characterized by dysfunctional glycoprotein (GP) lb and severely reduced amounts of GPIX and GPV. Br J Haematol 1998;103:1004–1013.
90. Stine KC, Becton DL. DDAVP therapy controls bleeding in Ehlers-Danlos syndrome. J Pediatr Hematol Oncol 1997;19:156–158.
91. Castaman G, Ruggeri M, Rodeghiero F. Clinical usefulness of desmopressin for prevention of surgical bleeding in patients with symptomatic heterozygous factor XI deficiency. Br J Haematol 1996;94:168–170.
92. Lind SE. The bleeding time does not predict surgical bleeding. Blood 1991;77:2547–2552.
93. de Franchis R, Arcidiacono PG, Carpinelli L, et al. Randomized controlled trial of desmopressin plus terlipressin vs. terlipressin alone for the treatment of acute variceal hemorrhage in cirrhotic patients: a multicenter, double-blind study. New Italian Endoscopic Club. Hepatology 1993;18:1102–1107.
94. Levi M, Cromheecke ME, de Jonge E, et al. Pharmacological strategies to decrease excessive blood loss in cardiac surgery: a meta-analysis of clinically relevant endpoints. Lancet 1999;354:1940–1947.
95. Cattaneo M, Harris AS, Stromberg U, et al. The effect of desmopressin on reducing blood loss in cardiac surgery—a meta-analysis of double-blind, placebo-controlled trials. Thromb Haemost 1995;74:1064–1070.
96. Gratz I, Koehler J, Olsen D, et al. The effect of desmopressin acetate on postoperative hemorrhage in patients receiving aspirin therapy before coronary artery bypass operations. J Thorac Cardiovasc Surg 1992;104:1417–1422.
97. Sheridan DP, Card RT, Pinilla JC, et al. Use of desmopressin acetate to reduce blood transfusion requirements during cardiac surgery in patients with acetylsalicylic-acid-induced platelet dysfunction. Can J Surg 1994;37:33–36.
98. Flordal PA, Sahlin S. Use of desmopressin to prevent bleeding complications in patients treated with aspirin. Br J Surg 1993;80:723–724.
99. Flordal PA. Pharmacological prophylaxis of bleeding in surgical patients treated with aspirin. Eur J Anaesthesiol Suppl 1997;14:38–41.
100. Weinbaum PJ, Cassidy SB, Campbell WA, et al. Pregnancy management and successful outcome of Ehlers-Danlos syndrome type IV. Am J Perinatol 1987;4:134–137.
101. Kadir RA. Women and inherited bleeding disorders: pregnancy and delivery. Semin Hematol 1999;36:28–35.
102. Ray JG. DDAVP use during pregnancy: an analysis of its safety for mother and child. Obstet Gynecol Surv 1998;53:450–455.
103. Castaman G, Rodeghiero F. Failure of DDAVP to shorten the prolonged bleeding time of two patients with congenital afibrinogenemia. Thromb Res 1992;68:309–315.
104. DiMichele DM, Hathaway WE. Use of DDAVP in inherited and acquired platelet dysfunction. Am J Hematol 1990;33:39–45.
105. Kobrinsky NL, Tulloch H. Treatment of refractory thrombocytopenic bleeding with 1-desamino-8-D-arginine vasopressin (desmopressin). J Pediatr 1988;112:993–996.
106. Kohler M, Hellstern P, Miyashita C, et al. Comparative study of intranasal, subcutaneous and intravenous administration of desamino-D-arginine vasopressin (DDAVP). Thromb Haemost 1986;55:108–111.

107. Dunn AL, Powers JR, Ribeiro MJ, et al. Adverse events during use of intranasal desmopressin acetate for haemophilia A and von Willebrand disease: a case report and review of 40 patients. Haemophilia 2000;6:11–14.
108. Humphries JE, Siragy H. Significant hyponatremia following DDAVP administration in a healthy adult. Am J Hematol 1993;44:12–15.
109. Mannucci PM, Lusher JM. Desmopressin and thrombosis [letter]. Lancet 1989;2:675–676.
110. Flordal PA, Ljungstrom KG, Fehrm A. Desmopressin and postoperative thromboembolism. Thromb Res 1992;68:429–433.
111. Mannucci PM, Carlsson S, Harris AS. Desmopressin, surgery and thrombosis [letter]. Thromb Haemost 1994;71:154–155.
112. Federici AB, Sacco R, Stabile F, et al. Optimising local therapy during oral surgery in patients with von Willebrand disease: effective results from a retrospective analysis of 63 cases. Haemophilia 2000;6:71–77.
113. Collen D. On the regulation and control of fibrinolysis. Thromb Haemost 1980;43:77–89.
114. Verstraete M. Clinical application of inhibitors of fibrinolysis. Drugs 1985;29:236–261.
115. Hedner CL, Hirsh J, Marder VJ. Therapy with antifibrinolytic agents. In Colman RW, Hirsh J, Marder VJ, Clowes AW, George JN (Eds): Hemostasis and Thrombosis: Basic Principles and Clinical Practice, 4th ed. Philadelphia, Lippincott Williams & Wilkens, 2001, pp. 795–814.
116. Dunn CJ, Goa KL. Tranexamic acid: a review of its use in surgery and other indications. Drugs 1999;57:1005–1032.
117. Okamoto S, Sato S, Takada Y, Okamato U. An active stereoisomer (transform) of AMCHA and its antifibrinolytic (antiplasmic) action in vitro and in vivo. Keio J Med 1964;13:177.
118. Kane MJ, Silverman LR, Rand JH, et al. Myonecrosis as a complication of the use of epsilon amino-caproic acid: a case report and review of the literature. Am J Med 1988;85:861–863.
119. Seymour BD, Rubinger M. Rhabdomyolysis induced by epsilon-aminocaproic acid. Ann Pharmacother 1997;31:56–58.
120. Aoki N, Saito H, Kamiya T, et al. Congenital deficiency of alpha 2-plasmin inhibitor associated with severe hemorrhagic tendency. J Clin Invest 1979;63:877–884.
121. Nilsson IM. Local fibrinolysis as a mechanism for haemorrhage. Thromb Diath Haemorrh 1975;34:623–633.
122. Gardner FH, Helmer RE. Aminocaproic acid. Use in control of hemorrhage in patients with amegakaryocytic thrombocytopenia. JAMA 1980;243:35–37.
123. Bartholomew JR, Salgia R, Bell WR. Control of bleeding in patients with immune and nonimmune thrombocytopenia with aminocaproic acid. Arch Intern Med 1989;149:1959–1961.
124. Shpilberg O, Blumenthal R, Sofer O, et al. A controlled trial of tranexamic acid therapy for the reduction of bleeding during treatment of acute myeloid leukemia. Leuk Lymphoma 1995;19:141–144.
125. Fricke W, Alling D, Kimball J, et al. Lack of efficacy of tranexamic acid in thrombocytopenic bleeding. Transfusion 1991;31:345–348.
126. Ratnoff OD. Epsilon aminocaproic acid—a dangerous weapon. N Engl J Med 1969;280:1124–1125.
127. Williams EC. Plasma alpha 2-antiplasmin activity. Role in the evaluation and management of fibrinolytic states and other bleeding disorders. Arch Intern Med 1989;149:1769–1772.
128. Butterworth J, James RL, Lin Y, et al. Pharmacokinetics of epsilon-aminocaproic acid in patients undergoing aortocoronary bypass surgery. Anesthesiology 1999;90:1624–1635.
129. Horrow JC, Van Riper DF, Strong MD, et al. The dose-response relationship of tranexamic acid. Anesthesiology 1995;82:383–392.
130. Karski JM, Dowd NP, Joiner R, et al. The effect of three different doses of tranexamic acid on blood loss after cardiac surgery with mild systemic hypothermia (32 degrees C). J Cardiothorac Vasc Anesth 1998;12:642–646.
131. Leipzig TJ, Redelman K, Horner TG. Reducing the risk of rebleeding before early aneurysm surgery: a possible role for antifibrinolytic therapy. J Neurosurg 1997;86:220–225.
132. Chakrabarti S, Varma S, Singh S, et al. Low dose bolus aminocaproic acid: an alternative to platelet transfusion in thrombocytopenia? [letter]. Eur J Haematol 1998;60:313–314.
133. Ong YL, Hull DR, Mayne EE. Menorrhagia in von Willebrand disease successfully treated with single daily dose tranexamic acid. Haemophilia 1998;4:63–65.
134. Tauber PF, Wolf AS, Herting W, et al. Hemorrhage induced by intrauterine devices: control by local proteinase inhibition. Fertil Steril 1977;28:1375–1377.
135. Singh I, Laungani GB. Intravesical epsilon aminocaproic acid in management of intractable bladder hemorrhage. Urology 1992;40:227–229.
136. Crouch ERJ, Williams PB, Gray MK, et al. Topical aminocaproic acid in the treatment of traumatic hyphema. Arch Ophthalmol 1997;115:1106–1112.
137. Bell WR. Platelets and coagulation factors. In Spivak J, Bell WR (Eds): Yearbook of Hematology. Baltimore, MD, Mosby, 1991, pp. 245–246.
138. Hiippala ST, Strid LJ, Wennerstrand MI, et al. Tranexamic acid radically decreases blood loss and transfusions associated with total knee arthroplasty. Anesth Analg 1997;84:839–844.
139. Kaspar M, Ramsay MA, Nguyen AT, et al. Continuous small-dose tranexamic acid reduces fibrinolysis but not transfusion requirements during orthotopic liver transplantation. Anesth Analg 1997;85:281–285.
140. Casati V, Guzzon D, Oppizzi M, et al. Hemostatic effects of aprotinin, tranexamic acid and epsilon-aminocaproic acid in primary cardiac surgery. Ann Thorac Surg 1999;68:2252–2256.
141. Bennett-Guerrero E, Sorohan JG, Gurevich ML, et al. Cost-benefit and efficacy of aprotinin compared with epsilon-aminocaproic acid in patients having repeated cardiac operations: a randomized, blinded clinical trial. Anesthesiology 1997;87:1373–1380.
142. Harmon DE. Cost/benefit analysis of pharmacologic hemostasis. Ann Thorac Surg 1996;61:S21–S25.
143. Munoz JJ, Birkmeyer NJ, Birkmeyer JD, et al. Is epsilon-aminocaproic acid as effective as aprotinin in reducing bleeding with cardiac surgery?: a meta-analysis. Circulation 1999;99:81–89.
144. Murkin JM. Con: tranexamic acid is not better than aprotinin in decreasing bleeding after cardiac surgery. J Cardiothorac Vasc Anesth 1994;8:474–476.
145. Guenther CR. Pro: tranexamic acid is better than aprotinin in decreasing bleeding after cardiac surgery. J Cardiothorac Vasc Anesth 1994;8:471–473.
146. Royston D. Aprotinin versus lysine analogues: the debate continues. Ann Thorac Surg 1998;65:S9–19.
147. Henry DA, O'Connell DL. Effects of fibrinolytic inhibitors on mortality from upper gastrointestinal haemorrhage. BMJ 1989;298:1142–1146.
148. Cooke I, Lethaby A, Farquhar C. Antifibrinolytics for heavy menstrual bleeding. Cochrane Database Syst Rev 2000;2:CD000249.
149. Vermeulen M, Lindsay KW, Murray GD, et al. Antifibrinolytic treatment in subarachnoid hemorrhage. N Engl J Med 1984;311:432–437.
150. Roos Y. Antifibrinolytic treatment in subarachnoid hemorrhage: a randomized placebo-controlled trial. STAR Study Group. Neurology 2000;54:77–82.
151. Schisano G, Nina P. Antifibrinolytic therapy [letter]. J Neurosurg 1997;87:486–487.
152. Saba HI, Morelli GA, Logrono LA. Brief report: treatment of bleeding in hereditary hemorrhagic telangiectasia with aminocaproic acid. N Engl J Med 1994;330:1789–1790.

153. Poon MC, Kloiber R, Birdsell DC. Epsilon-aminocaproic acid in the reversal of consumptive coagulopathy with platelet sequestration in a vascular malformation of Klippel-Trenaunay syndrome. Am J Med 1989;87:211–213.
154. Ortel TL, Onorato JJ, Bedrosian CL, et al. Antifibrinolytic therapy in the management of the Kasabach Merritt syndrome. Am J Hematol 1988;29:44–48.
155. Cooper DL, Sandler AB, Wilson LD, et al. Disseminated intravascular coagulation and excessive fibrinolysis in a patient with metastatic prostate cancer. Response to epsilon-aminocaproic acid. Cancer 1992;70:656–658.
156. De Bonis M, Cavaliere F, Alessandrini F, et al. Topical use of tranexamic acid in coronary artery bypass operations: a double-blind, prospective, randomized, placebo-controlled study. J Thorac Cardiovasc Surg 2000;119:575–580.
157. Sindet-Pedersen S, Ramstrom G, Bernvil S, et al. Hemostatic effect of tranexamic acid mouthwash in anticoagulant-treated patients undergoing oral surgery. N Engl J Med 1989;320:840–843.
158. Walsh PN, Rizza CR, Matthews JM, et al. Epsilon-aminocaproic acid therapy for dental extractions in haemophilia and Christmas disease: a double blind controlled trial. Br J Haematol 1971;20:463–475.
159. Wahl MJ. Dental surgery in anticoagulated patients. Arch Intern Med 1998;158:1610–1616.
160. Blinder D. Manor Y, Martinowitz U, et al. Dental extractions in patients maintained on continued oral anticoagulant: comparison of local hemostatic modalities. Oral Surg Oral Med Oral Pathol Oral Radiol Endod 1999;88:137–140.
161. Tibbelin A, Aust R, Bende M, et al. Effect of local tranexamic acid gel in the treatment of epistaxis. ORL J Otorhinolaryngol Relat Spec 1995;57:207–209.
162. Stefanini M, English HA, Taylor AE. Safe and effective, prolonged administration of epsilon aminocaproic acid in bleeding from the urinary tract. J Urol 1990;143:559–561.
163. Schultz M, van der Lelie H. Microscopic haematuria as a relative contraindication for tranexamic acid. Br J Haematol 1995;89:663–664.
164. Johnson AL, Skoza L, Claus E. Observations on epsilon aminocaproic acid [abstract]. Thromb Diath Haemorrh 1962;7:203.
165. Lindoff C, Rybo G, Astedt B. Treatment with tranexamic acid during pregnancy, and the risk of thrombo-embolic complications. Thromb Haemost 1993;70:238–240.
166. Longstaff C. Studies on the mechanisms of action of aprotinin and tranexamic acid as plasmin inhibitors and antifibrinolytic agents. Blood Coagul Fibrinol 1994;5:537–542.
167. Royston D, Bidstrup BP, Taylor KM, et al. Effect of aprotinin on need for blood transfusion after repeat open-heart surgery. Lancet 1987;2:1289–1291.
168. van Oeveren W, Jansen NJ, Bidstrup BP, et al. Effects of aprotinin on hemostatic mechanisms during cardiopulmonary bypass. Ann Thorac Surg 1987;44:640–645.
169. Porte RJ, Molenaar IQ, Begliomini B, et al. Aprotinin and transfusion requirements in orthotopic liver transplantation: a multicentre randomised double-blind study. EMSALT Study Group. Lancet 2000;355:1303–1309.
170. Diefenbach C, Abel M, Limpers B, et al. Fatal anaphylactic shock after aprotinin reexposure in cardiac surgery. Anesth Analg 1995;80:830–831.
171. Shampo MA, Kyle RA. Henrik Dam—Discoverer of vitamin K. Mayo Clin Proc 1998;73:46.
172. Dam H, Glavind J. Vitamin K in human pathology. Lancet 1938;1:720–721.
173. Alperin JB. Coagulopathy caused by vitamin K deficiency in critically ill, hospitalized patients. JAMA 1987;258:1916–1919.
174. Chakraverty R, Davidson S, Peggs K, et al. The incidence and cause of coagulopathies in an intensive care population. Br J Haematol 1996;93:460–463.
175. Spector I, Corn M. Laboratory tests of hemostasis. The relationship to hemorrhage in liver disease. Arch Intern Med 1967;119:577–582.
176. Shearer MJ. Vitamin K metabolism and nutriture. Blood Rev 1992;6:92–104.
177. Vermeer C, Schurgers LJ. A comprehensive review of vitamin K and vitamin K antagonists. Hematol Oncol Clin North Am 2000;14:339–353.
178. Furie B, Bouchard BA, Furie BC. Vitamin K-dependent biosynthesis of gamma-carboxyglutamic acid. Blood 1999;93:1798–1808.
179. Blanchard RA, Furie BC, Jorgensen M, et al. Acquired vitamin K-dependent carboxylation deficiency in liver disease. N Engl J Med 1981;305:242-248.
180. Van der Meer J, Hemker HC, Loeliger EA. Pharmacological aspects of vitamin K1. A clinical and experimental study in man. Thromb Diath Haemorrh Suppl 1968;29:1–96.
181. Hirsh J, Dalen JE, Anderson DR, et al. Oral anticoagulants. Mechanism of action, clinical effectiveness, and optimal therapeutic range. Chest 2001;119:8S–21S.
182. Nee R, Doppenschmidt D, Donovan DJ, et al. Intravenous versus subcutaneous vitamin K1 in reversing excessive oral anticoagulation. Am J Cardiol 1999;83:286–287.
183. Raj G, Kumar R, McKinney WP. Time course of reversal of anticoagulant effect of warfarin by intravenous and subcutaneous phytonadione. Arch Intern Med 1999;159:2721–2724.
184. Soedirman JR, De Bruijn EA, Maes RA, et al. Pharmacokinetics and tolerance of intravenous and intramuscular phylloquinone (vitamin K1) mixed micelles formulation. Br J Clin Pharmacol 1996;41:517–523.
185. Taylor CT, Chester EA, Byrd DC, et al. Vitamin K to reverse excessive anticoagulation: a review of the literature. Pharmacotherapy 1999;19:1415–1425.
186. Third ACCP consensus conference on antithrombotic therapy. Chest 1992; 102(suppl):303S–549S.
187. Guyatt G, Schunemann H, Cook D, et al. Grades of recommendation for antithrombotic agents. Chest 2001;119:3S–7S.
188. Hirsh J. Reversal of the anticoagulant effects of warfarin by vitamin K1 [editorial]. Chest 1998;114:1505–1508.
189. Cosgriff SW. The effectiveness of an oral vitamin K1 in controlling excessive hypoprothrombinemia during anticoagulant therapy. Ann Intern Med 1956;45:14–22.
190. White RH, McKittrick T, Hutchinson R, et al. Temporary discontinuation of warfarin therapy: changes in the international normalized ratio. Ann Intern Med 1995;122:40–42.
191. Wentzien TH, O'Reilly RA, Kearns PJ. Prospective evaluation of anticoagulant reversal with oral vitamin K1 while continuing warfarin therapy unchanged. Chest 1998;114:1546–1550.
192. Palareti G, Legnani C. Warfarin withdrawal. Pharmacokinetic-pharmacodynamic considerations. Clin Pharmacokinet 1996;30:300–313.
193. Lousberg TR, Witt DM, Beall DG, et al. Evaluation of excessive anticoagulation in a group model health maintenance organization. Arch Intern Med 1998;158:528–534.
194. Perry DJ, Kimball DBJ. Low dose vitamin K for excessively anticoagulated prosthetic valve patients. Mil Med 1982;147:836–837.
195. Shetty HG, Backhouse G, Bentley DP, et al. Effective reversal of warfarin-induced excessive anticoagulation with low dose vitamin K1. Thromb Haemost 1992;67:13–15.
196. Brophy MT, Fiore LD, Deykin D. Low-dose vitamin K therapy in excessively anticoagulated patients: a dose-finding study. J Thromb Thrombolysis 1997;4:289–292.
197. Andersen P, Godal HC. Predictable reduction in anticoagulant activity of warfarin by small amounts of vitamin K. Acta Med Scand 1975;198:269–270.
198. Fredriksson K, Norrving B, Stromblad LG. Emergency reversal of anticoagulation after intracerebral hemorrhage. Stroke 1992;23:972–977.

199. Kitchens CS. Efficacy of intravenous vitamin K in a case of massive warfarin overdosage (letter). Thromb Haemost 2001;86:719–720.
200. Monagle PT, Andrew M. Hemorrhagic and thromboembolic complications during infancy and childhood. In Colman RW, Hirsh J, Marder VJ, Clowes AW, George JN (Eds): Hemostasis and Thrombosis: Basic Principles and Clinical Practice, 4th ed. Philadelphia, Lippincott Williams & Wilkens, 2001, pp. 1053–1070.
201. Furukawa M, Nakanishi T, Okuda H, et al. Changes of plasma des-gamma-carboxy prothrombin levels in patients with hepatocellular carcinoma in response to vitamin K. Cancer 1992;69:31–38.
202. Ansell JE, Kumar R, Deykin D. The spectrum of vitamin K deficiency. JAMA 1977;238:40–42.
203. Weitzel JN, Sadowski JA, Furie BC, et al. Surreptitious ingestion of a long-acting vitamin K antagonist/rodenticide, brodifacoum: clinical and metabolic studies of three cases. Blood 1990;76:2555–2559.
204. Lipsky JJ. Antibiotic-associated hypoprothrombinaemia. J Antimicrob Chemother 1988;21:281–300.
205. Breen GA, St Peter WL. Hypoprothrombinemia associated with cefmetazole. Ann Pharmacother 1997;31:180–184.
206. Rich EC, Drage CW. Severe complications of intravenous phytonadione therapy. Two cases, with one fatality. Postgrad Med 1982;72:303–306.
207. Elenbaas JK. Phytonadione-induced cardiovascular collapse. Micromedex Inc., 1988, 83.
208. Havel M, Muller M, Graninger W, et al. Tolerability of a new vitamin K1 preparation for parenteral administration to adults: one case of anaphylactoid reaction. Clin Ther 1987;9:373–379.
209. Labatut A, Sorbette F, Virenque C. [Shock states during injection of vitamin K (letter)]. Therapie 1988;43:58.
210. Barash P, Kitahata LM, Mandel S. Acute cardiovascular collapse after intravenous phytonadione. Anesth Analg 1976;55:304–306.
211. Whitling AM, Bussey HI, Lyons RM. Comparing different routes and doses of phytonadione for reversing excessive anticoagulation. Arch Intern Med 1998;158:2136–2140.
212. Lefrere JJ, Girot R. Acute cardiovascular collapse during intravenous vitamin K1 injection [letter]. Thromb Haemost 1987;58:790.
213. Verstraete M, Vermylen J, Tyberghein J. Double blind evaluation of the haemostatic effect of adrenochrome monosemicarbazone, conjugated estrogens and epsilonaminocaproic acid after adenotonsillectomy. Acta Haematol 1968;40:154–161.
214. Alperin JB. Estrogens and surgery in women with von Willebrand's disease. Am J Med 1982;73:367–371.
215. Weinstein P. Treatment of ophthalmic hemorrhage by premarin. Int Z Klin Pharmakol Ther Toxikol 1969;2:72–73.
216. Livio M, Mannucci PM, Vigano G, et al. Conjugated estrogens for the management of bleeding associated with renal failure. N Engl J Med 1986;315:731–735.
217. Ambrus JL, Schimert G, Lajos TZ, et al. Effect of antifibrinolytic agents and estrogens on blood loss and blood coagulation factors during open heart surgery. J Med 1971;2:65–81.
218. Pluss J. Hemostasis by premedication with estrogen in hair-transplant surgery. J Dermatol Surg Oncol 1977;3:320–321.
219. van Cutsem E, Rutgeerts P, Vantrappen G. Treatment of bleeding gastrointestinal vascular malformations with oestrogen-progesterone. Lancet 1990;335:953–955.
220. Frenette L, Cox J, Arnall M, et al. Effectiveness of conjugated estrogen in orthotopic liver transplantation. South Med J 1998;91:365–368.
221. Vigano G, Gaspari F, Locatelli M, et al. Dose-effect and pharmacokinetics of estrogens given to correct bleeding time in uremia. Kidney Int 1988;34:853–858.
222. Jacobs P, Jacobson J, Kahn D. Perioperative administration of a single dose of conjugated oestrogen to uraemic patients is ineffective in improving haemostasis. Am J Hematol 1994;46:24–28.
223. Shemin D, Elnour M, Amarantes B, et al. Oral estrogens decrease bleeding time and improve clinical bleeding in patients with renal failure. Am J Med 1990;89:436–440.
224. Sloand JA, Schiff MJ. Beneficial effect of low-dose transdermal estrogen on bleeding time and clinical bleeding in uremia. Am J Kidney Dis 1995;26:22–26.
225. Harrison RL, McKee PA. Estrogen stimulates von Willebrand factor production by cultured endothelial cells. Blood 1984;63:657–664.
226. Kroon UB, Tengborn L, Rita H, et al. The effects of transdermal oestradiol and oral progestogens on haemostasis variables. Br J Obstet Gynaecol 1997; 104 (Suppl 16):32–37.
227. Carr JA, Silverman N. The heparin-protamine interaction. A review. J Cardiovasc Surg (Torino) 1999;40:659–666.
228. Byun Y, Singh VK, Yang VC. Low molecular weight protamine: a potential nontoxic heparin antagonist. Thromb Res 1999;94:53–61.
229. Dietrich CP, Shinjo SK, Moraes FA, et al. Structural features and bleeding activity of commercial low molecular weight heparins: neutralization by ATP and protamine. Semin Thromb Hemost 1999; 25 (Suppl 3):43–50.
230. Crowther MA, Ginsberg JS, Hirsh J. Practical aspects of anticoagulant therapy. In Colman RW, Hirsh J, Marder VJ, Clowes AW, George JN (Eds): Hemostasis and Thrombosis: Basic Principles and Clinical Practice, 4th ed. Philadelphia, Lippincott Williams & Wilkens, 2001, pp. 1497–1516.
231. Despotis GJ, Gravlee G, Filos K, et al. Anticoagulation monitoring during cardiac surgery: a review of current and emerging techniques. Anesthesiology 1999;91:1122–1151.

CHAPTER 26

Topical Hemostatic Agents for Localized Bleeding

Mark R. Jackson, M.D.

For many years topical hemostatic agents have consisted primarily of various forms of animal collagen and gelatin. These commercially prepared products have been used by surgeons in the operating room as adjuncts to surgical hemostasis. A limitation of these products is the lack of any significant inherent coagulation mechanism, so that they function as a means of tamponade and a scaffold upon which the patient's own clotting mechanisms play out. Newer products, such as fibrin sealant, are now available as commercial preparations. These materials are combinations of highly purified, virally inactivated human thrombin and fibrinogen, and as such, mimic the final step in the coagulation cascade. Other newer products include combinations of gelatin matrix with bovine thrombin that possess some of the properties of the older agents and also provide some inherent coagulation properties. In this chapter, we will review these products, their intended and potential future uses, and the clinical scenarios that lead to their use.

INTRAOPERATIVE AND POSTOPERATIVE BLEEDING

The most common cause of significant intraoperative bleeding is inadequate surgical hemostasis, so-called silk deficiency. There are no pharmacologic or blood bank substitutes for a careful dissection and attention to technical detail. Application of digital pressure to an area of active bleeding is a useful maneuver while more definitive steps are in progress. Even what seems like trivial bleeding from skin edges and subcutaneous tissue can add up, and such bleeding can account for up to 100 to 200 mL of blood loss if unattended.[1] Dissection using electrocautery rather than a scalpel reduces blood loss.[2,3]

Intraoperative disorders of hemostasis can be acquired for a number of reasons. Coagulopathy in vascular-trauma patients has been shown to be related more to hypotension and hypoperfusion than to dilutional factors.[4] Tissue hypoxia can cause release of plasminogen activators thereby stimulating fibrinolysis. Hypothermia may be another contributing factor, particularly in the trauma patient. Dilutional thrombocytopenia may occur in the massively transfused patient, particularly following 20 or more units of banked or cell salvage blood.[5]

In order to successfully manage hemostasis at the local level, systemic factors contributing to coagulopathy should be corrected first. Restoration of hemodynamic stability and normal temperature must be accomplished. Dilutional coagulopathy must be corrected with platelet or factor replacement as indicated by laboratory markers of hemostasis. Disorders of hemostasis secondary to antiplatelet agents and anticoagulation introduce an additional layer of complexity for many patients, particularly those undergoing cardiac or vascular surgery, for which withdrawal or reversal of antithrombotic therapy might be undesirable. In situations where local bleeding persists despite all reasonable efforts to restore systemic coagulation mechanisms, and despite the use of sutures and electrocautery as needed, topical hemostatic agents may provide a useful adjunct to securing adequate hemostasis.

AVAILABLE TOPICAL AGENTS

Collagen-Based

A number of absorbable bovine collagen products are available commercially for use as topical hemostatic agents (Table 26–1). These materials are often packaged

Table 26-1 • COMPARISON OF TOPICAL HEMOSTATIC MATERIALS

Material	Absorption Time	Hemostatic Mechanism Inherent to Preparation
Bovine collagen (Helistat, Colla-Tec, Inc., Plainsboro, NJ)	8–12 weeks	Minimal
Purified gelatin (Gelfoam, The Upjohn Company, Kalamazoo, MI)	4–6 weeks	No
Oxidized regenerated cellulose (Surgicel, Johnson & Johnson Medical Inc., Arlington, TX)	1–2 weeks	No
Fibrin sealant (Tisseel, Immuno AG, Vienna, Austria)	8 weeks	Yes
Bovine gelatin matrix, bovine thrombin (FloSeal, Fusion Medical Technologies, Mountain View, CA)	6–8 weeks	Yes (relies on patient's plasma fibrinogen in shed blood)

as sheets that can be cut to various sizes once opened and placed on the sterile surgical field. These materials are somewhat stiff, so they often can be more easily used and manipulated if they are moistened with saline solution or blood from the wound. Also, when these materials are dry they are somewhat "sticky" and are not as easily handled. Many surgeons will moisten these products with solutions of bovine thrombin. Once moistened, these sheets have the consistency of wet felt and can be easily wrapped around a vascular anastomosis, or placed in a single layer upon a relatively flat bleeding wound surface. Such materials can be useful on small capsular tears of the spleen, for example. Collagen based topical agents are absorbable and therefore may be left in the wound if necessary.

Microfibrillar collagen has a consistency similar to sawdust and is packaged as a powder. Like other collagen products, it absorbs surrounding blood and basically functions as a mechanical template upon which the patient's own hemostatic mechanisms form clot. Microfibrillar collagen has a tendency to adhere to the surgeon's gloves and instruments as well as to the wound. Because of its powder-like consistency, it can be placed easily within irregular surfaces and crevices of deep wounds.

Collagen materials have demonstrated hemostatic efficacy in preclinical and clinical studies.[6,7] Early preclinical studies of the hemostatic properties of microcrystalline collagen in a canine model of arterial injury demonstrated a 93% rate of early hemostasis when collagen was applied to a carotid artery puncture made with a 17-gauge trocar.[6] Hemostasis was far superior with microcrystalline collagen than with either oxidized cellulose or pressure alone. An interesting finding from these experiments was observed with the use of collagen in animals anticoagulated with intravenously administered heparin (300 IU/kg). Twenty-four percent in this group had delayed bleeding during the 1-hour experiment, suggesting that intact coagulation mechanisms are instrumental for the effectiveness of collagen topical agents.

Cellulose-Based

Topical hemostatic agents composed of oxidized regenerated cellulose are also available. These agents are available in a fabric-like product and a fibrillar (powder-like) product. The cellulose fabric can be cut to conform to the wound or to wrap a vascular anastomosis. Since it is softer than collagen and gelatin products, wetting is optional. The cellulose fabric is also thinner than most collagen products and is knitted in a manner that produces interstices. A potential advantage of the cellulose over collagen and gelatin-based agents is that oxidized regenerated cellulose has demonstrated antibacterial properties in vitro.[8,9] Like collagen, oxidized regenerated cellulose is absorbable and can be left in the wound.

Gelatin-Based

Purified gelatin of bovine origin is also used as a topical hemostatic agent. It is prepared as a thin, wafer-like sheet that has the consistency of Styrofoam. Once moistened, it is pliable and easily conforms to the shape of a wound or a vascular anastomosis. As with collagen and cellulose-based agents, gelatin-based materials are also absorbable and can be left in the wound after closure. Many surgeons will use bovine thrombin as the wetting agent. Gelatin-based topical hemostatic agents have been compared to collagen-based agents in a number of animal models of hemostasis. While some studies indicate superiority of the collagen products,[10,11] others have shown equivalency.[12,13]

Recently, another gelatin-based hemostatic agent has been approved by the U. S. Food and Drug Administration (FDA) (FloSeal Matrix, Fusion Medical Technologies, Mountain View, CA). This product is composed of bovine-source gelatin granules and bovine thrombin. These two ingredients are mixed together and placed in a single-barrel syringe prior to use. The gelatin and thrombin mixture is then applied to the site of bleeding. The final product has a granular, gel-like consistency, and is easily applied using the accompanying syringe. Recently, investigators at Columbia University College of Physicians and Surgeons reported results of a cohort group of 93 patients experiencing hemorrhage in a multicenter, randomized clinical trial evaluating this hemostatic agent in a total of 309 patients undergoing cardiac, vascular, and spinal surgery.[14] Patients were randomized to receive either FloSeal or bovine thrombin-soaked Gelfoam (Upjohn and Pharmacia, Kalamazoo, MI) applied at sites of bleeding that required topical hemostatic agents. Hemostasis at 10 minutes was achieved in 94% of patients with FloSeal, and only 60% in the control group ($p = 0.001$). All patients were tested for the development of antibodies to bovine thrombin and factor V preoperatively and at 6 to 8 weeks. Although there was no evidence of antibody-related hemorrhage in either group, bovine thrombin antibodies were detected by enzyme-linked immunosorbent assay in 9 FloSeal patients and in 12 control patients ($p = 0.76$). Bovine factor V antibodies were detected in 11 FloSeal patients and in 15 controls ($p = 0.43$).

COMBINATIONS OF THROMBIN AND FIBRINOGEN

Cryoprecipitate-Based

The use of fibrin-based topical hemostatic products was reported as early as 1909.[15] Subsequent developments allowed the purification of thrombin and fibrinogen, which eventually led to the development of fibrin sealant products in the 1970s. Because of concerns of transmission of viral blood-borne infection, the FDA revoked the license for commercial fibrinogen concentrates in 1978. Since then, careful donor selection and the development of a variety of viral-inactivation methods have largely resolved the viral safety issue (Table 26–2).

Until the recent approval of Tisseel VH (Baxter Healthcare Corporation), the use of fibrin sealant in the United States was restricted to the so-called homebrews of bovine thrombin and human pooled cryoprecipitated plasma as the source of fibrinogen. Such preparations are limited by the lack of viral inactivation methods. Single donor and autologous cryoprecipitate have also been used in an effort to minimize infectious risk. Additional limitations of these preparations include a relatively low fibrinogen concentration and induction of antibodies against bovine factor V.[16–18] The bovine thrombin preparation having the lowest concentration of bovine factor V is produced by Jones Medical Industries, St. Louis, MO.[19]

Antibodies to bovine factor V and thrombin can result in coagulopathy and bleeding, and are not merely a laboratory abnormality (see Chapter 6). The classic feature of such an acquired factor V deficiency caused by antibody formation is excessive bleeding that is not responsive to administration of vitamin K or fresh frozen plasma.[19] Laboratory findings include a prolonged prothrombin time (PT) and activated partial thromboplastin time (aPTT) that are not corrected by mixing patient and normal plasma in vitro and reduced factor V activity, which is usually less than 30%.[19] Bleeding patients should be treated with fresh frozen plasma or platelet transfusion for factor V replacement. Immunosuppression with steroids has also been used effectively.[19] For patients requiring continued anticoagulation, it should not be assumed that the elevated PT and aPTT indicate a state of "autoanticoagulation."[20] Nonetheless, the probability of increased risk of bleeding with continued anticoagulation must be weighed against the risk of thrombosis, and as such the decision for or against anticoagulation must be individualized for each patient. Cessation of pharmacologic anticoagulation with monitoring for thrombus by serial echocardiography has been used successfully in one such patient with a prosthetic aortic valve.[21]

Cryoprecipitate-based fibrin glue is prepared using equal volumes of thawed cryoprecipitated plasma as the source of fibrinogen, and bovine thrombin with calcium chloride (Table 26–3).[22] These solutions are placed in separate syringes and then mixed together to form a layer of fibrin polymer. The consistency of such home brews varies widely for two primary reasons. First, the fibrinogen concentration of cryoprecipitate varies considerably, ranging from approximately 4 mg/mL to 25 mg/mL.[23] Fibrinogen concentration has been shown to

Table 26–2 • EXAMPLES OF FIBRIN SEALANT IN THE UNITED STATES AND OTHER COUNTRIES

Source	Human Fibrinogen (mg/mL)	Human Thrombin (U/mL)	Virus-Inactivated Fibrinogen	Virus-Inactivated Thrombin
Baxter/Immuno AG (United States and Europe)[a]	70–115	500	Two-step vapor heat at 60° and 80°C	Two-step vapor-heat at 60° and 80°C
Baxter/American Red Cross (United States)	100	300	SD[b]	SD, nanofilter
Blood bank	10–15 (cryoppt)	1000 (bovine)	None	None (bovine)
Centeon Pharma GmbH (Germany)	65–115	400–600	Wet heat, 10 hours, at 60°C	Wet heat, 10 hours, at 60°C
LFB-Lille (France)	115	500	SD	SD
SNBTS (Scotland)	40	200	Dry heat, 72 hours at 80°C	SD
Haemacure Biotech (Canada)	50–70	150–250	SD, nanofilter, dry heat, 1 hour and 100°C	SD, nanofilter dry heat, 1 hour and 100°C

Modified from Alving BM, Weinstein MJ, Finlayson JS, et al. Fibrin sealant: summary of a conference on characteristics and clinical uses. Transfusion 1995; 35:783–790, with permission.
[a] Only product approved in the United States.
[b] Solvent-detergent treatment.

Table 26-3 • INGREDIENTS FOR "HOME-MADE" FIBRIN GLUE

Materials
- Bovine thrombin (1000 IU/mL)
- Thawed cryoprecipitate (20 to 30 mL or more depending upon surface area of bleeding wound(s) to be treated)
- One ampule calcium chloride (10%)
- Triple-lumen catheter, cut to 10 cm
- Two syringes (size appropriate for one-half of the intended volume of fibrin glue)
- Two sterile containers (urine specimen cups work well)

Directions
1. Draw equal volumes of thrombin solution and cryoprecipitate into *separate* containers.
2. Add calcium chloride (10%) solution to the thrombin solution for a final volume ratio of 1:10 (CaCl$_2$:thrombin).
3. Draw each solution into *separate* syringes, the volume of which is appropriate for the total volume of fibrin glue.
4. Attach each syringe to separate ports of the triple-lumen catheter. Cap the unused port.
5. A coordinated effort of two providers is then required for application of the fibrin glue. One provider depresses the plungers of the syringes while the other directs the "stream" of liquid fibrin glue to the site(s) of bleeding. The cryoprecipitate is considerably more viscous than the thrombin. This can result in premature depletion of the thrombin. Awareness of these properties is all that is required for the mixing to be done correctly. As an added measure, one can secure the two plungers of the syringes by drilling a sterile orthopedic drill bit through the plungers at their ends. Alternatively, the Micromedics device can be used if available.

Modified from Cohn SM, Feinstein AJ, Nicholas JM, et al. Recipe for poor man's fibrin glue. J Trauma 1998, 44:907, with permission.

correlate with the tensile and adhesive strength of fibrin sealant.[15] Another limitation that can compromise the final material properties of the fibrin polymer is the method of fibrinogen/thrombin mixture. The tensile strength of the fibrin polymer is less when incomplete or inadequate mixture occurs.[24] A dual-syringe delivery device similar to that used to apply the two components of epoxy glue is commercially available and can simplify the simultaneous administration and mixing of the fibrinogen and thrombin solutions (Micromedics, Inc., St. Paul, MN). The two syringes are connected and are joined at their tips by a "Y" connector through which the two solutions mix as they are applied to the wound. Catheter and spray tips are also available to allow different delivery methods depending upon the nature of the bleeding. Catheter tips work well where precise application is important, such as to the suture line of a vascular anastomosis. Spray tips are better suited for application over a large surface area.

Commercially Prepared

In 1978 the FDA revoked the license for commercial fibrinogen concentrates because of high rates of hepatitis resulting from virally contaminated blood used for their preparation. Although commercial development of fibrin sealant products continued in Europe, it was abandoned in the United States. Renewed interest in commercial development occurred with the onset of improved viral inactivation methods and careful donor screening. Most manufacturers utilize two different viral inactivation methods in processing their protein concentrates. These processes include solvent-detergent treatment, two-step vapor heat, wet heat, dry heat, nanofiltration, and ultraviolet light.[25]

The FDA recently approved one commercial fibrin sealant product for use, the Tisseel VH Kit (Baxter Healthcare Corporation). This two-component fibrin sealant product contains two separate vials for a purified human fibrinogen concentrate, and a purified human thrombin concentrate (Table 26-4). In addition to several filtration steps and freeze-drying, the protein concentrates are subjected to a two-step vapor heat treatment for viral inactivation. Aprotinin, an antifibrinolytic agent of bovine origin, is present in the fibrinogen component of Tisseel. Several other commercial fibrin sealant products are currently in clinical trials.

In addition to viral inactivation, advantages of commercial fibrin sealants over "home-brew" fibrin glue include higher fibrinogen concentration (50 to 150 mg/mL),[25] and ready availability without the need to thaw cryoprecipitate from the blood bank. Most commercial preparations require warming to 37°C prior to use. Warming devices are available to facilitate this step.

A number of fibrin sealant products have been evaluated in both prospective and retrospective studies. In a randomized clinical trial evaluating the hemostatic efficacy of fibrin sealant (Tisseel, Immuno AG, Vienna, Austria) during cardiac reoperations, 92.6% of patients randomized to receive fibrin sealant had complete hemostasis at 5 minutes, compared with only 12.4% of patients treated with conventional topical agents.[26] At 1 year of follow-up there was no evidence of inflammation in response to fibrin sealant. A post-hoc analysis of the data showed improved survival, a shorter hospital stay, and less blood loss at 12 hours in the group treated with fibrin sealant.[27] In another randomized clinical trial, fibrin sealant prepared by the Scottish National Blood Transfusion Service was evaluated in vascular surgery procedures.[28] Seventeen patients undergoing carotid endarterectomy with adjunctive polytetrafluoroethylene (PTFE) patch angioplasty were randomized to re-

Table 26-4 • COMPONENTS OF FIBRIN SEALANT (TISSEEL VH KIT, BAXTER HEALTHCARE CORPORATION)

Fibrinogen Component		Thrombin Component	
Fibrinogen (human)	75–115 mg/mL	Thrombin (human)	500 IU/mL
Aprotinin (bovine)	3000 KIU/mL	Calcium chloride	40 μmol/mL

ceive either fibrin sealant or nothing on the PTFE patch suture holes. Suture holes in PTFE graft material have an inherent tendency to bleed and can be associated with hemorrhagic complications.[29] Fibrin sealant was prepared using heat-treated fibrinogen from pooled donor plasma cryoprecipitate and solvent-detergent-treated human thrombin. The fibrinogen concentration ranged from 29 to 39 mg/mL. The fibrin sealant was administered using a dual-syringe technique. There was a statistically significant reduction in time to achieve hemostasis in the fibrin sealant group (5.5 minutes) compared to controls (19 minutes, $p < 0.005$). No difference was noted in survival or measured blood loss. No thrombotic or neurologic complications occurred in patients treated with fibrin sealant.

Most of the attention focused on fibrin sealant products concerns issues of safety and hemostatic efficacy of the sealant itself. While this is both understandable and appropriate, the development of customized delivery devices that allow optimal application of fibrin sealant for different clinical uses is an important and sometimes overlooked issue. Although the standard dual syringe technique is adequate for most applications, there are limitations. For example, the tips that attach to the "Y" connector frequently become plugged with fibrin, such that their replacement is generally required for repeat administration from the same dual-syringe device. The current Tisseel VH Kit does not contain a spray tip, thereby limiting the ability to apply a thin layer of sealant over a large surface area wound, such as a skin graft harvest site or full-thickness burn tangential excision wound. Currently available catheter tips are not long enough to reach into deep wounds, and a longer single-channel tip might be more predisposed to plugging problems than the short tips.

Another issue related to the importance of the delivery device is the cost of using large volumes of fibrin sealant. There would be considerable advantage to a device that would allow efficient use of a limited volume of fibrin sealant to cover larger wounds. For example, a stellate liver fracture from blunt trauma would likely require multiple kits for complete application. The maximum total volume of the Tisseel VH Kit is 10 mL of sealant. While this, or smaller amounts, will be adequate for many indications, it is likely that several kits would be necessary for some wounds. The development of application devices that would release a finer spray might allow a more cost-effective use of a given volume of sealant.

Fibrin sealant products are best used for diffuse, nonsurgical bleeding, such as suture hole bleeding at a vascular anastomosis, parenchymal bleeding after suture of vessels, and general oozing of blood from wound edges in patients with hemostatic defects. More significant bleeding sources should be sutured or treated with electrocautery, as appropriate. Although fibrin sealant appears to be a useful adjunct to surgical hemostasis, it is not a substitute. If fibrin sealant is applied to an actively bleeding wound, the sealant will usually "float off" the area of bleeding without achieving hemostasis. Moreover, current forms of liquid fibrin sealant make application of pressure, an often vital maneuver, somewhat problematic. The application of pressure can disrupt the adhesive bond of the sealant to the wound, and can cause the sealant to adhere more to the surgeon's glove or gauze material, resulting in disruption of the sealant when pressure is removed. These material properties of liquid fibrin sealant present limitations to its use in wounds that are associated with significant or active bleeding.

The use of fibrin sealant incorporated into a dry dressing offers the potential of addressing some of these material property limitations associated with actively bleeding wounds. Commercially prepared fibrin sealant dressings consisting of a thin layer of lyophilized human thrombin and fibrinogen applied to one side of a sheet of equine collagen have been used clinically in Europe, but currently are not approved for use in the United States. Clinical reports on the use of such fibrin sealant dressings are encouraging,[30] although randomized clinical trials are needed. A dry dressing of lyophilized fibrinogen and thrombin mounted on an absorbable backing delivers a higher concentration of fibrin to the wound and permits the application of pressure, a critically important adjunctive maneuver in surgical hemostasis. The mass effect of the backing material might also be important in order to maintain contact of the fibrin sealant with the bleeding wound. Such materials easy to handle and, once wet with blood in the wound, easily flexible to the contour of the wound surface.[31] Preclinical studies indicate superior hemostasis with fibrin sealant dressings compared to controls consisting of collagen fleece,[31] Silastic and Immunoglobulin G,[32] and surgical gauze.[33,34] In a study evaluating the hemostatic efficacy of a fibrin sealant dressing in a porcine model of femoral artery injury, the use of a fibrin sealant dressing with 15 minutes of minimal pressure was effective in achieving complete hemostasis at femoral artery lacerations 4 mm in length.[32] It is unlikely that use of liquid fibrin sealant alone, particularly when used without adjunctive pressure application, would be effective on brisk arterial bleeding as encountered in this study.

SUMMARY

Although topical hemostatic agents are no substitute for precise surgical technique in the treatment of localized bleeding disorders, there are a number of products that can serve as useful adjuncts in these situations. Historically, collagen, cellulose, and gelatin-based products have been most frequently used in the United States as topical hemostatic agents, but with the recent FDA approval of fibrin sealant, this may change. As more manufacturers bring fibrin sealant products to market, it is likely that newer application devices and fibrin sealant formulations will be developed that are more closely tailored to specific clinical needs. Newer agents based upon gelatin and collagen are now available with more under development. These products will add an additional level to our present array of topical agents. The ultimate best uses and clinical indications for these products will require results from appropriately designed clinical trials. The development of better delivery devices for the application of these sealant materials is continuing and will greatly improve the clinical usefulness of these hemostatic agents.

REFERENCES

Chapter 26 References

1. Spence RK. Bleeding and the vascular surgery patient. Semin Vasc Surg 1994;7:104–113.
2. Miller E, Paull DE, Morrissey K, et al. Scalpel versus electrocautery in modified radical mastectomy. Am Surg 1988;54:284–286.
3. Pearlman NW, Stiegmann GV, Vance V, et al. A prospective study of incisional time, blood loss, pain and healing with carbon dioxide laser, scalpel and electrosurgery. Arch Surg 1991; 126:1018–1020.
4. Collins JA. Recent developments in the area of massive transfusion. World J Surg 1987;11:75–81.
5. Leslie S, Toy P. Laboratory hemostatic abnormalities in massively transfused patients given red blood cells and crystalloid. Am J Clin Pathol 1991;96:770–773.
6. Abbott WM, Austen WG. The effectiveness and mechanism of collagen-induced topical hemostasis. Surgery 1975;78:723–729.
7. Morgenstern L. Microcrystalline collagen used in experimental splenic injury: a new surface hemostatic agent. Arch Surg 1974; 109:44–47.
8. Dineen P. Antibacterial activity of oxidized regenerated cellulose. Surg Gynecol Obstet 1976;142:481–486.
9. Dineen P. The effect of oxidized regenerated cellulose on experimental infected splenotomies. J Surg Res 1977;23:114–116.
10. Hanisch ME, Baum N, Beach PD, et al. A comparative evaluation of Avitene and gelfoam for hemostasis in experimental canine prostatic wounds. Invest Urol 1975;12:333–336.
11. Coln D, Horton J, Ogden ME, et al. Evaluation of hemostatic agents in experimental splenic lacerations. Am J Surg 1983; 145:256–259.
12. Sanfilippo JS, Barrows GH, Yussman MA. Comparison of avitene, topical thrombin, and gelfoam as sole hemostatic agent in tuboplasties. Fertil Steril 1980;33:311–316.
13. Benoit PW, Hunt LM. Comparison of a microcrystalline collagen preparation and gelatin foam in extraction wounds. J Oral Surg 1976;34:1079–1083.
14. Cosgrove DM, Badduke BR, Hill JD, et al. Controlled clinical trial of a novel hemostatic agent in cardiac surgery. The Fusion Matrix Study Group. Ann Thorac Surg, 2000;69:1376–1382.
15. Sierra DH. Fibrin sealant adhesive systems: a review of their chemistry, material properties and clinical applications. J Biomat Applicat 1993;7:309–352.
16. Zehnder JL, Leung LLK. Development of antibodies to thrombin and factor V with recurrent bleeding in a patient exposed to topical bovine thrombin. Blood 1990;76:2011–2016.
17. Banninger H, Hardegger T, Tobler A, et al. Frequent development of inhibitors of bovine thrombin and human factor V. Br J Haematol 1993;85:528–532.
18. Nichols WL, Daniels TM, Fisher PK, et al. Antibodies to bovine thrombin and coagulation factor V associated with surgical use of topical bovine thrombin or fibrin "glue": a frequent finding. Blood 1993;82:59 (abstr).
19. Christie RJ, Carrington L, Alving B. Postoperative bleeding induced by topical bovine thrombin: report of two cases. Surgery 1997;121:708–710.
20. Ortel TL, Charles LA, Keller FG, et al. Topical thrombin and acquired coagulation factor inhibitors: clinical spectrum and laboratory diagnosis. Am J Hematol 1994;45:128–135.
21. Zumberg MS, Waples JM, Kao KJ, et al. Management of a patient with a mechanical aortic valve and antibodies to both thrombin and factor V after repeat exposure to fibrin sealant. Am J Hematol 2000;64:59–63.
22. Cohn SM, Feinstein AJ, Nicholas JM, et al. Recipe for poor man's fibrin glue. J Trauma 1998;44:907.
23. Ness PM, Perkins HA. Cryoprecipitate as a reliable source of fibrinogen replacement. JAMA 1979;241:1690–1691.
24. Redl H, Schlag G, Dinges HP. Methods of fibrin seal application. Thorac Cardiovasc Surg 1982; 30:223–227.
25. Jackson MR, Alving BM. Fibrin sealant in preclinical and clinical studies. Curr Opin Hematol 1999;6:415–419.
26. Rousou J, Levitsky S, Gonzalez-Lavin L, et al. Randomized clinical trial of fibrin sealant in patients undergoing resternotomy or reoperation after cardiac operations. A multicenter study. J Thorac Cardiovasc Surg 1989;97:194–203.
27. Levitsky S. Randomized clinical trial of Immuno's fibrin sealant in patients undergoing resternotomy or reoperation after cardiac operations: a multicenter study (letter). Transfusion 1996;36:845.
28. Milne AA, Murphy WG, Reading SJ, et al. Fibrin sealant reduces suture line bleeding during carotid endarterectomy: a randomised trial. Eur J Vasc Endovasc Surg 1995;10:91–94.
29. McCready RA, Siderys H, Pittman JN, et al. Delayed postoperative bleeding from polytetrafluoroethylene carotid artery patches. J Vasc Surg 1992;15:661–663.
30. Agus GB, Bono AV, Mira E, et al. Hemostatic efficacy and safety of TachoComb in surgery. Ready to use and rapid hemostatic agent. Int Surg 1996;81:316–319.
31. Jackson MR, Taher MM, Burge JR, et al. Hemostatic efficacy of a fibrin sealant dressing in an animal model of kidney injury. J Trauma 1998;45:662–665.
32. Jackson MR, Friedman SA, Carter AJ, et al. Hemostatic efficacy of a fibrin sealant-based topical agent in a femoral artery injury model: a randomized, blinded, placebo-controlled study. J Vasc Surg 1997;26:274–280.
33. Larson MJ, Bowersox JC, Lim RC Jr, et al. Efficacy of a fibrin hemostatic bandage in controlling hemorrhage from experimental arterial injuries. Arch Surg 1995;130:420–422.
34. Holcomb J, MacPhee M, Hetz S, et al. Efficacy of a dry fibrin sealant dressing for hemorrhage control after ballistic injury. Arch Surg 1998;133:32–35.

PART V

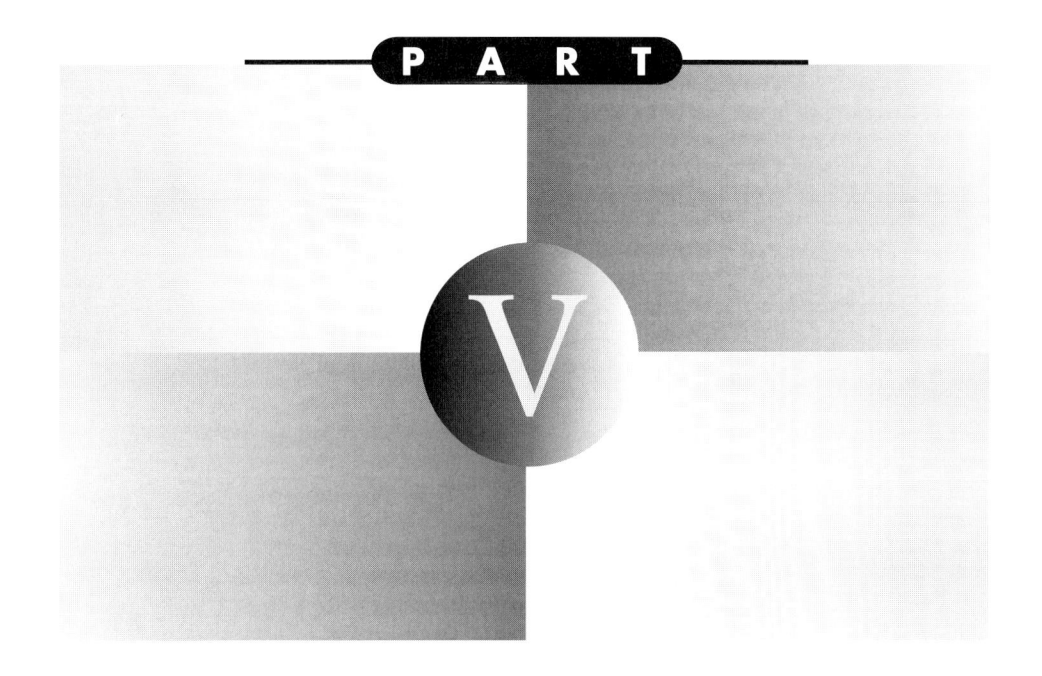

WOMEN'S ISSUES

CHAPTER 27

Thrombotic Risk of Oral Contraceptives, Postmenopausal Hormone Replacement, and Selective Estrogen Receptor Modulators (SERMs)

Steven Stein, M.D.
Barbara A. Konkle, M.D.

Hormones are used in various forms: for contraception, postmenopausal hormone replacement, treatment of hormone-responsive cancers, and, recently, breast cancer risk reduction. This chapter will focus on the association of hormone therapy with thromboembolic disease. The benefits of these drugs will be discussed in less detail. In deciding whether to prescribe hormone therapy, one must try to assess the risk:benefit ratio in each individual patient. While much still needs elucidation, the goal of this chapter is to provide the available data with which to make these decisions.

BASIC SCIENCE

Although there are numerous studies on the effect hormones have on the coagulation system, there are no clear findings that explain the increased risk of thrombosis associated with the use of these agents. Several studies have shown that estrogen activates the coagulation system. Caine and coworkers showed that the administration of 0.625 or 1.25 mg of conjugated equine estrogen to 29 healthy postmenopausal women (average age 57 years) for 3 months increased an index of thrombin generation (prothrombin fragments 1+2) in a dose-dependent manner.[1] The generation of fibrinopeptide A was also increased and levels of inhibitors of thrombin generation (protein S) and activity (antithrombin) were decreased relative to placebo. With menopause the levels of several coagulation factors increase (factors VII and VIII and fibrinogen); these changes are due to both estrogen status and aging.[2] Levels of plasminogen activator inhibitor-1, a critical inhibitor of fibrinolysis, are higher in postmenopausal women.[3] There are conflicting data about estrogen and its effect on the fibrinolytic system but on the whole there seems to be heightened fibrinolytic activity in women taking estrogens, although this effect may be secondary to increased coagulation pathway activity.[4]

Estrogens have both rapid and longer-term effects on the blood vessel wall. Estrogen influences the bioavailability of endothelial-derived nitric oxide and causes the relaxation of vascular smooth muscle cells.[5] The longer-term effects of estrogen are due, at least in part, to changes in gene and protein expression, which lead to the inhibition of the response to vascular injury and to the preventive effect of estrogen against atherosclerosis.

Although the slight increased risk of thrombosis in association with the use of oral contraceptive pills (OCPs) is well established, no clear causal relations within the hemostatic system have been reported. In general, the effects of OCPs on coagulation are modest, and several reports suggest that OCPs induce changes in the procoagulant and anticoagulant pathways that may counterbalance each other.[6]

ORAL CONTRACEPTIVE USE AND THROMBOSIS

Since their introduction, OCPs have been linked to an increased incidence of thromboembolic events.[7] First-generation OCPs included at least 50 μg of ethinylestradiol or mestranol and a progestogen, typically norethindrone. Because estrogen was suspected of increasing the risk for thromboembolism, contraceptives that contained less than 50 μg of estrogen and a new progestogen, levonorgestrel, were introduced—second-generation OCPs. More recently, the newest progestogens (desogestrel, gestodene, and norgestimate) in combination with no more than 35 μg of ethinylestradiol have become available—third-generation OCPs (see Table 27–1 for OCPs available in the United States). In 1988, 82% of prescriptions for OCPs were for formulations that contained less than 50 μg of estrogen.[8] Compared with non-OCP users, women who take second-generation OCPs have a risk for venous thrombosis that is increased about four-fold.[9] Recently, concern has been raised that third-generation OCPs further increase the risk of thromboembolims.[10] The small but definite increase in the incidence of thromboembolism in OCP users becomes more manifest when other thrombotic risk factors are present. This will be discussed later in this chapter.

Myocardial Infarction

The current use of OCPs increases the risk for myocardial infarction (MI), but most of the excess risk is attributable to a synergistic interaction with cigarette smoking.[11] Taken together, case-control and cohort studies suggest that current users of OCPs who are younger than 40 years of age and do not smoke have little or no increased risk for MI. In the United States the baseline risk for fatal ischemic heart disease ranges from 1 to 2 per 100,000 persons in women younger than 35 years of age to 4.1 per 100,000 persons in women 35 to 39 years of age and to 10 to 21 per 100,000 persons for women in their 40s.[12] Thus, most studies have been too small to address whether the risk for MI from OCP use differs according to coronary risk factors other than smoking. The data consistently show that past use of OCPs is not associated with increased risk. In a meta-analysis of 13 studies, Stampfer and coworkers estimated that past users of OCPs had a pooled relative risk for MI of 1.01 (confidence interval [CI] 0.91 to 1.13).[13] The above findings suggest that any increase in

Table 27–1 • ORAL CONTRACEPTIVES AVAILABLE IN THE UNITED STATES

Monophasic	**Estrogen (μg)**	**Progestin (mg)**
Genora 1/50, Nelova 1/50M, Norinyl 1+50, Ortho-Novum 1/50	50 mestranol	1 norethindrone
Ovcon-50	50 ethinyl estradiol	1 norethindrone
Demulen 1/50, Zovia 1/50E	50 ethinyl estradiol	1 ethynodiol
Ovral	50 ethinyl estradiol	0.5 norgestrel
Genora 1/35, NEE 1/35, Nelova 1/35E, Norethrin 1/35E, Norinyl 1+35, Ortho-Novum 1/35	35 ethinyl estradiol	1 norethindrone
Brevicon, Modicon, Genora & Nelova 0.5/35E	35 ethinyl estradiol	0.5 norethindrone
Ovcon-35	35 ethinyl estradiol	0.4 norethindrone
Ortho-Cyclen	35 ethinyl estradiol	0.25 norgestimate
Demulen 1/35, Zovia 1/35E	35 ethinyl estradiol	1 ethynodiol
Loestrin 21 1.5/30, Loestrin Fe 1.5/30	30 ethinyl estradiol	1.5 norethindrone
Lo/Ovral	30 ethinyl estradiol	0.3 norgestrel
Desogen, Ortho-Cept	30 ethinyl estradiol	0.15 desogestrel
Levlen, Levora, Nordette	30 ethinyl estradiol	0.15 levonorgestrel
Loestrin 21 1/20, Loestrin Fe 1/20	20 ethinyl estradiol	1 norethrindrone
Alesse, Levlite	20 ethinyl estradiol	0.1 levonorgestrel
Progestin-Only		
Micronor, Nor-Q.D.	None	0.35 norethindrone
Ovrette	None	0.075 norgestrel
Triphasic		
Tri-Norinyl, Ortho-Novum 7/7/7	Ethinyl estradiol	Norethindrone
Tri-Levlen, Triphasil	Ethinyl estradiol	Levonorgestrel
Ortho Tri-Cyclen	Ethinyl estradiol	Norgestimate
Other		
Estrostep, Estrostep Fe	20/30/35 ethinyl estradiol	1 norethindrone
Mircette	Ethinyl estradiol	0.15 desogestrel

Norethindrone containing OCP—First-generation OCP.
Levonorgestrel containing OCP—Second-generation OCP.
Norgestimate and desogestrel containing OCP—Third-generation OCP.

risk for MI due to OCP use occurs only with current use and probably acts through an acute prothrombotic synergism with cigarette smoking. This statement is supported by the finding that angiographic studies of young women with MI tend to show an absence of atherosclerosis in cases associated with current or recent use of OCPs.[14]

Stroke

Most recent prospective studies have not shown an increased risk for stroke among past users of OCPs and studies of stroke in current users have yielded inconsistent results.[11] Available studies are often small, do not differentiate between hemorrhagic and thromboembolic stroke, and often do not control for other major risk factors. In studies that have shown an increased risk, the interaction with smoking does not seem to be as great as that associated with myocardial infarction.

The Nurses' Health Study[15] found no statistically significant increase in risk for stroke among past users (ischemic stroke and subarachnoid hemorrhage were combined in the study). In the Royal College of General Practitioners' Oral Contraception Study,[16] past users who were smokers had an increased relative risk for stroke of 1.8 (CI 1.1 to 2.8). The World Health Organization case-control study[17] also suggested that an interaction between smoking and contraceptives was associated with ischemic stroke.

Taken together, studies of low-dose OCP suggest that these drugs produce little increase in risk for ischemic stroke, but a two- to threefold increase in risk cannot be ruled out. Occlusive stroke in young women has an estimated rate of 5.4 per 100,000 person-years.[18] Fatal occlusive stroke is even rarer, with rates less than 0.5 per 100,000 for women less than 45 years of age.[12] Therefore any attributable risk for death from occlusive stroke associated with the use of OCPs is small at most, although smokers may be more susceptible. Current studies provide no persuasive evidence of any increase in risk for hemorrhagic stroke among young women without risk factors who use low-dose OCPs.[11]

Venous Thromboembolic Disease

Soon after the introduction of OCPs, their use was associated with an increase in risk for venous thromboembolism (VTE). These were with preparations containing 50 μg of estrogen or more. The true risk with that dose is unclear as studies varied in the methods used to diagnose VTE.[19,20]

There is evidence that efforts to reduce the risk for VTE by reducing the estrogen content have proven successful. Gerstman and colleagues[21] showed a dose-response relationship between estrogen and VTE by comparing OCPs that contain high levels of estrogen (more than 50 μg) with OCPs that contain intermediate levels of estrogen (50 μg) and low levels of estrogen (less than 50 μg). A Swedish study by Böttiger and colleagues[22] noted a marked decline of approximately 80% in reports of nonfatal VTE per 100,000 users when low-dose estrogen OCPs replaced high-dose preparations. Data from prospective studies are sparse, reflecting the rarity of VTE in young women. In the Oxford Family Planning Study[23] lower incidence rates were noted among users of low-dose contraceptives (39 per 100,000 person-years) compared with users of high-dose contraceptives (62 per 100,000 person-years).

Recent studies have suggested that there is an increased risk of VTE for users of the newer progestogens (desogestrel and gestodene) compared with persons who do not use OCPs. This risk is approximately double the risk of preparations containing levonorgestrel, a progestogen in the second-generation OCPs. The World Health Organization, in a hospital-based case-control study in nine countries, found a higher incidence of VTE (relative risk 2.6 [CI 1.4 to 4.8]) in patients using the newer progestogens compared to users of second-generation (levonorgestrel) progestogens.[24] Another case-control study,[10] conducted by Spitzer and coworkers in 10 centers in Germany and the United Kingdom, found a modest increase in risk with products containing the newest progestins compared with products containing the earlier progestogens (relative risk 1.5 [CI 1.1 to 2.13]). Farmer and coworkers, in a community-based case-control study,[25] reported a relative risk of 1.76 (CI 0.91 to 3.48) and a relative risk of 1.32 (CI 0.7 to 2.69) for users of desogestrel and gestodene, respectively, compared with users of levonorgestrel. There are problems with some of the studies particularly concerning confounding variables and bias, and there are varying results; however, overall, the data are consistent with a pattern of increased risk.

Thrombophilia

Other risk factors may interact with OCP use to increase the risk of VTE. For example, women who are carriers of the factor V Leiden mutation and who use OCPs have a considerably increased risk of thrombosis.[26] Vandenbroucke and coworkers showed that the risk for thromboembolic events was increased more than 30-fold in women with the factor V Leiden mutation who also used OCPs (relative risk 34.7 [CI 7.8 to 154]).[26] Bloemenkamp and colleagues have reported that women who use OCPs containing a third-generation progestagen and who are heterozygous for the factor V Leiden mutation have a 50-fold increased risk of VTE compared with nonusers without the mutation.[27] About 4% of the West-European population appears to be heterozygous for the factor V Leiden mutation[28] and this abnormality is found in 20% to 50% of patients with venous thrombosis.[29] In a recent study by Bloemenkamp and coworkers, women who developed VTE in their first few months of OCP use were more likely to have an inherited thrombophilic state[30] than women who developed VTE after longer periods of OCP use. Among women with thrombophilia, the risk of developing deep venous thrombosis (DVT) during the first 6 months of

OCP use (compared with prolonged use) was increased 19-fold (95% CI 1.9 to 175.7) and in the first year of use, it was increased 11-fold (95% CI 2.1 to 57.3). Patients and controls in this study were considered thrombophilic if they had protein C deficiency, protein S deficiency, antithrombin deficiency, or heterozygosity for the factor V Leiden mutation or prothrombin 20210 A mutation.

Martinelli and coworkers in a small study showed that individuals heterozygous either for the 20210A mutation or for factor V Leiden are at an increased risk for cerebral venous thrombosis.[31] The use of OCPs is also strongly and independently associated with this disorder. This study found that women who were taking OCPs and who also had the prothrombin gene mutation, the odds ratio for cerebral vein thrombosis rose to 149.3 (95% CI 31 to 711). One must view this increased risk in light of the fact that cerebral venous thrombosis is a rare condition. The incidence of cerebral venous thrombosis is not precisely known, but it is much lower than the incidence of approximately 1 per 1000 persons per year reported for DVT (see Chapter 15).

It appears that women with thrombophilia who use OCPs develop VTE not only more often but also sooner after initiation of use than do women without thrombophilia. At present it is not considered cost effective to screen young healthy women for thrombophilia wanting to use OCP; however, screening could be considered in those with a family history of thromboses or inherited thrombophilia.[32,33] Price and Ridker have calculated that to protect one woman from fatal pulmonary embolism, almost 500,000 women would have to be screened to identify the 20,000 to 25,000 who would test positive for factor V Leiden. These women would then be denied the use of OCP.[34] If an OCP user develops a VTE, particularly during the first year of OCP use, then testing for thrombophilia is appropriate. While testing should be guided by family and personal history, laboratory assessment could include testing for factor V Leiden, the prothrombin 20210 mutation, lupus anticoagulant, and for protein C, protein S, and antithrombin III deficiency.

Whether or not to prescribe OCPs to women who have had VTE will depend partly on whether the VTE were idiopathic or acquired secondary to an identifiable and avoidable provocation. In the latter case, one may well decide to proceed with OCP use. For those women who are known to have an inherited thrombophilic trait or who have had idiopathic VTE, one will have to consider other means of birth control, such as barrier methods or medroxyprogesterone acetate at a dose of 150 mg intramuscularly every 3 months.

Summary

Defining risks for arterial and venous thrombosis is difficult, as events in young women on OCPs are rare and the formulations of OCPs have changed over time. Even in large cohorts, cardiovascular events are rare and thus the estimates of effect are often statistically unreliable. OCP use by nonsmokers does not seem to increase the risk for MI and the lack of an effect of past use is well documented. There may be a small to moderate increase in risk for ischemic stroke in women who use current preparations of low-dose OCPs, although no evidence supports an increased risk among past users. The newest progestogens are less androgenic, have less effect on carbohydrate and lipid metabolism, and may be associated with stronger suppression of ovarian activity. These properties have allowed a further reduction in the estrogen dose. This is no evidence that further estrogen dose reductions provide any added benefit and indeed there is some evidence that users of these newer progestogens have a higher risk of VTE than do users of other OCPs (although this relationship awaits confirmation). Many believe that second-generation OCPs are the choice for all women who use OCPs. Despite possible bias in the data showing an increased risk for VTE with third-generation OCPs, these should not be first-choice preparations. In addition, for women with known or suspected thrombophilia who choose to use OCPs, third-generation OCPs should be avoided and only second-generation OCPs should be used.

Cardiovascular diseases occur mainly among OCP users who smoke or have predisposing factors. Every effort should be made to encourage smoking cessation among potential users of OCPs. At present it is not cost effective to screen potential OCP users for the known thrombophilic gene mutations. However, should a known asymptomatic thrombophilic gene carrier want to start the OCP this should be done with the necessary caution, with strong consideration given to alternative methods of contraception.

HORMONE REPLACEMENT THERAPY AND THROMBOSIS

In the United States and other developed countries, more women die from cardiovascular disease than from any other disease. The Nurses' Health Study, among others, has suggested that postmenopausal women who take estrogen have fewer cardiovascular events over time compared with untreated women.[35] After cessation of menses (menopause), the average circulating estrogen levels eventually fall to less than 10% of premenopausal levels. This state of estrogen deficiency contributes to the acceleration of several age-related health problems in women, including cardiovascular disease, osteoporosis, and possibly dementia. Despite a large and growing body of information on the use of long-term hormone replacement therapy (HRT) to prevent or treat some of the disorders associated with menopause, whether to take postmenopausal hormones is a difficult decision and remains an area of significant therapeutic controversy and study.

Conjugated equine estrogen is by far the most widely used estrogen in the United States and has the most epidemiologic data available on its use. Because of the increased risk of endometrial hyperplasia and carcinoma with estrogen alone, most women who have not undergone hysterectomy are treated with a progestogen in addition to estrogen.

Information critical for the optimal use of HRT should be provided by large-scale, controlled clinical trials such as the U.S. National Institutes of Health-sponsored Women's Health Initiative (WHI). The WHI is a placebo-controlled long-term trial of HRT, calcium/vitamin D supplementation, and dietary modification, evaluating the effects of these interventions on many end points, including the incidence of cardiovascular disease, osteoporotic fractures, and breast cancer. The Women's International Study of Long Duration Oestrogen after Menopause (WISDOM), coordinated by the U.K. Medical Research Council, will also examine the effects of HRT during a 10-year placebo-controlled trial followed by a 10-year observation phase. The complete WHI trial will not be analyzed until at least 2005.

Cardiovascular Disease

Atherosclerosis accelerates after menopause, especially among women who have undergone surgical oophorectomy.[36] Retrospective data from case-control studies of women treated with estrogen (mostly unopposed conjugated equine estrogens) generally support the concept of a cardioprotective effect. Most of the prospective (usually nonrandomized) studies of estrogen therapy in postmenopausal women indicate a clear benefit in terms of coronary artery disease, especially a lower rate of death. It is generally believed that estrogen therapy is associated with a 40% to 50% reduction in the risk of coronary heart disease among postmenopausal women (i.e., primary prevention). This enthusiasm for HRT must be tempered by recent data, discussed below, that imply no benefits for HRT use in women with established coronary artery disease (i.e., secondary prevention).

Many of the observational studies that report reduced mortality for women taking hormones have had methodologic flaws that limit firm conclusions. Women for whom estrogens are prescribed are often healthier initially, and those who continue to take hormones tend to be free of disease. Thus lower mortality among hormone users may be attributed erroneously to the hormone itself. The benefits of postmenopausal hormone use may also be underestimated since the decrease in cardiovascular disease appears to be limited largely to current users, yet studies often combine current and past use into an "ever" category. The most frequently used and most studied replacement regimen has been estrogen alone; the recent addition of progestogen provides a more nearly physiologic replacement regimen, but this agent may oppose some of the benefits of estrogen, particularly with respect to cardiovascular disease. However, Grodstein and coworkers, using data from the Nurses' Health Study, reported that the addition of progestin did not appear to attenuate the cardioprotective effects of postmenopausal estrogen therapy.[37] In this large prospective study the risk of major coronary disease was substantially decreased among users of estrogen and progestin, as well as among current users of estrogen alone.

In the Heart and Estrogen/Progestin Replacement Study (HERS), the first large clinical trial to examine the effects of HRT on risk for cardiovascular disease, 2763 women with established coronary disease were randomly assigned to receive daily conjugated equine estrogen plus medroxyprogesterone acetate or to placebo.[38] After a mean of 4.1 years of follow-up, no differences were seen in the primary composite outcome of nonfatal MI or death from coronary heart disease (HRT group, 179 events; placebo group, 182 events; relative hazard, 0.99 [95% CI 0.81 to 1.22]) or any of the secondary clinical outcomes. This null result has shaken a foundation on which recommendations for widespread use of estrogen replacement have been built—that estrogen reduces a woman's risk for heart disease. On the basis of these results assertions regarding secondary prevention of coronary heart disease can no longer be made with confidence. However, more detailed analysis of the HERS results reveals that within the overall null effect, risk for coronary heart disease was reduced in years 3 to 5, but this reduction was offset but the unexpected 50% increase in risk during year 1. There are at least two possible explanations for the surprising data. One is that the regimen used in the HERS has no effect on risk for heart disease, and the pattern of changing risk over time is simply the result of chance. The other possible explanation is that the pattern of early increase and late reduction in risk is due to real but opposing effects of the regimen used. The HERS data indicate the need to conduct properly designed prospective randomized clinical trials to evaluate both the benefits and risks of new therapies over time. It is hoped that data from WHI and WISDOM will further elucidate these controversial areas. Herrington and coworkers[39] randomly assigned a total of 309 women with angiographically verified coronary disease to receive either 0.625 mg of conjugated estrogen plus 2.5 mg of medroxyprogesterone acetate per day, or placebo. They found that at a mean of 3.2 years, neither estrogen alone nor the combination affected the progression of coronary atherosclerosis in women with established disease.

The data on stroke and HRT use are unclear. The Leisure World Study reported that the relative risk of mortality from stroke was 0.3 among current estrogen users as compared with women who had never used estrogen.[40] Falkeborn and coworkers reported that the relative risk of stroke was 0.72 among women taking estrogen and 0.61 among those taking combined hormones.[41] Neither estrogen alone nor combined therapy substantially affected the risk of stroke in the study by Grodstein and coworkers mentioned above.[37] Similarly, a large prospective study in Copenhagen, Denmark,[42] found little association between the risk of stroke and hormone use (relative risk 0.8; 95% CI 0.4 to 1.4). At present the data on stroke are still too sparse to clarify the effect of hormones on reducing the risk of this event.

Venous Thromboembolic Disease

The use of HRT appears to increases the risk for VTE two- to three-fold; the data supporting this statement are discussed below. Daly and coworkers[43] showed that the adjusted odds ratio for VTE in current users of HRT compared with nonusers (never users and past users combined) was 3.5 (95% CI 1.8 to 7.0; $p < 0.001$). In that study no association was found with past use, and the risk of VTE appeared to be highest among short-term current users. In the conclusion of that study the authors make the point that the number of extra cases is about 1 in 5000 users per year and this should be weighed against the many documented benefits of long-term use of HRT.

Jick and coworkers in 1996 reported a case-control study of women aged 50 to 74 years in the Group Health Cooperative of Puget Sound[44] who were hospitalized for idiopathic VTE. The study reported a matched relative risk estimate of 3.6 (95% CI 1.6 to 7.8) for current users of estrogens compared to nonusers; the higher the dose of estrogen used, the higher the risk estimate for VTE. The authors of this study indicated that the absolute risk for VTE was so low that the increased risk for VTE accounted for only a modest increase in morbidity in women using HRT.

Data from the Nurses' Health study[45] showed that current users of postmenopausal hormones had an increased risk of primary pulmonary embolism (no identified antecedent cancer, trauma, surgery, or immobilization). The relative risk adjusted for multiple risk factors was 2.1 (95% CI 1.2 to 3.8); there was no association with past use. Among postmenopausal women aged 50 to 59 years in this cohort, five additional cases of PE would be expected for 100,000 person-years of HRT use.

The two- to threefold increased relative risk for thromboembolic events reported in observational studies have been confirmed by clinical trial data from the HERS.[38] In the HERS, confirmed VTE occurred in 34 women in the hormone group (6.2/1000 woman-years) and in 13 women in the placebo group (2.3/1000 woman-years). This translated to a relative hazard ratio of 2.7 (95% CI 1.4 to 5.0) for users of the estrogen/progestin combination. The excess risk was 3.9 per 1000 women years (CI 1.4 to 6.4 per 1000 woman-years) and the number needed to treat for harm was 256 (CI 157 to 692).[46] More women in the hormone group experienced DVTs (25 vs. 9; relative hazard 2.8; CI 1.3 to 6.0; $p = 0.008$) and pulmonary emboli (11 vs. 4; relative hazard 2.8; CI 0.9 to 8.7; $p = 0.08$); for two women, both in the hormone group, pulmonary emboli were fatal. Recent observational studies have reported similar relative risks for idiopathic VTE among users of both unopposed estrogen and estrogen plus progestin therapy.

Whether or not the relative risk of VTE with HRT is higher in women with underlying thrombophilia phenotypes was recently addressed.[47] The combination of HRT use and thrombophilias (especially if multiple) increased the relative risk of VTE substantially. For example, the combination of HRT use and activated protein C (APC) resistance increased the risk about 13-fold compared with women of similar age without APC resistance or HRT use (odds ratio [OR] 13.27; 95% CI 4.30 to 40.97).

In April 2000, Claude Lenfant, the director of the National Heart, Lung, and Blood Institute, released a statement concerning preliminary trends in the Women's Health Initiative (WHI). The WHI Data and Safety Monitoring Board (DSMB) noted that sufficient data had accumulated in the first 2 years of study to indicate that women in WHI who were taking hormones had somewhat more cardiovascular events than those taking placebo, yet the increases did not meet statistical criteria for stopping the trial and may have occurred by chance. All participants were informed of the trends and reminded that a similar association between HRT use and an early increase in cardiovascular risk had also been found in the HERS.

SELECTIVE ESTROGEN RECEPTOR MODULATORS AND THROMBOSIS

Selective estrogen receptor modulators (SERMs) are nonsteroidal antiestrogens. The potential value of SERMs is their combination of estrogenic and antiestrogenic activity, i.e., the ability to provide antitumor activity in the breast without antiestrogenic side effects such as decreased bone density and increased risk of cardiovascular disease. Two agents (tamoxifen and raloxifene) are discussed further below but a number of compounds are in development. These include nonsteroidal agents related to tamoxifen (toremifene, idoxifene, droloxifene and TAT-59), novel nonsteroidal agents (raloxifene, LY-353381), and pure steroidal antiestrogen agents (ICI 182,780 and EM 800). Most SERMs, including tamoxifen, are based on a triphenylethylene structure; raloxifene and LY-353381 are benzothiophenes. Newer compounds in development tend to have less agonist (estrogenic) and more antagonist (antiestrogenic) activity than tamoxifen; agents with the strongest antiestrogenic activity are raloxifene and idoxifene. In contrast, pure antiestrogens are analogs of 17-β-estradiol. These agents are generally devoid of estrogenic activity and lack cross-resistance with tamoxifen.

The estrogen agonist/antagonist tamoxifen is widely used in the management of breast cancer. Currently this drug is used in the adjuvant setting after local therapy for early-stage breast cancer that is hormone receptor positive, in the treatment of metastatic breast cancer, and prophylactically in women deemed to be at high risk for the development of invasive breast cancer. Several case reports have described women with breast cancer who developed DVT or pulmonary embolism while being treated with tamoxifen.[48] There is also growing evidence from randomized clinical trials that the incidence of VTE is higher among women exposed to tamoxifen than in comparison groups.[49]

Data from the National Surgical Adjuvant Breast and Bowel Project (NSABP) published in 1996 demonstrated a 1.7% VTE rate in tamoxifen-treated women as compared to 0.4% in the placebo-treated group.[50] Saphner and coworkers retrospectively analyzed the 10-year experience of 2673 women with breast cancer in multicenter trials conducted by the Eastern Cooperative Oncology Group (ECOG); there was an increase in VTE associated with tamoxifen therapy alone and a substantial increase in patients allocated to combined treatment with tamoxifen plus chemotherapy compared with untreated controls or those who received chemotherapy alone.[51] Specifically their data showed that premenopausal patients who received chemotherapy and tamoxifen had more venous events than those who received chemotherapy without tamoxifen (2.8% vs. 0.8%, $p = 0.03$). Postmenopausal patients who received tamoxifen and chemotherapy had more venous thrombi than those who received tamoxifen alone (8.0% vs. 2.3%, $p = 0.03$) or those who were observed (8.0%, vs. 0.4%, $p < 0.0001$). These findings and those from other studies suggest that chemotherapy contributes to thrombosis in patients with breast cancer.[52] A large U.K.-based General Practice Research Database study concluded that the relative risk estimate for VTE for current tamoxifen exposure, as compared with never and past use as a reference group, was 7.1 (95% CI 1.5 to 33).[53]

In the National Surgical Adjuvant Breast and Bowel Project (NSABP) P-1 study,[54] a randomized clinical trial of 13,388 women to evaluate the effectiveness of tamoxifen in the prevention of breast cancer in women considered to be at increased risk for the disease, the use of tamoxifen was associated with an increased risk of VTE. Pulmonary emboli were observed in almost three times as many women in the tamoxifen group as in the placebo group (18 vs. 6; RR, 3.01; 95% CI, 15 to 9.27). More women who received tamoxifen developed DVTs than did women who received placebo (35 vs. 22 cases, respectively). The average annual rates per 1000 women treated were 1.34 versus 0.84 (RR, 1.60; 95% CI, 0.91 to 2.86).

In the NSABP B24 randomized trial, in which the use of tamoxifen after lumpectomy and radiation therapy for ductal carcinoma in situ was compared to placebo, there was a slight excess of pulmonary embolism and DVTs in the treatment arm: of 891 women in the tamoxifen group, nine DVTs (1%) and two pulmonary emboli (0.2%) occurred while in the placebo arm of 890 women, two had DVTs (0.2%), and one had a pulmonary embolus (0.1%).

Increased relative risk estimates from studies published to date on the use of tamoxifen range from no effect up to a seven times increased incidence. Most authorities in the field quote a two to four times increased relative risk for VTE with the use of tamoxifen as compared to patients not receiving the drug. Again, as has often been discussed in this chapter, the absolute risk of VTE in a patient on tamoxifen may be so low as to not impact on the decision to use the agent in the management of a patient with breast cancer. There are emerging data on the increased risk for VTE that the known thrombophilic mutations, like factor V Leiden, impose on patients treated with tamoxifen, but at the present time these data are mainly in the form of case reports.[56]

Raloxifene hydrochloride is a SERM, chemically distinct from tamoxifen and estradiol, that has antiestrogenic effects on breast and endometrial tissue and estrogenic effects on bone, lipid metabolism, and the coagulation system. Currently raloxifene is U.S. Food and Drug Administration approved for the treatment of postmenopausal osteoporosis. The Multiple Outcomes of Raloxifene Evaluation (MORE) study, which treated a total of 7705 postmenopausal women with osteoporosis, was the pivotal trial leading to the drug's approval.[57] In the MORE study the use of raloxifene increased the risk of VTE (RR 3.1 [95% CI 1.5 to 6.2]). By 40 months of follow-up, there was a higher rate of DVT (38 cases) and pulmonary embolus (17 cases) in the combined raloxifene groups (60- and 120-mg doses were used) than in the placebo groups (5 and 3 cases, respectively). One case of VTE occurred for every 155 women treated with raloxifene for 3 years.

As can be ascertained from this chapter, raloxifene and tamoxifen increase the risk of VTE to a similar degree. At present, it is considered prudent not to prescribe either tamoxifen or raloxifene to a woman with a history of VTE, but the decision should be individualized based on the woman's clinical history and known underlying risk factors. There are scenarios, especially in metastatic breast cancer patients who are hormone receptor positive, when the use of tamoxifen is clearly indicated in the management of the disease, even with coexistent VTE. In these cases, such patients resonably can be placed on concomitant anticoagulation therapy.

SUMMARY

Although there are numerous studies dealing with the thrombogenic potential for the agents discussed in this chapter, data are still insufficient to confirm the true risks for VTE. We have provided a table (Table 27-2) that contains our best estimates from the available literature of the relative risks associated with these agents. Often, the absolute risks for adverse events are so low

Table 27-2 • ESTIMATED RELATIVE RISKS ASSOCIATED WITH THE USE OF HORMONAL AGENTS[a]

	OCP[b] (Smoker)	OCP (Nonsmoker)	HRT[c]	Tamoxifen/Raloxifene
MI	2	1	Decrease	No data
Stroke	1–3	No data	No data	? Increase
VTE	4	4	2–3	2–4

[a] Authors' opinions based on available literature.
[b] OCP, oral contraceptive.
[c] HRT, hormone replacement therapy.

as not to impact on the risk:benefit calculations that are estimated when deciding whether or not to use these agents. As is almost always the case in clinical medicine, decisions have to be highly individualized, as the benefits of these agents to the patient and society may be large and the risks may be small. With the expanding use of hormonal agents, including SERMs, the need to better define risks for thrombotic events in women with a remote history of thrombosis or a laboratory-defined hypercoagulable state are needed. Additionally, an understanding of the pathogenesis of hormonally induced thrombosis would aid in the development of new therapies without this side effect.

REFERENCES

Chapter 27 References

1. Caine YG, Bauer KA, Barzegar S, et al. Coagulation activation following estrogen administration to postmenopausal women. Thromb Haemost 1992;68:392–395.
2. Meade TW, Imerson JD, Haines AP, et al. Menopausal status and hemostatic variables. Lancet 1983;1:22–24.
3. Gebara OCE, Mittleman MA, Sutherland P, et al. Association between increased estrogen status and increased fibrinolytic potential in the Framingham Offspring Study. Circulation 1995;91:1952–1958.
4. Scarabin PY, Plu-Bureau G, Bara L, et al. Haemostatic variables and menopausal status: influence of hormonal replacement therapy. Thromb Haemost 1993;70:584–587.
5. Joswig M, Hach-Wunderle V, Ziegler R, et al. Postmenopausal hormone replacement and the vascular wall: mechanism of 17 beta-estradiol's effects on vascular biology. Exp Clin Endocrinol Diabetes 1999;107:477–487.
6. Speroff L, DeCherney A. Evaluation of a new generation of oral contraceptives. The Advisory Board for the New Progestins. Obstet Gynecol 1993;81:1034–1047.
7. Jordan WM. Pulmonary embolism. Lancet 1961;2:1146–1147.
8. Gerstman BB, Gross TP, Kennedy DL, et al. Trends in the content and use of oral contraceptives in the United States, 1964–88. Am J Public Health 1991;81:90–98.
9. World Health Organization Collaborative Study of Cardiovascular Disease and Steroid Hormone Contraception. Venous thromboembolic disease and combined oral contraceptives: results of international multicenter case-control study. Lancet 1995;346:1575–1582.
10. Spitzer WO, Lewis MA, Heinemann LAJ, et al. Third generation oral contraceptives and risk of venous thromboembolic disorders: an international case-control study. Transnational Research Group on Oral Contraceptives and the Health of Young Women. Br Med J 1996;312:83–88.
11. Chasan-Taber L, Stampfer MJ. Epidemiology of oral contraceptives and cardiovascular disease. Ann Intern Med 1998;128:467–477.
12. Vital statistics of the United States, 1992. vol. 1. Mortality, part B. Hyattsville, MD; U.S. Dept. of Health and Human Services, Centers for Disease Control and Prevention, National Center for Health Statistics, 1996; pp. 24–27.
13. Stampfer MJ, Willett WC, Colditz GA, et al. Past use of oral contraceptives and cardiovascular disease: a meta-analysis in the context of the Nurses' Health Study. Am J Obstet Gynecol 1990;163:285–291.
14. Jugdutt BI, Stevens GF, Zacks DJ, et al. Myocardial infarction, oral contraception, cigarette smoking, and coronary artery spasm in young women. Am Heart J 1983;106:757–761.
15. Stampfer MJ, Willett WC, Colditz GA, et al. A prospective study of past use of oral contraceptive agents and risk of cardiovascular diseases. N Engl J Med 1988;319:1313–1317.
16. Hannaford PC, Croft PR, Kay CR. Oral contraception and stroke: Evidence from the Royal College of General Practitioners' Oral Contraception Study. Stroke 1994;25:935–942.
17. Ischaemic stroke and combined oral contraceptives: results of an international, multicentre, case-control study. WHO Collaborative Study of Cardiovascular Disease and Steroid Hormone Contraception. Lancet 1996;348:498–505.
18. Petitti DB, Sidney S, Bernstein A, et al. Stroke in users of low-dose oral contraceptives. N Engl J Med 1996;335:8–15.
19. Huisman MV, Buller HR, ten Cate JW, et al. Serial impedance plethysmography for suspected deep venous thrombosis in outpatients. The Amsterdam General Practitioners Study. N Engl J Med 1986;314:823–828.
20. Lensing AW, Prandoni P, Brandjes D, et al. Detection of deep-vein thrombosis by real-time B-mode ultrasonography. N Engl J Med 1989;320:342–345.
21. Gerstman BB, Piper JM, Tomita DK, et al. Oral contraceptive estrogen dose and the risk of deep venous thromboembolic disease. Am J Epidemiol 1991;133:32–37.
22. Böttiger LE, Boman G, Eklund G, et al. Oral contraceptives and thromboembolic disease: effects of lowering oestrogen content. Lancet 1989;1178:1097–1101.
23. Vessey M, Mant D, Smith A, et al. Oral contraceptives and venous thromboembolism: findings in a large prospective study. Br Med J (Clin Res Ed) 1986;292:526.
24. Effect of different progestagens in low oestrogen oral contraceptives on venous thromboembolic disease. World Health Organization Collaborative Study of Cardiovascular Disease and Steroid Hormone Contraception. Lancet 1995;346:1582–1588.
25. Farmer RD, Lawrenson RA, Thompson CR, et al. Population-based study of risk of venous thromboembolism associated with various oral contraceptives. Lancet 1997;349:83–88.
26. Vandenbroucke JP, Koster T, Briet E, et al. Increased risk of venous thrombosis in oral-contraceptive users who are carriers of factor V Leiden mutation. Lancet 1994;344:1453–1457.
27. Bloemenkamp KWM, Rosendaal FR, Helmerhorst FM, et al. Enhancement by factor V Leiden mutation of risk of deep-vein thrombosis associated with oral contraceptives containing a third generation progestagen. Lancet 1995;346:1593–1596.
28. Rosendaal FR, Koster T, Vandenbroucke JP, et al. High risk of thrombosis in patients homozygous for factor V Leiden. Blood 1995;85:1504–1508.
29. Svensson PJ, Dahlback B. Resistance to activated protein C as a basis for venous thrombosis. N Engl J Med 1994;330:517–522.
30. Bloemenkamp KWM, Rosendaal FR, Helmerhost FM, et al. Higher risk of venous thrombosis during early use of oral contraceptives in women with inherited clotting defects. Arch Intern Med 2000;160:49–52.
31. Martinelli I, Sacchi E, Landi G, et al. High risk of cerebral-vein thrombosis in carriers of a prothrombin-gene mutation and in users of oral contraceptives. N Engl J Med 1998;338:1793–1797.
32. Rosendaal FR. Oral contraceptives and screening for factor V Leiden. Thromb Haemost 1996;75:524–525.
33. Vandenbroucke JP, van der Meer FJM, Helmerhost FM, et al. Factor V Leiden: should we screen oral contraceptive users and pregnant women? Br Med J 1996;313:1127–1130.
34. Price, DT, Ridker PM. Factor V Leiden mutation and the risk of thromboembolic disease: A clinician's perspective. Ann Intern Med 1997;127:895–903.
35. Stampfer MJ, Colditz GA, Willett WC, et al. Postmenopausal estrogen therapy and cardiovascular disease: ten-year follow-up from the Nurses' Health Study. N Engl J Med 1991; 325:756–762.
36. Colditz GA, Willett WC, Stampfer MJ, et al. Menopause and the risk of coronary heart disease in women. N Engl J Med 1987; 316:1105–1110.

37. Grodstein F, Stampfer MJ, Manson JE, et al. Postmenopausal estrogen and progestin use and risk of cardiovascular disease. N Engl J Med 1996;335:453–461.
38. Hulley S, Grady D, Bush T, et al. Randomized trial of estrogen plus progestin for secondary prevention of coronary heart disease in postmenopausal women. Heart and Estrogen/progestin Replacement Study (HERS) Research Group. JAMA 1998;280:605–613.
39. Herrington DM, Reboussin DM, Brosnihan KB, et al. Effects of estrogen replacement on the progression of coronary-artery atherosclerosis. N Engl J Med 2000;343:522–529.
40. Henderson BE, Paganini-Hill A, Ross RK. Decreased mortality in users of estrogen replacement therapy. Arch Intern Med 1991;151:75–78.
41. Falkeborn M, Persson I, Terent A, et al: Hormone replacement therapy and the risk of stroke: follow-up of a population-based cohort in Sweden. Arch Intern Med 1993;153:1201–1209.
42. Boysen G, Nyboe J, Appleyard M, et al. Stroke incidence and risk factors for stroke in Copenhagen, Denmark. Stroke 1988;16:1345–1353.
43. Daly E, Vessey MP, Hawkins MW, et al. Risk of venous thromboembolism in users of hormone replacement therapy. Lancet 1996;348:977–980.
44. Jick H, Derby LE, Myers MW, et al. Risk of hospital admission for idiopathic venous thromboembolism among users of postmenopausal estrogens. Lancet 1996;348:981–983.
45. Grodstein F, Stampfer MJ, Goldhaber SZ, et al. Prospective study of exogenous hormones and risk of pulmonary embolism in women. Lancet 1996;348:983–987.
46. Grady D, Wenger NK, Herrington D, et al. Postmenopausal hormone therapy increases risk for venous thromboembolic disease. Ann Intern Med 2000;132:689–696.
47. Lowe G, Woodward M, Vessey M, et al. Thrombotic variables and risk of idiopathic venous thromboembolism in women aged 45–64 years: Relationship to hormone replacement therapy. Thromb Haemost 2000;83:530–535.
48. Nevasaari K, Heikkinen M, Taskinen PJ. Tamoxifen and thrombosis. Lancet 1978;2:946–947.
49. Fisher B, Costantino J, Redmond C, et al. A randomized clinical trial evaluating tamoxifen in the treatment of patients with node-negative breast cancer who have estrogen-receptor positive tumors. N Engl J Med 1989;320:479–484.
50. Fisher B, Dignam J, Bryant J, et al. Five versus more than five years of tamoxifen therapy for breast cancer patients with negative lymph nodes and estrogen-positive tumors. J Natl Cancer Inst 1996;88:1529–1542.
51. Saphner T, Tormey DC, Gray R. Venous and arterial thrombosis in patients who received adjuvant therapy for breast cancer. J Clin Oncol 1991;9:286–294.
52. Levine MN, Gent M, Hirsh J, et al. The thrombogenic effect of anticancer drug therapy in women with stage II breast cancer. N Engl J Med 1988;318:404–407.
53. Meier CR, Jick H. Tamoxifen and risk of idiopathic venous thromboembolism. Br J Clin Pharmacol 1998;45:608–612.
54. Fisher B, Constantino JP, Wickerham DL, et al. Tamoxifen for the prevention of breast cancer: report of the National Surgical Adjuvant Breast and Bowel Project P-1 study. J Natl Cancer Inst 1998;90:1371–1388.
55. Fisher B, Dignam J, Wolmark N, et al. Tamoxifen in treatment of intraductal breast cancer: National Surgical Adjuvant Breast and Bowel Project B-24 randomised controlled trial. Lancet 1999;353:1993–2000.
56. Weitz IC, Israel VK, Liebman HA. Tamoxifen-associated venous thrombosis and activated protein C resistance due to factor V Leiden. Cancer 1997;79:2024–2027.
57. Ettinger B, Black DM, Mitlak BH, et al. Reduction of vertebral fracture risk in postmenopausal women with osteoporosis treated with raloxifene: results from a 3-year randomized clinical trial. Multiple Outcomes of Raloxifene Evaluation (MORE) Investigators. JAMA 1999;282:637–645.

CHAPTER 28

Management of Bleeding Disorders in Pregnancy

Stephanie Seremetis, M.D.
Victoria Afshani, M.D.

Bleeding disorders during pregnancy and the puerperium pose specific and sometimes difficult management problems for both the obstetrician and the consulting hematologist. Issues relating to diagnosis and management may relate to both the mother and her unborn child. The various bleeding disorders can be categorized into several distinct categories. First are the inherited disorders, including the relatively common von Willebrand disease (vWD), the less common factor deficiencies, and the inherited platelet disorders. The second category comprises acquired disorders that typically manifest prior to pregnancy, including immune thrombocytopenic purpura (ITP) and clotting factor inhibitors, but may also first occur in the context of pregnancy. Finally there are disorders related directly to the physical or pathophysiologic mechanisms that can occur in pregnancy. The alterations in the normal hematologic responses to pregnancy that lead to disregulation of the clotting cascade include both disseminated intravascular coagulation (DIC) and the hemolysis with elevated liver functions and low platelets (HELLP) syndrome. Obstetric and anatomic causes include placental issues such as placenta previa and abruption, ectopic pregnancy, abortion and miscarriage, and retained products of conception. For management of these presentations, the reader is referred to a textbook of obstetrics and gynecology. Occasionally medications are implicated when a bleeding tendency develops during pregnancy. The use of aspirin and heparin in women who have cardiac disease, including coronary artery disease and coronary valve replacement with mechanical prostheses, as well as in women with systemic lupus erythematosus (SLE) with or without circulating anticoagulants or with known venous or arterial thromboses, has the potential to cause increased bleeding during pregnancy.

INHERITED DISORDERS OF BLEEDING IN PREGNANCY

Coagulation Factor Changes During Normal Pregnancy

Normal pregnancy is a relatively procoagulant state, as coagulation and fibrinolytic pathways undergo major changes that lead to a net increased propensity for clotting. The concentrations of some coagulation factors increase significantly, as do the concentrations of plasminogen activation inhibitors, which decrease the activity of the fibrinolytic system. Both factor VIII and von Willebrand factor (vWF) increase steadily throughout gestation.[1-5] Factors VII and X and fibrinogen also rise significantly.[4,6] Other factors in the clotting cascade, factors II, IX, XII, and XIII, show no difference in levels throughout pregnancy.[6] Controversial data regarding factor XI levels have been published, with reports of an increase or a fall in the levels with advancing gestation.[6,7] Additionally, the platelet count may decrease slightly in the third trimester during normal pregnancy, but not to a degree that will pose a risk of bleeding during delivery.[8,9] The bleeding time, which reflects primary hemostasis, remains normal throughout pregnancy or may shorten, reflecting the increased platelet–endothelium interactions of pregnancy. The prothrombin time (PT) and activated partial thromboplastin time (aPTT) may decrease to the lower limits of normal or be slightly shortened in plasma from women in the third trimester, suggesting a low-grade process of intravascular coagulation.[9]

Coagulation Factor Changes in Inherited Bleeding Disorders

In pregnant women with inherited bleeding disorders, the data regarding coagulation factor levels are less mature. Women with type 1 von Willebrand disease (vWD) or who are carriers of hemophilia A sustain a significant rise in levels of factor VIII and both the antigen and activity of vWF in the second half of pregnancy. These women therefore rarely need hemostatic treatment later in pregnancy or during delivery. Factor IX levels, in contrast, remain relatively constant during gestation. Factor XI levels have not been measured prospectively during pregnancy in patients deficient in factor XI.

Von Willebrand Disease

Von Willebrand disease (vWD) is the most common inherited bleeding disorder, with prevalence estimated at 1% to 3% in the general population[4] (see Chapter 7 for a detailed discussion of vWD). The precise frequency of vWD is difficult to determine, as there is considerable genotypic and clinical heterogeneity in this disorder. The majority of cases of vWD are inherited in an autosomal dominant pattern; thus the implications for women of childbearing age are significant. The disorder is classified into three major types, types 1, 2, and 3, based on the specific pathophysiologic mechanisms involved. The classification of vWD was recently the subject of a consensus committee of the International Society on Thrombosis and Haemostasis,[10] which proposed a revised system that retains the three major types of vWD, and further classifies type 2 into four subtypes, based on laboratory and clinical data. Type 1 vWD, which comprises 70% to 80% of all cases, usually causes only mild bleeding. Type 2 accounts for another 10%. Type 3 vWD, which is the only form inherited in an autosomal recessive pattern, makes up an additional 10% of cases, and causes the most severe bleeding manifestations. Correct determination of the specific subtype of vWD becomes important for both counseling and therapy during pregnancy and delivery.[10]

Clinical Presentation of vWD at Diagnosis

The clinical manifestations of vWD classically are mucocutanaeous hemorrhage, in contrast to the deep-tissue hemorrhage associated with hemophilia A. Many cases, particularly of the milder forms, go undiagnosed until the pathways of coagulation are exposed to the stress of trauma, surgery, or administration of antiplatelet agents. Increasingly, menorrhagia has been identified as a sentinel symptom of an inherited coagulopathy in menstruating women.[11] Menorrhagia of long-standing duration, specifically from onset of menarche, recently has been shown to be a valuable predictor of a systemic bleeding disorder, and may be the first clue to milder forms of these disorders.[12] In one study, menorrhagia was defined objectively and measured and then used as a screening method for bleeding disorders; 17% of women with this complaint were subsequently diagnosed as having a coagulopathy. Conversely, almost 75% of women with a defined coagulopathy reported menorrhagia as a presenting complaint.[11,12]

Changes in Factor Levels With Gestation

Among the original observations made by von Willebrand regarding the disease named for him was that obstetric patients with this disorder were at less risk of hemorrhage during pregnancy than at any other times. He also observed that these patients were at increased risk for postpartum bleeding episodes.[13] Type 1 vWD, which is a quantitative disorder resulting from an absolute deficiency of vWF, typically has equivalently low plasma levels of all three aspects of the factor VIII complex: factor VIII coagulant activity (FVIII:C), vWF antigen (vWF:Ag), and vWF activity (vWF:Ac), usually in the range of 5 to 40 IU/dL. During pregnancy in type 1 patients, factor levels of both vWF and factor VIII increase steadily, beginning in the second trimester, to levels that reach three to four times her nonpregnant baseline by the time of delivery in the majority of women. Levels may increase even further during active labor.[2] Immediately postpartum the levels begin to fall rapidly and within several weeks reach prepregnancy levels.

Type 2A is a qualitative disorder caused by mutations in the vWF gene that result in a variable decrease in plasma vWF:Ag, marked decrease in vWF:Ac measured as the vWF ristocetin cofactor (RcoF), and absence of high and intermediate molecular weight vWF forms on gel electrophoresis.[14] The severity of the bleeding risk is proportional to the level of vWF:RcoF.[15] vWF levels increase throughout pregnancy, but the abnormal multimers remain, thus the benefit of the increase may not be as significant as for type 1 disease. Type 2B is further characterized by a mutation in the vWF gene that causes increased affinity for the platelet membrane glycoprotein Ib. Thrombocytopenia results from the enhanced binding of platelets to vWF, and as the vWF levels rise during pregnancy, thrombocytopenia may worsen.[16] The increased platelet aggregation, even in the setting of thrombocytopenia, may paradoxically predispose to thrombosis.

Type 3 vWD, the most severe and least common form, results from total absence of vWF:Ag and vWF:Ac, due to gross mutations of the vWF gene, with resultant severe decrease (i.e., 2% to 5% of normal) in FVIII:C. The levels do not rise during pregnancy, and therefore pregnant women with this form of vWD remain at severe risk of hemorrhage throughout pregnancy as well as during the postpartum period.

General experience suggests that low RcoF levels are the most important determinant of abnormal surgical or peripartum bleeding. Bleeding risk for the majority of women with vWD appears to be greatest in the immediate postpartum or postabortion period when factor VIII and vWF levels may drop precipitously.[3] Monitoring of factor levels should occur at least every 8 to 12 weeks beginning at the confirmation of pregnancy and continuing 6 to 8 weeks postpartum.[17] More frequent testing may be necessary during the puerperium. Factor levels of 50 IU/dL, which reflect the lower end of the normal range, generally are considered to be a safe threshold above which there is no increased risk of bleeding complications, and is the usual therapeutic goal for replacement therapy when such intervention is indicated.

First-trimester vaginal bleeding occurs in women with vWD at a rate of 33% in one study, which is twice the incidence of 16% in all pregnant women. However, the overall spontaneous miscarriage rate is the same (21%) in both groups, reflecting no evidence of increased pregnancy loss in this population. The increased documentation of even minor vaginal bleeding may reflect a reporting bias in women who have a heightened awareness to the significance of gestational bleeding in their circumstance. Furthermore, the incidence of antepartum hemorrhage was not increased in vWD.[5]

Therapy During Labor and Delivery

It is useful to recheck the factor levels at 34 to 36 weeks' gestation, to prepare for delivery. At coagulation factor levels of 50 IU/dL and above, uncomplicated vaginal deliveries are unlikely to be associated with abnormal bleeding. If labor is prolonged, or if a caesarian section is planned or becomes necessary, then factor levels should ideally exceed 50 IU/dL to minimize bleeding. A planned delivery date either by induction or by caesarian section may facilitate the timing of administration of factors. Many patients with type 1 vWD and some with type 2A do not require additional intervention prior to delivery because of the increases in factor levels. Table 28–1 outlines therapies for different procedures that are performed during pregnancy or at parturition. Typically factor concentrates such as Humate-P, Alphanate, or Koate-DVI,[18,19] which contain both factor VIII and vWF, are used to replace the deficient factors in type 2B and type 3, as well as in those few patients with type 1 or 2A who do not reach acceptable factor levels. Parturient women with type 2B or type 3 probably should receive factor replacement to a level greater than 50 IU/dL for at least 3 to 4 days to minimize hemorrhage. Specific dosing with clotting factor concentrates during pregnancy as distinct from other surgical prophylaxis in vWD has not been established. Data are available only from anecdotal reports and must be generalized from larger experience in the use of these clotting factor concentrates in surgery.[15] Dosing recommendations are made in terms of RcoF units with the caution that only one of the currently available clotting factor concentrates containing vWF (Humate-P) is labeled specifically with reference to RcoF units (see product insert, Aventis-Behring). Delivery should be regarded as a moderate or severe challenge to hemostasis and be treated by analogy as minor or major surgical episodes are treated. Thus, in major hemostatic challenges (e.g., caesarian section) a dose of 50 to 75 IU/kg vWF should be given, with subsequent dosing of 40 to 60 IU/kg every 8 to 12 hours for 3 days, the goal being to maintain the nadir level of RcoF greater than 50 IU/dL.[15] Therapy can be changed to daily administration of 50 IU/kg for a total of up to 7 days of treatment. Again, it is difficult to establish clear norms for use of this intervention in that very little to no data are available. It is widely assumed that caesarean section presents the same stresses as a major surgical procedure, while episiotomy or a low-degree tear during delivery would present a minor surgical stress.

DDAVP in Pregnancy

Intravenous administration of DDAVP (desmopressin) results in an increase in FVIII:C and vWF concentrations by stimulating V_2 receptors. This rise lasts for more than 6 hours and the biologic half-life is only marginally shorter than that of exogenous factor VIII and vWF from plasma concentrates.[20] DDAVP has also been shown to prevent bleeding in mild or moderate hemophilia or vWD. Some hematologists and obstetricians are reluctant to use it during pregnancy because of the

Table 28–1 • SUGGESTED TREATMENT OF vWD DURING PREGNANCY

Type	1	2A	2B	3
Change expected with pregnancy	Usually normalize	May normalize	vWF rises, platelets fall	No change
Therapy for antenatal procedures (<50 IU/dL)	Humate-P, Alphanate, or Koate DVI for 2–3 days	Humate-P, Alphanate, or Koate DVI for 2–3 days	Humate-P, Alphanate, or Koate DVI for 2–3 days	Humate-P, Alphanate, or Koate DVI for 2–3 days
Vaginal delivery	No replacement if >50 IU/dL[a]	No replacement if >50 IU/dL[a]	Factor concentrate	Factor concentrate
C-section	No replacement if >50 IU/dL[a]	No replacement if >50 IU/dL[a]	Factor conc. for 7 days	Factor conc. for 7 days
Postpartum	DDAVP/factor conc. 3–4 days	DDAVP/factor conc. 3–4 days	Factor conc. for 3–4 days	Factor conc. for 3–4 days

[a] If no factor replacement, monitor factor levels for 2 to 4 days after delivery.

risk of inducing uterine contractions and preterm labor. However, DDAVP is very specific to V_2 receptors and has little effect on smooth muscle V_1 receptors and consequently does not cause uterine contraction.[21] The other concern regarding antenatal use of DDAVP regards a possible decrease in blood flow from the placenta and subsequent intrauterine growth retardation; however, DDAVP's vasopressor effect is weak.[21] There are several publications on the management of diabetes insipidus[22] and Ehlers-Danlos syndrome[23] in pregnant women with no harm to the fetus. While the theoretical risk of uterine contraction may be a contraindication to use during pregnancy, this should not be a problem for a patient in labor. The use of DDAVP is indicated in the immediate postpartum period in type 1 and type 2A, generally for a period of 3 to 4 days, to minimize the risk of postpartum hemorrhage, which has occurred in as many as 25% of parturients in some series.[24] When DDAVP is used in the postpartum period, hyponatremia has been reported and thus serum sodium concentration should be monitored during DDAVP therapy. The use of hypotonic intravenous fluids should be minimized, and oral fluids somewhat restricted. Women who present with spontaneous miscarriage or elective termination are also at increased risk for hemorrhage, and should also empirically receive DDAVP therapy (if type 1 or 2A) or clotting factor concentrate for several days following the event. Women who exhibit evidence of bleeding despite DDAVP therapy should also receive a factor concentrate such as Humate-P.

Therapy During Prenatal Diagnostic Testing and for Anesthesia

Prenatal diagnosis of the fetus usually occurs within the first trimester of pregnancy, either by chorionic villus sampling or by amniocentesis. It is therefore possible, but less likely than would be the case later in pregnancy, that the coagulation factors involved will have risen to a safe range for invasive procedures. Measurement of maternal FVIII:C should be obtained within 1 week of the procedure, and adequate therapy administered for factor VIII levels below 50 IU/dL. As this procedure represents a minor hemostatic challenge, correction should continue for 48 to 72 hours after the procedure. Clotting factor concentrates may be used; in this instance, too, there is disagreement as to the role of DDAVP. Anecdotes describe its use and there is no published evidence of a specific contraindication in early pregnancy. It is our practice to have a comprehensive discussion with the patient about risks and benefits of each of the approaches, and to individualize therapy.

The use of regional anesthesia must be decided for each woman, as recommendations remain controversial. In one series, patients with type 1 or 2A vWD underwent epidural catheter placement with factor VIII levels 50 IU/dL or higher without untoward consequences.[25] Some centers recommend that the bleeding time also be checked and believe that if it is below 15 minutes, there is no increased risk for hemorrhagic complications.

Hemophilias

Hemophilia A (factor VIII deficiency) and hemophilia B (factor IX deficiency) are both inherited in an X-linked recessive pattern. Women from hemophilia-affected families are most commonly asymptomatic carriers. However, 10% to 20% of female carriers may be at risk for significant bleeding complications due to extreme lyonization and subsequent reduction of factor VIII or IX to levels below the minimal amount to maintain hemostatic equilibrium. Hemophilia carriers would be expected on average to have factor levels of 50% of normal, with normal ranging from 50 to 150 IU/dL, as only one chromosome is affected. However, levels as low as 5% have been reported as a result of lyonization, the random inactivation of one of each pair of X chromosomes.[26] Factor levels below 30 IU/dL could lead to clinical bleeding analogous to that seen in classical mild hemophilia A.[27]

Two unusual conditions may result in factor VIII levels low enough to be of concern during pregnancy. The first, vWD type 2N (Normandy), consists of distinct missense mutations that inactivate the binding site of factor VIII on vWF. The platelet function and multimer patterns are normal, but FVIII:C levels are low, frequently less than 10%, which causes these patients to resemble mild hemophilia A patients. Because of the qualitative defect in the vWF protein, these patients have short-lived factor VIII responses to DDAVP or to highly purified or recombinant factor VIII products. The management of choice during pregnancy is a plasma-derived vWF product such as Humate-P, which contains normal vWF as well as factor VIII.[28,29]

In the second, Turner syndrome (gonadal dysgenesis), the 45, X karyotype seen in 50% of cases, will result in streak gonads and infertility. However, 25% of affected individuals will have (46, XX/45, X) mosaicism and 25% will have a (46, XX) structurally abnormal X chromosome.[30] A small number of these women will have sufficient follicles to become pregnant, and if they are from hemophilia A-affected families, they may exhibit severe factor deficiencies, and must be managed accordingly during pregnancy.

There is limited literature regarding the changes of clotting factors during pregnancy in patients with bleeding disorders. However, a significant rise in FVIII:C, vWF:Ag, and vWF:Ac has been reported in normal women, in carriers of hemophilia A, and, as previously discussed, in patients with vWD of the various subtypes. These increases generally begin during the late first trimester and gradually levels continue to increase until the end of pregnancy. It is therefore extremely rare for women, even those who as a consequence of extreme lyonization have low factor VIII levels at baseline, to require treatment during late pregnancy or at parturition. However, consideration of prophylaxis for bleeding at the time of prenatal diagnostic testing must be undertaken; carriers with low factor VIII levels (whose levels may still be less than 50 IU/dL at term) are at considerable risk of bleeding and will require prophylactic treatment. In contrast to factor VIII and vWF, factor

IX levels do not increase through pregnancy although controversial results have been published regarding changes in this plasma protein. The hemostatic challenges of pregnancy, such as invasive prenatal diagnostic techniques, termination of pregnancy, spontaneous abortion, normal spontaneous vaginal delivery, and delivery by caesarian section, can all be complicated by excessive and prolonged hemorrhage. It is important, therefore, that factor levels be checked before any of these procedures are undertaken and that prophylactic treatment be arranged when factor levels are less than 50 IU/dL for factor VIII and factor IX. Because it may not be possible to measure factor levels in emergency situations, we recommend that these should be assayed at regular intervals during the gestation, at least once per trimester. Usually carriers of hemophilia A will normalize factor VIII levels during pregnancy to well above 50 IU/dL and thus do not require therapeutic intervention. However, women who are carriers of factor IX deficiency will often require consideration of prophylactic treatment with clotting factor concentrate, as levels do not significantly change during pregnancy.

For women who are carriers of hemophilia A, DDAVP may be considered as an appropriate pharmacologic intervention to increase the factor VIII level above 50 IU/dL. The provisos with regard to the use of this agent were outlined in the section on treatment of vWD during pregnancy and will not be repeated here. If inadequate response to DDAVP is noted, or if there is discomfort on the part of the physician or patient with regard to the use of DDAVP after a comprehensive discussion of risks and benefits of this therapeutic approach, then treatment with recombinant factor VIII concentrates should be undertaken in the context of prophylaxis of excessive bleeding either during invasive procedures or at the time of delivery (Table 28–2). Again, the interventions at the time of prenatal diagnostic testing are generally regarded as minor surgical interventions requiring 3 days of therapy at levels allowing the achievement of a nadir of 50 IU/dL. Calculations of the dose to be administered are based on the baseline clotting factor available and desired goal of therapy. Women who are carriers of hemophilia B would be at increased risk of bleeding in the context of diagnostic interventions during pregnancy or at the time of labor and delivery. If the patient requires correction of the baseline concentration of factor IX, the use of recombinant factor IX concentrates would be indicated (Table 28–2). The goal would be to maintain a nadir of 50 IU/dL or higher; most diagnostic interventions would be considered as minor surgical procedures and caesarian section a major surgical procedure.

Factor XI Deficiency

Factor XI deficiency is a prevalent genetic disorder among the Ashkenazi Jewish population, with a heterozygous frequency of 8%.[31] Its frequency in non-Jews is unknown. The inheritance pattern is autosomal, with severe deficiency in homozygotes and partial deficiency in heterozygotes. Normal plasma levels are 70 to 150 IU/dL. Homozygotes typically have factor levels below 15 IU/dL, while the range for heterozygotes is 15 IU/dL to the lower range of normal.[32] Unlike forms of vWD and hemophilia, factor XI-deficient patients do not have spontaneous pathologic bleeding, but may have significant hemorrhage after a hemostatic challenge. Menstruation may represent the first such challenge for women of childbearing age. Importantly, there is poor correlation between the factor XI level and bleeding tendency,[32–34] and even homozygotes with undetectable levels may have never experienced hemorrhage even with surgery, trauma, or previous pregnancies. Such patients are usually discovered during family studies or by evaluation of a prolonged aPTT. Additionally, the tendency to bleed following hemostatic challenge may also vary over time in individuals with this deficiency. Furthermore, the presence of additional coagulation defects, the most common of which is vWD, in a factor XI-deficient patient can further influence the bleeding risk.

Factor XI Deficiency in Pregnancy

The changes in plasma factor XI levels in factor XI-deficient women during pregnancy have not been studied extensively. Results in normal women have been

Table 28–2 • SUGGESTED FACTOR REPLACEMENT FOR SELECTED INHERITED BLEEDING DISORDERS

	Prenatal Procedure/Labor and Delivery	**Postpartum Care**
Hemophilia A carrier	Factor >50 IU/dL No therapy Factor <50 IU/dL DDAVP or rFVIII × 3 d	No therapy DDAVP or rFVIII conc. for 3–4 days
Hemophilia B carrier	Factor >50 IU/dL No therapy Factor <50 IU/dL rFIX conc. × 3 days	No therapy rFIX conc. 3–4 days
Factor XI	Factor XI conc. to goal 40 IU/dL × 1 dose (10–15 mL/kg) or FFP	FXI conc. q 48h × 3–5 days (10–15 mL/kg) or FFP
Factor XIII	Treatment throughout pregnancy with cryoprecipitate	3–4 days of cryoprecipitate

FFP, fresh frozen plasma; rFVIII, recombinant factor VIII; rFIX, recombinant factor IX.

conflicting, with some studies showing an increase[6] and others a fall in levels during pregnancy.[7,35] The one available study evaluating factor XI-deficient women showed inconsistent changes in the second and third trimesters of pregnancy. Four women had some increase and four had a slight decrease in the factor XI levels from baseline.[36] Prospective studies of changes in factor XI levels during pregnancy and postpartum need to be conducted.

Therapy During Pregnancy

Conventional treatment for factor XI deficiency employs fresh frozen plasma. This therapy potentially is problematic for both the usual risks of transmission of infectious agents and volume challenge, the latter of which is partially balanced by the long half-life of infused factor XI (50 hours). Factor XI concentrate, currently in development but not available in the United States, permits correction of the isolated factor deficiency with less risk of viral exposure.[37] Several case reports of factor XI-related thromboses have been reported. This complication occurred only in a population with known pre-existing thrombotic or vascular disease.[34,38] While there is a potential risk due to the hypercoagulable state induced by pregnancy, no reports of thrombotic complications in pregnant women deficient in factor XI have been reported. If prescribing factor XI replacement, the goal of therapy should be a factor level of approximately 40 IU/dL,[36] to minimize bleeding, for a period of 3 to 4 days after a vaginal delivery and 4 to 5 days after a caesarian section (see Table 28–2). It is important to maintain factor levels as close to the target level of 40 IU/dL as possible, and to avoid levels in excess of 100 IU/dL, as this theoretically may increase the thrombotic risk. The dose should not exceed 30 IU/kg.[37] If the woman has other risk factors in addition to pregnancy for a hypercoagulable state (e.g., obesity, increased age, or vascular disease), then fresh frozen plasma should be employed instead. In patients without any prior hemorrhagic history regardless of factor XI level, it is reasonable to not infuse any fresh frozen plasma or factor XI concentrate but to be prepared to do so should hemorrhage result.

Preconception Counseling

Once the factor XI level has been determined in a patient who is suspected of having factor XI deficiency, the probability of heterozygosity may be determined, using pedigree analysis to assess prior probability, from an available chart.[32] Patients from factor XI-deficient families may receive genetic counseling prior to conception on the risk of vertical transmission of severe deficiency. Factor XI-deficient patients who are attempting to conceive should be counseled properly in advance of the risks of pregnancy and delivery, and advised on the utility of hepatitis B vaccination should blood products become necessary. If pregnancy occurs prior to immunization, the vaccine can be given safely in pregnancy.

Once a factor XI-deficient woman has become pregnant, the potential risks and benefits of prenatal testing must be addressed. Invasive procedures during pregnancy may be desirable for individual patients, but they must be evaluated on an individual patient basis, because of the potential for significant accidental maternal, fetal, or placental bleeding.

Rare Inherited Bleeding Disorders

The rare inherited bleeding disorders include several other hereditary disorders of blood coagulation that may be associated with excessive bleeding in pregnancy. These include deficiencies in prothrombin, fibrinogen, and factors V, VII, X, and XIII (see Chapter 5). These disorders have a frequency of 1 to 2 per million persons and usually become manifest in childhood.[39] Because of the rarity of these conditions, there is very limited experience in the specific management of obstetric problems in women with these bleeding disorders. Factor XIII-deficient women routinely spontaneously miscarry if not treated throughout pregnancy, as factor XIII seems necessary for successful and durable implantation of the fertilized ovum in the uterus. In addition, hereditary afibrinogenemia and hypofibrinogenemia (especially if the level is below 50 mg/dL) also have been reported to be associated, if untreated, with recurrent pregnancy loss. Therapy for the rare inherited bleeding disorders is based on knowledge of the half-life and volume of distribution of the factor in question, as well as on replacement therapy currently available. Factor VII-deficient patients may now be treated with recombinant factor VIIa. Dosing is yet to be established but is clearly less than the recommended dose for the treatment of hemorrhaging patients with inhibitors to coagulation factors. Factor V-deficient patients, factor X-deficient patients, prothrombin-deficient patients, and those with factor XIII deficiency may be treated with fresh frozen plasma.[39] Cryoprecipitate is useful for the treatment of hypo- and dysfibrinogenemias and is useful in the treatment of factor XIII deficiency as well (see Table 28–2). Again, in none of these cases are specific recommendations available for the prophylaxis of bleeding during pregnancy and delivery. Therapeutic recommendations are based entirely on experience and the treatment of surgery and other bleeding episodes generically in patients with these disorders.

Preconception Counseling

Women from families with known inherited bleeding disorders should be assessed whenever possible prior to pregnancy to ascertain carrier status for the particular disease in question. The purpose of early identification is several-fold. First, the degree to which a woman is affected is a major factor in decisions regarding the safety of conceiving and carrying a pregnancy to term, as well as developing appropriate and realistic expectations. Management of the disorder during pregnancy may require serial monitoring of factor levels, with baseline levels obtained prior to conception. Immunization against hepatitis A and B should be undertaken in patients who could require blood product transfusion during pregnancy or delivery. In certain disorders (e.g., vWD), it may be appropriate to treat patients and monitor response of plasma levels prior to pregnancy, to confirm efficacy of therapy. Genetic counseling should be offered to all affected and carrier women from affected families to provide adequate information of inheritance enabling the patient and her partner to make decisions regarding pregnancy and prenatal diagnosis.

THROMBOCYTOPENIA

The normal platelet count in nonpregnant women varies from 150,000 to 300,000/μL. Relative thrombocytopenia is a normal physiologic response to pregnancy and the mean platelet count has been found to decrease successively in each trimester of normal, uncomplicated pregnancies. The maternal plasma volume expansion with increasing gestational age is believed to be the principal factor leading to a decrease in the platelet count. In one study of healthy gravidas, the mean platelet counts for each successive trimester were 322,000 ± 75,000; 298,000 ± 55,000; and 278,000 ± 75,000/μL.[40] Although a mild relative thrombocytopenia is common and even expected in pregnancy, bleeding is rare with platelet counts above 50,000 to 75,000/μL unless a qualitative platelet defect is also present. Generally, platelet counts below 100,000/μL should prompt a hematologic evaluation to exclude reversible or potentially life-threatening causes of thrombocytopenia.[40,41] Events and platelet counts of prior pregnancies very accurately predict the course in future pregnancies.

The most frequent cause of thrombocytopenia occurring during pregnancy is incidental thrombocytopenia of pregnancy, also referred to as gestational thrombocytopenia. In one large series of pregnant women, 74% of patients with thrombocytopenia had incidental thrombocytopenia, with the second most common cause being hypertensive disorders of pregnancy, in 21%. An immune disorder such as ITP or SLE was implicated in fewer than 5% of thrombocytopenic gravidas, and fewer than 2% were found to have DIC, thrombotic thrombocytopenic purpura (TTP), HELLP syndrome, or other related syndromes as the cause of the thrombocytopenia.[42]

Incidental thrombocytopenia of pregnancy was first described in 1988, when pregnant women considered to have ITP were distinguished from typical ITP patients based on their clinical course and that of their infants. In women for whom prepregnancy data were available, platelet counts were in the normal range. When platelet counts in these women were followed in the puerperium, the counts returned to normal within 6 weeks of delivery,[43] consistent with normalization of plasma volume and other hemostatic factors altered during pregnancy. The mechanism for the decrease in platelet count remains unknown, but it has been reported that mean platelet volumes are higher than in pregnant women with platelet counts in the normal range, suggestive of a nonimmunologic destructive process.[44]

Incidental thrombocytopenia of pregnancy typically is mild, with platelet counts usually ranging from 100,000 to 150,000/μL, with counts as low as 70,000/μL less commonly seen. The diagnosis is considered after the exclusion of prior history of bleeding or known thrombocytopenia, as well as in the absence of other hemostatic or systemic abnormalities that may alter the platelet count. Laboratory studies that may be helpful include liver function tests, coagulation tests, and human immunodeficiency virus (HIV) testing. A recent normal platelet count obtained prior to conception, or a mild thrombocytopenia in a prior pregnancy that resolved spontaneously in the postpartum period can be very useful in ascertaining the diagnosis of incidental thrombocytopenia. The definition of incidental thrombocytopenia that has been established is that of a platelet count of 70,000 to 150,000/μL in an otherwise healthy gravida.[43] It is recognized that platelet counts less than 70,000/μL may still represent incidental thrombocytopenia, and that patients with mild ITP may have platelet counts in the 70,000 to 100,000/μL range. The implications of confusion in the diagnosis of these two disorders are generally not clinically significant, as the obstetric management of the patient with mild ITP or gestational thrombocytopenia remains the same as for a hematologically normal patient. Epidural anesthesia is not contraindicated for platelet counts above 70,000/μL, and there is no benefit to choosing caesarian section over vaginal delivery in these women. Transfusion of platelets, likewise, is not indicated in the absence of overt bleeding.

The hypertensive disorders of pregnancy, which are the second most common cause of a low platelet count during pregnancy, are discussed in more detail elsewhere in this chapter. Serial measurements of blood pressure (as well as tests of liver function and coagulation) should be obtained at the time of diagnosis of thrombocytopenia, and at suitable intervals during the remainder of the pregnancy, determined by clinical course and presence of continued platelet decline.

As with nonpregnant individuals, the causes of thrombocytopenia in the gravida may be categorized as problems of decreased production, increased destruction, or sequestration. The initial evaluation of thrombocytopenia must include review of the peripheral smear. The laboratory platelet count should be confirmed manually, and the platelet and red blood cell morphology evaluated for clues to the cause of the thrombocytopenia. Pseudothrombocytopenia is a laboratory artifact due to platelet clumping of normal platelets at the time of collection, and is of no clinical significance except for the confusion and ill treatment it may produce. The presence of megathrombocytes in the peripheral smear suggests a compensation of the bone marrow for a state of increased peripheral removal of platelets. If the process is one of immune-mediated platelet removal, the red blood cell morphology is typically normal. Evidence of erythrocyte trauma in combination with decreased platelet counts may be indicative of a microangiopathic process, such as DIC, HELLP, or ITP. The presence of teardrop or nucleated red blood cells on the smear suggests a problem of primary bone marrow production. The leukocytes may also provide information of the cause of the thrombocytopenia, suggesting a nutritional deficiency, or malignant process.

Initial corroborative laboratory studies that should be obtained in all pregnant women with confirmed thrombocytopenia include blood coagulation studies to evaluate for the presence of DIC. The PT, aPTT, fibrinogen, and levels of fibrin split products (FSPs) will provide information to rule out DIC. Addition of liver function studies will aid in the evaluation of the HELLP syndrome discussed below in this chapter. Other laboratory evaluation will depend on the clinical history, and may include tests for collagen vascular disease including SLE or rheumatoid arthritis (RA), and testing for HIV infection.

A careful drug history may exclude possible toxic exposures. The possible offending agent should be discontinued and the platelet count monitored for recovery.

IMMUNE THROMBOCYTOPENIC PURPURA

Diagnosis

Immune thrombocytopenic purpura (ITP) is a relatively uncommon cause of thrombocytopenia in pregnancy, occurring in less than 4% of thrombocytopenic gravidas, or 1 to 2 per 1000 live births overall[42] (see Chapter 9). ITP is typically a chronic condition in adults. A long clinical history of easy bruising suggestive of a mild hemostatic impairment already may have led to the discovery of a mild thrombocytopenia that was diagnosed as ITP prior to pregnancy. Routine complete blood cell counts obtained early in pregnancy identify the majority of cases of ITP undiagnosed prior to pregnancy. The finding of a moderate asymptomatic thrombocytopenia as low as 50,000 to 70,000/μL in the absence of a hypertensive disorder of pregnancy during the first trimester is most likely to be chronic ITP.[43] ITP is three times more prevalent in women than men, and typically affects women in the second and third decades of life. Because ITP is a condition of young women, it is not an uncommon diagnosis during pregnancy. Practice guidelines recently set forth by the American Society of Hematology on the management of ITP include specific recommendations for the care of pregnant women and their newborn infants.[44] There is *currently no reliable basis for distinguishing* ITP from incidental thrombocytopenia of pregnancy. The diagnosis is determined on the basis of clinical data for each patient. A history of thrombocytopenia or bleeding consistent with ITP (petechiae or epistaxis) prior to conception suggests the diagnosis of ITP. Platelet counts below 50,000/μL also are more commonly found to be secondary to ITP. Current recommendations of confirmatory testing include measurement of blood pressure to rule out preeclampsia, liver function tests to exclude HELLP, and HIV testing. As in the case of nonpregnant women, the diagnosis of ITP rests on the exclusion of other systemic disorders as the cause of the low platelets, the presence of normal white and red blood cell indices, the absence of splenomegaly, and the absence of toxic or drug exposures. Antiplatelet antibody testing is not routinely recommended as the assay has high false-positive and false-negative rates.

Management During Pregnancy

Management of ITP in pregnancy is distinguished from that of nonpregnant women by several considerations.[44] First, attention must be paid to the potential adverse effects of standard ITP treatments on fetal development and on the course of pregnancy. Second, the incidence of thrombocytopenia is increased in newborns of mothers with documented ITP, which may affect obstetric management. The most commonly used initial therapy in ITP diagnosed in nonpregnant individuals is glucocorticoid administration, which is nonteratogenic to fetuses, but may induce or exacerbate gestational diabetes mellitus and postpartum psychiatric disorders. Intravenous immunoglobulin (IVIg) is considered safe for the fetus but may cause maternal side effects. The use of immunosuppressive or cytotoxic agents, including cyclophosphamide, the vinca alkaloids, and azothioprine, is relatively contraindicated as the harmful effects on the fetus are unpredictable. As with any intra-abdominal surgical procedure, the use of splenectomy in refractory cases of ITP has been reported to increase preterm labor and pregnancy loss in the first trimester, and may be technically difficult in the third trimester because of the size of the uterus. Last, adequate hemostasis is required at the time of delivery to reduce the risk of maternal postpartum bleeding complications.

Timing of Intervention

Gravidas with the diagnosis of ITP (either confirmed as chronic or presumed as a first presentation given the timing of detection during the pregnancy and absence of other causes) with platelet counts greater than 50,000/μL at any time during pregnancy and those with platelet counts of 30,000 to 50,000/μL during the first two trimesters and no evidence of bleeding should be observed. For women with platelet counts less than 10,000/μL at any time during pregnancy, or with counts of 10,000 to 30,000/μL in the latter two trimesters, or with bleeding, intervention should be undertaken. The goal of therapy for ITP in the gravida is to maintain a safe (as distinct from normal) platelet count, particularly with regard to labor and delivery.

In gravidas requiring treatment of the thrombocytopenia, glucocorticoids, usually prednisone at a dose of 1 mg/kg/day, is the first choice for therapy in women with platelet counts between 10,000 and 30,000/μL. The platelet count should rise to greater than 50,000/μL within approximately 1 week of initiation of therapy. The dose should then be tapered slowly to the minimum effective dose required to maintain the platelet count in an acceptable range. Too-rapid lowering of the steroid dose often results in recurrence of the thrombocytopenia. Women with severe thrombocytopenia (below 10,000/μL) should receive IVIg as initial treatment, at a dose of 0.4 g/kg/day for 5 days, or 1 g/kg daily for 2 days, with platelet transfusions administered if significant bleeding is present. IVIg often requires repeat administration every 2 to 4 weeks to maintain the platelet count at an acceptable level, particularly near term. IVIg is also appropriate second-line treatment for women who have failed glucocorticoid therapy. Splenectomy in gravidas is rarely undertaken because of the increased risks of the surgery to both the mother and the fetus as compared to a nonpregnant individual. Current recommendations for the use of surgical intervention are the presence of ITP refractory to both steroids and IVIg with platelet counts below 10,000/μL in the second trimester, and overt bleeding. When possible, pneumococcal vaccine should be administered 2 weeks prior to splenectomy.

The medical management recommendations of ITP in the pregnant woman differ from those in nongravidas in the lower threshold for the use of IVIg in pregnancy, and in the less frequent use of splenectomy for refractory cases, due to the increased maternal and fetal risks with surgery.

Impact of Maternal ITP on the Fetal Platelet Count

The autoantibodies produced in ITP are of the IgG class, and therefore readily cross the placenta. The manifestation of this phenomenon is variable in terms of the fetal platelet counts. The severity of the maternal thrombocytopenia does not correlate with that of the fetus,[45] and moreover the pharmacologic interventions used to raise the maternal platelet count may not necessarily result in an elevation in the fetal platelet count.[46,47] Refractory severe maternal thrombocytopenia despite splenectomy and previous history of delivery of a thrombocytopenic infant are both predictors for neonatal thrombocytopenia with the current pregnancy.[48]

There are currently two methods available to determine the fetal platelet counts (in utero), and both are problematic. Fetal scalp sampling, which involves removal of blood via a heparinized capillary tube from a small scalp laceration, requires that the woman be in active labor, with ruptured membranes and a dilated cervix. The fetal head must be engaged in the pelvis to allow access to the scalp. The platelet count obtained in this fashion may be grossly inaccurate because of contamination with amniotic fluid or maternal blood, or platelet clumping. Additionally, there is a risk of scalp hematoma. A platelet count above 50,000/μL obtained in this fashion is reassuring for a vaginal delivery. The second method, cordocentesis, or percutaneous umbilical cord sampling (PUBS), provides a more accurate platelet count, but requires an experience with the technique to minimize the potential risks of postpuncture bleeding of the fetus, which is usually self-limited but may necessitate emergency caesarian section or may result in fetal death in 1% of cases, a figure similar to the fetal death rate without PUBS testing.[49] The risks to the fetus appear to be least problematic after 35 weeks gestation.[45] For women who have maintained a platelet count above 50,000/μL at term, cordocentesis may guide the decision to permit a vaginal delivery, by reassuring that the fetal count is also adequate for that method of delivery. Infants born to mothers with ITP may experience further decline in the platelet count during the first week postpartum.[45] If the thrombocytopenia is severe, IVIg is recommended, with platelet transfusional support for evidence of active bleeding.

ALLOIMMUNE THROMBOCYTOPENIA

Alloimmune thrombocytopenia (AIT) is a clinical entity distinct from ITP, in that the maternal platelet counts are usually normal or only mildly decreased, yet the fetus may suffer a severe, life-threatening thrombocytopenia.[50] It results from maternal sensitization to fetal platelet antigens, and may be considered as the platelet equivalent to red blood cell Rh sensitization and hemolytic disease of the fetus and neonate. Fetal platelets apparently cross the placental barrier, and are recognized as foreign by the maternal immune system. The IgG antiplatelet antibodies are directed against platelet-specific antigens inherited from the father, yet absent from the mother's platelets. It has an incidence of approximately 1 in 1000 fetuses.[50] The most frequent abnormality causing this disorder is an incompatibility in the polymorphism affecting the P1A (HPA-1) antigen encoded on the gene for platelet glycoprotein IIIa. Alloantibodies from a sensitized P1A1-negative mother cross the placenta and cause immune-mediated thrombocytopenia in a P1A1-positive fetus. The P1A antigen polymorphism also causes the most severe form of the reported cases of alloimmune thrombocytopenia.[51] The diagnosis is usually first made after the birth of a child with unexpected severe thrombocytopenia. The chief complication of AIT is intracranial hemorrhage (ICH), which occurs in 10% to 20% of such severely affected neonates, with 25% to 50% of the ICH occurring in utero.[51] In contrast to Rh sensitization of red blood cells, AIT may occur with a first pregnancy. Efforts to screen mothers at risk to deliver affected infants are complicated by the fact that only 1 in 20 P1A1-negative mothers with antigen-incompatible partners ever become sensitized despite repeated pregnancies. Thus the incidence is not well predicted on the basis of antigen screening tests. However, once an affected fetus or neonate has been diagnosed, the maternal risk of subsequent affected pregnancies ranges from 50% to 100%, dependent on homozygosity or heterozygosity of the father for the allele even with different mates. It is suggested that in cases of paternal heterozygosity for the P1A1 allele, amniocentesis be performed at 15 to 18 weeks to allow platelet–antigen genotyping of the fetus. If the incompatible antigen is not present then the fetal platelet count will be unaffected, and normal delivery without further intervention may occur. If the antigen is present, then PUBS at 20 to 24 weeks should be undertaken, with transfusion of maternal platelets to minimize the risk to the fetus of hemorrhage during this procedure. If the fetus is found to be thrombocytopenic with a platelet count less than 100,000/µL, then maternal treatment with IVIg at a dose of 1 g/kg/week should be instituted immediately and continued for the duration of the pregnancy, as an increase or lack of further decrease of the fetal platelet count has been documented using this therapy in 62% to 85% of affected fetuses. Addition of low-dose steroid therapy has not been proven to increase response rates over IVIg alone. A repeat PUBS should be undertaken 3 to 6 weeks after instituting therapy to document an improvement in the platelet count. If the counts remain low, high-dose prednisone at 60 mg/day added to weekly IVIg will result in a rise in the platelet count in approximately half of the remaining cases.[52] PUBS should again be performed in 3 to 6 weeks to determine the platelet count. If the count remains below 50,000/µL then caesarian section should be performed. Delivery prior to 34 weeks for severe thrombocytopenia of less than 20,000/µL is of questionable utility, as prematurity alone may also lead to intracranial hemorrhage.

THE HELLP SYNDROME

The HELLP syndrome was first described in 1954 by Pritchard and coworkers, and was given the acronym in 1982 by Weinstein[53] on the basis of the three cardinal manifestations of the syndrome. The "H" stands for *H*emolysis, the "EL" for *E*levated *L*iver enzymes, and the "LP" for *L*ow *P*latelets. It is considered in conjunction with the disorders of pre-eclampsia and eclampsia to comprise a spectrum of heterogeneous hypertensive disorders occurring in the latter half of pregnancy and is one of the leading causes of maternal morbidity and mortality in the Western world. The diagnosis of the HELLP syndrome is based on hematologic and serum chemistry abnormalities, but there continues to be variation among centers for the criteria to establish the diagnosis. The University of Tennessee uses strict laboratory criteria, which include an abnormal peripheral smear with evidence of microangiopathic hemolytic anemia, total bilirubin above 1.2 mg/dL, lactate dehydrogenase (LDH) above 600 IU/L, aspartate aminotransferase (AST) above 70 IU/L, and platelets below 100,000/µL.[54] A recent study of uncomplicated singleton pregnancies followed to delivery found that a small fraction of gravidas experienced an asymptomatic gradual decline of the platelet count to less than 150,000/µL. These women were more than seven times as likely to develop AST elevation as those without thrombocytopenia; this suggests that the fall in platelets precedes the elevation of the liver enzyme tests.[55]

The earliest clinical signs and symptoms of this disorder are protean, and thus it may be mistaken for other conditions, from the benign to the life-threatening. The diagnosis may often be delayed if the symptoms, including shoulder, neck, and upper-body pain, malaise, nausea, vomiting, and headaches, are attributed to a viral syndrome, gastritis, or a musculoskeletal problem. The disorder, in more severe presentation, can be difficult to distinguish from other severe hepatic or hematologic syndromes seen in pregnancy. Severe pre-eclampsia, hemolytic uremic syndrome (HUS), TTP, SLE, and acute fatty liver of pregnancy can all produce clinical manifestations and laboratory studies similar to the HELLP syndrome. The target organs in all the above diseases include the kidney, the liver, and the vascular endothelium, and as the possibility for two syndromes to occur in the same individual also exists, the diagnosis can be extremely difficult. The subtle differences in these conditions can guide diagnosis of the correct clinical entity, and correct diagnosis is essential, because the management during pregnancy may be significantly different for each disorder. Several key characteristics for each of the above disorders have been characterized that may be useful in differentiation of the various syndromes. These features are depicted in Table 28–3.[56] Thrombocytopenia is the earliest and most common coagulation abnormality in the HELLP syndrome and is seen in all gravidas with this diagnosis. Abnormalities of the coagulation cascade, manifested by elevated PT, aPTT, and decreased fibrinogen level, and derangement of liver enzymes do not occur until very late in the course. LDH is frequently elevated much earlier than any liver abnormalities become apparent, suggesting the initial source is hemolyzed red cells. In contrast, acute fatty liver of pregnancy typically displays high serum bilirubin concentrations, prolongation of the PT and aPTT, hypoglycemia, and only modestly diminished platelet counts. Both TTP and HUS can imitate HELLP in many of the clinical features. All three syndromes share microangiopathic hemolytic anemia, thrombocy-

Table 28–3 • DIFFERENTIATION OF HELLP FROM SIMILAR DISEASES[a]

	Platelets	PT/aPTT	LDH	Bilirubin	Glucose	SBP	Proteinuria
HELLP	↓↓	N	↑↑↑	N	N	N/↑	↑
AFLP	↓	↑↑	N/↑	↑↑↑	↓	N	N
Pre-eclampsia	N	N	N	N	N	↑↑	↑↑
TTP	↓↓	N	↑↑	N	N	N	↑
HUS	N	N	↑	N	N	↑	↑↑

[a] Early in disease course.
HELLP, hemolysis, elevated liver tests, low platelets; AFLP, acute fatty liver of pregnancy; TTP, thrombotic thrombocytopenic purpura; HUS, hemolytic uremic syndrome; SBP, systemic blood pressure; N, normal or no change.

topenia, proteinuria, increased serum LDH, and renal compromise. However, TTP typically does not cause marked derangement of hepatic function as manifest by AST and alanine transferase elevations. In HELLP, the degree of renal dysfunction is usually correlated with the level of hepatic impairment, whereas in HUS, the renal failure is elevated out of proportion to the liver enzymes. Both TTP and HUS are managed with plasma exchange.

Pre-eclampsia is a well-defined clinical triad of hypertension, proteinuria, and nondependent edema, which can be mild or severe. The criteria for mild and severe disease have recently been established by the American College of Obstetrics and Gynecology.[56] The presence of grand-mal seizures is classified as eclampsia, and is a life-threatening condition with a high risk of both maternal and fetal mortality. The most efficacious treatment is prevention in a woman with identified pre-eclampsia. Immediate delivery of the fetus is mandatory once the syndrome has progressed to eclampsia. Measures that may be used to mitigate the sequelae of pre-eclampsia include control of the blood pressure with intravenous hydralazine at doses of 5 to 10 mg every 30 minutes, or labetalol or less commonly sodium nitroprusside, because of the concern for fetal cyanide toxicity at doses above 10 μg/kg/min.[56] Seizure prophylaxis should be initiated in patients with pre-eclampsia in active labor and in HELLP patients in labor, or at any time that epigastric pain is present. Intravenous magnesium sulfate, administered as a bolus and then by continuous infusion, is the treatment of choice, with the toxicity monitored by patellar reflexes and serum magnesium levels. The infusion may need to continue into the postpartum period until evidence of resolution of the hypertensive disorder is apparent.[56]

Once the diagnosis of the HELLP syndrome has been considered, some centers find it useful to further classify the disorder by severity to assist in prognosis and management in the peripartum period. A three-class system was created based on the maternal platelet count nadir. Class 1 is a platelet count below 50,000/μL; class 2, 50,000 to 100,000/μL; and class 3 above 100,000 but less than 150,000/μL. Regardless of the course during pregnancy and in the immediate peripartum period, HELLP syndrome may further worsen postpartum, and eventuate in pathologic thrombosis. Prophylactic administration of heparin is probably reasonable postpartum in most cases of HELLP syndrome; there is no published documentation of the use of low-molecular-weight heparin in this clinical situation.

REFERENCES

Chapter 28 References

1. Bennett B, Oxnard SC, Douglas AS, et al. Studies on antihemophilic factor (AHF, factor VIII) during labor in normal women, in patients with premature separation of the placenta, and in a patient with von Willebrand's disease. J Clin Lab Med 1974;84:851–860.
2. Bennett B, Ratnoff OD. Changes in antihemophilic factor (AHF, factor VIII) procoagulant activity and AHF-like antigen in normal pregnancy, and following exercise and pneumoencephalography. J Clin Lab Med 1972;80:256–263.
3. Conti M, Mari D, Conti E, et al. Pregnancy in women with different types of von Willebrand disease. Obstet Gynecol 1986;68:282–285.
4. Economides DL, Kadir RA, Lee CA. Inherited bleeding disorders in obstetrics and gynecology. Br J Obstet Gynaecol 1999;106:5–13.
5. Kadir RA, Lee CA, Sabin CA, et al. Pregnancy in women with von Willebrand's disease or factor XI deficiency. Br J Obstet Gynaecol 1998;105:314–321.
6. Condie RG. A serial study of coagulation factors XII, XI, and X in plasma in normal pregnancy and in pregnancy complicated by pre-eclampsia. Br J Obstet Gynaecol 1976;93:636–639.
7. Hilgartner MW, Smith CH. Plasma thromboplastin antecedent (factor XI) in the neonate. J Paediatr 1965;66:747–752.
8. Burrows RF, Kelton JG. Thrombocytopenia at delivery: a prospective survey of 6715 deliveries. Am J Obstet Gynecol 1990;162:731–734.
9. Forbes CD, Greer JA. Physiology of haemostasis and the effect of pregnancy. In Greer IA, Turpie AG, Forbes CD (Eds.): Haemostasis and Thrombosis in Obstetrics and Gynecology, London, UK, Chapman & Hall, 1992, pp. 1–26.
10. Sadler JE. A revised classification of von Willebrand disease. Thromb Haemost 1994;71:520–525.
11. Lee CA. Women and inherited bleeding disorders: Menstrual issues. Semin Hematol 1999;36(suppl 4):21–27.
12. Kadir RA, Economides DL, Sabin CA, et al. Frequency of inherited bleeding disorders in women with menorrhagia. Lancet 1998;351:485–489.
13. von Willebrand E. Hereditar pseudo-hemofili. Finska Lakarsallskapets Handl 1926;67:7–112.
14. Lyons SE, Bruck NE, Bowie EJ, Ginsburg D. Impaired intracellular transport produced by a subset of type IIa von Willebrand disease mutations. J Biol Chem 1992;267:4424–4430.
15. Phillips MD, Santhouse A. von Willebrand disease: Recent advances in pathophysiology and treatment. Am J Med Sci 1998;316:77–86.
16. Rick ME, Williams SB, Sacher RA, et al. Thrombocytopenia associated with pregnancy in a patient with type IIB von Willebrand's disease. Blood 1987;69:786–789.
17. Walker ID. Investigation and management of haemorrhagic disorders in pregnancy. J Clin Pathol 1994;47:100–108.
18. Metzner HJ, Hermentin P, Cuesta-Linker T, et al. Characterization of factor VIII/von Willebrand factor concentrates using a modified method of von Willebrand factor multimer analysis. Haemophilia 1998, 4 (Suppl 3), 25–32.
19. Dobrkovska A, Krzensk U, Chediak JR. Pharmacokinetics, efficacy and safety of Humate-P in von Willebrand disease. Haemophilia 1998, 4 (Suppl 3) 33–39.
20. Mannucci PM, Canciani MT, Rota L, et al. Response of factor VIII/von Willebrand factor to DDAVP in healthy subjects and patients with haemophilia A and von Willebrand's disease. Br J Haematol 1981;47:283–293.
21. Mannucci PM. Desmopressin. A nontransfusional form of treatment for congenital and acquired bleeding disorders. Blood. 1988;72:1449–1455.
22. Burrow GN, Wassenaar W, Robertson GL, et al. DDAVP treatment of diabetes insipidus during pregnancy and the post-partum period. Acta Endocrinol (Copenh) 1981;97:23–25.
23. Rochelson B, Caruso R, Davenport D, et al. The use of prophylactic desmopressin (DDAVP) in labor to prevent hemorrhage in a patient with Ehlers-Danlos syndrome. NY State J Med 1991;91:268–269.
24. Greer IA, Lowe GD, Walker JJ, et al. Haemorrhagic problems in obstetrics and gynaecology in patients with congenital coagulopathies. Br J Obstet Gynaecol 1991;98:909–918.
25. Sage DJ. Epidurals, spinals and bleeding disorders in pregnancy: review. Anaesth Intensive Care 1990;18:319–326.

26. Lyon M. Sex chromatin and gene action in the mammalian X chromosome. Am J Hum Genet 1962;14:135–148.
27. Bunschoten EPM, van Houwelingen JC, Visser SEJM, et al: Bleeding symptoms in carriers of hemophilia A and B. Thromb Haemost 1988;59:349–352.
28. Sadler JE, Blinder M. von Willebrand Disease: Diagnosis, classification, and treatment. In Colman RW, Hirsh J, Marder VJ, Clowes AW, George JN (eds.) Hemostasis and Thrombosis, 4th ed. Philadelphia, Lippincott Williams & Wilkins, 2001, pp. 825–837.
29. Nishino M, Nishino S, Sugimoto M, et al. Changes in factor VIII binding capacity of von Willebrand factor and factor VIII coagulant activity in two patients with type 2N von Willebrand disease after hemostatic treatment and during pregnancy. Int J Hematol 1996;64:127–34.
30. Wilson JD, Griffin JE. Disorders of sexual differentiation. In Fauci AS, Braunwald E, Isselbacher KJ, et al. (Eds.): Harrison's Principles of Internal Medicine, 14th ed. New York, McGraw-Hill, 1998; pp. 2119–2131.
31. Seligsohn U. Factor XI deficiency. Thromb Haemost 1993;70:68–71.
32. Bolton-Maggs PHB, Young Wan-Nin B, McCraw AH, et al. Inheritance and bleeding in factor XI deficiency. Br J Haemotol 1988;69:521–528.
33. Kitchens CS. Factor XI: A review of its biochemistry and deficiency. Semin Thromb Hemost 1991;17:55–72.
34. Bolton-Maggs PHB, Colvin BJ, Satchi G, et al. Thrombogenic potential of factor XI concentrate. Lancet. 1994;344:748–749.
35. Nossel HL, Lanzkowsky P, Levy S, et al. A study of coagulation factor levels in women during labour and in their newborn infants. Thromb Diath Haemorrh 1966;16:185–197.
36. Kadir RA, Economides DL, Lee CA. Factor XI deficiency in women. Am J Hematol 1999;60:48–54.
37. Kadir RA. Women and inherited bleeding disorders: Pregnancy and delivery. Semin Hematol 1999;36 (Suppl 4):28–35.
38. Collins PW, Lilley P, Guldman E, et al. Clinical experience of factor XI deficiency. The use of fresh frozen plasma and factor XI concentrate. Thromb Haemost 1995;73:1441 (2070a).
39. Lusher J. Women and inherited bleeding disorders. Semin Hematol 1999;36 (Suppl 4):10–20.
40. Pitkin RM, Witte DL. Platelet and leukocyte counts in pregnancy. JAMA 1979;242:2696–2698.
41. Pritchard JA, Weisman R Jr, Ratnoff OD, Vasburgh GJ. Intravascular hemolysis, thrombocytopenia, and other hematologic abnormalities associated with severe toxemia of pregnancy. N Engl J Med 1954;250:89–98.
42. Burrows RF, Kelton JG. Fetal thrombocytopenia and its relation to maternal thrombocytopenia. N Engl J Med 1993;329:1463–1466.
43. Shehata N, Burrows RF, Kelton JG. Gestational thrombocytopenia. Clin Obstet Gynecol 1999;42:327–334.
44. George JN, Woolf SH, Raskob GE, et al. Idiopathic thrombocytopenic purpura: A practice guideline developed by explicit methods for the American Society of Hematology. Blood 1996;88:3–40.
45. Kelton JG. Management of the pregnant patient with idiopathic thrombocytopenic purpura. Ann Intern Med 1983;99:796–800.
46. McCrae KR, Samuels P, Schreiber AD. Pregnancy-associated thrombocytopenia: Pathogenesis and management. Blood 1992;80:2697–2714.
47. Kaplan C, Daffos F, Forestier F, et al. Fetal platelet counts in thrombocytopenic pregnancy. Lancet 1990;336:979–982.
48. Sharon R, Tatarsky I. Low fetal morbidity in pregnancy associated with acute and chronic idiopathic thrombocytopenic purpura. Am J Hematol 1994;46:87–90.
49. Moise KJ Jr, Carpenter RJ Jr, Cotton DB, et al. Percutaneous umbilical cord sampling in the evaluation of fetal platelet counts in pregnant patients with autoimmune thrombocytopenic purpura. Obstet Gynecol 1988;72 (3 Pt 1):346–350.
50. Hohlfeld P, Forestier F, Kaplan C, et al. Fetal thrombocytopenia: a retrospective survey of 5,194 fetal blood samplings. Blood 1994;84:1851–1856.
51. Bussel JB, Zabusky MR, Berkowitz RL, et al. Fetal alloimmune thrombocytopenia. N Engl J Med 1997;337:22–26.
52. Skupski DW, Bussel JB. Alloimmune thrombocytopenia. Clin Obstet Gynecol 1999;42:335–348.
53. Weinstein L. Syndrome of hemolysis, elevated liver enzymes, and low platelet count: A severe consequence of hypertension in pregnancy. Am J Obstet Gynecol 1982;142:159–167.
54. Sibai BM. The HELLP syndrome (hemolysis, elevated liver enzymes, and low platelets): Much ado about nothing? Am J Obstet Gynecol 1990;162:311–316.
55. Minakami H, Sato I. HELLP syndrome. JAMA 1999;281:703–704.
56. Magann EF, Martin JN. Twelve steps to optimal management of HELLP syndrome. Clin Obstet Gynecol 1999;42:532–550.

CHAPTER 29

Management of Thrombophilia and Antiphospholipid Syndrome During Pregnancy

Prof. Amiram Eldor*

There is great interest in the hereditary and acquired thrombophilias because of a high prevalence of patients presenting with thromboembolic disorders. Recent evidence shows that hereditary thrombophilia and the occurrence of acquired antiphospholipid syndrome (APLS) underlie many of the thrombotic events seen in pregnancy, and these disorders are now major issues in the management of pregnant women.

Several molecular risk factors for venous thromboembolism (VTE) are recognized.[1-9] Deficiencies of the natural coagulation inhibitors protein C, protein S, and antithrombin III (AT III) predispose to thromboembolic events.[2,3] Mutations in coagulation factors increase the risk of thrombosis and appear to have a high prevalence in the general population.[1] The mutation in the gene encoding factor V (G1691A), factor V Leiden, is associated with resistance to activated protein C.[1] The prothrombin gene mutation G20210A is associated with elevated plasma factor II levels, and is associated with an increased risk of thromboembolism.[4-7] Mild hyperhomocysteinemia, frequently associated with homozygosity for a common mutation (C677T) in the enzyme 5,10-methylenetetrahydrofolate reductase (MTHFR), is associated with an enhanced risk of both arterial and venous thrombosis.[10,11] Similarly, acquired antiphospholipid antibody (APLA) constitutes a risk factor for both venous and arterial thrombosis.[12]

The risk of VTE associated with acquired and inherited thrombophilias is further amplified by other risk factors, for example, the postsurgical state and immobilization. Recent evidence suggests that the risk of maternal VTE in cases with underlying thrombophilia is increased substantially. The risk of VTE in pregnant women may be amplified further by the type of underlying genetic predisposition, for example, homozygosity for a mutation, the presence of multiple mutations (multigenic defects), or thrombophilic anomalies.[13-15]

VENOUS THROMBOEMBOLISM IN PREGNANCY

The risk of VTE in pregnancy is approximately six times greater than in nonpregnant women, and VTE is a major cause of death among women during pregnancy and the puerperium. Pulmonary embolism (PE) occurs in approximately 16% of patients with untreated deep venous thrombosis (DVT), and is the most common cause of maternal death (Table 29–1).[12,16-18] The overall risk of DVT in pregnancy (0.05% to 1.8%)[16] is higher in women with a previous history of VTE, with a recurrence rate of about 1 case in 71 women.[19] Maternal DVT is more common in the left leg (accounting for about 85% of leg thromboses), occurs more commonly in iliofemoral veins than in calf veins (72% compared with 9%, respectively), and is more often associated with PE.[20]

Underlying factors increasing the risk of VTE in pregnant women include obstruction of venous return by the enlarging uterus, venous atonia due to hormonal effects,[21] and the acquired prothrombotic changes that occur in hemostatic proteins (Table 29–2). The physiologic changes in the hemostatic system include elevation of fibrinogen levels and factor VIII activity, acquired functional resistance to activated protein C, a decrease in protein S, increases in plasminogen activator inhibitors 1 and 2 (PAI-1, PAI-2) that decrease fibrinolysis, and platelet activation.[12,17,22,23] All contribute to the hypercoagulable state that occurs in normal pregnancy.

The form of delivery is an important risk factor for VTE. The incidence of clinical DVT is estimated at 0.08% to 1.2% following vaginal delivery, rising to 2.2% to 3.0% following caesarean section.[24] Emergency caesarean section is associated with the highest risk, and maternal age and weight are also important risk factors.[25] A high proportion of both postpartum DVT and

---

*Deceased

Table 29-1 • VENOUS THROMBOEMBOLIC EVENTS DURING PREGNANCY: DVT AND PE RATES

DVT Rates	PE Rates
Incidence six times higher in pregnant women	Most common cause of maternal death. 16% PE rate if DVT is not treated
Risk estimated between 0.05 and 1.80	
Risk increases if previous VTE	
Recurrence rate 1 in 71	

DVT, deep venous thrombosis; PE, pulmonary embolism; VTE, venous thromboembolism.

PE manifests after discharge from hospital,[25] highlighting the need for careful continued surveillance in the puerperium.[17]

If venous thrombosis is suspected during pregnancy, an objective diagnosis must be obtained. With proper precautions, the radiation dose from the necessary investigations is small, and the risk to the fetus is negligible.[26] If VTE is suspected but unconfirmed by test results, treatment should be started and tests repeated within 7 days; therapy is discontinued if findings remain negative.[18]

Table 29-2 • VENOUS THROMBOEMBOLIC EVENTS DURING PREGNANCY: ETIOLOGY AND RISK FACTORS

Etiology
Mechanical
   Enlarging uterus obstructs venous return
   Venous atonia due to hormonal effects
Hemostatic
   Elevated factor II, factor V, factor VII, factor VIII, factor X activities
   Elevated von Willebrand factor level
   Elevated fibrinogen level
   Reduced fibrinolysis due to increases in PAI-1 and -2
   Reduced free protein S activity
   Acquired functional resistance to activated protein C
   Platelet activation

Risk Factors
Maternal characteristics
   Age
   Obesity
   Immobilization
   Thrombophilia
   Protein C deficiency
   Protein S deficiency
   AT III deficiency
   Factor V Leiden mutation
   Factor II 20210 mutation
   MTHFR mutation
   Antiphospholipid syndrome
Route of delivery
   Vaginal
   Caesarean

PAI-1, PAI-2, plasminogen activator inhibitor 1 and 2

The third trimester or the postpartum period is the most likely time for PE to occur. Diagnosis during pregnancy is difficult as many of the signs and symptoms also occur in healthy pregnant women, and pulmonary emboli may arise from the pelvic veins while the leg veins remain normal.[24] The elevation of plasma levels of D-dimers during pregnancy may be unrelated to VTE.[23] In many cases anticoagulant therapy is initiated justifiably on the basis of clinical awareness and suspicion only; however, in view of potential hazards, an objective diagnosis is then mandatory.

HEREDITARY THROMBOPHILIAS AND VENOUS THROMBOSIS DURING PREGNANCY

The risk of venous thrombosis in women with an inherited or acquired thrombophilia is increased in pregnancy. However, not all women with thrombophilia will develop VTE during pregnancy, suggesting the existence of additional, yet unidentified, environmental factors. The fact that a patient has been pregnant before without manifesting VTE does not rule out the risk of VTE in subsequent pregnancies. The risk of VTE depends on the type of thrombophilia and the existence of additional risk factors.

AT III deficiency is the most thrombogenic of the hereditary thrombophilias, with a 50% lifetime chance of thrombosis.[27] The frequency of AT III deficiency in the general population is 0.02% to 0.17% and is higher in patients with VTE (1.1%). The risk of thromboembolism in AT III-deficient pregnant women not receiving anticoagulant therapy is about 50%.[2]

Abnormalities of the protein C and protein S system are present in 0.14% to 0.5% of the general population and 3.2% of patients with thrombosis. The risk of thrombosis in pregnancy is 3% to 10% for patients with protein C deficiency and 0% to 6% for those with protein S deficiency, substantially lower than for AT III-deficient women. In postpartum women, the thrombosis risk is 7% to 19% for protein C deficiency and 7% to 22% for protein S deficiency.[3,12,28,29] While antigenic and functional assays of protein C levels during pregnancy remain unchanged, there is a marked decrease in protein S levels (free or functional protein S). Protein S levels are frequently decreased in 25% of healthy women in the first trimester, 60% in the second, and 83% to 100% in the third trimester.[23] Hence, when protein S deficiency is suspected during pregnancy, reliable assay results are obtainable only in the first months of pregnancy. An alternative approach is to test the parents of the patient.

Activated protein C resistance (APCR) is present in 3% to 7% of healthy Caucasians and in 20% to 30% of patients with thrombosis. In the vast majority of the patients, APCR is due to the factor V Leiden mutation. APCR has been found in up to 78% of women investigated for venous thrombosis in pregnancy,[8] whereas the factor V Leiden genotype was found in up to 46% of cases.[9,15]

Recently Gerhardt and coworkers described the prevalence of congenital thrombophilia in 352 women, 119 of whom had a VTE during pregnancy or the puerpurium.[14] In the women with VTE, the prevalence of factor V Leiden was 43.7%, compared with 7.7% among the age-matched normal women (relative risk [RR] 9.3; 95% confidence interval [CI] 5.1 to 16.9). The prevalence of the G20210A prothrombin-gene mutation was 16.9% in women with VTE as compared with 1.3% in the control group (RR 15.2; 95% CI 4.2 to 52.6). The prevalence of the combined defects of both factor V Leiden and G20210A prothrombin-gene mutation was 9.3%, as compared with zero in the control group. The presence of both mutations substantially increased the risk for VTE, with an odds ratio estimated at 107 for the combination of mutations. Additional risk factors, such as AT III deficiency or protein C and protein S deficiencies, were present in 25% of the women with a history of VTE, as compared with 11% of the women with no history.

Further insight into the risk of thrombosis in previously symptom-free women with factor V Leiden mutation has been provided in a study of 43 women from symptomatic families. Overall, the incidence of pregnancy-associated thrombosis was 14%,[28] and it appears the risk may be higher postpartum. McColl and colleagues estimated the risk of VTE in pregnancy to be 1 in 437 for factor V Leiden, 1 in 113 for protein C deficiency, 1 in 28 for type I (quantitative) AT III deficiency, and 1 in 42 for type II (qualitative) AT III deficiency.[7]

APCR can be caused by disorders other than factor V Leiden mutation, including APLS and other genetic defects in the factor V molecule. The resistance can also be acquired during the second and third trimester of normal pregnancy as a result of increases in factor V and factor VIII and decreased protein S levels.[1,2,20,26] The precise mechanism for this "physiologic" APCR is still not known, nor its contribution to the higher risk of VTE during pregnancy.[1,2,20,26]

The prothrombin G20210A mutation is associated with elevated plasma prothrombin levels (factor II activity above 130%) and is present in about 2% to 5% of healthy individuals. This mutation has been associated with a threefold increased risk of VTE. As would be predicted, higher risk of thrombosis was found in women using oral contraceptives and in women with obstetric complications.[4,5,7,30]

Gerhardt and coworkers demonstrated that the G20210A prothrombin-gene mutation and factor V Leiden mutation are individually associated with an increased risk of VTE during pregnancy and the puerperium, and that the risk among women with both mutations is disproportionately higher than that among women with only one mutation.[14] A calculation of the positive predictive value for each genetic defect, assuming an underlying rate of VTE of 0.67 per 1000 pregnancies in Western populations, gave values of 1:500 for factor V Leiden mutation, 1:200 for the G20210A prothrombin-gene mutation, and 4.6:100 for the combination of the two defects.

Hyperhomocysteinemia is frequently associated with homozygosity for the thermolabile variant of MTHFR (C677T)[2] and is present in about 8% to 10% of otherwise healthy individuals.[10,11] Pregnancy is associated with decreased concentrations of homocysteine and folic acid supplementation will further lower homocysteine concentrations. However, the contribution of homocysteine to VTE in pregnancy is as yet unclear. Gerhardt and coworkers revealed that homozygosity for the C677T MTHFR mutation was not associated with an increase in risk for VTE during pregnancy.[14] This may be explained by the fact that plasma homocysteine concentrations decrease during pregnancy and most pregnant women take folic acid supplements, which ameliorate hyperhomocysteinemia.[15]

Interestingly, an inherited thrombophilia in a pregnant woman may have salubrious effects. Factor V Leiden mutation has been associated with a reduced risk of intrapartum bleeding complications, conferring a possible survival advantage for carriers.[31]

THE MANAGEMENT OF THROMBOPHILIA DURING PREGNANCY

The management of thrombophilia during pregnancy encompasses primary thromboprophylaxis in asymptomatic women, secondary prophylaxis of recurrences in women who have previously developed thrombosis, and the treatment of an acute thrombotic episode. It is rather difficult to establish guidelines for antithrombotic therapy because of the paucity of relevant, well-controlled trials. Thus the recommendations regarding prophylactic and therapeutic strategies in pregnancy are largely based on clinical trials in nonpregnant populations.[32] An additional problem in assessing the response to antithrombotic therapy during pregnancy is the danger of imaging procedures. An objective diagnosis of VTE during pregnancy is crucial.[32] The diagnosis has serious implications, not only for the immediate management of the pregnancy, but also for the management of future pregnancies.

Heparin is currently the drug of choice for the prevention and treatment of VTE during pregnancy, though it is gradually being replaced by low-molecular-weight heparins (LMWHs). LMWHs exhibit a number of advantages over unfractionated heparin (UFH), including improved bioavailability, a longer half-life, ease of administration, no monitoring requirement, and fewer side-effects (Table 29–3).[32–37] Animal and human studies have shown that heparins are not teratogenic or fetotoxic and do not cross the placenta.[38] Oral anticoagulants (OACs) are rarely employed during pregnancy because of substantial side-effects (Table 29–3).[12,17,32] Coumarin derivatives cross the placenta and are associated with embryopathy in 4% to 5% of exposed fetuses, especially during the first trimester.[32] Central nervous system anomalies can occur in any trimester. OACs are reserved for conditions in which the effectiveness of heparin and LMWH may be limited. These may include the management of women with artificial heart valves and in cases where heparin therapy is contraindicated, including cases of heparin-induced thrombocytopenia (HIT) or skin allergy. Heparin, LMWH, and coumarin

Table 29-3 • A COMPARISON OF ANTITHROMBOTIC THERAPIES DURING PREGNANCY

	Advantages	Disadvantages
Heparin (UFH)	Traditionally drug of choice Doesn't cross the placenta Not secreted in breast milk Cost	Two to three times daily subcutaneous injections Unpredictable dosing aPTT monitoring necessary Injection site pain Significant osteoporosis Thrombocytopenia 1%–2% Induces hair loss
Warfarin	Administered weeks 13–36 and postpartum Not secreted in breast milk Cost	Contraindicated weeks 6–12 Crosses the placenta Significant risk to fetus with malformation Intracranial hemorrhage
LMWH	Convenient administration: once daily, self-administered injection No monitoring requirement Suitable for prolonged administration Does not cross the placenta Not secreted in breast milk No evidence of mutagenic or teratogenic effects Low risk of thrombocytopenia and skin allergy	Epidural anesthesia should be delayed for 6–12 hours Occasional decrease in bone density Rare allergic skin reactions Cost

derivatives are not secreted in the breast milk and can be given safely to nursing mothers.[32]

Primary Prophylaxis of Thrombosis in Asymptomatic Women

In asymptomatic women with a known protein C deficiency, protein S deficiency, or factor V Leiden or G20210A prothrombin mutation who have never experienced VTE, we recommend either clinical surveillance or prophylactic therapy during the last weeks of pregnancy and 2 to 6 weeks in the puerperium. Subcutaneous heparin 5000 IU twice daily, or a LMWH (enoxaparin, 40 mg once daily, or dalteparin, 5000 U daily) is used. This thromboprophylactic treatment is firmly indicated in women undergoing caesarean section. In women with AT III deficiency, the risk may be substantially greater and prophylactic therapy may be indicated throughout the pregnancy.

Clinical and ultrasonic surveillance is usually reserved for women who are allergic to heparin, who refuse to use heparin or LMWH, or who have experienced a previous VTE in association with a transient risk factor.[32] The effectiveness of a surveillance approach is dependent on the early detection and treatment of VTE disease, especially before the development of PE. Compression stockings, which are effective in women with recurrent DVT, may be useful in pregnancy and should be recommended to women with previous DVT or varicose veins.[39]

In a recent review, Greer recommends that all patients with thrombophilia be referred to a unit that specializes in the management of thrombophilia in pregnancy,[12] supporting the view that there is a clear need for randomized, placebo-controlled trials of thromboprophylaxis to establish evidence-based clinical practice.[15,32]

Secondary Prophylaxis in Women With Previous Thrombosis

All patients with a personal or family history of VTE should be considered for antenatal prophylaxis and be screened for a thrombophilia. The two general approaches recommended for pregnant women with previous VTE are active prophylactic therapy with heparin or LMWH and clinical surveillance.[15,32] Thromboprophylaxis is firmly indicated for women who exhibit additional risk factors such as hyperemesis, obesity, immobilization, or surgery, and particularly if they have pre-eclampsia or concurrent medical conditions associated with thrombosis, such as nephrotic syndrome, inflammatory bowel disease, or infection.

Women with thrombophilia and a history of previous VTE should receive thromboprophylaxis during pregnancy and the puerperium. Symptom-free carriers of thrombophilia require special consideration. The risk of thrombosis varies with the type of thrombophilia and currently no controlled guidelines are available. Some investigators find it useful to risk stratify patients as low risk or high risk to help guide clinical evaluation. Asymptomatic patients at high risk of VTE may be defined as those with AT III deficiency, those with more than one thrombophilic anomaly or a homozygote mutation, and those with first-degree relatives who have experienced severe VTE. Management also requires careful discussion with the patient and her relatives as personal concerns and preferences will impact risk:benefit decisions. All other patients are considered low risk.

The Treatment of Acute Thrombotic Episode

Acute DVT during pregnancy in women with or without thrombophilia is usually treated with full-dose intravenous heparin for 5 to 10 days, followed by maintenance subcutaneous heparin given twice daily, adjusted to prolong the activated partial thromboplastin time (aPTT) into the therapeutic range.[32] Changes in the metabolism and clearance of heparin during pregnancy complicate dosing and equivalent doses of subcutaneous heparin produce lower plasma concentrations in pregnant women than in nonpregnant women.[40] It is not clear whether the dose of heparin should be adjusted with increasing weight.[41] Although some centers advocate weight-adjusted doses, others recommend frequent aPTT testing or measurements of anti-factor Xa taken 4 hours after injection as a guide to reaching the desired level of 0.3 to 1.0 U/mL.[32] Heparin is given until term, discontinued shortly before delivery, and restarted in conjunction with initiation of warfarin therapy postpartum. Heparin is subsequently discontinued when the international normalized ratio (INR) is 2 to 3.

The optimal duration of postpartum warfarin therapy in women with thrombophilia who have developed DVT during pregnancy is currently undefined, and no guidelines are available based on clinical trials. In our opinion, the duration of therapy depends on the magnitude of risk of a recurrent VTE. Individual risk assessment should be performed, taking into consideration the type of thrombophilia, the presence of multigenic defects, the extent and site of thrombosis, the time frame of occurrence, the history of VTE, and the family history. Low-risk mothers are given prophylactic therapy for a further 4 to 6 weeks, and patients at high risk should receive extended thromboprophylaxis. Patients with APLS or AT III deficiency who have experienced a VTE appear to require indefinite treatment because of the high risk of recurrence.

LMWHs continue to replace UFH in the management of acute VTE. The dose required for the treatment of acute DVT is derived from controlled studies in medical patients. No adequate clinical trials have assessed DVT treatment in pregnancy. The recommended doses for the treatment of VTE are shown in Table 29–4.[42] LMWH should be injected subcutaneously into the abdominal wall, and in later months of pregnancy, the anterior aspect of the thigh. These simple, once-daily treatment regimens offer the potential for home or outpatient treatment of DVT, with obvious resource implications, and are feasible in patients with proximal DVT who do not require hospitalization. However, treatment of acute VTE in the pregnant patient with LMWH has not undergone official approval by the U.S. Food and Drug Administration.

After therapeutic administration of LMWH for 10 to 14 days, a prophylactic dose of LMWH should be continued throughout the pregnancy and then heparin or warfarin for 6 to 8 weeks postpartum as described for UFH.[12,33,37] Published studies indicate that the effective maintenance prophylactic dose of enoxaparin is 40 mg once daily and of dalteparin, 5000 U once daily.[33–37,43,44] However, in certain thrombophilic conditions these doses should be increased depending on the risk of recurrent VTE. Plasma levels of enoxaparin, given at 40 mg once daily, are not affected by gestational age.[34] Monitoring of LMWH levels is not required, but some investigators advocate measurements of peak anti-factor Xa concentrations 3 to 6 hours after the last injection, with the goal of achieving target plasma levels of 0.4 to 0.6 U/mL.[45] The dose of LMWH should be reduced during delivery, and the timing of administration adjusted to allow epidural or spinal anesthesia (see Chapter 39). Epidural anesthesia may be managed by omitting the last dose of LMWH or by delaying placement of the epidural catheter for 6 to 12 hours.[28] LMWH can be restarted 2 hours after catheter removal.[12] Warfarin should be used postpartum, particularly to avoid the risk of osteoporosis associated with prolonged LMWH administration.[45]

A recent systematic review of all published clinical reports (mostly unblinded or uncontrolled) employing LMWH in at-risk pregnancies, and data from an international interest group (21 studies in total), reported the incidence of recurrent VTE as 3 of 486 pregnancies.[33] No congenital malformations in the newborns were observed. Adverse effects generally were uncommon, and the most frequently described were minor hemorrhagic complications. The number of adverse fetal outcomes was significantly higher in women with comorbid conditions (mostly the presence of APLAs) compared with those without (Table 29–5).

The risk of osteoporosis is lower in pregnant women treated with LMWH than with UFH.[35] However, in a study of 34 women who received dalteparin, one woman without other risk factors for osteoporosis developed osteoporotic vertebral collapse postpartum. However, it was noted that this patient had received higher than usual maintenance doses of LMWH.[28] Densitometer evaluations or prophylactic therapy for osteoporosis have not been recommended routinely for women treated for long periods with LMWH.

Insertion of a vena caval filter may rarely be indicated in pregnant women with VTE. Patients who may benefit are those with PE despite adequate antithrombotic therapy, iliofemoral DVT in the weeks prior to delivery, or severe femoropopliteal DVT (see Chapters 37 and 38). Placement of a filter does not negate the need for anticoagulation. The clinical impression is that filters prevent PE, but some patients develop significant leg swelling

Table 29–4 • TREATMENT OF VTE DURING PREGNANCY: RECOMMENDED LMWH DOSES FROM CONTROLLED STUDIES IN MEDICAL PATIENTS

LMWH	Commercial Name	Recommended Dose
Dalteparin	Fragmin	200 anti-factor Xa units/kg once daily
Enoxaparin	Clexane, Lovenox	1.0 mg/kg twice daily or 1.5 mg/kg once daily
Nadroparin	Fraxiparin	200 anti-factor Xa units/kg once daily
Tinzaparin	Innohep	175 anti-factor Xa units/kg once daily

From Hirsh J. Low-molecular-weight heparin for the treatment of venous thromboembolism. Am Heart J 1998;135:S336–S342, with permission.

Table 29-5 • SAFETY OF LMWH IN PREGNANCY: A SYSTEMATIC REVIEW

Women With Comorbidity			Women Without Comorbidity		
Indication	Patients (n)	Adverse Outcome[a]	Indication	Patients (n)	Adverse Outcome*
APLS	163	27	Previous VTE	149	5
Recent fetal loss	93	10	Acute VTE	19	0
Pre-eclampsia	28	0	Thrombophilia	14	0
Miscellaneous	6	2	Previous arterial thrombosis	8	0
Mechanical heart valve	3	1	Miscellaneous	3	0
Total	293	40 (13.6%)	Total	193	5 (2.5%)

[a] The adverse outcomes were 41 conceptus deaths and 4 unhealthy premature births.
From Sanson BJ, Lensing AW, Prins MH, et al. Safety of low-molecular-weight heparin in pregnancy: A systematic review. Thromb Haemost 1999;81:668–672, with permission.

despite adequate maintenance with low-dose subcutaneous heparin. There does not appear to be any fetal morbidity or mortality associated with filter insertion.[46] Surgical thrombectomy does not appear to offer any advantage over anticoagulation treatment in terms of the long-term outcome of VTE during pregnancy or the puerperium.

THE ANTIPHOSPHOLIPID SYNDROME

The diagnosis of the antiphospholipid syndrome, also known as lupus anticoagulant syndrome or Hughes syndrome, is dependent on the occurrence of clinical events in association with the unequivocal demonstration of APLA, either lupus anticoagulant (LAC) positivity in a coagulation test, or anticardiolipin detected by immunoassay.[47] Testing for APLA requires assessment of the three antibody idiotypes, IgG, IgA, and IgM. The presence of the antibody alone, in the absence of clinical symptoms, is not sufficient for diagnosis.

The clinical manifestations of APLS include DVT and PE, coronary or peripheral artery thrombosis, cerebrovascular or retinal vessel thrombosis, and pregnancy morbidity.[47] The vast majority of miscarriages (94%) in women with APLS occur in the first trimester, and there is a correlation between the APLA titers and the risk of recurrent thrombotic events and spontaneous abortions.[48] The diagnosis of APLS should be considered if there are three or more unexplained consecutive miscarriages without anatomic, genetic, or hormonal causes, one or more unexplained deaths of a morphologically normal fetus after the 10th week of gestation, or one or more premature births of a morphologically normal neonate before the 34th week of gestation associated with severe pre-eclampsia or severe placental insufficiency.

A recent review of APLS and reproduction summarized the findings of a number of studies. APLA was reported in 5.3% of 7726 pregnancies of normal women, in 20% of 2226 women with recurrent pregnancy loss and in 37% of 1579 women with systemic lupus erythematosus (SLE).[49] Mild thrombocytopenia is a regular finding in APLS pregnancies and usually remits at the conclusion of the pregnancy.

Although newborns do not usually develop APLS, the transplacental passage of antibody with associated thrombosis has been reported.[50] Following delivery, growth-restricted infants rapidly gain weight and short-term surveys suggest that such children develop in the same fashion as other infants born at a similar stage of prematurity.

Maternal and Fetal Monitoring During Pregnancy

Monitoring consists of measuring platelet counts, APLA and LAC titers in early pregnancy. Serial antibody testing is unnecessary, as a decrease in titer does not permit a relaxation of vigilance. The platelet counts should be repeated, since thrombocytopenia may occur at any time. Monthly monitoring of fetal growth and development is essential (Table 29–6). Slowed fetal growth may indicate a need to intervene and, for viable infants, to deliver if fetal distress is clearly identified. Unexplained elevations of α-fetoprotein and maternal human chorionic gonadotrophic (hCG) hormone have been reported in women with APLS.

Primary Prophylaxis of Thrombosis in Asymptomatic Women

Women with no history of thrombosis or prior fetal losses who are found to have APLA during a first pregnancy do not need prophylactic therapy although it is common to offer them low-dose aspirin (0.1 g/day). The same approach is usually appropriate for women with previous early (less than 8 weeks) pregnancy losses, or women with low or intermittent APLA titer (Table 29–6).

Secondary Prophylaxis in Women With Previous Thrombosis or Recurrent Pregnancy Complications

Women with APLA or LAC titers who have had prior thromboses, whether or not associated with pregnancy,

Table 29-6 • MONITORING AND TREATMENT RECOMMENDATIONS FOR PREGNANT WOMEN WITH ANTIPHOSPHOLIPID ANTIBODY

Monitoring
Maternal and fetal monitoring:
  APLA and LAC titers in early pregnancy
  Platelet counts (monthly)
  Fetal growth and development (monthly)

Treatment
Primary prophylaxis of thrombosis in asymptomatic women (APLA):
  Prophylactic therapy unnecessary
  Low-dose aspirin (0.1 g/day)
Secondary prophylaxis in women with previous thrombosis or recurrent pregnancy complications (APLS):
  Heparin (5000 U bid or LMWH 1 mg/kg qd or bid) and low-dose aspirin (0.1 g/day) throughout pregnancy and the postpartum period
Treatment of acute thrombotic episode (7–14 days):
  Heparin (aPTT—adjusted dose, SC or IV) or LMWH (1 mg/kg bid)
Maintenance until delivery:
  Heparin (5000 U bid, SC) or LMWH (1 mg/kg qd or bid)
  Aspirin (0.1–0.3 g/day) for severe cases including stroke or transient ischemic attack
Postpartum:
  OACs (INR 2.5–3.5) ± aspirin, for an extended period

should receive thromboprophylactic therapy throughout pregnancy and the postpartum period. The recommended therapy is low-dose aspirin (0.1 g/day) and either heparin (5000 U bid) or LMWH.[51] The dose of LMWH depends on the risk of thrombosis. In "high-risk" patients we usually recommend LMWH at therapeutic doses, such as those used for the treatment of DVT (enoxaparin, 1mg/kg bid). Postpartum, LMWH is replaced by warfarin. Because of the complexity and danger of pregnancy in such women, decisions should be deliberated between the patient, her partner, the obstetrician, and the hematologist before pregnancy. This is especially true for women who have previously developed an arterial thrombosis or stroke.

Women who have had at least two fetal losses, and who are unequivocally positive for APLA or LAC, should receive low-dose aspirin (0.1 g/day) and prophylactic heparin (5000 U bid), or LMWH. This management strategy is documented by well-controlled, small, prospective studies.[51-53] Treatment should start after confirmation of pregnancy and continue until 8 weeks postdelivery. Corticosteroids give no additional benefit and should be administered only to women with APLS secondary to SLE, or women with APLS and severe thrombocytopenia. Despite the progress made by employing the current therapeutic regimens, complications still occur in a significant number of pregnant women with APLS. In a study conducted by Rai and coworkers, a quarter of successful pregnancies were delivered prematurely,[53] suggesting that the optimal therapeutic regimen has not yet been established. Intravenous infusions of immune globulin (IVIg) (400 mg/kg for 5 days, once a month), have been used in a limited number of patients and have been beneficial. Patients have included those with severe APLS refractory to the standard treatments, cases with severe and early onset pre-eclampsia that has complicated a previous pregnancy, and patients undergoing in-vitro fertilization.[54,55] IVIg has been associated with more positive pregnancy outcomes, a gradual decline in APLA and increases in platelet counts.[56,57] However, a controlled trial using IVIg to prevent pregnancy loss recently demonstrated no benefit.[57]

The Treatment of Acute Thrombotic Episodes

The treatment of an acute venous thrombosis in an APLA carrier is similar to that for women with other types of thrombophilia (described above). However, in our opinion there are differences in the maintenance doses and duration of prophylactic therapy required. In women with APLS, we tend to administer higher doses of LMWH depending on the severity of the thrombotic event, the history of previous thromboembolic events, and the antibody titer. LMWH or UFH is given until term and discontinued shortly before delivery. After delivery, the heparin therapy is reinstated with concomitant OAC, which are then administered for an extended period of time. In women with APLS it is usual to recommend low-dose aspirin (0.1 g/day) in addition for the prevention of arterial thrombosis (cerebral events). For women with APLS who present with recurrent arterial or venous thrombotic events during pregnancy, aspirin, at a dose of 0.3 to 0.5 g/day, and full therapeutic doses of UFH or LMWH may be considered (Table 29-6). Aspirin therapy alone is not considered sufficient for APLS.

POSTPARTUM OVARIAN VEIN THROMBOSIS

Postpartum ovarian vein thrombosis (POVT) is a relatively rare complication that occurs within a few days of labor in 1:500 to 1:2000 women[58] (see Chapter 15 also). Presentation is characterized by fever and abdominal pain, and occasionally by an abdominal mass that occasionally requires explorative laparotomy. The pathogenesis of POVT has been attributed to bacterial spread from the uterus or vagina to the right ovarian veins, and to the stasis and hypercoagulability associated with the postpartum period (Table 29-7).[58]

In a recent study, investigation of 22 women with POVT revealed thrombophilia in 11 cases. Of these, 8 developed POVT after caesarean section.[59] With the advent of modern imaging, the correct diagnosis of POVT can be made relatively easily and therefore surgical exploration is now rarely needed. The sensitivities of computed tomography (CT), magnetic resonance imaging (MRI), and Doppler ultrasonography are 100%, 92%, and 50%, respectively.[60] Treatment of POVT includes heparin during the acute episode, followed by OACs. The duration of OAC therapy is determined by presence and type of thrombophilia (Table 29-7).

Table 29-7 • POSTPARTUM OVARIAN VEIN THROMBOSIS

Characteristics
Estimated risk 1 : 500–1 : 2000
Occurs within a few days of labor
Fever, abdominal pain, with or without abdominal mass
Rarely requires laparotomy
Frequently associated with caesarean section

Pathogenesis
Bacterial spread from uterus or vagina to right ovarian vein
Stasis and postpartum hypercoagulability
High incidence of thrombophilia

Diagnosis
CT
MRI
Doppler

Treatment
Heparin or LMWH followed by oral anticoagulants

CT, computed tomography; MRI, magnetic resonance imaging.

ARTERIAL THROMBOSIS DURING PREGNANCY

Stroke carries a high mortality and morbidity, and is a severe complication during pregnancy and the puerperium. Among 50 million deliveries in the United States, 17.7 cases of stroke and 11.4 cases of intracranial venous thrombosis occurred per 100,000 deliveries.[61] Stroke was strongly associated with pregnancy-related hypertension and eclampsia[62] and its incidence was increased after delivery (8.7) but not during pregnancy per se.[63] Intracranial venous thrombosis has been associated with maternal age.[61] The association of thrombotic cerebral events and inherited thrombophilia is still controversial. Several studies have reported that patients with prothrombin or factor V Leiden mutations are at an increased risk for developing cerebral venous thrombosis.[23,25,64] However, other studies have failed to show a significant link between thrombophilia and the occurrence of cerebral venous or arterial thrombosis.[1,2,17,18,24,25,26,65] No studies have described the association between thrombophilia and cerebral ischemic events during pregnancy. We have recently investigated 12 previously healthy pregnant women who had transient cerebral ischemic events during pregnancy.[66] The incidence of inherited thrombophilia was significantly higher in the 12 women with neurologic symptoms (83%) compared with healthy pregnant women matched for age, ethnicity, and smoking habits (17%). Hence it is possible that pregnancy and the puerperium may precipitate arterial thrombotic events in patients with inherited thrombophilia, similar to the effects of smoking and the use of oral contraceptives. These agents were found to substantially increase the relative risk of myocardial infarction and cerebral venous thrombosis in patients with the factor II and factor V mutations.[67] We suggest that women with transient neurologic events appearing during pregnancy should be investigated for inherited thrombophilia and a right-to-left shunt.

Women who develop stroke or transient focal neurologic deficits during pregnancy should be treated for a prolonged period with aspirin, 0.3 to 0.5 g/day. Women with APLS should be treated with a combination of aspirin and either heparin or LMWH.[68] No guidelines are available for the women with other types of thrombophilia and the decision whether to add heparin or LMWH should be made individually on the basis of the type of thrombophilia, additional known risk factors, and recurrence of thrombotic events, and their severity.

THROMBOPHILIA AND OBSTETRIC COMPLICATIONS

Recurrent pregnancy loss (RPL) is a common health problem affecting 1% to 2% of women of reproductive age. APLS is commonly associated with RPL and with the presence of placental infarctions and thrombotic changes in decidual microvessels.[12,68] Hereditary thrombophilias appear to play a role in the pathogenesis of RPL. RPL, particularly in the second trimester, has been associated with a higher prevalence of factor V Leiden and MTHFR mutations, possibly leading to thrombotic events in the placenta.[69–73]

Recently, Brenner and colleagues examined a group of 76 women with RPL of no apparent cause.[74] Significantly more women with RPL (49%) had some form of thrombophilia compared with the control group (21%). In particular, factor V Leiden mutation was significantly more common in the RPL group, present in 24 cases compared with the 11 of 106 cases in the control group. A further study of combined thrombophilic anomalies again revealed a higher number of cases in the RPL patient group. Significantly more cases with thrombophilia were documented in the RPL patients (6 of 76 cases) compared with controls (1 of 106 cases).

A large European study (The European Prospective Cohort on Thrombophilia, EPCOT) analyzed the risk of fetal loss in a cohort of 571 women with a variety of known inherited thrombophilias. The study described odds ratios of 3.6 for stillbirths and 1.3 for miscarriages.[75] Women with factor V Leiden mutation had odds ratios of 2.0 (0.5 to 1.77) for stillbirth and 0.9 (0.5 to 1.5) for miscarriages.

Various other studies have examined the incidence of RPL in women with thrombophilia. A case control study of 60 women with documented thrombophilias revealed an increased risk of RPL.[76] Miscarriage occurred in 42 of 188 pregnancies (22%) in women with thrombophilia compared with 23 of 202 (11%) in the controls. Ridker and coworkers reported a 2.3-fold increased prevalence of factor V Leiden mutation in women with RPL.[77] Lindqvist and coworkers described a prospective study of 2480 women in early pregnancy.[78] The overall prevalence of the factor V Leiden mutation was 11% (270 of 2480). Pregnancy complications did not occur more frequently in factor V Leiden carriers, but carriers did experience an eight-fold higher risk of VTE (3 of 270 cases compared with 3 of 2210). The discrepancies among these various studies may be partially explained by differences in selection criteria, including the ethnic origins of the study populations and the study methodology.

Several recent studies have evaluated the potential role of the prothrombin G20210A mutation in RPL. No difference in the prevalence of the mutation between women with RPL and controls was described.[79] However, a further study demonstrated an odds ratio of 2.2 (95% CI 0.6 to 8.0, $p = 0.23$) for prothrombin G20210A in the RPL group compared to controls.[74] These small-scale studies do not rule out the possibility that prothrombin G20210A mutation is a mild risk factor for RPL.

Other obstetric complications have been associated with thrombosis of placental capillaries. The pathologic features of pre-eclampsia include thrombosis of the spiral arteries, impairing placental perfusion. Intrauterine growth retardation (IUGR) is associated with villous infarctions, avascular villi, and atheromatosis and thrombosis of uteroplacental vessels.[80] Severe abruptio placentae is found in about 50% of cases with low birth weight,[81] and stillbirth also is associated with impaired placental development and compromised uteroplacental vessels.[82] Although the pathophysiology of these complications generally remains undefined, all have been associated with the presence of thrombophilia.

We recently compared 110 women with one of the obstetric complications described above with 110 women who had successfully completed one or more apparently normal pregnancies. The prevalence of the factor V Leiden mutation, homozygosity for the MTHFR mutation, and the prothrombin G20210A mutation was significantly higher in women with obstetric complications compared with the control group. Overall, 57 women with obstetric complications (52%) had a thrombophilic mutation as compared with 19 normal women (17%, $p < 0.001$). Furthermore, deficiencies of protein S, protein C, or AT III or the presence of ACLA were detected in an additional 14 women with obstetric complications, compared with one case in the control group.[83]

We recently investigated the majority of the 110 women described above for a genetic polymorphism in the PAI-1 gene as a possible determinant of obstetric complications.[84] PAI-1 functions as a fast-acting inhibitor of tissue plasminogen activator activity, and elevated levels of PAI-1 increase thrombotic risk in both the venous and arterial circulation.[85–88] PAI-1 contains several polymorphic loci, including a 4G/5G insertion deletion.[89] Homozygous 4G individuals appear to be at increased risk of thrombosis.[90] Ninety-four women with obstetric complications and 95 "control" women with normal pregnancies were investigated for the hypofibrinolytic 4G/5G polymorphism in the PAI-1 gene.[84] Patients with complications were significantly more likely than controls to be 4G/4G homozygotes (30 of 94 compared with 18 of 95, odds ratio [OR] 2, 95% CI 1.02 to 3.9, $p = .041$). Heterozygosity or homozygosity for factor V Leiden was present only in the cases with a PAI-1 4G/4G polymorphism (33% compared with zero).[84]

These findings suggest that thrombophilia, and genetic hypofibrinolysis manifesting as an increased incidence of the 4G/4G polymorphism of the PAI-1 gene, may facilitate thrombosis in placental capillaries and contribute to the high recurrence rate (20% to 60%) of obstetric complications.

The role of hyperhomocysteinemia with and without the MTHFR mutation in pregnancy complications has also been investigated. In one study, hyperhomocysteinemia was documented in 26% of women with placental abruption, in 11% of the cases with intrauterine fetal death and in 38% of women delivering babies with birth weights below the fifth percentile. This compares with an estimated incidence of 2% to 3% in a control population.[91] In another study, hyperhomocysteinemia was found in 26 of 84 (31%) women with previous placental infarcts or abruption as compared to 4 of 46 (9%) control cases.[92] The Hordaland Homocysteine Study evaluated plasma homocysteine levels in 5883 women with 14492 gestations. High levels of homocysteine were found to be related to an increased risk for pre-eclampsia, stillbirth, early labor, and placental abruption (OR 1.33, 2.11, 1.41, and 3.03, respectively).[93]

Combinations of thrombophilic states may further increase the risk for RPL. The EPCOT study showed a high odds ratio for stillbirth (OR 14.3, 95% CI 2.4 to 86) in patients with combined thrombophilic defects.[75]

Based on these observations, it is recommended that women who experience recurrent pregnancy loss, or one of the obstetric complications listed above, should be screened for thrombophilia.[12] A history of obstetric complications may act as a marker for thrombophilic mutations, providing a useful predictor of an elevated risk of thromboembolism throughout life.

ANTITHROMBOTIC AGENTS FOR PREVENTING OBSTETRIC COMPLICATIONS

Women with a history of obstetric complications are commonly treated with low-dose aspirin throughout subsequent pregnancies. However, a recent large multicenter study revealed that low-dose aspirin did not reduce the incidence of pre-eclampsia significantly or improve perinatal outcomes in pregnant women at high risk for pre-eclampsia.[94] Thus, alternative or additional antithrombotic drugs may be indicated in the management of preeclampsia. In this context, it may be that the findings of studies investigating the role of aspirin and heparin in women with APLS can be extrapolated. The addition of heparin to aspirin resulted in a successful outcome in 83 of 93 (89%) gestations in women with RPL, and in all 28 gestations in women who experienced pre-eclampsia during a previous pregnancy.[51] Administration of enoxaparin, 20 mg once daily, to women with primary early RPL and an impaired fibrinolytic capacity produced positive results. The women experienced a normalization of impaired fibrinolysis, conception occurred in 16 of 20 cases (80%), and a successful live birth in 13 of 16 cases (81%).[95]

Brenner reported the effective use of LMWH as treatment for 42 women with thrombophilia who had previously presented with thromboembolism and/or RPL. Women received enoxaparin, 40 mg once daily, or, in the case of a combined thrombophilia or abnormal Doppler velocimetry (suggesting decreased placental perfusion), enoxaparin, 40 mg twice daily. Forty-five of the 63 pregnancies (71%) resulted in live births. In women with inherited thrombophilia and RPL, the percentage of live births increased from 20% without therapy to 75% following LMWH treatment.[96]

We have recently treated with enoxaparin 32 thrombophilic women who previously had experienced severe complications of pregnancy. Enoxaparin (40 mg once daily) and aspirin (100 mg/day) were administered from the 12th week of gestation until 6 weeks postpartum. There was significantly increased mean gestational age (32.2 ± 4.9 weeks compared with 37.7 ± 4.9 weeks) and birth weight (1123 ± 655 g compared with 2795 ± 540 g) in the treated pregnancies compared with the previous untreated pregnancies.[97] Pregnancy complications occurred in three of the treated pregnancies and all the newborns survived with no morbidity. In a similar study, 26 patients with documented thrombophilia and a history of pre-eclampsia and/or IUGR, were treated with the LMWH nadroparin (7500 U twice daily) and aspirin (80 mg once daily) throughout pregnancy. The birth weight of babies born to these women was higher than that recorded in women with no thrombotic predisposition.[98] These encouraging preliminary results on the efficacy of LMWH in the prevention of recurrent obstetric complications should be further substantiated in controlled clinical trials.

Hyperhomocysteinemia in pregnancy is usually managed with folate supplementation (1 mg/day). Although such an approach seems logical, there is no evidence that lowering homocysteine concentration is beneficial for the mother or the child in terms of lowering the risk of thromboembolic complications.

REFERENCES

Chapter 29 References

1. Dahlback B. Molecular genetics of venous thromboembolism. Ann Med 1995;27:187–192.
2. Conard J, Horellou MH, Van Dreden P, et al. Thrombosis and pregnancy in congenital deficiencies in AT III, protein C or protein S: Study of 78 women. Thromb Haemost 1990;63:319–320.
3. De Stefano V, Leone G, Mastrangelo S, et al. Thrombosis during pregnancy and surgery in patients with congenital deficiency of antithrombin III, protein C, protein S. Thromb Haemost 1994; 71:799–800.
4. Poort SR, Rosendaal FR, Reitsma PH, et al. Common genetic variation in the 3′-untranslated region of the prothrombin gene is associated with elevated plasma prothrombin levels and an increase in venous thrombosis. Blood 1996;88:3698–3703.
5. Rosendaal FR, Siscovick DS, Schwartz SM, et al. A common prothrombin variant (20210 G to A) increases the risk of myocardial infarction in young women. Blood 1997;90:1747–1750.
6. Simioni P, Prandoni P, Lensing AWA, et al. Risk of subsequent venous thromboembolic complications in carriers of the prothrombin or the factor V mutation with the first episode of deep-vein thrombosis. Blood 2000;96:3329–3333.
7. McColl MD, Walker ID, Greer IA. A mutation in the prothrombin gene contributing to venous thrombosis during pregnancy. Br J Obstet Gynaecol 1998;105:923–925.
8. Hallak M, Senderowicz J, Cassel A, et al. Activated protein C resistance (factor V Leiden) associated with thrombosis in pregnancy. Am J Obstet Gynecol 1997;176:889–893.
9. Bokarewa ML, Bremme K, Blomback M. Arg506-Gln mutation in factor V and risk of thrombosis during pregnancy. Br J Haematol 1996;92:473–478.
10. Frosst P, Blom HJ, Milos R, et al. A candidate genetic risk factor for vascular disease: A common mutation in methylenetetrahydrofolate reductase. Nat Genet 1995;10:111–113.
11. den Heijer M, Koster T, Blom HJ, et al. Hyperhomocysteinemia as a risk factor for deep-vein thrombosis. N Engl J Med 1996; 334:759–762.
12. Greer IA. Thrombosis in pregnancy: maternal and fetal issues. Lancet 1999;353:1258–1265.
13. Seligsohn U, Zivelin A. Thrombophilia as a multigenic disorder. Thromb Haemost 1997;78:297–301.
14. Gerhardt A, Scharf RE, Beckmann MW, et al. Prothrombin and factor V mutations in women with a history of thrombosis during pregnancy and the puerperium. N Engl J Med 2000;342:374–380.
15. Greer IA. The challenge of thrombophilia in maternal–fetal medicine. N Engl J Med 2000;342:424–425.
16. Turnball A, Tindall VR, Beard RW. Report on confidential enquiries into maternal death in England and Wales 1982–1984. London, HMSO, 1989, Report No. 28.
17. Greer IA. Epidemiology, risk factors and prophylaxis of venous thrombo-embolism in obstetrics and gynaecology. Baillières Clin Obstet Gynaecol 1997;11:403–430.
18. Ferrari E, Jambou D, Fischer F, Appert-Flory A. Maladie thromboembolique veineuse chez la femme enceinte. Sang Thrombose Vaisseaux 1999;11:16.
19. Badaracco MA, Vessey M. Recurrence of venous thromboembolism and the use of oral contraceptives. BMJ 1974;2:215–217.
20. Ginsberg JS, Brill-Edwards P, Burrows RF, et al. Venous thrombosis during pregnancy: Leg and trimester of presentation. Thromb Haemost 1992;67:519–520.
21. Macklon NS, Greer IA, Bowman AW. An ultrasound study of gestational and postural changes in the deep venous system of the leg in pregnancy. Br J Obstet Gynaecol 1997;104:191–197.
22. Clark P, Brennand J, Conkie JA, et al. Activated protein C sensitivity, protein C, protein S and coagulation in normal pregnancy. Thromb Haemost 1998;79:1166–1170.
23. Greer IA. Haemostasis and thrombosis in pregnancy. In: Bloom AL, Forbes CD, Thomas DP, Tuddenham EGD Edinburgh, Churchill Livingstone, 1994, p. 987.
24. Friend JR, Kakkar VV. The diagnosis of deep venous thrombosis in the puerperium. J Obstet Gynaecol Br Commonw 1970;77: 820–823.
25. Macklon NS, Greer IA. Venous thromboembolic disease in obstetrics and gynaecology: The Scottish experience. Scott Med J 1996;41:83–86.
26. Ginsberg JS, Hirsh J, Rainbow AJ, Coates G. Risks to the fetus of radiologic procedures used in the diagnosis of maternal venous thromboembolic disease. Thromb Haemost 1989;61:189–196.
27. Finazzi G, Barbui T. Different incidence of venous thrombosis in patients with inherited deficiencies of antithrombin III, protein C and protein S. Thromb Haemost 1994;71:15–18.
28. Hunt BJ, Doughty HA, Majumdar G, et al. Thromboprophylaxis with low molecular weight heparin (Fragmin) in high risk pregnancies. Thromb Haemost 1997;77:39–43.
29. Friederich PW, Sanson BJ, Simioni P, et al. Frequency of pregnancy-related venous thromboembolism in anticoagulant factor-deficient women: implications for prophylaxis. Ann Intern Med 1996;125:955–960.
30. Martinelli I, Sacchi E, Landi G, et al. High risk of cerebral-vein thrombosis in carriers of a prothrombin-gene mutation and in users of oral contraceptives. N Engl J Med 1998;338:1793–1797.

31. Lindqvist PG, Svensson PJ, Dahlback B, Marsal K. Factor V Q506 mutation (activated protein C resistance) associated with reduced intrapartum blood loss—a possible evolutionary selection mechanism. Thromb Haemost 1998;79:69–73.
32. Ginsberg JS, Greer I, Hirsh J. Use of antithrombotic agents during pregnancy. Chest 2001;119:122S–131S.
33. Sanson BJ, Lensing AW, Prins MH, et al. Safety of low-molecular-weight heparin in pregnancy: a systematic review. Thromb Haemost 1999;81:668–672.
34. Nelson-Piercy C, Letsky EA, De Swiet M. Low-molecular-weight heparin for obstetric thromboprophylaxis: experience of sixty-nine pregnancies in sixty-one women at high risk [see comments]. Am J Obstet Gynecol 1997;176:1062–1068.
35. Melissari E, Parker CJ, Wilson NV, et al. Use of low molecular weight heparin in pregnancy. Thromb Haemost 1992;68:652–656.
36. Gillis S, Shushan A, Eldor A. Use of low molecular weight heparin for prophylaxis and treatment of thromboembolism in pregnancy. Int J Gynaecol Obstet 1992;39:297–301.
37. Fejgin MD, Lourwood DL. Low molecular weight heparins and their use in obstetrics and gynecology. Obstet Gynecol Surv 1994;49:424–431.
38. Harenberg J, Schneider D, Heilmann L, Wolf H. Lack of antifactor Xa activity in umbilical cord vein samples after subcutaneous administration of heparin or low molecular mass heparin in pregnant women. Haemostasis 1993;23:314–320.
39. Macklon NS, Greer IA. Technical note: compression stockings and posture: A comparative study of their effects on the proximal deep veins of the leg at rest. Br J Radiol 1995;68:515–518.
40. Brancazio LR, Roperti, KA, Stierer, R, Laifer SA. Pharmacokinetics and pharmacodynamics of subcutaneous heparin during the early third trimester of pregnancy. Am J Obstet Gynecol 1995;173:1240–1245.
41. Barbour LA, Smith JM, Marlar RA. Heparin levels to guide thromboembolism prophylaxis during pregnancy. Am J Obstet Gynecol 1995;173:1869–1873.
42. Hirsh J. Low-molecular-weight heparin for the treatment of venous thromboembolism. Am Heart J 1998;135:S336–S342.
43. Rasmussen C, Wadt J, Jacobsen B. Thromboembolic prophylaxis with low molecular weight heparin during pregnancy. Int J Gynaecol Obstet 1994;47:121–125.
44. Dulitzki M, Pauzner R, Langevitz P, et al. Low-molecular-weight heparin during pregnancy and delivery: Preliminary experience with 41 pregnancies. Obstet Gynecol 1996;87:380–383.
45. Thomson AJ, Walker ID, Greer IA. Low-molecular-weight heparin for immediate management of thromboembolic disease in pregnancy. Lancet 1998;352:1904.
46. Aburahma AF, Boland JP. Management of deep vein thrombosis of the lower extremity in pregnancy: a challenging dilemma. Am Surg 1999;65:164–167.
47. Greaves M. Antiphospholipid antibodies and thrombosis [Letter; Comment]. Lancet 1999;354:1031.
48. Lockshin MD. Pregnancy loss in the antiphospholipid syndrome. Thromb Haemost 1999;82:641–648.
49. Kutteh WH. Antiphospholipid antibodies and reproduction. J Reprod Immunol 1997;35:151–171.
50. Navarro F, Dona-Naranjo MA, Villanueva I. Neonatal antiphospholipid syndrome. J Rheumatol 1997;24:1240–1241.
51. Kutteh WH, Ermel LD. A clinical trial for the treatment of antiphospholipid antibody-associated recurrent pregnancy loss with lower dose heparin and aspirin. Am J Reprod Immunol 1996;35:402–407.
52. Kutteh WH. Antiphospholipid antibody-associated recurrent pregnancy loss: treatment with heparin and low-dose aspirin is superior to low-dose aspirin alone. Am J Obstet Gynecol 1996;174:1584–1589.
53. Rai R, Cohen H, Dave M, Regan L. Randomised controlled trial of aspirin and aspirin plus heparin in pregnant women with recurrent miscarriage associated with phospholipid antibodies (or antiphospholipid antibodies). BMJ 1997;314:253–257.
54. Clark AL, Branch DW, Silver RM, et al. Pregnancy complicated by the antiphospholipid syndrome: Outcomes with intravenous immunoglobulin therapy. Obstet Gynecol 1999;93:437–441.
55. Cowchock S. Treatment of antiphospholipid syndrome in pregnancy. Lupus 1998;7 Suppl 2:S95–S97.
56. Sher G, Matzner W, Feinman M, et al. The selective use of heparin/aspirin therapy, alone or in combination with intravenous immunoglobulin G, in the management of antiphospholipid antibody-positive women undergoing in vitro fertilization. Am J Reprod Immunol 1998;40:74–82.
57. Branch DW, Peaceman AM, Druzin M, et al. A multicenter, placebo-controlled pilot study of intravenous immune globulin treatment of antiphospholipid syndrome during pregnancy. Am J Obstet Gynecol 2000;182:122–127.
58. Dunnihoo DR, Gallaspy, JW, Wise RB, Otterson WN. Postpartum ovarian vein thrombophlebitis: A review. Obstet Gynecol Surv 1991;46:415–427.
59. Salomon O, Apter S, Shaham D, et al. Risk factors associated with postpartum ovarian vein thrombosis. Thromb Haemost 1999;82:1015–1019.
60. Twickler DM, Setiawan AT, Evans RS, et al. Imaging of puerperal septic thrombophlebitis: Prospective comparison of MR imaging, CT, and sonography. Am J Roentgenol 1997;169:1039–1043.
61. Lanska DJ, Kryscio, RJ. Stroke and intracranial venous thrombosis during pregnancy and puerperium. Neurology 1998;51:1622–1628.
62. Mas JL, Lamy C. Stroke in pregnancy and the puerperium. J Neurol 1998;245:305–313.
63. Kittner SJ, Stern BJ, Feeser, BR, et al. Pregnancy and the risk of stroke. N Engl J Med 1996;335:768–774.
64. Rizk B, Meagher S, Fisher AM. Severe ovarian hyperstimulation syndrome and cerebrovascular accidents. Hum Reprod 1990;5:697–698.
65. Kaaja R, Siegberg R, Tiitinen A, Koskimies A. Severe ovarian hyperstimulation syndrome and deep venous thrombosis [Letter]. Lancet 1989;2:1043.
66. Kupferminc MJ, Yair D, Bornstein NM, Lessing JB. Transient focal neurological deficits during pregnancy in carriers of inherited thrombophilia. Stroke 2000;31:892–895.
67. Bertina RM, Rosendaal FR. Venous thrombosis—the interaction of genes and environment. N Engl J Med 1998;338:1840–1841.
68. Lima F, Khamashta MA, Buchanan NM, et al. A study of sixty pregnancies in patients with the antiphospholipid syndrome. Clin Exp Rheumatol 1996;14:131–136.
69. Rai RS, Regan L, Chitolie A, et al. Placental thrombosis and second trimester miscarriage in association with activated protein C resistance. Br J Obstet Gynaecol 1996;103:842–844.
70. Grandone E, Margaglione M, Colaizzo D, et al. Factor V Leiden, C > T MTHFR polymorphism and genetic susceptibility to preeclampsia. Thromb Haemost 1997;77:1052–1054.
71. Dizon-Townson DS, Meline L, Nelson LM, et al. Fetal carriers of the factor V Leiden mutation are prone to miscarriage and placental infarction. Am J Obstet Gynecol 1997;177:402–405.
72. Grandone E, Margaglione M, Colaizzo D, et al. Factor V Leiden is associated with repeated and recurrent unexplained fetal losses. Thromb Haemost 1997;77:822–824.
73. Brenner B, Mandel H, Lanir N, et al. Activated protein C resistance can be associated with recurrent fetal loss. Br J Haematol 1997;97:551–554.
74. Brenner B, Sarig G, Weiner Z, et al. Thrombophilic polymorphisms are common in women with fetal loss without apparent cause. Thromb Haemost 1999;82:6–9.
75. Preston FE, Rosendaal FR, Walker ID, et al. Increased fetal loss in women with heritable thrombophilia. Lancet 1996;348:913–916.
76. Sanson BJ, Friederich PW, Simioni P, et al. The risk of abortion and stillbirth in antithrombin-, protein C-, and protein S-deficient women. Thromb Haemost 1996;75:387–388.

77. Ridker PM, Miletich JP, Buring JE, et al. Factor V Leiden mutation as a risk factor for recurrent pregnancy loss. Ann Intern Med 1998;128:1000–1003.
78. Lindqvist PG, Svensson PJ, Marsaal K, et al. Activated protein C resistance (FV:Q506) and pregnancy. Thromb Haemost 1999;81:532–537.
79. Deitcher SR, Park VM, Kutteh WH. Prothrombin 20210 GA mutation analysis in Causcasian women with early first trimester recurrent pregnancy loss. Blood 1998;92[Suppl 1]:118b
80. Salafia CM, Minior VK, Pezzullo JC, et al. Intrauterine growth restriction in infants of less than thirty-two weeks' gestation: associated placental pathologic features. Am J Obstet Gynecol 1995;173:1049–1057.
81. Green JR. Placenta previa and abruptio placentae. In: Maternal Fetal Medicine: Principles and Practice. Philadelphia, WB Saunders, 1994, p. 609.
82. Infante-Rievard C, Davis M, Gauthier R, Ribard GE. Lupus anticoagulants, anticardiolipin antibodies and fetal loss. N Engl J Med 1991;325:1063–1066.
83. Kupferminc MJ, Eldor A, Steinman N, et al. Increased frequency of genetic thrombophilia in women with complications of pregnancy. N Engl J Med 1999;340:9–13.
84. Glueck CJ, Wang P, Fontaine RN, et al. Plasminogen activator inhibitor activity: an independent risk factor for the high miscarriage rate during pregnancy in women with polycystic ovary syndrome. Metabolism 1999;48:1589–1595.
85. Eriksson P, Kallin B, 't Hooft FM, et al. Allele-specific increase in basal transcription of the plasminogen-activator inhibitor 1 gene is associated with myocardial infarction. Proc Natl Acad Sci USA 1995;92:1851–1855.
86. Ossei-Gerning N, Mansfield MW, Stickland MH, et al. Plasminogen activator inhibitor-1 promoter 4G/5G genotype and plasma levels in relation to a history of myocardial infarction in patients characterized by coronary angiography. Arterioscler Thromb Vasc Biol 1997;17:33–37.
87. Sartori MT, Wiman B, Vettore S, et al. 4G/5G Polymorphism of PAI-1 gene promoter and fibrinolytic capacity in patients with deep vein thrombosis. Thromb Haemost 1998;80:956–960.
88. Grancha S, Estelles A, Tormo G, et al. Plasminogen activator inhibitor-1 (PAI-1) promoter 4G/5G genotype and increased PAI-1 circulating levels in postmenopausal women with coronary artery disease. Thromb Haemost 1999;81:516–521.
89. Dawson SJ, Wiman B, Hamsten A, et al. The two allele sequences of a common polymorphism in the promoter of the plasminogen activator inhibitor-1 (PAI-1) gene respond differently to interleukin-1 in HepG2 cells. J Biol Chem 1993;268:10739–10745.
90. Stegnar M, Uhrin P, Peternel P, et al. The 4G/5G sequence polymorphism in the promoter of plasminogen activator inhibitor-1 (PAI-1) gene: Relationship to plasma PAI-1 level in venous thromboembolism. Thromb Haemost 1998;79:975–979.
91. de Vries JI, Dekker GA, Huijgens PC, et al. Hyperhomocysteinaemia and protein S deficiency in complicated pregnancies. Br J Obstet Gynaecol 1997;104:1248–1254.
92. Goddijn-Wessel TA, Wouters MG, van de Molen EF, et al. Hyperhomocysteinemia: A risk factor for placental abruption or infarction. Eur J Obstet Gynecol Reprod Biol 1996;66:23–29.
93. Vollsett SE, Bjorke-Monsen AAL, Igrens LM. Plasma total homocysteine and previous pregnancies: The Hordaland homocysteine study. Proceedings of the 2nd International Symposium on Homocysteine. Neth J Med 1998;52:S54.
94. Caritis S, Sibai B, Hauth J, et al. Low-dose aspirin to prevent preeclampsia in women at high risk. N Engl J Med 1998;338:701–705.
95. Gris JC, Neveu S, Tailand ML, et al. Use of low-molecular-weight heparin (enoxaparin) or of a phenformin-like substance (moroxydine chloride) in primary early recurrent aborters with an impaired fibrinolytic capacity. Thromb Haemost 1995;73:362–367.
96. Brenner B. Inherited thrombophilia and pregnancy loss. Thromb Haemost 1999;82:634–640.
97. Kuperminc MJ, Fait G, Many A, et al. Low molecular weight heparin for the prevention of obstetric complications in women with thrombophilia. Hypertens Pregnancy. 2001;20:35–44.
98. Riyazi N, Leeda M, de Vries JI, et al. Low-molecular-weight heparin combined with aspirin in pregnant women with thrombophilia and a history of preeclampsia or fetal growth restriction: a preliminary study. Eur J Obstet Gynecol Reprod Biol 1998;80:49–54.

PART VI

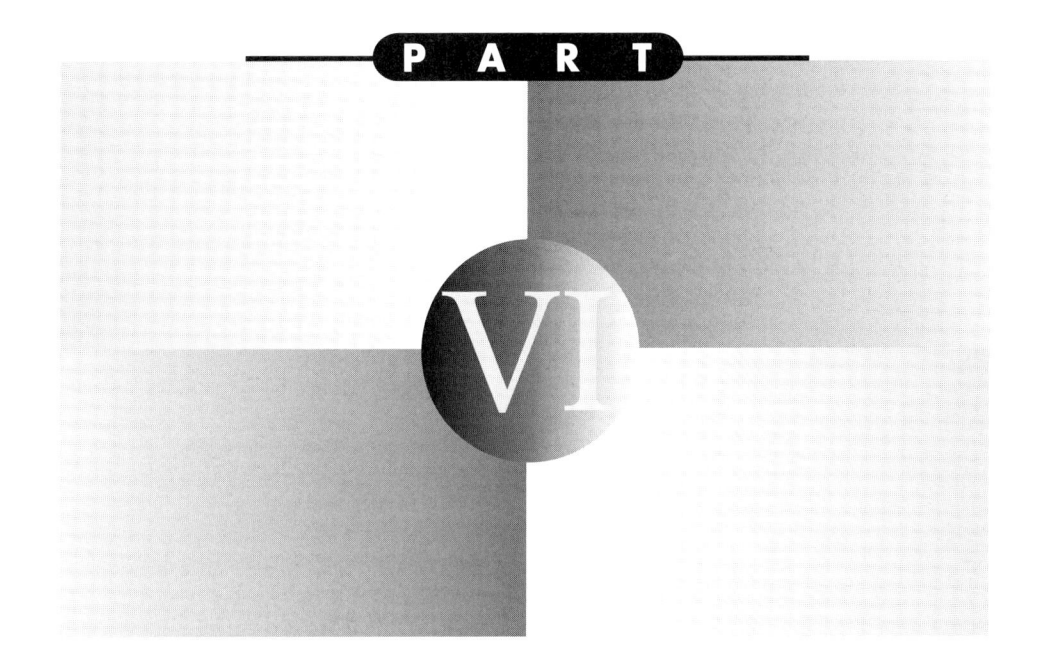

SPECIAL CONSIDERATIONS

CHAPTER 30

Surgery and Hemostasis

Craig S. Kitchens, M.D.

Blood coagulation exists to halt excessive blood loss, with surgery and trauma being the major challenges to hemostasis. While Kearon and Hirsh estimated that surgery and trauma increase the baseline risk of thrombosis up to a hundred-fold,[1] patients with mild hemophilia who have never bled from stresses of everyday life may bleed vigorously from surgical procedures.[2]

The history of the discovery of blood coagulation has been well reviewed by Ratnoff,[3] while the maturation of our understanding of and management of traumatic and surgical wounds has been reviewed by Majno.[4] The concept of pressure dressings and ligature of blood vessels to control excessive bleeding was not described until 300 to 200 BC by physicians in Alexandria. It was not until the 18th century that the French surgeon Petit deduced that the clotting of blood had something to do with the control of hemorrhage following surgery; prior to then, it was thought that constriction and retraction of vessels were the only mechanisms of hemostasis.[4] Not until the end of the 19th century did Wright observe that blood from hemophiliacs clotted more slowly than normal blood and that perhaps this observation was related to the hemorrhage characteristics of hemophilia.

By observing and studying the effects of surgery and trauma on hemostasis—including physiologic as well as hypocoagulable and hypercoagulable hemostasis—our understanding of the interrelationship between hemostasis and trauma has been advanced.

This chapter contains six sections:

1. Surgery for patients with congenital hemostatic defects.
2. The effects of surgery on hemostasis (with particular attention to cardiopulmonary bypass and orthotopic liver transplantation).
3. Preoperative hemostatic testing.
4. Invasive procedures for patients with abnormal coagulation studies.
5. Invasive procedures for patients on anticoagulant therapy.
6. Consultation on patients with intraoperative or postoperative hemorrhage.

SURGERY FOR PATIENTS WITH CONGENITAL HEMOSTATIC DEFECTS

That hemophiliacs bleed abnormally has been known since antiquity.[5] Because uncontrolled bleeding occurred in daily life, surgical procedures were generally avoided. Any surgery that was performed on hemophiliacs was usually done as a heroic measure; the results were expectedly disastrous and many patients bled to death.

Transfusion science was essentially nonexistent until World War II. Whole blood was available for hemophiliacs but it is now clear that while whole blood improved the hematocrit value, it was unable to raise the level of either factor VIII or factor IX by more than about 10% to 20%. Acute hemorrhagic mortality dropped from 50% before any blood banking to about 25%. Cryoprecipitate was discovered by Dr. Judith Pool in the 1960s, allowing factor VIII levels to reach briefly any level desired. Hemorrhagic mortality dropped to 2%. After factor VIII and factor IX concentrates became available in the 1970s, factor VIII and factor IX levels could be raised to any level desired, theoretically indefinitely, and surgical mortality approached zero.[6] Patients still experience nonfatal hemorrhage at an overall rate of approximately 18%.[6-9]

Factor levels should be maintained in the patient undergoing surgery as high and as long as indicated. The prescribed factor is infused the morning prior to surgery and the factor level is measured before anesthesia induction in order to confirm both that the factor has been appropriately administered and that no unexpectedly low increment of factor resulted (i.e., less than about 60% calculated), which could be the first sign of an occult inhibitor.

For fairly minor surgical procedures (including such procedures such as endoscopy with biopsy, arthroscopic surgery, skin or breast biopsies, lymph node biopsies, and complicated dental work), the factor level is kept at a minimum (trough) of approximately 30% and a maximum (peak) of about 60% for 3 to 4 days, with longer amounts being necessary if there is significant traction along the incision line. For more invasive surgery such as open abdominal or orthopedic surgery and particularly cardiovascular or neurologic surgery, a minimum concentration of 80% with a maximum of 150% is advised. "Peak and trough" levels are followed once a day for several days. Most hemostatic wounds are well healed from a hemostatic point of view by the 4th or 5th day and therefore factor levels can be allowed to drift down to about half the levels required at the time of surgery. The most notable exceptions to these are procedures that are characterized by significant tension along the incision line such as open abdominal operations or operations through the muscles of posture. Therapy is often quite prolonged at a slightly lower level (50% to 60%) following major orthopedic surgery during rehabilitation and aggressive physical therapy. We rarely give factor longer than 7 to 10 days following surgical procedures. Table 30–1 provides general guidelines for surgical procedures in hemophiliacs.

If one wishes to use continuous infusion of factor concentrates, a more even level of factor concentration results with less severe peaks and troughs. Less factor administration is possible and overall costs are decreased as less factor is consumed. Therapeutic levels closer to 60% to 70% are sufficient accordingly.[15,16]

Table 30–1 • GUIDELINES FOR SUCCESSFUL SURGERY IN PATIENTS WITH CONGENITAL HEMOSTATIC DISORDERS

- Establish the correct hemostatic diagnosis.
- Confirm the inhibitor, hepatitis, and human immunodeficiency virus status of the patient.
- Assume that surgical indications are the same as in hemostatically normal patients.
- Develop and follow a surgical plan.
- Consult with the blood bank concerning logistics; minimize the number of lots of factor.
- Consult with the anesthesiologist.
- Prohibit intramuscular medications, especially preoperatively.
- Avoid aspirin, aspirin-containing medications, and other platelet-inhibiting medications.
- Determine and administer the appropriate preoperative clotting factor dosage, and measure the plasma level before induction of anesthesia.
- Monitor appropriate hemostatic tests frequently.
- Sustain a hemostatic level of the patient's deficient factor as long as needed by repeated intravenous infusions of the appropriate agent.
- Consider whether adjunctive agents, e.g., antifibrinolytic drugs or hypotensive anesthesia, might enhance hemostasis.

Extracorporeal shock-wave lithotripsy (ESWL) can be performed safely using factor replacement levels of 50% to 60% before the treatments and for 3 to 5 days post-treatment. As in normal patients undergoing ESWL, hematuria is common but serious (capsular or retroperitoneal) hematomas were not encountered in a series of 11 hemophiliacs so managed.[12]

Cardiovascular surgery can be done successfully in hemophiliacs. Best results are obtained if the surgeons, anesthesiologists, and perfusion technicians all use their routine protocol based on the dictum that a hemophiliac with near 100% replacement therapy can and should undergo diagnostic and therapeutic cardiac catheterization receiving heparin, protamine, and aprotinin as would any other patient. Monitoring the appropriate factor concentration, probably best managed by the hematologist so that others can focus on their tasks, is the only difference.[13,14] An advantage of bioprosthetic heart valves for those patients requiring valve replacement is that the chronic use of warfarin postoperatively can be avoided. The use of aspirin chronically for ischemic heart disease is uncertain and must be approached on a case-by-case basis,[14] although its low-dose (81 mg/day) usage following coronary artery bypass grafting (CABG) appears rational and safe.

In the rarer contact factor deficiencies (factor XII, high-molecular-weight kininogen, and prekallikrein), replacement therapy for surgery is not indicated. In order to monitor adequate heparin levels during cardiopulmonary bypass, the patient's baseline activated clotting time cannot be used as it is 600 to 800 seconds before heparin infusion and is not "corrected" by factor replacement therapy. Davidson and coworkers successfully used heparin levels to monitor such a patient and also documented typical levels of thrombin generation during the CABG despite the inherited defect.[15]

It is essential to discuss with the surgeon (or other proceduralist) that during treatment hemostasis will be normal and therefore the surgical procedure should be carried out as completely and fully as it would be in a normal patient.

Bleeding may be more obstinent following oral surgical procedures or following prostate surgery because of profibrinolytic agents in saliva and urine that bathe the wounds dissolving hemostatic clots. For patients undergoing either prostate or oral surgery, an antifibrinolytic agent (ε-aminocaproic acid, [EACA], 2 g every 8 hours orally, or tranexamic acid, 20 mg/kg orally every 8 hours for approximately a week) helps prevent otherwise stable clots from becoming lysed.[16]

Special attention may be required in patients with von Willebrand's disease undergoing invasive procedures. In patients undergoing fairly minor procedures (such as dental procedures, colonoscopies, arthroscopic examinations, and most biopsies) DDAVP, 0.3 μg/kg intravenously, suffices for patients with type 1 von Willebrand disease (vWD). This dose of DDAVP can be given daily or twice daily for about 3 days before the agent typically becomes ineffective because of tachyphylaxis. Hyponatremia can be troubling and can cause seizures; accordingly free water intake must be minimized during DDAVP therapy. However, this time period usually suffices for hemostasis with such operations. Antifibrinolytic agents in doses mentioned above is advised concomitantly for mucosal procedures.

In patients with type 2 or type 3 vWD or in patients with type 1 vWD who are undergoing larger procedures requiring hemostatic control longer than the 3 days that can be provided by DDAVP, factor VIII concentrates that contain von Willebrand factor (vWF; Alphanate or Humate) work well. Many clinicians have noticed that it is much easier to correct the factor VIII clotting activity or vWF level to desirable levels (i.e., 30% to 50% or higher) than it is to correct the bleeding time; most experts have deduced that it is best to monitor the factor VIII activity or vWF level rather than the bleeding time as it often does not correct and failure to correct the bleeding time does not predict bleeding.[17-19]

For patients with inhibitors needing surgery it is advisable to be quite cautious, especially regarding elective surgery. Refer to Chapter 6 for general comments regarding hemorrhage in patients who have inhibitors. Porcine factor VIII has been effectively employed for hemostasis.[20] The newly released recombinant factor VIIa (NovoSeven)[21] has proven effective for surgical procedures in patients with factor VIII or factor IX inhibitors, usually infused initially at 90 µg/kg intravenously every 2 to 3 hours for 48 hours followed by dose reduction during a total of 5 days of treatment.[22]

EFFECT OF SURGERY ON HEMOSTASIS

Large-vessel hemorrhage (in general, named arteries or veins) tends to require physical methods such as pressure, ligature, or tamponade to control blood loss, whereas microcirculatory hemorrhage depends on an intact hemostatic system. Tissue factor (TF) is released from damaged blood vessels and initiates the extrinsic arm of the coagulation system.[23, 24] Thrombin generation should be sufficient that enough platelets are stimulated to adhere to denuded areas of the open endothelium and then recruit, through release of their attractants enough platelets to begin aggregation in order to breach the leak. Any compromise in this elaborate system such as a factor deficiency, thrombocytopenia, or excessive anticoagulation therapy might well result in hemorrhage. The system designed to regain hemostatic control of the open system may result potentially in an equally devastating thrombotic condition.

Initiators of coagulation include TF and other cytokines, particularly tumor necrosis factor (TNF) and interleukin 6 (IL-6) if inflammation or infection is present.[25,26] These cytokines rapidly accelerate the extrinsic system. Tissue destruction and TF release also occur in medical situations such as myocardial infarction,[27] sepsis,[28] and malignancy (see Chapter 21). During the first several hours following surgery or significant trauma there is an increase to approximately twice normal in circulating tissue plasminogen activator (tPA) levels and a rapid decrease toward normal levels by the end of the first 24 hours. Beginning approximately 2 hours after the trauma, levels of plasminogen activator inhibitor type I (PAI-1) begin to rapidly rise approaching levels four to five times normal and then gradually decrease over a day or so only to have a secondary peak at about day 7.[25,26,29,30] During that period, these high levels of PAI-1 dampen the fibrinolytic system, a process that has been termed "fibrinolytic shutdown."[29]

While thrombin is being generated, antithrombin is consumed as it neutralizes thrombin by forming thrombin : antithrombin complexes (T : AT).[31] Antithrombin levels acutely can become severely reduced during surgery, particularly with trauma and burns.[32]

Levels of these mediators will fluctuate rapidly and their degree of perturbation as measured by static laboratory tests will be a function not only of the type, degree, and duration of trauma, but also timing of blood sample collection. Experimental evidence in reproducible trauma in animals validates that graduated degrees of trauma results in graduated amounts of hypercoagulability.[33]

Shock and stasis often follow trauma. Stasis and venodilation is induced in surgery by various anesthetic agents. General anesthetics cause more systemic venostasis than local anesthetics used in epidural anesthesia. General anesthesia is associated with higher levels of PAI-1 generation 24 hours after the surgery and a higher incidence of thrombosis when compared in a controlled manner to patients undergoing the same procedure using epidural anesthesia. These higher levels of PAI-1 correlated well with subsequent thrombosis.[34] Comerota and colleagues[35] studied the degree of venodilation of arm veins in patients undergoing total hip replacement. In patients who experienced a postoperative DVT, the mean degree of venous dilation was 29% over presurgical diameters, whereas the mean dilation of those who did not experience a DVT was only 12%. All patients who experienced over 20% dilation of their arm veins experienced a DVT. Venodilation created microtears in the endothelial lining that exposed underlying collagen and may very well have served as the nidus or initiating trigger for thrombosis associated with surgery. These theories of surgically induced hypercoagulability are summarized in Table 30–2.

Prophylaxis against DVT and pulmonary embolism (PE) are discussed thoroughly in Chapter 14 as well as in a recent consensus.[36] The role of mechanical and similar adjuncts in prophylaxis against venous thromboembolism (VTE) verifies their use. Westrich and co-workers[37] demonstrated that intermittent pneumatic compression (IPC) in total knee replacement surgery was, in their hands, more effective than low-molecular-

Table 30–2 • PUTATIVE CAUSES OF HYPERCOAGULABILITY IN SURGERY AND TRAUMA

- Generation of large amounts of procoagulant factors
- Generation of high concentrations of PAI-1 ("fibrinolytic shutdown")
- Venous stasis
  Pooling of blood
  Venous microtears

weight heparin (LMWH) and far more effective than aspirin alone in reducing both DVT and PE. However, they did note only a 33% compliance rate with patients for whom IPC was prescribed. Others have demonstrated not only the effectiveness of IPC and similar devices but the additive effect of this methodology with chemical (heparin) prophylaxis.[38,39] The efficacy is theoretically due to a decrease in cross-sectional area of capacitance veins, thus generating both an increase in linear blood flow as well as protection of venous valve competency. Additionally, since the vein wall is less distended, one might speculate a decrease in microtears in the venous wall.[39]

Whereas there has been a general and increasing acceptance of chemical prophylaxis in surgical patients, there remains a reticence on the part of neurosurgeons for understandable fear of possible additional risk of hemorrhage. For many indications, IPC is probably effective.[38] However, several recent analyses of VTE prophylaxis in neurosurgical patients[40–42] have indicated not only is LMWH itself safe but, when combined with IPC, adds to the efficacy of VTE prophylaxis either without any additional risk of hemorrhage[40,41] or with such a small amount of increased risk that such risk of hemorrhage is easily absorbed by the decrease in overall morbidity and mortality from VTE.[41] In these last three studies, all prophylactic doses of LMWH were initiated postoperatively. In one small study involving only patients for brain tumor surgery, LMWH was given preoperatively with an increased risk (5 of 46 patients) of intracranial hemorrhage.[43]

The coagulation challenges associated with two surgical procedures, *cardiopulmonary bypass* (*CPB*) and *orthotopic liver transplant* (*OLT*), are more likely than not mediated by surges of endogenous tPA resulting in a brisk hyperfibrinolytic state.

The effects of CPB on blood have been thoroughly reviewed.[44] Whereas multiple platelet defects have been ascribed to CPB,[45] these are probably rather minor and transient. These aberrations are produced by partial activation of platelets coming in contact with the nonbiologic material of the CPB pump and oxygenator apparatus as well as binding and agglutination of platelets to such material. Platelet glycoprotein Ib (GpIb) is decreased on these platelets but it is doubtful whether this change itself is sufficient to cause a significant hemostatic challenge. Hemorrhage may be serious enough to result in re-exploration in 3% to 7%[46] of cases of CABG and is associated with a 30% increase in mortality.[44]

When excessive hemorrhage in CPB patients was thought due to acquired platelet defects, many studies examined the efficacy of DDAVP in managing those defects.[47,48] DDAVP was not uniformly efficacious in reducing mortality, re-exploration, and blood usage, and may have even contributed to a two-fold risk of perioperative acute myocardial infarction (Table 30–3). These data suggest that hemorrhage in the majority of CPB patients is not primarily due to a platelet defect or at least a platelet defect that could be reversed by the administration of DDAVP. DDAVP should not be used routinely in CPB patients but employed only when it is apparent that a patient is hemorrhaging and then it should be given in the routine dosage (0.3 μg/kg intravenously).[49,50] This approach may reverse hemorrhage in patients who took aspirin prior to their surgery.[51] Similarly the routine nonspecific use of platelet transfusions as well as fresh frozen plasma (FFP) infusion is not indicated.[52,53]

There is now general consensus that the majority of excessive bleeding following CPB is due to the surge of tPA that occurs during rewarming of the patient, which temporally correlates with coming off the CPB apparatus and closure of the mediastinum.[54,55] Until that time, circulating levels of tPA are not particularly high as the surge does not begin until the rewarming phase. Of interest, patients who undergo cardiothoracic surgery without CPB do not experience this tPA surge.[54]

Pharmacologic agents serve to block the effects of tPA. Aprotinin is a serpin isolated from bovine pancreas. It is a powerful inhibitor of plasmin and thus an effective blocker of fibrinolysis. It has little or no anti-tPA or platelet activity.[56,57] A meta-analysis of 72 trials including 8409 CPB patients concluded that of multiple hemostatic agents, aprotinin was associated with the greatest decrease in blood loss, mortality, rate of re-exploration, and overall blood usage[48] (see Table 30–3) whether the routine-dose aprotinin (2 million KIU as a bolus followed by 500,000 KIU every hour) or lower doses was employed. Others[58–60] have stated that other

Table 30–3 • META-ANALYSIS OF EFFICACY OF HEMOSTATIC AGENTS COMPARED TO PLACEBO FOR PERIOPERATIVE HEMORRHAGE ASSOCIATED WITH CARDIOPULMONARY BYPASS SURGERY

		Odds Ratio			
	Mean Decrease in Blood Loss, mL	Mortality	Re-exploration	Blood Product Usage	Perioperative AMI[a]
Aprotinin[b]	446	0.55	0.37	0.37	1.13
Antifibrinolytic agents[c]	264	0.78	0.44	0.46	0.48
DDAVP[d]	114	1.02	0.67	0.79	2.40

Data from Laupacis and Fergusson[47] and Levi et al.[48]
[a] AMI, acute myocardial infarction.
[b] Either "conventional" or "low" dose.
[c] Either EACA or tranexamic acid.
[d] DDAVP, desmopressin.

fibrinolytic agents are as good as and particularly less expensive than aprotonin.

Perioperative myocardial infarction occurred in 4% of patients receiving lower-dose aprotonin and in 8% of those receiving the conventional dose; however, the overall mortality rate was still half that of patients not receiving aprotonin. The overall perioperative myocardial infarction rate was essentially the same as placebo.[48]

Aprotonin has also been shown in both case reports and small studies to be efficacious in special situations requiring CPB such as patients undergoing hypothermic surgery,[61] heart transplantation,[62] aortic surgery,[63] CABG in patients with ITP,[64] or lung transplantation,[65] and in patients requiring a left ventricular assist device (LVAD) as a bridge while awaiting transplant.[66]

Re-exploration to assess hemorrhage is necessary in 3% to 7% of cases following CPB,[46] and 67% of the time a specific bleeding site responding to local measures is found.[44] Of interest, Pelletier[46] found for the 33% of cases in which they did not find a surgical or anatomic reason for hemorrhage, most hemorrhage simply stopped as though the re-exploration itself had a net hemostatic effect. Studying their hypothesis, various coagulation components of mediastinal blood were measured, and compared to systemic levels in the same patient. The fibrinogen and α_2-plasmin inhibitor levels were both significantly lower ($p \leq 0.05$), while the levels of PAI-1 and fibrin degradation products (FDPs) were both significantly higher ($p \leq 0.05$) in the shed mediastinal blood than in systemic blood. They used these data as evidence for increased fibrinolytic activity primarily in the mediastinal cavity itself and that drainage via exploration may have eliminated self-perpetuating local hyperfibrinolysis.

Recombinant factor VIIa has been anecdotally employed successfully in a few cases of uncontrolled hemorrhage following CPB[67]; however, its routine use for this indication cannot be supported at this time without further studies.

Aprotonin, EACA, and tranexamic acid[68,69] exert their primary procoagulant effects by blocking the action of plasmin, thereby greatly impeding fibrinolysis. Thrombotic events to include either arterial (myocardial infarction or stroke) or venous (DVT or PE) events do not appear increased using these agents.[55,70] As aprotonin is prepared from bovine pancreas, it could be expected to cause immunologic reactions, including anaphylaxis.[71] Dietrich and colleagues[72] studied 248 cases of re-exposure to aprotonin and found a 3% incidence of adverse reactions, which typically occurred on initiation of aprotinin administration and were characterized by an acute fall in blood pressure. All survived the reaction. Only 1.5% of patients experienced adverse reaction on re-exposure if more than 6 months had lapsed since their last exposure. Patients who had had re-exposure within 6 months had a reaction rate of 4.5%.

Drugs that block the platelet glycoprotein IIb/IIIa (GpIIb/IIIa) platelet receptor (see Chapter 19) are used in patients with acute coronary syndrome, a population that may undergo emergent CABG with CPB and attendant extra risk for hemorrhage. Following abciximab, the GpIIb/IIIa receptor blocker with the longest half-life, a 12-hour hiatus after the last infusion is recommended.[73] Because abciximab is very tightly bound to platelet membranes with negligible amounts of unbound circulating abciximab in the plasma, use of platelet transfusions is rational for preparation of the patient requiring emergent surgery prior to 12 hours since the last abciximab infusion.

Hyperfibrinolysis following CPB is associated with a tPA surge that may occur in response to enhanced procoagulant activity. Dietrich and colleagues[74] operated on patients at risk for post-CPB hyperfibrinolysis by first treating them with warfarin to a mean international normalized ratio (INR) of 2.4; their control group had an INR of 1.1. Those patients undergoing CPB at the therapeutic INR required less heparin to reach appropriate anticoagulation as determined by the activated clotting time (ACT) and in particular required less heparin during the operation to maintain an appropriate ACT value. These data suggest that warfarin pretreatment resulted in less thrombin (and therefore less fibrin) generation during CPB with subsequently a diminished tPA surge. Blood loss at 6 and 12 hours with warfarin-treated patients was 381 and 505 mL, respectively, whereas the control group lost 472 and 527 mL, respectively, reaching statistical significance ($p < 0.05$). They noticed no correlation with blood loss even with patients at the highest INRs, including up to 6.0. They neither reversed the warfarin nor administered FFP during the operation.[74]

Orthotopic liver transplantation (OLT) historically has been complicated by massive hemorrhage and heavy demands on the transfusion service. In the past 10 years our understanding of the hemorrhagic nature of OLT has increased to the point that effective therapy has greatly reduced both the incidence and severity of hemorrhage as well as impact on the blood bank.

OLT often is performed in patients with profound deterioration of their hemostatic system, even preoperatively, given the role of the liver in coagulation and fibrinolysis. The platelet count is often low because of hypersplenism. Accordingly, it previously had been regarded that these preoperative changes were the primary cause(s) of hemostatic failure in OLT.

Our understanding of hemostatic failure has been assisted by dividing OLT into four phases: the preoperative, anhepatic, and reperfusion phases with a convalescent phase occurring in the week or two following the transplantation. The hemostatic changes characteristic of OLT have been described by many[75–80] and are outlined in Table 30–4. In summary, the patient has impaired hemostasis that deteriorates during the anhepatic phase. During the reperfusion phase, the surge of tPA results from wash-out from the donor liver following anastomosis with the recipient. It is also during this phase that hemorrhage can become excessive. Those using thromboelastography (TEG) were instrumental in discovery of reperfusion hyperfibrinolysis.[75] In the convalescent period from postoperative day 1 through 14, procoagulant factors appear to replenish faster than anticoagulant factors (see Table 30–4). This may in part explain acute hepatic artery thrombosis that, if it happens, does so in this period.

Table 30–4 • HEMOSTATIC ALTERATIONS IN ORTHOTOPIC LIVER TRANSPLANTATION

	Preoperative	Anhepatic	Reperfusion	Convalescence* (Days)
Coagulation factors	50%	↓	↓	1–2
Antithrombin III	50%	→	→	7–14
Protein C	50%	→	→	7–14
Protein S	50%	→	→	7–14
Plasminogen	50%	↓	→	4–7
α_2PI	50%	↓	↓	4–7
tPA	↑	↑↑	↑↑↑	1–2
PAI-1	NI	↓↓↓	↓↓↓	1–2
FDP	↑	↑↑	↑↑	1–2
TAT	NI	→	↑	1–7
Platelet count	50%	→	→	1–7
Platelet function	NI	→	↓	1–2

*The convalescence period is the time required to return to normal adult levels. These data represent a theoretical case with hepatic dysfunction before surgery, resulting in a hypothetic situation in which hepatic proteins circulate at levels of 50% of normal. Data derived from Sato et al.,[75] Himmelreich et al.,[76] Sato et al.,[77] Grosse et al.,[78] Velasco et al.,[79] and Grosse et al.[80]

α_2PI, α_2-plasmin inhibitor; tPA, tissue plasminogen activator; PAI-1, rapid plasminogen activator inhibitor; FDP, fibrin(ogen) degradation products, TAT, thrombin-antithrombin complex; NI, normal.

→ indicates no change; ↑ indicates a mild increase; ↑↑ indicates a significant increase; ↑↑↑ indicates a marked increase.

Several groups infused aprotinin (using 2 million KIU as a loading dose followed by 500,000 KIU every hour until skin closure) at the time of reperfusion noting marked decrease in blood loss and transfusion requirements of red cells, FFP, and platelets.[81,82] Patients who did not require transfusion of any blood product increased from 17% in patients not receiving aprotinin to 39% in those who did receive aprotinin.[82] Although some studies have shown no benefit using the same aprotinin regimen,[83,84] a recent double-blind study[85] supports the use of aprotinin in OLT.

Aprotinin usage may also decrease blood loss and transfusion needs in patients undergoing total hip replacement,[86] total knee replacement,[87] orthopedic tumor surgery, or removal of infected orthopedic hardware.[88] Doses were less than those used with CPB or OLT yet blood loss was decreased by 40% to 60% without a major increase in DVT (although all patients received LMWH for these procedures). Aprotinin has not gained universal acceptance in orthopedics, perhaps because blood loss usually is much less for these surgical procedures than with CPB or OLT and a majority of orthopedic blood loss can be recovered by use of cell savers.[89]

PREOPERATIVE HEMOSTATIC TESTING

Screening for Hemostatic Defects

Approximately 3% of all surgical procedures will be accompanied by a degree of hemorrhage deemed by the surgeon to be excessive. In their large meta-analysis of over 50 randomized studies comparing low-dose heparin to placebo in DVT prophylaxis, Collins and colleagues noted that among the 7486 controls receiving placebo, 3.3% of patients were judged to have bled excessively by the surgeon and that 0.1% succumbed to bleeding.[90] Three papers[91–93] rendered a similar rate of hemorrhage among patients who are undergoing surgical procedures during studies of appropriateness of preoperative hemostatic testing. Of 4499 patients, 2% were deemed to bleed excessively. The sensitivity of hemostatic screening tests in these 4499 patients was 18%, the specificity was 90%, the positive predictive value was 3%, and the negative predictive value was 98%. There was no correlation between results of these preoperative screening tests for hemostatic competence and surgery-related hemorrhage. Of the 85 patients who bled,[91–93] 70% had completely normal tests. Of the 435 patients who had abnormal tests, only 15 bled, implying that 97% of patients potentially identified as those likely to bleed did not bleed. Nonetheless preoperative prothrombin time (PT), activated partial thromboplastin time (aPTT), and platelet counts are almost as common as any admission order and their use seems to have become a habit.[94,95]

Approximately $30 billion are spent in the United States for preoperative testing of all types,[96] and the worth of these tests is extremely limited. In studying over 1000 patients at the Mayo Clinic who underwent surgery without any preoperative tests, outcome analyses show that the death or major operative mortality rate was 0%. None required blood tranfusion.[97]

The routine use of the bleeding time as a predictor of hemostatic competency in patients without a bleeding history is without foundation.[98] However, if patients do have a bleeding history, the bleeding time is held as worthwhile in sorting out whether the abnormal bleeding is associated with platelet:endothelial dysfunction. Despite frequent use to the contrary, the bleeding time is not even effective to predict among patients taking aspirin preoperatively who is likely to bleed.[98] Newer

Table 30–5 • APPROPRIATE QUESTIONS TO SCREEN FOR POSSIBLE ABNORMAL HEMOSTASIS

- Have you or anyone in your family ever been labeled a "bleeder"? Has someone in the family ever sustained abnormal bleeding?
- Have you ever bled previously with surgery or following childbirth? What surgical procedures have you had, including major surgery, minor surgery, biopsies, and dental extractions?
- Did a surgeon or dentist ever have to re-explore the wound site or did you ever have to return to the operative suite for hemorrhagic control?
- Have you ever had excessive menstrual periods? How long do your periods last? How many pads or tampons are needed each day? Have you ever required iron supplementation for anemia due to menstrual blood loss?
- Do you bruise excessively? Are these bruises multiple? Are they confined only to the outer thighs or other areas that are subject to trauma? Are any of these bruises palpable (i.e., are they true hematomas) or are they level with the surface of the skin?
- Do you have nosebleeds now or was there ever a period of time in your life when you did have spontaneous nosebleeds?
- Have you ever required a blood or plasma transfusion and if so, why?
- Have you ever bruised or experienced hemorrhage following trauma, car wrecks, falls, organized or unorganized sporting activities, altercations, or any acts of violence?

platelet function assays (PFAs) may well replace the bleeding time (see Chapter 35).

The best method to determine hemorrhagic risk with surgery is an adequate history and physical examination[97–99] (Table 30–5). What is the role of hemostatic testing among individuals who have undiagnosed disorders of hemostasis? This small group of patients may or may not have abnormal hemostatic testing. However, far more specific and sensitive is the history of bleeding. Three papers examined the presentation of patients harboring mild hemophilia who could hemorrhage, perhaps even in a major fashion, following operative procedures.[2,100,101] The patients included in these papers are the very ones who are of concern to surgeons and other persons practicing invasive procedures yet represent less than 1% of the population. Of the patients described in these three papers, patients who had undergone dental extraction and/or tonsillectomy without subsequent bleeding, did not harbor an underlying heritable hemorrhagic diathesis indicative of the history's ability to accurately predict good hemostasis. A positive past medical history of bleeding is 12.5 times more likely to predict the true hemorrhagic potential than any battery of laboratory tests. In using newer tests to identify patients with vWD, Biron and colleagues found that while 1% of the population tested true positive, 10% tested false positive.[102] Naturally, patients may acquire causes of bleeding such as severe liver disease, administration of anticoagulant drugs, or the rare development of a spontaneous inhibitor of a coagulation factor (see Chapter 6).

What if hemostatic screening tests are abnormal? In one report,[91] abnormal studies were found in 1.9% of patients. If another sample were collected and the test repeated before the surgical procedure, results of half of those abnormal tests returned normal, showing that specimen collection, laboratory error, or laboratory variability explained many abnormalities.

When the cause of persistently prolonged aPTTs of unknown etiology[103] was determined, 67% of patients were not at actual risk for hemorrhage because the nature of the process leading to the prolongation (bad laboratory sample, laboratory error, lupus anticoagulant, and prelaboratory variability) would not be expected to result in postoperative hemorrhage. However, the other 33% were at very clear risk to bleed; however, 81% of these 33% had already given a clear, positive history of a hemorrhagic diathesis even before the nature of their laboratory abnormality was determined. There was a lack of correlation between the degree of prolongation of the aPTT and the risk of bleeding, a conclusion made by others[91]; the risk of bleeding rather is a function of the *cause* of the aPPT prolongation, not the degree of prolongation.

Of significant concern is the fact that often an abnormal result frequently is ignored or forgotten by the practitioner who ordered the tests.[95,104]

One might question why such laboratory tests are unable to define precisely which patients are likely to bleed following an invasive procedure. Table 30–6 gives lines of reasoning why this is true.

Hemostatic tests should be ordered much less frequently than they customarily are. They are indicated in patients who answer affirmatively to any of the questions in Table 30–5. Others have stated that indications of screening tests as determined by the history and physical examination should include those with malabsorption, trauma, a history of active hemorrhage, a history

Table 30–6 • LINES OF REASONING WHY HEMOSTATIC TESTING IS NOT USUALLY SUFFICIENT TO DETECT THOSE LIKELY TO EXPERIENCE OPERATIVE HEMORRHAGE

- Patients suffering the worst hemorrhagic disorders, classic hemophilia A or B, are identified very early in life and have established diagnoses for life. Accordingly, preoperative screening is not effective or even warranted as the diagnosis is already known.
- The great majority of postoperative bleeding is not due to hemostatic failure but to a surgical or technical problem more appropriately corrected by surgical maneuvers. Exhaustive preoperative screening cannot predict operative errors.
- Traditionally employed tests to screen for hemostatic disorders (PT, aPTT, platelet count) were designed primarily to detect static disorders of hemostasis. As such, they do not reflect accurately ongoing changes in a situation as dynamic as trauma or surgery.
- The most flagrant examples of hemostatic failure—disseminated intravascular coagulation, hyperfibrinolysis, and thrombocytopenia—develop during an operation and cannot be predicted by tests performed before the operation.
- The PT and aPTT are expected to give abnormal results approximately 2.3% of the time. If one is screening for mild defects in factor VIII or factor IX, these disorders occur in about 1 : 20,000 males and therefore the ratio of true positives to false positives is in the order of 1 : 500.*

*From Clarke JR, Eisenberg JM. A theoretical assessment of the value of the PTT as a preoperative screening test in adults. Med Decis Making 1981; 1:40–43, with permission.

of chemotherapy or radiotherapy, purpura, anemia, or the prior use of anticoagulants.[105] Some[106] have added patients with liver disease, operations characteristically associated with a blood loss of greater than 1500 mL or highly invasive procedures such as those included in Table 30-7. It would seem rational to include those patients refusing to accept blood or blood product infusion. Using criteria similar to these, four studies indicated that screening was appropriate in 11%,[91] 8%,[93] 23%,[105] and 19%[107] of patients, giving a mean of 15%, implying that 85% of preoperative hemostatic testing is without merit.

Table 30-7 offers a proposed schema for preoperative hemostatic evaluation that seems rational, defensible, and conscious of cost-containment.

Screening for Thrombotic Disorders

Bleeding is not the only complication that can follow operative procedures. Venous thromboembolism (VTE) can be a major or fatal complication of a surgical procedure. Whereas risk stratification and prophylactic measures to reduce these risks are covered in Chapter 14, suffice it to say that a history of a prior VTE places the patient at 30 to 40 times the risk of the normal population to experience yet another VTE and that risk is still further exacerbated perhaps 100-fold by surgery.[1] These patients may well deserve screening for the more common thrombophilic abnormalities, particularly if laboratory findings may alter therapy (see Chapter 13).

Routine coagulation or special tests (e.g., factor V Leiden and prothrombin 20210 mutations) are not indicated to screen the general population solely for the possibility of VTE following surgery.[107a] An abnormally short aPTT (less than 23 seconds) recently has been shown to predict for poor outcome, including death, thrombosis, or bleeding.[108]

An appropriately performed history and physical examination again is the best path to predict the possibility of these events. Particular attention should be paid to cancer, heart failure, use of estrogens, and especially a history of prior VTE.[109] These risks are not simply additive but increasing risk factors implies even more rapid escalation of overall risk for VTE following surgery. Over 30 years ago Kakkar and colleagues[110] showed that the risk factors most predictive for VTE were a previous VTE, varicose veins, and operations on patients with a malignancy or patients over 60 years old.

Special attention should be paid to those patients who recently experienced a VTE. Sarasin and Bounameaux[111] have determined that patients who recently have had a VTE are at extreme risk for the first 20 weeks following their VTE with a gradual decrease in this very high rate after that 20-week period. They suggested that patients are at such high risk for rethrombosis that any elective procedures should be postponed for several months. Similar conclusions were deduced by Kearon and Hirsh.[1]

INVASIVE PROCEDURES IN PATIENTS WITH ABNORMAL COAGULATION TESTS

Invasive procedures such as bronchoscopy, endoscopy, lumbar punctures, paracenteses, and the insertion of lines for central venous access are part of modern medical practice. Although many patients needing these procedures have abnormal coagulation studies, published data underscore their safety and acceptable outcome in cancer patients, transplant patients, and patients in intensive care units. There is no published evidence for increased risks of procedure-related hemorrhage, and there is no controlled study that indicates at what levels the PT, aPTT, and platelet count actually represent contraindications to invasive procedures or that prophylactic replacement of blood products reduces risk of hemorrhage resulting from an invasive procedure.

General surgery in patients with thrombocytopenia from acute leukemia was far safer than hematologists' or surgeons' preconceived notions.[112] Bishop and colleagues performed 130 invasive procedures on patients whose platelet count was less than 50,000/μL (and usually remained less than 50,000/μL despite platelet transfusion therapy because of refractoriness to platelet

Table 30-7 • A SCHEMA FOR PREOPERATIVE HEMOSTATIC EVALUATION

Level of Risk[a]	Screening History		Proposed Surgery	Recommended Tests
Minimal	Negative ± prior surgery	and	Minor	None
Low	Negative with prior surgery	and	Major	Platelet count, aPTT, or none
Moderate	Possible bleeding disorder	or	CNS	Above tests *plus*
			CPB	BT, PT
			Prostatectomy	
High	Highly suspicious or documented bleeding disorder	and	Major or minor	Above tests *plus* factor VIII, IX, XI levels, TT If these are negative, pursue diagnosis

[a] Level of risk is estimated by the product of the risk of bleeding times the clinical consequence of bleeding.
CNS, central nervous system; CPB, cardiopulmonary bypass; aPTT, activated partial thromboplastin time; BT, bleeding time; PT, prothrombin time; TT, thrombin time. The bleeding time may well be replaced by platelet function assays (see Chapter 35).
Modified from Rapaport SI. Preoperative hemostatic evaluation: Which tests, if any? Blood 1983;61:229-231; and Woodman RC, Harker LA. Bleeding complications associated with cardiopulmonary bypass. Blood 1990;76:1680-1687, with permission.

transfusion). Only 7% required more than four units of packed red cells at the time of major surgery and none died secondary to the operation or from resultant bleeding. They concluded that major surgery or invasive procedures had a positive risk : benefit ratio in such patients. In cancer patients, gastrointestinal endoscopies and biopsy for investigation of patients with gastrointestinal hemorrhage can be safely performed with platelet counts as low as 20,000/μL.[113]

Liver Biopsy

It is frequent practice to administer a few units of FFP prior to liver biopsy in patients with liver failure in order to decrease risk of hemorrhage. In patients having PTs greater than 3 seconds above normal, administration of three units of FFP failed to correct the PT; however, subsequent liver biopsy did not result in hemorrhage.[114] In a larger study, McGill and colleagues performed 9212 liver biopsies over a 21-year period[115] if patients' ratio of the PT to control (i.e., the prothrombin time ratio (PTR)) was less than 1.5 (corresponding now to an INR of approximately 1.8) and the platelet count was 55,000/μL or higher. Among the 32 patients who experienced significant postbiopsy hemorrhage, there was no correlation between any coagulation test results and hemorrhage. McVay and Toy[116] performed a similar study in which they limited liver biopsy to patients whose PT ratio was below 1.5, aPTT ratio below 1.5, and platelet count 50,000/μL or higher. They found that 6 of 175 (3.4%) patients were adjudged to have bled abnormally. They found no correlation between the hemorrhage and preprocedure hemostatic results. Additionally, they showed that of their patients who did experience hemorrhage, the only positive predictor was the presence of liver malignancy. They concluded that the infusion of FFP and/or platelets within these variables was not warranted. Boberg and colleagues questioned whether a prolonged bleeding time heralded increased risk of hemorrhage following liver biopsy. In their study they were unable to find that the risk of bleeding correlated with the bleeding time except, unexplainably, in patients who were bone marrow transplant patients. They also corroborated that there was no correlation between hemorrhage and platelet count, PT, or aPTT.[117] Ewe[118] studied the "liver bleeding time," meaning that, following laparoscopic liver biopsy, the site was directly observed to determine duration of bleeding. In 200 patients, 10 experienced prolonged bleeding yet the prebiopsy studies were unable to predict which of their patients would hemorrhage. These biopsies were performed on patients whose platelet counts were as low as 30,000/μL, PT ratios as high as 2.2 (implying an INR of at least 2.6), and whole blood clotting times markedly prolonged. Makris and colleagues[119] in a prospective study measured PT, aPTT, TT, fibrinogen concentration, bleeding time, and platelet count prior to liver biopsy. All patients were prospectively screened by computed tomography (CT) 24 hours after the biopsy. Over half the patients had at least one abnormal screening test and many had more than one with PTs as long as 19.5 seconds (INR of approximately 2.0), aPTTs as long as 67 seconds, or almost twice their control, and bleeding times as long as 19 minutes with platelet counts as low as 52,000/μL. Only two patients out of 104 bled abnormally as determined by the CT scan and these patients had completely normal prebiopsy screening tests. Quite recently Bravo and colleagues[120] extensively reviewed liver biopsy. They pointed out that the mortality of liver biopsy was 1 : 10,000 and that the vast majority of such mortality occurred in patients with cirrhosis or, especially, tumors. Inexplicably they listed as absolute contraindications patients with PTs prolonged greater than 3 seconds, platelet counts less than 50,000/μL, and a bleeding time over 10 minutes. No data are offered to support these contentions.

Evidence-based methodology has failed thus far to establish cutoff values of hemostatic tests beyond which liver biopsy is unsafe and additionally no trial has demonstrated that the administration of platelets or FFP before this procedure has clinical efficacy or rationale.[53,115,116] An alternative if one is concerned about hemostatic integrity is that such concern is an indication for performing transvenous liver biopsy as bleeding would be directly into the vascular system.

Esophagastroduodenoscopy and Colonoscopy

Concurrent aspirin or nonsteroidal anti-inflammatory drug (NSAID) administration increases the risk of minor bleeding following esophagastroduodenoscopy and colonoscopy with biopsy threefold, from 2.1% to 6.3%. However, major bleeding, defined as the need for hospitalization or for treatment directed toward the bleeding, occurred at the same rate, namely 0.6%, whether or not aspirin or NSAIDs were used.[121] There is great diversity in the approach of invasive gastroenterologic procedures and particularly of the perceived danger among different practitioners, Rutgeerts[122] presented four cases of colonoscopy with biopsy to three experts around the globe; one cannot help but be impressed by the wide ranges of responses on how they would go about managing (or whether they would even perform) the procedures in such patients.

Paracentesis and Thoracentesis

In 108 patients undergoing either paracentesis or thoracentesis, in patients whose PT and aPTT were at least twice normal and platelet counts were as low as 50,000/μL, 10 patients received four units of FFP prior to procedure, while the other 90% did not. There was no correlation between hemorrhage as defined by hemoglobin concentration dropping at least 2 g/dL and any preoperative hemostatic tests or especially the infusion of FFP.[123]

Bronchoscopy

Three studies are available regarding the safety of bronchoscopy with transbronchial biopsy in patients with abnormal coagulation studies. Kozak and Brath[124] studied bleeding in such patients and were unable to show correlation between hemostatic test results and the risk of hemorrhage. In a major bone marrow transplant unit where thrombocytopenia is common, Weiss and colleagues[125] performed 66 fiberoptic bronchoscopies and bronchoalveolar lavages; only 4 patients bled, with one event being major but not fatal. Thirteen of their patients underwent these studies with platelet counts less than 20,000/μL. Because a diagnosis was secured by their procedure in half the cases, they concluded that the risk : benefit ratio is strongly in favor of the procedure. In a prospective study, Bjortuft and colleagues[126] performed 105 consecutive biopsies on patients monitoring the PT, aPTT, bleeding time, and platelet count. They measured the actual blood loss by repeated suction and defined blood loss greater than 20 mL as worrisome. The mean blood loss for all patients was 7 mL but eight patients (8%) bled more than 20 mL; none of these bleeds were life threatening. Of interest, there was no correlation between the prebiopsy test results and the ability to predict blood loss. They also noted that none of 17 (16%) of their patients with a bleeding time longer than 10 minutes experienced excessive hemorrhage.

Lumbar Puncture

Although lumbar puncture has been studied less thoroughly, Howard and colleagues[127] examined the safety of lumbar puncture, which was commonly done for diagnostic and therapeutic purposes in patients with leukemia and thrombocytopenia. They performed 5223 consecutive lumbar punctures on patients whose platelet count was below 100,000/μL with 941 of those patients having platelet counts ranging from 0 to 50,000/μL (29 had counts below 10,000/μL). They observed no serious complications and correctly assumed that this procedure was indicated despite thrombocytopenia because of its favorable risk : benefit ratio. They also concluded prophylactic platelet transfusions may not be indicated for a lumbar puncture if the platelet count is 10,000/μL or higher.

Central Venous Access Devices

Six studies have addressed the role of preprocedure coagulation studies and outcome of insertion of central venous access devices, typically either subclavian vein (SC) or internal jugular vein (IJ) cannulation. Ray and Shenoy[128] divided a large cohort of patients into three groups, those having platelet counts less than 50,000/μL, those with platelet counts between 50,000 and 100,000/μL, and patients whose platelet count was greater than 100,000/μL. They observed no differences in bleeding or other complication rates although it was their practice to administer platelets routinely prior to insertion of such devices in patients with platelet counts less than 50,000/μL. Although the average platelet count increased by only 12,000/μL following transfusion, they proceeded with the cannulation, which caused them to question whether platelet transfusion was rational. Four patients having platelet counts less than 50,000/μL did not receive platelet transfusions yet did not experience abnormal bleeding. Goldfarb and Lebrec[129] performed 1000 consecutive IJ cannulations in patients with "coagulopathies" and experienced a bleeding rate of 1%. Fisher and Mutimer[130] performed either IJ or SC cannulation in 658 patients with severe liver disease whose INR averaged greater than 1.5 (median 2.4, range 1 to 16) and/or had platelet counts less than 150,000/μL (median 10,000, range 9000 to 1,088,000/μL). Patients received neither prophylactic FFP nor platelet transfusions. Among these 658 patients, there was one major event (a hemothorax occurring in a patient whose INR was 1.5 and platelet count was 68,000/μL), which was deemed due to inadvertent laceration of the subclavian artery. The risk of local hematoma formation (which rarely required any treatment other than pressure) was 6% in patients whose INR was 5 or less and 12% in patients whose INR was above 5. Four risk factors predicted minor bleeding; namely, that the IJ site tended to bleed more than the SC; a procedure requiring more than one pass with the needle to cannulate the vein; failure to easily insert the guidewire; and patients whose INR was above 5. Values of the INR or other coagulation factors were not contraindications to a central line placement, particularly if it was deemed that such placement was beneficial for the patient's overall care. Foster and colleagues[131] examined the advisability and safety of central venous catheterization insertion in 259 patients awaiting or having just undergone OLT. Their patients' mean platelet count was 47,000/μL (range 8000 to 79,000/μL), mean aPTT of 97 seconds (range 78 to 100 seconds) and estimated mean INR 2.0 (range 1.5 to 8.0). They administered no preprocedure FFP or platelets yet experienced no serious bleeding using their most experienced operator. They concluded that there are no data supporting fear of increased bleeding complications in central venous cannulation in patients with coagulopathy. DeLoughery and colleagues[132] examined the outcome of central line placement in critically ill patients as a function of hemostatic testing. They performed 938 procedures with 41% of the patients having at least one abnormal test, 27% having several abnormalities, and 17% having undergone no testing prior to the procedure. Thirty-seven percent of their patients received some blood product prior to the procedure. They found that 16 (1.7%) of patients experienced minor bleeding and that only 2 (0.2%) experienced serious bleeding (neither was fatal). They concluded that laboratory data did not predict bleeding and that, in retrospect, the infusion of blood products, particularly FFP, was inappropriate. Doerfler and colleagues[133] inserted 104 central lines in patients with abnormalities of coagulation. They judged that seven (6.5%) had some abnormal bleeding; all seven had a platelet count 37,000/μL or less. They had not infused platelets into patients prior to the procedure but used their most experienced operator. There was no predictive value of routine coagulation. In summary, all these studies show that there is no predictive value of routine tests prior to the insertion of central lines. FFP and platelets should not be administered routinely and the most experienced operator should insert lines in these challenging cases. Thus there is no reproducible laboratory value that serves as a cutoff for safe insertion and there is no value in delay caused by testing and costly, time-consuming infusion of blood or blood products. The bleeding rate appears to be extremely low, on the order of 1% to 2% and with no report of any fatality in these series. When one considers the benefit of such access, it is clear that the risk:benefit ratio favors performing the procedure. Especially noticeable is that no study has shown that the preprocedure infusion of FFP or platelets decreases any real or hypothetical increase in hemorrhage.[132,133]

INVASIVE PROCEDURES FOR PATIENTS ON ANTICOAGULANT THERAPY

More patients are chronically receiving oral anticoagulant therapy. Such patients are prescribed this therapy for legitimate reasons. Accordingly it is not advisable for another practitioner preparing a patient for surgery or an invasive procedure to unilaterally stop warfarin therapy because of fear of bleeding. Should the risk of bleeding be considerably less than the operator perceives (which is almost always the case), then the risk:benefit ratio of withholding warfarin might very well be unfavorable for the patient's overall care. The risk of stopping anticoagulant therapy obviously varies from patient to patient with the risks of thrombosis being often at an absolute fairly low risk (such as patients with atrial fibrillation who are on warfarin for prophylaxis of a stroke) to moderate risk (such as patients with modern prosthetic heart valves), to those with extremely high risk (such as patients who have had thromboses or have active antiphospholipid syndrome). There is substantial evidence[1,134] that a thromboembolic event (such as may result from withholding anticoagulants) has a 30-fold higher incidence for either death or permanent sequelae than does a hemorrhagic event that may occur from continuing a patient on anticoagulant therapy for a procedure. Kearon and Hirsh estimated that major surgery itself increases the risk of a thromboembolic event approximately 100 times, a factor to be incorporated in estimating the risk:benefit ratio regarding the wisdom of stopping or continuing anticoagulant therapy for a procedure. It is dangerous to perform any elective surgery in someone who has had a thrombotic event within the previous 90 days; in nearly all such cases, elective invasive procedures should be withheld unless anticoagulation is carried out at the lowest therapeutic intensity. Recommendations[1] have been made regarding feasible management strategies for patients who need to undergo invasive procedures who are receiving chronic oral anticoagulation. These are detailed in Table 34–4, Chapter 34.

A paper by Katholi and colleagues[135] frequently is cited claiming that for patients undergoing noncardiac surgery while remaining on anticoagulant therapy (estimated INRs in that time period of 2 to 7) that 50% experienced some bleeding with 10% having serious bleeding yet none fatal. However, they also reported that of 35 patients with prosthetic heart valves for whom anticoagulants were held, there were two fatal thromboembolic events. The hemorrhagic rate of procedures done at modern INRs (2 to 3) has yet to be determined.

A survey of ophthalmologists[136] showed that while most unilaterally stopped anticoagulant therapy before lens implantation, there were no hemorrhagic consequences reported by those who did not stop anticoagulant therapy. However, among those ophthalmologists who did discontinue therapy, there were nine thromboembolic events, including two fatal events.

Until recently it was standard dentistry practice to stop anticoagulant therapy for extractions or similar procedures. This practice was reviewed by Weibert,[137] who concluded that modern therapy with INRs of 2 to 3 does not result in any appreciable increased bleeding or, that if any bleeding occurred, it was never serious and was easily controlled by local measures. In a recent study[138] of dental patients on warfarin therapy, all patients continued their medication. Patients were randomized to receive Gelfoam sponges and sutures, those two measures plus tranexamic acid, or of the three above efforts plus fibrin glue. All patients fared the same and none bled significantly. Because the first option, namely Gelfoam sponges and suture, was the easiest to carry out, that was the method recommended. This entire subject has been thoroughly reviewed by Wahl,[139] who concludes that the risk:benefit ratio of maintaining patients on oral anticoagulants for any oral procedure greatly favors the patient remaining on warfarin and the risk for bleeding is greatly exaggerated or misunderstood.

Hip surgery for either fractured hips or total hip replacement has always been an operation fraught with thromboembolism, which is the major cause of death in such patients. In a very early (1959) controlled study, Sevitt and Gallagher[140] reported pinning fractured hips in patients either on no anticoagulant therapy or on phenindione. One hundred fifty patients were in the control group and 150 patients received full-dose phenindione. It is impossible to reconstruct what those patients' INRs were but they were likely approximately 5 to 8. Whereas one could have predicted at such INRs some major bleeding would occur (five in the phenindione group and two in the control group), deaths from pulmonary embolism were decreased by 80%. Later, in 1971, Salzman and colleagues[141] used warfarin anticoagulation to an estimated INR of 2.5 to 4.5 in a similar study and showed a 20% risk of bleeding, which was about the same as patients receiving aspirin or dextran as their control group yet with a decrease in VTE in the group on warfarin. In 1983 Francis and coworkers[142] began warfarin anticoagulant therapy to an estimated INR of 1.8 several days prior to total hip replacement or total knee replacement. Four percent of their patients bled, which was the same incidence as controls receiving dextran. Of the patients who were treated with warfarin compared to dextran, there was a 60% reduction in DVT and an 88% reduction in large proximal vein thrombosis. These papers served to show that major surgery is feasible with very acceptable bleeding, with INRs that are not so high as to provoke bleeding but high enough to result in excellent prophylaxis of VTE in very high-risk patients.

If a patient on chronic oral anticoagulant therapy undergoes surgery without warfarin, many practitioners will use a "heparin bridge" to protect the patient during the brief period of subtherapeutic INR during the surgery and particularly after the surgery while the INR returns to therapeutic levels. LMWH may be used for this purpose.[143]

Should a patient need emergent surgery (such as for trauma or an acute abdominal process), it may be advisable to reverse or at least partially reverse the effect of the warfarin prior to surgery. This can be done quite safely with very small doses of intravenous vitamin K, which will decrease the INR within 6 hours.[144] Intravenous administration is safe when small amounts, such as 0.5 to 1.0 mg, are administered in a diluted solution over approximately 30 minutes. Not only do higher doses far too often result in total reversal of the warfarin (which may not be desirable) but also doses greater than 1 to 2 mg frequently lead to warfarin resistance, making it difficult to reachieve a therapeutic INR. When vitamin K is given intravenously it is safe, faster, and more reliable than giving it subcutaneously or orally.[145-147] Should one overshoot and the INR become unacceptably subtherapeutic, the heparin bridge method can be employed until patients' INR returns to therapeutic range.

CONSULTATION ON PATIENTS WITH INTRAOPERATIVE OR POSTOPERATIVE HEMORRHAGE

Hematologists are called by surgeons, anesthesiologists, and critical care personnel for the evaluation of bleeding either during an operation or afterward. Surgery or major trauma is the ultimate test of the hemostatic system. Accordingly, it is possible for patients who have never hemorrhaged to any significant degree to bleed excessively.

Nearly all reviews of intraoperative and early postoperative bleeding[44,148] point out that 75% to 90% of all such bleeding is technical in nature because of a structural problem such as an undone ligature or cauterized vessel. It is very important to work with the surgeon as the cause of bleeding must be either surgical or hemostatic failure. Early in the consultation process it is advisable to have personnel draw blood samples for routine available coagulation tests. A sample of blood must be drawn from a fresh peripheral venipuncture. This may seem counterintuitive to the anesthesiologist, who may have several vascular devices from which blood could be drawn. Too frequently samples are adulterated by the infusion of heparin or even saline, erythrocytes, or plasma.[149] Therefore, the very sample that one needs for critical decision-making must not be suspect from the very beginning. It is advisable to call the coagulation laboratory so that technicians can be alerted to both the seriousness of these particular tests as well as to work with the hematologist in a sequential manner regarding subsequent tests, the indications for which will unfold as the laboratory consultation progresses. Assessment of all patients experiencing substantial hemorrhage should include a PT, aPTT, thrombin time (TT), platelet count, and measurements for FDPs. If the PT, aPTT, and TT are all prolonged with decreased platelets and positive assays for FDP, disseminated intravascular coagulation (DIC) is very high on the list for hemorrhage. If the FDPs are high but with the PT, aPTT, and platelet count fairly well preserved with a very long TT, hyperfibrinolysis is strongly suggested. Conversely if the TT is the sole test that is most prolonged, the culprit more often than not is excessive heparin. The coagulation laboratory can set up a 1:1 mix of patient plasma with normal plasma to repeat the PT, aPTT, and TT if any of these three tests are abnormal on initial testing of the patient's plasma. If the 1:1 mixture results in a previously abnormal test becoming normal, it strongly suggests a deficiency that can occur either congenitally, because of vitamin K deficiency or warfarin therapy, or from liver disease. Should the 1:1 mixture not correct the abnormal test(s) then an inhibitor, to include heparin, FDPs, or spontaneous acquired inhibitor, is strongly suggested. The use of the thromboelastogram by anesthesiologists has been discussed vigorously.[150,151] Whereas this test does not traditionally fit into hematologists' thinking, it clearly is one of the most accurate and rapid ways to detect hyperfibrinolysis in situations that are characterized by hyperfibrinolysis, namely CPB and OLT.

Next the consultant should ascertain if any preoperative coagulation tests were done and what the results were. Often preoperative tests were abnormal yet were either not seen or not acted upon. A slight prolongation of the aPTT could very well represent a mild previously undetected deficiency of factor VIII, IX, or XI, or if the PT and PTT are both prolonged while the level of albumin is low and bilirubin elevated, significant liver disease is suggested. If the preoperative and intraoperative coagulation tests mentioned are all normal, a local structural or technical problem is likely to be at fault.

Once laboratory studies are initiated, attention must be paid to the clinical features of hemorrhage. As Table 30–8 depicts, the nature of bleeding is very helpful. The concept that bleeding is due to a structural defect is greatly strengthened if there is bleeding from a single site while other potential sites are not bleeding. If bleeding is sudden and massive with bright red, pulsatile blood, arterial bleeding is probable. Clinical features that favor a basic hemostatic defect are multiple concurrent bleeding sites. Concomitant hemoglobinuria and hemoglobinemia strongly implicates transfusion reaction-induced DIC. Slow and persistent oozing, particularly several days after surgery, suggests a hemostatic defect.

Table 30–9 lays out an overall evaluation. Appropriate questions asked of the treatment team and review of the chart or any pre-existing data often are the best sources of information.

Table 30–10 lists several hemostatic aspects that may or may not affect postoperative hemorrhage. Low-dose prophylactic use of heparin does not increase bleeding

Table 30-8 • CLINICAL FEATURES OF HEMORRHAGE

Clinical Features Favoring Structural or Technical Defects
- Bleeding from a single site while other candidate sites are not bleeding
- Sudden onset of massive and/or rapid bleeding
- Bright red or pulsatile bleeding from an identifiable source

Clinical Features Favoring Hemostatic Defect
- Multiple simultaneous bleeding sites:
    Surgical incision
    Vascular access sites
    Mucosal membranes
    Skin
    Hematuria
    Hemoglobinuria or hemoglobinemia
- Slow persistent ooze of blood from a nonidentifiable source
- Delayed hemorrhage following adequate hemostasis

---

according to comprehensive meta-analyses.[90] Agents that may substantially impair coagulation are aspirin and NSAIDs, particularly ketorolac in the postoperative period. Recalling that perhaps 1% of the population may have von Willebrand syndrome, it is highly possible that the addition of aspirin or NSAIDs is enough to expose the underlying nature of that bleeding diathesis. Increasingly, antiplatelet agents, not only clopidogrel but GpIIb/IIIa inhibitors, are finding their way into patient care. By far the rarest abnormality is mild, previously undiagnosed hemophilia,[2] which is characterized by a slow ooze that usually starts on postoperative days 1 to 3 and is rarely of a brisk or alarming nature initially. Characteristically, hemostasis in mild hemophiliacs undergoing surgery is surprisingly normal for the first day

Table 30-9 • EVALUATION OF POSTOPERATIVE HEMORRHAGE

- Obtain fresh venipuncture sample of blood for:
    Thrombin time
    Prothrombin time
- Activated Partial thromboplastin time
    1 : 1 mix with normal plasma of the above if any are abnormal
    Blood smear for schistocytes and platelet count estimation
        Signs of sepsis such as leftward shift, toxic granulation, or vacuolization of granulocytes
- Note features of bleeding (see Table 30-8)
- Repeat directed history and physical examination
- Review patient's chart:
    Were preoperative liver and renal tests normal?
    Were preoperative coagulation screening tests normal?
    Were aspirin or NSAIDs administered?
- Is the patient septic?
- Was the patient transfused? With what? When?
- Was bovine thrombin or fibrin glue containing bovine thrombin used as hemostatic agent?
- What surgical procedure was performed?
- Was anesthesia time prolonged?
- Note type and rate of bleeding
- Estimate consequences of continued bleeding

Table 30-10 • FACTORS THAT AFFECT INTRAOPERATIVE OR POSTOPERATIVE HEMORRHAGE

Do Not Affect
- Low-dose heparin prophylaxis
- Low-dose warfarin prophylaxis
- Osler-Weber-Rendu syndrome
- Mild thrombocytopenia ($\geq 60,000/\mu L$)

Occasionally Affect
- Aspirin or NSAID administration
- Adjusted-dose heparin prophylaxis
- Poor metabolic/nutrition states[a]
- Moderate thrombocytopenia (30,000 to 60,000/μL)

Frequently Affect
- Ticlopidine, clopidogrel, or GpIIb/IIIa inhibitors
- Platelet defects, especially with concomitant aspirin or NSAID administration
- Factor VIII or IX levels <30% of normal
- Fibrinogen <60 mg/dL
- Severe thrombocytopenia (<30,000/μL)
- Multiorgan failure

[a] Prolonged use of glucocorticosteroids, malnutrition, inanition, bedridden state from chronic illness, septicemia, and chronic renal or hepatic failure.

---

or so during high levels of TF generation. The nature of hemophilic bleeding has been described exquisitely in the older literature; the interested reader is referred to such descriptive papers.[152-155]

Table 30-11 presents various causes of postoperative bleeding. The differential diagnosis is in part a function of time from the operation. Hyperfibrinolysis, while not limited to patients undergoing CPB or OLT, characteristically is very brisk but usually of short duration. In CPB and OLT in which the index of suspicion and prevalence is high, prompt administration of aprotonin or other fibrinolytic agent as covered in the earlier section of this chapter is strongly indicated. Thrombocytopenia

Table 30-11 • CAUSES OF INTRAOPERATIVE OR POSTOPERATIVE HEMORRHAGE

Intraoperative Hemorrhage[a]
- Structural/technical defects
- Disseminated intravascular coagulation
- Heparin overdosage
- Hyperfibrinolysis

Early Postoperative (Days 0 to 2)[a]
- Structural/technical defects
- Thrombocytopenia
- Qualitative platelet disorders
- Mid/moderate hereditary coagulation disorder

Delayed Postoperative Bleeding (Days 2 to 7)[a]
- Thrombocytopenia
- Aspirin or NSAID administration
- Vitamin K deficiency
- Multiorgan failure
- Antibodies to factor V following use of bovine thrombin in fibrin glue

[a] These times are those commonly encountered but are used only as approximations.

that begins postoperatively and becomes worse, particularly if it is associated with thrombosis, is highly suggestive of heparin-induced thrombocytopenia (see Chapter 23). Vitamin K deficiency of an acquired nature is surprisingly common in intensive care situations, particularly if the patient has been ill for some time and therefore malnourished from the onset; after several days/weeks in the intensive care unit, one becomes depleted of vitamin K-dependent factors. One clinical hallmark of this situation is that the PT tends to prolong comparatively earlier than the aPTT. Vitamin K deficiency is diagnosed and treated by the suspicion of this problem and the response of the patient to vitamin K administration.[156]

Table 30–12 offers several therapeutic options. Watching and waiting with the appropriate administration of red blood cells and fluid is often appropriate, particularly if the rate of bleeding seems to be decreasing. Re-exploration of the surgical site not only often will find the bleeding site but also may be therapeutic in itself as it may remove thromboplastic as well as fibrinolytic agents released from large collections of clotted blood.[46] If a specific diagnosis is made, therapy obviously is addressed toward that cause.

The use of topical surgical adjuvants including fibrin glue is covered thoroughly in Chapter 26. Bleeding that begins 4 to 14 days or even longer after surgery in which fibrin glue was employed raises the possibility of the induction of anti-bovine factor II and/or factor V, which may have cross-reactivity to their human counterparts. Management of such problems has been recently reviewed.[157]

The administration of DDAVP is effective for platelet dysfunction due to aspirin or NSAIDs. Administration of 0.3 μg/kg intravenously over 30 minutes is highly effective in bleeding due to platelet dysfunction.

The tempo, depth, and thoroughness of evaluation will be a function of the potential consequences of continued bleeding. A small amount of bleeding in a confined space upon which pressure cannot be applied (such as the brain or internal organ) is obviously of more immediate concern than bleeding outside the body such as from a wound on the extremities. Accordingly, a more conservative approach may be indicated for the latter. Attempts at surgical techniques to stop true hemostatic defects will not work. One is unable to suture adequately enough to replace the hemostatic function of a missing coagulation factor. In fact, the tighter one attempts to suture, the more inward the bleeding becomes, which continues and can dissect internally at an alarming rate and actually cause more damage than had the blood been allowed to escape the confines of the body.

Not all excessive hemorrhage is necessarily due to hemostatic failure. Bleeding in large named vessels, particularly arteries, requires surgical repair. Bleeding from those vessels is rarely if ever due to a defect in the hemostatic system. Massive amounts of clotting factors, plasma, and platelets will not correct large structural lesions.

A peculiar massive intracranial bleeding can occur at the time of takedown of central nervous system arteriovenous malformations (AVMs). This has been termed *"normal perfusion pressure breakthrough syndrome"*.[158,159] It can cause considerable hemorrhage despite an absolutely normal coagulation system. Normal perfusion pressure breakthrough syndrome is thought to result from the loss of vascular autoregulation due to the chronic hypotension that vessels distal to the AVM have experienced until the reduction of the AVM. It is believed that the sudden return of normal pressure and perfusion into these vessels results in this brisk hemorrhagic syndrome, which may persist until the vessels reset their autoregulatory function. Treatment for this syndrome during hemorrhage is directed toward high-dose barbiturate anesthesia, pharmacologically induced hypotension, controlled hyperventilation, and the administration of glucocorticosteroids and osmotic dehydrating agents.[158,159]

■ REFERENCES

Chapter 30 References

1. Kearon C, Hirsh J. Management of anticoagulation before and after elective surgery. N Engl J Med 1997;336:1506–1511.
2. Kitchens CS. Occult hemophilia. Johns Hopkins Med J 1980;146:255–259.
3. Ratnoff OD. Why do people bleed? Chapter 18. In Wintrobe MM (Ed): Blood, Pure and Eloquent. McGraw-Hill, New York, 1980, pp. 600–657.
4. Majno G. The Healing Hand. Man and Wound in the Ancient World. Harvard University Press, Cambridge, Mass, 1975, pp. 1–571.
5. Rosner F. Hemophilia in the Talmud and rabbinic writings. Ann Intern Med 1969;70:833–837.
6. Kitchens CS. Surgery in hemophilia and related disorders. A prospective study of 100 consecutive procedures. Medicine 1986;65:34–45.
7. Rudowski WJ, Scharf R, Ziemski JM. Is major surgery in hemophiliac patients safe? World J Surg 1987;11:378–386.
8. Brown B, Steed DL, Webster MW, et al. General surgery in adult hemophiliacs. Surgery 1986;99:154–159.
9. Kasper CK, Boylen AL, Ewing NP, et al. Hematologic management of hemophilia after surgery. JAMA 1985;253:1279–1283.
10. Mortinowitz U, Schulman S, Gitel H, et al. Adjusted dose continuous infusion of factor VIII in patients with haemophilia A. Br J Haematol 1992;82:729–734.
11. Tagariello G, Davoli PG, Gaso GB, et al. Safety and efficacy of high-purity concentrates in haemophiliac patients undergoing surgery by continuous infusion. Haemophilia 1999;5:426–430.

Table 30–12 • THERAPEUTIC OPTIONS IN INTRAOPERATIVE OR POSTOPERATIVE HEMORRHAGE

- Acute volume and red cell administration as indicated
- Angiography with or without arterial embolization
- Watchful waiting
- Re-exploration of bleeding site
- Limited use of FFP, cryoprecipitate, and platelet transfusion, except for precise diagnoses and indications
- DDAVP
- Antifibrinolytic agents

12. Czaplicki M, Jakubczyk T, Judycki J, et al. ESWL in hemophiliac patients. Eur Urol 2000;38:301–302.
13. Palanzu DA, Sadr FS. Coronary artery bypass grafting in a patient with haemophilia B. Perfusion 1995;10:265–270.
14. MacKinlay N, Taper J, Renisson F, et al. Cardiac surgery and catheterization in patients with haemophilia. Haemophilia 2000; 6:84–88.
15. Davidson SJ, Burman JF, Rutherford LC, et al. High molecular weight kininogen deficiency: a patient who underwent cardiac surgery. Thromb Haemost 2001;85:195–197
16. Zanon E, Martinelli F, Bacci C, et al. Proposal of a standard approach to dental extraction in hemophilia patients: a case-control study with good results. Haemophilia 2000;6:533–536.
17. Hanna W, Bona RD, Zimmerman CE, et al. The use of intermediate and high purity factor VIII products in the treatment of von Willebrand disease. Thromb Haemost 1994;71:173–179.
18. Foster P. A perspective on the use of FVIII concentrates and cryoprecipitate prophylactically in surgery or therapeutically in severe bleeding in patients with von Willebrand disease unresponsive to DDAVP: results of an international study. Thromb Haemost 1995;74:1370–1378.
19. Nitu-Whalley IC, Griffioen A, Harrington C, et al. Retrospective review of the management of elective surgery with desmopressin and clotting factor concentrates in patients with von Willebrand disease. Am J Hematol 2001;66:280–284.
20. Scharf R, Kucharski W, Nowak T. Surgery in hemophilia A patients with factor VIII inhibitor: 10 year experience. World J Surg 1996;20:1171–1181.
21. Arkin S, Blei F, Fetten J, et al. Human coagulation factor FVIIa (recombinant) in the management of limb-threatening bleeds unresponsive to alternative therapies: results from the NovoSeven® emergency-use programme in patients with severe haemophilia or with acquired inhibitors. Blood Coagul Fibrinol 2000; 11:255–259.
22. Shapiro AD. Prospective, randomized trial of two doses of rFVIIa (NovoSeven) in haemophilia patients with inhibitors undergoing surgery. Thromb Haemost 1999;80:773–778.
23. Blomback M, Eklund J, Hellgren M, et al. Blood coagulation and fibrinolytic factors as well as their inhibitors in trauma. Scand J Clin Lab Invest (Suppl) 1985;178:15–23.
24. Boisclair MD, Lane DA, Philippou H, et al. Mechanisms of thrombin generation during surgery and cardiopulmonary bypass. Blood 1993;82:3350–3357.
25. Koh SC, Pua HL, Tay DH, et al. The effects of gynaecological surgery on coagulation activation, fibrinolysis and fibrinolytic inhibitor in patients with and without ketorolac infusion. Thromb Res 1995;79:501–514.
26. Sorensen JV. Levels of fibrinolytic activators and inhibitors in plasma after severe trauma. Blood Coagul Fibrinol 1994;5: 43–49.
27. Moschos CB, Khan MI, Regan TJ. Thrombogenic properties of blood during early ischemic and nonischemic injury. Am J Physiol 1971;220:1882–1884.
28. Voss R, Matthias FR, Borkowsk G, et al. Activation and inhibition of fibrinolysis in septic patients in an internal intensive care unit. Br J Haematol 1990;75:99–105.
29. Kluft C, Verheijen JH, Jie AF, et al. The postoperative fibrinolytic shutdown: a rapidly reverting acute phase pattern for the fast acting inhibitor of tissue type plasminogen activator after trauma. Scand J Clin Lab Invest 1985;45:605–610.
30. Kambayashi J, Sakon M, Yokota M, et al. Activation of coagulatin and fibrinolysis during surgery, analyzed by molecular markers. Thromb Res 1990;60:157–167.
31. Kowal-Vern A, Gamelli RL, Walenga RJM, et al. The effect of burn wound size on hemostasis: a correlation of the hemostatic changes to the clinical state. J Trauma 1992;33:50–57.
32. Gorman R, Gordan L, Zumberg M, Kitchens C. Successful use of argatroban as an anticoagulant in burn-related severe acquired antithrombin III deficiency after heparin failure. Thromb Haemost 2001;86:1596–1597.
33. Borgstrom S, Gelin LE, Zederefeldt B. The formation of vein thrombi following tissue injury: an experimental study in rabbits. Acta Chir Scand 1951;247:1–14.
34. Rosenfeld BA, Beattie C, Christopherson R, et al. The effects of different anesthetic regimens on fibrinolysis and the development of postoperative arterial thrombosis. Anesthesiology 1993;79:435–443.
35. Comerota AJ, Stewart GJ, Alburger PD, et al. Operative venodilation: a previously unsuspected factor in the cause of postoperative deep vein thrombosis. Surgery 1989;106:301–309.
36. Geerts WH, Heit JA, Clagett GP, et al. Prevention of venous thromboembolism. Chest 2001;119:132S–175S.
37. Westrich GH. The role of mechanical and other adjuncts. Am J Knee Surg 1999;12:55–60.
38. Hull RD, Pineo GF. Intermittent pneumatic compression for the prevention of venous thromboembolism. Chest 1996;109:6–9.
39. Agu O, Hamilton G, Baker D. Graduated compression stockings in the prevention of venous thromboembolism. Br J Surg 1999; 86:992–1004.
40. Nurmohamed MT, van Riel AM, Henkens CMA, et al. Low molecular weight heparin and compression stockings in the prevention of venous thromboembolism in neurosurgery. Thromb Haemost 1996;75:233–238.
41. Agnelli G, Piovella F, Buoncristiani P, et al. Enoxaparin plus compression stockings compared with compression stockings alone in the prevention of venous thromboembolism after elective neurosurgery. N Engl J Med 1998;339:80–85.
42. Agnelli G. Prevention of venous thromboembolism after neurosurgery. Thromb Haemost 1999;82:925–930.
43. Dickinson LD, Miller LD, Patel CP, et al. Enoxaparin increases the incidence of postoperative intracranial hemorrhage when initiated preoperatively for deep venous thrombosis prophylaxis in patients with brain tumors. Neurosurgery 1998;43:1074–1081.
44. Bevan DH. Cardiac bypass haemostasis: putting blood through the mill. Br J Haematol 1999;104:208–219.
45. Harker L, Malpass TW, Branson HE, et al. Mechanism of abnormal bleeding in patients undergoing cardiopulmonary bypass: Acquired transient platelet dysfunction associated with selective α-granule release. Blood 1980;56:824–834.
46. Pelletier MP, Solymoss S, Lee A, et al. Negative reexploration for cardiac postoperative bleeding: can it be therapeutic? Ann Thorac Surg 1998;65:999–1002.
47. Laupacis A, Fergusson D. Drugs to minimize perioperative blood loss in cardiac surgery: meta-analyses using perioperative blood transfusions as the outcome. Anesth Analg 1997;85:1258–1267.
48. Levi M, Cromheecke ME, deJonge E, et al. Pharmacological strategies to decrease excessive blood loss in cardiac surgery: meta-analysis of clinically relevant endpoints. Lancet 1999; 354:1940–1947.
49. Cattaneo M, Harris A-S, Stromberg U, et al. The effect of desmopressin on reducing blood loss in cardiac surgery—a meta-analysis of double-blind, placebo-controlled trials. Thromb Haemost 1995;74:1064–1070.
50. Czer LSC, Bateman TM, Gray RJ, et al. Treatment of severe platelet dysfunction and hemorrhage after cardiopulmonary bypass: reduction in blood product usage with desmopressin. J Am Coll Cardiol 1987;9:1139–1147.
51. Gratz I, Koehler J, Olsen D, et al. The effect of desmopressin acetate on postoperative hemorrhage in patients receiving aspirin therapy before coronary artery bypass operations. J Thorac Cardiovasc Surg 1992;104:1417–1422.
52. NIH Consensus Conference: Platelet transfusion therapy. JAMA 1987;257:1777–1780.
53. NIH Consensus Conference: Fresh-frozen plasma: Indications and risks. JAMA 1985;253:551–553.

54. Hunt BJ, Parratt RN, Segal HC, et al. Activation of coagulation and fibrinolysis during cardiothoracic operations. Ann Thorac Surg 1998;65:712–718.
55. Smith CR. Management of bleeding complications in redo cardiac operations. Ann Thorac Surg 1998;65(4 Suppl):S2–8; discussion S27–28.
56. Wahba A, Black G, Koksch M, et al. Aprotinin has no effect on platelet activation and adhesion during cardiopulmonary bypass. Thromb Haemost 1996;75:844–848.
57. Ray MJ, Marsh NA. Aprotinin reduces blood loss after cardiopulmonary bypass by direct inhibition of plasmin. Thromb Haemost 1997;78:1021–1026.
58. Casati V, Guzzon D, Oppizzi M, et al. Hemostatic effects of aprotinin, tranexamic acid and epsilon-aminocaproic in primary cardiac surgery. Ann Thorac Surg 1999;68:2252–2256.
59. Munoz JJ, Birkmeyer NJ, Birkmeyer JD, et al. Is epsilon-aminocaproic acid as effective as aprotinin in reducing bleeding with cardiac surgery? A meta-analysis. Circulation 1999;99:81–89.
60. Slaughter TF, Faghih F, Greenberg CS, et al. The effects of epsilon-aminocaproic acid on fibrinolysis and thrombin generation during cardiac surgery. Anesth Analg 1997;85:1221–1226.
61. Rooney SJ, Bonser RS. The management of bleeding following surgery requiring hypothermic circulatory arrest. J Card Surg 1997;12:238–242.
62. Prendergast TW, Furukaa S, Beye AJ 3rd, et al. Defining the role of aprotinin in heart transplantation. Ann Thorac Surg 1996;62:670–674.
63. Okita Y, Takamoto S, Ando M, et al. Is use of aprotinin safe with deep hypothermic circulatory arrest in aortic stenosis? Investigations on blood coagulation. Circulation 1996;94:177–181.
64. Whitten CW, Allison PM, Latson TW, et al. Management of the thrombocytopenic cardiac surgical patient—a role for aprotinin. Anesth Analg 1994;79:796–800.
65. Gu YJ, de Haan J, Brenken UP, et al. Clotting and fibrinolytic disturbance during lung transplantation: effect of low-dose aprotinin. Groningen Lung Transplant Group. J Thorac Cardiovasc Surg 1996;112:599–606.
66. Goldstein DJ, Seldomridge JA, Chen JM, et al. Use of aprotinin in LVAD recipients reduces blood loss, blood use, and perioperative mortality. Ann Thorac Surg 1995;59:1063–1067.
67. Al Douri M, Shafi T, Al Khudairi D, et al. Effect of the administration of recombinant activated factor VII (rFVIIa; NovoSeven) in the management of severe uncontrolled bleeding in patients undergoing heart valve replacement surgery. Blood Coagul Fibrinolysis 2000;11(Suppl 1):S121–127.
68. Slaughter TF, Greenberg CS. Antifibrinolytic drugs and perioperative hemostasis. Am J Hematol 1997;56:32–36.
69. Dunn CJ, Goa KL. Tranexamic acid: a review of its use in surgery and other indications. Drugs 1999;57:1005–1032.
70. Schmaier AH. Aprotinin: can its benefits be offset by harmful effects? Transfusion 1997;37:1105–1107.
71. Cohen DM, Norberto J, Cartabuke R, et al. Severe anaphylactic reaction after primary exposure to aprotinin. Ann Thorac Surg 1999;67:837–838.
72. Dietrich W, Spath P, Ebell A, et al. Prevalence of anaphylactic reactions to aprotinin: analysis of two hundred forty eight reexposures to aprotinin in heart operations. J Thorac Cardiovasc Surg 1997;113:194–201.
73. Dyke C, Gammie JS. Surgical implications of platelet glycoprotein IIb-IIIa inhibition. J Thorac Cardiovasc Surg 1998;116:1083–1084.
74. Dietrich W, Dilthey G, Spannagl M, et al. Warfarin pretreatment does not lead to increased bleeding tendency during cardiac surgery. J Cardiothorac Vasc Anesth 1995;9:250–254.
75. Sato M, Nasha B, Ringe B, et al. Coagulation disorder during liver transplantation. Blood Coagul Fibrinolysis 1991;2:25–31.
76. Himmelreich G, Hundt K, Nevhaus P, et al. Decreased platelet aggregation after reperfusion in orthotopic liver transplantation. Transplantation 1992;53:582–586.
77. Sato M, Nashan B, Grosse H, et al. Hemostatic studies of ex situ hepatic surgery. Jpn J Surg 1991;21:561–565.
78. Grosse H, Lobbes W, Sato M, et al. Systemic fibrinogenolysis in liver transplantation. Transplant Proc 1990;22:2303–2304.
79. Velasco F, Villalba R, Fernandez M, et al. Diminished anticoagulant and fibrinolytic activity following liver transplantation. Transplantation 1992;53:1256–1261.
80. Grosse H, Lobbes W, Frambach M, et al. The use of high dose aprotinin in liver transplantation: the influence on fibrinolysis and blood loss. Thromb Res 1991;63:287–297.
81. Llamas P, Cabrera R, Gomez-Arnau J, et al. Hemostasis and blood requirements in orthotopic liver transplantation with and without high-dose aprotinin. Haematologica 1998;83:338–346.
82. Lentschener C, Benhamou D, Mercier FJ, et al. Aprotinin reduces blood loss in patients undergoing elective liver resection. Anesth Analg 1997;84:875–881.
83. Kufner RP. Antifibrinolytics do not reduce transfusion requirements in patients undergoing orthotopic liver transplantation. Liver Transpl Surg 1997;3:668–674.
84. Garcia-Huete L, Domenech P, Sabate A, et al. The prophylactic effect of aprotinin on intraoperative bleeding in liver transplantation: a randomized clinical study. Hepatology 1997;26:1143–1148.
85. Porte RJ, Molenaar IQ, Begliomini B, et al. Aprotinin and transfusion requirements in orthotopic liver transplantation: a multicentre randomized double-blind study. Lancet 2000;355:1303–1309.
86. D'Ambrosio A, Borghi B, Damato A, et al. Reducing perioperative blood loss in patients undergoing total hip arthroplasty. Int J Artif Organs 1999;22:47–51.
87. Hiippala ST, Strid LJ, Wennerstrand MI, et al. Tranexamic acid radically decreases blood loss and transfusions associated with total knee arthroplasty. Anesth Analg 1997;84:839–844.
88. Capdevia X, Calvet Y, Biboulet P, et al. Aprotinin decreases blood loss and homologous transfusions in patients undergoing major orthopedic surgery. Anesthesiology 1998;88:50–57.
89. Kasper SM, Schmidt J, Rutt J. Is aprotinin worth the risk in total hip replacement? Anesthesiology 1994;81:517–519.
90. Collins R, Scrimgeour A, Yusuf S, et al. Reduction in fatal pulmonary embolism and venous thrombosis by perioperative administration of subcutaneous heparin. Overview of results of randomized trials in general, orthopedic and urologic surgery. N Engl J Med 1988;318:1162–1173.
91. Burk CD, Muller L, Handler SD. Preoperative history and coagulation screening in children undergoing tonsillectomy. Pediatrics 1992;89:691–695.
92. Haberman SD II, Shattuck TG, Dion NM. Is outpatient suction cautery tonsillectomy safe in a community hospital setting? Laryngoscope 1990;100:551–555.
93. Suchman AL, Mushlin AL. How well does the activated partial thromboplastin time predict postoperative hemorrhage? JAMA 1986;256:750–753.
94. Kitchens CS. Preoperative PT's, PTT's, cost-effectiveness, and health care reform. Radical changes that make good sense. Chest 1994;106:661–662.
95. Schein OD, Katz J, Bass EB, et al. The value of routine preoperative medical testing before cataract surgery. N Engl J Med 2000;342:168–175.
96. Roizen MF. More preoperative assessment by physicians and less by laboratory tests. N Engl J Med 2000;342:204–205.
97. Narr, BJ, Warner ME, Schroeder DR, et al. Outcomes of patients with no laboratory assessment before anesthesia and a surgical procedure. Mayo Clin Proc 1997;72:505–509.
98. Peterson P, Hayes TE, Arkin CF, et al. The preoperative bleeding time lacks clinical benefits. Arch Surg 1998;133:134–139.
99. Bowie EJW, Owen CA Jr. The significance of abnormal preoperative hemostatic tests. Prog Hemost Thromb 1980;5:179–209.

100. Aggeler PM, Hoag MS, Wallerstein RO, et al. The mild hemophilias. Occult deficiencies of AHF, PTC and PTA frequently responsible for unexpected surgical bleeding. Am J Med 1961; 30:84–94.

101. Bachmann F. Diagnostic approach to mild bleeding disorders. Semin Hematol 1980;17:292–305.

102. Biron C, Mahieu B, Rochette A, et al. Preoperative screening for von Willebrand disease type 1: low yield and limited ability to predict bleeding. J Lab Clin Med 1999;134:605–609.

103. Kitchens CS. Prolonged activated partial thromboplastin time of unknown etiology: A prospective study of 100 consecutive cases referred for consultation. Am J Hematol 1988;27:38–45.

104. Golub R, Cantu R, Sorrento JJ, et al. Efficacy of preadmission testing in ambulatory surgical patients. Am J Surg 1992;163: 565–571.

105. Kaplan EB, Sheiner LB, Boeckmann AJ, et al. The usefulness of preoperative laboratory screening. JAMA 1985;253:3576–3581.

106. Litaker D. Preoperative screening. Med Clin North Am 1999; 83:1565–1581.

107. Eisenberg JM, Clarke JR, Sussman SA. Prothrombin and partial thromboplastin times as preoperative screening test. Arch Surg 1982;117:48–51.

107a. Bauer KA. The thrombophilias. Well-defined risk factors with uncertain therapeutic implications. Ann Intern Med 2001;135: 367–373.

108. Reddy NM, Hall SW, MacKintosh FR. Partial thromboplastin time. Prediction of adverse events and poor prognosis by low abnormal values. Arch Intern Med 1999;159:2706–2710.

109. Lowe GD. Prediction of postoperative deep-vein thrombosis. Thromb Haemost 1997;78:47–52.

110. Kakkar VV, Howe CT, Nicolaides AN, et al. Deep vein thrombosis of the leg: is there a "high risk" group? Am J Surg 1970; 120:527–530.

111. Sarasin FP, Bounameaux H. Duration of oral anticoagulant therapy after proximal deep vein thrombosis in a decision analysis. Thromb Haemost 1994;71:286–291.

112. Bishop JF, Schiffer CA, Aisner J, et al. Surgery in acute leukemia: a review of 167 operations in thrombocytopenic patients. Am J Hematol 1987;26:147–155.

113. Chu DZJ, Shivshanker K, Stroehlein JR, et al. Thrombocytopenia and gastrointestinal hemorrhage in the cancer patient: prevalence of unmasked lesion. Gastrointest Endosc 1983; 29:269–272.

114. Gazzard BG, Henderson JM, Williams R. The use of fresh frozen plasma or a concentrate of factor IX as replacement therapy before liver biopsy. Gut 1975;16:621–625.

115. McGill DB, Rakela J, Zinsmeister AR, et al. A 21-year experience with major hemorrhage after percutaneous liver biopsy. Gastroenterology 1990;99:1396–1400.

116. McVay PA, Toy PTCY. Lack of increased bleeding after liver biopsy in patients with mild hemostatic abnormalities. Am J Clin Pathol 1990;94:747–753.

117. Boberg KM, Brosstad F, Egeland T, et al. Is a prolonged bleeding time associated with an increased risk of hemorrhage after liver biopsy? Thromb Haemost 1999;81:378–381.

118. Ewe K. Bleeding after liver biopsy does not correlate with indices of peripheral coagulation. Dig Dis Sci 1981;26:388–393.

119. Makris M, Nakielny R, Toh CH, et al. A prospective investigation of the relationship between haemorrhagic complications of percutaneous needle biopsy of the liver and coagulation screening tests. Br J Haematol 1992;81:51(abstr).

120. Bravo AA, Sheth SG, Chopra S. Liver biopsy. N Engl J Med 2001;344:495–500.

121. Shiffman ML, Farrel MT, Yee YS. Risk of bleeding after endoscopic biopsy or polypectomy in patients taking aspirin or other NSAIDs. Gastrointest Endosc 1994;40:458–462.

122. Rutgeerts P, Wang T-H, Llorens PS. Gastrointestinal endoscopy and the patient with a risk of bleeding disorder. Gastrointest Endosc 1999;49:134–136.

123. McVay PA, Toy PTCY. Lack of increased bleeding after paracentesis and thoracentesis in patients with mild coagulation abnormalities. Transfusion 1991;31:164–171.

124. Kozak EA, Brath LK. Do "screening" coagulation tests predict bleeding in patients undergoing fiberoptic bronchoscopy with biopsy? Chest 1994;106:703–705.

125. Weiss SM, Hert RC, Gianola FJ, et al. Complications of fiberoptic bronchoscopy in thrombocytopenic patients. Chest 1993;104: 1025–1028.

126. Bjortuft O, Brosstad F, Boe J. Bronchoscopy with transbronchial biopsies: measurement of bleeding volume and evaluation of the predictive value of coagulation tests. Eur Respir J 1998;12:1025–1027.

127. Howard SC, Gajjar A, Ribeiro RC, et al. Safety of lumbar puncture for children with acute lymphoblastic leukemia and thrombocytopenia. JAMA 2000;284:2222–2224.

128. Ray CE Jr, Shenoy S. Patients with thrombocytopenia: outcome of radiologic placement of central venous access devices. Radiology 1997;204:97–99.

129. Goldfarb G, Lebrec D. Percutaneous cannulation of the internal jugular vein in patients with coagulopathies: an experience based on 1000 attempts. Anesthesiology 1982;56:321–323.

130. Fisher NC, Mutimer DJ. Central venous cannulation in patients with liver disease and coagulopathy—a prospective audit. Intensive Care Med 1999;25:481–485.

131. Foster PF, Moore LR, Sankary HN, et al. Central venous catheterization in patients with coagulopathy. Arch Surg 1992;127: 273–275.

132. DeLoughery TG, Liebler JM, Simonds V, et al. Invasive line placement in critically ill patients: do hemostatic tests matter? Transfusion 1996;36:827–831.

133. Doerfler ME, Kaufman B, Goldenberg AS. Central venous catheter placement in patients with disorders of coagulation. Chest 1996;110:185–188.

134. Eckman MH, Beshansky JR, Durand-Zaleski I, et al. Anticoagulation for noncardiac procedures in patients with prosthetic heart valves: Does low risk mean high cost? JAMA 1990;263:1513–1521.

135. Katholi RE, Nolan SP, McGuire LD. Living with prosthetic heart valves. Subsequent noncardiac operations and the risk of thromboembolism or hemorrhage. Am Heart J 1976;92:162–167.

136. Stone LS, Kline OR Jr, Sklar C. Intraocular lenses and anticoagulation and antiplatelet therapy. Am Intra-ocular Implant Soc J 1985;11:165–168.

137. Weibert RT. Oral anticoagulant therapy in patients undergoing dental surgery. Clin Pharm 1992;11:857–864.

138. Blinder D, Manor Y, Martinowitz U, et al. Dental extractions in patents maintained on continued oral anticoagulant: comparison of local hemostatic modalities. Oral Surg Oral Med Oral Pathol Oral Radiol Endod 1999;88:137–140.

139. Wahl MJ. Dental surgery in anticoagulated patients. Arch Intern Med 1998;158:1610–1616.

140. Sevitt S, Gallagher NG. Prevention of venous thrombosis and pulmonary embolism in injured patients. A trial of anticoagulant prophylaxis with phenindione in middle-aged and elderly patients with fractured necks of femur. Lancet 1959;2:981–989.

141. Salzman EW, Harris WH, DeSanctis RW. Reduction in venous thromboembolism by agents affecting platelet function. N Engl J Med 1971;284:1287–1292.

142. Francis CW, Marder VJ, Evarts CMC, et al. Two-step warfarin therapy. Prevention of postoperative venous thrombosis without excessive bleeding. JAMA 1983;249:374–378.

143. Spandorfer JM, Lynch S, Weitz HH, et al. Use of enoxaparin for the chronically anticoagulated patient before and after procedure. Arch Intern Med 1998;158:1610–1616.

144. Shetty HGM, Backhouse G, Bentley DP, et al. Effective reversal of warfarin-induced excessive anticoagulation with low dose vitamin K. Thromb Haemost 1992;67:13–15.

145. Whitling AM, Bussey HI, Lyons RM. Comparing different routes and doses of phytonadione for reversing excessive anticoagulation. Arch Intern Med 1998;158:2136–2140.
146. Raj G, Kumar R, McKinney WP. Time course of reversal of anticoagulant effect of warfarin by intravenous and subcutaneous phytonadione. Arch Intern Med 1999;159:2721–2724.
147. Shields RC, McBaive RD, Kuiper JD, et al. Efficacy and safety of intravenous phytonadione (vitamin K_1) in patients on long-term oral anticoagulant therapy. Mayo Clin Proc 2001;76:260–266.
148. Woodman RC, Harker LA. Bleeding complications associated with cardiopulmonary bypass. Blood 1990;1680–1687.
149. Manco-Johnson MJ, Nuss R, Jacobson LJ. Heparin neutralization is essential for accurate measurement of factor VIII activity and inhibitor assays in blood samples drawn from implanted venous access devices. J Lab Clin Med 2000;136:74–79.
150. Mallett SV, Cox DJ. Thromboelastography. Br J Anaesth 1992;69:307.
151. Wang JS, Lin CY, Hung WT, et al. Thromboelastogram fails to predict postoperative hemorrhage in cardiac patents. Ann Thorac Surg 1992;53:435.
152. Edmonds AR. Death from respiratory obstruction in haemophilia. Med J Aust 1951;1:227–228.
153. MacDonald AC, Robson JB, Waapshaw H. Haemophilia with respiratory obstruction. Br Med J 1953;1:1144–1146.
154. Pappas AM, Barr JS, Salzman EW, et al. The problem of unrecognized "mild hemophilia." JAMA 1964;187:772–774.
155. Coy J, Bivins BA, Belin RP. Surgical procedures in unsuspected hemophilia. Arch Surg 1974;109:835–836.
156. Alperin JB. Coagulopathy caused by vitamin K deficiency in critically ill, hospitalized patients. JAMA 1987;258:1916–1919.
157. Zumberg MS, Waples, JM, Kao KJ, et al. Management of a patient with a mechanical aortic valve and antibodies to both thrombin and factor V after repeat exposure to fibrin sealant. Am J Hematol 2000;64:59–63.
158. Day AL, Friedman WA, Sypert GW, et al. Successful treatment of normal perfusion pressure breakthrough syndrome. Neurosurgery 1982;11:625–630.
159. Young WL, Pile-Spellman J, Prohovnik I, et al. Evidence for adaptive autoregulatory displacement for hypotensive cortical territories adjacent to arteriovenous malformations. Neurosurgery 1994;34:601–610.

CHAPTER 31

Liver Disease, Organ Transplantation, and Hemostasis

Margaret V. Ragni, M.D., M.P.H.

In patients with chronic liver disease, adequate hemostatic function usually is preserved until 80% or more of functional hepatic tissue is lost. Once this critical juncture is reached, there is profound compromise of hemostatic function, including decreased synthesis and decreased degradation of activated coagulation factors, platelet functional defects and thrombocytopenia associated with portal hypertension, activation of fibrinolysis, and, rarely, disseminated intravascular coagulation (DIC). These profound coagulation changes are not always associated with a clinical bleeding tendency: they may lead to spontaneous or traumatic bleeding that may be life-threatening, they may recur, and they may require blood product replacement. In those in whom chronic liver disease progresses to end-stage liver disease, transplantation may become a consideration. This procedure, in which the old liver is removed and a new liver is implanted, may acutely and transiently worsen the coagulopathy of chronic liver disease, and may result in significant blood loss.

Patients with chronic liver disease may develop spontaneous bleeding, such as epistaxis, dental or gum bleeding, and bruising. Alternatively, bleeding may arise from anatomic abnormalities associated with end-stage liver disease, such as varices; bleeding may also be induced by trauma, such as with shunting procedures for control of ascites. Specific coagulation abnormalities are not predictive of clinical bleeding, and, moreover, treatment modalities available for management of the profound hemostatic abnormalities of chronic liver disease are suboptimal. Fresh frozen plasma, while providing coagulation factor replacement, is limited by volume constraints, the brevity of its efficiency due to the short half-life of infused clotting factors, and potential transmissible disease, such as hepatitis. Platelet transfusions provide hemostatic support, but this is only temporary, as platelets do not reverse the pathophysiology of portal hypertension; and cryoprecipitate may provide fibrinogen replacement, but does not reverse the consumptive coagulopathy or fibrinolysis of end-stage liver disease.

For patients who undergo transplantation, management of the associated acute perioperative coagulopathy, which is superimposed on the coagulation abnormalities of chronic liver disease, is an even greater therapeutic challenge. Future goals in the management of chronic liver disease are to develop better predictors of bleeding, to elucidate the role of cytokines and tissue mediators of inflammation that trigger the coagulopathy of liver disease, and to promote clinical trials to determine safer, more specific products to improve and maintain hemostasis in patients with a failing liver.

HISTORICAL OVERVIEW

From ancient times, the liver was regarded as the seat of life. Clay models of livers of sacrificed animals in ancient Mesopotamia in 900 BC and, similarly, bronze models of livers by the Etruscans in 300 BC were used to divine the prognosis of illness[1] (Figs. 31–1 and 31–2). Divining was considered a sacred act, and religious leaders, imbued with heavenly authority, studied animal entrails to understand the meaning of disease and to predict disease outcome. Liver disease was among the earliest of recorded diseases, with the first description of hepatitis by Hippocrates in 400 BC.[1] Over the centuries, the liver came to be regarded for its important role not only in protein synthesis, digestion, degradation of wastes, and immunologic defense against disease, but also in clot formation. Following the identification of coagulation factors and their role in hemostasis in the

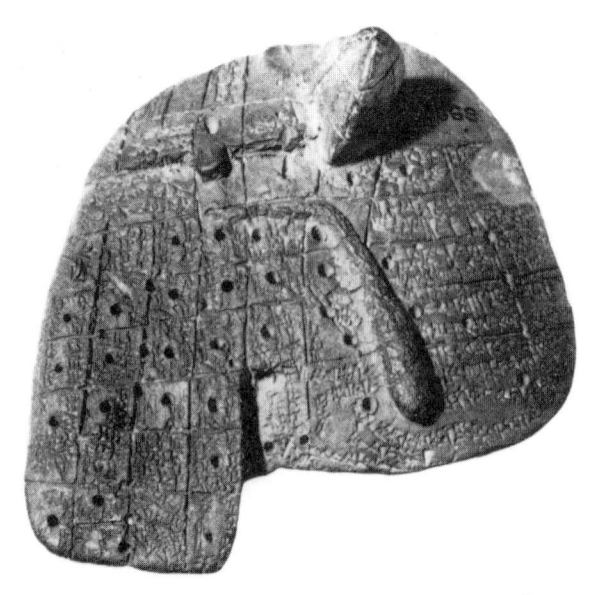

Figure 31–1. Clay model of the liver of a sheep used by 19th century B.C. Babylonians in divination to determine disease outcome. (From Medicine: An Illustrated History. Ancient Civilization, Mesopotamia (59) Albert S. Lyons. Figure 98, page 65, with permission.)

late 19th and first half of the 20th century, the liver was recognized as the site of synthesis of coagulation factors, and liver disease became recognized as an important cause of clinical bleeding.

The essential role of the liver in hemostasis was confirmed by the pioneering work of Starzl in liver transplantation, beginning in the 1960s.[2–4] Removal of the liver was shown to have a profound effect on the coagulation system, resulting in severe coagulation abnormalities and massive blood loss.[5] Subsequently, in the 1980s, implantation of a normal liver was shown to provide phenotypic correction of the congenital disorder hemophilia,[6,7] demonstrating the restorative effect of the normal liver on the coagulation system.

Prospective studies of patients with chronic liver disease and those undergoing transplantation led to the identification of specific coagulation abnormalities and to transfusion support tailored to the specific defects.[8–13] The judicious use of blood product replacement therapy, tailored to correct specific coagulation abnormalities of chronic liver disease and during transplantation, led to reduction in blood loss and blood product usage, as well as in complications of the procedure, resulting in improved transplantation outcomes. Yet, the triggers of the coagulopathy of liver disease and bleeding are not known, and, thus, management of the coagulopathy of liver disease remains reactive rather than preventive.

PATHOPHYSIOLOGY OF COAGULOPATHY ASSOCIATED WITH LIVER DISEASE

Liver disease constitutes an important acquired disorder of both primary hemostasis and secondary hemostasis. Primary hemostasis, that is, platelet plug formation, may be compromised in patients with liver disease as a result of thrombocytopenia and/or qualitative defects in platelet function. Thrombocytopenia may result from either portal hypertension with splenic sequestration of platelets or decreased thrombopoietin production,[14] or both. Secondary hemostasis, or fibrin clot formation, may be limited in patients with chronic liver disease because of defects in clotting factor synthesis and increased degradation. These changes may lead to clinical bleeding, yet, because of its remarkable regenerative capacity, the liver is able to sustain significant injury before clinical manifestations of hemostatic decompensation occur.

Clinically, patients may experience bruising, epistaxis, bleeding from venipuncture sites, oozing from dental and oral mucosa, and bleeding from gastrointestinal mucosa or varices. The proposed mechanism of the coagulopathy of liver disease[15,16] includes (1) decreased synthesis of coagulation factors, (2) synthesis of abnormal coagulation factors, (3) decreased degradation of activated coagulation factors, (4) activation of fibrinolysis, and (5) consumptive coagulopathy or DIC (Table 31–1). Each of these will be considered separately.

Decreased Synthesis of Coagulation Factors

Deficiencies in levels of coagulation factors in both the intrinsic and extrinsic coagulation pathways occur, with

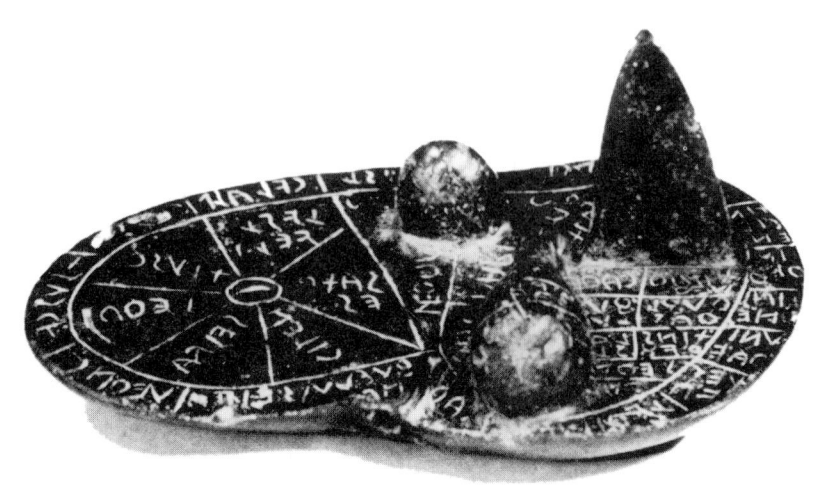

Figure 31–2. Bronze model of a sheep liver used by 3rd century B.C. Etruscans in divination. (From Medicine: An Illustrated History. Greece and Rome, Medicine in Roman Times (231) Albert S. Lyons. Figure 340, page 232, with permission.)

Table 31-1 • HEMOSTATIC CONSEQUENCES OF LIVER DISEASE

- Decreased synthesis of coagulation factors
- Synthesis of abnormal coagulation factors
    Abnormal fibrinogen sialic acid moiety—dysfibrinogen
- Vitamin K deficiency
    Dietary deficiency
    Impaired synthesis of vitamin K-dependent factors
    Lack of bile salts—obstructive jaundice
- Hypersplenism with platelet sequestration—thrombocytopenia
- Decreased degradation of activated coagulation factors
    Increased activated coagulation factors—DIC
    Increased activation of fibrinolytic system—Fibrinolysis

associated prolongation of the prothrombin time (PT) and activated partial thromboplastin time (aPTT). The liver is the major site of synthesis of fibrinogen and factors II, V, VII, IX, X, XI, and XII; factor VIII is also synthesized in the endothelium.[15,16] Progressive loss of hepatocytes and liver parenchymal cells results in a functional synthetic defect with worsening factor deficiencies. The importance of the liver in factor VIII synthesis is underscored by the demonstration that liver transplantation in a hemophilic patient with end-stage liver disease resulted in a phenotypic cure of his hemophilia.[6,7] Factor VIII and fibrinogen are also acute-phase reactants and may increase in liver disease, as they increase in other situations of chronic inflammation[17] Deficiency of factor V is common in chronic liver disease and, because it is not a vitamin K-dependent factor, is regarded as a better predictor of overall synthetic impairment than factors II, VII, IX, or X. Although fibrinogen is an acute-phase reactant, its measurement may be useful in end-stage liver disease: when the fibrinogen level falls below 100 mg/dL in patients with chronic liver disease, the risk of acute liver failure markedly increases.[18]

Predicting the outcome of a patient with liver disease or whether a patient will have bleeding complications is difficult, as there are no noninvasive markers that are predictive of liver disease outcome. The presence and severity of coagulation abnormalities do not appear to be predictive of bleeding in this setting.[19] In one study of alcoholic cirrhotic patients, however, those with bleeding symptoms demonstrated significantly lower factor VII, plasminogen, antithrombin III, and albumin levels than did those with no bleeding symptoms.[19] These findings suggest that the severity of hepatocellular damage may be an important determinant of bleeding tendency. It is unknown, however, whether liver biopsy, the gold standard for determining liver disease progression,[20] is predictive of bleeding tendency or of the severity of the coagulopathy of liver disease.

Synthesis of Abnormal Coagulation Factors

Patients with liver disease may produce a dysfibrinogen,[21] which contains excessive sialic acid residues,[22] resulting in abnormal fibrin polymerization.[19,21,22] The dysfibrinogen is not as efficient as normal fibrinogen in the formation of a fibrin clot, and thus conversion from fibrinogen to fibrin, the last step in fibrin clot formation, is slowed, resulting in prolongation of the thrombin time and reptilase times. Despite the abnormal polymerization and slowing in fibrin formation, the dysfibrinogenemia of liver disease is not associated with clinical bleeding symptoms. The dysfibrinogen, however, is among the earliest coagulation abnormalities of liver disease,[12,19] and among the last coagulation abnormalities to correct following transplantation.[10,12,13] An abnormally synthesized fibrinogen may also be detected in patients with hepatocellular carcinoma.[23]

Patients with advanced liver disease may also produce an abnormal prothrombin, known as des-γ-carboxy prothrombin.[24,25] This dysprothrombin is caused by an acquired defect in carboxylation of vitamin K-dependent proteins. Specifically, this defect involves the γ-carboxylation of the glutamic acid residues in the N-terminal region of these proteins by a vitamin K-dependent carboxylase.[25] Clinically, the proportion of prothrombin that is synthesized in this defective form is small, and the dysprothrombin is not associated with clinical bleeding symptoms. This des-carboxylated prothrombin is also detected in individuals who develop hepatoma.[26]

Vitamin K Deficiency

In liver disease, deficiencies of the vitamin K-dependent factors may occur by several mechanisms. These factors may be reduced as part of the overall reduction in all coagulation factor synthesis in the diseased liver. If there is extrahepatic obstructive (cholestatic) liver disease, there may be reduced absorption of bile salts required for absorption of vitamin K.[24] In addition, poor oral intake or treatment with antibiotics that destroy the gut bacteria that synthesize vitamin K may also contribute to vitamin K deficiency. Thus, vitamin K deficiency is a common concomitant of chronic liver disease.

Vitamin K is a fat-soluble vitamin necessary for the synthesis of functional clotting proteins, factors II, VII, IX, and X and of functional clot regulatory proteins, protein C and S. Vitamin K is a cofactor in the enzymatic conversion of glutamic acid into γ-carboxyglutamic acid. The oral anticoagulants known as coumarins inhibit vitamin K at this step of clotting factor synthesis, thereby simulating vitamin K deficiency. The γ-carboxyglutamic acid residues are necessary for calcium (Ca^{++}) and metal ion binding by vitamin K-dependent proteins to phospholipid and cell membranes, which is essential to many coagulation reactions in the coagulation cascade.[24,25]

Thrombocytopenia and Platelet Functional Defects

In patients with chronic liver disease, progressive hepatic dysfunction leads to portal hypertension and congestive splenomegaly with splenic pooling of platelets and thrombocytopenia.[27,28] As many as a third of patients with chronic liver disease develop thrombocytopenia,[19] which is usually mild to moderate (e.g., 70,000 to 90,000/μL), and among those who progress to end-stage liver disease, over 90% develop thrombocytopenia.[8] As chronic liver disease progresses, there is increasing distortion of hepatocyte architecture with reversal of blood flow from the high-pressure portal circulation to the low-pressure systemic circulation and development of portal-systemic collaterals, such as hemorrhoidal veins and esophageal varices, from which bleeding may occur. Bleeding via portal collaterals may worsen with pooling of platelets in the spleen and splenic sinusoids and onset of thrombocytopenia.[27,28]

The bleeding time in patients with liver disease is prolonged out of proportion to the decrease in platelet count, suggesting the presence of platelet functional defects, as well (see Chapter 10). These abnormalities include nonspecific platelet aggregation defects[19] and a shortened platelet survival.[28] Alcohol may lead to direct toxic effects on the platelet and megakaryocytes in the marrow[29]; nutritional deficiencies or complicating infections may further suppress marrow production of platelets. Reduced thrombopoietin levels in liver disease may also contribute to thrombocytopenia.[14] Less commonly, thrombocytopenia may be part of the consumptive coagulopathy and DIC in some patients with end-stage liver disease.[30]

Accelerated Fibrinolysis

Fibrinolysis, the mechanism by which a clot, once formed, is dissolved and eliminated from the circulation, may be accelerated in chronic liver disease. Fibrinolysis specifically involves local conversion of the inactive enzyme, plasminogen, to plasmin, which cleaves fibrin and fibrinogen to fibrin split (degradation) products (FDPs). This reaction is triggered primarily by tissue plasminogen activator (tPA), which is released from vascular endothelium when a thrombus is formed; this reaction occurs locally at the site of the thrombus.[31]

In liver disease, fibrinolysis may be accelerated as a result of several defects, including reduced synthesis of the plasmin inhibitor, α_2-plasmin inhibitor,[31] decreased degradation of activated coagulation factors,[32,33] and increased consumption of activated clotting factors[30,34] which, when liver degradation mechanisms are exhausted, accumulate in excess.[30-34] There is some evidence that the likely mechanism of hyperfibrinolysis in end-stage liver disease is clotting activation, as elevated levels of D-dimer and tPA activity are usually found in association with increased generation of thrombin and high circulating levels of prothrombin fragment F1+2.[35]

Fibrinolysis, as evidenced by hypofibrinogenemia, elevated levels of FDPs, and a shortened euglobulin clot lysis time, may occur alone or with DIC; this is important to determine prior to treatment (see below).

Disseminated Intravascular Coagulation

Rarely, DIC may occur in the setting of chronic liver disease. The diagnosis of DIC in the setting of chronic liver disease may be difficult, however, because coagulation changes that occur in DIC may be similar to or indistinguishable from those occurring in chronic liver disease.[34] The mechanism by which DIC occurs in advanced liver disease is through entrance into the circulation of activated clotting factors, which are not cleared because of defective hepatic degradation. These activated factors activate the coagulation mechanism.[30,34] The coagulation changes that occur in DIC reflect excess thrombin action.[30,34] Specifically, there is excess thrombin-mediated conversion of fibrinogen to fibrin, with consumption of fibrinogen, resulting in hypofibrinogenemia, and excess fibrinolysis of fibrin to FDPs, which increase as do fibrin monomer (FM) and fibrin dimer (FD).[30,34] As the concentration of FDPs increases, they deposit in the microcirculation and circulating red cells may fragment into burr cells or schistocytes,[30,34] giving rise to a microangiopathic hemolytic anemia (MAHA). There is excess thrombin-induced platelet aggregation, leading to further thrombocytopenia, and excess thrombin-induced activation and deactivation of coagulation factors, leading to factor deficiencies.[30,34] Excess consumption of antithrombin III (AT III), which complexes with thrombin to inhibit further clot formation, leads to deficiency of AT III[36] (see Chapter 12).

CLINICAL DIAGNOSIS

In individuals suspected of having liver disease, the history should include questions about past jaundice, hepatitis, previous blood transfusions, intravenous drug use, use of other medications (prescription or over-the-counter), alcohol or liquor consumption, a family history of liver disease, mental or psychiatric symptoms, diabetes, and symptoms of autoimmune disease. The examination should include an assessment of the skin for ecchymoses, discoloration, spider angioma, palmar erythema, the musculoskeletal system for muscle wasting, careful ophthalmologic exam for Kayser-Fleischer rings, evaluation of liver and spleen size, and evaluation for ascites and peripheral edema. There should be screening for subtle changes in mood, behavior, or sleep, and evidence of apraxia or agraphia. The laboratory screening should include liver function tests, including levels of albumin, alanine aminotransferase (ALT [SGPT]), aspartate aminotransferase (AST [SGOT]), alkaline phosphatase; a complete blood count (CBC); iron studies for hemochromatosis; and serologies for hepatitis A, B, and C. Coagulation screening should include a PT, aPTT, and platelet count: if the latter screening tests are abnormal, specific coagulation factor levels and coagulation factor inhibitors may be measured. The bleeding time and platelet aggregation tests may be abnormal in liver disease but are neither specific nor predictive of clinical bleeding,[37] and, thus, other than to exclude aspirin use, are not helpful.

Once a diagnosis of liver disease is confirmed, an assessment of hemorrhagic tendency should be made, as hemorrhage is a common complication of chronic liver disease and contributes significantly to morbidity and mortality in chronic liver disease.[15,16,19,38] Despite this, there is poor correlation between clinical bleeding

Table 31-2 • CLINICAL BLEEDING SYMPTOMS WITH LIVER DISEASE COAGULOPATHY

- Ecchymoses
- Gastrointestinal bleeding
- Variceal bleeding
- Epistaxis
- Oozing from venipuncture sites
- Bleeding with procedures

and coagulation findings.[15,16,19,38] This is, in part, due to the fact that hemorrhage in such patients is the result of not only hemostatic failure but also structural defects (e.g., ulcers, gastritis, or varices) and abnormally high venous pressure from portal hypertension. The role of the classic hemostatic system, as measured in the coagulation laboratory, in controlling high pressure hemorrhage in large-vessel bleeds is actually minimal. For example, patients may have large variceal bleeds and chronic hepatitis C with essentially normal coagulation factor levels. Typical bleeding symptoms observed in a series of carefully studied alcoholic cirrhotic patients include bruising, purpura, epistaxis, oozing from venipuncture, gastrointestinal bleeding, genitourinary bleeding, and bleeding with procedures and surgery (Table 31-2).

It is not unusual for individuals with advanced liver disease to go unrecognized until tests of coagulation (PT and/or aPTT) are found to be prolonged prior to a procedure or surgery. Minor ecchymoses, epistaxis, or dental bleeding may be an early sign of the liver disease coagulopathy, but, in many, a gastrointestinal bleed or variceal bleed may be the first evidence that the coagulopathy of liver disease has developed, indicating the advanced level of their disease and progressive nature of their liver dysfunction.

The bleeding associated with liver disease may be mucosal, reflecting the primary hemostatic defect, specifically the inability to form a platelet plug because of thrombocytopenia and qualitative platelet defects. The bleeding associated with liver disease may also occur in soft tissues, reflecting the secondary hemostatic defect, specifically the inability to form and sustain a fibrin clot as a result of depressed synthesis of coagulation factors. With advanced liver disease, generalized oozing from venipuncture sites and with procedures may occur after multiple coagulation abnormalities develop, including, usually extremely late in the course, hypofibrinogenemia.

Bleeding in chronic liver disease is often due not to one but to multiple coagulation abnormalities, with or without an anatomic defect. It is known that varices are present at least 50% of the time at diagnosis of cirrhosis.[39] Thus, while a patient with mild to moderate vitamin K deficiency may not necessarily bleed because of that defect alone, if that same patient also has thrombocytopenia, multiple coagulation factor deficiencies, excessive fibrinolysis, and an anatomic defect (e.g., gastric varices), the likelihood of hemorrhage escalates. This underscores the importance of screening patients with chronic liver disease for coagulation defects in order to anticipate bleeding problems with procedures and surgery before they occur. For example, surgery should be avoided in patients with DIC and advanced liver disease, as such will result in worsening of the DIC and increase the probability a fatal outcome.[40]

LABORATORY DIAGNOSIS OF COAGULOPATHY ASSOCIATED WITH LIVER DISEASE

Prolongation of the PT and the aPTT are perhaps the most common abnormal coagulation tests in patients with chronic liver disease. The specific coagulation laboratory tests diagnostic of the coagulopathy of liver disease are found in Table 31-3. These tests may reflect synthetic deficiency of factors, vitamin K deficiency, or, less likely, DIC or fibrinolysis. Yet, the presence of an abnormal test does not necessarily require intervention. In the nonbleeding patient, no correction is required; however, in the bleeding patient or the patient anticipating surgery, specific coagulation factor assays should be obtained and specific treatment recommended (see below).

In addition to obtaining specific coagulation tests, the physician should know the patient's type of liver disease, that is, hepatocellular versus extrahepatic obstructive disease. Hepatocellular disease is usually associated with more severe coagulation abnormalities than extrahepatic obstructive disease. Further, with progression of hepatocellular liver disease, as compared with extrahepatic obstructive liver disease, there is a generally greater severity and frequency of coagulation factor de-

Table 31-3 • LABORATORY FEATURES OF LIVER DISEASE COAGULOPATHY

- Prolonged PT and normal aPTT
    Deficiency of factor VII
- Prolonged PT and prolonged aPTT
    Deficiency of factors I, II, V, X, IX, XI, XII
- Prolonged thrombin and reptilase times
    Dysfibrinogen
    Hypofibrinogenemia
- Thrombocytopenia
    Platelet sequestration—hypersplenism, portal hypertension
    Platelet consumption—disseminated intravascular coagulation
    Decreased thrombopoietin production
- Platelet functional defects
    Nonspecific platelet aggregation abnormalities
- Shortened euglobulin lysis time
    Decreased plasminogen activator inhibitor
    Decreased α_2 plasmin inhibitor
- Special features associated with transplantation
    Dilutional effect of organ preservation solution
    Activation of fibrinolysis
    Tissue plasminogen activator release from hepatic vasculature
    Loss of hepatic clearance of activated factors
    Endogenous heparin release from engrafted liver

ficiencies, and a greater frequency of thrombocytopenia, fibrinolysis, and/or DIC.[12]

In one study of cirrhotic patients without sepsis, infection, malignancy, or recent surgery, no one coagulation test was predictive of bleeding; however, bleeding was significantly associated with four tests; namely, lower factor VII, AT III, plasminogen, and albumin levels.[19] High serum levels of FDPs, specifically measured as D-dimer, have also been shown, along with tPA, to be highly associated with bleeding tendency in cirrhotic patients.[41] Because D-dimer is a readily available test, it often is used, in addition to the PT and aPTT, to screen for bleeding risk in end-stage liver disease.

The Child-Pugh score, which measures severity of liver decompensation,[39] was found in another study of bleeding tendency to correlate with prolongation of the PT: bleeding tendency in Child-Pugh class 1 was based on PT less than 5 seconds prolonged; class 2 on PT 5 to 6 seconds prolonged, and class 3 on PT greater than 6 seconds prolonged.[39] Prospective studies of larger cohorts are needed to determine better and earlier predictors of the bleeding tendency, and to determine the correlation among liver pathologic classification schemas, cytokine levels, and coagulation factor levels in order to develop ultimately better and earlier interventions to reduce clinical bleeding.

If a liver biopsy is performed as part of the evaluation of liver disease, the less-invasive transjugular biopsy approach may be safer than the percutaneous approach, especially in the patient with active bleeding. Moreover, the transjugular approach provides adequate tissue specimens for diagnostic purposes with fewer than 1% bleeding or other complications.[42]

Impaired Synthesis of Coagulation Factors

Depressed factor V activity is considered a good marker of liver disease, as factor V is synthesized almost entirely in the liver.[15,16] By comparison, factor VIII and fibrinogen are acute-phase reactants that increase with inflammation. Factors II, VII, IX, and X are vitamin K dependent, and deficiencies may also reflect vitamin K deficiency, such as with extrahepatic obstructive liver diseases, or may reflect treatment with antibiotics that destroy gut flora producing vitamin K. The contact factors, including factors XI, XII, prekallikrein, and high-molecular-weight kininogen, are usually only mildly decreased in liver disease and, thus, are not as helpful in diagnosis of liver disease.

Examples of impaired synthesis of inhibitors in liver disease include the typically reduced levels of AT III[36] and heparin cofactor II.[43] Deficiencies of coagulation factor inhibitors are not typically associated with thrombosis. This may be due to the concomitant reduced levels of many coagulation factors. On the other hand, a prolonged PT and aPTT in a patient with liver disease does not result in "auto-anticoagulation" and, as such, for example, does not protect a patient with atrial fibrillation from having a stroke.

Synthesis of Abnormal Proteins

Diagnosis of the dysfibrinogen of liver disease is based on the presence of both a prolonged thrombin time and a prolonged reptilase time. These assays measure the time required for conversion of fibrinogen to fibrin. The reptilase time prolongation is specific for the dysfibrinogen: by comparison, heparin effect is distinguished by its prolongation of the thrombin time but absence of any effect on the reptilase time.[21,22] Diagnosis of the dysprothrombin associated with liver disease is based on the presence of des-γ-carboxyl prothrombin.[24] The latter defect is due to defective carboxylation of glutamic residues in prothrombin. Neither the dysfibrinogen nor the dysprothrombin are usually associated with clinical bleeding, but may serve as useful markers of liver disease.

Vitamin K Deficiency

The best coagulation screening test for vitamin K deficiency is the PT, which measures the extrinsic coagulation pathway. Because factor VII has the shortest half-life, about 7 hours, it is the first vitamin K-dependent factor to decrease, and, once vitamin K replacement is given, the earliest to correct.[24] Thus, early vitamin K deficiency is characterized by a prolonged PT, and as vitamin K deficiency worsens, there is progressive depletion of factors II, IX, and X, and both the PT and aPTT are prolonged. With vitamin K administration, levels of factor VII, with the shortest half-life, correct first, with slower correction of factors II, IX, and X and the prolonged aPTT and PT.

Thrombocytopenia and Platelet Dysfunction

Patients with chronic liver disease may have thrombocytopenia for several reasons. By far, the most common reason for thrombocytopenia is portal hypertension and splenic sequestration of platelets. Rarely, patients may have evidence of DIC with a consumption of platelets (see below). Platelet function abnormalities in chronic liver disease include abnormal clot retraction, abnormal platelet adhesion, measured by glass-bead column retention; and abnormal platelet aggregation with ADP, collagen, epinephrine, ristocetin, and thrombin.[19,27–29]

Activation of Fibrinolysis

Laboratory abnormalities of fibrinolytic activity include hypofibrinogenemia with associated prolongation of the PT, aPTT, thrombin time, and reptilase times, increased FDPs, decreased plasminogen, and a shortened euglobulin clot lysis time.[32,33] There may also be decreased α_2-plasmin inhibitor,[31,32] the major inhibitor of plasmin, correlating with severity of liver disease.[32]

The thromboelastograph (TEG), an ancillary test that measures the quality and dynamics of clot formation,[11] may be abnormal in chronic liver disease. Specifically, there may be a decrease in the amplitude and width of the TEG trace, and delay in onset of clot formation.[11,13] Although the TEG does not correlate with coagulation abnormalities,[11,13] TEG traces are used by some to aid in early, rapid recognition of excessive fibrinolysis or thrombocytopenia.[11]

Disseminated Intravascular Coagulation

In the absence of infection, sepsis, surgical procedures, or malignancy, patients with chronic liver disease may be unlikely to develop DIC.[19] In studies in which strict criteria were applied to enrollment, specifically excluding patients with sepsis, infection, or malignancy, DIC and fibrinolysis were not detected.[19] In end-stage liver disease, however, some patients may develop DIC or laboratory studies that mimic DIC[30,34]: with the trigger for DIC and markers predictive of DIC obscure. Yet, the associated morbidity and mortality make a diagnosis of DIC, while controversial, an important one in the management of patient with liver disease.

In order to make a diagnosis of DIC, there must be evidence of excess thrombin action in several coagulation pathways (i.e., factor deficiencies, thrombocytopenia, hypofibrinogenemia, FDPs, depletion of AT III, or MAHA).[30,34] Usually, at least three of these six criteria should be present, the first three of which are more specific for a diagnosis of DIC. Bleeding with or without concomitant thrombosis is nearly universal in such patients with DIC, but more often not present in liver disease patients whose coagulation studies only mimic DIC.

It may be difficult to distinguish DIC from chronic liver disease. One helpful approach is to attempt to establish the time of onset of the coagulation abnormalities. Specifically, the clinician should establish whether changes in the PT, aPTT, fibrinogen, or platelets have occurred recently, for example, within the several weeks prior to the current evaluation, indicating an acute consumptive process, or whether the changes have been present chronically, supporting chronic liver disease.

LIVER TRANSPLANTATION

Liver transplantation is indicated for individuals with decompensated end-stage liver disease, manifested by intractable ascites, recurrent variceal bleeding, encephalopathy, recurrent spontaneous bacterial peritonitis, and hepatorenal syndrome.[4] Although liver transplantation is associated with massive blood loss, advances in understanding the coagulopathy that develops during and after the procedure have greatly improved perioperative management and survival.

The liver transplantation procedure is divided into three stages: stage 1, the preimplant stage; stage 2, the anhepatic phase, in which the diseased liver is excised; and stage 3, the reimplantation stage, in which the new liver is placed and perfusion re-established.[12,44] Coagulation abnormalities that reflect the underlying chronic liver disease are present from the very beginning of the transplantation procedure. The coagulopathy worsens acutely as the procedure progresses through the three stages, and is especially profound during the anhepatic stage; it persists, but improves in the last stage, and resolves slowly during the postoperative period.[9,13,44] Specific coagulation changes that occur in each of the stages of the transplantation procedure will be considered (Table 31–4).

During the first stage, coagulation changes are modest, with only minor worsening of the baseline coagulopathy associated with the underlying liver disease. Coagulation changes in this stage reflect surgical blood loss associated with dissection of adhesions, transection of collaterals at sites of inflammation or previous procedures, and removal of the diseased liver.[9,44] The amount of blood loss correlates most closely to the skill of the surgeon[44] and to the extent of anatomic abnormalities from previous procedures. There may be a dilutional coagulopathy associated with blood product replacement, although it is usually minimal in this stage.

During the second, or anhepatic, stage, the coagulopathy arises primarily from removal of the liver, rather than from surgical bleeding, as most of the larger and smaller vessels have already been clamped and the collaterals ligated. With removal of the native liver, hepatic synthetic and degradative functions cease, resulting in a profound coagulopathy, and, in some patients, fibrinolysis and DIC. Whether DIC or fibrinolysis occurs in the setting of transplantation is controversial,[45–49] and many suspect the occurrence of either DIC or fibrinolysis heralds a complication, such as sepsis, infection, pancreatitis, or acute respiratory distress syndrome (ARDS).[19] Fibrinolysis is highly associated with bleeding in the anhepatic stage.[9,44] Very high levels of tPA are generated within 10 minutes after the donor liver is placed: the tPA activity arises from both its increased release and decreased clearance. Some have suggested the tPA arises from the graft, although an active signaling process has not been excluded. Evidence of fibrinolysis, including a decrease in levels of α_2-antiplasmin and fibrinogen with elevated FDP levels, may be detected following the escape of tPA into the general

---

Table 31–4 • HEMOSTATIC CHANGES WITH LIVER TRANSPLANTATION

Preimplant Phase—Stage 1
- Dilutional coagulopathy
- Mild fibrinolysis
- Prolonged thrombin and reptilase times (due to dysfibrinogen)

Anhepatic Phase—Stage 2
- Absence of hepatic synthetic and clearance function
- Release of tissue plasminogen activator: fibrinolysis
- Consumptive coagulopathy due to poor clearance of activated factors
- Reperfusion coagulopathy: fibrinolysis, heparin release from graft

Reimplantation Phase—Stage 3
- Restoration of coagulation factor and coagulation inhibitor synthesis
- Resolution of dysfibrinogenemia

circulation, which is highly correlated with clinical bleeding and oozing during this period.[11] With aggressive blood product replacement, including fresh frozen plasma (FFP), red cells, platelets, and cryoprecipitate, potential blood loss during active fibrinolysis may be minimized.[44] Additional findings may include a decrease in coagulation factor inhibitors such as AT III,[50] but this does not lead to a thrombotic event, likely because the decrease is offset by the severe synthetic defect and resulting deficiencies of coagulation factors occurring in this stage. Thrombocytopenia, which may also occur during this stage, is caused by increased platelet consumption.

During the third, or reimplantation, stage, restoration of coagulation factor and coagulation factor inhibitor synthesis begins. Fibrinolysis, which peaks as the donor liver is implanted, begins to resolve, with improvement in levels of fibrinogen and plasminogen, and reduction in FDPs, as the functioning donor liver engrafts.[9,13] Of the many laboratory changes occurring with transplantation, the aPTT, whether measured as part of an overall coagulation score[8] or alone,[51] appears to predict survival following transplantation better than the PT, thrombin time, fibrinogen levels, platelet count, or liver function tests.[51]

TREATMENT OF TRANSPLANTATION COAGULOPATHY

Liver transplantation is associated with significant loss of blood volume: it is not uncommon for patients to receive 10 units of red cells, as well as FFP and platelets (Table 31–5). Postoperative outcome following transplantation is highly correlated with blood loss and transfusion requirement.[8] However, pretransplantation coagulation abnormalities do not predict intraoperative blood requirements, likely because they can not predict the accelerated fibrinolysis that occurs during transplantation.[12,13,19]

The approach to hemostatic management of liver transplantation is specific for each stage. In stage 1, the predominant coagulation abnormalities are those of the underlying end-stage liver disease. Management is focused on controlling bleeding that arises from surgical dissection, which may vary with the extent of adhesions, inflammation, and past surgeries.[44]

During stage 2, ensuing fibrinolysis is managed by aggressive blood product replacement, cryoprecipitate for hypofibrinogenemia, and protamine sulfate.[11,13,44] Until recently, the role of protamine and antifibrinolytic therapy in transplantation[30,52,53] was considered controversial. However, in 1998, Kettner and coworkers using TEG, reported the presence of a significant endogenous heparin effect in patients undergoing transplantation, both before and after reperfusion of newly engrafted livers.[54] These investigators postulated that this heparin effect was caused by release of heparin-like substances from the liver graft. The potential role of heparin, as well as of tPA,[13] in the excessive blood loss during transplantation, thus provided rationale for the use of antifibrinolytic therapy. Recently, Porte and coworkers, in a randomized double-blind study of liver transplant recipients, showed that treatment with the antifibrinolytic serine protease inhibitor, aprotonin, significantly reduced blood loss with no increase in thrombosis or mortality.[55]

In stage 3, the coagulopathy is directly related to the quality of the donor liver and its successful engraftment.[44] An ischemic transplanted organ or an organ with damaged vascular endothelium may trigger activation of the coagulation system and, potentially, DIC.[44] Antifibrinolytic therapy may be continued for up to 2 hours after reperfusion,[55] as fibrinolysis usually does not resolve until then. The role of antihemorrhagic agents such as AT III concentrates,[56] tranexamic acid,[52] and estrogen,[57] although advocated by some, will require clinical trials to establish their utility in treatment of individuals undergoing transplantation.

TREATMENT OF LIVER DISEASE COAGULOPATHY

Management of the coagulopathy of liver disease is difficult. Treatment is directed at replacing the factor deficiencies, replacing dysfunctional or decreased platelets, and replacing fibrinogen if there is hypofibrinogenemia and/or excessive fibrinolysis (Table 31–5). FFP is indicated to replace coagulation factor deficiencies that may arise from the liver synthetic defect, either in patients who are actively bleeding or in preparation for upcoming procedures or surgery. The dosing of FFP depends on plasma volume and clinical presence of edema or ascites, which may limit volume considerations. In general, five 200-cc bags of FFP are sufficient to achieve a 10% to 20% correction of coagulation factor deficiencies,[9,12,13] with subsequent monitoring of the PT and aPTT for adjustment of repeated dosing for ongoing blood loss. FFP is also indicated to avoid dilutional depletion of factors following administration of packed red cells and volume expansion during treatment of acute bleeding or for procedures. In general, two units

---

Table 31–5 • TREATMENT OF COAGULOPATHY ASSOCIATED WITH LIVER DISEASE/TRANSPLANTATION

- Fresh frozen plasma—replacement for factor deficiencies
- Platelets—replacement for thrombocytopenia
- Vitamin K—replacement for vitamin K-dependent factor deficiencies
- Cryoprecipitate—replacement for fibrinogen deficiency
- DDAVP—amelioration of platelet functional defects
- Packed red cells—replacement for blood loss
- Aprotonin—control of hyperfibrinolysis
- Controversial:
  α_2-antiplasmin
  ε-Aminocaproic acid
  Tranexamic acid
  AT III concentrates
  Estrogens

of FFP are replaced for each unit of packed red blood cells given.

The use of activated clotting factor concentrates for replacement of coagulation factor deficiencies in patients with chronic liver disease who are bleeding is generally discouraged because significant risks chiefly, thrombosis may be associated with use of these activated products.

Platelet transfusions are indicated in patients who are bleeding and have a platelet count below 10,000/μL. When other coagulation abnormalities are present, as is typical in chronic liver disease, and the patient is bleeding, transfusion may be initiated at a higher platelet count. In order to determine the efficacy of platelet transfusion, a 1-hour post-transfusion platelet count should be obtained. Patients with large spleens will not likely respond with a high increment in their platelet count following transfusion, because of increased platelet sequestration. If platelet functional defects contribute to clinical bleeding, intravenous DDAVP, at a dose of 0.3 μg/kg, may be tried. Alternatively, estrogens may also be tried, but are generally considered less useful.[57]

Vitamin K deficiency may be treated with oral or subcutaneous vitamin K. In general, if the PT and/or aPTT are prolonged, a trial of vitamin K is warranted, beginning with a dose of 10 mg administered subcutaneously. Responses occur quite rapidly and partial correction of levels may be reached within 24 to 48 hours. If complete correction of the PT and aPTT does not occur after 3 days, the abnormalities likely indicate concomitant hepatic synthetic defects of liver disease.

Cryoprecipitate is recommended for hypofibrinogenemia resulting from activation of fibrinolysis, or from consumptive coagulopathy with DIC, or rarely from synthetic deficiency. Replacement of fibrinogen loss should begin with an infusion of about 1200 mg of fibrinogen provided by six bags of cryoprecipitate for a 60- to 70-kg patient daily, with prospective monitoring of the PT and aPTT for subsequent dosing adjustment.

Fibrinolysis is difficult to treat in end-stage liver disease. While cryoprecipitate is an excellent source of fibrinogen, it does not correct the underlying defect, that is, the deranged degradative function and enhanced fibrinolytic activity. Antifibrinolytic agents such as ε-aminocaproic acid,[13] tranexamic acid,[52] and aprotonin[52,53,55] have been reported to reduce bleeding associated with fibrinolysis in chronic liver disease and intraoperative blood loss during transplantation and to reduce the requirement for plasma, platelets, and cryoprecipitate transfusion.[13,33,52,53] However, the benefits of such treatment are not known, as there have been no controlled trials to assess the role of antifibrinolytic agents in liver disease. Thus, firm recommendations regarding the role of antifibrinolytics in liver disease and transplantation must await confirmation in prospective trials. In the presence of DIC, antifibrinolytic agents for fibrinolysis may be harmful and are contraindicated.[38] Estrogens[57] have also been used in the setting of bleeding in chronic liver disease and during transplantation, and although helpful in some, recommendations await demonstrated efficacy in clinical trials.

Patients with DIC complicating chronic liver disease have overall poor survival, despite treatment. Therapy is aimed at treating the underlying disease, that is, maximizing hemostasis in advanced liver disease, including platelet transfusion for severe thrombocytopenia, FFP for severe factor deficiencies, cryoprecipitate for hypofibrinogenemia, and antibiotics for infection or sepsis. Use of AT III concentrates is not routinely recommended in DIC: in some studies, its use has been associated with some improvement in fibrinogen levels due to enhanced synthesis.[36] In the setting of transplantation, AT III concentrates have not resulted in any consistent reduction in transfusion requirement or mortality.[56] Heparin and antiplatelet agents may increase bleeding in DIC in the setting of chronic liver disease or during transplantation and are not generally recommended for DIC.

In patients with gastrointestinal bleeding, FFP, cryoprecipitate, and platelets may be prescribed to replace missing factors, fibrinogen, and platelets. To achieve hemostasis, in general, factor levels may be maintained above 0.40 to 0.50 U/mL, fibrinogen above 100 mg/dL, and the platelet count 50,000/μL or higher. For refractory and/or recurrent variceal bleeding, consideration may be given to sclerotherapy,[58] transjugular intrahepatic portosystemic shunt (TIPS),[59] or octreotide,[60] somatostatin, or vasopressin[61] administration.

Drugs that may worsen thrombocytopenia or remaining liver function should be avoided,[62] especially drugs that inhibit platelet function, such as nonsteroidal anti-inflammatory agents (NSAIDs), acetylsalicylic acid and heparin flushes in intravenous lines and catheters.

Recurrent bleeding may lead to other hematologic problems, for example, iron deficiency anemia due to recurrent gastrointestinal or variceal bleeding, or chronic epistaxis or gum bleeding occurring with qualitative platelet dysfunction and thrombocytopenia. In those patients who are alcoholic, folic acid and other vitamin supplementation is essential.

FUTURE ADVANCES

Future goals in the diagnosis and management of chronic liver disease include the exploration of the role of inflammatory mediators, such as cytokines, in the coagulopathy of liver disease. The cytokines interleukin-6 and transforming growth factor-β are upregulated in patients with cirrhosis, fibrosis, and liver disease progression,[63,64] yet the role of these cytokines and other proinflammatory cytokines in the coagulopathy of chronic liver disease and end-stage liver disease is not known.[63,64] The study of tissue factors and cytokines involved in the coagulopathy of liver disease could potentially lead to identification of markers predictive of bleeding in chronic liver disease or open new avenues for treatment.

For example, investigation of mediators of tissue inflammation and tissue damage that trigger the tPA surge, fibrinolysis, and massive bleeding during the second stage of transplantation could potentially lead to reduction in blood loss, blood usage, and morbidity associated with transplantation. Further, such studies could lead to the development of safer, more specific agents to improve and maintain hemostasis.

Finally, development of recombinant activated clotting factors without thrombogenic potential or transmissible infection potential would potentially provide more specific, effective therapy than is now possible with FFP in the management of end-stage liver disease. In that regard, preliminary data suggest that recombinant factor VIIa (rFVIIa) is safe and corrects the prothrombin time in nonbleeding cirrhotic patients.[65] Whether rFVIIa is efficacious in the treatment of the bleeding patient with end-stage liver disease awaits the results of future trials.

REFERENCES

Chapter 31 References

1. Lyons AS, Petrucelli RJ. Medicine: An Illustrated History. New York, Harry N. Abrams, 1978, pp 63–67, 231–233.
2. Starzl TE. Marchioro TL, von Kaulla KN, et al. Homotransplantation of the liver in humans. Surg Gynecol Obstet 1963;117:659–676.
3. Starzl TE, Iwatsuki S, van Thiel DH, et al. Evolution of liver transplantation. Hepatology 1982;2:614–636.
4. Starzl TE, Demetris A, van Thiel DH. Liver transplantation. N Engl J Med 1989;321:1014-22, 1092–1099.
5. Mann FD, Shonyo ES, Mann FC. Effect of removal of the liver on blood coagulation. Am J Physiol 1951;164:111–116.
6. Lewis JH, Bontempo FA, Spero JA, et al. Liver transplantation in a hemophiliac. N Engl J Med 1985;312:1189–1190.
7. Bontempo FA, Lewis J, Gorenc TJ, et al. Liver transplantation in hemophilia A. Blood 1987;62:1721–1724.
8. Bontempo FA, Lewis JH, van Thiel DH, et al. The relation of preoperative coagulation findings to diagnosis, blood usage, and survival in adult liver transplantation. Transplantation 1985;39:532–536.
9. Porte RJ, Bontempo FA, Knot EA, et al. Systemic effects of tissue plasminogen activator-associated fibrinolysis and its relation to thrombin generation in orthotopic liver transplantation. Transplantation 1989;47:978–984.
10. Porte RJ, Knot EA, Bontempo FA. Hemostasis in liver transplantation. Gastroenterology 1989;97:488–501.
11. Kang YG, Martin DJ, Marquez J, et al. Intraoperative changes in blood coagulation and thromboelastographic monitoring in liver transplantation. Anesth Analg 1985;64:888–896.
12. Lewis JH, Bontempo FA, Awad SA, et al. Liver transplantation: Intraoperative changes in coagulation factors in 100 first transplants. Hepatology 1989;9:710–714.
13. Kang YG, Lewis JH, Novalgund A, et al. Epsilon aminocaproic acid for treatment of fibrinolysis during liver transplantation. Anesthesiology 1987;66:766–773.
14. Martin TG, Somberg KA, Meng YG, et al. Thrombopoietin levels in patients with cirrhosis before and after orthotopic liver transplantation. Ann Intern Med 1997;127:286–288.
15. Walls WD, Losowsky MS. The hemostatic defect of liver disease. Gastroenterology 1971;60:108–119.
16. Roberts HR, Cedarbaum AI. The liver and blood coagulation physiology and pathology. Gastroenterology 1972;63:297–320.
17. Green AJ, Ratnoff OD. Elevated antihemophilic factor (AHF, factor VIII) procoagulant activity and AHF-like antigen in alcoholic cirrhosis of the liver. J Lab Clin Med 1974;83:189–197.
18. Dymock IW, Tucher JS, Woolf IL, et al. Coagulation studies as a prognostic index in acute liver failure. Br J Haematol 1975;29:385–395.
19. Ragni MV, Lewis JH, Spero JH, et al. Bleeding and coagulation abnormalities in alcoholic cirrhotic liver disease. Alcohol Clin Exp Res 1982;6:267–274.
20. Perrillo RP. The role of liver biopsy in hepatitis C. Hepatology 1997;26 (Suppl 1):57S–61S.
21. Palascak J, Martinez J. Dysfibrinogenemia associated with liver disease. J Clin Invest 1977;60:89–95.
22. Martinez J, Palascak JE, Kwasniak D. Abnormal sialic acid content of the dysfibrinogenemia associated with liver disease. J Clin Invest 1978;61:535–538.
23. von Felten A, Straub PW, Frick PD. Dysfibrinogenemia in a patient with primary hepatoma: first observation of an acquired abnormality of fibrin monomer aggregation. N Engl J Med 1969;280:405–409.
24. Blanchard RA, Furie BC, Jorgenson MJ, et al. Acquired vitamin K-dependent carboxylation deficiency in liver disease. N Engl J Med 1981;305:242–248.
25. Stenflo J, Fernlund P, Egan W, et al. Vitamin K-dependent modifications of glutamic acid residues in prothrombin. Proc Natl Acad Sci USA 1974;71:2730–2733.
26. Liebman HA, Furie BC, Tong MJ, et al. Des-γ-carboxy prothrombin as a serum marker of primary hepatocellular carcinoma. N Engl J Med 1984;310:1427–1431.
27. Aster RH. Pooling of platelets in the spleen: role in the pathogenesis of "hypersplenic" thrombocytopenia. J Clin Invest 1966;45:645–657.
28. Cowan DH. Effect of alcoholism on hemostasis. Semin Hematol 1980;17:137–147.
29. Sullivan LW, Herbert V. Suppression of hematopoiesis by ethanol. J Clin Invest 1964;43:2048–2055.
30. Carr JM. Disseminated intravascular coagulation in cirrhosis. Hepatology 1989;10:103–110.
31. Fletcher AP, Biederman O, Moore D, et al. Abnormal plasminogen-plasmin system activity (fibrinolysis) in patients with hepatic cirrhosis: its cause and consequences. J Clin Invest 1964;43:681–695.
32. Aoki N, Yamanaka T. The α_2-plasmin inhibitor levels in liver disease. Clin Chim Acta 1978;84:99–105.
33. Tytgat GN, Collen D, Verstraete M. Metabolism of fibrinogen in cirrhosis of the liver. J Clin Invest 1971;50:1690–1701.
34. Bloom AL. Intravascular coagulation in cirrhosis. Br J Hematol 1975;30:1–7.
35. Violi F, Ferro D, Basili S, et al. Hyperfibrinolysis resulting from clotting activation in patients with different degrees of cirrhosis. Hepatology 1993;17:78–83.
36. Schipper HG, ten Cate JW. Anti-thrombin III transfusion in patients with hepatic cirrhosis. Br J Haematol 1982;52:25–33.
37. Basili S, Ferro D, Leo R, et al. Bleeding time does not predict gastrointestinal bleeding in patients with cirrhosis. J Hepatol 1996;24:574–580.
38. Ratnoff OD. Hemostatic defects in liver and biliary tract disease. In: Ratnoff OD, Forbes CD (Eds). Disorders of Hemostasis. Philadelphia, WB Saunders, 1996, p 422.
39. Pugh RN, Murray-Lyon IM, Dawson JL, et al. Transection of the oesophagus for bleeding oesophageal varices. Br J Haematol 1973;60:646–649.
40. Ragni MV, Lewis JH, Spero JA. Ascites-induced LeVeen shunt coagulopathy. Ann Surg 1983;198:91–95.
41. Violi F, Basili S, Ferro D, et al. Association between high values of D-dimer and tissue-plasminogen activator activity and first gastrointestinal bleeding in cirrhotic patients. Thromb Haemost 1996;76:177–183.
42. Little AF, Zajko AB, Orons PD. Transjugular liver biopsy: a prospective study in 43 patients with the Quick-Core biopsy needle. JVIR 1996;7:127–131.

43. Tollefsen DM, Pestka CA. Heparin cofactor II activity in patients with disseminated intravascular coagulation and hepatic failure. Blood 1985;66:769–774.
44. Porte RJ. Coagulation and fibrinolysis in orthotopic liver transplantation. Semin Thromb Hemostas 1993;19:191–196.
45. Sporn P, Mauritz W, Schindler I, et al. Zur Problematik des Blutersatzesbei Libertransplantationen. Infusionstherapie 1985;12:187–191.
46. Owen CA, Rettke SR, Bowie EJW, et al. Hemostatic evaluation of patients undergoing liver transplantation. Mayo Clin Proc 1987;62:761–777.
47. Bellani KG, Estrin JA, Ascher NL, et al. Reperfusion coagulopathy during human liver transplantation. Transplant Proc 1987;19:71–72.
48. Dzik WH, Arkin CF, Jenkins RL, et al. Fibrinolysis during liver transplantation in humans: role of tissue-type plasminogen activator. Blood 1988;71:1090–1095.
49. Ascher NL, Lake JR, Emond JC, et al. Liver transplantation for fulminant hepatic failure. Arch Surg 1993;128:677–682.
50. Lewis JH, Bontempo FA, Ragni MV, et al. Antithrombin III during liver transplantation. Transplant Proc 1989;21:3543–3544.
51. Moia M, Martinelli I, Gridelli B, et al. Prognostic value of hemostatic parameters after liver transplantation. J Hepatol 1992;15:125–128.
52. Boylan JF, Klinck JR, Sandler AN, et al. Tranexamic acid reduces blood loss, transfusion requirements, and coagulation factor use in primary orthotopic liver transplantation. Anesthesiology 1996;85:1043–1048.
53. Neuhaus P, Bechstein WO, Lefebre B, et al. Effect of aprotinin on intraoperative bleeding and fibrinolysis in liver transplantation. Lancet 1989;2:924–925.
54. Kettner SC, Gonano C, Seebach F, et al. Endogenous heparin-like substances significantly impair coagulation in patients undergoing orthotopic liver transplantation. Anesth Analg 1998;86:691–695.
55. Porte RJ, Molenaar B, Groenland THN, et al. Aprotonin and transfusion requirements in orthotopic liver transplantation: a multicenter randomised double-blind study. Lancet 2000;355:1303–1309.
56. Palareti G, Legagni C, Maccaferri M, et al. Coagulation and fibrinolysis in liver transplantation: the role of the recipient's disease and the use of antithrombin III concentrates. Haemostasis 1991;21:68–76.
57. Frenette L, Cox J, McArdle P, et al. Conjugated estrogen reduces transfusion and coagulation factor requirements in orthotopic liver transplantation. Anesth Analg 1998;86:1183–1186.
58. Steigmann GV, Goff JS, Michaletz-Onody PA, et al. Endoscopic sclerotherapy as compared with endoscopic ligation for bleeding esophageal varices. N Engl J Med 1992;326:1527–1532.
59. Shiffman ML, Jeffers L, Hoofnagle JH, et al. The role of transjugular intrahepatic porto-systemic shunt for treatment of portal hypertension and its complications: a conference sponsored by the National Digestive Diseases Advisory Board. Hepatology 1995;22:1591–1597.
60. Besson I, Ingrand P, Person B, et al. Sclerotherapy with or without octreotide for acute variceal bleeding. N Engl J Med 1995;333:555–560.
61. Imperiale TF, Teran JC, McCullough AJ. A meta-analysis of somatostatin versus vasopressin in the management of acute esophageal variceal hemorrhage. Gastroenterol 1995;109:1289–1294.
62. Lee WM. Drug-induced hepatotoxicity. N Engl J Med 1995;333:1118–1128.
63. Matsumoto K, Fuji H, Michalopoulis G, et al. Human biliary epithelial cells secrete and respond to cytokines and hepatocyte growth factors: IL-6, HGF, and EGF promote DNA synthesis in vitro. Hepatology 1994;20:376–382.
64. Castilla A, Prieto J, Fausto N. Transforming growth factors $\beta 1$ and α in chronic liver disease: effects of interferon alfa therapy. N Engl J Med 1991;324:933–940.
65. Bernstein DE, Jeffers L, Erhardtsen E, et al. Recombinant factor VIIa corrects prothrombin time in cirrhotic patients: a preliminary study. Gastroenterology 1997;113:1930–1937.

CHAPTER 32

Hemorrhagic and Thrombotic Disorders in the Intensive Care Setting

Thomas G. DeLoughery, M.D.

One of the greatest challenges for the consultant is the critically ill patient. Patients require critical care units for a multitude of reasons, ranging from postoperative care to management of overwhelming sepsis. Hemostatic and thrombotic complications in the critically ill may be due to underlying disease or to complications of therapy.

This chapter presents an approach to hemostatic and thrombotic problems in critically ill patients. Initial evaluation and laboratory testing are discussed, and then specific entities such as disseminated intravascular coagulation (DIC), liver disease, and thrombocytopenia are described. Finally, thrombosis is addressed. Several of these topics are discussed in detail in other chapters of this book; thus, the emphasis will be on critical care aspects of these coagulation disorders.

BLEEDING PROBLEMS

Patients in intensive care units (ICU) often develop coagulation defects. Bleeding due to coagulation defects is seen in 16% of ICU patients and abnormal coagulation tests are found in 66%.[1] Thrombocytopenia is very common, with platelet counts below 100,000/μL occurring in 25% to 38% of ICU patients and counts fewer than 10,000/μL seen in 2% to 3%.[1-4]

The immediate priorities for these patients are to establish the veracity, tempo, and severity of the coagulation defects, evaluate for life-threatening processes such as heparin-induced thrombocytopenia (HIT), and initiate therapy. In the critical care setting, therapeutic decisions are often made before a definitive cause of the coagulation defect is established.

INITIAL EVALUATION

The initial assessment is rapid, focusing on whether the patient is bleeding or experiencing thrombosis, the underlying disorder that leads to the ICU admission, current medications, and (if available) past medical history.

During the bleeding and thrombosis assessment one should determine whether the patient is suffering from "structural" causes of bleeding (e.g., bleeding from a gastric ulcer) or generalized bleeding (suggesting a coagulation defect). One should inspect sites of instrumentation such as intravenous line sites, chest tube drainage, or mucosa for bleeding. The fingertips and toes should be examined for evidence of emboli, ischemia, or vasculitis.

Exposure to medicines is a common cause of thrombocytopenia and can exacerbate certain coagulation defects.[5,6] One should carefully review the medication sheets and note all the medicines the patient has received and quiz the family about medication (prescribed, over the counter, and herbal[7-9]) the patient is taking (Tables 32-1 and 32-2).

Laboratory Testing

Defects of hemostasis can present either as prolongation of routine coagulation laboratory values or as a serious bleeding diathesis.

The first step in evaluation is to obtain a prothrombin time (PT) and an activated partial thromboplastin time (aPTT).[10] One should ensure the sample is obtained from a peripheral vein. Drawing samples through heparin-containing catheters, even with elaborate ma-

Table 32-1 • DRUGS AND HEMOSTASIS

Action	Drug	Action	Drug
Increases activity of warfarin	**Acetaminophen** Allopurinol **Aminodarone*** (may last for months after drug is stopped) Anabolic steroids* **Aspirin*** Cephalosporins (N-methylthiotetrazole group) **Cimetidine*** Ciprofloxacin Clofibrate* Cyclophosphamide **Disulfiram** Erythromycin* **Fluconazole*** Furosemide Gemfibrozil Isoniazid **Itraconazole*** **Ketoconazole*** **Metronidazole*** **Micronase*** Omeprazole **Propafenone** Propranolol Quinidine* Quinine* Quinolones Serotonin uptake inhibitors **Sulfinpyrazone*** Sulfonylureas* Tamoxifen* Tetracycline* **Thyroid hormones*** Tricyclics Vitamin E*	Decreases activity of warfarin Increase prothrombin time TTP/HUS Hemolysis/DIC syndrome Thrombocytopenia	Alcohol **Barbiturates*** Carbamazepine **Cholestyramine** Corticosteroids Dicloxacillin Estrogens **Griseofulvin** Nafcillin **Phenytoin** (may potentiate warfarin with initiation of drug) Rifampin Sucralfate Vitamin K (often in protein/calorie supplement drinks) N-methylthiotetrazole group-containing antibiotics: cefamandole, cefoperazone, cefotetan, cefmenoxime, and cefmetazole Mitomycin C, cyclosporine, FK 506, carboplatin or cis-platinum, ticlopidine, clopidogrel Quinine Second- and third-generation cephlosporins See Table 32-10

Asterisk indicates major effect; boldface indicates strongest evidence for effect.
Adapted from Tiede DJ, Nishimura RA, Gastineau DA, et al. Modern management of prosthetic valve anticoagulation. Mayo Clin Proc 1998;73:665–680; Hirsh J, Dalen JE, Anderson DR, et al. Oral anticoagulants: mechanism of action, clinical effectiveness, and optimal therapeutic range. Chest 2001;119:8S–21S; DeLoughery TG. Anticoagulant therapy in special circumstances. Curr Cardiol Reports 2000; 2:74–79.

nipulation to prevent contamination, can result in elevation of clotting times. Three patterns of defects can be seen (Table 32-3). Isolated elevations of the PT are indicative of an isolated factor VII deficiency. Isolated elevations of the aPTT in the ICU setting are unusual and typically are due to heparin contamination, lupus inhibitors, isolated defects of factors VIII, IX, or XI, or of the contact pathway. Mixing studies can provide information to narrow the list of possible diagnoses (Table 32-4). Prolongation of both the PT and aPTT suggest multiple defects or deficiency of factors II, V, or X. Marked prolongation of the PT and aPTT can also be seen with low levels of fibrinogen (below 50 mg/dL). Patients with hematocrits more than 60% may have spurious elevations of the PT and aPTT due to improper plasma:anticoagulant ratio in the sample tube.[11] Further coagulation tests are ordered based on the PT and aPTT to better define the defect if the reason for the coagulation deficiency is not apparent by the history (e.g., in severe liver disease).

In the patient with thrombocytopenia, examination of the blood smear can quickly reveal whether pseudothrombocytopenia (artifactual platelet clumping)[12] is present and verify the degree of thrombocytopenia. The smear should be carefully reviewed for the presence of fragmented red cells (schistocytes). Laboratory assessment of liver and renal functions also should be reviewed. A markedly elevated level of lactate dehydrogenase (LDH) out of proportion to other liver function abnormalities is often seen in thrombotic thrombocytopenia purpura (TTP) and hantavirus pulmonary syndrome.[13,14] If there is any suspicion of HIT, all heparin administration should be stopped and laboratory confirmation initiated.[15–17]

Table 32-2 • HERBAL MEDICINES AND HEMOSTASIS

Possible Increase in Risk of Bleeding
Angelica root
Horse chestnut
Arnica flower
Licorice root
Anise
Lovage root
Asafoetida
Meadowsweet
Bogbean
Onion
Borage seed oil
Parsley
Bromelian
Passionflower herb
Ginkgo
Celery
Quassia
Chamomile
Red clover
Clove
Rue
Fenugreek
Sweet clover
Feverfew
Turmeric
Garlic
Willow bark
Ginger
Capsicum
Poplar

Possible Increase in Warfarin Effect
Danshen
Dong quai
Devil's claw
Papain

Possible Decrease in Warfarin Effect
Coenzyme Q10
Green tea
Ginseng

Adapted from Heck AM, DeWitt BA, Lukes AL. Potential interactions between alternative therapies and warfarin. Am J Health Syst Pharm 2000;57:1221–1230.

Diagnostic Clues

The reason for the ICU admission is a very important indicator in the evaluation of any coagulation defect (Tables 32-5 and 32-6).[18] For example, thrombocytopenia in patients who present with multiorgan system failure may be a clue to TTP or sepsis. In long-term critical care patients, new-onset thrombocytopenia may be a manifestation of HIT, drug-induced thrombocytopenia, occult sepsis, or bacteremia.

IMMEDIATE THERAPY: TRANSFUSION THERAPY

Five laboratory values reflect the basic parameters essential for both blood volume and hemostasis[19,20]:

Table 32-3 • COMMON CAUSES OF ABNORMAL LABORATORY TESTS

Elevated PT, Normal aPTT
Factor VII deficiency
  Vitamin K deficiency
  Warfarin
  Sepsis

Normal PT, Elevated aPTT
Isolated factor deficiency (VIII, IX, XI, XII, contact pathway factors)
Specific factor inhibitor
High hematocrit (>60%, is spurious)
Heparin
Lupus inhibitor

Elevated PT, Elevated aPTT
Multiple coagulation factor deficiencies
  Liver disease
  Disseminated intravascular coagulation
Isolated factor X, V, or II deficiency
Factor V inhibitors
High heparin levels
Warfarin
Low fibrinogen (< 50 mg/dl)
Dysfibrinogemia
Dilutional

1. Hematocrit
2. Platelet count
3. Prothrombin time
4. Activated partial thromboplastin time
5. Fibrinogen level

Replacement therapy is based on the results of these laboratory tests and the clinical situation of the patient (Table 32-7).

The transfusion threshold for low hematocrit depends on the stability of the patient. If the hematocrit is below 30% and the patient is bleeding or hemodynamically unstable, one should transfuse packed red cells. Stable patients can tolerate lower hematocrits while an aggressive transfusion policy may be detrimental.[21,22]

The "transfusion trigger" for platelets can be 10,000/μL if the patient is stable without signs of bleeding, is not on platelet inhibitors, has preserved renal function, and does not have DIC.[23] If the patient is bleeding, has

Table 32-4 • INTERPRETATION OF MIXING STUDIES

Mixing Study Result	Diagnosis
aPTT completely corrects to normal ranges	Coagulation factor deficiency
aPTT does not completely correct to normal range	Lupus inhibitor, heparin contamination, coagulation factor inhibitor
aPTT initially corrects to normal range but then prolongs with incubation	Coagulation factor inhibitor

Mixing study is performed by combining equal parts of patient's plasma and control plasma and performing an aPTT.

Table 32-5 • DIAGNOSTIC CLUES TO THROMBOCYTOPENIA

Clinical Setting	Differential Diagnoses
Cardiac surgery	Cardiopulmonary bypass, HIT, dilutional thrombocytopenia
Interventional cardiac procedure	Abciximab or other GP IIb/IIIa blockers, HIT
Sepsis syndrome	DIC, ehrlichiosis, sepsis hemophagocytosis syndrome, drug-induced, misdiagnosed TTP, mechanical ventilation, pulmonary artery catheters
Pulmonary failure	DIC, hantavirus pulmonary syndrome, mechanical ventilation, pulmonary artery catheters
Mental status changes/seizures	TTP, ehrlichiosis
Renal failure	TTP, dengue, HIT, DIC
Cardiac failure	HIT, drug-induced, pulmonary artery catheter
Postsurgery	Dilutional, drug-induced, HIT
Pregnancy	HELLP syndrome, fatty liver of pregnancy, TTP/HUS
Acute liver failure	Splenic sequestration, HIT, drug-induced, DIC

HIT, heparin-induced thrombocytopenia; DIC, disseminated intravascular coagulation; TTP, thrombotic thrombocytopenic purpura; HELLP, hemolysis, elevated liver function tests, and low platelets.

Table 32-6 • DIAGNOSTIC CLUES TO COAGULATION DEFECTS

Clinical Setting	Differential Diagnoses
Cardiac surgery	Factor V inhibitor, heparin excess or rebound, protamine excess, fibrinolysis
Sepsis syndrome	Isolated factor VII deficiency, DIC, vitamin K deficiency,
Recent use of quinine, second- or third-generation cephalosporin	Drug-induced hemolysis/DIC syndrome
Postsurgery	Dilutional, DIC, thrombin inhibitors
Pregnancy	HELLP syndrome, fatty liver of pregnancy, vitamin K deficiency
Acute liver failure	Consumption, DIC, fibrinolysis, vitamin K deficiency (biliary obstruction)

DIC, disseminated intravascular coagulation; HELLP, hemolysis, elevated liver function tests, and low platelets.

Table 32-7 • MANAGEMENT OF COAGULATION DEFECTS IN BLEEDING PATIENTS

- Platelets <50,000 to 75,000/μL: give platelet concentrates or six to eight packs of single-donor platelets
- Fibrinogen <100 mg/dL: give 10 units of cryoprecipitate
- Hematocrit <30%: give red cells
- Prothrombin time >INR 2.0 and aPTT abnormal: give two to four units of FFP

---

florid DIC, or has received platelet-aggregation inhibitors, keeping the count more than 50,000/μL is reasonable. Data do exist from the literature regarding massive transfusion indicating that, at least in those patients, keeping the count at 50,000/μL or higher results in less microvascular bleeding.[19,24] The dose of platelets to be transfused should be six to eight platelet concentrates or one plateletpheresis unit. Low platelet counts are the strongest determinant of microvascular bleeding in massively transfused patients.

For a fibrinogen level less 100 mg/dL, transfusions of 10 units of cryoprecipitate will increase the plasma fibrinogen level by 100 mg/dL.

In patients with a PT demonstrating an INR greater than 2 and an abnormal aPTT, one should give two to four units of fresh frozen plasma (FFP). For an aPTT greater than 1.5 times normal, two to four units of FFP should be given. Elevations of the aPTT above 1.8 times normal are associated with microvascular bleeding in trauma patients.[25] Patients with marked abnormalities such as an aPTT more than two times normal may require aggressive therapy with at least four units of FFP. Minor abnormalities of PT and aPTT should be judiciously treated with lesser amounts of FFP or none at all.

The basic five laboratory tests should be repeated after administering the blood products. This allows one to ensure adequate replacement therapy was given for the coagulation defects. Frequent checks of the coagulation tests also allow rapid identification and therapy of new coagulation defects in a timely fashion. A flow chart of the test and the blood products administered should also be maintained.

Occasionally empiric therapy of the severely bleeding patient is required. One should considering starting with platelet transfusions. In patients likely also to have DIC (i.e., head trauma patients[26]), empiric administration of 10 units of cryoprecipitate is rational.

Correcting Coagulation Defects Before Procedures

Procedures such as central venous line placement are very frequently performed successfully on patients with coagulation defects.[27-30] One study found the risk was not related to the degree of hemostatic defects.[31] In this study, the risk of hemorrhage was higher when inexperienced operators attempted line placement. For urgent line placement, use of an experienced operator is prudent instead of waiting on attempts of transfusion therapy to correct laboratory abnormalities.[31] In a nonurgent situation, increasing the platelet count to 30,000 to 50,000/μL and attempting to lower the aPTT to less than 1.5 times normal may be reasonable goals, but one should not delay a necessary procedure by trying to achieve arbitrary targets for laboratory values.

COAGULATION DEFECTS

Disseminated Intravascular Coagulation

Disseminated intravascular coagulation, the clinical manifestation of inappropriate and uncompensated thrombin activation,[32] can be due to multiple causes, such as sepsis or obstetric complications.[33-35] The activation of thrombin leads to (1) conversion of fibrinogen to fibrin, (2) activation and consumption of platelets, (3) activation of factors V and VIII, (4) activation of protein C (and degradation of factors Va and VIIIa), (5) activation of endothelial cells, and (6) activation of fibrinolysis.

Patients with DIC can present in one of four ways[32,34]:

1. **Asymptomatic**. Patients can present with laboratory evidence of DIC but no clinical problems. This is often seen in patients with sepsis or cancer. However, with further progress of the underlying disease, these patients can rapidly become symptomatic.
2. **Bleeding**. Many patients with DIC bleed. The bleeding is due to combinations of factor depletion, platelet dysfunction, thrombocytopenia, and excessive fibrinolysis.[32] These patients may present with diffuse bleeding from intravenous line sites, surgical wounds, and mucosa.
3. **Thrombosis**. Despite the general activation of the coagulation process, thrombosis is unusual in most patients with acute DIC. The exceptions include cancer patients, trauma patients, and certain obstetric patients. Most often the thrombosis is venous but arterial thrombosis and nonbacterial thrombotic endocarditis have been reported.[36]
4. **Purpura fulminans**. This cutaneous manifestation is described in more detail below.

There is no one test that will diagnose DIC, rather, one must match the test results to the clinical situation.[35] The usual screening tests of coagulation lack sensitivity and specificity.[37,38] The PT and aPTT are usually prolonged in severe DIC but may be normal, even shortened, in chronic forms. One may also see a shortened aPTT in severe acute DIC because of the rapid generation of activated coagulation factors. The platelet count is usually decreased but may be normal in 25% of patients with DIC.[37] Low plasma fibrinogen levels are specific for DIC but are decreased in only 25% of patients.[37]

When plasmin acts on the fibrin/fibrinogen molecule, it cleaves the molecule in specific sites. Accordingly, fibrin degradation product levels (FDPs) will be raised in situations of increased fibrin/fibrinogen destruction (DIC, fibrinolysis). FDPs are typically mildly elevated in renal and liver disease.[39] A specific FDP, D-dimer, is produced by thrombin activation of factor XIII to cross-link the D-domain of the fibrin monomer by a plasmin-resistant bond. The D-dimer assay has the higher positive predictive value for DIC.[37]

The best way to treat DIC is to treat the underlying causes.[32,33,35,40] However, one must replace factors if depletion occurs and bleeding ensues. General guidelines for replacement are given above (see Transfusion Therapy) (Table 32–8). Plasma replacement is needed to correct multiple factor deficiencies.[33] Past concerns about "feeding the fires" have not been shown to be clinically valid.[38,41] One should strive for decreasing the aPTT to less than 1.5 times normal if possible. Keeping the fibrinogen level over 100 mg/dL also is reasonable.

Heparin therapy is reserved for patients who have thrombosis as a component of their DIC.[33,41,42] Chronic DIC in association with malignancy should be aggressively treated with therapeutic doses of heparin. Reliance on the aPTT to follow heparin therapy may lead to over- or undertreatment of patients; one should follow heparin levels in these patients.[43,44]

Table 32–8 • THERAPY OF COAGULATION DEFECTS ASSOCIATED WITH BLEEDING IN LIVER DISEASE

- Prothrombin time >INR 2.0 and aPTT abnormal: plasma
- Platelets <50,000 to 70,000/μL: platelet concentrates
- Fibrinogen <100 mg/dL: 10 units of cryoprecipitate
- Hematocrit <30%: packed red cells
- Euglobulin clot lysis time < 1 hour: antifibrinolytic therapy if patient is bleeding and does not have DIC

Antifibrinolytic therapy
- ε-Aminocaproic acid: bolus 4 to 5 g over 1 hour followed by 1 g/h for 8 hours
- Tranexamic acid: 10 mg/kg IV bolus followed by either 10 mg/kg IV every 6 to 8 hours or 25 mg/kg orally every 6 to 8 hours.

Purpura Fulminans

DIC in association with symmetric limb ecchymosis and necrosis of the skin is seen in two situations.[45] *Primary* purpura fulminans is most often seen after a viral infection.[46] In these patients the purpura fulminans starts with a painful red area on an extremity that rapidly progresses to a black ischemic area. In many patients, acquired deficiency of protein S is found along with laboratory evidence of DIC.[45,47]

Secondary purpura fulminans is most often associated with meningococcemia infections but can be seen in any patient with an overwhelming infection. Postsplenectomy sepsis syndrome patients also are at risk.[48] Patients present with signs of sepsis and the skin lesions often involve the extremities, which can lead to amputations.

Therapy for purpura fulminans is controversial. Patients with primary purpura fulminans, especially those with postvaricella autoimmune protein S deficiency, have responded to plasma infusion titrated to keep the protein S level more than 25% of normal levels.[45] Heparin has been reported to control the DIC and extent of necrosis.[49] A reasonable starting dose in these patients is 5 to 8 units/kg/h.[33]

Very ill patients with secondary purpura fulminans have been treated with plasma infusions, plasmapheresis, and continuous plasma ultrafiltration.[49-51] Heparin therapy alone has not been shown to improve survival.[52]

Much attention has been given to replacement of natural anticoagulants such as protein C and antithrombin III (AT III) as therapy for purpura fulminans. A series of small randomized trials have shown mostly negative results for the use of AT III, but a large multicenter trial is in progress.[45,47,53-55] Trials using both zymogen protein C and activated protein C have shown more promise in controlling the coagulopathy of purpura fulminans and improving outcomes in sepsis.[50,56-58]

Drug-Induced Hemolytic-DIC Syndromes

A severe variant of the drug-induced immune complex hemolysis associated with DIC has been recognized. Rare patients who receive certain second- and third-generation cephalosporins such as cefotetan, ceftriaxone, cefoxitin, and ceftizoxime have been reported to develop this syndrome.[59-62] The most common agents are cefotetan and ceftriaxone.[63] The clinical syndrome starts 7 to 10 days after receiving the drug. Often the patient has received the antibiotic only for surgical prophylaxis. The patient will develop severe Coombs-positive hemolysis with hypotension and DIC. The patients are often believed to have sepsis and are often re-exposed to the cephalosporin, resulting in worsening of the clinical picture. Massive hemolysis and thrombosis often result in death.[61,64-66]

Quinine is associated with a unique syndrome of drug-induced DIC.[67-70] Approximately 24 to 96 hours after quinine exposure, the patient becomes acutely ill with nausea and vomiting. The patient then develops a microangiopathic hemolytic anemia, DIC, and renal failure. Some patients, besides having antiplatelet antibodies, also have antibodies binding to red cells and neutrophils that may lead to the more severe syndrome. Despite therapy, patients with quinine-induced TTP have a high incidence of chronic renal failure.

Treatment of drug-induced hemolytic-DIC syndromes is anecdotal. Patients have responded to aggressive therapy, including plasma exchange, dialysis, and prednisone. Early recognition of the hemolytic anemia and suspicion that it is drug related are important for early diagnosis and discontinuation of the implicated drug.

Liver Disease

Patients with severe liver disease have multiple coagulation defects.[71-74] With the exception of factor VIII and von Willebrand factor, all major coagulation factors and inhibitors are synthesized solely in the liver. The liver is the source of thrombopoietin, and lack of this platelet growth factor may worsen thrombocytopenia.[75,76] Patients may have platelet dysfunction due to the increase in FDPs and circulating plasmin.[77] Patients with liver disease appear to have an increase in consumption of clotting factors, perhaps due to delay in clearance of activated enzymes. Finally, liver disease is the most common cause of primary fibrinolysis due to a decrease in plasma levels of fibrinolytic inhibitors and delayed clearance of plasmin: evidence of fibrinolysis can be found in 30% of patients with end-stage liver disease.

The coagulation defects in patients with liver disease will lead to a variety of laboratory abnormalities. The PT will be prolonged as a result of decreased levels of factor VII. As other factor levels decrease, the aPTT will also prolonged. Another cause of prolonged aPTT in patients with liver disease is antiphospholipid antibodies, which are a frequent occurrence, especially in patients with hepatitis C.[78]

Initial screening of the bleeding patient with liver disease should consist of a hematocrit, platelet count, PT, aPTT, plasma fibrinogen level, and D-dimer assay. If available, the euglobulin clot lysis time can help indicate the presence of excessive fibrinolysis. Values less than 60 minutes (normal, more than 60 minutes) indicate a fibrinolytic state.

Since DIC can commonly complicate liver disease, evaluation for DIC should be done on unstable patients with liver disease. Levels of FDPs often are increased in liver disease. This may be due to impaired clearance of the FDPs by the diseased liver. Also, some patients with liver disease will have acquired dysfibrinogenemia that can artifactually raise the levels of FDPs. The D-dimer assay is a more reliable assay for DIC than is measurement of FDPs in patients with liver disease.[39]

In the acutely hemorrhaging patient, therapy is guided by five key tests: hematocrit, PT, aPTT, platelet count, and plasma fibrinogen level (see Table 32-8).

It is important to not overtreat the patient with liver disease by trying to correct the PT to normal or near-normal levels. Attempting to normalize the PT is often difficult because of the short half-life of factor VII and the minimal increases one achieves with FFP (approximately 3% to 5% increase per unit infused for each clotting factor).[79] With a normal aPTT, a prolonged PT only indicates decreased factor VII levels. Since only 5% to 15% of factor VII is needed for hemostasis, isolated minor elevations of the PT (INR less than 3) do not require further plasma therapy.[80] Overzealous attempts to correct totally the INR are unproductive and will result in volume overload. Also, the increased plasma volume may increase portal pressures.[81]

Abnormal fibrinolysis is an often-overlooked cause of bleeding in patients with liver disease. Bleeding in these patients tends to be characterized by diffuse oozing from sites of minor trauma. Often these patients are futilely treated with massive amounts of FFP before the fibrinolytic defect is discovered. Diagnosis is made either clnically or, if possible, by demonstrating a shortened euglobulin clot lysis time in the setting of excessive bleeding.

In the patient who is bleeding from fibrinolysis, a trial of antifibrinolytic therapy is warranted. The patient should be screened for DIC and significant urinary tract bleeding. The dose of ε-aminocaproic acid (EACA) is a bolus of 4 to 5 g given over 1 hour followed by a continuous infusion of 1 g/h for 8 hours.[72,82,83] The oral dosing of EACA is 4 g every 4 hours. The dosing for tranexamic acid is 10 mg/kg IV bolus followed either by 10 mg/kg IV every 6 to 8 hours or 25 mg/kg every 6 to 8 hours orally.[84]

Vitamin K Deficiency

Vitamin K is crucial in the synthesis of coagulation factors II, VII, IX, and X, protein C, and protein S. Humans obtain vitamin K from food sources and from metabolism by intestinal flora. Despite being a fat-soluble vitamin, body stores of vitamin K are low and the daily requirement is 40 to 80 μg/day.

Vitamin K deficiency can present dramatically.[85] Once the body stores of vitamin K are depleted, production of the vitamin K-dependent proteins ceases and the PT increases rapidly to high levels. This is demonstrated in patients with poor nutrition, who have a mildly prolonged INR going into surgery but several days postoperatively have a marked elevation of the PT; the aPTT will also begin to lengthen a day or two later.

Antibiotics affect vitamin K metabolism by two mechanisms. Most antibiotics with activity against anaerobic bacteria can sterilize the gut, eliminating flora production of vitamin K.[86,87] Certain cephalosporins that contain the N-methylthiotetrazole group can inhibit vitamin K epoxide reductase.[88-90] This prevents the normal recycling of vitamin K. The most commonly implicated antibiotics are cefamandole, cefoperazone, cefotetan, cefmenoxime, and cefmetazole.[91,92] The use of prophylactic vitamin K, 10 mg weekly, during chronic antibiotic administration has dramatically reduced the incidence of vitamin K deficiency.

The diagnosis is suspected when there is a history of prolonged antibiotic use, biliary obstruction, or pre-existing malnourishment.[85,93,94] One must also suspect vitamin K deficiency in a previously healthy patient who presents with a prolonged PT that corrects with administration of a 50:50 mix of normal plasma. This is a common presentation of accidental or surreptitious warfarin or rat poison ingestion.[95,96]

Treatment (and a diagnostic test of vitamin K deficiency) is by replacement of vitamin K. Most patients will respond rapidly to 10 mg orally. For a more rapid (6 to 8 hours) and reliable response, 5 to 10 mg may be given intravenously over 30 to 60 minutes. However, anaphylaxis has been reported with rapid infusion of vitamin K. Alternatively, plasma can be used for the patient with life- or limb-threatening bleeding and marked elevation of the PT. At least three to four units of FFP may be needed until the administered vitamin K takes effect.

Therapy of the Bleeding Patient on Warfarin

For the ICU patient who is receiving warfarin, therapy for an elevated INR is based on the risk of bleeding and the indication for warfarin therapy. INRs can vary greatly in ICU patients because of variations in nutritional status, medications, and other illnesses.[97,98] In these patients it may be more practical to change over to heparin therapy for anticoagulation.

For the nonbleeding patient with an INR above the therapeutic range but less than 5, one can simply omit or lower the dose of warfarin. For INRs in the 5 to 9 range, one can hold the next one or two doses. However, in one study, a 4% risk of severe bleeding was seen in older patients with INRs in this range.[99] In patients at risk of bleeding, one can administer orally 1 to 2.5 mg of vitamin K.[100] For INRs of more than 9, one should prescribe 5 to 10 mg of vitamin K orally with the expectation that the INR will be lowered in 24 to 48 hours.[101,102]

If the patient requires rapid reversal when the INR is greater than 5, one can give 5 to 10 mg of vitamin K with the expectation that the INR will be lowered in 24 hours if the vitamin K is given orally or in 6 to 8 hours if given parenterally. If there is an urgent need for reversal this dose of vitamin K can be augmented by FFP.

For immediate management of intracranial bleeding, one should rapidly reverse the warfarin effect.[103] This can be done by giving both vitamin K (10 mg intravenously slowly over 1 hour) and two to four units of FFP. Intravenous vitamin K is associated with a slight risk of anaphylaxis and many reserve its use for life-threatening bleeding. Ideally the patient should receive prothrombin concentrates such as Konyne or Profilnine at a dose of a 50 units/kg, which can result in very rapid reversal, but these are not often readily available.[104] In patients with very strong indications for anticoagulation (mechanical heart valves, etc.) recent data suggest omission of warfarin for 1 to 2 weeks is unlikely to result in thrombosis.[105-107]

Factor V Inhibitors

Factor V inhibitors may develop in patients exposed to topical thrombin.[108,109] The frequency has been reported as high as 10%.[110] Topical thrombin is derived from bovine plasma and is contaminated with bovine factor V. Starting about 1 week after surgery, some patients will demonstrate antibodies to the bovine thrombin and also an antibody to the bovine factor V. This antibody readily cross-reacts with human factor V, leading to lower plasma levels. Rarely antibodies to human thrombin will also be seen.

Patients may present with severe bleeding or the inhibitor may simply be detected on routine laboratory screening. The thrombin time is prolonged if it is performed with bovine thrombin. If factor V antibodies are present, the PT and aPTT will also be prolonged and not show correction with the 50:50 mix with normal plasma. Because of presence of the inhibitor, plasma factor V levels are decreased.

Many patients with factor V antibodies do not bleed.[109] One reason may be that platelet factor V, residing inside the platelet α granule, is protected from circulating antibodies. For the bleeding patient, therapy with plasma and platelets may be used. The antibodies disappear in several weeks without therapy. For the rare patient with severe bleeding, there is anecdotal evidence that immune globulin or steroids may speed removal of the antibody.[108]

Massive Transfusions

The massively transfused patient is defined as one who receives greater than one blood volume in 24 hours or less.[111] It is more practically defined as receiving one blood volume in 2 hours or less. The most common settings for massive transfusion are trauma or gastrointestinal bleeding.[112] Management of blood products is outlined above. The use of a laboratory-guided transfusion therapy has helped to reduce the mortality in patients requiring massive transfusions.[113,114]

Coagulation defects are common in massively transfused patients.[115] These can be due to dilution of the plasma by massive fluid resuscitation or by red cell transfusions. Packed red cell units contain little plasma and massive replacement of blood volume with packed red blood cells and crystalloids can lead to a dilutional coagulopathy. Patients may also develop a coagulopathy as a result of their underlying medical or surgical conditions.

One cannot predict the degree of coagulopathy from the amount of blood transfused.[116] Some patients may receive 20 units of packed red cells and still have adequate hemostatic functions; others may have florid coagulopathies due to injuries before the first unit of blood is administered. Therefore, monitoring the patient's coagulation status during massive transfusions is crucial.

Two common problems that arise in the massively transfused patient are isolated elevations of the PT and a greatly prolonged aPTT. Factor VII is labile and often patients will have a mildly prolonged PT with normal aPTTs for hours to days after massive transfusions. As mentioned before, this minor prolongation of the PT is irrelevant to bleeding risk and should not be treated. If both the PT and aPTT are very prolonged (longer than 100 seconds), plasma fibrinogen level should be measured. Fibrinogen levels below 50 to 80 mg/dL interfere with the endpoints of the PT/aPTT determinations and will lead to prolonged results. A very prolonged aPTT with only a minor elevation of the PT suggests heparin contamination, especially if confirmed by a prolonged thrombin time. This can be a common occurrence in the hectic management of massive transfusions.

Critical Illness and Pregnancy

One should consider three syndromes in the critically ill pregnant woman who presents with a coagulation defect. These are the HELLP syndrome, acute fatty liver of pregnancy (AFLP), and TTP (Table 32-9). TTP is discussed in the section on TTP in this chapter.[117]

The acronym HELLP (*h*emolysis, *e*levated *l*iver tests, *l*ow *p*latelets) describes a variant of pre-eclampsia. Classically, HELLP syndrome occurs after 28 weeks of gestation in a patent suffering from pre-eclampsia.[118,119] The pre-eclampsia need not be severe. The first sign is a decrease in the platelet count followed by abnormal liver function tests. Signs of hemolysis are present, with abundant schistocytes on the smear and a high serum LDH level. HELLP can progress to liver failure and deaths are also reported due to hepatic rupture. Unlike TTP, fetal involvement is present in the HELLP syndrome, with fetal thrombocytopenia reported in 30% of cases. In severe cases, elevated D-dimers consistent with DIC are also found. Delivery of the baby will most often result in cessation of the HELLP syndrome, but refractory cases will require dexamethasone and plasma exchange.[120] Patients should be closely observed for 1 to 2 days after delivery as the hematologic picture can transiently worsen before improving.[121] A pernicious variant of HELLP syndrome is seen in patients with antiphospholipid antibody disease who may present at 20 to 24 weeks with HELLP. These patients may have continuing thrombosis refractory to heparin and require delivery to stop the process.

AFLP also occurs late in pregnancy and is associated with pre-eclampsia in only 50% of cases.[122,123] Patients first present with nonspecific symptoms of nausea and vomiting but can progress to fulminant liver failure. Patients develop thrombocytopenia early in the course but in the later stages can develop DIC and very low fibrinogen levels. Mortality rates without therapy can be a high as 90%. Low glucose and high ammonia levels

Table 32-9 • PREGNANCY-RELATED DISEASES: TTP/HUS, HELLP SYNDROME, AND AFLP

	HELLP	TTP/HUS	AFLP
Hypertension	Always present	Sometimes present	Sometimes present
Proteinuria	Always present	Sometimes present	Sometimes present
Thrombocytopenia	Always	Always	Always
LDH elevation	Present	Marked	Present
Fibrinogen	Normal to Low	Normal	Normal to very low
Schistocytes	Present	Present	Absent
Liver tests	Elevated	Normal	Elevated
Ammonia	Normal	Normal	Elevated
Glucose	Normal	Normal	Low

HELLP, hemolysis, elevated liver tests, and low platelets; TTP/HUS, thrombotic thrombocytopenic purpura/hemolytic uremia syndrome; AFLP, acute fatty liver of pregnancy.
Adapted from Egerman RS, Sibai BM. Imitators of preeclampsia and eclampsia. Clin Obstet Gynecol 1999;42:551-562; Esplin MS, Branch DW. Diagnosis and management of thrombotic microangiopathies during pregnancy. Clin Obstet Gynecol 1999;42:360-367.

can help distinguish AFLP from other pregnancy complications.[117] Treatment consists of prompt delivery of the child and blood product support.

THROMBOCYTOPENIA AND PLATELET DYSFUNCTION

Heparin-Induced Thrombocytopenia

Heparin-induced thrombocytopenia (HIT) is suspected when there is a sudden onset of thrombocytopenia with either a 50% drop in the platelet count or a drop in the platelet count to less than 100,000/μL in a patient receiving heparin in *any* form.[15,124–126] HIT occurs 5 to 10 days after starting heparin therapy but may occur suddenly in patients with recent (3 to 4 months) exposure.[127] An often-overlooked feature of HIT is recurrent thrombosis in a patient receiving heparin despite having a normal platelet count.[128] The clinical diagnosis of HIT can be challenging in the very ill critical care patient who has multiple reasons for being thrombocytopenic. In this situation a laboratory assay for HIT may be helpful. Given the operator dependence of platelet-based assays for HIT, the ICU physician needs to be very familiar with the nuances of the particular laboratory's assay.[16,17,127]

Therapy of HIT consists of stopping all heparin. Two particular problems occur in the critical care setting. First, many catheters are kept open with heparin; this practice is very common and is often overlooked as a source of heparin for patients with HIT. Also, many central venous catheters and intra-aortic balloon pumps are coated with heparin. Because the presence of heparin-coated catheters is enough to perpetuate the HIT process, these must be changed to nonheparin coated devices[129,130] (see Chapter 23).

Patients with HIT and active thrombosis are difficult to manage. Obviously these patients cannot receive heparin. Since low-molecular-weight heparin (LMWH) products cross-react with the HIT antibodies, these agents are also contraindicated.[127] Institution of warfarin therapy alone has been associated with an increased risk of thrombosis.[127] For therapy of HIT patients, three new antithrombotic agents are available.[131,132]

Hirudin is derived from leech saliva; a recombinant form (lepirudin) is FDA approved for therapy of patients with HIT. Lepirudin, a direct inhibitor of thrombin, is monitored by using the commonly available aPTT. Although not widely available, more precise monitoring of lepirudin may be obtained by using either the ecarin time or the quantitative thrombin time.[133,134] The half-life of lepirudin is short, but the drug accumulates in renal insufficiency, with the half-life increasing to more than 50 hours. There is no antidote for lepirudin. Patients with even slight renal insufficiency must have their lepirudin doses adjusted to avoid overanticoagulation.[135] Lepirudin prolongs the PT, making initiation of warfarin therapy difficult. If available, the chromogenic factor X assay can be used to adjust warfarin therapy.[136] Up to 80% of patients receiving long-term lepirudin therapy will develop antibodies.[137,138] These antibodies reduce the metabolism of hirudin and *increase* the therapeutic effect of lepirudin. Patients on long-term (longer than 6 days) lepirudin therapy should still continue to have monitoring to avoid over-anticoagulation.

Argatroban is a synthetic thrombin inhibitor.[132,139] Like lepirudin, it has a short half-life. Dosing is 2 μg/kg/min, with the infusion adjusted to keep the aPTT 1.5 to 3 times normal. One advantage of argatroban is that it is not renally excreted and no dose adjustment is necessary in renal failure.[140] These characteristics make it the most useful agent for patients in the critical care unit. However, it must be used with caution in patients with liver disease.

Also available is danaparoid, a mixture of various glycosaminoglycans.[141,142] Unfortunately, its half-life is 25 hours, there is no antidote, and monitoring must be done by specific danaparoid levels. It is renally cleated. These factors greatly limit the use of this agent.

Even with the best of therapy, patients with HIT are at high risk of complications. In one therapeutic trial 18% of patients with HIT died and another 11% had amputations, with 11% of patients having major bleeding complications.[140]

As mentioned above, initiation of warfarin alone has been associated with limb gangrene and should not be initiated as the sole agent in HIT. In patients receiving specific antithrombin therapy, warfarin can be started with small initial doses (2 to 5 mg). These very ill patients tend to have a very dramatic response to warfarin therapy, and excessive anticoagulation can easily occur. One should overlap warfarin and parental therapy by 2 to 3 days.

Patients with HIT but without evidence of thrombosis are at a high risk of thrombosis (53% in one study)[143] and should be considered for antithrombotic therapy.[132,144] Patients with HIT should also be carefully screened for any thrombosis. It is unknown whether prophylactic doses are necessary or therapeutic doses of anticoagulants are needed. Since the risk lasts for at least 1 month after the diagnosis of HIT, any therapy should be at least this long.

Thrombotic Thrombocytopenic Purpura

Thrombotic thrombocytopenic purpura should be suspected when any patient presents with any combination of renal insufficiency, thrombocytopenia, and central nervous system symptoms.[145,146] Critical care patients with TTP most often present with altered mental status, intractable seizures, strokes, or sequelae of renal insufficiency. Many patients who present to the critical care unit with TTP have been misdiagnosed as having sepsis or vasculitis. A syndrome of TTP occurring 1 to 2 weeks after surgery is increasingly being recognized[147] (see Chapter 22).

There is currently no one diagnostic test for TTP; rather, the diagnosis is based on the clinical presentation.[145,146] Patients uniformly will have a microangiopathic hemolytic anemia with the presence of schistocytes on the peripheral smear. Renal insufficiency and not frank renal failure is the most common renal manifestation. Thrombocytopenia may range from a mild decrease in platelet number to platelets being undetectable. The LDH level is often extremely elevated and is a prognostic factor in TTP.

Untreated, TTP is rapidly fatal. Mortality before the plasma exchange era ranged from 95% to 100%. Today plasma exchange therapy is the cornerstone of TTP treatment and has reduced mortality to less than 20%.[14,146,148]

Intravenous glucocorticosteroid therapy is often given to patents presumed to have TTP. This should be continued until the patient has fully recovered and perhaps longer given the presumed autoimmune nature of the disease and the high relapse rates. Plasma infusion is beneficial, perhaps because of replenishing deficient von Willebrand factor-cleaving protease.[149] Plasma exchange has been shown to be superior to simple plasma infusion in therapy of TTP.[148] In patients who cannot be exchanged immediately, plasma infusions should be started at a dose of one unit every 4 hours. Recent evidence indicates that FFP is equivalent to cryoprecipitate-poor plasma in the initial therapy of TTP.[150] Patients with all but the mildest cases of TTP should receive one-volume plasma exchange each day for at least 5 days.[146] Plasma exchange should be continued daily until the LDH level has normalized. Frequency of exchange may be tapered starting with every-other-day exchange. If the platelet count falls or LDH level rises, daily exchange should be reinstated.[145] Since the platelet count can be affected by a variety of external influences, the LDH level tends to be a reliable marker of disease activity.

Platelet transfusions are contraindicated in most patients with TTP,[151] and in most patients with TTP there is very little justification for platelet transfusion. In severely thrombocytopenic patients, line placement for plasma exchange should be performed by an experienced person. Platelet transfusion should be limited to truly life-threatening situations such as intracranial hemorrhage.

Therapy-Related Thrombotic Thrombocytopenic Purpura/Hemolytic-Uremic Syndrome

Thrombotic thrombocytopenic purpura/hemolytic-uremic syndrome (TTP/HUS) can complicate a variety of therapies.[152] TTP/HUS can be associated with medications such as cyclosporine, mitomycin, and ticlopidine. Commonly, TTP/HUS occurs within days after cyclosporine is started, with the appearance of a falling platelet count, falling hematocrit, and rising serum LDH level. Some cases have been fatal but often the TTP/HUS resolves with decreasing the cyclosporine dose or changing to another agent. The newer immunosuppressant agent, FK 506, has been implicated in TTP/HUS.[153] The etiology seems to be direct endothelial or renal damage caused by these drugs.

TTP/HUS is most commonly seen with the antineoplastic agent mitomycin C, with an incidence of 10% when a cumulative dose of more than 60 mg/m^2 is used.[154] The onset is slow, with the first sign being a falling platelet count months after therapy has been stopped. This is followed by a relentless course of renal failure and death. A characteristic feature of mitomycin C TTP/HUS is the occurrence of a noncardiac pulmonary edema with red cell transfusions. Anecdotal reports state that treatment with staphylococcal A columns may be useful for this condition. Since advanced cancer itself can be associated with a TTP-like syndrome, it may be due to the cancer and not active cancer treatment.

Although TTP/HUS have been reported with other drugs, including carboplatin and gemcitabine, the newest drug now featured in case reports is ticlopidine, with an incidence of 1:1600.[152,155] Since this drug is often prescribed for patients with vascular disease, these patients may be initially misdiagnosed as having strokes. Patients seem to respond to plasma exchange but mortality rates of up to 50% have been reported. TTP/HUS is also reported with clopidogrel, but with a lower incidence.[156]

TTP/HUS can complicate both autologous and allogenic bone marrow transplants.[157,158] The incidence ranges widely depending on the criteria used to diagnosis TTP/HUS but it is in the range of 15% for allogeneic and 5% for autologous bone marrow transplants. Several types of TTP/HUS are recognized in bone marrow transplantation.[158] One is "multiorgan fulminant," which occurs early (20 to 60 days), has multiorgan system involvement, and is often fatal. This has also been associated with severe cytomegalovirus (CMV) infections. Another type of TTP/HUS is similar to cyclosporine/FK 506 HUS. A "conditioning" TTP/HUS occurs 6 months or more after total-body irradiation, and is associated with primary renal involvement. Finally, patients with systemic CMV infections will present with TTP/HUS related to vascular infection with CMV. The etiology of bone marrow transplant-related TTP appears to be different from that of "classic" TTP. Alterations of the von Willebrand factor cleaving protease have not been found in bone marrow transplant-related TTP implicating therapy-related vascular damage.[159] The therapy of bone marrow transplant TTP/HUS is uncertain. Patients should have their cyclosporine or FK506 doses decreased. Although plasma exchange is often tried, patients with fulminant or conditioning-related TTP/HUS do not respond.[160]

Pregnancy-Related TTP

Thrombotic thrombocytopenic purpura can occur anytime during pregnancy, often leading to diagnostic confusion because of the overlap of symptoms between TTP and HELLP syndrome.[117] There does appear to be a unique presentation of TTP that occurs in the second trimester at 20 to 22 weeks.[161] The fetus is uninvolved, with no evidence of infarction or thrombocytopenia if the mother survives. The pregnancy appears to promote the TTP since the TTP will resolve with termination of the pregnancy and may recur with the next pregnancy.[162] Therapy includes termination of the pregnancy or attempts to support the patient with plasma exchange until delivery. Many patients will have relapses with future pregnancies, so this information must be weighed in planning future pregnancies. An unusual complication of pregnancy is a HUS-type syndrome seen up to 28 weeks postpartum. This form of HUS is severe, and permanent renal failure often results despite aggressive therapy.[162]

Drug-Induced Thrombocytopenia

In patients with a possible drug-induced thrombocytopenia, the standard therapy is to stop the suspect drug.[163] In a critical care patient receiving 10 to 20 drugs, this is often impractical. In a recent review, drugs were implicated in less than 1% of cases of ICU thrombocytopenia.[3] There is now also an evidence-based list of drugs implicated in drug-induced thrombocytopenia.[6] One approach is to stop any drug started in the past 7 days that is strongly associated with thrombocytopenia[164] (Table 32–10). One also can change the drug class of the drug being administered, such as substituting sucralfate or a proton-pump inhibitor in the patient receiving histamine H_2 blockers. Unfortunately, often the patient is receiving many therapeutic agents known (rarely) to cause thrombocytopenia but essential for treatment. In this situation one option is to support the patient with platelet transfusions until the agent can be discontinued.

Immune globulin, corticosteroids, and intravenous anti-D have been suggested as useful in drug-related thrombocytopenia. However, since most of these thrombocytopenic patients recover when the agent is cleared from the body, these therapies are probably not necessary.

Severe thrombocytopenia has been reported in 0.5% of patients receiving abciximab and in 0.5% to 2% of patients receiving other specific glycoprotein (GP) IIb/IIIa inhibitors.[165,166] However, recent data suggest the incidence may be as high as 7.8% when these agents are used outside of the setting of clinical trials.[167] The thrombocytopenia can occur within 2 hours after the drug is started.[168] The mechanism of thrombocytopenia is unknown but may be related to conformational changes in the GP IIb/IIIa site induced by binding of the inhibitors. Experience with abciximab has shown that infusion of immune globulin is not helpful.[169,170] Platelet transfusions result in a prompt rise in platelet count as the drug is cleared from the plasma.

Sepsis

A frequent finding in patients with sepsis syndrome is thrombocytopenia.[171–173] Classically, this has been ascribed to DIC or immune destruction. One mechanism receiving increasing attention is cytokine-driven hemophagocytosis of platelets.[174–178] In two studies, examination of bone marrow obtained from septic critical care patients indicated that 60% to 68% had evidence of hemophagocytosis.[174,176] These patients had lower platelet counts (60,000 versus 72,000/μL), higher serum ferritin levels (1822 versus 399 μg/L), and higher LDH levels than those without evidence of bone marrow hemophagocytosis. The patients with hemophagocytosis had higher rates of multiple organ system failure and higher mortality rates. Inflammatory cytokines, especially monocyte colony-stimulating factor (M-CSF), are thought responsible for inducing the hemophagocytosis.[172,177]

Thrombocytopenia may be a diagnostic clue to infection with unusual organisms. Three members of the *Ehrlichia* family have been reported to cause infections in humans.[178] They are transmitted by ticks and the diseases that they produce are similar. Most patients have a febrile illness, with high fevers, headaches, and myalgias.[178,179] Patients may have central nervous system signs and marked elevation of the serum levels of liver enzymes. Rarely, patients may present with a toxic shock-like syndrome.[180] Although many cases are mild, severe disease is common and the case fatality rate is 2% to 5%.[179] The typical hematologic picture is leukopenia (1300 to 4000/μL) and mild thrombocytopenia (30,000 to 60,000/μL). In many patients the buffy coat reveals the organisms bundled in a 2- to 5-μm morula in the cytoplasm of the granulocytes or monocytes. Consideration of ehrlichiosis is important because its highly specific therapy is doxycycline, which is a drug not routinely used for therapy of sepsis syndromes.

Table 32–10 • COMMON CRITICAL CARE DRUGS IMPLICATED IN THROMBOCYTOPENIA

Antiarrythmics
    Procainamide
    Quinidine
Anti-GPIIb/IIIa agents
    Abciximab
    Eptifibatide
    Tirofiban
Antimicrobial agents
    Amphotericin B
    Linazolid
    Rifampin
    Trimethoprim-sulfamethoxazole
    Vancomycin
Histamine H_2 blockers
    Cimetidine
    Ranitidine
Acetaminophen
Amirone
Carbamazepine
Gold
Heparin
Hydrochlorothiazide
Nonsteroidal anti-inflammatory agents
Quinine

Adapted from DeLoughery T. Drug induced immune hematological disease. Allergy Immunol Clin 1998;18:829–841; DeLoughery TG. Thrombocytopenia in the critical care patient. In: Alving BM (Ed): Blood Components and Pharmacologic Agents. Bethesda: AABB Press, 2001, pp. 83–98; George JN, Raskob GE, Shah SR, et al. Drug-induced thrombocytopenia: a systematic review of published case reports. Ann Intern Med 1998;129:886–890.

Hantavirus pulmonary syndrome (HPS) was described in 1993. Patients suffer a flu-like prodrome and then rapidly develop a noncardiac pulmonary edema resulting in profound respiratory failure.[13,181] Ventilatory support is required in 75% of cases and the mortality is approximately 50%. A powerful indicator of the presence of hantavirus is found on the peripheral smear.[13,182] The triad of thrombocytopenia, increased and left-shifted white cell count, and more than 10% circulating immunoblasts can identify all cases of HPS and was seen in only 2.6% of non-HPS controls in a recent study.[13] Marked hemoconcentration is also present because of the capillary leak syndrome, with the hematocrit reaching in some patients as high as 68%.

Thrombocytopenia can also be a major complication of dengue and rickettsial infections.[183–185] In the patient with an exotic travel history, the viral hemorrhagic syndromes such as yellow fever or Rift Valley fever must be considered.[186,187]

Catastrophic Antiphospholipid Antibody Syndrome

Rarely, patients with antiphospholipid antibody syndrome can present with fulminant multiorgan system failure.[188–190] Catastrophic antiphospholipid antibody syndrome (CAPS) is caused by widespread microthrombi in multiple vascular fields. These patients will develop renal failure, encephalopathy, adult respiratory distres syndrome (often with pulmonary hemorrhage), cardiac failure, dramatic livido reticularis, and worsening thrombocytopenia. Many of these patients have pre-existing autoimmune disorders and high-titer anticardiolipin antibodies. It appears that the best therapy for these patients is aggressive immunosuppression with plasmapheresis, perhaps followed by intravenous cyclophosphamide monthly. Early recognition of this syndrome can lead to quick therapy and resolution of the multiorgan system failure. The relationship of CAPS to "thrombotic storm" is not yet certain.[191]

Post-Transfusion Purpura

Patients with this disorder will have the onset of severe thrombocytopenia (less than 10,000/μL) 1 to 2 weeks after receiving blood products.[192–194] Post-transfusion purpura (PTP) occurs in patients who lack common platelet antigens, usually PL^{A1}. For unknown reasons, exposure of the antigens from the transfusion leads to rapid destruction of the patient's own platelets. Unlike most immune thrombocytopenias, bleeding may be severe in PTP.[195] The diagnostic clue is thrombocytopenia in a patient, typical female, who has received a red cell or platelet blood product in the past 7 to 10 days. Another feature is severe reaction to transfused platelets. Treatment consists of administration of intravenous immunoglobulin.[196] Rare patients may require plasmapheresis. The thrombocytopenia will resolve in a few months. If patients with a history of PTP require further transfusions, the red cells should be washed and only PL^{A1}-negative platelets should be given.

Cardiac Bypass

Cardiac bypass results in very complex and still poorly defined defects in all aspects of hemostasis.[197,198] Exposure of flowing of blood over artificial surfaces results in activation of both the contact coagulation system and the tissue factor pathway.[199,200] Platelets can be activated by contact with the artificial surfaces in the bypass machine.[201] Excessive activation of platelets depletes their granules, leading to the circulation of "spent platelets." Platelet function is also inhibited by loss of their key receptors, GP Ib and GP IIb/IIIa. This is due in part to cleavage of platelet GP IIb/IIIa by activated proteolytic enzymes and in part to binding of the receptor GP Ib to the artificial surface. Finally, there is activation of the fibrinolytic system both via the contact pathway and by release of endothelial tissue-type plasminogen activator due to the stress of surgery and hypothermia.[202] Large amounts of heparin are used for the bypass machine to prevent formation of clots in the filters. Levels of heparin can reach as high as 5 units/mL. These large doses need to be reversed at the end of surgery to prevent bleeding. Since protamine has a shorter half-life than heparin, patients rarely may experience "heparin rebound." High doses of protamine can lead to coagulation defects or the inhibition of platelet function.

If the patient is still in the operating suite and starts to have microvascular bleeding, one should check a full panel of coagulation tests, including the platelet count, PT, aPTT, and fibrinogen level. Patients who have had multiple transfusions of cell-saver blood or of packed red cells may have dilutional coagulation defects that need to be treated. In the bleeding patient still on bypass, an infusion of DDAVP is indicated. Given the platelet defect, if the PT and aPTT are in an acceptable range and the patient is still bleeding after administration of DDAVP, transfusion of platelets is indicated.

If bleeding occurs in the postoperative setting, coagulation tests should be obtained and surgical hemostasis achieved. Again, attention should be paid to the PT/aPTT and fibrinogen level. Often patients will respond to empiric transfusions of platelets. In the immediate postoperative state, a thrombin time should be checked to ensure the patient is not experiencing "heparin rebound."

Uremia

Before the advent of dialysis, bleeding was a common late complication of uremia.[203–206] Life-threatening bleeding is now uncommon but dialysis patients have a high incidence of gastrointestinal bleeding and subdural hematomas. The defect in uremia appears to be a platelet function defect.[205] The bleeding time is usually prolonged. Blood coagulation factors appear not to be affected and unless other problems are present, and the PT and aPTT are not prolonged.

Uremic patients who are bleeding should have a PT, aPTT, and platelet count performed. Patients with uremia are prone to vitamin K deficiency so assessment of the PT is important. The half-life of both unfractionated heparin, and especially LMWH is increased in renal failure. Patients usually receive a bolus of heparin with dialysis and rare patients will have a persistently prolonged anticoagulant effect. LMWH products are cleared in the kidneys and if the dose is not adjusted, levels can greatly increase above therapeutic goals. Bleeding times are prolonged in renal disease. Unfortunately, there is little correlation between prolongation of the bleeding time and actual bleeding, especially following procedures.

Multiple treatment options exist for uremic bleeding (Table 32–11). Patients who are severely uremic and are bleeding may respond to aggressive dialysis.[207] Cryoprecipitate is not effective in some patients and its use exposes the patient to the risk of transfusions transmitted viral disease.[207–209]

DDAVP is effective in uremic patients, with the bleeding time shortening for at least 4 hours after infusion. The reason DDAVP works in uremia is unknown.[209] It has been speculated that the DDAVP effect is through platelet aggregation-promoting properties or increasing the level of functional von Willebrand factor. Patients can exhibit tachyphylaxis with DDAVP; thus this agent is not useful for continued dosing.

For chronic bleeding, an infusion of conjugated estrogens will shorten the bleeding time. The dose is 0.6 mg/kg/day intravenously for 5 days. The onset of action takes up to 1 day but is of long duration, lasting for 2 weeks after the series of infusions.[210] For patients with chronic gastrointestinal bleeding from telangiectasias, chronic therapy with oral combinations of estrogen and progesterone may be helpful.[211]

Raising the hematocrit above 30% will shorten the bleeding time in uremic patients. This can be done either by transfusion or chronically with the use of erythropoietin.[212] It is speculated that increasing the red cell mass will increase platelet–vessel wall interactions. There is also some evidence that erythropoietin may have effects on the platelet independent of the hematocrit. It has been shown that the number of reticulated platelets, indicative of platelets newly released from the bone marrow, increases with erythropoietin infusion. For purposes of hemostasis, the target hematocrit with the use of erythropoietin should be 27% to 30%. Uremic patients who present with severe bleeding may benefit from transfusion of red cells.

Drug-Induced Platelet Dysfunction

Sophisticated testing of platelet function has revealed that acquired abnormalities are extremely common, but the clinical significance, if any, of these abnormalities is controversial.[213] Of the many agents and diseases that result in impaired platelet performance, only the few reviewed below appear to be of clinical consequence. Many of these proposed abnormalities are only reflected in an increased bleeding time, a test of uncertain clinical value.[214]

Multiple drugs have been shown to inhibit platelet function in vitro but clinical bleeding has only been associated with a few. Aspirin has been shown associated with increased risk of bleeding in clinical trials.[213] Ketorolac (Toradol) has also been associated with significant clinical bleeding. This is especially true with combined use of ketorolac and heparin or in patients with other bleeding defects such as von Willebrand disease.

Acquired platelet dysfunction was first seen with carbenicillin therapy but has been reported with multiple antibiotics, especially early antipseudomonal penicillin derivatives.[89,215,216] Infusions of therapeutic doses of ticarcillin and carbenicillin into normal volunteers will reproducibly prolong the bleeding time by the third or fourth day of drug administration.[217] In some patients this increase in bleeding time will persist for up to 2 weeks.[89,217,218] The newer antibiotics against *Pseudomonas* do not appear to have significant antiplatelet effects.

VENOUS THROMBOEMBOLISM

Incidence

Patients in ICUs are at high risk for venous thromboembolism. Studies have documented a venous thrombosis rate of 12% to 33%.[219–221] Certain patients are at higher risk of thrombosis.[222,223] Trauma patients have venous thrombosis rates of up to 60%. Stroke patients will develop thrombosis at a rate of 60% and patients with traumatic spinal cord damage have thrombosis rates that approach 80% (see Chapter 36).

Diagnosis

Diagnosis of venous thrombosis is best accomplished by venous ultrasonography. In patients with suggestive symptoms, Doppler ultrasound has a sensitivity of 95%.[224] However, Doppler ultrasonography will miss sites of some thromboses, especially iliac vein and inferior vena cava thrombosis.[225] Further imaging such as venography or computed tomography (CT) is suggested in patients with clinical signs of thrombosis but a negative Doppler exam.

Table 32–11 • THERAPY FOR UREMIC BLEEDING

Acute
Aggressive dialysis
DDAVP 0.3 μg/kg IV Q 12 h × 1–2 days
Cryoprecipitate 10 units

Long Term
Conjugated estrogen 0.6 mg/kg IV for 5 days
Erythropoietin to increase hematocrit > 30%

Diagnosis of pulmonary embolism in ICU patients presents many challenges. Respiratory compromise can occur for many reasons and pulmonary embolism must always be kept in mind as a diagnosis. Due to pre-existent pulmonary problems, ventilation/perfusion scans are extremely unlikely to provide useful information.[226,227] Also, transport of the patient to and from the critical care unit presents a formidable challenge. Pulmonary angiography is an effective and rapid method of detecting pulmonary embolism. Although associated with some risk, these hazards are less than that of empiric heparin therapy or missing the diagnosis of pulmonary embolism. Another strategy is to look for venous thrombosis in the legs of patients suspected of having pulmonary embolism.[228,229] If thrombosis is found, this establishes the need for anticoagulation and avoids the need for angiography.

Recently newer testing methodologies have been introduced to try to ease the problem of diagnosing pulmonary embolism.[230] Studies using the cumbersome enzyme-linked immunosorbant assay method have shown that detecting elevated levels of D-dimer is a sensitive (but not specific!) method of screening for thrombosis.[231,232] It must be strongly emphasized that in most clinic laboratories D-dimer assays are *not* sensitive for thrombosis and cannot be used to screen for thrombosis.[233,234] Point-of-care devices have been introduced to screen for thrombosis. In some studies sensitivities for detection of thrombosis by the newer assays ranged from 95% to only 70% in cancer patients.[233,235,236] New semiquantitative methods appear to be more sensitive to thrombosis.[237,238] The elevation in D-dimers is proportional to the thrombotic burden, and patients with small pulmonary emboli are more likely to have normal D-dimers.[239] One study in ICU patients found that most have elevated D-dimer, rendering the test not useful for screening in this population.[240]

In many institutions CT is rapidly replacing other methods of diagnosing pulmonary embolism.[241] CT has high specificity for pulmonary embolism but is only highly sensitive to central and segmental pulmonary arterial embolism.[242] The overall sensitivity of CT for pulmonary embolism may be as low as 70%.[243,244] Thus, especially in a very ill critical care patient, a negative CT scan does not rule out the diagnosis of pulmonary embolism. It must also be remembered that to date there still has been no rigorously controlled trial with long-term follow-up comparing CT to other diagnostic methods for pulmonary embolism. Thus, it is still unknown how accurate CT will be when compared with more traditional methods of diagnosing pulmonary embolism.

Given the lack of an ideal testing approach, the diagnostic evaluation of an ICU patient suspected of having a pulmonary embolism must be individualized. Lower-extremity Doppler ultrasonography performed at the bedside may rapidly confirm deep venous thrombosis, obviating the need to transport the patient to the radiology department. A CT scan may be useful in evaluation of respiratory failure and can be extended to examine other areas of the body. However, in many patients, pulmonary angiography will be the final arbitrator of thrombosis.

Treatment

Treatment of newly diagnosed venous thromboembolism is rapid initiation of heparin in therapeutic doses. One can chose from either LMWH products or standard unfractionated heparin.[245] Therapy with unfractionated heparin is initiated with a bolus of 5000 units (10,000 for larger thrombi or pulmonary embolism) followed by a continuous infusion of 1400 units/h. The tradition of starting with 1000 units/h results in inadequate anticoagulation in the vast majority of patients. The administration of heparin based on the patient's weight is useful in achieving therapeutic anticoagulation.[246,247] The aPTT is checked 6 hours after the bolus and the drip is adjusted accordingly. Since a supratherapeutic aPTT may just reflect the bolus, one should not decrease the drip until two consecutive aPTTs are supratherapeutic. Because of binding of heparin to acute-phase proteins, some patients may require as much as 2000 to 2400 units/h.

Laboratories should standardize their therapeutic aPTT ranges for heparin against heparin levels based on anti-factor Xa activity.[43,44,248] Thus, one should not use an arbitrary target aPTT of "60 to 90" seconds or 2 to 2.5 times control aPTT, but should instead use an aPTT range that corresponds to anti-Xa levels of 0.3 to 0.9 anti-Xa units, a range considered to be therapeutic. In one study, the therapeutic aPTT range varied from 1.8 to 2.5 to as high as 2.6 to 4.2 times control.[43]

Because of standard heparin's unfavorable and unpredictable pharmacokinetics, there is increased use of LMWH for treatment and prevention of thrombotic disorders.[132,245] LMWH products are derivatives of heparin with improved anti-Xa effect and less antiplatelet effect.[245,249–251] Several trials have shown that the LMWH products have an improved risk–benefit ratio over unfractionated heparin. Since LMWH products do not bind to acute-phase proteins or endothelial cells, their pharmacokinetics are more predictable than standard heparin. There is now abundant evidence that using LMWH for therapy in both deep venous thrombosis and pulmonary embolism treatment is as (and perhaps more[252]) effective as unfractionated heparin.[245,253–255]

For therapy, one can use any of the several brands of LMWH.[132,245] For most patients, laboratory monitoring is not needed. Monitoring should be considered for patients who are very obese (more than two times ideal body weight), who have severe liver or heart failure, who are pregnant, or who require long-term therapy. Very obese patients still require weight-based dosing without "capping" the dose at an arbitrary figure, but documenting a level the second day of therapy is prudent.[256] Levels are drawn 4 to 6 hours after injections and the therapeutic range in 0.7 to 1.2 anti-Xa units.[131]

LMWH is cleared by a renal mechanism and will accumulate in patients with renal failure. In patients with renal failure, dosing should reduced by 50% or more. One approach is to use enoxaparin, 0.75 mg/kg/

day. Monitoring with heparin levels is strongly encouraged.

Thrombolytic therapy for pulmonary embolism remains controversial.[257,258] No prospective study has shown meaningful clinical benefit in patients who have received thrombolytic therapy. Furthermore, the intracranial hemorrhage rate is substantially higher in patients receiving thrombolytic therapy for pulmonary embolism than for cardiac indications.[259] Advocates of thrombolytic therapy would argue that clinical trials of thrombolysis were not structured to examine the highest-risk patients (those with hypotension or right heart failure) who may benefit from rapid reduction in thrombus burden. Thrombolytic therapy may be considered for the patient with documented pulmonary embolism who remains hypotensive despite maximal medical management.

Another contentious treatment modality is the use of inferior vena cava (IVC) filters.[260] The sole randomized clinical trial demonstrated less pulmonary embolism but no reduction in mortality with the use of IVC in high-risk patients with thrombosis.[261] It does appear that filters double the long-term thrombosis risk of patients.[260,262] Reasonable indications for filters include deep venous thrombosis in a patient with an absolute contraindication to anticoagulation and deep venous thrombosis in a very ill patient in whom even a small embolism may be fatal (see Chapters 37 and 38).

Prevention

In high-risk surgical patients such as neurosurgical, orthopedic, and trauma patients, LMWH is superior to other forms of prophylaxis.[222,263,265] Medical patients at risk for thrombosis have not been studied for thrombosis prevention as extensively as surgical patients. LMWH has been shown to be useful for stroke patients. Evidence is accumulating that LMWH is effective in patients with severe respiratory infections or heart disease.[265,266,266a]

CATHETER THROMBOSIS

Central venous catheters are frequently placed in ICU patients. The clinically apparent thrombosis incidence for catheters is estimated to be 5% to 30%.[267–269] The signs of catheter thrombosis are nonspecific and the incidence of thrombosis is underestimated. Central venous catheters are often coated with sheaths of fibrin soon after introduction.[270] Pulmonary artery catheters directly visualized at surgery 1 to 2 hours after insertion were all found to be coated with thrombus.[271] Catheter thrombosis can also be a sign of HIT.[146]

Therapy is not well defined. Intuitively, removing the catheter will remove the nidus of thrombosis and, if possible, should be done. If the patient is stable, one should consider anticoagulation for 4 to 6 weeks. Given the low risk of long-term sequelae, there is little indication for thrombolytic therapy.

Prevention of catheter thrombosis is difficult. Two trials with long-term tunnelled catheters have shown that low-dose unmonitored warfarin (1 mg/day) or LMWH may prevent thrombosis.[272,273] However, applicability of these trials to ICU patients is unknown.

■ REFERENCES

Chapter 32 References

1. Chakraverty R, Davidson S, Peggs K, et al. The incidence and cause of coagulopathies in an intensive care population. Br J Haematol 1996;93:460–463.
2. Hanes SD, Quarles DA, Boucher BA. Incidence and risk factors of thrombocytopenia in critically ill trauma patients. Ann Pharmacother 1997;31:285–289.
3. Bonfiglio MF, Traeger SM, Kier KL, et al. Thrombocytopenia in intensive care patients: a comprehensive analysis of risk factors in 314 patients. Ann Pharmacother 1995;29:835–842.
4. Stéphan F, Hollande J, Richard O, et al. Thrombocytopenia in a surgical ICU. Chest 1999;115:1363–1370.
5. DeLoughery T. Drug induced immune hematological disease. Allergy Immunol Clin 1998;18:829–841.
6. George JN, Raskob GE, Shah SR, et al. Drug-induced thrombocytopenia: a systematic review of published case reports. Ann Intern Med 1998;129:886–890.
7. Heimpel H. When should the clinician suspect a drug-induced blood dyscrasia, and how should he proceed?. Eur J Haematol Suppl 1996;60:11–15.
8. Forsyth PD, Davies JM. Pure white cell aplasia and health food products. Postgrad Med J 1995;71:557–558.
9. Heck AM, DeWitt BA, Lukes AL. Potential interactions between alternative therapies and warfarin. Am J Health Syst Pharm 2000;57:1221–1230.
10. Goodnight SH, Hathaway WE. Evaluation of Bleeding in the Hospitalized Patient. Disorders of Hemostasis and Thrombosis. New York, McGraw-Hill, 2001, pp. 61–69.
11. Peterson P, Gottfried EL. The effects of inaccurate blood sample volume on prothrombin time (PT) and activated partial thromboplastin time (aPTT). Thromb Haemost 1982;47:101–103.
12. Bizzaro N. EDTA-dependent pseudothrombocytopenia: a clinical and epidemiological study of 112 cases, with 10-year follow-up. Am J Hematol 1995;50:103–109.
13. Mertz GJ, Hjelle BL, Bryan RT. Hantavirus infection. Dis Mon 1998;44:89–138.
14. Bell WR, Braine HG, Ness PM, Kickler TS. Improved survival in thrombotic thrombocytopenic purpura-hemolytic uremic syndrome—Clinical experience in 108 patients. N Engl J Med 1991;325:398–403.
15. Warkentin TE. Heparin-induced thrombocytopenia- pathogenesis, frequency, avoidance and management. Drug Saf 1997;17:325–341.
16. Warkentin TE, Greinacher A. Laboratory testing for heparin-induced thrombocytopenia. In: Warkentin TE, Greinacher A (Eds): Heparin-Induced Thrombocytopenia. New York, Marcel Dekker, 2000, pp. 211–244.
17. Baglin TP. Heparin induced thrombocytopenia thrombosis (HIT/T) syndrome: diagnosis and treatment. J Clin Pathol 2001;54:272–274.
18. DeLoughery TG. Thrombocytopenia in the Critical Care Patient. In: Alving BM (Ed): Blood Components and Pharmacologic Agents. Bethesda: AABB Press, 2001, pp. 83–98.
19. Counts RB, Haisch C, Simon TL, et al. Hemostasis in massively transfused trauma patients. Ann Surg 1979;190:91–99.
20. Stainsby D, MacLennan S, Hamilton PJ. Management of massive blood loss: a template guideline. Br J Anaesth 2000;85:487–491.

21. Hébert PC, Wells G, Blajchman MA, et al. A multicenter, randomized, controlled clinical trial of transfusion requirements in critical care. N Engl J Med 1999;340:409–417.
22. Blair SD, Janvrin SB, McCollum CN, Greenhalgh RM. Effect of early blood transfusion on gastrointestinal haemorrhage. Br J Surg 1986;73:783–785.
23. Rebulla P, Finazzi G, Marangoni F, et al. The threshold for prophylactic platelet transfusions in adults with acute myeloid leukemia. N Engl J Med 1997;337:1870–1875.
24. Miller RD, Robbins TO, Tong MJ, Barton SL. Coagulation defects associated with massive blood transfusions. Ann Surg 1971;174:794–801.
25. Ciavarella D, Reed RL, Counts RB, et al. Clotting factor levels and the risk of diffuse microvascular bleeding in the massively transfused patient. Br J Haematol 1987;67:365–368.
26. Goodnight SH, Kenoyer G, Rapaport SI, et al. Defibrination after brain-tissue destruction. A serious complication of head injury. N Engl J Med 1974;290:1043–1047.
27. Goldfarb G, Lebrec D. Percutaneous cannulation of the internal jugular vein in patients with coagulopathies: An experience based on 1,000 attempts. Anesthesiology 1982;56:321–323.
28. Foster PF, Moore LR, Sankary HN, et al. Central venous catheterization in patients with coagulopathy. Arch Surg 1992;127:273–275.
29. VanDervort A, Kopec I, Groeger J, Carlon G. Venous access hemorrhage in critically ill cancer patients. Chest 1987;92:1185 (abstr).
30. Fisher NC, Mutimer DJ. Central venous cannulation in patients with liver disease and coagulopathy—a prospective audit. Intensive Care Med 1999;25:481–485.
31. DeLoughery TG, Liebler JM, Simonds V, et al. Invasive line placement in critically ill patients: Do hemostatic defects matter? Transfusion 1996;36:827–831.
32. Carey MJ, Rodgers GM. Disseminated intravascular coagulation: Clinical and laboratory aspects. Am J Hematol 1998;59:65–73.
33. De Jonge E, Levi M, Stoutenbeek CP, Van Deventer SJH. Current drug treatment strategies for disseminated intravascular coagulation. Drugs 1998;55:767–777.
34. Baker WF Jr. Clinical aspects of disseminated intravascular coagulation: a clinician's point of view. Semin Thromb Hemost 1989;15:1–57.
35. Levi M, ten Cate H. Disseminated intravascular coagulation. N Engl J Med 1999;341:586–592.
36. Sharma S, Mayberry JC, DeLoughery TG, Mullins RJ. Fatal cerebroembolism from nonbacterial thrombotic endocarditis in a trauma patient: case report and review. Mil Med 2000;165:83–85.
37. Carr JM, McKinney M, McDonagh J. Diagnosis of disseminated intravascular coagulation. Role of D-dimer. Am J Clin Pathol 1989;91:280–287.
38. Rocha E, Paramo JA, Montes R, Panizo C. Acute generalized, widespread bleeding. Diagnosis and management. Haematologica 1998;83:1024–1037.
39. Wilde JT, Kitchen S, Kinsey S, et al. Plasma D-dimer levels and their relationship to serum fibrinogen/fibrin degradation products in hypercoagulable states. Br J Haematol 1989;71:65–70.
40. Hoffman JN, Faist E. Coagulation inhibitor replacement during sepsis: useless? Crit Care Med 2000;28(9:Suppl): S74–S76.
41. Feinstein DI. Diagnosis and management of disseminated intravascular coagulation: the role of heparin therapy. Blood 1982;60:284–287.
42. Callander N, Rapaport SI. Trousseau's syndrome. West J Med 1993;158:364–371.
43. Brill-Edwards P, Ginsberg JS, Johnston M, Hirsh J. Establishing a therapeutic range for heparin therapy. Ann Intern Med 1993;119:104–109.
44. Olson JD, Arkin CF, Brandt JT, et al. College of American Pathologists Conference XXXI on Laboratory Monitoring of Anticoagulant Therapy: Laboratory monitoring of unfractionated heparin therapy. Arch Pathol Lab Med 1998;122:782–798.
45. Darmstadt GL. Acute infectious purpura fulminans: pathogenesis and medical management. Pediatr Dermatol 1998;15:169–183.
46. Spicer TE, Rau JM. Purpura fulminans. Am J Med 1976;61:566–571.
47. Smith OP, White B. Infectious purpura fulminans: diagnosis and treatment. Br J Haematol 1999;104:202–207.
48. Carpenter CT, Kaiser AB. Purpura fulminans in pneumococcal sepsis: case report and review. Scand J Infect Dis 1997;29:479–483.
49. Duncan A. New therapies for severe meningococcal disease but better outcomes? Lancet 1997;350:1565–1566.
50. Smith OP, White B, Vaughan D, et al. Use of protein-C concentrate, heparin, and haemodiafiltration in meningococcus-induced purpura fulminans. Lancet 1997;350:1590–1593.
51. Branson HE, Katz J. A. structured approach to the management of purpura fulminans. J Natl Med Assoc 1983;75:821–825.
52. Manios SG, Kanakoudi F, Maniati E. Fulminant meningococcemia. Heparin therapy and survival rate. Scand J Infect Dis 1971;3:127–133.
53. Giudici D, Baudo F, Palareti G, et al. Antithrombin replacement in patients with sepsis and septic shock. Haematologica 1999;84:452–460.
54. Fourrier F, Jourdain M, Tournoys A. Clinical trial results with antithrombin III in sepsis. Crit Care Med 2000;28(9:Suppl):S38–43.
55. Levi M, De Jonge E, van der PT, ten Cate H. Novel approaches to the management of disseminated intravascular coagulation. Crit Care Med 2000;28(Suppl):1–4.
56. Rivard GE, David M, Farrell C, Schwarz HP. Treatment of purpura fulminans in meningococcemia with protein C concentrate. J Pediatr 1995;126:646–652.
57. White B, Livingstone W, Murphy C, et al. An open-label study of the role of adjuvant hemostatic support with protein C replacement therapy in purpura fulminans-associated meningococcemia. Blood 2000;96:3719–3724.
58. Bernard GR, Vincent J-L, Laterre PF, et al. Efficacy and safety of recombinant human activated protein C for severe sepsis. N Engl J Med 2001;344:699–709.
59. Garratty G. Immune cytopenia associated with antibiotics. Transfus Med Rev 1993;7:255–267.
60. Chenoweth CE, Judd WJ, Steiner EA, Kauffman CA. Cefotetan-induced immune hemolytic anemia. Clin Infect Dis 1992;15:863–865.
61. Garratty G, Nance S, Lloyd M, Domen R. Fatal immune hemolytic anemia due to cefotetan. Transfusion 1992;32:269–271.
62. Endoh T, Yagihashi A, Sasaki M, Watanabe N. Ceftizoxime-induced hemolysis due to immune complexes: case report and determination of the epitope responsible for immune complex-mediated hemolysis. Transfusion 1999;39:306–309.
63. Arndt PA, Leger RM, Garratty G. Serology of antibodies to second- and third-generation cephalosporins associated with immune hemolytic anemia and/or positive direct antiglobulin tests. Transfusion 1999;39:1239–1246.
64. Bernini JC, Mustafa MM, Sutor LJ, Buchanan GR. Fatal hemolysis induced by ceftriaxone in a child with sickle cell anemia. J Pediatr 1995;126:813–815.
65. Borgna-Pignatti C, Bezzi TM, Reverberi R. Fatal ceftriaxone-induced hemolysis in a child with acquired immunodeficiency syndrome. Pediatr Infect Dis J 1995;14:1116–1117.
66. Lascari AD, Amyot K. Fatal hemolysis caused by ceftriaxone. J Pediatr 1995;126:816–817.
67. Gottschall JL, Elliot W, Lianos E, et al. Quinine-induced immune thrombocytopenia associated with hemolytic uremic syndrome: a new clinical entity. Blood 1991;77:306–310.

68. Gottschall JL, Neahring B, McFarland JG, et al. Quinine-induced immune thrombocytopenia with hemolytic uremic syndrome: clinical and serological findings in nine patients and review of literature. Am J Hematol 1994;47:283–289.

69. Crum NF, Gable P. Quinine-induced hemolytic-uremic syndrome. South Med J 2000;93:726–728.

70. Vesely T, Vesely JN, George JN. Quinine-induced thrombotic thrombocytopenic purpura-hemolytic uremic syndrome (TTP-HUS): Frequency, clinical features, and long-term outcomes. Blood 2000;96:629a.

71. DeLoughery TG. Management of bleeding with uremia and liver disease. Curr Opin Hematol 1999;6:329–333.

72. Carr JM. Hemostatic disorders in liver disease. In: Schiff L, Schiff ER (Eds): Disease of the Liver. Philadelphia, JB Lippincott, 1993, pp. 1061–1076.

73. Kelly DA, O'Brien FJ, Hutton RA, et al. The effect of liver disease on factors V, VIII and protein C. Br J Haematol 1985;61:541–548.

74. Spector I, Corn M. Laboratory tests of hemostasis. The relation to hemorrhage in liver disease. Arch Intern Med 1967;119:577–582.

75. Martin TG3, Somberg KA, Meng YG, et al. Thrombopoietin levels in patients with cirrhosis before and after orthotopic liver transplantation. Ann Intern Med 1997;127:285–288.

76. Peck-Radosavljevic M, Zacherl J, Meng YG, et al. Is inadequate thrombopoietin production a major cause of thrombocytopenia in cirrhosis of the liver? J Hepatol 1997;27:127–131.

77. Thorsen LI, Brosstad F, Gogstad G, et al. Competitions between fibrinogen with its degradation products for interactions with the platelet-fibrinogen receptor. Thromb Res 1986;44:611–623.

78. Giordano P, Galli M, Del Vecchio G, et al. Lupus anticoagulant, anticardiolipin antibodies and hepatitis C virus infection in thalassaemia. Br J Haematol 1998;102:903–906.

79. Spector I, Corn M, Ticktin HE. Effect of plasma transfusions on the prothrombin time and clotting factors in liver disease. N Engl J Med 1966;275:1032–1037.

80. Roberts HR, Bingham MD. Other Coagulation Factor Deficiencies. In: Loscalozo JL, Schafer AI (Eds): Thrombosis and Hemorrhage. Baltimore, Williams & Wilkins, 1998, pp. 773–802.

81. Elizalde JI, Moitinho E, Garcia-Pagan JC, et al. Effects of increasing blood hemoglobin levels on systemic hemodynamics of acutely anemic cirrhotic patients. J Hepatol 1998;29:789–795.

82. Palascak JE, Martinez J. Dysfibrinogenemia associated with liver disease. J Clin Invest 1977;60:89–95.

83. Bolan CD, Alving BM. Pharmacologic agents in the management of bleeding disorders. Transfusion 1990;30:541–551.

84. Mannucci PM. Hemostatic drugs. N Engl J Med 1998;339:245–253.

85. Ansell JE, Kumar R, Deykin D. The spectrum of vitamin K deficiency. JAMA 1977;238:40–42.

86. Antimicrobials and haemostasis. Lancet 1983;1:510–511.

87. Sattler FR, Weitekamp MR, Sayegh A, Ballard JO. Impaired hemostasis caused by beta-lactam antibiotics. Am J Surg 1988;155:30–39.

88. Shevchuk YM, Conly JM. Antibiotic-associated hypoprothrombinemia: a review of prospective studies, 1966–1988. Rev Infect Dis 1990;12:1109–1126.

89. Brown CH, III, Natelson EA, Bradshaw W, et al. The hemostatic defect produced by carbenicillin. N Engl J Med 1974;291:265–270.

90. Matsubara T, Touchi A, Harauchi T, et al. Depression of liver microsomal vitamin K epoxide reductase activity associated with antibiotic-induced coagulopathy. Biochem Pharmacol 1989;38:2693–2701.

91. Breen GA, St Peter WL. Hypoprothrombinemia associated with cefmetazole. Ann Pharmacother 1997;31:180–184.

92. Williams KJ, Bax RP, Brown H, Machin SJ. Antibiotic treatment and associated prolonged prothrombin time. J Clin Pathol 1991;44:738–741.

93. Alperin JB. Coagulopathy caused by vitamin K deficiency in critically ill, hospitalized patients. JAMA 1987;258:1916–1919.

94. Pineo GF, Gallus AS, Hirsh J. Unexpected vitamin K deficiency in hospitalized patients. CMAJ 1973;109:880–883.

95. Chua JD, Friedenberg WR. Superwarfarin poisoning. Arch Intern Med 1998;158:1929–1932.

96. Routh CR, Triplett DA, Murphy MJ, et al. Superwarfarin ingestion and detection. Am J Hematol 1991;36:50–54.

97. Hulse ML. Warfarin resistance: diagnosis and therapeutic alternatives. Pharmacotherapy 1996;16:1009–1017.

98. Demirkan K, Stephens MA, Newman KP, Self TH. Response to warfarin and other oral anticoagulants: effects of disease states. South Med J 2000;93:448–454.

99. Hylek EM, Chang YC, Skates SJ, et al. Prospective study of the outcomes of ambulatory patients with excessive warfarin anticoagulation. Arch Intern Med 2000;160:1612–1617.

100. Crowther MA, Julian J, McCarty D, et al. Treatment of warfarin-associated coagulopathy with oral vitamin K: a randomised controlled trial. Lancet 2000;356:1551–1553.

101. Penning-van Beest FJ, Rosendaal FR, Grobbee DE, et al. Course of the International Normalized Ratio in response to oral vitamin K1 in patients overanticoagulated with phenprocoumon. Br J Haematol 1999;104:241–245.

102. Wentzien TH, O'Reilly RA, Kearns PJ. Prospective evaluation of anticoagulant reversal with oral vitamin K1 while continuing warfarin therapy unchanged. Chest 1998;114:1546–1550.

103. Butler AC, Tait RC. Management of oral anticoagulant-induced intracranial haemorrhage. Blood Rev 1998;12:35–44.

104. Makris M, Greaves M, Phillips WS, et al. Emergency oral anticoagulant reversal: the relative efficacy of infusions of fresh frozen plasma and clotting factor concentrate on correction of the coagulopathy. Thromb Haemost 1997;77:477–480.

105. Wijdicks EF, Schievink WI, Brown RD, Mullany CJ. The dilemma of discontinuation of anticoagulation therapy for patients with intracranial hemorrhage and mechanical heart valves. Neurosurgery 1998;42:769–773.

106. Butler AC, Tait RC. Restarting anticoagulation in prosthetic heart valve patients after intracranial haemorrhage: a 2-year follow-up. Br J Haematol 1998;103:1064–1066.

107. Phan TG, Koh M, Wijdicks EFM. Safety of discontinuation of anticoagulation in patients with intracranial hemorrhage at high thromboembolic risk. Arch Neurol 2000;57:1710–1713.

108. Ortel TL, Charles LA, Keller FG, et al. Topical thrombin and acquired coagulation factor inhibitors: Clinical spectrum and laboratory diagnosis. Am J Hematol 1994;45:128–135.

109. Zumberg MS, Waples JM, Kao KJ, et al. Management of a patient with a mechanical aortic valve and antibodies to both thrombin and factor V after repeat exposure to fibrin sealant. Am J Hematol 2000;64:59–63.

110. Dorion RP, Hamati HF, Landis B, et al. Risk and clinical significance of developing antibodies induced by topical thrombin preparations. Arch Pathol Lab Med 1998;122:887–894.

111. Hiippala S. Replacement of massive blood loss. Vox Sang 1998;74 Suppl 2:399–407.

112. Sawyer PR, Harrison CR. Massive transfusion in adults. Diagnoses, survival and blood bank support. Vox Sang 1990;58:199–203.

113. Cinat ME, Wallace WC, Nastanski F, et al. Improved survival following massive transfusion in patients who have undergone trauma. Arch Surg 1999;134:964–968.

114. Faringer PD, Mullins RJ, Johnson RL, Trunkey DD. Blood component supplementation during massive transfusion of AS-1 red cells in trauma patients. J Trauma 1993;34:481–5.

115. Leslie SD, Toy PTCY. Laboratory hemostatic abnormalities in massively transfused patients given red blood cells and crystalloid. Am J Clin Pathol 1991;96:770–773.

116. Harvey MP, Greenfield TP, Sugrue ME, Rosenfeld D. Massive blood transfusion in a tertiary referral hospital. Clinical outcomes and haemostatic complications. Med J Aust 1995;163:356–359.

117. Egerman RS, Sibai BM. Imitators of preeclampsia and eclampsia. Clin Obstet Gynecol 1999;42:551–562.

118. Egerman RS, Sibai BM. HELLP syndrome. Clin Obstet Gynecol 1999;42:381–389.

119. Saphier CJ, Repke JT. Hemolysis, elevated liver enzymes, and low platelets (HELLP) syndrome: a review of diagnosis and management. Semin Perinatol 1998;22:118–133.

120. Martin JN Jr, Perry KG Jr, Blake PG, et al. Better maternal outcomes are achieved with dexamethasone therapy for postpartum HELLP (hemolysis, elevated liver enzymes, and thrombocytopenia) syndrome. Am J Obstet Gynecol 1997;177:1011–1017.

121. Magann EF, Martin JN Jr. Twelve steps to optimal management of HELLP syndrome. Clin Obstet Gynecol 1999;42:532–550.

122. Jwayyed SM, Blanda M, Kubina M. Acute fatty liver of pregnancy. J Emerg Med 1999; 17:673–677.

123. Bacq Y. Acute fatty liver of pregnancy. Semin Perinatol 1998;22:134–140.

124. Nand S, Wong W, Yuen B, et al. Heparin-induced thrombocytopenia with thrombosis: Incidence, analysis of risk factors, and clinical outcomes in 108 consecutive patients treated at a single institution. Am J Hematol 1997;56:12–16.

125. Fabris F, Luzzatto G, Stefani PM, et al. Heparin-induced thrombocytopenia. Haematologica 2000;85:72–81.

126. Warkentin TE. Clinical Picture of Heparin-Induced Thrombocytopenia. In: Warkentin TE, Greinacher A (Eds): Heparin-Induced Thrombocytopenia. New York, Marcel Dekker, 2000, pp. 43–80.

127. Warkentin TE. Heparin-induced thrombocytopenia: A ten-year retrospective. Annu Rev Med 1999;50:129–147.

128. Hach-Wunderle V, Kainer K, Krug B, et al. Heparin-associated thrombosis despite normal platelet counts. Lancet 1994;344:469–470.

129. Laster JL, Nichols WK, Silver D. Thrombocytopenia associated with heparin-coated catheters in patients with heparin-associated antiplatelet antibodies. Arch Intern Med 1989;149:2285–2287.

130. Laster J, Silver D. Heparin-coated catheters and heparin-induced thrombocytopenia. J Vas Surg 1988;7:667–672.

131. Laposata M, Green D, Van Cott EM, et al. College of American Pathologists Conference XXXI on Laboratory Monitoring of Anticoagulant Therapy: The clinical use and laboratory monitoring of low-molecular-weight heparin, danaparoid, hirudin and related compounds, and argatroban. Arch Pathol Lab Med 1998;122:799–807.

132. Hirsh J, Warkentin TE, Shaughnessy SG, et al. Heparin and low molecular weight heparin. Chest 2001;119:64S–94S.

133. Reid TJ, III, Alving BM. A quantitative thrombin time for determining levels of hirudin and Hirulog. Thromb Haemost 1993;70:608–616.

134. Berry CN, Lunven C, Girardot C, et al. Ecarin clotting time: a predictive coagulation assay for the antithrombotic activity of argatroban in the rat. Thromb Haemost 1998;79:228–233.

135. Greinacher A, Janssens U, Berg G, et al. Lepirudin (recombinant hirudin) for parenteral anticoagulation in patients with heparin-induced thrombocytopenia. Heparin-Associated Thrombocytopenia Study (HAT) investigators. Circulation 1999;100:587–593.

136. Moll S, Ortel TL. Monitoring warfarin therapy in patients with lupus anticoagulants. Ann Intern Med 1997;127:177–185.

137. Song X, Huhle G, Wang L, et al. Generation of anti-hirudin antibodies in heparin-induced thrombocytopenic patients treated with r-hirudin. Circulation 1999;100:1528–1532.

138. Huhle G, Hoffmann U, Song X, et al. Immunologic response to recombinant hirudin in HIT type II patients during long-term treatment. Br J Haematol 1999;106:195–201.

139. Lewis BE, Wallis MD, Berkowitz SD, et al. Argatroban anticoagulant therapy in patients with heparin induced thrombocytopenia. Circulation 2001;103:1838–1843.

140. Swan SK, Hursting MJ. The pharmacokinetics and pharmacodynamics of argatroban: effects of age, gender, and hepatic or renal dysfunction. Pharmacotherapy 2000;20:318–329.

141. Tardy-Poncet B, Tardy B, Reynaud J, et al. Efficacy and safety of danaparoid sodium (ORG 10172) in critically ill patients with heparin-associated thrombocytopenia. Chest 1999;115:1616–1620.

142. Wilde MI, Markham A. Danaparoid. A review of its pharmacology and clinical use in the management of heparin-induced thrombocytopenia. Drugs 1997;54:903–924.

143. Warkentin TE, Levine MN, Hirsh J, et al. Heparin-induced thrombocytopenia in patients treated with low-molecular-weight heparin or unfractionated heparin [see comments]. N Engl J Med 1995;332:1330–1335.

144. Warkentin TE. Heparin-induced thrombocytopenia and its treatment. J Thromb Thrombolysis 2000;9:S29–S35.

145. Medina PJ, Sipols JM, George JN. Drug-associated thrombotic thrombocytopenic purpura-hemolytic uremic syndrome. Curr Opin Hematol 2001;8:286–293.

146. George JN. How I treat patients with thrombotic thrombocytopenic purpura-hemolytic uremic syndrome. Blood 2000;96:1223–1229.

147. Chang JC, Shipstone A, Llenado-Lee MA. Postoperative thrombotic thrombocytopenic purpura following cardiovascular surgeries. Am J Hematol 1996;53:11–17.

148. Rock GA, Shumak KH, Buskard NA, et al. Comparison of plasma exchange with plasma infusion in the treatment of thrombotic thrombocytopenic purpura. N Engl J Med 1991;325:393–397.

149. Furlan M, Robles R, Galbusera M, et al. Von Willebrand factor-cleaving protease in thrombotic thrombocytopenic purpura and the hemolytic-uremic syndrome. N Engl J Med 1998;339:1578–1584.

150. Zeigler ZR, Shadduck RK, Gryn JF, et al. Cryoprecipitate poor plasma does not improve early response in primary adult thrombotic thrombocytopenic purpura (TTP). J Clin Apheresis 2001;16:19–22.

151. Gordon LI, Kwaan HC, Rossi EC. Deleterious effects of platelet transfusions and recovery thrombocytosis in patients with thrombotic microangiopathy. Semin Hematol 1987;24:194–201.

152. Moake JL, Byrnes JJ. Thrombotic microangiopathies associated with drugs and bone marrow transplantation. Hematol Oncol Clin North Am 1996;10:485–497.

153. Gharpure VS, Devine SM, Holland HK, et al. Thrombotic thrombocytopenic purpura associated with FK506 following bone marrow transplantation. Bone Marrow Transplant 1995;16:715–716.

154. Wu DC, Liu JM, Chen YM, et al. Mitomycin-C induced hemolytic uremic syndrome: a case report and literature review. Jap J Clin Onc 1997;27:115–118.

155. Bennett CL, Connors JM, Carwile JM, et al. Thrombotic thrombocytopenic purpura associated with clopidogrel. N Engl J Med 2000;342:1773–1777.

156. Moussa I, Oetgen M, Roubin G, et al. Effectiveness of clopidogrel and aspirin versus ticlopidine and aspirin in preventing stent thrombosis after coronary stent implantation. Circulation 1999;99:2364–2366.

157. Schriber JR, Herzig GP. Transplantation-associated thrombotic thrombocytopenic purpura and hemolytic uremic syndrome. Semin Hematol 1997;34:126–133.

158. Clark RE. Thrombotic microangiopathy following bone marrow transplantation. Bone Marrow Transplant 1994;14:495–504.

159. Van der Plas RM, Schiphorst ME, Huizinga EG, et al. von Willebrand factor proteolysis is deficient in classic, but not in bone marrow transplantation-associated, thrombotic thrombocytopenic purpura. Blood 1999;93:3798–3802.

160. Sarode R, McFarland JG, Flomenberg N, et al. Therapeutic plasma exchange does not appear to be effective in the management of thrombotic thrombocytopenic purpura/hemolytic ure-

mic syndrome following bone marrow transplantation. Bone Marrow Transplant 1995;16:271–275.

161. Esplin MS, Branch DW. Diagnosis and management of thrombotic microangiopathies during pregnancy. Clin Obstet Gynecol 1999;42:360–367.

162. Dashe JS, Ramin SM, Cunningham FG. The long-term consequences of thrombotic microangiopathy (thrombotic thrombocytopenic purpura and hemolytic uremic syndrome) in pregnancy. Obstet Gynecol 1998;91:1–8.

163. DeShazo RD, Kemp SF. Allergic reactions to drugs and biologic agents. JAMA 1997;278:1895–1906.

164. Pedersen-Bjergaard U, Andersen M, Hansen PB. Drug-induced thrombocytopenia: clinical data on 309 cases and the effect of corticosteroid therapy. Eur J Clin Pharmacol 1997;52:183–189.

165. Berkowitz SD. Thrombocytopenia caused by platelet glycoprotein IIb/IIIa receptor antagonist. Hematology 1998: Washington D.C., American Society of Hematology, 1998, pp. 374–379.

166. Jubelirer SJ, Koenig BA, Bates MC. Acute profound thrombocytopenia following C7E3 Fab (abciximab) therapy: case reports, review of the literature and implications for therapy. Am J Hematol 1999;61:205–208.

167. Arshad A, Hashem M, Rehan A, et al. Beyond randomized trials: safety of platelet glycoprotein IIb/IIIa receptor antagonists in real life. Circulation 2000;102[Suppl II]: 666.

168. Bhatt DL, Topol EJ. Current role of platelet glycoprotein IIb/IIIa inhibitors in acute coronary syndromes. JAMA 2000; 284:1549–1558.

169. Berkowitz SD, Harrington RA, Rund MM, Tcheng JE. Acute profound thrombocytopenia after c7E3 Fab (abciximab) therapy. Circulation 1997;95:809–813.

170. Kereiakes DJ, Essell JH, Abbottsmith CW, et al. Abciximab-associated profound thrombocytopenia: therapy with immunoglobulin and platelet transfusion. Am J Cardiol 1996;78:1161–1163.

171. Harris RL, Musher DM, Bloom K, et al. Manifestations of sepsis. Arch Intern Med 1987;147:1895–1906.

172. van Gorp EC, Suharti C, ten Cate H, et al. Review: infectious diseases and coagulation disorders. J Infect Dis 1999;180: 176–186.

173. Tiab M, Mechinaud F, Harousseau JL. Haemophagocytic syndrome associated with infections. Baillieres Clin Haematol 2000;13:163–178.

174. Francois B, Trimoreau F, Vignon P, et al. Thrombocytopenia in the sepsis syndrome: role of hemophagocytosis and macrophage colony-stimulating factor. Am J Med 1997;103:114–120.

175. Risdall RJ, Brunning RD, Hernandez JI, Gordon DH. Bacteria-associated hemophagocytic syndrome. Cancer 1984;54:2968–2972.

176. Stephan F, Thioliere B, Verdy E, Tulliez M. Role of hemophagocytic histiocytosis in the etiology of thrombocytopenia in patients with sepsis syndrome or septic shock. Clin Infect Dis 1997; 25:1159–1164.

177. Baker GR, Levin J. Transient thrombocytopenia produced by administration of macrophage colony-stimulating factor: Investigations of the mechanism. Blood 1998;91:89–99.

178. Dumler JS, Bakken JS. Human ehrlichiosis: Newly recognized infections transmitted by ticks. Annu Rev Med 1998;49:201–213.

179. Bakken JS, Krueth J, Wilson-Nordskog C, et al. Clinical and laboratory characteristics of human granulocytic ehrlichiosis. JAMA 1996;275:199–205.

180. Fichtenbaum CJ, Peterson LR, Weil GJ. Ehrlichiosis presenting as a life-threatening illness with features of the toxic shock syndrome. Am J Med 1993;95:351–357.

181. Butler JC, Peters CJ. Hantaviruses and hantavirus pulmonary syndrome. Clin Infect Dis 1994;19:387–394.

182. Nolte KB, Feddersen RM, Foucar K, et al. Hantavirus pulmonary syndrome in the United States: a pathological description of a disease caused by a new agent. Hum Pathol 1995;26:110–120.

183. Rigau-Perez JG, Clark GG, Gubler DJ, et al. Dengue and dengue haemorrhagic fever. Lancet 1998;352:971–977.

184. Cowan G. Rickettsial diseases: the typhus groups of fevers—a review. Postgrad Med J 2000;76:269–272.

185. Srichaikul T, Nimmannitya S. Haematology in dengue and dengue haemorrhagic fever. Baillieres Clin Haematol 2000; 13:261–276.

186. Enria DA, Pinheiro F. Rodent-borne emerging viral zoonosis. Hemorrhagic fevers and hantavirus infections in South America. Infect Dis Clin North Am 2000;14:167–184.

187. Barry M. Viral Hemorrhagic fevers, in, Hematology 2000: Educational Program Book. Washington D.C., American Society of Hematology, 2000, pp. 414–423.

188. Asherson RA. The catastrophic antiphospholipid syndrome. J Rheumatol 1992;19:508–512.

189. Asherson RA, Piette JC. The catastrophic antiphospholipid syndrome 1996: Lupus 1996;5:414–417.

190. Asherson RA, Cervera R. Catastrophic antiphospholipid syndrome. Curr Opin Hematol 2000;5:325–329.

191. Kitchens CS. Thrombotic storm: When thrombosis begets thrombosis. Am J Med 1998;104:381–385.

192. Mollison PL, Engelfriet CP, Contreras M. Some unfavourable effects of transfusions. In: Mollison PL, Engelfriet CP, Contreras M (Eds): Blood Transfusion in Clinical Medicine. Oxford, Blackwell Science, 1997, 487–508.

193. Jenner PW, Holland PV. Diagnosis and management of transfusion reactions. In: Petz LD, Kleinman S, Swisher SN, et al. (Eds). Clinical Practice of Transfusion Medicine. New York, Churchill Livingstone, 1996, pp. 905–930.

194. Mueller-Eckhardt C. Post-transfusion purpura. Br J Haematol 1986;64:419–424.

195. Lubenow N, Eichler P, Albrecht D, et al., Very low platelet counts in post-transfusion purpura falsely diagnosed as heparin-induced thrombocytopenia: Report of four cases and review of literature. Thromb Res 2000;100:115–125.

196. Mueller-Eckhardt C, Kiefel V. High-dose IgG for post-transfusion purpura—revisited. Blut 1988;57:163–167.

197. Woodman RC, Harker LA. Bleeding complications associated with cardiopulmonary bypass. Blood 1990;76:1680–1697.

198. Bevan DH. Cardiac bypass haemostasis: putting blood through the mill. Br J Haematol 1999;104:219.

199. Gallimore MJ, Jones DW, Wendel HP. A chromogenic substrate assay kit for factor XII: evaluation and use for the measurement of factor XII levels in cardiopulmonary bypass patients. Thromb Res 1999;94:103–109.

200. Parratt R, Hunt BJ. Direct activation of factor X by monocytes occurs during cardiopulmonary bypass. Br J Haematol 1998; 101:40–46.

201. Weerasinghe A, Taylor KM. The platelet in cardiopulmonary bypass. Ann Thorac Surg 1998;66:2145–2152.

202. Hunt BJ, Parratt RN, Segal HC, et al. Activation of coagulation and fibrinolysis during cardiothoracic operations. Ann Thor Surg 1998;65:712–718.

203. Livio M, Benigni A, Remuzzi G. Coagulation abnormalities in uremia. Semin Nephrol 1985;5:82–90.

204. Rabelink TJ, Zwaginga JJ, Koomans HA, et al. Thrombosis and hemostasis in renal disease. Kidney Int 1994;46:287–296.

205. Weigert AL, Schafer AI. Uremic bleeding: pathogenesis and therapy. Am J Med Sci 1998;316:94–104.

206. Sagripanti A, Barsotti G. Bleeding and thrombosis in chronic uremia. Nephron 1997;75:125–139.

207. Andrassy K, Ritz E. Uremia as a cause of bleeding. Am J Nephrol 1985;5:313–319.

208. Triulzi DJ, Blumberg N. Variability in response to cryoprecipitate treatment for hemostatic defects in uremia. Yale J Biol Med 1990;63:1–7.

209. Mannucci PM. Desmopressin (DDAVP) in the treatment of bleeding disorders: The first 20 years. Blood 1997;90:2515–2521.
210. Vigano G, Gaspari F, Locatelli M, et al. Dose-effect and pharmacokinetics of estrogens given to correct bleeding time in uremia. Kidney Int 1988;34:853–858.
211. Bronner MH, Pate MB, Cunningham JT, Marsh WH. Estrogen-progesterone therapy for bleeding gastrointestinal telangiectasias in chronic renal failure. An uncontrolled trial. Ann Intern Med 1986;105:371–374.
212. Moia M, Mannucci PM, Vizzotto L, et al. Improvement in the haemostatic defect of uraemia after treatment with recombinant human erythropoietin. Lancet 1987;2(8570):1227–1229.
213. George JN, Shattil SJ. The clinical importance of acquired abnormalities of platelet function. N Engl J Med 1991;324:27–39.
214. Lind SE. Prolonged bleeding time. Am J Med 1984;77:305–312.
215. Andrassy K, Weischedel E, Ritz E, Andrassy T. Bleeding in uremic patients after carbenicillin. Thromb Haemost 1976;36:115–126.
216. Wisloff F, Godal HC. Prolonged bleeding time with adequate platelet count in hospital patients. Scand J Haematol 1981;27:45–50.
217. Brown CH III, Natelson EA, Bradshaw MW, et al. Study of the effects of ticarcillin on blood coagulation and platelet function. Antimicrob Agents Chemother 1975;7:652–657.
218. Sattler FR, Weitekamp MR, Ballard JO. Potential for bleeding with the new beta-lactam antibiotics. Ann Intern Med 1986;105:924–931.
219. Hirsch DR, Ingenito EP, Goldhaber SZ. Prevalence of deep venous thrombosis among patients in medical intensive care. JAMA 1995;274:335–337.
220. Marik PE, Andrews L, Maini B. The incidence of deep venous thrombosis in ICU patients. Chest 1997;111:661–664.
221. Legere BM, Dweik RA, Arroliga AC. Venous thromboembolism in the intensive care unit. Clin Chest Med 1999;20:367–384.
222. Clagett GP, Anderson FA Jr, Geerts W, et al. Prevention of venous thromboembolism. Chest 1998;114 Suppl:531S–560S.
223. Thorborg P. Bleedings and thrombosis in critical care patients—an update. Crit Care Shock 2000;1:4–10.
224. Kearon C, Ginsberg JS, Hirsh J. The role of venous ultrasonography in the diagnosis of suspected deep venous thrombosis and pulmonary embolism. Ann Intern Med 1998;129:1044–1049.
225. Birdwell BG, Raskob GE, Whitsett TL, et al. The clinical validity of normal compression ultrasonography in outpatients suspected of having deep venous thrombosis. Ann Intern Med 1998;128:1–7.
226. Hull RD, Raskob GE. Low-probability lung scan findings: a need for change. Ann Intern Med 1991;114:142–143.
227. PIOPED Investigators. Value of the ventilation/perfusion scan in acute pulmonary embolism. JAMA 1990;263:2753–2759.
228. Stein PD, Hull RD, Pineo G. Strategy that includes serial noninvasive leg tests for diagnosis of thromboembolic disease in patients with suspected acute pulmonary embolism based on data from PIOPED. Arch Intern Med 1995;155:2101–2104.
229. Hull RD, Raskob GE, Ginsberg JS, et al. A noninvasive strategy for the treatment of patients with suspected pulmonary embolism. Arch Intern Med 1994;154:289–297.
230. Riedel M. Acute pulmonary embolism 1: pathophysiology, clinical presentation, and diagnosis. Heart 2001;85:229–240.
231. Quinn DA, Fogel RB, Smith CD, et al. D-dimers in the diagnosis of pulmonary embolism. Am J Respir Crit Care Med 1999;159:1445–1449.
232. Anderson DR, Wells PS. D-dimer for the diagnosis of venous thromboembolism. Curr Opin Hematol 2000;5:296–301.
233. Janssen MCH, Heebels AE, De Metz M, et al. Reliability of five rapid D-dimer assays compared to ELISA in the exclusion of deep venous thrombosis. Thromb Haemost 1997;77:262–266.
234. Kutinsky I, Blakley S, Roche V. Normal D-dimer levels in patients with pulmonary embolism. Arch Intern Med 1999;159:1569–1572.
235. Farrell S, Hayes T, Shaw M. A negative SimpliRED D-dimer assay result does not exclude the diagnosis of deep vein thrombosis or pulmonary embolus in emergency department patients. Ann Emerg Med 2000;35:121–125.
236. Lee AY, Julian JA, Levine MN, et al. Clinical utility of a rapid whole-blood D-dimer assay in patients with cancer who present with suspected acute deep venous thrombosis. Ann Intern Med 1999;131:417–423.
237. van der GF, van den BH, van der KM, et al. Exclusion of deep venous thrombosis with D-dimer testing—comparison of 13 D-dimer methods in 99 outpatients suspected of deep venous thrombosis using venography as reference standard. Thromb Haemost 2000;83:191–198.
238. Freyburger G, Trillaud H, Labrouche S, et al. D-dimer strategy in thrombosis exclusion—A gold standard study in 100 patients suspected of deep venous thrombosis or pulmonary embolism: 8 DD methods compared. Thromb Haemost 1998;79:32–37.
239. Sijens PE, Van Ingen HE, Van Beek EJR, et al. Rapid ELISA assay for plasma D-dimers in the diagnosis of segmental and subsegmental pulmonary embolism. Thromb Haemost 2000;84:156–159.
240. Kollef MH, Zahid M, Eisenberg PR. Predictive value of a rapid semiquantitative D-dimer assay in critically ill patients with suspected venous thromboembolic disease. Crit Care Med 2000;28:414–420.
241. Garg K, Welsh CH, Feyerabend AJ, et al. Pulmonary embolism: diagnosis with spiral CT and ventilation-perfusion scanning—correlation with pulmonary angiographic results or clinical outcome. Radiology 1998;208:201–208.
242. Beigelman C, Chartrand-Lefebvre C, Howarth N, et al. Pitfalls in diagnosis of pulmonary embolism with helical CT angiography. Am J Roentgenol 1998;171:579–585.
243. Rathbun SW, Raskob GE, Whitsett TL. Sensitivity and specificity of helical computed tomography in the diagnosis of pulmonary embolism: a systematic review. Ann Intern Med 2000;132:227–232.
244. Hartmann IJ, Hagen PJ, Melissant CF, et al. Diagnosing acute pulmonary embolism. Effect of chronic obstructive pulmonary disease on the performance of d-dimer testing, ventilation/perfusion scintigraphy, spiral computed tomographic angiography, and conventional angiography. Am J Respir Crit Care Med 2000;162:2232–2237.
245. Hyers TM, Agnelli G, Hull RD, et al. Antithrombotic therapy for venous thromboembolic disease. Chest 2001;119:176S–193S.
246. De Groot MR, Büller HR, ten Cate JW, Kooy MV. Use of a heparin nomogram for treatment of patients with venous thromboembolism in a community hospital. Thromb Haemost 1998;80:70–73.
247. Bernardi E, Piccioli A, Oliboni G, et al. Nomograms for the administration of unfractionated heparin in the initial treatment of acute thromboembolism—an overview. Thromb Haemost 2000;84:22–26.
248. Kitchen S. Problems in laboratory monitoring of heparin dosage. Br J Haematol 2000;111:397–406.
249. Simonneau G, Sors H, Charbonnier B, et al. A comparison of low-molecular-weight heparin with unfractionated heparin for acute pulmonary embolism. N Engl J Med 1997;337:663–669.
250. Pineo GF, Hull RD. Low-molecular-weight heparin: Prophylaxis and treatment of venous thromboembolism. Annu Rev Med 1997;48:79–91.
251. Weitz JI. Low-molecular-weight heparins. N Engl J Med 1997;337:688–698.
252. Gould MK, Dembitzer AD, Sanders GD, Garber AM. Low-molecular-weight heparins compared with unfractionated heparin for treatment of acute deep venous thrombosis—A cost-effectiveness analysis. Ann Intern Med 1999;130:789–799.

253. Koopman MMW, Prandoni P, Piovella F, et al. Treatment of venous thrombosis with intravenous unfractionated heparin administered in the hospital as compared with subcutaneous low-molecular-weight heparin administered at home. N Engl J Med 1996;334:682–687.

254. Raskob GE. Heparin and low molecular weight heparin for treatment of acute pulmonary embolism. Curr Opin Pulm Med 1999;5:216–221.

255. Pineo GF, Hull RD. Heparin and low-molecular-weight heparin in the treatment of venous thromboembolism. Baillieres Clin Haematol 1998;11:621–637.

256. Yee JYV, Duffull SB. The effect of body weight on dalteparin pharmacokinetics—A preliminary study. Eur J Clin Pharmacol 2000;56:293–297.

257. Arcasoy SM, Kreit JW. Thrombolytic therapy of pulmonary embolism—A comprehensive review of current evidence. Chest 1999;115:1695–1707.

258. Riedel M. Acute pulmonary embolism 2: treatment. Heart 2001;85:351–360.

259. Kanter DS, Mikkola KM, Patel SR, et al. Thrombolytic therapy for pulmonary embolism—frequency of intracranial hemorrhage and associated risk factors. Chest 1997;111:1241–1245.

260. Streiff MB. Vena cava filters: a comprehensive review. Blood 2000;95:3669–3677.

261. Decousus H, Leizorovicz A, Parent F, et al. A clinical trial of vena caval filters in the prevention of pulmonary embolism in patients with proximal deep-vein thrombosis. N Engl J Med 1998;338:409–415.

262. White RH, Zhou H, Kim J, Romano PS. A population-based study of the effectiveness of inferior vena cava filter use among patients with venous thromboembolism. Arch Intern Med 2000;160:2033–2041.

263. Geerts WH, Jay RM, Code KI, et al. A comparison of low-dose heparin with low-molecular-weight heparin as prophylaxis against venous thromboembolism after major trauma. N Engl J Med 1996;335:701–707.

264. Agnelli G, Piovella F, Buoncristiani P, et al. Enoxaparin plus compression stockings compared with compression stockings alone in the prevention of venous thromboembolism after elective neurosurgery. N Engl J Med 1998;339:80–85.

265. Haas S. Recommendations for prophylaxis of venous thromboembolism: International consensus and the American College of Chest Physicians Fifth Consesus Conference on Antithrombotic Therapy. Curr Opin Pulm Med 2000;6:314–320.

266. Geerts WH, Heit JA, Clagett GP, et al. Prevention of venous thromboembolism. Chest 2001;119:132S–175S.

266a. Mismetti P, Laporte-Simitsidis S, Tardy B, et al. Prevention of venous thromboembolism in internal medicine with unfractionated or low-molecular-weight heparins: A meta-analysis of randomised clinical trials. Thromb Haemost 2000;83:14–19.

267. Timsit JF, Farkas JC, Boyer JM, et al. Central vein catheter-related thrombosis in intensive care patients: incidence, risks factors, and relationship with catheter-related sepsis. Chest 1998;114:207–213.

268. Cobos E, Dixon S, Keung YK. Prevention and management of central venous catheter thrombosis. Curr Opin Hematol 1998;5:355–359.

269. Durbec O, Viviand X, Potie F, et al. A prospective evaluation of the use of femoral venous catheters in critically ill adults. Crit Care Med 1997;25:1986–1989.

270. Hoshal VL, Ause RG, Hoskins PA. Fibrin sleeve formation on indwelling subclavian central venous catheters. Arch Surg 1971;102:353–358.

271. Hoar PF, Stone G, Wicks AE, et al. Thrombogenesis associated with Swan-Ganz catheters. Anesthesiology 1978;48:445–447.

272. Bern MM, Lokich JJ, Wallach SR, et al. Very low doses of warfarin can prevent thrombosis in central venous catheters. A randomized prospective trial. Ann Intern Med 1990;112:423–428.

273. Boraks P, Seale J, Price J, et al. Prevention of central venous catheter associated thrombosis using minidose warfarin in patients with haematological malignancies. Br J Haematol 1998;101:483–486.

CHAPTER 33

Hemostatic Aspects of Patients with Human Immunodeficiency Virus/Acquired Immunodeficiency Syndrome

Bruce L. Evatt, M.D.
W. Craig Hooper, Ph.D.

Infection with human immunodeficiency viruses (HIV) initiates a chronic, progressive disease process that usually advances to acquired immunodeficiency syndrome (AIDS), a syndrome characterized clinically by a low CD4 count, opportunistic infections, and excess immunologic damage. The time interval from the initial infection by HIV to the clinical presentation of AIDS can be as short as 1 year or as long as 20 years. Clinical managment with newer treatment modalities that include protease inhibitors and other antiviral and antifungal drugs can significantly alter the course of the disease, improving the quality of life and increasing survival. However, the longer life spans associated with increased survival will require that physicians understand and have the capacity to manage the chronic manifestations of HIV/AIDS or those that develop as a consequence of therapy.[1]

The hematologic manifestations of HIV infection and AIDS, which are common, may present confusion clinical problems and if untreated, can be life threatening. For instance, bone marrow failure due to depletion or inhibition of progenitor cells, ineffective hematopoiesis, and decreased survival of hemopoietic cell lines can lead to well-recognized anemia, neutropenia, and thrombocytopenia, conditions that often limit appropriate antiviral therapy and necessitate frequent transfusion.[2,3] In addition, infection with blood-borne viruses such as cytomegalovirus (CMV), parvovirus,[4] and hepatitis viruses may further suppress hematopoiesis, while other infections either directly or indirectly may interfere with proper hemostasis, producing both bleeding and thrombosis. Decreased plasma levels of protein S and the presence of lupus-like inhibitors or protease inhibitors may foster thrombosis. Thrombotic thrombocytopenic purpura (TTP) may result from events subsequent to damage to the endothelium by infection or from other mechanisms. Furthermore, drugs and autoantibodies may also result in complications by causing platelet dysfunction and thrombocytopenia. For the consulting physician, these effects of HIV/AIDS on the coagulation system can be especially challenging because they usually do not occur in isolation. Several effects occurring simultaneously often cause a departure from typical clinical presentations of these bleeding disorders. To successfully diagnose and manage these patients, the physician must be aware of how these possible complications may alter progression of HIV/AIDS in the individual patient.

HIV/AIDS-ASSOCIATED THROMBOCYTOPENIA

HIV-associated thrombocytopenia, a serious complication of HIV infection, is a consequence of several factors, including: (1) immune-mediated platelet destruction due to immune complexes on the surface of the platelet or antibodies against platelets[5]; (2) decreased and defective platelet production due to infection of megakaryocytes with HIV-1[6–8]; and (3) megakaryocyte dysplastic changes that appear to reduce platelet formation, drug-induced myelosuppression, or HIV-associated neoplasms. Among persons with clinical AIDS, the 1-year incidence of thrombocytopenia is 8.6%,[9] and its prevalence among all HIV-infected patients is 9% to 37%, varying in accordance with the study population. For example, thrombocytopenia is more frequently observed among white males, older persons, or persons who have a history of intravenous drug use. Spontaneous remissions occur in about 20% of persons with HIV-related thrombocytopenia, a higher remission rate than that observed among non-HIV-infected persons with immune thrombocytopenic purpura (ITP).[10] However, HIV-related thrombocytopenia may herald an accelerated progression to AIDS and decreased survival rates; thus, recognition of the condition in such individuals is crucial.[10]

Management of Thrombocytopenia

Recognition of symptomatic thrombocytopenia and prompt therapeutic intervention are essential to prevent severe complications. Patients normally have no bleeding problems unless their platelet counts drop below 50,000/μL and thus most patients generally do not require treatment. Treatment is usually indicated in all patients with platelet counts below 20,000 to 30,000/μL and those patients with counts below 50,000/μL who exhibit significant mucous membrane bleeding or have risk factors for bleeding (e.g., peptic ulcer disease or hypertension).[11] Patients with significant mucous membrane bleeding and platelet counts below 20,000/μL should be hospitalized and those with life-threatening bleeding should receive the necessary critical care measures.

Since multiple factors often are responsible for producing thrombocytopenia in patients with HIV infection, the most appropriate treatment is still subject to some debate. Antiviral therapy with zidovudine has been associated with improved platelet counts in 60% to 70% of patients with HIV-associated thrombocytopenia[12-14] and the addition of protease inhibitor-based antiretroviral drugs may offer an additional small advantage.[15] These drugs are thought to exert their effect by an antiviral effect in the bone marrow cells or by decreasing viral load.[16] Improvement may not be immediate, and treatment with other modalities will be necessary in patients with symptomatic bleeding. Since a large component of thrombocytopenia may be due to immune-mediated platelet destruction, the use of steroids (prednisone 1 to 2 mg/kg/d)[11] is effective in 60% to 80%[11] of the cases; however, concerns have been expressed that glucocorticosteroid use may lead to further immunosuppression or that they may accelerate disease in persons with Kaposi's sarcoma.[17] If life-threatening bleeding occurs or if a bleeding patient fails to respond to prednisone, intravenous immunoglobulin (IVIg) in doses of 400 mg/kg daily should be given for 5 days. High doses of immune globulin are effective even in the most refractory of cases, but the expense and availability may limit the extent of their use.[18] However, the duration of response is between 3 and 5 weeks. In addition, prophylactic IVIg or oral glucocorticosteroid treatment is indicated for patients with platelet counts below 20,000/μL.[11] Some recent studies have suggested that Anti-Rh$_0$(D) immune globulin can be effective in the nonsplenectomized Rh$_0$(D)-positive patient.[19] Though not widely used, vincristine has been shown in some studies to be an effective treatment modality.[20] Splenectomy is often appropriate if the patient has had bleeding symptoms during the clinical course and platelets remain below 30,000/μL after 4 to 6 weeks of medical treatment. Splenectomy does not appear to accelerate the progression of HIV/AIDS.[21] Plasmapheresis has been proven to have no therapeutic benefit. For a thorough discussion of management and other treatment options, the reader is referred to Chapter 9 or to the American Society of Hematology Practice Guidelines on ITP.[11]

BLEEDING COMPLICATIONS IN HIV-INFECTED HEMOPHILIA PATIENTS TREATED WITH PROTEASE INHIBITORS

HIV-infected hemophiliacs treated with protease inhibitors often experience excessive bleeding. Reports have included increased frequency of hemorrhage into sites commonly encountered, (i.e., joints, muscle/soft tissues, and brain), and less common sites (i.e., small joints of hands and feet, including soles and palms); in addition, mucocutaneous bleeding and genitourinary bleeding occur commonly.[22-26] The underlying pathophysiology of this increased bleeding is unknown. Ritonavir, saquinavir, and indiavir have all been associated with and implicated in this increased bleeding. The cause may be related to the ability of the drugs to inhibit cytochrome P450, which has an important role in arachidonic acid metabolism, thereby affecting normal platelet function on which the hemophiliac depends. Even though prolonged bleeding times have been reported in some patients,[22] the heightened bleeding tendency is not accompanied by any consistent laboratory abnormality of the coagulation system.

Management

Protease inhibitors are of proven importance in the modern effective management of patients with HIV infection. Since there is no way to predict risk factors for the increased hemorrhagic tendency among patients with hemophilia, those who are being treated with these medications should be observed for increased bleeding tendencies and treated prophylactically with additional

Table 33-1 • SIGNIFICANT HEMATOLOGIC COMPLICATIONS IN HIV/AIDS

- Bone marrow supression
- Anemia
- Idiopathic thrombocytopenic purpura (ITP)
- Thrombotic thrombocytopenic purpura (TTP)
- Protein S deficency
- Anticardiolipin antibodies

factor concentrate if clinically indicated (e.g., 25 IU/kg on alternate days in factor VIII-deficient patients).[24]

THROMBOSIS

An increased incidence of thrombosis (2.6/1000 person-years) has been observed in patients with HIV/AIDS.[27] Besides expected risk factors for thrombosis such as being older than 45 years, having a coexisting opportunistic infection, or being hospitalized, there have been a number of other possible risk factors identified that result from conditions associated with HIV/AIDS.[27] These include acquired protein S deficiency, high levels of anticardiolipin antibodies, heparin cofactor II deficiency, continual use of venous catheters, coexistence of other conditions such as Kaposi sarcoma (KS), infection with cytomegalovirus (CMV), and the use of protease inhibitors. On the other hand, other factors such as race, sex, or mode of HIV exposure have no apparent relationship to the risk for developing thrombosis.

Acquired Protein S Deficiency

The vitamin K-dependent coagulation inhibitor, protein S, serves as a cofactor for activated protein C in the proteolytic degradation of clotting factors Va and VIIIa. Deficiency of protein S increases the risk for venous thrombosis by prolonging the half-life of these activated coagulation factors. The prevalence of hereditary heterozygous protein S deficiency in the general population is about 1 in 30,000; however, acquired protein S deficiency has been reported in 27% to 73% of HIV-infected adults, and as many as 12% of these may develop thrombotic complications.[28,29] No increased levels of the C4b-binding protein were found in any of the patients with decreased protein S levels.[28] However, Bissuel and coworkers did find a correlation between decreased protein S levels and HIV disease progression.[30] Their data suggested that the decrease in protein S levels that they found in 65% of their HIV/AIDS patients occurred during the transition period from HIV infection to clinical AIDS. Lafeuillade and coworkers[31] have observed similar results, though to a smaller magnitude, but have also extended those findings to correlate decreased protein S with the presence of protein S auto-antibodies in HIV-infected patients.[32] In support of these findings, Sorice and coworkers have reported that the association with anti-protein S antibodies was more prevalent in patients with protein S levels below 50%.[33] There have been no reports of decreased protein C levels in these patients. Though the mechanism for decreased protein S levels in HIV/AIDS patients is not clear, it has been suggested that endothelial cell and/or cytokine dysfunction may be contributing factors.[34]

The type of assay used to determine the level of free protein S can affect the number of protein S-deficient patients identified.[35] Some assays use polyethylene glycol precipitation to remove the protein S bound to C4b-binding protein, and the residual unbound (free) protein S is measured in the supernatant. In the presence of high levels of anticardiolipin antibodies, the plasma may contain large amounts of cell-derived microparticles, which also bind free protein S, and are precipitated by the polyethylene glycol. This artifact results in an underestimation of the level of free protein S in plasma and an overestimation of the number of persons with free protein S deficiency. Thus, deficiency of free protein S should be confirmed in other assays. Deficiency of free protein S in HIV-infected patients is correlated with poor prognosis.[35]

Antiphospholipid Antibodies

Antiphospholipid antibodies (including lupus anticoagulants and anticardiolipin antibodies) are associated with thrombotic events in non-HIV-infected patients, and reports of avascular necrosis, skin necrosis, strokes, and other thrombotic events have been reported in HIV/AIDS patients having these antibodies. However, the role of these antibodies in producing thrombosis in patients with HIV/AIDS is unclear. The prevalence of either anticardiolipin antibodies or lupus anticoagulants is 20% to 80% among HIV/AIDS patients.[36,37] No consistent relationship has been established between anticardiolipin antibody titers and active disease, CD4 count,[38] thrombocytopenia,[39] or progression from HIV seropositivity to AIDS.[38] The mechanism responsible for the increased frequency of the antiphospholipid antibodies in HIV/AIDS patients is unknown.

Protease Inhibitors

It has been suggested that the risk for both venous and arterial thrombosis is increased following the initiation of protease inhibitor therapy for HIV. There have been several case reports of premature coronary artery disease and peripheral vascular disease ascribed to protease inhibitor-induced hypercholesterolemia.[40,41] In addition, thromboembolism has been reported within 124 days following initiation of therapy with four different protease inhibitors (ritonavir, indinavir, nelfinavir, and saquinavir).[42] Some of the patients were reported to have required unusually high doses of warfarin (up to 30 mg daily) to maintain a therapeutic International Normalized Ratio (INR) of greater than 2. Because a substantial proportion of the reported patients had historical risk factors for thrombosis, it seems prudent to closely observe patients with a history of risk factors for thromboembolism following the initiating of protease inhibitor therapy.[42]

Management of Thrombosis in Patients With HIV/AIDS

Regardless of the underlying cause, the management of the acute thrombotic event is similar for HIV-infected and noninfected patients. Although the reported frequency of thrombosis in HIV-infected patients is only

2.6/1000 patient-years, many episodes may not be diagnosed because they may simulate complications of AIDS. For example, pulmonary infiltrates may be attributed to infection; occlusion of vessels within the central nervous system may be thought to be related to infection or tumors; and leg swelling may be attributed to malnutrition or low circulating albumin. A high degree of suspicion for thrombosis in patients with such symptoms should be maintained. Signs such as leg swelling or tenderness should be investigated by Doppler ultrasound scanning and ascending venography when indicated. Magnetic resonance imaging may be used as an alternative form of imaging, particularly if no abnormality has been detected on Doppler.

Anticoagulants are normally well tolerated in patients with HIV infection. The duration of anticoagulation in patients with venous thrombosis should be dictated by a number of factors, including the site and extent of the thrombus, a history pulmonary embolus and/or thrombosis,[43] and overall status of the patient.

Initial treatment of an acute venous thrombotic episode should be heparin or low-molecular-weight heparin if no contraindications to anticoagulation exist. The dosage should be adequate to prevent pulmonary embolus or recurrent venous thrombosis. A heparin level that achieves an activated partial thromboplastin time (aPTT) that is equivalent to 0.2 to 0.4 U/mL by protamine titration or 0.3 to 0.6 anti-factor Xa U/mL is recommended.[44] This range is usually achieved with an average daily dose of about 32,000 units by infusion or 35,000 U/day by twice-daily subcutaneous injections. Low-molecular-weight heparin has greater bioavailability and a longer half-life than heparin, thus giving a more predictable response. As it is cleared by the kidneys, the dose should be adjusted in patients with renal dysfunction. Limited data suggest that the therapeutic range is 0.5 to 1.2 anti-factor Xa U/mL.[45] Heparin is given for 5 days along with warfarin at an oral dose of 5 mg daily, which is usually started within 24 hours of the initiation of heparin treatment. Heparin is usually discontinued when the INR measured by the prothrombin time has been therapeutic (i.e., INR of at least 2.0) for 2 consecutive days.[46] Patients with extensive iliofemoral thrombosis or massive pulmonary embolus may benefit from longer courses of heparin.[47]

All patients should receive at least 3 to 6 months of secondary prophylaxis with oral anticoagulants. However, the duration of anticoagulation should be determined after considering a number of factors, including whether the patient has a prior history of thrombosis or pulmonary embolus. In addition, since 9.3% of patients with KS, 9.8% of patients with CMV infection, and as many as 5% to 6% of patients receiving megesterol therapy have been reported to have developed thrombosis,[48] these conditions or situations may be considered additional risk factors. It should be noted that some patients with AIDS who are receiving antiviral therapy may require substantially larger doses of warfarin,[42,49] which should be adjusted to achieve a therapeutic INR. Decisions concerning the use of other higher-risk treatment modalities such as thrombolytic therapy, intracaval filter, or surgical embolectomy or thromboectomy should be made by the physician after considering the individual circumstances of the affected patient.

Consensus guidelines for the use of long-term prophylactic anticoagulation for an individual patient are not yet available. There is growing evidence that the risk for thrombosis is multifactorial, and the relative risks of individual factors are not yet defined. For the time being, decisions concerning prophylaxis against thrombosis remain at the discretion of the clinician. However, the decision needs to be based upon assessing the patient characteristics that are independent risk factors for thrombosis. Besides the risk factors discussed above, others include increasing age, family history, surgery, trauma, hospital or nursing home confinement, malignancy, central vein catheterization, presence of a transvenous pacemaker, and neurologic disease with extremity paresis.

HIV-ASSOCIATED THROMBOTIC MICROANGIOPATHY: THROMBOTIC THROMBOCYTOPENIC PURPURA AND HEMOLYTIC-UREMIC SYNDROME

The two conditions, thrombotic thrombocytopenic purpura (TTP) and hemolytic-uremic syndrome (HUS), that comprise the syndromes of thrombotic microangiopathy (TMA) represent potentially fatal complications of HIV infection that can be managed if correctly diagnosed and promptly treated. Physicians should be alert for the development of TMA. For the most part, the pentad of signs and symptoms that accompany TMA (i.e., thrombocytopenia, microangiopathic hemolytic anemia, neurological deficit, renal dysfunction, and fever) are rarely seen until the disease is well advanced and at a stage when patients do not respond as well to therapy. In addition, thrombocytopenia and anemia are common features of other complications of HIV infection and often complicate the ability to make the appropriate diagnosis. HIV-infected patients who develop TMA before they have progressed to AIDS have a better prognosis, similar to that of the general population who develop TMA. The more common development of TMA among persons with at least one prior

---

Table 33–2 • RISK FACTORS FOR THROMBOEMBOLIC EVENTS IN HIV/AIDS

- Age > 45 years
- Opportunistic infections
- Megestrol acetate
- Indinavir (an inhibitor of HIV protease)
- Hospitalization

AIDS-defining illness[50] carries a much worse prognosis despite any therapeutic attempt.

TTP, the more common TMA condition associated with AIDS, begins with intravascular platelet clumping that often produces reversible obstruction of the capillaries and arterioles of the brain, kidneys, and other organs. Endothelial cell injury is thought to be the initial event and may be mediated by bacterial toxins, antibodies, immune complexes, oxidative injury, or certain drugs. As a result of the injury, there are extraordinary increases in circulating levels of unusually large, highly adhesive, multimers of von Willebrand factor (vWF) that induce platelet agglutination.[51,52] The rise in these levels may be due to either the massive release of the highly polymeric vWF or a reduction of a circulating vWF-cleaving protease (which normally clear the large multimers) either by antibody or reduced production. The exact mechanism of the disease process associated with HIV infection is yet to be defined (see Chapter 22).

Management of AIDS-Associated Thrombotic Microangiopathy

Current management of AIDS-related TMA is directed at removing or reducing the amount of the large species of vWF in the circulation. Plasma infusion or plasma exchange using fresh frozen plasma (FFP), cryoprecipitate-depleted fraction of plasma (cryosupernatant), or solvent/detergent-treated plasma for replacement is considered to be the treatment of choice for TTP.[5,50] It is presumed that such therapy provides supplemental quantities of the proteinase as well as physically removing both the large forms and proteinase antibodies by the plasmapheresis procedure. Survival rates have been dramatically improved even though many patients may remain refractory to therapy. Early recognition of such patients is important since they may benefit from additional complementary therapies. In a review of patients who developed TTP, approximately 73% responded to intensive plasma exchange therapy. This compares to an approximate 19% response rate with other forms of therapy.[50] If plasmapheresis is not immediately available, it has been recommended that an infusion of normal FFP be instituted at 30 mL/kg/day until plasma exchanges can be arranged. Recommended plasma exchanges at the rate of 35 to 40 mL/kg/exchange should be continued for more than 3 days after patients attain complete remission as demonstrated by normal neurologic status, platelet count above 150,000/μL, rising hemoglobin value, and improving serum lactate dehydrogenase levels (below 700 IU/dL). In patients with a partial response, plasma exchanges should continue for additional days to determine if a complete remission is obtainable. In such patients or those with no response, complementary therapy may be considered. Some physicians recommend the addition of glucocorticosteroids in a dosage of 200 mg/day.[54] Red cell transfusions may be required, and, if bleeding is a primary problem as a result of thrombocytopenia, platelet transfusion may be necessary. Platelet transfusions do pose a risk, however, by exacerbating microcirculatory thrombosis in the central nervous system if the process has not been brought under control. Other forms of therapy have been tried with various degrees of success. They include the use of vincristine,[55] splenectomy,[56–60] and other immunosuppressive agents.[56,61] The use of antiplatelet agents such as aspirin[54,56,62–64] and ticlopidine[65,66] remain controversial, and the effectiveness of intravenous dextran has not be established.[57,60,67]

■ REFERENCES

Chapter 33 References

1. Cohen PT, Sande MA, Volberding PA (Eds). The AIDS Knowledge Base, 3rd edition. Philadelphia, Lippincott Williams & Wilkins, 1999.
2. Frontiera M, Myers AM. Peripheral blood and bone marrow abnormalities in the acquired immunodeficiency syndrome. West J Med 1987;147:157–160.
3. Zon LI, Groopman JE. Hematologic manifestations of the human immune deficiency virus (HIV). Semin Hematol 1988;66:25: 208–218.
4. Brown KE, Young NS. Parvovirus B19 infection and hematopoiesis. Blood Rev 1995;9:176–182.
5. Karpatkin S, Nardi MA, Hymes KB. Immunologic thrombocytopenic purpura after heterosexual transmission of human immunodeficiency virus. Ann Intern Med 1988;109:190–193.
6. Zucker-Franklin D, Cao YZ. Megakaryocytes of human immunodeficiency virus-infected individuals express viral RNA. Proc Natl Acad Sci USA 1989;86:5595–5599.
7. Lauache F, Bettaieb A, Henri A, et al. Infection of megakaryocytes by human immunodeficiency virus seropositive patients with immune thrombocytopenic purpura. Blood 1991;78:1697–1705.
8. Kunzi MS, Groopman JE. Identification of a novel human immunodeficiency virus strain cytopathic to megakaryocytic cells. Blood 1993;81:3336–3342.
9. Sullivan PS, Hanson DL, Chu SY, et al. Surveillance for thrombocytopenia in persons infected with HIV; Results from the Multistate Adult and Adolescent Spectrum of Disease Project. J Acquir Immune Defic Syndr 1997;14:374–379.
10. Lord RV, Coleman MJ, Milliken ST. Splenectomy for HIV-related immune thrombocytopenia: comparison with results of splenectomy for non-HIV immune thrombocytopenic purpura. Arch Surg 1998;133:205–210.
11. George JN, Woolf SH, Raskob GE, et al. Idiopathic thrombocytopenic purpura: A practice guideline developed by explicit methods for the American Society of Hematology. Blood 1996;88:3–40.
12. Landonio G, Cinque P, Nosari A, et al. Comparison of two dose regimens of zidovudine in an open, randomized, multicentre study for severe HIV-related thrombocytopenia. AIDS 1993;7:209–212.

Table 33–3 • POSSIBLE THERAPEUTIC MODALITIES FOR THE TREATMENT OF THROMBOCYTOPENIA[a]

- Antiviral therapy with zidovudine
- Glucocorticosteroid therapy
- IVIg therapy
- Anti-Rh₀(D) immune globulin for the nonsplenectomized, Rh₀(D)-positive patient
- Splenectomy

[a] These therapeutic options are listed only to serve as a general guide; complete evaluation of the patient is necessary before any treatment regiment is initiated.

13. Ehmann WC, Rabkin CS, Eyster ME, Goedert JJ. Thrombocytopenia in HIV-infected and uninfected hemophiliacs. Multicenter Hemophilia Cohort study. Am J Hematol 1997;54:296–300.
14. Coyle TE. Hematologic complications of human immunodeficiency virus infection and the acquired immunodeficiency syndrome. Med Clin North Am 1997;81:449–470.
15. Carbonara S, Ingravallo G, Fiorentino G, et al. Efficacy of protease inhibitor-based anti-retroviral therapy in severe HIV-associated thrombocytopenia unresponsive to AZT [letter]. Br J Haematol. 1999;105:1147–1149.
16. Ballem PJ, Belzberg A, Devine DV, et al. Kinetic studies of the mechanisms of thrombocytopenia in patients with human immunodeficiency virus infection. N Engl J Med 1992;327:1779–1784.
17. Guo WX, Antakly T. AIDS-related Kaposi's sarcoma: evidence for direct stimulatory effect of glucocorticoid on cell proliferation. Am J Pathol 1995;146:727–734.
18. Bussel JB, Haimi JS. Isolated thrombocytopenia in patients infected with HIV: treatment with intravenous gammaglobulin. Am J Hematol 1988;28:79–84.
19. Scaradavov A, Woo B, Woloski BM, et al. Intravenous anti-D treatment of immune thrombocytopenic purpura: experience in 272 patients. Blood 1997;89:2689–2700.
20. Mintzer DM, Real FX, Jovino L, Krown SE. Treatment of Kaposi's sarcoma and thrombocytopenia with vincristine in patients with the acquired immunodeficiency syndrome. Ann Intern Med 1985;102:200–202.
21. Oskenhendler E, Berling P, Cheveret S, et al. Splenectomy is safe and effective in human immunodeficiency virus related immune thrombocytopenia. Blood 1993;82:29–32.
22. Wilde JT, Lee CA, Collins P, et al. Increased bleeding associated with protease inhibitor therapy in HIV-positive patients with bleeding disorders. Br J Haematol 1999;107:556–559.
23. Ginsberg JS. Management of venous thromboembolism. N Engl J Med 1996;335:1816–1828.
24. Pollmann H, Richter H, Jürgens H. Platelet dysfunction as the cause of spontaneous bleeding in two haemophilic patients taking HIV protease inhibitors. Thromb Haemost 1998;79:1213–1214.
25. Stanworth SJ, Bolton MJ, Hay CR, Shiach CR. Increased bleeding in HIV-positive haemophiliacs treated with antiretroviral protease inhibitors. Haemophilia 1998;4:109–114.
26. Hagerty SL, Ascher DP. Spontaneous bleeding associated with the use of the protease inhibitor ritonavir in a hemophiliac patient with human immunodeficiency virus infection. Pediatr Infect Dis J 1998;17:929–930.
27. Sullivan PS, Dworkin MS, Jones JL, Hooper WC. Epidemiology of thrombosis in HIV-infected individuals. The Adult/Adolescent Spectrum of HIV Disease project. AIDS 2000;14:321–324.
28. Stahl CP, Wideman CA, Spira TJ, et al. Protein S deficiency in men with long-term human immunodeficiency virus infection. Blood 1993; 81:1801–1807.
29. Sugerman RW, Church JA, Goldsmith JC, et al. Acquired protein S deficiency in children infected with human immunodeficiency virus. Pediatr Infect Dis J 1996;15:106–111.
30. Bissuel F, Berruyer M, Causse X, et al. Acquired protein S deficiency: correlation with advanced disease in HIV-1-infected patients. J Acquir Immune Defic Syndr 1992;5:484–489.
31. Lafeuillade A, Alessi MC, Poizot-Martin I. Protein S deficiency and HIV infection. (letter) N Engl J Med 1991;324:1220.
32. Lafeuillade A, Sorice M, Griggi T. Role of autoimmunity in protein S deficiency during HIV-1 infection. Infection 1994;22: 201–203.
33. Sorice M, Griggi T, Archieri P, et al. Protein S and HIV infection. The role of anticardiolipin and anti-protein S antibodies. Thromb Res 1994;73:165–175.
34. Hooper WC, Phillips DJ, Riberio MJA, et al. Tumor necrosis factor-alpha downregulates protein S secretion in human microvascular and umbilical vein endothelial cells but not in the HepG-2 hepatoma cell line. Blood 1994;84:483.
35. Gris JC, Toulon P Brun S, et al. The relationship between plasma microparticles, protein S and anticardiolipin antibodies in patients with human immunodeficiency virus infection. Thromb Haemost 1996;76:38–45.
36. Cohen AJ, Phillips TM, Kessler CM. Circulating coagulation inhibitors in the acquired immunodeficiency syndrome. Ann Intern Med 1986;104:175.
37. Stimmler MM, Quismorio FP, McGehee WG, et al. Anticardiolipin antibodies in acquired immunodeficiency syndrome. Arch Interm Med 1989;149:1833–1835.
38. Panzer S, Stain C, Hartl H, et al. Anticardiolipin antibodies are elevated in HIV-1 infected hemophiliacs but do not predict for disease progression. Thromb Haemost 1989;61:81–85.
39. Intrator L, Oksenhendler E, Desforges L, Bierling P. Anticardiolipin antibodies in HIV-infected patients with or without thrombocytopenia purpura. Br J Haematol 1988;68:269–270.
40. Vittecoq D, Escaut L, Monsuez JJ. Vascular complications associated with use of HIV protease inhibitors. Lancet 1998;351:1959.
41. Teitel J. A side effect of protease inhibitors. CMAJ 1998;158: 1129–1130.
42. George SL, Swindells S, Knudson R, Stableton JT. Unexplained thrombosis in HIV-infected patients receiving protease inhibitors: Report of seven cases. Am J Med 1999;107:624–626.
43. Geerts WH, Heit JA, Clagett GP, et al. Prevention of venous thromboembolism. Chest 2001;119:132S–175S.
44. Hirsh J, Fuster V. Guide to anticoagulant therapy. Part 1: Heparin. Circulation 1994;89:1449–1468.
45. Weitz JI. Treatment of venous thromboembolism. In Schecter GP, Hoffman R, Schrier SL (eds). Hematology 1999. American Society of Hematology, Washington, DC, pp. 218–222.
46. Kearon C. Initial treatment of venous thromboembolism. Thromb Haemost 1999;82:887–891.
47. Gallus A, Jackaman J, Tillet J, et al. Safety and efficacy of warfarin started early after submassive venous thrombosis or pulmonary embolism. Lancet 1986;ii:1293–1296.
48. Laing RBS, Brettle RP, Leen CLS. Venous thrombosis in HIV infection. Int J STD AIDS 1996;7:82–85.
49. Knoell KR, Young TM, Cousins ES. Potential interaction involving warfarin and ritonavir. Ann Pharmacother 1998;32:1299–1302.
50. Viale P, Pagani L, Alberici F. Clinical features and prognostic factors of HIV-associated thrombotic microangiopathies. Eur J Haematol 1998;60:262–263.
51. Moake JL, Chow TW. Thrombotic thrombocytopenic purpura: Understanding a disease no longer rare. Am J Med Sci 1998; 316:105–119.
52. Furlan M, Robles R, Galbusera M, et al. Von Willebrand factor-cleaving protease in thrombotic thrombocytoopenic purpura and the hemolytic-uremic syndrome. N Engl J Med. 1998;339:1578–1584.
53. Furlan M, Lämmle B. von Willebrand factor in thrombotic thrombocytopoenic purpura. Thromb Haemost 1999;82:592–600.
54. Bell WR, Braine HG, Ness PM, Kickler TS. Improved survival in thrombotic thrombocytopenic purpura-hemolytic uremic syndrome: clinical experience in 108 patients. N Engl J Med 1991; 325:398–402.
55. Gutterman LA, Stevenson TD. Treatment of thrombotic thrombocytopenic purpura with vincristine. JAMA. 1982;247:1433–1436.
56. Bukowski RM, Hewlett JS, Reimer RR, et al. Therapy of thrombotic thrombocytopenic purpura: an overview. Semin Thromb Hemost 1981;7:1–8.
57. Byrnes JJ, Moake JL. Thrombotic thrombocytopenic purpura and the hemolytic-uremic syndrome: evolving concepts of pathogenesis and therapy. Clin Haematol 1986;15:413–442.
58. Moake JL, McPherson PD. von Willebrand factor in thrombotic thrombocytopenic purpura and the hemolytic-uremic syndrome. Transfus Med 1990;4:163–168.

59. Rowe JM, Francis CW, Cyran EM, Marder VJ. Thrombotic thrombocytopenic purpura: recovery after splenectomy associated with persistence of abnormally large von Willebrand factor multimers. Am J Hematol 1985;20:161–168.
60. Thompson CE, Damon LE, Ries CA, Linker CA. Thrombotic microangiopathies in the 1980s: clinical features, response to treatment, and the impact of the human immunodeficiency virus epidemic. Blood 1992;80:1890–1895.
61. Moake JL, Rudy CK, Troll JH, et al. Therapy of chronic relapsing thrombotic thrombocytopenic purpura with prednisone and azathioprine. Am J Hematol 1985;20:73–79.
62. Kamat SG, Turner NA, Konstantopoulos K, et al. Effects of Integrelin on platelet function in flow models of arterial thrombosis. J Cardiovasc Pharmacol 1997;29:156–163.
63. Moake JL. von Willebrand factor abnormalities in thrombotic thrombocytopenic purpura and the hemolytic uremic syndrome. In: Kaplan B, Trompeter R, Moake J (Eds): Hemolytic Uremic Syndrome and Thrombotic Thrombocytopenic Purpura. New York, Marcel Dekker, 1992, pp. 459–471.
64. Moake JL, Eisenstaedt RS. Thrombotic thrombocytopenic purpura and the hemolytic-uremic syndrome. In: Coleman RW, Hirsh J, Marder VJ, Salzman EW (Eds): Hemostatasis and Thrombosis: Basic Principles and Clinical Practices, 3rd edition. Philadelphia, JB Lippincott, 1994, pp. 1064–1075.
65. Gachet C, Cattaneo M, Ohlmann P, et al. Purinoceptors on blood platelets: further pharmacological and clinical evidence to suggest the presence of two ADP receptors. Br J Haematol 1995;91:434–444.
66. Cattaneo M, Lombardi R, Bettega D, et al. Shear-induced platelet aggregation is potentiated by desmopressin and inhibited by ticlopidine. Arterioscler Thromb 1993;13:393–397.
67. Bobbio-Pallavicini E, Porta C, Tacconi F, et al. Intravenous prostacyclin (as epoprostenol) infusion in thrombotic thrombocytopenic purpura: four case reports and review of the literature. Haematologica 1994;79:429–437.

CHAPTER 34

Outpatient Anticoagulant Therapy

Jack E. Ansell, M.D.

The coumarin-type oral anticoagulants have been in use for over 50 years and are well-established weapons in the armamentarium against thrombotic disease.[1] Their discovery evolved from investigations into a hemorrhagic disease of cattle occuring early in the twentieth century attributed to the consumption of spoiled sweet clover. Karl P. Link,[2] a biochemist at the University of Wisconsin, eventually isolated the responsible agent in spoiled sweet clover, dicoumarol (3-3' methyl-bis-4-hydroxy coumarin), which quickly entered the clinical arena through work at the Mayo Clinic in 1941. Link subsequently synthesized a related compound (warfarin), initially popularized as a rodenticide in the late 1940s, that entered clinical practice in the 1950s and quickly became the major oral anticoagulant in clinical use. Little has changed in the formulation of oral anticoagulants. They have remained critically important drugs in the primary and secondary prevention of thromboembolism. In the last 20 years, the use of oral anticoagulants has grown considerably, commensurate with the increased understanding of the important role of thromboembolism in cardiovascular disorders.

MECHANISM OF ACTION

Vitamin K_1 is an essential cofactor in the post-translational γ-carboxylation of several glutamic acid residues in the vitamin K-dependent coagulation factors II, VII, IX, and X (Fig. 34–1). In the absence of γ-carboxylation, these proteins are unable to bind calcium and phospholipid, and depending on the level of carboxylation, they manifest a reduced coagulant (i.e., enzymatic) potential. Warfarin produces its anticoagulant effect by interfering with the cyclic interconversion of vitamin K and its 2,3 epoxide (vitamin K epoxide).[3,4] Warfarin exerts this effect by inhibiting one of two vitamin K epoxide reductases (Fig. 34–1). Dietary vitamin K_1 enters the body in a partially reduced state bypassing the warfarin-sensitive reductase, and thus, replenishing fully reduced vitamin K_1 stores in the presence of warfarin therapy.

PHARMACOKINETICS

Because of its excellent bioavailability and favorable pharmacokinetics, warfarin is the most commonly used oral anticoagulant in North America. It is highly water soluble and rapidly absorbed from the gastrointestinal tract after oral ingestion.[5,6] Peak absorption occurs in 60 to 90 minutes. Food may delay the rate of absorption but is said not to reduce the extent of absorption.

Warfarin is a racemic mixture of stereoisomers known as the R and S forms; each has distinctive metabolic pathways, half-lives, and potencies. Racemic warfarin has an average half-life of 36 to 42 hours, with ranges from 15 to 60 hours. Variability in warfarin half-life, due either to natural differences in metabolism or to disease and/or drug-induced alterations in metabolic fate, account for the marked variations in an individual's initial response to, or maintenance requirement for warfarin. The S form of warfarin (the more potent isomer) is metabolized primarily by the cytochrome P450 system, specifically, the enzyme CYP2C9.[7] A number of genetic polymorphisms in this enzyme have been described that influence both the dose required to achieve a therapeutic level and the bleeding risk with warfarin therapy.[8] Specifically, the CYP2C9*2 and CYP2C9*3 alleles are associated with lower dose requirements and higher bleeding complication rates compared to the wild-type enzyme CYP2C9*1.[8] Warfarin's effect also varies inversely with the amount of vitamin K_1 absorbed (from the diet and from metabolic byproducts of gastrointestinal bacteria) and directly with the amount of warfarin absorbed or available to exert its anticoagulant effect.

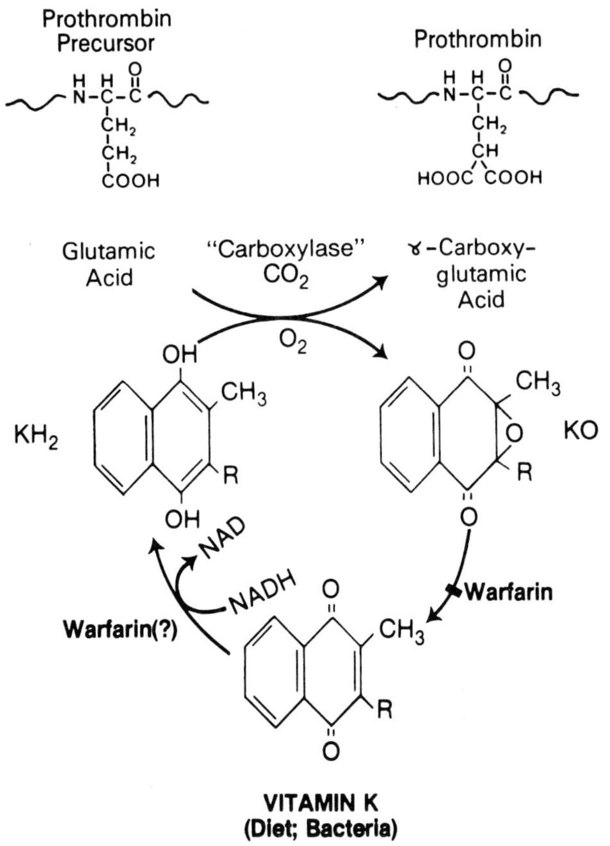

Figure 34-1 Reduced vitamin K is oxidized in the formation of γ-carboxyglutamic acid. Warfarin interferes with the recycling (reduction) of oxidized vitamin K.

WARFARIN AND DRUG INTERACTIONS

Drug interactions commonly occur by affecting the pharmacokinetic or pharmacodynamic behavior of warfarin.[5,9] Drug interactions may interfere with gastrointestinal absorption of warfarin resulting in a reduction in plasma levels, or interfere with the metabolism of warfarin leading to a reduction or increase in clearance, and consequently, higher or lower plasma warfarin levels. The latter effects may be stereospecific in that only one of the stereoisomers may be affected or it may be nonspecific in that both isomers may be affected. Interference in the metabolism of the S isomer, usually by affecting the P450 cytochrome system (CYP2C9 enzyme), is more common and has a greater potential for enhancing the intensity of anticoagulation since the S isomer is several times more potent than the R isomer. Drugs may also decrease plasma warfarin levels by enhancing the metabolic clearance of racemic warfarin.

The pharmacodynamics of warfarin may also be altered when drugs interfere with other aspects of hemostasis or vitamin K_1 homeostasis. Third-generation cephalosporins containing an N-methyl-thiotetrazole side chain are an example in that they interfere with the regeneration of reduced vitamin K_1 from the 2,3 epoxide form. Some drugs or disease states (liver disease, hyperthyroidism) can alter the metabolism of coagulation factors, inhibit coagulation factor interactions by other mechanisms (heparin), or inhibit other aspects of hemostasis (aspirin's effect on platelet function) and lead to a greater risk of bleeding. In general, such interactions are most problematic when interacting drugs are added or deleted (or a dose change is made) from a patient's regimen. Once a patient is stabilized on warfarin and an interacting medication, there should be little problem in maintaining stability of warfarin dosing.

A new problem of recent development is the widespread use of dietary supplements and herbal preparations. Unlike drug products, dietary supplements are not tested prior to marketing for safety, efficacy, dosing requirements, or interactions with other medications. They are not required to meet quality standards for labeling, nor are they required to meet U.S. Pharmacopeia standards for tablet content uniformity. Consequently, patients may be exposed to different ingredients as well as different doses of those ingredients among similar products produced by different manufacturers and among batches from the same manufacturer. There are a growing number of case reports describing interactions between warfarin and dietary supplements, but virtually none of these interactions has been systematically substantiated. Because of the uncertainty that exists, it is wise for patients on warfarin to avoid the use of dietary supplements, or at best, to be carefully observed when beginning or stopping a supplement. For a listing of various drug interactions or reported herbal interactions, the reader is referred elsewhere.[9]

THERAPEUTIC RANGE AND MONITORING OF ORAL ANTICOAGULANTS

The concept of a safe and effective therapeutic range developed largely as a consequence of trial and error and clinical empiricism in the 1940s and 1950s.[1] A prothrombin time (PT) ratio of 2.0 to 2.5 or 3.0, using a human brain thromboplastin reagent sensitive to a reduction in the vitamin K-dependent coagulation factors, was thought to represent this therapeutic range. In North America, manufacturers switched to a less sensitive rabbit brain thromboplastin reagent in the 1950s and 1960s, resulting in the need for a higher average warfarin dose to achieve the same prolongation of the PT.[10] This change was subtle, occurring over years, and physicians did not adjust their treatment by lowering the therapeutic range. Consequently, patients were more intensely anticoagulated. Hull and coworkers[11] demonstrated the consequences of this situation in a study of patients with deep venous thrombosis treated with warfarin by documenting a higher incidence of bleeding in those monitored with the less sensitive rabbit brain thromboplastin, yet no increase in recurrent thromboembolism in those monitored by the more sensitive reagent, when both groups were maintained in a similar therapeutic range.

To correct for differences in thromboplastin sensitivity the World Health Organization recommended the use of an international standard PT.[12] This is achieved

Table 34-1 • USE OF ISI TO CALCULATE AN INR

To convert a prothrombin time (PT) ratio to an INR equivalent:
$$INR = PT\ ratio^x\ (x = ISI)$$
Example:
  PT = 17.9 sec
  Mean of normal range = 12.2 sec
  ISI of thromboplastin = 2.3
Then:
  17.9 ÷ 12.3 = 1.47 PT Ratio
  $1.47^{2.3}$ = 2.4 INR

ISI, International Sensitivity Index; a comparative rating of different thromboplastins
INR, International Normalized Ratio; a comparative rating of prothrombin time ratios for individuals with stable therapeutic anticoagulation

by equilibrating all thromboplastins against a sensitive international reference thromboplastin and then using that equilibration factor (the International Sensitivity Index, or ISI) to convert PT ratios (PT divided by the mean of the normal range) to an international ratio (the International Normalized Ratio, or INR). The INR is essentially the PT ratio one would obtain if the international reference thromboplastin had been used to measure the PT. Table 34–1 demonstrates how a local PT ratio is converted to an INR, which is now performed automatically by laboratory instrumentation. By converting all PT ratios to INRs one can interpret a patient's PT result regardless of where it is performed and then follow the guidelines of international consensus groups for therapeutic effectiveness as outlined in Table 34–2.[13] Use of the INR does not eliminate all discrepancies in PT reporting,[14] but it significantly improves reporting PT results using raw seconds or the PT ratio when monitoring patients on warfarin.

Table 34-2 • INDICATIONS FOR ORAL ANTICOAGULATION AND RECOMMENDED INTENSITY OF TREATMENT

Indication	Target INR (Range)
Prophylaxis of venous thrombosis	2.5 (2.0–3.0)
Treatment of venous thrombosis	2.5 (2.0–3.0)
Treatment of pulmonary embolism	2.5 (2.0–3.0)
Prevention of systemic embolism	
Atrial fibrillation	2.5 (2.0–3.0)
Recurrent systemic embolism	2.5 (2.0–3.0)
Postmyocardial infarction[a]	3.0 (2.5–3.5)
Bioprosthetic heart valves (M or Ao position)[b]	2.5 (2.0–3.0)
Mechanical prosthetic heart valves	
Bileaflet valve[c] in Ao position	2.5 (2.0–3.0)
Bileaflet or tilting valve in M position	3.0 (2.5–3.5)
Mechanical valve + AF (any position)	3.0 (2.5–3.5)
Mechanical valve + additional risk factors	3.0 (2.5–3.5) + aspirin(80 mg/d)

[a] For prevention of recurrent MI, an INR of 3.0 (2.5–3.5) is recommended.
[b] M, mitral valve; Ao, aortic valve.
[c] For St. Jude or Carbomedics bileaflet or Medtronic-Hall tilting disc valve.
From Hirsh J, Dalen JE, Anderson DR, et al. Oral anticoagulants: mechanism of action, clinical effectiveness, and optimal therapeutic range. Chest 2001;119(Suppl):8S-21S, 220S–227S, with permission.

PRACTICAL ASPECTS OF ORAL ANTICOAGULATION MANAGEMENT

Initiation and Maintenance Dosing

The use of a loading dose of warfarin to initiate therapy is of historical interest only. A loading dose induces a rapid, but excessive reduction in factor VII activity, the factor with the shortest half-life, predisposing patients to hemorrhage in the first few days of therapy, while it fails to achieve a more rapid decline of the other vitamin K_1-dependent coagulation factors (II, IX, and X).[15,16] Therefore, therapy is properly initiated using an average maintenance dose (5 mg) for the first 2 or 3 days.[16] When an immediate effect is required, such as in the treatment of acute venous thrombosis, heparin should be given concurrently with warfarin for at least 5 days. Warfarin should overlap with heparin therapy for a period of 4 to 5 days, since it takes that long to lower to vitamin K_1-dependent coagulation factors with a longer half-life. Heparin is usually discontinued when the INR has been in the therapeutic range on two measurements at least 24 hours apart. If treatment is not urgent (e.g., chronic stable atrial fibrillation), warfarin can be commenced out-of-hospital with an anticipated maintenance dose of 4 to 5 mg/d, which usually achieves a therapeutic anticoagulant effect in about 5 days, although a stable INR may take longer to achieve. The fear of creating a hypercoagulable state in patients with unrecognized protein C deficiency who are not simultaneously heparinized has not been substantiated. However, in patients with a known protein C deficiency or other thrombophilic state, it would be prudent to begin heparin before or at the same time as warfarin. There is room for flexibility in selecting a starting dose of warfarin. Some clinicians prefer to use a larger starting dose (e. g., 7.5 to 10 mg). Additionally, lower than 5 mg starting doses might be appropriate in the elderly, in patients with impaired nutrition or liver disease, and in patients at high risk of bleeding. The physician should be aware of factors that influence the response to anticoagulation in the elderly. The dose required to maintain a therapeutic range for patients above the age of 60 years has been shown to decrease with increasing age,[17] and older patients are more likely to have other factors that might influence INR stability or might influence the risk of bleeding such as a greater number of other medical conditions or concurrent drug use.[17] Consequently, it is advisable to monitor older patients more carefully in order to maximize their time in therapeutic range.[18]

Estimation of the maintenance dose is often based on observations of the INR response following a fixed dose of warfarin over a few days interval. An individual who rapidly achieves a high therapeutic PT (INR above 2.0) after two doses of warfarin is likely to require a low maintenance dose. The opposite holds for those who show little elevation of the PT (INR below 1.5) after two doses.

Prothrombin time monitoring is usually performed daily until the therapeutic range has been achieved and maintained for at least 2 consecutive days, then two or three times weekly for 1 to 2 weeks, then less often, depending on the stability of PT results. Immediately after hospital discharge is often the most unstable and dangerous time for patients. Therefore, monitoring should be performed frequently for the first 1 to 2 weeks after discharge. If the PT response remains stable, the frequency of testing can be reduced to intervals as long as every 4 weeks, although there is growing evidence to suggest that more frequent testing will lead to a greater time in therapeutic range. If adjustments to the dose are required, then the cycle of more frequent monitoring is repeated until a stable dose response is again achieved.

Outpatient management of warfarin therapy should aim for simplicity and clarity to avoid patient confusion, poor compliance, and dosing errors that may result in complications.[1] It is recommended that a limited number of warfarin tablet strengths be used in clinical practice and that patients clearly understand the various dosing patterns that are used, such as alternate-day doses or dosing levels based on days of the week.[1]

Management of Nontherapeutic INRs

Patients receiving long-term warfarin therapy often have unexpected fluctuations in dose response that require careful management. These may be due to inaccuracy in PT testing, changes in vitamin K_1 intake (increased or decreased vitamin K_1 in the diet), changes in vitamin K_1 or warfarin absorption (gastrointestinal factors or drug effects), changes in warfarin metabolism (liver disease or drug effects), changes in vitamin K_1-dependent coagulation factor synthesis or metabolism (liver disease, drug effects, other medical conditions), or patient compliance issues (surreptitious self-medication, missed doses, miscommunication about dose adjustment, etc.).

A nontherapeutic (e. g., elevated) INR can be managed by discontinuing warfarin, administering vitamin K_1, or infusing fresh frozen plasma or prothrombin concentrate, although the latter may be difficult to obtain.[19] Recombinant factor VII_a is currently under study as a therapeutic intervention for correcting warfarin-induced anticoagulation.[20] The choice is based largely on the severity of the clinical situation (e. g., the degree of elevation of the INR or the presence of severe bleeding). When warfarin is interrupted, it takes about 4 to 5 days for the INR to return to the normal range in patients whose INR is between 2.0 and 3.0.[21] After treatment with oral vitamin K_1 the INR declines substantially within 24 hours. Since the absolute daily risk of bleeding is low even when the INR is excessively prolonged, many physicians manage patients with INR values of 4.0 to 9.0 by stopping warfarin and monitoring more frequently,[22] unless the patient is at a higher risk of bleeding or bleeding has already developed. Vitamin K_1 can be administered by the intravenous, subcutaneous or oral routes. Intravenous injection may be associated with anaphylactic reactions, yet can reverse even very high INRs in 6 to 8 hours. The response to subcutaneous vitamin K_1 may be unpredictable and sometimes delayed.[23] Recent studies confirm earlier reports that oral administration is predictably effective, and has the advantages of safety and convenience over parenteral routes. Ideally, vitamin K_1 should be administered in a dose that will quickly lower the INR into a safe but not subtherapeutic range without causing resistance once warfarin is reinstated.[24,25] High doses of vitamin K_1, though effective, may lower the INR more than is necessary and lead to warfarin resistance for up to a week.

Table 34-3 • RECOMMENDATIONS FOR MANAGING ELEVATED INRs OR BLEEDING IN PATIENTS RECEIVING ORAL ANTICOAGULANTS BASED ON THE 2001 ACCP RECOMMENDATIONS

INR above therapeutic but less than 5.0 No significant bleeding	Lower dose or omit dose and resume at lower dose when INR therapeutic; if only minimally above therapeutic range, no dose reduction may be required.
INR > 5.0 but < 9.0 No significant bleeding	Omit next one or two doses, monitor more frequently and resume at lower dose when INR therapeutic. Alternatively, omit dose and give vitamin K_1 (1–2.5 mg) orally, particularly if at increased risk of bleeding. If more rapid reversal is required because the patient requires urgent surgery, vitamin K_1 (2–4 mg) orally can be given with the expectation that a reduction of the INR will occur in 24 hours. If the INR is still high, additional vitamin K_1 (1–2 mg) orally can be given.
INR > 9.0 No significant bleeding	Hold warfarin and give higher dose of vitamin K_1 (3–5 mg) orally with the expectation that the INR will be reduced substantially in 24–48 hours. Monitor more frequently and use additional vitamin K_1 if necessary. Resume therapy at lower dose when INR therapeutic.
INR > 20 and/or serious bleeding	Hold warfarin and give vitamin K_1 (10 mg) by slow IV infusion and supplement with fresh plasma or prothrombin complex concentrate depending on the urgency of the situation. Vitamin K_1 can be repeated every 12 hours.
Life-threatening bleeding	Hold warfarin and give prothrombin complex concentrate supplemented with vitamin K_1, 10 mg by slow IV infusion; repeat if necessary depending on INR.

Note: If continuing warfarin therapy is indicated after high doses of vitamin K_1, then heparin can be given until the effects of vitamin K_1 have been reversed and the patient becomes responsive to warfarin therapy.
From Ansell J, Hirsh J, Dalen J, et al. Managing oral anticoagulant therapy. Chest 2001; 119(Suppl):22S-38S, with permission.

Table 34–3 outlines the 2001 American College of Chest Physicians recommendations for managing patients on coumarin anticoagulants who need their INR lowered because of actual or potential bleeding.[19]

Management of Oral Anticoagulation During Invasive Procedures

Clinicians are often confronted with the challenge of managing anticoagulation in individuals requiring noncardiac surgery or other invasive procedures, especially in individuals with prosthetic heart valves. There is a paucity of critical studies examining the alternative choices for anticoagulation in this setting. Physicians must assess the risk of bleeding from a procedure if anticoagulation is continued versus the risk of thrombosis if anticoagulation is discontinued, as well as the cost of alternative anticoagulation options. This subject has been reviewed recently with suggested alternative options based on an estimate of the pre-and postoperative daily risk of bleeding or thrombosis.[26] Traditionally, full-dose, intravenous unfractionated heparin has been the standard for patients who need full anticoagulant protection that is readily reversible before a procedure. Its major drawback is the complexity and cost associated with intravenous heparin therapy and hospitalization. Low-molecular-weight heparin (LMWH) offers another, less complex alternative in that it requires no monitoring and can be given at home.[27–29] Warfarin is usually discontinued 4 days before the procedure and the INR allowed to decline. Two days before the procedure LMWH is started, usually at a full treatment dose (100 to 150 antiX$_a$ units/kg subcutaneously) once or twice daily depending on the risk of thrombosis, with the last dose given the night before the procedure (approximately 12 hours prior to the procedure). It is then restarted about 12 hours after the procedure along with warfarin. When the INR becomes therapeutic, LMWH is stopped. Studies suggest that LMWH is a simple and less costly alternative for full anticoagulation protection, but randomized, controlled trials are still needed to identify the best means of alternative anticoagulation. Table 34–4 summarizes the 2001 ACCP Chest Consensus Conference recommendations for management of oral anticoagulation during invasive procedures.[19]

Dental procedures represent a particularly common intervention for patients on anticoagulants. A recent comprehensive review of the subject indicated that in most cases no change in the intensity of anticoagulation is needed.[30] If there is need to control local bleeding, tranexamic acid or ε-amino caproic acid (EACA) mouthwash have been used successfully without interrupting anticoagulant therapy.[31,32]

Diagnostic Evaluation of Bleeding

When bleeding occurs, especially from the gastrointestinal or urinary tract, it is important to consider the possibility of a serious, underlying occult lesion as the source of bleeding. A number of descriptive studies indicate the probability of finding such a lesion.[33–36] Coon and Willis[34] identified occult lesions responsible for bleeding in 11% of 292 patients with hemorrhage. Jaffin and coworkers[35] found a 12% prevalence of positive stool occult blood tests in 175 patients on warfarin or heparin compared with 3% in 74 controls. There was no difference between the mean PT or aPTT in patients with or without lesions. In 16 patients evaluated, 15 had a lesion not previously suspected and 4 had neoplastic disease. Landefeld and coworkers[33] found 14 of 41 patients with gastrointestinal bleeding to have important remediable lesions of which 2 were malignant. This limited informa-

Table 34–4 • RECOMMENDATIONS FOR MANAGING ANTICOAGULATION IN PATIENTS REQUIRING INVASIVE PROCEDURES BASED ON THE 2001 ACCP RECOMMENDATIONS

Low risk of thromboembolism[a]	Stop warfarin ~4 days before surgery, allow the INR to return to near normal, briefly use postoperative prophylaxis (if the intervention itself creates a higher risk of thrombosis) with low-dose heparin, 5000 units SC, and simultaneously begin warfarin therapy.
Intermediate risk of thromboembolism	Stop warfarin ~4 days before surgery, allow the INR to fall, cover the patient beginning 2 days preoperatively with low-dose heparin, 5000 units SC, or a prophylactic dose of LMWH and then commence low-dose heparin (or LMWH) and warfarin postoperatively.
High risk of thromboembolism[b]	Stop warfarin ~4 days before surgery, allow the INR to return to normal; begin therapy with full-dose heparin or full-dose LMWH as the INR falls (~2 days preoperatively). Heparin can be given as a SC injection as an outpatient; it can then be given as a continuous IV infusion after admission in preparation for surgery and discontinued 5 hours before surgery with the expectation that the anticoagulant effect will have worn off at the time of surgery. It is also possible to continue with SC heparin or LMWH and to stop therapy 12–24 hours before surgery with the expectation that the anticoagulant effect will be very low or have worn off at the time of surgery.
With low risk of bleeding	Continue warfarin at a lower dose and operate at an INR of 1.3–1.5, an intensity that has been shown to be safe in randomized trials of gynecologic and orthopedic surgical patients. The dose of warfarin can be lowered 4 or 5 days before surgery. Warfarin therapy can then be restarted postoperatively, supplemented with low-dose heparin (5000 units SC), if necessary.

[a] Low risk of thromboembolism: examples include no recent venous thromboembolism (> 3 months); atrial fibrillation without a history of stroke; bileaflet mechanical cardiac valve in aortic position.
[b] High risk of thromboembolism: examples include recent (< 3 months) history of venous thromboembolism; mechanical cardiac valve in mitral position; old model of cardiac valve (ball/cage).
From Ansell J, Hirsh J, Dalen J, et al. Managing oral anticoagulant therapy. Chest 2001; 119(Suppl):22S–38S, with permission.

tion supports the need for investigation, since if occult blood is found in the stool, there may be a 5% to 25% chance of finding a malignant source.

In a randomized controlled study, Culclasure and coworkers[37] found microscopic hematuria at a prevalence of 3.2% in a warfarin-treated group compared with a prevalence of 4.8% in their nonanticoagulated control group. There was no difference in the rate of hematuria with therapeutic or high INRs. Following a second episode of hematuria, 43 patients (32 anticoagulated and 11 control) were investigated; 27 of 32 (84%) of the anticoagulated and 8 of 11 (73%) of the control patients were found to have significant underlying diseases with a total of 3 patients (from both groups) having cancers (7%). These findings are in contrast to results of other case series identifying a much higher likelihood of finding underlying lesions in patients who develop hematuria while receiving anticoagulant therapy.[38–40]

MANAGING THE RISKS OF ORAL ANTICOAGULANT THERAPY

Over the last 20 years several developments have improved the safety and efficacy of oral anticoagulation. These include defining the optimal intensity of therapy by well-designed randomized trials and standardizing the reporting of PTs using the INR, leading to more appropriate and standardized therapy. Less, however, has occurred until recently to substantially improve the management of oral anticoagulation. There is growing evidence that coordinated programs focused on anticoagulant management achieve a high rate of maintaining patients in therapeutic range leading to good outcomes. Time in therapeutic range (TTR) is an important measure of the quality of anticoagulation care. A strong relationship between time in therapeutic range (TTR) and bleeding or thrombosis rates has been observed across a large number of studies with different patient populations, different target ranges, different scales for measuring intensity of anticoagulation (i.e., PT, PT ratio, and INR), and different models of dose management.[41–48] In a large, representative study by Cannegieter and coworkers,[41] the relationship between TTR and major bleeds was approximately exponential—that is, small increases above the target range were associated with small-to-moderate increases in bleeding rates, while large increases above the target range were associated with large increases in bleeding rates. A similar relationship holds for decreases below the target therapeutic range and thromboembolism rates.

Anticoagulation Management Services

A coordinated and focused approach to the management of therapy by specialized programs (anticoagulation clinics) significantly improves clinical outcomes by improving therapeutic control and TTR, lessening the frequency of hemorrhage or thrombosis, and decreasing the use of medical resources, leading to more cost-effective therapy. These programs are characterized by a knowledgeable provider who manages therapy, an organized system of follow-up, rapid and reliable INR monitoring, and good patient communication and education.

Most patients receiving chronic oral anticoagulation today are managed by their personal physician along with all other patients in their physician's practice without an organized program of management, education, or follow-up.[19,49] There are only a few studies assessing clinical outcomes in this "usual care" model of management (Table 34–5).[50–52] These studies indicate a rate of major hemorrhage of at least 7% to 8% per patient-year of therapy. There is a similar rate of recurrent or de novo thromboembolism for an overall serious adverse event rate of at least 15% per patient-year of therapy. These adverse events are generally a consequence of poor therapeutic control with hemorrhage or thrombosis occuring as a consequence of excessive or subtherapeutic anticoagulation.

These outcomes can be contrasted to the rates identified in a large number of retrospective and some prospective studies of care delivered by an anticoagulation management service (Table 34–6).[41,43,44,53–61] These mostly observational studies indicate a more than 50% reduction in both major hemorrhage and thrombosis compared to usual care.

Lastly, Table 34–7 summarizes studies examining both models of management where coordinated care is measured against a control group of usual care within each study.[62–65] These mostly nonrandomized, retrospective analyses provide further evidence for the benefit of coordinated care.

A few studies also suggest a significant cost benefit to coordinated compared to usual care by a reduction

Table 34–5 • FREQUENCY OF MAJOR HEMORRHAGE/THROMBOEMBOLISM IN PATIENTS MANAGED UNDER A USUAL CARE MODEL OF MANAGEMENT

Study/Year	No. Patients	No. Patient Years	Years of Data Collection	New or Established Patients	Indications	Maj Hem[a]	Fatal Hem[a]	Rec TE[a]
Landefeld and Goldman[50] 1989	565	876	1977–1983	New	Ven & Art	7.4	1.1	NA
Gitter et al.[51] 1995	261	221	1987–1989	Estab	Ven & Art	8.1	0.45	8.1
Beyth et al.[52] 1998	264	440	1986–1993	New	Ven & Art	5.0	0.68	NA

[a] Major and fatal hemorrhage and thromboembolism rates expressed as percent per patient-year of therapy; fatal hemorrhagic events also included with major hemorrhage. Ven & Art, mixed indications in the venous and arterial system; NA, not available; TE, thromboembolism.

Table 34-6 • FREQUENCY OF MAJOR HEMORRHAGE/THROMBOEMBOLISM IN PATIENTS MANAGED UNDER AN ANTICOAGULATION MANAGEMENT SERVICE

Study/Year	No. Patients	No. Patient Years	Years of Data Collection	New or Established Patients	Indications	Target PTR/INR	Maj Hem[a]	Fatal Hem[a]	Rec TE[a]
Forfar[44] 1982	541	1,362	1970–1978	N & E	Ven & Art	1.8–2.6^{PTR}	4.2	0.14	NA
Errichetti et al.[53] 1984	141	105	1978–1983	N & E	Ven & Art	1.3–2.0^{PTR}	6.6	NA	NA
Conte et al.[54] 1986	140	153	1975–1984	N & E	Ven & Art	1.7–2.5^{PTR}	2.6	NA	8.4
Petty et al.[55] 1988	310	385	1977–1980	N & E	Ven & Art	NA	7.3	0.77	NA
Charney et al.[56] 1988	73	77	1981–1984	N & E	Ven & Art	1.5–2.5^{PTR}	0	0	5.0
Bussey et al.[57] 1989	82	199	1977–1986	N	Ven & Art	NA	2.0	NA	3.5
Seabrook et al.[58] 1990	93	158	1981–1988	N	Ven & Art	1.5–2.0^{PTR}	3.8	0	2.5
Fihn et al.[59] 1993	928	1,950	NA	N	Ven & Art	1.3–1.5^{PTR} 1.5–1.8^{PTR}	1.7	0.2	7.5
van der Meer et al.[43] 1993	6,814	6,085	1988	N & E	Ven & Art	2.4–5.3^{INR}	3.3	0.64	NA
Cannegieter et al.[41] 1995	1,608	6,475	1985–	N & E	Mech Valves	3.6–4.8^{INR}	2.5	0.33	0.7
Palareti et al.[60,61] 1996, 1997	2,745	2,011	1993–1995	N	Ven & Art	2.0–3.0^{INR} 2.5–4.5^{INR}	1.4	0.24	3.5

[a] Major and fatal hemorrhage and thromboembolism rates expressed as percent per patient year of therapy; fatal hemorrhagic events also included with major hemorrhage. Ven & Art, mixed indications in the venous and arterial systems; NA, not available; TE, thromboembolism.

in adverse events and reduced utilization of hospital services. Gray and coworkers[66] estimated a savings of $860 per patient-year of therapy as a result of reduced hospital days per patient-year. Chiquette and coworkers[65] reported cost savings through a coordinated approach compared to usual care of approximately $1320 per patient-year of therapy.

PATIENT SELF-TESTING AND PATIENT SELF-MANAGEMENT (See Chapter 35)

As a result of technological advances in PT measurement, there is potential for further simplifying and improving anticoagulation management by point-of-care (POC) testing. POC testing allows for the determination of a PT from a fingerstick sample of whole blood, and consequently, opens the possibility for patient self-testing. Portability of instrumentation means that INR measurements are no longer confined to the physician's office, a private laboratory, or a nearby hospital, but can be moved into the patient's home or even taken with the patient when travelling. Standardization of reagents and instruments, as well as reliance on the INR, further reduces the inaccuracies of multiple reagents and laboratories.

Since the late 1980s, a number of instruments have been introduced or are in development (Table 34–8).[67] These instruments are based on clot detection methodology using thromboplastin to initiate clot formation, while the endpoint of clot detection varies from instrument to instrument. The validity of this methodology was initially established in 1987 by Lucas and cowork-

Table 34-7 • FREQUENCY OF MAJOR HEMORRHAGE/THROMBOEMBOLISM IN PATIENTS MANAGED UNDER USUAL MEDICAL CARE VERSUS ANTICOAGULATION MANAGEMENT SERVICE

Study/Year	Model of Care	No. Patients	No. Patient Years	Years of Data Collection	Indications	Target PT/INR	Maj Hem[a]	Fatal Hem[a]	Rec TE[a]	Comb Hem/TE[a]	Cost Savings[a]
Garabedian-Ruffalo et al.[62] 1985	UC	26	64.3	1977–1980	Ven & Art	1.5–2.5^{PTR}	12.4	0	6.2	18.6	
	AMS	26	41.9	1980–1983	Ven & Art	1.5–2.5^{PTR}	2.4	0	0	2.4	$860
Cortelazzo et al.[63] 1993	UC	271	677	1982–	Mech Valves	25–35%[b]	4.7	0	6.6	11.3	
	AMS	271	669	1987–1990	Mech Valves	3.0–4.5^{INR}	1.0	0	0.6	1.6	
Wilt et al.[64] 1995	UC	44	28	1988–1993	Ven & Art	NA	17.8	0	42.8	60.6	
	AMS	68	60	1988-1993	Ven & Art	NA	0	0	0	0	$4,072
Chiquette et al.[65] 1998	AMS	82	199	1977–1986	Ven & Art	NA	2.0	NA	3.5	5.5	
	UC	142	102	1991–1992	Ven & Art	NA	3.9	0.9	11.8[c]	15.7	
	AMS	176	123	1992-1994	Ven & Art	NA	1.6	0	3.3	4.9	$1,621

[a] Major and fatal hemorrhage, thromboembolism, and cost savings rates expressed as percent per patient year of therapy; fatal hemorrhagic events included with major hemorrhage.
[b] Prothrombin activity.
[c] Two TE events fatal.
Ven & Art, mixed indications in the venous and arterial systems; UC, usual care; AMS, anticoagulation management service; TE, thromboembolism.

Table 34-8 • CAPILLARY WHOLE BLOOD (POINT-OF-CARE) PT INSTRUMENTS

Instrument	Clot Detection Methodology	Home Use Approval	Type of Sample
Protime Monitor 1000 Coumatrak[a] Ciba Corning 512 Coagulation Monitor[a] CoaguChek Plus[a] CoaguChek Pro[a] CoaguChek Pro/DM[a]	Clot initiation: Thromboplastin Clot detection: Cessation of blood flow through capillary channel		Capillary WB Venous WB
CoaguChek Thrombolytic Assessment System	Clot initiation: Thromboplastin Clot detection: Cessation of movement of iron particles	Yes (CoaguChek only)	Capillary WB Venous WB Plasma
ProTIME Monitor Hemochron Jr[b] GEM PCL[b]	Clot initiation: Thromboplastin Clot detection: Cessation of blood flow through capillary channel	Yes	Capillary WB Venous WB
Avosure Pro + Avosure Pro Avosure PT	Clot initiation: Thromboplastin Clot detection: Thrombin generation detected by fluorescent thrombin probe	Yes	Capillary WB Venous WB Plasma

[a] All instruments in this category are based on the original Biotrack model (Protime Monitor 1000) and licensed under different names. The latest version available is the CoaguChek Pro and Pro/DM (as models evolved they acquired added capabilities). Earlier models no longer available.
[b] Hemochron Jr and GEM PCL are simplified versions of the ProTIME Monitor.

ers[68] using the Biotrack instrument (Biotrack; Biotrack Inc; Freemont, CA) showing a correlation coefficient of 0.96 between reference plasma PTs and capillary whole blood PTs. Within-day precision using two different levels of controls revealed coefficient of variations of 4.9% and 2.9%. The accuracy of the instrument was not compromised by hematocrit measurements ranging from 23% to 54%. Similar results have been obtained by others,[69,70] but some investigators have identified limits of comparability because of the high ISI (i.e., low sensitivity) of one company's thromboplastin, as well as the inability to determine a true geometric mean normal PT for the instrument.[71,72] Studies by McCurdy and White[73] indicated that the INR correlation was adequate within an INR range of 2.0 to 3.0 (the therapeutic range for most indications), but it began to lose its comparabil-

Table 34-9 • PATIENT SELF-TESTING/PATIENT SELF-MANAGEMENT STUDIES

Study/Year	Study Design	Study Groups	No. Patients	Time in Range (% of days)	Major Hemorrhage (%/pt-yr)	Thromboembolism (%/pt-yr)	Indications
White et al,[80] 1989	RCT	PST AMS	23 23	93 75	0 0	0 0	Mixed Mixed
Anderson et al.[81] 1993	Inception Cohort	PST	40	2.3	0	0	Mixed
Beyth and Landefeld[82] 1997	RCT	PST UC	162 163	56 33	5.7 12	9 13	Mixed Mixed
Ansell et al.[83,84] 1989, 1995	Obs Matched cont	PSM AMS	20 20	89 68	0 0	0 0	Mixed Mixed
Bernardo[85] 1996	Obs	PSM	216	83	NA	NA	Heart Valves
Horstkotte et al.[86] 1996	RCT	PSM UC	75 75	92 59	4.5[a] 10.9[a]	0.9 3.6	Heart Valves Heart Valves
Hasenkam et al.[87] 1997	Obs Matched cont	PSM UC	20 20	77 53	NA NA	NA NA	Heart Valves Heart Valves
Sawicki[88] 1999	RCT	PSM UC	90 89	57/53[b] 34/43[b]	2.2 2.2	2.2 4.5	Mixed Mixed
Koertke et al.[89] 2000	RCT	PSM UC	581 567	78 60	1.8 2.7	2.4 4.5	Mixed Mixed

[a] Major and minor bleeding.
[b] Time in range at 3 months and 6 months.
RCT, randomized controlled trial; Obs, observational; PST, patient self-testing; PSM, patient self-management; AMS, anticoagulation management service; UC, usual care; Mixed, mixed indications.

ity as the INR increased above 4.5. These limitations suggest that there is room for further improvement, but they do not negate the potential advantages. Although the appropriate studies have not been done, it is possible that this new system is significantly more reliable and consistent than the variable and haphazard PT monitoring often employed in the usual care of most patients on oral anticoagulants.[74] These POC instruments have been tested in a number of different clinical settings and their accuracy and precision are considered to be more than adequate for the monitoring of oral anticoagulant therapy in both adults and children.[75-79]

A number of studies have demonstrated the ability of patients to perform self-testing and obtain an accurate result.[80-82] Patients can then call their physician and obtain instructions for warfarin dose adjustment. Table 34–9 summarizes those studies where clinical outcomes, either time in therapeutic range or adverse events, have been reported. Patient self-testing can also incorporate patient self-management of warfarin dosing, and a number of studies have shown this model of care to be safe and effective as well.[83-89] These studies are also summarized in Table 34–9.

Based on the foregoing, POC PT monitors offer the potential to lower the risk/benefit profile of anticoagulant therapy; to improve patient satisfaction and possibly patient compliance; and by reducing the labor intensity of physician management, to encourage the more widespread use of warfarin. The cost-effectiveness of such therapy needs to be studied.

REFERENCES

Chapter 34 References

1. Ansell J. Oral anticoagulant therapy: Fifty years later. Arch Intern Med 1993;153:586–596.
2. Link KP. The discovery of dicumarol and its sequels. Circulation 1959;19:97–107.
3. Stenflo J, Fernlund P, Egan W, et al. Vitamin K dependent modifications of glutamic acid residues in prothrombin. Proc Natl Acad Sci USA 1974;71:2730–2733.
4. Nelsestuen GL, Zytkovicz TH, Howard JB. The mode of action of vitamin K: Identification of gamma carboxyglutamic acid as a component of prothrombin. J Biol Chem 1974;249:6347–6350.
5. Hirsh J. Oral anticoagulant drugs. N Engl J Med 1991;324:1865–1875.
6. Wittkowsky AK. Warfarin pharmacology. In: Ansell JE, Oertel LB, Wittkowsky AK (Eds): Managing Patients on Oral Anticoagulants: Clinical and Operational Guidelines. Gaithersburg, Md, Aspen Publishers, 1997.
7. Miners JO, Birkett DJ. Cytochrome P4502C9: an enzyme of major importance in human drug metabolism. Br J Clin Pharmacol 1998;45:525–538.
8. Aithal GP, Day CP, Kesteven PJ, et al. Association of polymorphisms in the cytochrome P450 CYP2C9 with warfarin dose requirement and risk of bleeding complications. Lancet 1999;353:717–719.
9. Hansten P, Wittkowsky AK. Warfarin drug interactions. In: Ansell JE, Oertel LB, Wittkowsky AK (Eds): Managing Patients on Oral Anticoaglants: Clinical and Operational Guidelines. Gaithersburg, Md, Aspen Publishers, 1997.
10. Hirsh J, Levine MN. The optimal intensity of oral anticoagulant therapy. JAMA 1987;258:2723–2726.
11. Hull R, Hirsh J, Jay R, et al. Different intensities of anticoagulation in the long-term treatment of proximal venous thrombosis. N Engl J Med 1982;307:1676–1681.
12. Kirkwood TBL. Calibration of reference thromboplastins and standardization of the prothrombin time ratio. Thromb Haemost 1983;49:238–244.
13. Hirsh J, Dalen JE, Anderson DR, et al. Oral anticoagulants: mechanism of action, clinical effectiveness, and optimal therapeutic range. Chest 2001;119(Suppl):8S–21S.
14. Hirsh J, Poller L. The International Normalized Ratio: A guide to understanding and correcting its problems. Arch Intern Med 1994;154:282–288.
15. O'Reilly RA, Aggeler PM. Studies on coumarin anticoagulant drugs: initiation of warfarin therapy without a loading dose. Circulation 1968;38:169–177.
16. Harrison L, Johnston M, Massicotte MP, et al. Comparison of 5 mg and 10 mg loading doses in initiation of warfarin therapy. Ann Intern Med 1997;126:133–136.
17. Gurwitz JH, Avorn J, Ross-Degnan D, et al. Aging and the anticoagulant response to warfarin therapy. Ann Intern Med 1992;116:901–904.
18. McCormick D, Gurwitz JH, Goldberg J, et al. Long-term anticoagulation therapy for atrial fibrillation in elderly patients: Efficacy, risk, and current patterns of use. J Thromb Thrombolysis 1999;7:157–163.
19. Ansell J, Hirsh J, Dalen J, et al. Managing oral anticoagulant therapy. Chest 2001;119(Suppl):22S–38S.
20. Berntorp E, Stigendal L, Lethagen S, et al. NovoSeven in warfarin-treated patients. Blood Coagul Fibrinolysis 2000;11(Suppl 1):S113–S116.
21. White RH, McKittrick T, Hutchinson R, et al. Temporary discontinuation of warfarin therapy: Changes in the international normalized ratio. Ann Intern Med 1995;122:40–42.
22. Lousberg TR, Witt DM, Beall DG, et al. Evaluation of excessive anticoagulation in a group model health maintenance organization. Arch Intern Med 1998;158:528–534.
23. Raj G, Kumar R, McKinney P. Time course of reversal of anticoagulant effect of warfarin by intravenous and subcutaneous phytonadione. Arch Intern Med 1999;159:2721–2724.
24. Weibert RE, Le DT, Kayser SR, et al. Correction of excessive anticoagulation with low dose oral vitamin K_1. Ann Intern Med 1997;125:959–962.
25. Crowther MA, Donovan D, Harrison L, et al. Low dose oral vitamin K reliably reverses over anticoagulation due to warfarin. Thromb Haemost 1998;79:1116–1118.
26. Kearon C, Hirsh J. Management of anticoagulation before and after elective surgery. N Engl J Med 1997;336:1506–1511.
27. Johnson J, Turpie AGG. Temporary discontinuation of oral anticoagulants: Role of low molecular weight heparin. Thromb Haemost 1999;Suppl(Aug):62–63.
28. Tinmouth A, Kovacs MJ, Cruickshank M, et al. Outpatient peri-operative and peri-procedure treatment with dalteparin for chronically anticoagulated patients at high risk for thromboembolic complications. Thromb Haemost 1999;Suppl(Aug):662.
29. Spandorfer JM, Lynch S, Weitz HH, et al. Use of enoxaparin for the chronically anticoagulated patient before and after procedures. Am J Cardiol 1999;84:478–480.
30. Wahl MJ. Dental surgery in anticoagulated patients. Arch Intern Med 1998;158:1610–1616.
31. Sindet-Pedersen S, Ramstrom G, Bernvil S, et al. Hemostatic effect of tranexamic mouthwash in anticoagulant-treated patients undergoing oral surgery. N Engl J Med 1989;324:840–843.
32. Soute JC, Oliver A, ZuaZu-Jausoro I, et al. Oral surgery in anticoagulated patients without reducing the dose of oral anticoagulant: a prospective randomized study. J Oral Maxillofac Surg 1996;54:27–32.
33. Landefeld CS, Rosenblatt MW, Goldman L. Bleeding in outpatients treated with warfarin: Relation to the prothrombin time and important remedial lesions. Am J Med 1989;87:153–159.

34. Coon WW, Willis PW. Hemorrhagic complications of anticoagulant therapy. Arch Intern Med 1974;133:386–392.
35. Jaffin BW, Bliss CM, Lamont JT. Significance of occult gastrointestinal bleeding during anticoagulation therapy. Am J Med 1987;83:269–272.
36. Wilcox CM, Truss CD. Gastrointestinal bleeding in patients receiving long-term anticoagulant therapy. Am J Med 1988;84:683–690.
37. Culclasure TF, Bray VJ, Hasbargen JA. The significance of hematuria in the anticoagulated patient. Arch Intern Med 1994;154:649–652.
38. Caralis P, Gelbard M, Washer J, et al. Incidence and etiology of hematuria in patients on anticoagulant therapy. Clin Res 1989;37:791A.
39. Schuster GA, Lewis GA. Clinical significance of hematuria in patients on anticoagulant therapy. J Urol 1987;137:923–925.
40. van Savage JG, Fried FA. Anticoagulant associated hematuria: a prospective study. J Urol 1995;153:1594–1596.
41. Cannegieter SC, Rosendaal FR, Wintzen AR, et al. The optimal intensity of oral anticoagulant therapy in patients with mechanical heart valve prostheses: the Leiden artificial valve and anticoagulation study. N Engl J Med 1995;333:11–17.
42. European Atrial Fibrillation Trial Study Group. Optimal oral anticoagulant therapy in patients with nonrheumatic atrial fibrillation and recent cerebral ischemia. N Engl J Med 1995;333:5–10.
43. van der Meer FJM, Rosendaal FR, Vandenbroucke JP, et al. Bleeding complications in oral anticoagulant therapy: An analysis of risk factors. Arch Intern Med 1993;153:1557–1562.
44. Forfar JC. Prediction of hemorrhage during long-term oral coumarin anticoagulation by excessive prothrombin ratio. Am Heart J 1982;103:445–446.
45. Ezekowitz MD, Bridgers SL, James KE, et al. Warfarin in the prevention of stroke associated with nonrheumatic atrial fibrillation. N Engl J Med 1992;327:1406–1412.
46. Boston Area Anticoagulation Trial for Atrial Fibrillation Investigators. The effect of low dose warfarin on the risk of stroke in patients with nonrheumatic atrial fibrillation. N Engl J Med 1990;323:1505–1511.
47. Connoly SJ, Laupacis A, Gent M, et al. Canadian atrial fibrillation anticoagulation (CAFA) study. J Am Coll Cardiol 1991;18:349–355.
48. Petersen P, Boysan G, Godtfredsen J, et al. Placebo-controlled, randomized trial of warfarin and aspirin for prevention of thromboembolic complications in chronic atrial fibrillation: the Copenhagen AFASAK Study. Lancet 1989;1:175–179.
49. Ansell JE, Hughes R. Evolving models of warfarin management: Anticoagulation clinics, patient self-monitoring, and patient self-management. Am Heart J 1996;132:1095–1100.
50. Landefeld CS, Goldman L. Major bleeding in outpatients treated with warfarin. Incidence and prediction by factors known at the start of outpatient therapy. Am J Med 1989;87:144–152.
51. Gitter MJ, Jaeger TM, Petterson TM, et al. Bleeding and thromboembolism during anticoagulant therapy: A population based study in Rochester, Minnesota. Mayo Clin Proc 1995;70:725–733.
52. Beyth RJ, Quinn LM, Landefeld S. Prospective evaluation of an index for predicting the risk of major bleeding in outpatients treated with warfarin. Am J Med 1998;105:91–99.
53. Errichetti AM, Holden A, Ansell J. Management of oral anticoagulant therapy: Experience with an anticoagulation clinic. Arch Intern Med 1984;144:1966–1968.
54. Conte RR, Kehoe WA, Nielson N, et al. Nine-year experience with a pharmacist-managed anticoagulation clinic. Am J Hosp Pharm 1986;43:2460–2464.
55. Petty GW, Lennihan L, Mohr JP, et al. Complications of long-term anticoagulation. Ann Neurol 1988;23:570–574.
56. Charney R, Leddomado E, Rose DN, et al. Anticoagulation clinics and the monitoring of anticoagulant therapy. Int J Cardiol 1988;18:197–206.
57. Bussey HI, Rospond RM, Quandt CM, et al. The safety and effectiveness of long-term warfarin therapy in an anticoagulation clinic. Pharmacotherapy 1989;9:214–219.
58. Seabrook GR, Karp D, Schmitt DD, et al. An outpatient anticoagulation protocol managed by a vascular nurse-clinician. Am J Surg 1990;160:501–504.
59. Fihn SD, McDonell M, Martin D, et al. Risk factors for complications of chronic anticoagulation: a multicenter study. Ann Intern Med 1993;118:511–520.
60. Palareti G, Leali N, Coccheri S, et al. Bleeding complications of oral anticoagulant treatment: An inception-cohort, prospective collaborative study (ISCOAT). Lancet 1996;348:423–428.
61. Palareti G, Manotti C, D'Angelo A, et al. Thrombotic events during anticoagulant treatment: results of the inception-cohort, prospective, collaborative ISCOAT study. Thromb Haemost 1997;78:1438–1443.
62. Garabedian-Ruffalo SM, Gray DR, Sax MJ, et al. Retrospective evaluation of a pharmacist-managed warfarin anticoagulation clinic. Am J Hosp Pharm 1985;42:304–308.
63. Cortelazzo S, Finazzi G, Viero P, et al. Thrombotic and hemorrhagic complications in patients with mechanical heart value prosthesis attending an anticoagulation clinic. Thromb Haemost 1993;69:316–320.
64. Wilt VM, Gums JG, Ahmed OI, et al. Pharmacy operated anticoagulation service: improved outcomes in patients on warfarin. Pharmacotherapy 1995;15:732–779.
65. Chiquette E, Amato MG, Bussey HI. Comparison of an anticoagulation clinic and usual medical care: anticoagulation control, patient outcomes, and health care costs. Arch Intern Med 1998;158:1641–1647.
66. Gray DR, Garabedian-Ruffalo SM, Chretien SD. Cost justification of a clinical pharmacist-managed anticoagulation clinic. Drug Intel Clin Pharm 1985;19:575–580.
67. Leaning KE, Ansell JE. Advances in the monitoring of oral anticoagulation: point-of-care testing, patient self-monitoring, and patient self-management. J Thromb Thrombolysis 1996;3:377–383.
68. Lucas FV, Duncan A, Jay R, et al. A novel whole blood capillary technique for measuring prothrombin time. Am J Clin Pathol 1987;88:442–446.
69. Yano Y, Kambayashi J, Murata K, et al. Bedside monitoring of warfarin therapy by a whole blood capillary coagulation monitor. Thromb Res 1992;66:583–590.
70. Weibert RT, Adler DS. Evaluation of a capillary whole blood prothrombin time measurement system. Clin Pharm 1989;8:864–867.
71. Jennings I, Luddington RJ, Baglin T. Evaluation of the Cibra Corning Biotrack 512 coagulation monitor for the control of oral anticoagulation. J Clin Pathol 1991;44:950–953.
72. Tripodi A, Arbini AA, Chantarangkul V, et al. Are capillary whole blood coagulation monitors suitable for the control of oral anticoagulant treatment by the international normalized ratio? Thromb Haemost 1993;70:921–924.
73. McCurdy SA, White RH. Accuracy and precision of a portable anticoagulation monitor in a clinical setting. Arch Intern Med 1992;152:589–592.
74. Mennenmeyer ST, Winkelman JW. Searching for inaccuracy in clinical laboratory testing using Medicare data: evidence for prothrombin time. JAMA 1993;269:1030–1033.
75. Tripodi A, Chantarangkul V, Clerici M, et al. Determination of the international sensitivity index of a new near-patient testing device to monitor oral anticoagulant therapy. Thromb Haemost 1997;78:855–858.
76. Kaatz AA, White RH, Hill J, et al. Accuracy of laboratory and portable monitor international normalized ratio determinations. Arch Intern Med 1995;155:1861–1867.
77. Ansell J, Becker D, Andrew M, et al. Accurate and precise prothrombin time measurement in a multicenter anticoagulation trial employing patient self-testing. Blood 1995;86(Suppl 1):864a.

78. Andrew M, Marzinotto V, Adams M, et al. Monitoring of oral anticoagulant therapy in pediatric patients using a new microsample PT device. Blood 1995;86(suppl 1):863a.
79. Ansell JE, Zweig S, Meyer B, et al. Performance of the Avocet$_{PT}$ prothrombin time system. Blood 1998;92(Suppl 1):112b.
80. White RH, McCurdy A, Marensdorff H, et al. Home prothrombin time monitoring after the initiation of warfarin therapy: a randomized, prospective study. Ann Intern Med 1989;111:730–737.
81. Anderson D, Harrison L, Hirsh L. Evaluation of a portable prothrombin time monitor for home use by patients who require long-term oral anticoagulant therapy. Arch Intern Med 1993; 153:1441–1447.
82. Beyth RJ, Landefeld CS. Prevention of major bleeding in older patients treated with warfarin: results of a randomized trial. J Gen Intern Med 1997;12:66 (abstr).
83. Ansell J, Holden A, Knapic N. Patient self-management of oral anticoagulation guided by capillary (fingerstick) whole blood prothrombin times. Arch Intern Med 1989;149:2509–2511.
84. Ansell J, Patel N, Ostrovsky D, et al. Long-term patient self-management of oral anticoagulation. Arch Intern Med 1995; 155:2185–2189.
85. Bernardo A. Experience with patient self-management of oral anticoagulation. J Thromb Thrombolysis 1996;2:321–325.
86. Horstkotte D, Piper C, Wiemer M, et al. Improvement of prognosis by home prothrombin estimation in patients with life-long anticoagulant therapy. Eur Heart J 1996;17(suppl):230 (abstr).
87. Hasenkam JM, Kimose HH, Knudsen L, et al. Self-management of oral anticoagulant therapy after heart valve replacement. Eur J Cardiothorac Surg 1997;11:935–942.
88. Sawicki PT, Working Group for the Study of Patient Self-Management of Oral Anticoagulation. A structured teaching and self-management program for patient receiving oral anticoagulation. A randomized controlled trial. JAMA 1999;281:145–150.
89. Koertke H, Minami K, Breymann T, et al. INR self-management following mechanical heart valve replacement. Are education level and therapeutic compliance connected? J Thromb Thrombolysis 2000;9(Suppl 1):S41–S46.

Near-Site Testing in Hemostatic Disorders

B. Gail Macik, M.D.

With the consolidation of centralized testing to buildings often miles away from the patient, the "turn-around time" for a laboratory result is lengthening. For routine tests, consolidation improves cost effectiveness and is unlikely to be detrimental to patient care. However, for the bleeding patient or the patient receiving a hemostatic drug, delayed testing cannot accurately monitor the rapidly changing clinical situation. Several coagulation test systems are available that perform whole-blood prothrombin time (PT), activated partial thromboplastin time (aPTT), heparin monitoring, platelet function tests, and other tests of hemostatic function near the site of patient care.[1] Some point-of-care (POC) technologies offer testing superior to that performed in the centralized laboratory or that is otherwise unavailable. Others are not as precise as those available in the laboratory, but provide clinically equivalent results that expedite care.

In 1999, a survey reported the availability of 16 analyzers manufactured by 10 companies for measuring hemostasis at the point of patient care.[1] Are these instruments necessary for the care of patients? Hematologists for years have relied on centralized testing and concentrated on diagnostic testing. The POC market has grown primarily in response to the demands of cardiologists, interventional radiologists, surgeons, and anesthesiologists. As interventions have become more complex and utilize a cadre of new antiplatelet and anticoagulant drugs, real-time monitoring of rapidly changing hemostatic parameters become an important component of care. Diagnosis is less of an issue than following the course of a pharmacologic manipulation. In order to function as a consultant to the procedure-oriented specialties, the hematologist must become familiar with the technologies that are emerging to monitor patients during procedures.

In addition, the practicing hematologist must also become familiar with new regulations governing the use of laboratory instruments. The Clinical Laboratories Improvement Act (CLIA) is a set of guidelines outlining the training and regulatory requirements necessary to operate any laboratory instrument. Instruments are rated as low or high complexity depending on the level of expertise required to operate the instrument and interpret the results. A special "waived" category exists for very simplistic tests that require little expertise. Any individual or institution engaged in using laboratory instruments must register for CLIA approval unless the only instruments or tests performed are in the "waived" category.

When is a POC test indicated? The most obvious answer is when the test does not exist in the central laboratory. For example, most centralized laboratories offer no equivalent to the activated clotting time (ACT) for monitoring high-dose heparin during cardiac interventions and surgery. The need for time-sensitive information is another potential indication for POC testing. If a drug or clinical condition is of brief duration, waiting even 1 or 2 hours for a result from the central laboratory indicates only what *was* happening and not what *is* happening to the patient. On the other hand, obtaining a test result within minutes if no clinical decision will be made for hours is not appropriate use of POC testing. Finally, a POC instrument may improve care by enabling patient self-testing and management. For example, monitoring of warfarin by home PT instruments has the potential to improve anticoagulation control.

What are the cost implications and medical-legal ramifications of POC testing? POC tests usually cost more per test than similar automated batch testing performed in the central laboratory. Cost effectiveness, however, must take into account the effect on all aspects of care. Does rapid testing lead to improved outcome and fewer complications? Does the patient spend less time in the operating room or the hospital? Is the medical professional able to work more efficiently and cost effectively?

Is the patient spared unnecessary blood transfusions or medical interventions? Currently clinical trials are looking at answering the above questions and validating the perceived benefit of POC testing. Since all the POC tests discussed in this chapter have U.S. Food and Drug Administration (FDA) approval, medical-legal questions regarding the use of these instruments has not been an active concern.

OVERVIEW OF HEMOSTATIC NEAR-SITE TESTING

Evaluating the array of instruments for near-site testing (NST) is a daunting experience. Knowing the characteristics and limitations of the technology improves the chance of selecting an appropriate test system.[2] The ideal POC test system is rapid, accurate, easy to use, transportable, and low cost. Additional desirable features include sample recognition software, continuous electronic monitoring of the system, electronic quality control, a program for transferring results to an information system, and a compact design to compete for space in the crowded workplace.[1-3] Fresh fingerstick samples are popular because of the ease and rapidity of collection, but citrated samples allow repeat testing and addition of other tests to the same sample. Choice of sample, adaptation of quality-control procedures, correlation to plasma-based assays, and determination of reference ranges are particular challenges for coagulation POC test systems. New instruments have appeared, and older systems have been given new names as technology and distributors change. All systems in this review are FDA cleared for marketing. Other technologies are available for "research use only," but they are "not for use in diagnostic procedures." No specific endorsement or ranking of tests is implied. To expedite inquiries regarding a product, Table 35–1 lists the contact information for manufacturers and distributors discussed in this chapter. To help follow the course of a technology, earlier generations of the same instrument that have different names than the current model are listed also.

OVERVIEW OF PLATELET FUNCTION ANALYZERS

Bruising and oozing patients are the bane of the surgeon and internist alike. Poor platelet function, congenital or drug induced, and von Willebrand disease (vWD) are common culprits. Traditional laboratory assessment is complicated, delayed, and limited in scope. New POC technologies are available that provide global assessment of primary hemostasis. The instruments are easy to use, provide results in less than an hour, and in some cases provide information not available from larger laboratory instruments. As with most NST, monitoring of therapy, either blood product replacement or antiplatelet drugs, is the most common reason for requesting a platelet analyzer. Table 35–2 lists the POC analyzers available. The instrument systems differ in the ease of use, parameters tested, and applicability of the test for detecting platelet and/or von Willebrand factor (vWF) abnormalities.[4] Compared to the bleeding time and platelet aggregation studies, the results of NST may prove more clinically relevant than existing test methods.

Ultegra Rapid Platelet Function Assay

The Ultegra Rapid Platelet Function Assay (RPFA) (Accumetrics, San Diego, California) assesses abciximab-induced glycoprotein (GP) IIb/IIIa receptor blockade by performing a semiquantitative, whole-blood platelet function assay.[5-7] A turbidimetric-based optical system detects platelet-induced agglutination of microparticles. Platelets are activated to express GP IIb/IIIa receptors that bind to the fibrinogen-coated beads and induce agglutination. Abciximab blocks GP IIb/IIIa receptors, decreasing the ability of platelets to bind and agglutinate the microparticles. The result is reported as a platelet aggregation unit (PAU). A post-drug infusion PAU is compared to the pre-drug infusion PAU to determine the percentage of platelet inhibition.

The analyzer measures $9.5 \times 9.25 \times 4$ inches and weighs 4 pounds. No external computer connection is required, but an optional printer is available. The cartridge contains a lyophilized preparation of human fibrinogen-coated beads, thrombin receptor activating peptide (iso-TRAP), preservative, and buffer. The analyzer reads from the encoded cartridge the assay type and specific lot number. The quality control system includes an electronic control cartridge, two levels of assayed "wet" controls, an in-cartridge humidity sensor, and a test for concurrence of the two assay channels. The analyzer performs electronic self-diagnostics and stores information including patient identification and assay results. No data management is available.

The assay requires a citrated whole blood sample tested within 15 minutes of collection. The evacuated blood-draw tube attaches directly to the instrument. The analyzer automatically dispenses blood into the cartridge. The result is available in less than 2 minutes. Concomitant medications that do not alter results include aspirin, ticlopidine, clopidogrel, heparin, warfarin, acetaminophen and other nonsteroidal anti-inflammatory drugs, β-adrenergic blockers, calcium channel blockers, "statins," and nitrates. Variable platelet counts between 100,000 and 350,000/μL, hematocrits between 25% and 45%, and fibrinogen levels between 200 and 600 mg/dL do not affect the assay results. Other GP IIb/IIIa inhibitors, including tirofiban and eptifibatide, do affect the baseline PAU. Clinical trials report that the Ultegra RPFA is equivalent to a radiolabeled abciximab receptor blockade assay or platelet aggregometry for monitoring abciximab therapy.[5-7] The Ultegra RPFA offers streamlined technology with a rapid result, but it is limited to monitoring GP IIb/IIIa receptor blockers and is lacking a data management package.

Whole Blood Aggregation

The Whole Blood Aggregometer (WBA) is a modified version of the larger platelet aggregometer manufac-

Table 35-1 • COAGULATION POINT-OF-CARE INSTRUMENTS

Company	Instrument and Tests	Names of Earlier Versions/ Alternate Names
Accumetrics, San Diego, CA 800-643-1641 www.accumetrics.com	Ultegra Rapid Platelet Function Assay (RPFA): monitors GP IIb/IIIa blockers	
Bayer Diagnostics, Medfield, MA 800-255-3232 www.bayerdiag.com	Rapidpoint Coag: PT ONE, PT NC, PT, aPTT, HMT, HMT low range (LHMT)	Thrombolytic Assessment System (TAS) (Pharmanetics, formerly Cardiovascular Diagnostics, Inc.)
Chrono-log Corporation, Havertown, PA 800-247-6665 www.chronolog.com	Whole Blood Aggregometer (WBA): Platelet function test	
Dade Behring, Deerfield, IL 800-241-0420 www.dadebehring.com	PFA-100: platelet function analyzer	
Haemoscope, Inc., Skokie, IL	Thromboelastogram (TEG)	
Instrumentation Laboratory, Lexington, MA 800-955-9525 www.ilww.com	GEM PCL: PT, aPTT, ACT, LR-ACT	Similar to Hemochron Jr.
International Technidyne Corporation, Edison, NJ 800-631-5945 www.itcmed.com	Hemochron Jr. Signature: PT, aPTT, ACT, ACTLR ProTime: home PT Hemochron Response: aPTT, TT, HNTT, HiTT, HRT, PRT, RXDX	Hemochron 401 Hemochron 801 Hemochron 8000
LifeScan, Inc., Milpitas, CA 800-972-2699 www.lifescan.com	Harmony INR Monitoring System	
Medtronic Perfusion Systems, Minneapolis, MN www.medtronic.com/cardiac/perfusion	ACT II: ACT, high-range heparinase test (HRHTC), PT, general-purpose cartridge (GPC) Hepcon HMS analyzer: same as ACT II and heparin management package; HemoSTATUS assay	HemTec ACT
Pharmanetics, Raleigh, NC www.pharmanetics.com	Thrombolytic Assessment System: heparin management panel (HMP)	Rapidpoint Coag: distributor heparin tests
Roche Diagnostics Corporation, Indianapolis, IN 800-329-8566 www.roche.com	CoaguChek S: PT CoaguChek: home PT CoaguChek Pro-DM: PT, aPTT, ACT	CoaguChek Pro CoaguChek Plus Biotrack (512) Coumatrak
Sienco Inc., Wheat Ridge, CO 800-432-1624 www.sienco.com	SonoClot	

Table 35-2 • PLATELET FUNCTION ANALYZERS FOR NEAR-SITE TESTING

Company	Instrument	Test Method	Procedure
Accumetrics	Ultegra Rapid Platelet Function Assay (RPFA)	Monitors abciximab only Optical detection of fibrin-coated bead agglutination; drug decreases agglutination	Simple—no pipetting or sample prep
Chrono-log Corporation	Whole Blood Aggregometer (WBA)	Platelet aggregation detected by whole blood electrical impedance Arachidonic acid, collagen, ristocetin, ADP agonists may be used	Moderate—pipet and dilute sample, pipet agonist, each agonist 6 min
Dade-Behring	PFA-100 platelet function analyzer	Occlusion of an aperture in a collagen/ADP or collagen/Epi cartridge Tests platelet adhesion (vWF), activation, aggregation in a flow system	Simple—pipet sample
Medtronic Perfusion System	HemoSTATUS: special cartridges and software for the Hepcon HMS analyzer	Indirect test of platelet function related to platelet activating factor (PAF)-induced shortening of the ACT	Simple—but requires Hepcon HMS system

tured by Chrono-log Corporation (Havertown, Pennsylvania). Both systems use electrical impedance to study platelet aggregation in whole blood. A citrated whole blood sample is diluted with an equivalent volume of isotonic saline and incubated at 37°C. Platelet aggregation is detected by passing a small electrical current between two electrodes immersed in the sample and measuring the impedance between the electrodes. Platelet aggregation occurs at the electrodes, increasing the impedance. The increase in impedance is directly proportional to the platelet mass deposited on the electrode probe. The final increase in ohms is displayed as a numeric LED readout.

Measuring $6 \times 13 \times 9$ inches and weighing 10 pounds, the WBA was designed to be smaller, simpler, and more portable.[8] One or two test channels are available. Automated calibration and readout functions and electronic quality control are provided. An optional printer and data management software are offered. Limitations include the lack of a positive identification system for the patient specimen and the lack of an onboard system for automatic error detection.

The WBA performs all the studies available using the larger instruments, but the smaller design makes it best suited for perioperative or antiplatelet drug monitoring. Like the parent model, the WBA may be used to detect platelet function abnormalities that increase bleeding risk during surgery.[9,10] For drug monitoring, Mascelli and coworkers[8] report that the WBA predicts the amount of GP IIb/IIIa receptor blockade induced by the drug abciximab. Difficulties associated with the system include the need to rinse the electronic probe in water and saline between samples, the requirement for strict pipetting, and the length of the testing—6 minutes for each agonist. Overall, it is more labor intensive than other POC tests, but the technology is well proven in the original, larger WBAs.

PFA-100 Platelet Function Analyzer

The PFA-100 Platelet Function Analyzer (Dade-Behring, Deerfield, Illinois) is an automated alternative to existing techniques for assessing platelet function.[11–13] The PFA-100 measures platelet function under flow conditions that mimic the process of primary hemostasis in a damaged blood vessel. Whole blood passes through an aperture cut into a membrane coated with collagen and either epinephrine or ADP. The system measures the ability of platelets to occlude the aperture and reports the closure time. The biologic stimuli and the high shear rates generated by the standardized flow result in platelet attachment, activation, and aggregation; therefore, the system can detect defects at any stage of platelet function.

The analyzer measures $15.1 \times 9 \times 14.2$ inches, weighs 24 pounds, and is best classified as a bench-top instrument. The disposable test cartridges contain all components for test performance. The collagen/epinephrine (CEPI) cartridge is used first to screen for platelet dysfunction induced by intrinsic platelet defects, vWF defects, or inhibitory drugs or substances. The collagen/ADP (CADP) cartridge does not detect aspirin and it is used with the CEPI to exclude an aspirin-like effect. Citrated whole blood, 800 μL, is transferred into the sample reservoir of the cartridge by pipet. Results are reported as closure times in seconds. Platelet counts of less than 100,000/μL affect the closure time, but the time is not significantly impacted by the hematocrit until it decreases to 15% to 20%. Heparin and oral anticoagulants do not affect the closure time, but antiplatelet drugs do.[12–14] Neither electronic nor wet quality control materials are available, so fresh control blood is required each day. Systems for automatic error detection and for identification of patient specimen and reagent are provided. Patient data can be transferred to an information system, but data management capability is lacking.

Several studies support the PFA-100's utility in a variety of clinical settings.[11–21] The instrument can be used to help diagnose vWD,[15,16] monitor antiplatelet drugs including ReoPro,[11,14,17] detect aspirin effects,[11–14,18] and uncover congenital[19] and acquired[20] platelet function defects. The instrument has also been used to evaluate platelet-induced hemostasis in the pediatric population.[21]

In a representative study by Ortel and coworkers,[12] 305 patients from 12 different clinical settings were enrolled in a study to evaluate the PFA-100 in a population typical of a tertiary care practice. Of these patients, 29% reported a previous blood transfusion, 29% reported taking aspirin, and 19% were on oral anticoagulants. Of this population, 37% had a prolongation of the closure time. Isolated prolongation of the CEPI closing time for patients on aspirin was the most common abnormality (69%). Conversely, only 68% of patients who reported taking aspirin had a prolonged closure time. The study was not designed to correlate bleeding risk with closure times, and indeed there was no correlation between results with hemorrhagic symptoms or a history of blood transfusions. In all, 93.5% of the patients with a prolonged closure time were found to have a specific quantitative or qualitative abnormality in platelet or vWF function. Other studies report 88% to 100% sensitivity for uncovering an underlying defect.[11–21] The PFA-100 advantages include its rapidity (results in 5 minutes), simplicity (three-step procedure), and global assessment of primary hemostatic function. Disadvantages include open sample handling, pipetting, lack of defined quality controls, and negative effect of moderately decreased platelet counts. More studies designed to correlate bleeding with closure times are needed.

HemoSTATUS Platelet Activated Clotting Test

The HemoSTATUS assay is a family of cartridges used to measure platelet function using the Hepcon HMS analyzer (Medtronic® Perfusion Systems, Minneapolis, Minnesota). The Hepcon HMS platform is discussed in a later section. The system is used during cardiopulmonary bypass to determine pre-, intra-, and postoperative hemostasis. The test is a modified clotting time study that is designed to isolate and test platelet function.

Platelet activating factor (PAF) is a potent, endogenous platelet activator that stimulates in-vitro clot formation. Increasing concentrations of PAF are present in channels 3 to 6 of the cartridge, while channels 1 and 2 serve as controls. A kaolin-activated clotting time (k-ACT) is determined for each channel. Platelet procoagulant activity is determined by measuring the PAF-induced shortening of the k-ACT.

A whole blood sample is collected in a 3-mL syringe that is then secured to the Hepcon HMS instrument. The instrument automatically distributes a 0.35-mL volume to each of the six channels in the self-contained test cartridge. Results are shown as a percentage of normal function. Based on these results, the HemoSTATUS test results are interpreted as low incidence of platelet-related bleeding (80% to 120%); moderate incidence of platelet-related bleeding (60% to 80%); and high incidence of platelet-related bleeding (0% to 60%).

The HemoSTATUS test has been reported to correlate with blood loss after cardiac bypass surgery,[22] but other investigators have found no correlation.[23] The test has been used to evaluate the effect of DDAVP during surgery,[24] to detect GP IIb/IIIa blockade by abciximab,[25,26] and to determine the need for platelet transfusion perioperatively.[27] ε-Aminocaproic acid (EACA) and aspirin do not affect the HemoSTATUS test.[25,27] Platelet counts must be above 50,000 to 70,000/μL and the white blood count must be between 4,000 and 9,000/μL.[26] The controlled, reproducible test procedure is an advantage that is offset by the need for a large, expensive instrument.

OVERVIEW OF CLOT-DETECTION ANALYZERS

When is a second not a second? When it is used to report the result of a coagulation test. Clotting time is determined by assay design, not clinical condition. For example, 300 seconds actual time may indicate a high heparin concentration for an ACT assay or it may be a normal clotting time for a whole blood aPTT system. Simply put, clotting times are "man-made" and there is nothing "physiological" about a 300-second clotting time. The result of a PT, aPTT, or ACT test must be interpreted using the normal and therapeutic ranges determined specifically for the assay method.[28-32]

Technology designed for POC testing must provide clinical information equal to that obtained with a standard laboratory method. Equality does not imply identical form or numerical result.[2] However, most manufacturers of POC testing systems succumb to clinical pressure and convert their results to a "plasma equivalent time" to mimic laboratory ranges. Satisfying clinical demand masks the true differences between testing systems. Results differ because of the sample type, reagent, or detection method used by an instrument.[2,28-30] Freshness of the sample may also affect the result, as clotting factors degrade and drug effects decay. Mathematical conversion of data cannot correct for all these variables. A new test method is compared to an existing technology to provide a frame of reference. Dissimilar numerical results may correlate better than results altered to give the illusion of being the same number. The take-home message is, look for correlation between methods, but do not expect identical results when comparing different testing systems.

For the PT, the International Normalized Ratio (INR) improves comparability between results obtained using different reagents and assay systems. However, the INR fails to "normalize" whole blood results reliably, cannot overcome inherent differences in clot detection methods, and cannot completely offset the effect of reagents with markedly different sensitivities (ISI).[28-30] Heparin monitoring with an aPTT or ACT test has become an even greater challenge as new reagents and detection methods have entered the market. No INR-like system exists to even attempt to "normalize" differences in heparin response curves observed with different reagents and testing systems.[31,32] Against these obstacles the following POC instruments are striving to be accepted as accurate and reliable alternatives to standard laboratory testing.

Home PT Test Systems

Self-testing and self-management of warfarin are slowly emerging as reliable alternatives to traditional provider-based care. Over 40,000 patients in Europe and North America are using a PT monitor at home. Several studies report that patients can test, adjust dosage, and achieve therapeutic goals as well as or better than healthcare providers or an anticoagulation clinic.[33-38] Complications of warfarin therapy decrease by as much as 76% if values remain in the therapeutic range.[36] A prospective, controlled trial reported by Watzke and coworkers[35] is representative of other studies. The investigators compared the quality of anticoagulation based on self-testing versus management by a physician-directed anticoagulation clinic in 113 consecutive patients. The self-management group performed four times more tests, made a significantly greater number of dose adjustments, and achieved an 84.5% success rate for keeping the PT in the target range compared to 73.8% for the control group. Complications included a severe gastrointestinal hemorrhage (INR 2.9) and a transient ischemic attack (INR 2.6), both occurring at therapeutic INR levels in the self-management group. The improved testing outcome is likely due to the increased number of INR determinations and dose adjustments performed, but the impact of patient motivation cannot be ignored. Additionally, less time is spent out of therapeutic range because of the immediate feedback of results. Table 35–3 lists the home PT test systems. For home testing, the instrument must be extremely easy to use with no pipetting and a limited number of steps. Long-term studies to verify the clinical impact of home management are needed, but a new standard for anticoagulation control is on the horizon.

ProTime Microcoagulation System

The ProTime microcoagulation analyzer is a CLIA-waived home-testing system. (International Techni-

Table 35–3 • PT HOME TESTING MONITORS

Company	Instrument	Test Method	Procedure
International Technidyne Corporation	ProTime	Optical detection of clot formation by interruption of blood flow. High and low controls are included on test cartridge	Simple—fingerstick
LifeScan, Inc.	Harmony	Optical detection of clot formation	Simple—fingerstick
Roche Diagnostics	CoaguChek S CoaguChek	Optical detection of cessation of movement of paramagnetic iron particles as clot forms	Simple—fingerstick

dyne, Edison, New Jersey). The analyzer is a table-top device measuring 2.5 × 4.5 × 9 inches and weighing 3 pounds. The system uses a fingerstick sample and the sample cup must be completely filled or an error message is generated. There is no electronic control, but the test card has integrated quality-control reaction chambers that allow controls to be run with every patient sample. It takes approximately 6 minutes to generate a test result. The instrument sends data to a printer, but data management and automated transfer of data to an information system are not available.

The ProTime uses an optical method to detect clot formation. Blood is added to a sample cup on the test cartridge. The sample is drawn into five parallel reaction channels and mixed with the appropriate reagents. When the blood clots, it no longer flows past the optical detector and a clotting time is generated. The result is reported as a plasma equivalent clotting time with calculated INR. The two outside channels serve as high and low controls with appropriate modifiers added to the channels to produce a clotting time within a predetermined value. The three middle reaction channels test the patient's blood in triplicate and a mean value is reported.

The ProTime has been evaluated at many clinical sites and compared in several studies with laboratory and other POC devices.[30,39–41] A representative correlation coefficient compared to a laboratory standard is 0.93 and imprecision studies reveal coefficients of variation of 3% to 6%. As for other POC PT monitors, the INR result shows a positive bias (i.e, overestimation on the lower end of the therapeutic range) when compared to standard laboratory methods.[30,41] Biasiolo and coworkers[39] studied 150 patients presenting to the anticoagulation clinic in a 15-day period. The average difference between the NST and the laboratory method was 0.2 INR. A difference of more than 1.0 INR was obtained in 5 of 150 (3%) patients. In four of five discordant patients, the difference was clinically relevant and in two of five the error was noted to be due to delay in filling the sample chamber. On a smaller number of patients ($n = 30$), Chapman and coworkers[40] reported far more variation between the ProTime and a standard laboratory value with a mean INR difference of 0.56 and 50% discordance in clinical management prompted by the result. The majority of studies, however, find the ProTime equivalent to other methods for managing anticoagulation therapy. The integrated high and low controls are a clear advantage for the ProTime. The relatively large volume of fresh whole blood required to fill the cuvette may provide some testing difficulty.

CoaguChek and CoaguChek S

The CoaguChek PT monitoring system (Roche Diagnostics Corporation, Indianapolis, Indiana) is commonly sited in the literature.[30,34,40–43] Recently, the CoaguChek has been updated to the CoaguChek S, a more user-friendly model. Despite similar sounding names, CoaguChek S (a.k.a. CoaguChek) and CoaguChek Pro-DM (a.k.a. CoaguChek Plus or CoaguChek Pro) are two different operating systems with different characteristics. Only the CoaguChek is approved for home use. The CoaguChek measures 8.8 × 5.5 × 2.2 inches and weighs 1.51 pounds. A fingerstick sample is required. The system has onboard error control and an electronic quality control. A lyophilized wet quality control material may be used. The CoaguChek S provides a test result in about 1 minute. The system does not have data management or download capability, but 60 tests may be stored (30 with CoaguChek). The CoaguChek S is available in multiple languages and results are reported as an INR, Quick %, or ratio.

Blood (approximately 10 μL) is applied to the sample well on the test strip and drawn by capillary action into a reaction chamber, where it is mixed with a dry PT reagent. Paramagnetic iron particles are present in the reaction chamber and they move in response to a magnetic field. Reflectance photometry detects change in particle movement with clot formation and the time is converted into a plasma equivalent clotting time and INR.

The system is a proven POC device, widely used in clinical trials.[35,40–43] Numerous studies have found the imprecision to be between 3% and 6% and the representative correlation coefficients range from 0.9 to 0.97. Chapman and coworkers[40] reported a 0.28 INR average difference between the CoaguChek and the laboratory value, with a 8.3% discordance rate in clinical management decisions. The instrument is reliable and is proving itself adept in the home market.

Harmony INR Monitoring System

The newest instrument to enter the market for home protime monitoring is the Harmony INR Monitoring

System (LifeScan, Inc., Milpitas, California). In the fall of 2001, the FDA cleared the product for use by patients at home and by healthcare professional in their medical offices. The new system is expected to be available for purchase in 2002 by healthcare professionals and by prescription to patients who have completed a training program on the use of the device. The instrument is small (approximately 8 × 2 × 3 inches) and weighs only 355 grams. A 20 µL whole blood sample is added to the test strip, the blood is drawn into the reaction cells and mixed with recombinant human thromboplastin reagent. The clot is detected by a change in light transmission through the blood sample. The result is ready in 90 seconds. There are two levels of quality control material integrated into the test strip, eliminating the need for separate quality control tests. The instrument has been compared to other POC PT monitors and found equivalent. Publications outlining clinical performance should be available soon.

Multitest Systems: PT, aPTT, ACT

Table 35–4 lists the analyzers offering a broader testing menu. These instruments are used primarily for monitoring anticoagulation therapy, or for guiding blood product replacement for the perioperative or bleeding patient. Heparin monitoring is a particular strong suit of several of these test systems. Despite the growing use of low-molecular-weight heparin, unfractionated heparin remains the standard of care for many clinical settings. For high-dose anticoagulation during cardiopulmonary bypass and invasive vascular procedures, heparin has no current rival. Table 35–5 lists the heparin tests available. These instruments are rated as moderate CLIA complexity and are designed for use by healthcare professionals.

Rapidpoint Coag Analyzer

The Rapidpoint Coag Analyzer (Bayer Diagnostics, Medfield, Massachusetts) offers six different tests for various clinical situations and sample types. The PT-ONE card (ISI approximately 1.0) is used with citrated whole blood or plasma samples. The PT NC card (ISI approximately 1.0) accepts fingerstick, and whole blood samples. The PT card (ISI approximately 1.6) is a second option for use with citrated whole blood or plasma. The aPTT test card accepts either citrated whole blood or plasma and is used to detect clotting factor deficiencies or to monitor low-range heparin therapy (heparin concentration 0 to 0.8 U/mL). The heparin management test (HMT) is an alternative to the ACT for monitoring patients receiving high dose heparin (heparin concentration 1.0 to 10.0 U/mL). Either citrated or noncitrated whole blood samples are appropriate for the HMT. Finally, the low-range heparin management test (LRHMT) is available to monitor patients receiving low- to moderate-range heparin (heparin concentration 0.25 to 3.0) during interventional radiology or cardiology procedures. Samples may be either citrated or fresh whole blood.

The Rapidpoint Coag analyzer measures 3.9 × 6 × 10.5 inches and weighs 4.25 pounds. It is an easily portable tabletop analyzer. An encoded test card provides information to the analyzer regarding type of test, card

Table 35–4 • MONITORS THAT PERFORM MULTIPLE TESTS

Company	Instrument	Tests Performed and Samples Used
Bayer Diagnostics	Rapidpoint Coag	PT NC—fingerstick
		PT, PT-ONE, aPTT—venous whole blood, citrated whole blood, citrated plasma (35 µL)
		HMT, low-range HMT (LRHMT)—venous whole blood, citrated whole blood (35 µL)
Instrumentation Laboratory	GEM PCL	PT, aPTT—fingerstick, citrated or venous whole blood (50 µL)
		ACT, low-range ACT (LRACT)—fingerstick or venous whole blood (50 µL)
International Technidyne Corporation	Hemochron Jr. Signature	PT, aPTT—fingerstick, citrated or venous whole blood (50 µL)
		ACT, (LRACT)—fingerstick or venous whole blood (50 µL)
International Technidyne Corporation	Hemochron Response: RxDx heparin management	aPTT, TT, heparin neutralizing thrombin time (HNTT), high thrombin time (HiTT), heparin response test (HRT), protamine response test (PRT)—venous whole blood (1.5 mL)
Medtronic Perfusion System	ACT II	ACT, high-range heparinase test (HRHTC), PT, general-purpose cartridge (GPC)—venous whole blood (400 µL)
	Hepcon HMS: software for the heparin dose response (HDR) heparin protamine titration (HPT)	ACT, HDR, HPT—venous whole blood (3 mL)
Pharmanetics	Heparin management panel and accent microprocessor accessory	HMT, LHMT, heparin titration test (HTT), protamine response test (PRT)—citrated or venous whole blood (35 µL)
Roche Diagnostics Corporation	CoaguChek Pro-DM (Pro and Plus)	PT, aPTT, ACT—fingerstick or venous whole blood (25 µL)

Table 35-5 • HEPARIN MONITORING POINT OF CARE TESTS

Level of Heparin	Tests Available
Low-range heparin (heparin concentration < 1 U/mL)	aPTT—Rapidpoint Coag analyzer aPTT—GEM PCL aPTT—Hemochron Jr. Signature aPTT, TT—Hemochron Response General-purpose cartridge—ACT II aPTT—CoaguChek Pro-DM (Pro, Plus)
Intermediate range heparin (heparin concentration 0-3 U/mL)	Low-range heparin management test (LRHMT)—Rapidpoint Coag analyzer (0-3) U/mL) Low-range ACT (LRACT)—GEM PCL (0-2.5 U/mL) Low-range ACT (LRACT)—Hemochron Jr. Signature (0-2.5 U/mL)
High-range heparin (heparin concentration > 3 U/mL)	HMT—Rapidpoint Coag (1-10 U/mL) ACT—GEM PCL (1.0-6.0 U/mL) ACT—Hemochron Jr. Signature (1.0-6.0 U/mL) ACT—Hemochron Response (1.0-6.0 U/mL) ACT—ACT II (1.0-8.0 U/mL) and Hepcon HMS ACT—CoaguChek Pro-DM
Heparin management tests	Heparin neutralizing thrombin time (HNTT), high thrombin time (HiTT), heparin response test (HRT), protamine response test (PRT)—Hemochron Response and RxDx system High-range heparinase test (HRHTC)—ACT II Heparin dose response test (HDR), heparin assay by heparin/protamine titration test (HPT)—Hepcon HMS Heparin management panel—Heparin titration test (HTT), protamine response test (PRT), HMT, ACCENT accessory—Rapidpoint/Thrombolytic Assessment System (TAS)

lot characteristics, and other test parameters. The reaction chamber on the card contains test-specific reagents and paramagnetic particles. Depending on the test, results are available in about 5 minutes, slightly longer for high-range results. Electronic and bilevel liquid quality controls are available. Features include quality-control lockout, identification for patient and operator, continuous electronic surveillance and 1000-test memory linking results to patient, test type, and time. Options include a data management system and interface for transfer of patient and quality-control data to an information system.

One drop of blood (approximately 35 µL) is applied to the sample well on the test card for dispersion to the reaction chamber. An electromagnet pulses on and off, causing the particles to move until they are stopped by clot formation. An optical analyzer detects the change in movement and the time to clot formation is converted into the appropriate test result form.[44]

All versions of the PT test compare favorably to other POC and standard laboratory methods [30,41,44,45] with $r = 0.93$ or better. The HMT correlates well with the ACT ($r = 0.9$) during cardiac bypass surgery and correlates better than the ACT to anti-Xa levels ($p < 0.01$).[46,47] Information regarding performance of aPTT and LRHMT is primarily provided by package inserts. The versatility offered by the test menu and assortment of test types makes this test system well suited for use at multiple sites in a clinical center.

GEM Portable Coagulation Laboratory

The GEM Portable Coagulation Laboratory (PCL) is a small whole blood analyzer that is available freestanding or as a component of the IL Synthesis or IL GEM Premier 3000 comprehensive, compact portable laboratory systems for NST (Instrumentation Laboratory (IL), Lexington, Massachusetts). International Technidyne (ITC) and IL have formed a partnership to codevelop the coagulation component. The GEM PCL offers PT, aPTT, ACT (heparin concentration 1.0 to 6.0 U/mL), and low-range ACT (LRACT) (heparin concentration below 2.5 U/mL) tests. The ACT and LRACT report results in "celite-equivalent" clotting times.

The instrument is a portable handheld device measuring $5.5 \times 2 \times 3.5$ and weighing 0.75 pounds. The GEM PCL accepts fingerstick or venous whole blood for all tests and citrate whole blood for the PT and aPTT. The technology for clot detection is identical to the Hemochron Jr., discussed below, but the software for the clot detection algorithms differ. The analyzer reads the encoded cartridges to determine test type. One drop of blood (approximately 50 µL) is applied to the sample well. The system will display a low sample error if the sample well is not adequately filled. The system is equipped with electronic quality control or wet quality control material. Outboard error management is present. A comprehensive data management system, downloading, and printing capabilities are available as part of the larger workstation. Results are available in less than 5 minutes for PT but may require longer for aPTT and ACT. Results (234 test memory) are stored automatically with time and date. The advantages of the system include the connection to a comprehensive POC testing workstation, the expanded menu of coagulation tests, and a comprehensive onboard data management system. The instrument may be disconnected from the workstation and carried to the bedside.

Hemochron Jr. Signature

The Hemochron Jr. Signature is the smallest of the line of multitask analyzers manufactured by International Technidyne Corporation (ITC) (Edison, New Jersey). The system performs the same panel of tests described for the GEM PCL—PT, aPTT, ACT (celite), and LRACT—but the reagents and test interpretation may differ. The PT and aPTT are available using either citrated or noncitrated whole blood; the ACT and LRACT accept fresh whole blood.

The instrument is a portable, handheld device measuring 2 × 7.5 × 3.75 inches and weighing 12 ounces. The test cartridge is composed of a waste channel and a test channel and is encoded with test type and other parameters. The PT and aPTT assays are available in about 2 minutes, with slightly longer times for ACT. Electronic control and wet quality control material are available. The Signature package provides a keypad and onboard data management, including the ability to identify, store, date, time stamp, and print patient and quality-control test results. Transfer of the data to an information system is available. No positive identification of patient specimens is available, but the system does have an onboard system for error control.

Blood (approximately 50 µL) is placed in the sample well of the cartridge and a 15-µL aliquot is drawn into the test channel that contains test-specific reagents. Excess blood from the sample well is directed to a waste channel. The test sample is pumped back and forth across a window, blocking light transmission between an LED and a light detector. Clot formation is signaled when the blood ceases to move. Clotting times are converted to test specific results.

The test system compares favorably to the ACT performed on the larger Hemochron instrument and to the laboratory aPTT.[48] Correlation of the PT with several other POC instruments found the PT to be adequate, but it had the lowest correlation coefficient with the routine laboratory method ($r = 0.89$) and tended to underestimate PT INR above 3.0.[30] This instrument is not approved for home use. The advantages include a variety of test options, and an onboard data management program.

Hemochron Response

A Hemochron analyzer (International Technidyne Corporation, Edison, New Jersey) has been monitoring heparin for the past 30 years as one of the first portable, rapid, whole blood coagulation analyzers.[49] Several versions of the instrument, including single-well (401), double-well (801), and data management-equipped (8000) models, have been marketed. The newest version, the Hemochron Response, uses fresh or citrated whole blood, offers an expanded test menu, and provides additional software for warfarin, protamine, and heparin management.

The system offers a full package for heparin management. The ACT monitors high-dose heparin therapy (heparin concentration 1.0 to 6.0). To supplement the ACT, other heparin tests are available, including an aPTT, a thrombin time (TT), the heparin-neutralizing thrombin time (HNTT), the high thrombin time (HiTT), the heparin response test (HRT), and the protamine response test (PRT). The HNTT and HiTT determine circulating heparin effect. The HRT and PRT together with patient specific determinants (age, weight, baseline ACT) are used by the on-board RxDx management program to determine heparin and protamine dosage.

The 401 measures 12.5 × 18 × 23 inches and weighs 3.75 pounds. The 801 measures 15 × 25 × 28 inches and weighs 5.75 pounds. The 8000 and the Response are about the same in size as the 801, but weigh in heavier at 12 pounds. A 1.5-mL sample must be accurately pipetted into the sample test tube or an evacuated tube must be used. Test results are available in 1 to 5 minutes depending on the test. Electronic quality control, an onboard system for instrument error detection, and wet quality control material are available on all instruments. The Response offers several features, including quality control lockout, identification for patient and operator, downloading capabilities, and a bar-code reader to identify reagent tubes.

The technology for clot detection is the same for all versions. Clot formation is detected by a sensitive electromagnetic method. A magnet is located in the sample test tube. The magnet aligns with a magnet detector within the instrument test well. The test well(s) slowly rotates and incubates the test tube during the coagulation test. The magnet and magnet detector remain aligned until the formation of a clot displaces the magnet, signifying test completion. The time to clot formation is converted into a plasma equivalent time for PT, aPTT and TT.

A recent study demonstrated coefficients of variation on whole blood for the ACT of 0.6% to 11.2% (celite) and 2.4% to 7.0% (kaolin).[50] Varying results have been reported with the heparin management programs.[51] Many comparison studies are available.[31,46,47,52,53] The PT and aPTT are rarely mentioned in the literature, especially since the arrival of easier to use, smaller-volume analyzers. Advantages of the Hemochron include the rapid, easy to perform ACT, the heparin package, and the years of testing experience. The need for a measured, large-volume sample is the most important disadvantage as the newer, small-volume instruments gain popularity.

ACT II Automated Coagulation Timer

The ACT II Automated Coagulation Timer (Medtronic Perfusion System, Minneapolis, Minnesota) is another work-horse of the operating room and catheterization laboratory. Tests include ACT, high-range heparinase test (HRHTC), PT, and a general-purpose cartridge (GPC) used as an aPTT. The analyzer measures 6.5 × 6.5 × 9.5 inches, weighs 8 pounds, and has two reaction wells that allow for either duplicate testing or testing of two separate samples. The cuvette consists of reaction chamber and plunger assembly with a "daisy" on one end and a flag on the other. A result is available in 5 to 12 minutes, slightly longer for high ACT values. The instrument displays individual test results, or the average or difference in seconds between duplicate tests. Electronic quality control and wet quality control material are available. The system does not differ data management or a data transfer system.

Citrated or fresh whole blood or citrated plasma (400 µL) is added to the test cuvette by syringe or pipette. Reagent is released from the reagent chamber when sample is added to the fill-line. The flag movement through the reaction chamber is timed by a photo optical detector. The endpoint is established when fibrin forms on the "daisy" and thus slows the flag movement. The clot detection time is converted to the appropriate test result form. Numerous studies compare the test system with other POC heparin monitors.[52,53] The ACT II allows duplicate testing to improve precision. However, sample volume and application are tedious.

Hepcon HMS Hemostasis Management System

The Hepcon HMS (Medtronic Perfusion System, Minneapolis, Minnesota) is the big brother to the ACT II. The clot detection method is the same, but the Hepcon is fully automated. The system offers complex testing programs including the HemoStatus platelet function assay (above) and a heparin management program. The heparin studies use four- to six-chambered cartridges that contain varying concentrations of heparin or protamine. Patient specific parameters (sex, weight, height) and the concentration of heparin desired are entered in to the management program and an initial heparin dose is suggested. ACT is followed to monitor the patient's response and to adjust the dose. For heparin reversal, the protamine dose is determined in a similar manner. A protamine assay to determine the concentration of heparin is also possible.

The Hepcon HMS is the largest analyzer in the category of POC instruments and is more transportable than portable. It measures 14.5 × 16.5 × 9.5 inches and weighs 30 pounds. A 3-mL syringe is used to collect a fresh venous sample. The syringe is attached to the instrument and the sample is automatically dispensed to each of the wells within a cartridge. The instrument has electronic quality control and uses a wet quality-control material. A minimum of 12 minutes is required for a test result. The analyzer does not have data management capability and it cannot transfer data to an information system. An onboard error detection system guides the automatic pipetting. The major disadvantages are the size, price, and long test generation times. Clinical studies have been mixed regarding the utility of several of the management programs.[54,55]

Thrombolytic Assessment System

The Thrombolytic Assessment System (TAS) is manufactured by Pharmanectics (Raleigh, North Carolina). Bayer distributes the platform as the Rapidpoint Coag with the PT and aPTT test cards and codistributes the HMT and the LHMT. Pharmanetics also markets the Accent, an accessory to the TAS/Rapidpoint Coag analyzer that is used in conjunction with the heparin management panel (HMP). The HMP is composed of the heparin titration test (HTT) and the protamine response test (PRT). The HTT is used to predict a patient's response to heparin and the PRT is used in combination with the HMT test card to determine the neutralizing dose of protamine. The platform and clot detection system are described in the Rapidpoint Coag section. No literature is available to assess the heparin management program.

CoaguChek Pro-DM, CoagChek Pro, CoaguChek Plus

The CoaguChek Pro-DM (Roche Diagnostics Corporation, Indianapolis, Indiana) is the newest version in a very long line of POC analyzers. The CoaguChek Plus, CoaguChek Pro and Coumatrak will continue to be supported but no new analyzers are available. These instruments are the offspring of the original handheld whole blood PT and aPTT monitor.[56] All of the analyzers use the same clot detection system with improvements in the microprocessor, data entry, and data management systems. The CoaguChek Pro-DM performs PT, aPTT, and ACT (heparin concentration below 3 U/mL) in less than 3 minutes. Data storage is available for 1000 tests. Data can be downloaded with the Accu-Chek HDM software or transferred to an LIS using the RALS-Plus network based interface. A keypad and optional bar code reader are available.

The new instrument measures 8.1 × 4.5 × 2 inches and weighs 1.5 pounds. A fingerstick or fresh whole blood sample is required. An error message generates if the sample volume is inadequate. The result is available in less than 3 minutes. Electronic quality control and wet control material are available. The CoaguChek Pro-DM has an upgraded onboard computer with data management, automatic lockout for quality control, and the ability to automatically transfer patient and quality-control data to an information system, including an interface with AccuChek HDM 3.2.

A drop of blood (approximately 25 μL) is placed in the sample well of the test cartridge. The blood moves into the reagent chamber and mixes with the test-specific reagents. The blood–reagent mixture travels along the reaction path, a coiled capillary tube, until clot forms. The cessation of flow is detected by a laser optical system that uses a property called "coherence." The movement of red blood cells in the flowing blood creates a specific speckled pattern on the photodetector. When the blood clots, the speckled pattern is altered by the lack of movement of the cells. The monitor interprets this change in pattern as clot formation and converts the endpoint into a quantitative plasma-equivalent PT, INR, or aPTT.

The laser photometer line of CoaguChek instruments has been the focus of many clinical studies over the last decade describing the acceptable performance of the instrument as a warfarin monitor, a heparin monitor, and a monitor of perioperative changes in a patient's coagulation status.[30,31,33,52,57,58] In several studies, transfusion protocols have been derived incorporating the POC result as a decision-making tool for determining the appropriate timing of transfusions.[57] The advantages of the monitor include the small size, the extensive clinical experience, and the new data management system.

The fingerstick sample application may be difficult with same patients.

GLOBAL ASSESSMENT OF CLOT FORMATION

Two POC instruments are significantly different from the rest; they do not mimic existing laboratory tests, but monitor the viscoelastic properties of clot formation. The Thromboelastogram (TEG) has experienced many face-lifts since its debut in the 1940s. The SonoClot Coagulation and Platelet Function Analyzer debuted in the late 1980s. Both of these instruments provide a clot signature that traces the processes of clot formation and clot resolution. By analyzing the tracing produced by the instruments, a global assessment can be made of the function of platelets, the soluble clotting proteins, anticoagulants present, and fibrinolysis. The major disadvantages of these systems are the skills required to perform and interpret the test.

Thromboelastogram

The complexity of the Thromboelastogram (Haemoscope, Skokie, Illinois) has been a major deterrent to routine use of this system for patient monitoring. In recent years, the technology has been automated and computerized to provide more reproducible and interpretable measurements. The test is performed by placing a small amount of whole blood (approximately 360 μL) into a cylindrical cup. A pin is suspended in the blood. The cup remains stationary and the pin is rotated though an angle of 4° 45'. As clot forms the rotary motion of the pin is progressively inhibited. Characteristic tracings are developed based on the motion of the pin. The components of the tracing have been ascribed to various counterparts of physiologic clot development and resolution. The maximal amplitude (MA) of the tracing is thought to be a function of platelet activity and fibrinogen concentration. In nonactivated blood, more than 30 minutes is required for the generation of the maximal amplitude; however, an activator (e.g., celite) shortens the time to maximal amplitude by inducing more rapid blood clotting. The major advantage of the TEG is the development of a full clot signature from initial platelet activation to eventual clot lysis. The major disadvantage has been the prolonged time required to see full development of the tracing. Several new reports are available regarding the use of the TEG for monitoring platelet and coagulation parameters.[59,60]

Sonoclot Coagulation Analyzer

The SonoClot Coagulation Analyzer (Sienco Inc., Wheat Ridge, Colorado) differs in design from the TEG, but both systems measure the clot's physical properties. Whole blood (approximately 400 μL) is placed in a cylindrical cuvette in which a vertically vibrating probe is suspended. The change in mechanical impedance extended on the probe by the viscoelastic properties of the forming clot produces a characteristic clot tracing. Reduced platelet function causes a decreased slope from inflection to peak, a lower peak, and a reduced contraction rate. Several clinical trials have been reported using the Sonoclot.[61,62] The advantage of this test is the more rapid completion, usually within 15 minutes, and the global testing of the blood elements of primary hemostasis.

■ REFERENCES

Chapter 35 References

1. Aller RD. Coagulation analysis at the point-of-care. CAP Today 1999;13:65–70.
2. Macik BG. Designing a point-of-care program for coagulation testing. Arch Pathol Lab Med 1995;119:929–938.
3. Jensen R. Near-patient hemostasis testing. Clin Hemost Rev 1994;8:1–4.
4. McKenzie ME, Gurbel PA, Levine DJ, Serebruany VL. Clinical utility of available methods for determining platelet function. Cardiology 1999;92:240–247.
5. Smith JW, Steinhubl SR, Lincoff AM, et al. Rapid platelet-function assay an automated and quantitative cartridge-based method. Circulation 1999;99:620–625.
6. Kereiakes DJ, Mueller M, Howard W, et al. Efficacy of abciximab induced platelet blockade using a rapid point of care assay. J Thromb Thrombolysis 1999;7:265–275.
7. Steinhubl SR, Kottke-Marchant K, Molitemo DJ, et al. Attainment and maintenance of platelet inhibition through standard dosing of abciximab in diabetic and non-diabetic patients undergoing percutaneous coronary intervention. Circulation 1999;100:1977–1982.
8. Mascelli MA, Worley S, Veriabo NJ, et al. Rapid assessment of platelet function with a modified whole blood aggregometer in percutaneous transluminal coronary angioplasty patients receiving anti-GP IIb/IIIa Therapy. Circulation 1997;96:3860–3866.
9. Kabakibi A, Vamvakas EC, Cannistraro PA, et al. Collagen-induced whole blood platelet aggregation in patients undergoing surgical procedures associated with minimal to moderate blood loss. Am J Clin Pathol 1998;109:392–398.
10. Ray MJ, Marsh NA, Just SJE, et al. Preoperative platelet dysfunction increases the benefit of aprotinin in cardiopulmonary bypass. Ann Thorac Surg 1997; 63:57–63.
11. Mammen EF, Comp PC, Gosselin R, et al. PFA-100 system: a new method for assessment of platelet dysfunction. Semin Thromb Hemost 1998;24:195–202.
12. Ortel TL, James AH, Thames EH, et al. Assessment of primary hemostasis by PFA-100® analysis in a tertiary care center. Thromb Haemost 2000;84:94–97.
13. Harrison P, Robinson MS, Mackie IJ, et al. Performance of the platelet function analyzer PFA-100 in testing abnormalities of primary haemostasis. Blood Coagul Fibrinolysis 1999;10:25–31.
14. Kottke-Marchant K, Powers JB, Brooks L, et al. The effect of antiplatelet drugs, heparin, and pre-analytical variables on platelet function detected by the platelet function analyzer (PFA-100). Clin Appl Thromb Hemost 1999;5:122–130.
15. Fressinaud E, Veyradier A, Truchaud F, et al. Screening for von Willebrand disease with a new analyzer using high shear stress: a study of 60 cases. Blood 1998;91:1325–1331.
16. Cattaneo M, Federici AB, Lecchi A, et al. Evaluation of the PFA-100 system in the diagnosis and therapeutic monitoring of patients with von Willebrand disease. Thromb Haemost 1999;82:35–39.

17. Hezard N, Metz D, Nazeyrollas P, et al. Use of the PFA-100 apparatus to assess platelet function in patients undergoing PTCA during and after infusion of c7E3 Fab in the presence of other antiplatelet agents. Thromb Haemost 2000;83:540–544.
18. Homoncik M, Jilma B, Hergovich N, et al. Monitoring of aspirin (ASA) pharmacodynamics with the platelet function analyzer PFA-100. Thromb Haemost 2000;83:316–321.
19. Cattaneo M, Lecchi A, Agati B, et al. Evaluation of platelet function with the PFA-100 system in patients with congenital defects of platelet secretion. Thromb Res 1999;96:213–217.
20. Escolar G, Cases A, Vinas M, et al. Evaluation of acquired platelet dysfunction in uremic and cirrhotic patients using the platelet function analyzer (PFA-100): influence of hematocrit elevation. Haematologica 1999;84:614–619.
21. Rand ML, Carcao MD, Blanchette VS. Use of the PFA-100 in the assessment of primary, platelet-related hemostasis in a pediatric setting. Semin Thromb Hemost 1998;24:523–529.
22. Despotis GJ, Levine V, Filos KS, et al. Evaluation of a new point-of-care test that measures PAF-mediated acceleration of coagulation in cardiac surgical patients. Anesthesiology. 1996;85:1311–1323.
23. Ereth MH, Nuttall GA, Santrach PJ, et al. The relation between the platelet-activated clotting test (HemoSTATUS) and blood loss after cardiopulmonary bypass. Anesthesiology. 1998;88:962–969.
24. Despotis GJ, Levine V, Saleem R, et al. Use of point-of-care test in identification of patients who can benefit from desmopressin during cardiac surgery: a randomised controlled trial. Lancet. 1999;354:106–110.
25. Coiffic A, Cazes E, Janvier G, et al. Inhibition of platelet aggregation by abciximab but not by aspirin can be detected by a new point-of-care test, the hemoSTATUS. Thromb Res 1999;95:83–91.
26. Despotis GJ, Ikonomakiou S, Levine V, et al. Effects of platelets and white blood cells and antiplatelet agent C7E3 (Reopro) on a new test of PAF procoagulant activity of whole blood. Thromb Res. 1997;86:205–219.
27. Saleem R, Bigham M, Spitznagel E, Despotis GJ. The effect of epsilon-aminocaproic acid on HemoSTATUS and kaolin-activated clotting time measurements. Anesth Analg 2000;90:1281–1285.
28. Becker DM, Humphries JE, Walker FB, et al. Standardizing the prothrombin time: calibrating coagulation instruments as well as thromboplastin. Arch Pathol Lab Med 1993;117:602–605.
29. Hirsh J, Dalen JE, Anderson DR, et al. Oral anticoagulants: Mechanism of action, clinical effectiveness, and optimal therapeutic range. Chest 2001;119:22S–38S.
30. Gosselin R, Owings JT, White RH, et al. A comparison of point-of-care instruments designed for monitoring oral anticoagulation with standard laboratory methods. Thromb Haemost 2000; 83:698–703.
31. Solomon HM, Mullins RE, Lyden P, et al. The diagnostic accuracy of bedside and laboratory coagulation: procedures used to monitor the anticoagulation status of patients treated with heparin. Am J Clin Pathol 1998;109:371–378.
32. Brill-Edwards P, Ginsberg JS, Johnston M, Hirsh J. Establishing a therapeutic range for heparin therapy. Ann Intern Med. 1993;119:104–109.
33. Ansell JE, Patel N, Ostrovsky D, et al. Long-term patient self-management of oral anticoagulation. Arch Intern Med. 1995; 155:2185–2189.
34. Jacobson, AK. Patient self-management of oral anticoagulation therapy: An international update. J Thromb Thrombolysis 1998; 5:25–28.
35. Watzke HH, Forberg E, Svolba G, et al. A prospective controlled trial comparing weekly self-testing and self-dosing with the standard management of patients on stable oral anticoagulation. Thromb Haemost. 2000;83:661–665.
36. Bussey H, Chiquette, E. Workshop on anticoagulation: clinic care versus routine medical care. A review and interim report. J Thromb Thrombolysis 1996;2:325–329.
37. Oral Anticoagulant Monitoring Study Group. Prothrombin measurement for professional and patient self-testing use: A multicenter clinical experience. Am J Clin Pathol 2001;115:288–296.
38. Macik BG. New concepts in management of thrombophilia—home PT monitoring. In Schechter GP, Broudy VC, Williams ME (eds). Hematology 2001. American Society of Hematology, Washington DC 2001, pp 330–338.
39. Biasiolo A, Rampazzo P, Furnari O, et al. Comparison between routine laboratory prothrombin time measurements and fingerstick determinations using a near-patient testing device (Pro-Time). Thromb Res 2000;97:495–498.
40. Chapman DC, Stephens MA, Hamann GL, et al. Accuracy, clinical correlation, and patient acceptance of two handheld prothrombin time monitoring devices in the ambulatory setting. Ann Pharmacother 1999;33:775–780.
41. Murray ET, Fitzmaurice DA, Allan TF, Hobbs FD. A primary care evaluation of three near patient coagulometers. J Clin Pathol 1999;52:842–845.
42. Van den Besselaar AM, Breddin K, Lutze G, et al. Multicenter evaluation of a new capillary blood prothrombin time monitoring system. Blood Coagul Fibrinolysis 1995;6:726–732.
43. Douketis JD, Lane A, Milne J, Ginsberg JS. Accuracy of a portable international normalization ratio monitor in outpatients receiving long-term oral anticoagulation therapy: comparison with a laboratory reference standard using clinically relevant criteria for agreement. Thromb Res 1998;92:11–17.
44. Rose VL, Dermott SC, Murray BF, et al. Decentralized testing for prothrombin time and activated partial thromboplastin time using a dry chemistry portable analyzer. Arch Pathol Lab Med 1993;117:611–617.
45. Cachia PG, McGregor E, Adlakha S, et al. Accuracy and precision of the TAS analyser for near-patient INR testing by non-pathology staff in the community. J Clin Pathol 1998;51:68–72.
46. Fitch JC, Geary KL, Mirto GP, et al. Heparin management test versus activated coagulation time during cardiovascular surgery: correlation with anti-Xa activity. J Cardiothorac Vasc Anesth 1999;13:53–57.
47. Helft G, Bartolomeo P, Zaman AG, et al. The heparin management test: a new device for monitoring anticoagulation during coronary intervention. Thromb Res 1999;96:481–485.
48. Carter AJ, Hicks K, Heldman AW, et al. Clinical evaluation of a microsample coagulation analyzer, and comparison with existing techniques. Cathet Cardiovasc Diagn 1996;39:97–102.
49. Esposito RA, Culliford AT, Colvin SB, et al. The role of the activated clotting time in heparin administration and neutralization for cardiopulmonary bypass. J Thorac Cardiovasc Surg 1983;85:174–185.
50. Zucker ML, Jobes C, Siegel M, et al. Activated clotting time (ACT) testing: analysis of reproducibility. J Extra Corpor Technol 1999;31:130–134.
51. Johnson HD, Morgan MS, Koenig GR, et al. Evaluation of the Hemochron 8000 Rx/Dx system for heparin management. J Extra Corpor Technol 1997;29:83–87.
52. O'Neill AI, McAllister C, Corke CF, Parkin JD. A comparison of five devices for the bedside monitoring of heparin therapy. Anaesth Intensive Care 1991;19:592–596.
53. Reich DL, Zahl K, Perucho MH, Thys DM. An evaluation of two activated clotting time monitors during cardiac surgery. J Clin Monit 1992;8:33–36.
54. Murray DJ, Brosnahan WJ, Pennell B, et al. Heparin detection by the activated coagulation time: a comparison of the sensitivity of coagulation tests and heparin assays. J Cardiothorac Vasc Anesth 1997;11:24–28.
55. Hardy JF, Belisle S, Robitaille D, et al. Measurement of heparin concentration in whole blood with the Hepcon/HMS device does not agree with laboratory determination of plasma heparin concentration using a chromogenic substrate for activated factor X. J Thorac Cardiovasc Surg 1996;112:154–161.

56. Lucas FV, Duncan A, Jay R, et al. A novel whole blood capillary technique for measuring the prothrombin time. Am J Clin Pathol 1987;88:442–446.
57. Despotis GJ, Joist JH, Goodnough LT. Monitoring of hemostasis in cardiac surgical patients: impact of point-of-care testing on blood loss and transfusion outcomes. Clin Chem 1997;43:1684–1696.
58. Becker RC, Ball SP Eisenberg P, et al. A randomized, multicenter trial of weight adjusted intravenous heparin dose titration and point of care coagulation monitoring in hospitalized patients with active thromboembolic disease. Antithrombotic Therapy Consortium Investigators. Am Heart J 1999;137:8–11.
59. Shore-Lesserson L, Manspeizer HE, DePerio M, et al. Thromboelastograpy-guided transfusion algorithm reduces transfusions in complex cardiac surgery. Anesth Analg 1999;88:312–319.
60. Stammers AH, Bruda NL, Gonano C, Hartmann T. Point-of-care coagulation monitoring: applications of the thromboelastograph. Anaesthesia 1998;53(Suppl 2):58–59.
61. Miyashita T, Kuro M. Evaluation of platelet function by Sonoclot analysis compared with other hemostatic variables in cardiac surgery. Anesth Analg 1998;87:1228–1233.
62. LaForce WR, Brudno DS, Kanto WP, Karp WB. Evaluation of the SonoClot analyzer for the measurement of platelet function in whole blood. Ann Clin Lab Sci 1992;22:30–33.

CHAPTER 36

Prevention and Treatment of Venous Thromboembolism in Neurologic and Neurosurgical Patients

David Green, M.D., Ph.D.

The headlines read, "Football mourns a hero."[1] A star pass-rusher is injured when his vehicle overturns on an icy highway. He sustains a cervical spine injury, resulting in tetraplegia. Surgery to stabilize his spine is successful, but 2 weeks postoperatively, as he is being transferred from his bed to a wheelchair, he utters something to his mother, his eyes roll back, and he has a cardiac arrest. Efforts at resuscitation are unsuccessful. The cause of death: massive pulmonary embolism.

Venous thromboembolism is a frequent occurrence in patients with neurologic and neurosurgical conditions. Table 36–1 lists the incidence of deep venous thrombosis (DVT) in patients not receiving prophylaxis who were in the acute phase of ischemic stroke[2] or spinal cord injury,[3] or undergoing neurosurgery.[2,4] The differences in the incidence figures are probably more related to the methods for detecting DVT than to actual differences in the frequency of thrombosis in the various conditions. However, it is clear that all these conditions are associated with a clinically important risk of thromboembolism. For example, fatal pulmonary embolism is reported in from 8% to 37% of patients with spinal cord injury,[5,6] and occurs in at least 5% of stroke and 1% of neurosurgical patients. In those patients who experience a proximal DVT, the hospital course is prolonged, and the exposure to therapeutic doses of anticoagulants may cause bleeding and other adverse effects. Lastly, patients with DVT may develop the post-thrombotic syndrome, a painful disorder accompanied by persistent leg edema, pigmentation, and ulceration (see Chapter 16). Therefore, in recognition of the frequency of thrombosis and its sequelae in this group of patients, effective prophylaxis is mandatory. In this chapter, methods for the prevention and treatment of venous thromboembolism will be discussed.

STROKE

Prophylaxis

As noted in Table 36–1, the frequency of DVT in patients with ischemic stroke is 55% (95% confidence intervals, 49% to 60%).[2] Turpie and coworkers[7,8] conducted two trials of thromboprophylaxis using a heparinoid (danaparoid) in patients with acute stroke. They first demonstrated that the drug was significantly more effective than placebo (venous thrombosis in 4% of anticoagulant-treated patients as compared with 28% of those receiving placebo, $p = 0.005$), with one major hemorrhage in the danaparoid group and one minor bleed in the placebo group.[7] They then went on to show that the drug was more effective than unfractionated heparin (UH). In a randomized, double-blind trial, 87 patients were treated with subcutaneous injections every 12 hours of either danaparoid, 750 mg, or UH, 5000 units. Venous thrombosis occurred in 9% of those receiving danaparoid and 31% of those receiving heparin ($p = 0.014$). The frequency of hemorrhage was 2% in each group.[8]

Following recovery from acute stroke, patients are usually transferred to a rehabilitation facility. Studies have shown that the risk of venous thromboembolism persists into the post stroke period.[9] Therefore, we performed a trial to determine whether relatively simple interventions would be safe and effective in preventing venous thrombosis in these patients.[10] Ninety patients were randomized to receive either pneumatic compression leggings, applied from 8 P.M. to 8 A.M. nightly, or low-molecular-weight heparin (LMWH), 50 U/kg, subcutaneously at bedtime. The frequency of DVT was

549

Table 30-1 • INCIDENCE OF DEEP VENOUS THROMBOSIS (DVT) IN PATIENTS IN THE ACUTE PHASE OF ISCHEMIC STROKE OR SPINAL CORD INJURY, AND IN THOSE UNDERGOING NEUROSURGERY

	No. of Patients	DVT	Incidence (%)
Ischemic stroke	346	190	55
Spinal cord injury	419	167	40
Neurosurgery	415	91	22

Data from Pierson,[1] Geerts et al.,[2] Consortium for Spinal Cord Medicine,[3] and Turpie et al.[4]

assessed by venography performed at the time of discharge from the rehabilitation facility, usually 2 to 4 weeks after admission. About a third of the patients had hemorrhagic strokes, and the majority had received some form of thromboprophylaxis during their acute hospital stay. Thrombosis occurred in two (5%) patients in the compression group and five (12%) in the LMWH group (p = NS). The thrombi were asymptomatic in most patients and in two were confined to the calf veins. No pulmonary emboli were detected. Six patients could not tolerate the compression devices and left the trial early. One patient assigned to the LMWH group had a positive stool examination for occult blood and the drug was discontinued. An economic analysis indicated that the two therapies were roughly equivalent in cost; the expense of the LMWH was mostly offset by the nursing time required for proper application and maintenance of the compression devices. The conclusion of the study was that use of either compression or LMWH is effective for the prevention of thromboembolism after stroke. The LMWH is better accepted, requires less nursing care, and is only marginally more expensive.

Treatment

While the general treatment of stroke is beyond the scope of this chapter, mention should be made of recent studies evaluating the use of heparins. In one of the largest stroke trials ever accomplished, 19,435 patients were randomized to receive UH, either 5000 units or 12,500 units twice daily, or no UH.[11] Patients were also randomized to receive aspirin, 300 mg daily, or no aspirin. Neither of the interventions, UH or aspirin, altered the mortality or dependency at 6 months. Patients allocated to UH had fewer recurrent ischemic strokes but this was offset by a similar-sized increase in hemorrhagic strokes. Furthermore, the higher dose of UH was associated with a significant excess of extracranial bleeds. On the other hand, there was a significant benefit from aspirin, without an increase in hemorrhagic strokes. The investigators concluded that if UH is given to patients with acute stroke, the dose should not exceed 5000 units twice daily. Aspirin is indicated for all patients with ischemic strokes.

Danaparoid was compared with placebo in a double-blind, multicenter trial of 1275 persons with acute stroke.[12] The heparinoid was given by continuous intravenous infusion for 7 days; doses were adjusted according to anti-factor Xa activity. The 7-day and 3-month outcomes were similar in the danaparoid- and placebo-treated groups, but there were significantly more serious bleeding events in the danaparoid-treated patients (15 versus 5, p = 0.05). Therefore, this aggressive anticoagulant approach cannot be recommended for the treatment of acute stroke.

Kay and coworkers[13] compared two doses of nadroparin (4100 units twice daily, 4100 units daily) with placebo in the treatment of acute stroke in 312 patients. The nadroparin was administered for 10 days. Death or dependency was observed in 45% of patients in the high-dose group, 52% in the low-dose group, and 65% of placebo patients (a statistically significant trend in favor of LMWH, p = 0.005). There was no increase in bleeding complications in the LMWH-treated patients. The data indicated a significantly better outcome for those patients receiving the LMWH.

In summary, LMWH in prophylactic doses is safe and effective for the prevention of thromboembolism in patients with acute ischemic stroke and for continued use during rehabilitation. Its administration in higher doses (by the subcutaneous route) early in acute ischemic stroke has some preliminary support. For patients with hemorrhagic strokes, our policy is to initiate LMWH prophylaxis when the patient is stable and imaging shows no progression of bleeding. This is usually a minimum of 1 to 2 weeks after the acute event. UH in doses of 5000 units twice daily is less effective, and higher doses of either UH or intravenous heparinoid appear to be both ineffective and dangerous. All patients with ischemic strokes should receive aspirin unless there is a contraindication to the use of this medication. Prophylactic doses of heparin can safely be given to patients receiving aspirin.

SPINAL CORD INJURY

Prophylaxis

A variety of methods for the prevention of thromboembolism in the spinal injury patient are available (Table 36-2). The use of compression boots alone has been shown to decrease the frequency of DVT by half.[14] There have been several theories as to why compression devices are effective. The rhythmic contractions may mechanically improve blood flow. Such a mechanism has been demonstrated for the foot pump, which empties the venous plexus on the sole of the foot, sending pulses of blood up the leg.[15] In addition, stimulation of the vascular endothelium promotes the release of tissue factor pathway inhibitor (TFPI). This potent endogenous anticoagulant blocks the activation of coagulation by inhibiting factor Xa and the tissue factor–factor VIIa complex. A variety of compression devices were recently shown to increase the levels of TFPI and reduce the concentrations of factor VIIa in normal subjects and patients with venous disease.[16]

Table 36–2 • METHODS FOR THE PREVENTION OF THROMBOEMBOLISM IN SPINAL CORD INJURY

Mechanical Methods
- Compression boots, calf and thigh
- Foot pump
- Elastic hose
- Vena caval filter

Pharmacologic Methods
- Unfractionated heparin
- Low-molecular-weight heparin
- Warfarin

Combined Modalities
- Compression device plus unfractionated heparin
- Graduated compression hose plus low-molecular-weight heparin
- Vena caval filter plus anticoagulants

The benefits of compression devices are limited by practical problems with their application and maintenance. The patient is required to be at bedrest; leaving the bed for any reason interrupts treatment and necessitates reapplication of the device. A study by Masri and coworkers[17] in patients having hip arthroplasty showed that interruptions decreased therapy time by 22%, and that pressures were within the prescribed range less than 10% of the time. In addition, failure to inspect the skin under a compression device may lead to abrasion and maceration, especially in patients with impaired sensation or cognition. The Consortium for Spinal Cord Medicine Clinical Practice Guidelines recommends that compression devices should be applied to the legs of all patients, but limited to the first 2 weeks after injury so that they will not interfere with the subsequent rehabilitative therapy of the patient.[3] During every nursing shift, the devices should be inspected to confirm that they are in proper position and that the underlying skin is free of abrasions or other damage. Lastly, it is recommended that if thromboprophylaxis has been delayed for more than 72 hours after injury, ultrasonography or other tests should be performed to exclude the possibility that thrombi have already formed. Such thrombi might be dislodged if disturbed by compression devices.

The usefulness of UH and LMWH have been examined in a few clinical trials of patients with traumatic spinal cord injury. Low-dose UH, 5000 units every 12 hours, was found to be less effective than giving heparin in doses adjusted to prolong the activated partial thromboplastin time into the upper range of normal ($p<0.05$), but the higher doses (mean, 13,200 units every 12 hours) were associated with significant bleeding.[18] In a subsequent trial by these same investigators, LMWH was found to be more effective than UH given in doses of 5000 units every 8 hours.[19] The LMWH used in this study was tinzaparin, and it was administered in a dose of 3500 anti-Xa units once daily. Not only was the LMWH more effective, but no patients receiving this dose had bleeding; on the other hand, two patients treated with UH had bleeding.

Geerts and coworkers[20] examined 344 patients with various degrees of severe trauma, including spinal cord injury. Patients were randomized to receive either UH, 5000 units every 12 hours, or LMWH (enoxaparin, 30 mg every 12 hours). Treatments were initiated within 36 hours of injury, and were continued for up to 14 days. At that point, contrast venography was performed. The LMWH was significantly more effective than the UH; the frequency of DVT was 31% in the former group and 44% in the latter group ($p = 0.014$). In addition, proximal vein thrombosis was also significantly decreased by LMWH (6% versus 15%, $p = 0.012$). Major bleeding occurred in only six patients: five in the LMWH group and one in the UH group ($p = 0.12$). Spinal cord injury was present in 23 of the patients entered into this trial; 8 were randomized to LMWH and 15 to UH. Four of the former but 10 of the latter developed DVT, and proximal vein thrombosis occurred only in the two patients receiving UH. The investigators concluded that LMWH was more effective than UH in preventing thromboembolism in patients having major trauma.

In a nonrandomized study, 105 consecutive patients with spinal cord injury were given LMWH (enoxaparin, 30 mg every 12 hours).[21] No patient developed clinical evidence of thromboembolism, and ultrasound studies were negative in the 60 patients who had this examination. Bleeding in three patients was attributed to the LMWH. Based on these and other reports, the Consortium for Spinal Cord Medicine Clinical Practice recommends that anticoagulation with LMWH should be initiated within 72 hours after spinal cord injury, provided there is no active bleeding, evidence of head injury, or coagulopathy.[3] The dose administered would depend on the drug selected; three LMWHs are currently approved for prophylaxis in the United States. Using a compression device along with the LMWH for the first 2 weeks would appear to maximize treatment efficacy.

Data on the optimal duration of thromboprophylaxis is fragmentary and anecdotal. The Consensus Conference on Spinal Cord Injury[22,23] reported that thromboembolism occurred 10 weeks or more after injury in an occasional patient whose prophylaxis was stopped at 8 weeks, suggesting that a longer duration of prophylaxis may be appropriate in some patients. One of these late thrombotic episodes was a fatal pulmonary embolism (PE). To examine the risk factors for fatal PE, we reviewed all autopsy-proven cases occurring in our center over a 5-year period.[24] Nine cases were encountered, eight men and one woman, whose ages ranged from 17 to 67. Cervical spine fracture with tetraplegia was present in 67% and obesity in 44%, and all had flaccid paralysis. These characteristics were significantly more common in the cases than in a concurrently selected control group. In addition, more of the control subjects than cases had received LMWH (60% versus 22%, $p = 0.07$). It was concluded that thromboprophylaxis needs to be especially aggressive in patients with cervical spine injuries, tetraplegia, and obesity.

The Consortium for Spinal Cord Medicine Clinical Practice recommends that treatment be individualized based on location of injury, presence and extent of paralysis, functional status, concomitant medical or surgical illness, age, obesity, and other factors.[3] They suggest that patients with incomplete motor paralysis receive prophylaxis until discharge from the hospital. For those with complete motor paralysis but no other risk factors, prophylaxis should continue for 8 weeks. Lastly, 12 or more weeks of treatment were recommended for those with high cervical spine injuries and tetraplegia, concomitant lower-limb fractures, obesity, age over 70, and history of prior thromboembolism. Patients should also be actively participating in a rehabilitation program before anticoagulants are terminated.

Should any studies to detect the presence of thrombosis be performed prior to discontinuing anticoagulant prophylaxis? The experience with routine ultrasonography has been disappointing. Ultrasonography had a sensitivity of 62% and a positive predictive value of 66% for detecting proximal thrombi when used to screen for DVT in patients after orthopedic surgery.[25] The D-dimer test may be more helpful in excluding the presence of thrombosis. In 67 patients with either paraplegia or tetraplegia, no patient with DVT had a negative D-dimer test, although 40 patients without thrombosis had positive tests.[26] The D-dimers were detected with either an enzyme-linked immunosorbent assay (Asserachrom D-Di) or a rapid automated turbidimetric test (STA-Liatest D-Di); the methods are important because some tests for D-dimer are more sensitive than others.

A reasonable strategy for deciding whether prophylactic anticoagulants should be discontinued is to measure D-dimer by a sensitive method. If the test is negative, prophylaxis is stopped. If the test is positive, prophylaxis should be continued and if clinical suspicion of thromboembolism is high, additional studies such as ultrasonography of the legs, ventilation/perfusion lung scans, or other evaluations would be warranted. If a thrombus is detected, full therapeutic doses of anticoagulants should be administered.

Inferior Vena Cava Filters

Inferior vena cava (IVC) filters are devices that can be introduced into the IVC to block the passage of thrombi from the lower extremities and pelvis into the lungs (see Chapters 37 and 38). If they were completely innocuous, there would be reason to insert them in every patient with DVT, because from 30% to 50% of such patients have evidence of pulmonary emboli.[27] However, their use is associated with a number of problems, including the need for expertise in their proper deployment, considerable expense, and certain risks. These include perforation of the vena cava, placement in the renal vein, migration of the device, or tilting of the filter allowing emboli to squeeze through. A previously unappreciated complication of IVC filters is an increase in the frequency of recurrent DVT. In a randomized trial of more than 400 patients with acute proximal DVT, Decousus and coworkers[28] observed an almost twofold risk of developing DVT in the 2 years after filter placement (Table 36–3). All patients received either UH or LMWH for the first 8 to 12 days after admission, and then were administered warfarin for at least 3 months.

Table 36–3 • OUTCOMES AFTER INFERIOR VENA CAVA FILTER PLACEMENT IN PATIENTS WITH PROXIMAL VEIN THROMBOSIS

Outcome	Filter n = 200	No Filter n = 200	p
PE, days 1–12	2	9	0.03
PE, 2 years	6	12	0.16
DVT, 2 years	37	21	0.02
Death	43	40	0.65

PE, pulmonary embolism; DVT, deep venous thrombosis.
Adapted from Decousus H, Leizorovicz A, Parent F, et al. A clinical trial of vena cava filters in the prevention of pulmonary embolism in patients with proximal deep-vein thrombosis. N Engl J Med 1998;338:409–415, with permission.

The authors concluded that vena caval filters were effective in preventing PE, but this benefit was counterbalanced by an excess of recurrent DVT without any difference in mortality.

The currently accepted indication for insertion of an IVC filter is the prevention of PE in patients with documented venous thrombus who are intolerant of systemic anticoagulation. Regarding prophylaxis, the Consensus Conference on Antithrombotic Therapy recommends that filters be used only in patients in whom other nonpharmacologic prophylaxis regimens are not possible.[29] Patients with lower-limb fractures who cannot be fitted with compression devices would be included in this category. Another potential indication for the use of an IVC filter is the patient with high cervical spinal cord injury who is ventilator dependent; even a small PE in such a patient could prove fatal. Finally, spinal cord injury patients who are unable to tolerate prophylactic doses of anticoagulants because of intracranial or other active bleeding, hemorrhagic diathesis, or history of heparin-induced thrombocytopenia might also be candidates for IVC filters.[3] A recent review of the literature on filters concluded that although filters represent a potentially important modality for the prevention of pulmonary emboli, further evaluation of outcomes in rigorous clinical trials is needed.[30]

Treatment

To date, no studies have compared long-term therapy with warfarin versus LMWH in this patient population. Furthermore, there are no data with regard to the duration of treatment after a patient has experienced a thromboembolic event. Lim and coworkers[31] examined the time to recanalization of thrombus in patients with tetraplegia, paraplegia, hemiplegia, and no paralysis. All patients received at least 3 months of anticoagulation prior to evaluation. Patients with tetraplegia and paraplegia took significantly longer for recanalization than nonparalyzed controls (54 days versus 33 days, $p = 0.04$); hemiplegic patients were intermediate. If persistent venous obstruction represents an ongoing risk factor for recurrent thrombosis, it would seem prudent to continue patients with paralysis on anticoagulants until complete recanalization of veins has been documented by ultrasonography or other techniques.

NEUROSURGERY

Prophylaxis

Nonpharmacologic methods of thromboprophylaxis traditionally have been preferred by neurosurgeons because of concerns about anticoagulant-induced bleeding. More than 20 years ago, Turpie and coworkers[32] reported that calf compression decreased the frequency of venous thrombosis from 20.8% in controls to 7.8% in patients given prophylaxis ($p = 0.01$). Subsequently, these investigators examined graduated compression stockings alone or with compression boots in another randomized trial of neurosurgical patients.[33] Again, the frequency of DVT was reduced from 19.8% in patients not receiving prophylaxis to 8.8% in those wearing stockings and 9% in those with stockings and compression. Thus, graduated compression stockings alone or combined with compression devices significantly decrease the risk of thromboembolism in neurosurgical patients.

With the demonstration that LMWH was safe and effective thromboprophylaxis for patients undergoing a variety of medical and surgical procedures, researchers became emboldened to evaluate these drugs in neurosurgical patients. In 1996, Nurmohamed and coworkers[34] randomized 485 neurosurgical patients to be fitted with compression stockings alone, or to have compression stockings plus nadroparin LMWH, 7500 units subcutaneously daily starting 18 to 24 hours postoperatively. Treatment was continued for up to 10 days. All patients then underwent bilateral venography and were followed for 8 weeks. Of the two thirds of the patients who had adequate venograms, thrombi were found in 26.3% of stocking alone patients and 18.7% stocking plus LMWH patients ($p = 0.065$). If one includes DVT detected in the follow-up period, the figures were 20.9% for stockings and 13.7% for LMWH ($p = 0.018$). Furthermore, the rates for proximal DVT and PE were 10.2% for the stockings and 5.8% for LMWH ($p = 0.036$). Major bleeding occurred in two stocking-alone patients and six LMWH patients ($p = 0.87$). The investigators concluded that adding LMWH to stockings resulted in a significant decrease in important venous thromboembolism without a significantly increased risk of major bleeding.

More recently, Agnelli and coworkers[35] compared stockings plus enoxaparin LMWH, 40 mg once daily, with compression stockings alone in 307 patients undergoing neurosurgery. All patients had venography on day 8, which was successful in 85%. The LMWH reduced the frequency of DVT from 32% (stocking group) to 17% (LMWH group) $p = 0.004$. Proximal vein thrombosis was also decreased significantly: 13% to 5%, $p = 0.04$. Two patients in the placebo group died of proven PE. Major bleeding occurred in 3% of patients in each group.

As in the previous study, this investigation also concluded that the combination of LMWH plus stockings was more effective than stockings alone, and does not cause excessive bleeding.

The studies described above, along with two earlier reports, were subjected to a meta-analysis.[36] A total of 187 thrombotic events were recorded in 827 patients (22.6%). Prophylaxis with heparins resulted in a 45% risk reduction for thrombosis. The number needed to harm was over 100, leading the investigators to conclude that heparins are effective in preventing venous thromboembolism in elective neurosurgery without excessive bleeding risk.

Treatment

The management of documented venous thromboembolism in the neurosurgical patient hinges on one key issue: the likelihood of the patient having a hemorrhage when exposed to full doses of anticoagulants. When does the risk of major intracranial bleeding subside in the patient who has had head trauma or surgery? The answer to this question hinges on several factors, including the time and extent of injury, the type of trauma, and the anatomic lesion. For most kinds of surgery, wounds are well sealed by 24 hours; exceptionally, a ligature will slip after this time and bleeding recurs. Crush injuries with large raw surfaces are more likely to ooze than cleanly severed tissue that has been reapproximated with sutures. Leaking aneurysms that cannot be fully embolized or ablated are another cause of potential bleeding.

The profile of the patient who can tolerate full-dose anticoagulant therapy is an individual who has sustained a well-demarcated wound more than 24 hours earlier and shows no signs of progressive neurologic deficit. A computed tomography (CT) scan or magnetic resonance imaging (MRI) scan of the head should reveal a stable pattern, with no suggestion of continued bleeding. Subarachnoid or subdural hemorrhages should be contained, and multiple metastatic lesions or aneurysms should not be in evidence. If these conditions are met, systemic anticoagulation for newly recognized venous thromboembolism is indicated. LMWH is preferred to UH for the following reasons:

1. Theoretically, the initial intravenous bolus dose of UH is more likely to promote bleeding than the initial subcutaneous dose of LMWH. This is because giving UH intravenously transiently makes the blood incoagulable, while the onset of anticoagulation with subcutaneous LMWH is more gradual, without the peak of incoagulability.
2. A meta-analysis of 13 clinical trials has concluded that LMWH is more effective and is associated with less bleeding than UH when used for the treatment of DVT.[37]
3. LMWH is easier to administer and generally does not require monitoring. However, under special circumstances, measurement of anti-factor Xa levels are suggested to ensure that the doses given

are neither excessive nor subtherapeutic. Monitoring is recommended in persons weighing less than 50 kg or more the 120 kg, in children and pregnant women, and in patients with renal failure.[38] Giving very high doses (for subjects weighing more than 120 kg), or treating patients with creatinine clearances of less than 30 mL/min, may result in anti-factor Xa levels exceeding 1.0 U/mL, and require dose reductions. The half-life of intravenously administered LMWH is only 3 to 4 hours, so that it is rarely necessary to try to reverse its action; however, LMWH given subcutaneously has a half-life of 16 to 24 hours. If life-threatening bleeding or surgical intervention is required in a patient who has just been given LMWH, efforts to combat its effects are justified. Protamine, in a dose of 50 to 100 mg depending on patient weight, is given intravenously at a rate not to exceed 5 mg/min, and with continuous monitoring of the blood pressure.

Where there is a contraindication to the use of systemic anticoagulation, IVC filter placement is appropriate. However, given the risk of subsequent DVT recurrence noted previously, anticoagulants should be started as soon as the danger of bleeding has subsided. The neurosurgical patient who has sustained either a DVT or a PE is at high risk for a recurrence; long-term anticoagulation is usually necessary. Warfarin is a safe and effective choice for patients who have a stable food intake and are cognitively intact; in such patients, the dose of warfarin can be adjusted to obtain an International Normalized Ratio (INR) in the accepted therapeutic range of 2 to 3. However, if the patient is not eating, is having frequent seizures and falls, or cannot be relied on to take the prescribed dose of warfarin, use of the drug is potentially hazardous. Warfarin-induced bleeding is often observed in neurosurgical patients whose food ingestion is variable, and in those requiring antibiotics for infection control. On the other hand, warfarin resistance is found in patients receiving anticonvulsant medications. Therefore, finding a safe and effective dose of warfarin may be challenging in many neurosurgical patients. In these persons, LMWH offers the advantages of safety and simplicity, since its effectiveness is not affected by diet or other medications, and it is given once or twice daily subcutaneously without the need for monitoring in most instances. The doses given are based on body weight, either 1.5 mg/kg or 175 to 200 U/kg once daily or 1 mg/kg or 100 U/kg twice daily.[39,40] Treatment should be continued until the risk of recurrent thromboembolism is low; for patients without filters, this may be 3 to 6 months depending on neurologic recovery, but for those with filters anticoagulation may be necessary for up to 2 years or more. When the patient is neurologically stable, cognitively intact persons may wish to switch from LMWH to an oral anticoagulant for reasons of convenience and cost.

Cost Containment

Venous thromboembolism in the neurologic and neurosurgical patient is a very costly complication, economically as well as in terms of morbidity and mortality. While UH and warfarin are inexpensive medications, giving heparin by continuous intravenous infusion is expensive and prolongs hospitalization. Giving warfarin so that the INR remains within the therapeutic range requires frequent blood tests and dose adjustments; lapses may be penalized by episodes of either thrombosis or bleeding, leading to recurrent hospitalization. LMWH is more expensive but can be given at home and does not require monitoring. Cost-effectiveness analyses of DVT treatment have shown that the use of LMWH compares very favorably with that of UH.[41]

Medical-Legal Aspects

Practicing thromboprophylaxis is good medicine. However, considerable judgment is required for the safe use of anticoagulants in neurologic and neurosurgical patients, and the medical literature is thin in this regard. Placebo-controlled studies have shown that some patients with neurologic or neurosurgical disease have new intracranial bleeding in the absence of anticoagulants. Nevertheless, when new bleeding occurs, it is usually attributed to these agents, and there may be litigation. The best defense is that most published reports stress that the benefit of antithrombotics outweighs the risks when the drugs are used in neurologically stable patients.

Role of the Consultant

A 66-year-old man becomes lightheaded and falls to the ground, sustaining a bruise on his left brow. A CT scan of the head shows no intracranial lesion or bleeding, but a scan of the chest shows a large pulmonary embolus extending into the left and right pulmonary arteries, which was probably the cause of the syncope. The consultant recommends that a catheter be inserted into the thrombus for catheter-directed thrombolysis, followed by the administration of a LMWH. However, the interventional radiologist believes that instrumenting the heart and pulmonary artery may cause an arrhythmia, and recommends systemic thrombolysis, which is initiated. After 2 hours of a planned 12-hour infusion, oozing is noted from the bruise on the scalp and a periorbital hematoma forms. The thrombolytic agent is discontinued and a continuous infusion of heparin is begun. After 12 hours, the patient states he feels well, and denies headache or shortness of breath. Two hours later, he suddenly become aphasic. A repeat CT scan of the head shows an extensive hemorrhage on the side opposite the original injury, suggesting the presence of a contracoup-type injury. Heparin therapy is stopped and a craniotomy is performed to evacuate the hematoma. Concurrently, an IVC filter is inserted and leg compression boots applied. Eleven days later, the patient is progressively regaining neurologic function and the consultant recommends that prophylactic doses of LMWH be started. However, the neurosurgeon is still concerned about bleeding and does not administer the drug. One week later, the patient has a new, extensive thrombosis extending from the iliac vein to the popliteal vein.

The role of the consultant is to recommend management based on the best medical evidence available. In this case, the suggestions of the consultant were not accepted; the interventional radiologist recommended a different approach and the attending neurosurgeon was uncomfortable with re-exposing the patient to anticoagulants. Consultants should be viewed as a member of the team caring for the patient; many voices are heard but ultimately the attending physician makes the difficult clinical decisions.

■ REFERENCES

Chapter 36 References

1. Pierson D. Football mourns a hero. Chicago Tribune, Wednesday, February 9, 2000, section 4, pp. 1 and 3.
2. Geerts W, Heit JA, Clagett GP, et al. Prevention of venous thromboembolism. Chest 2001;119:132S–175S.
3. Consortium for Spinal Cord Medicine. Prevention of thromboembolism in spinal cord injury. Washington, D.C. Paralyzed Veterans of America, 1997, p. 20.
4. Turpie ACC, Hirsh J, Gent M, et al. Prevention of deep vein thrombosis in potential neurosurgical patients. Arch Intern Med 1989;149:679–681.
5. Devivo MJ, Stover SL. Longterm survival and causes of death. In Stover SL, DeLisa JA, Whiteneck GG (Eds): Spinal Cord Injury: Clinical Outcomes from the Model Systems. Gaithersbug, MD, Aspen, 1995, pp. 289–316.
6. Tribe C. Cause of death in the early and late stages of paraplegia. Paraplegia 1963;1:19–47.
7. Turpie AGG, Levine MN, Hirsh J, et al. Double-blind randomised trial of ORG 10172 low-molecular-weight heparinoid in prevention of deep-vein thrombosis in thrombotic stroke. Lancet 1987;i:523–526.
8. Turpie AGG, Gent M, Cote R, et al. A low-molecular-weight heparinoid compared with unfractionated heparin in the prevention of deep vein thrombosis in patients with acute ischemic stroke. Ann Intern Med 1992;117:353–357.
9. Brandstater ME, Roth EJ, Siebens HC. Venous thromboembolism in stroke: literature review and implications for clinical practice. Arch Phys Med Rehabil 1992;73:S379–S391.
10. Green D, Akuhota V, Eiken M, et al. Prevention of thromboembolism in stroke rehabilitation patients. Top Stroke Rehabil 1998;5:68–74.
11. International Stroke Trial Collaborative Group. The international stroke trial (IST): a randomised trial of aspirin, subcutaneous heparin, both or neither among 19 435 patients with acute ischaemic stroke. Lancet 1997;349:1569–1581.
12. TOAST Investigators. Low molecular weight heparinoid, ORG 10172 (danaparoid), and outcome after acute ischemic stroke. JAMA 1998;279:1265–1272.
13. Kay R, Wong KS, Yu YUL, et al. Low-molecular-weight heparin for the treatment of acute ischemic stroke. N Engl J Med 1995;333:1588–1593.
14. Green D, Rossi EC, Yao JST, et al. Deep vein thrombosis in spinal cord injury: effect of prophylaxis with calf compression, aspirin, and dipyridamole. Paraplegia 1982;20:227–234.
15. Gardner AMN, Fox RH, Lawrence C, et al. Reduction of post-traumatic swelling and compartment pressure by impulse compression of the foot. J Bone Joint Surg 1990;72-B:810–815.
16. Chouhan VD, Comerota AJ, Sun L, et al. Inhibition of tissue factor pathway during intermittent pneumatic compression. Arterioscler Thromb Vasc Biol 1999;19:2812–2817.
17. Masri BA, McEwen J, Kerry RM, Duncan CP. Could patient outcome be affected by variations in delivered pneumatic compression therapy for prophylaxis of venous thromboembolism? American Academy of Orthopedic Surgeons, Anaheim, Feb 4–8, 1999.
18. Green D, Lee MY, Ito VY, et al. Fixed versus adjusted dose heparin in the prophylaxis of thromboembolism in spinal cord injury. JAMA 1988;260:1255–1258.
19. Green D, Lee MY, Lim AC, et al. Prevention of thromboembolism after spinal cord injury using low-molecular-weight heparin. Ann Intern Med 1990;113:571–574.
20. Geerts WH, Jay RM, Code KI, et al. A comparison of low-dose heparin with low-molecular-weight heparin as prophylaxis against venous thromboembolism after major trauma. N Engl J Med 1996;335:701–707.
21. Harris S, Chen D, Green D. Enoxaparin for thromboembolism prophylaxis in spinal injury. Am J Phys Med Rehabil 1996;75: 326–327.
22. Green D, Hull RD, Mammen EF, et al. Deep vein thrombosis in spinal cord injury: summary and recommendations. Chest 1992;102(suppl):633S–635S.
23. Green D. Prophylaxis of thromboembolism in spinal cord-injured patients. Chest 1992;102 (suppl):649S–651S.
24. Green D, Twardowski P, Wei R, Rademaker AW. Fatal pulmonary embolism in spinal cord injury. Chest 1994;105: 853–855.
25. Wells PS, Lensing AWA, Davidson BL, et al. Accuracy of ultrasound for the diagnosis of deep venous thrombosis in asymptomatic patients after orthopedic surgery. Ann Intern Med 1995;122: 47–53.
26. Roussi J, Bentolila S, Boudaoud L, et al. Contribution of d-dimer determination in the exclusion of deep venous thrombosis in spinal cord injury patients. Spinal Cord 1999;37:548–552.
27. Moser KM, Fedullo PF, LitteJohn KK, Crawford R. Frequent asymptomatic pulmonary embolism in patients with deep venous thrombosis. JAMA 1994;271:223–225.
28. Decousus H, Leizorovicz A, Parent F, et al. A clinical trial of vena cava filters in the prevention of pulmonary embolism in patients with proximal deep-vein thrombosis. N Engl J Med 1998; 338:409–415.
29. Clagett GP, Anderson FA Jr, Geerts WH, et al. Prevention of venous thromboembolism. Chest 1998;114:531S–560S.
30. Streiff MB. Vena caval filters: a comprehensive review. Blood 2000;95:3669–3677.
31. Lim AC, Roth EJ, Green D. Effect of lower limb paralysis on the recanalization of deep vein thrombosis. Arch Phys Med Rehab 1992;73:331–333.
32. Turpie AGG, Delmore T, Hirsh J, et al. Prevention of venous thrombosis by intermittent sequential calf compression in patients with intracranial disease. Thromb Res 1979;15:611–616.
33. Turpie AGG, Hirsh J, Gent M, et al. Prevention of deep vein thrombosis in potential neurosurgical patients. Arch Intern Med 1989;149:679–681.
34. Nurmohamed MT, van Riel AM, Henkens CMA, et al. Low molecular weight heparin and compression stockings in the prevention of venous thromboembolism in neurosurgery. Thromb Haemost 1996;75:233–238.
35. Agnelli G, Piovella F, Buoncristiani P, et al. Enozaparin plus compression stockings compared with compression stockings

alone in the prevention of venous thromboemblosim after elective neurosurgery. N Engl J Med 1998;339:80–85.
36. Iorio A, Agnelli G. Low-molecular-weight and unfractionated heparin for prevention of venous thromboembolism in neurosurgery. Arch Intern Med 2000;160:2327–2332.
37. Lensing AWA, Prandoni P, Prins MH, Buller HR. Deep-vein thrombosis. Lancet 1999;353:479–485.
38. Laposata M, Green D, Van Cott EM, et al. The clinical use and laboratory monitoring of low molecular weight heparin, danaparoid, hirudin and related compounds, and argatroban. Arch Pathol Lab Med 1998;122:799–807.
39. The Enoxaparin Clinical Trial Group. A multicenter clinical trial comparing once and twice-daily subcutaneous enoxaparin and intravenous heparin in the treatment of acute deep vein thrombosis. Blood 1997;90(suppl 1):295a.
40. Lensing AWA, Prins MH, Davidson BL, Hirsh J. Treatment of deep venous thrombosis with low-molecular-weight heparins. Arch Intern Med 1995;155:601–607.
41. Gould MK, Dembitzer AD, Sanders GD, Garber AM. Low-molecular-weight heparins compared with unfractionated heparin for treatment of acute deep venous thrombosis. A cost-effectiveness analysis. Ann Intern Med 1999;130:789–799.

CHAPTER 37

Inferior Vena Caval Interventions in Thromboembolic Disease—The Viewpoint of Vascular Radiology

Katan C. Davae, M.D.
Michael F. Meyerovitz, M.D.

The inferior vena cava is the major conduit of venous return from the lower extremities and pelvis. Eighty-five to ninety-five percent of pulmonary emboli originate in the lower extremities; others may occasionally arise in the deep veins of the upper extremities or in the right atrium. Lower-extremity deep venous thrombosis (DVT), with its associated complications, remains a major medical perplexity. Pulmonary embolism (PE), is the third leading cause of death in the United States, although the overall incidence has been decreasing. Current estimated mortality rates range from 2 to 6 per 100,000 per year.[1]

Although anticoagulation has over the last 50 years remained the treatment of choice for thromboembolic disease, there has been a dramatic change and evolution in treatment for those who cannot be readily anticoagulated. Surgical interruption of the cava has fallen by the wayside because of its inherent morbidity and mortality. The advent of the minimally invasive era has brought about smaller delivery systems, limiting postprocedure recovery as well as complications. Much has changed and developed since the introduction of the inferior vena caval (IVC) filter. New and elegant designs are constantly forthcoming with futuristic "memory" alloys, allowing lower profiles and improved strength. Sleek designs meant to be "invisible" maintain laminar flow within the cava, limiting turbulence, and thereby minimize thrombus formation.

Although the vast majority of filters are placed in the inferior vena cava, filters may rarely be placed in the superior vena cava, in cases of upper-extremity DVT.

Limited data exist as to filter placement in the pediatric population, benefits in terminal patients, use in tumor emboli, or prophylactic placement in patients at high risk for thromboembolic disease.

Concurrent use of anticoagulation when possible seems justified in order to treat the underlying DVT and to address any associated hypercoagulable disorders, since the filter merely prevents most large pulmonary emboli from occurring. Ortega and colleagues,[2] however, demonstrated that no early adverse effects are seen in those who are not anticoagulated after filter placement.

Most long-term data on IVC filters are based on clinical follow-up and therefore the true rates of recurrent PE or caval occulusion are anecdotal as discussed in a recent review of the literature by Streiff.[3] He demonstrated that of 3184 patients with filter placement from 40 different series, only 8.4% had actual vena cavography follow-up. Serial nuclear pulmonary perfusion scans on all patients would give a clearer understanding of the actual recurrent PE rate. In a clinical trial, Decousus and coworkers, in which 400 patients with proximal DVT were randomly assigned to receive an IVC filter or not in addition to either unfractionated or low-molecular-weight heparin, 2-year follow-up demonstrated an increased incidence of recurrent DVT in patients with IVC filters (20.8 % compared to 11.6%).[4] This counterbalanced the lower incidence of symptomatic or asymptomatic PE in the patients with IVC filters (1.1% compared to 4.8%).[4]

Much anticipated is the arrival of the temporary caval filters, which have been in use in Europe. Once available, these may change some of the current indications and limitations of the currently available permanent filters.

HISTORY OF IVC INTERRUPTION IN PREVENTION OF PULMONARY EMBOLISM

Most pulmonary emboli originate in the lower extremities. Mechanical obstruction proximal to the source of embolus was first postulated in the late 18th century,[5] although not applied in the United States until the late 1920s by Homans.[6] Anticoagulation was not available for use until 1935 (heparin) and 1948 (warfarin). Caval ligation, introduced by Ochsner and DeBakey[7] in the early 1940s, and bilateral common femoral vein ligation, proposed by Homans[8] in 1944 for patients with suspected PE, were complicated by venous stasis with lower-extremity swelling, pain, and venous ulceration, as well as their associated operative risks. IVC ligation was confounded by a 12% to 15% mortality rate,[9-11] albeit a reduced recurrent fatal PE rate. Ligation of the superficial femoral veins was attempted, but the complication rate remained high because of venous stasis as well as a 10% to 26% recurrent PE rate.[12] Temporary devices such as caval occlusion balloons (Moser[13]) or sieves (Eichelter[14]) were effective, but they were complicated by PE at the time of removal. In the late 1950s improved techniques were developed, allowing partial interruption of the cava, leaving small channels of flow to continue to reduce stasis, yet filtering out potentially devastating emboli. Suture plication, introduced by DeWeese and colleagues,[15] or modified clips, introduced by Moretz,[16] were used, allowing partial "filtered" flow through the cava. Venous stasis complications were reduced to 46% (compared to 76% for total caval ligation)[17] but the procedure itself was fairly invasive and mortality rates remained high.[18] In 1967, a new approach was developed to overcome the mortality associated with open laparotomy for caval interruption. A surgical cutdown of the right internal jugular vein was performed, allowing radiographically guided placement of an umbrella-shaped skeleton covered with an imperforate silicon skin, designated the Mobin-Uddin Umbrella[19] (Edwards Laboratories). Not surprising, late complications related to caval occlusion remained, so the design of the umbrella was altered, with channels in the membrane allowing flow through it while trapping the larger emboli, thus creating a true filter as opposed to an IVC occluder. Initially its use was limited as an adjunct to anticoagulation in patients who experienced recurrent pulmonary embolism despite adequate anticoagulation. Although the mortality rate of placement was less than 1%,[20] it remained plagued by high caval thrombosis rates, filter fracture, and filter migration. Modifications of this initial idea led in 1974 to the development of the Kimray-Greenfield filter, now known as the Greenfield filter (Boston Scientific, Natick, Massachusuts). Initially, it was limited by its large introducer size and inflexible delivery housing, and was placed for years via an internal jugular vein cutdown. In 1984, placement of the Kimray-Greenfield filter, via a percutaneous approach was described.[21] The large introducer size often resulted in insertion site thrombosis. Since then, new designs have been developed with smaller and smaller delivery systems truly designed for percutaneous insertion, exemplified by the newly commercially released 6F TrapEase filter (Cordis Corp, Miami, Florida). Newer alloys with flexibility, strength, and nonthrombogenic properties have been developed.

ANATOMY AND ANOMALIES OF THE INFERIOR VENA CAVA

The inferior vena cava is formed at the level of the forth or fifth lumbar vertebral body by the union of the common iliac veins. Table 37-1 gives a listing of major inferior vena cava tributaries. It ascends retroperitoneally, to the right of the abdominal aorta adjacent to the vertebral bodies. It extends upward through the posterior aspect of the liver, dividing right from left lobe, and through the central tendon of the diaphragm at the level of the eighth thoracic vertebral body to enter the right atrium. It has an average diameter of 25 mm. The union of the internal and external iliac veins in the pelvis forms the common iliac veins. Each common iliac vein receives an iliolumbar vein. The median sacral vein joins the left common iliac vein. The external iliac veins are a continuation of the common femoral veins, which are the combined deep and superficial drainage from the lower extremities. The third and fourth lumbar veins join the inferior vena cava at their respective levels. The first and second usually drain into the third lumbar vein or the azygos-hemiazygos veins. The right gonadal vein empties into the anterior aspect of the inferior vena cava just below the right renal vein. The left gonadal vein is a tributary to the left renal vein. The right adrenal vein empties into the inferior vena cava just above the right renal vein. The three hepatic veins drain into the anterior aspect of the inferior vena cava at the top of the liver just before it drains into the right atrium.

Anomalies of venous drainage are often seen and may dramatically change the technical aspects and positioning of the filter. Table 37-2 lists common anomalies of the inferior vena cava and the way they affect filter placement. An enlarged inferior vena cava, measuring greater than 28 mm (megacava) is seen in roughly 2% of the population and may be due to chronic pulmonary hypertension, congestive heart failure, or tricuspid insufficiency. A Bird's Nest filter is the only filter that can be successfully placed in an inferior vena cava with a diameter of greater than 28 mm, but to a maximum diameter of 40 mm. IVC anomalies such as azygous replacement, left inferior vena cava or double inferior

Table 37-1 • TRIBUTARIES OF THE INFERIOR VENA CAVA

- Common iliac veins
- Lumbar veins (third and fourth)
- Right gonadal vein
- Right adrenal vein
- Hepatic veins

Table 37-2 • INFERIOR VENA CAVA ANOMALIES AND FILTER DEPLOYMENT

- **Double inferior vena cava** (0.2%–3%)[22]: Bilateral standard filters are placed into infrarenal inferior venae cavae
- **Azygous continuation of the inferior vena cava** (absent inferior vena cava) (0.6%)[22]: The filter is placed into the azygous vein in an infrarenal location
- **Left inferior vena cava** (0.2%–0.5%)[23]: The filter is placed in the infrarenal left inferior vena cava as if it were right sided
- **Retroaortic left renal vein** (1.8%–2.4%)[22]: A suprarenal filter is placed to catch emboli from potential renal collaterals
- **Circumaortic left renal vein** (8.7%)[24]: A suprarenal filter is placed
- **Megacava** (rare): A Bird's Nest filter is placed for caval diameters up to 40 mm. If diameter is greater than 40 mm, bilateral common iliac filters or surgical interruption may be considered

vena cava may be encountered. Renal vein anomalies are included here because they can affect filter placement, and lead to recurrent pulmonary emboli if overlooked. Other renal anomalies that may influence IVC filter placement include horseshoe kidney or pelvic kidney, or anomalies of the ureter such as transcaval descent,[25] a rare anomaly in which the right ureter may pass through the cava prior to reaching the bladder.

INDICATIONS AND CONTRAINDICATIONS TO IVC FILTER PLACEMENT

The currently available U. S. Food and Drug Administration (FDA)-approved IVC filters are all permanent devices and should only be placed after careful consideration in the appropriate patient (Table 37–3). In the acute setting, a filter is an easy prescription, however, long-term sequelae must be considered in a patient with a long life expectancy. Systemic anticoagulation remains the pillar of treatment for DVT as well as PE. In a patient with a DVT, anticoagulation decreases the risk of lethal PE from 6%–14% to 0.14%–0.3%.[27–29] In patients who survive an initial PE, the risk of recurrent fatal PE is 18% to 26%, usually within 24 hours of the initial event.[30] Anticoagulation can decrease the risk of recurrent fatal PE to 0.9% to 1.3%.[27,29] Anticoagulation does, however, carry risks. The average frequency of fatal, major, or any bleeding as studied by Landefeld and Bleyth[31] was 0.05%, 0.8%, and 2% daily, respectively, for patients treated with heparin, and 0.6%, 3%, and 9.6% annually, respectively, for patients on warfarin. A second major problem is failure of anticoagulation. This includes recurrent PE, clot propagation despite adequate anticoagulation, or formation of a DVT. Technetium 99-labeled macroaggregated albumin perfusion imaging of the lungs provides objective evidence of recurrent PE in the symptomatic patient. Pulmonary angiography remains the gold standard for the diagnosis of PE, although with improving techniques in pulmonary CT angiography as well as new techniques in magnetic resonance imaging (MRI), proximal emboli may be adequately visualized. Noninvasive serial lower-extremity B-mode ultrasonography provides actual evidence of thrombus propagation. Patients with free-floating proximal iliofemoral DVT larger than 5 cm in length have a 60% chance of symptomatic PE within 10 days despite adequate anticoagulation.[26] Calf vein DVT is on the opposite end of the spectrum—because of their small size, emboli originating in the calf veins are unlikely to be fatal; however, if calf vein thrombosis propagates proximally, the risk of fatal PE increases substantially.[32] Noncompliant patients or patients whose anticoagulation levels are difficult to follow, as well as those patients in whom anticoagulation is contraindicated, are at higher risk for PE, a consideration in the decision making for filter placement. In patients with an IVC filter in place, who have evidence of recurrent PE, a full evaluation, just as in any other patient with a PE, is mandated. If filter failure is assumed, venous thrombosis from an upper-extremity or cardiac source may be completely overlooked. The inferior vena cava and indwelling filter may be occluded, and emboli may originate from the thrombosed cava above the filter. If the recurrent source is from the lower extremity, a second filter may be necessary. In patients who are considered at high risk for PE or its complications, or those in whom long-term anticoagulation may not be possible, prophylactic filters increasingly are being placed. These include neurosurgical and orthopedic patients, patients with a prior history of DVT, patients with multiple trauma, or patients with a low cardiopulmonary reserve at high risk for thrombosis and in whom a PE

Table 37-3 • INDICATIONS AND CONTRAINDICATIONS FOR IVC FILTER PLACEMENT

Indications
- Contraindication to anticoagulation
    - Recent stroke
    - Recent neurosurgical or ophthalmic procedure
    - Perioperative period
    - Active internal hemorrhage
    - Intracranial neoplasm
- Complication from anticoagulation
- Failure of anticoagulation
    - Recurrent PE
    - Propagation of DVT
- Postembolectomy for massive PE

Relative Indications
- Free-floating iliofemoral DVT
- Patients who cannot be adequately anticoagulated
- Prophylactic filter placement
    - Multitrauma patient
    - Neurological and orthopedic patients at high risk for thromboembolic disease
    - Poor cardiopulmonary reserve

Contraindications
- Thrombus at the available access site or between the access site and deployment site
- No safe deployment site
- Severe uncontrollable coagulopathy
- Early pregnancy (relative contraindication)

Table 37–4 • CHARACTERISTICS OF IDEAL IVC FILTER

- Efficient at trapping all potentially significant emboli
- Maintains caval patency
- Overall morbidity and mortality less than that of the thromboembolic disease itself
- Complete biocompatibility
- No impedance to caval flow
- Nonthrombogenic
- Easy to place
- Low cost
- Potentially retrievable at any time
- Resistant to fatigue and corrosion
- MRI compatible and without image distortion

would be deadly. In the high-risk trauma population, the incidence of PE is 6%, and 4.2% of these are fatal.[33] In a study by Khansarinia and coworkers,[33] of 108 trauma patients who received prophylactic Greenfield filters, none had symptomatic PE. In addition, 14% of trauma patients cannot be immediately anticoagulated because of their injuries, and of those who are, 10% still develop thromboembolic disease.[34–36] In a recent study of 385 trauma patients who had filters placed in their inferior venae cavae, 249 were prophylactic. Compared to the 136 filters placed for DVT or PE in these patients, event rates were similar.[37] Patients with massive PE who undergo emergency embolectomy are at high risk for immediate recurrent PE despite anticoagulation.[18] Long-term research still needs to determine the benefits of prophylactic filtration to form a conclusion on this topic. The prophylactic placement of temporary filters may be of particular benefit in this group of patients.

The contraindications to IVC filter placement are listed in Table 37–3. Contraindications include thrombus at all access sites, thrombus en route to the proposed deployment site, or thrombus at the proposed deployment site. Although there have been no proven cases of filter seeding in the literature, septic emboli trapped by a filter may create a permanent harbor for organisms. Nevertheless filter placement is safer than operative caval ligation when anticoagulation and antibiotics are inadequate.[18] Any patient who has an uncontrollable coagulopathy may be at undue risk of bleeding from the procedure, outweighing the benefit. Filter placement in the first trimester of pregnancy will lead to increased radiation exposure to the fetus during organogenesis, and this should be considered when weighing benefits versus risks.

APPROPRIATE FILTER SELECTION

The ideal filter should have most of the characteristics listed in Table 37–4. An ideal filter is impossible, since the principles of trapping all emboli and maintaining caval patency are inversely related. In practical terms, as long as a filter functions to trap all emboli of potentially lethal size, allowing harmless clots of smaller size through, antegrade caval flow can be maintained. This may be in large part dependent upon the patient's physical status, clot size, caval size, and so on, but filter design also plays a role. It may be impossible to predict the threshold clot size required to be lethal, but many studies have compared in-vitro clot trapping ability of the available filters and their hemodynamic characteristics. Counterintuitively, the Bird's Nest filter consistently showed the least flow turbulence of the available filters despite its freeform design.[38–40] Simon and Rabkin[39] demonstrated that the available filters vary significantly in their clot-capturing efficiency, depending on caval size, filter orientation, and size of emboli. The available filters trap 50% to 86% of 2 × 30-mm emboli, and 46% to 90% of 4 × 30-mm emboli; but efficiency may decrease at larger caval diameters.[39] Of course, other factors such as procedure-related morbidity and mortality of placing a filter should be less than that of thromboembolic disease itself. The filter should be biocompatible as well as magnetic resonance compatible (Table 37–5).

There are six currently available filter designs in the United States. The Stainless Steel Greenfield and Titanium Greenfield filters (Boston Scientific, Natick, Massachusetts), the Simon Nitinol filter (Bard Nitinol Medical Technologies, Woburn, Massachusetts), the Bird's Nest filter (Cook Inc., Bloomington, Indiana), the Vena Tech filter (Braun Medical Inc., Bethlehem, Pennsylvania), and the TrapEase filter (Cordis Corp., Miami, Florida). Although the currently available filters have similar efficacy and complications, there are certain differences between them that allow decisions to be made based on patient selection. The filters differ in shape, design, composition, and delivery size. These filters can all safely be placed into a cava with a diameter of up to 28 mm (24 mm in patients who will have general anesthesia within 2 weeks of placement); however, if the diameter of the vena cava is 28 to 40 mm, a Bird's Nest filter is the filter of choice. Although bilateral common iliac vein filters may be placed in this situation, the single Bird's Nest in the inferior vena cava is less occlusive and causes less flow

Table 37–5 • MRI GUIDELINES FOR IVC FILTERS

Placement
There have been no definitive guidelines for MRI timing after placement of a ferromagnetic IVC filter. No significant motion has been demonstrated in animal experiments soon after placement, although the potential exists. Based on stent incorporation into vessels, for a totally elective MRI examination, a 2-week interval after filter placement is suggested. However if the MRI examination needs to be done before the completion of this interval, we do not delay it. For filters made from nonferromagnetic metals, MRI may be performed at any time.

Artifact
Artifact from metallic devices may be subdivided into local field disturbances such as focal blackout of signal at the filter itself, or more extensive signal loss over the adjoining abdomen. The amount of ferromagnetic substance in the filter will be the main determinant. The large stainless steel Bird's Nest filter and the stainless steel Greenfield filter will cause larger areas of image distortion and should not be used if an MRI of the abdomen will be crucial in the future. The alloy filters, such as the Simon Nitinol, the Vena Tech, and the Titanium Greenfield, cause minimal distortion.

disturbance than bilateral iliac filters.[41] The Simon Nitinol filter has a low-profile, flexible design, allowing it to be placed via an arm vein if this is the only access available. If a compact space is involved, such as the superior vena cava or the suprarenal cava, a Vena Tech, Simon Nitinol, or Greenfield filter can be used. The Bird's Nest filter has a length of 7 cm and has a wire mesh, which may prolapse farther, and thus not be a good choice for use close to the heart. If the patient will require future abdominal MRI scans, then the steel filters should be avoided because their ferromagnetic properties (Table 37–5) will cause artifacts on the scans.

All filters currently available have similar caval patency rates and recurrent PE rates. A delicate balance exists between a highly effective filter that traps all emboli yet has a higher risk of caval occlusion and a filter that preserves caval patency yet allows emboli to pass to the lungs. Long-term filter data are limited and the data present are, unfortunately, dependent upon subjective follow-up. The adverse outcomes most commonly reported include death, symptomatic PE, and lower-extremity edema due to venous stasis. A study on 1765 filters placed over a 26-year period demonstrated a 3.7% fatal PE rate, mostly occurring soon after placement (mean 4 days); postfilter caval thrombosis was seen in 2.7%.[42] These adverse outcomes are, fortunately, relatively uncommon and so the lack of large-scale randomized trials limits the ability to differentiate the available filter designs. Randomized trials with follow-up serial imaging in all patients would be ideal since asymptomatic outcomes are more prevalent than symptomatic outcomes, but unfortunately there are no such published trials. Clinical follow-up underestimates caval thrombosis, which is usually asymptomatic.[9,41,43] Asymptomatic PE, which is seen in 35% to 51% of patients with DVT[44,45] will be overlooked as well. Other causes of venous stasis or shortness of breath or other sources of DVT (upper extremity) may also be reported in the adverse event clinical data. Clot-trapping ability of caval filters has been evaluated in in-vitro animal models, but no study can exactly duplicate human vena caval physiology. Once the venous thrombus becomes organized (which takes between 3 and 6 months[46]) it is unlikely to embolize, as it becomes incorporated into the venous wall. If a PE were to occur after this time period, it likely would be from a new thrombus.[47]

A comparison of major complications of the available filter designs is given in Table 37–6; this comparison is not reliable since it is merely a compilation of various studies most of which represent short-term and/or incomplete follow-up only. A complete list of potential filter complications is given in Table 37–7.

Table 37–7 • COMPLICATIONS OF IVC FILTER PLACEMENT

Local Entry Site Related
- Groin hematoma (2%)[a]
- AV fistula (1%–3%)[a]
- Arterial injury or nerve injury
- Pneumothorax from jugular insertion
- Local infection
- Insertion site thrombosis (2%–33%)[a]

Systemic
- Contrast reaction (5%)[a]
- Air embolus during jugular insertion (rare)[91]
- Death (0.16%)[86]

Filter Related
- Filter occlusion and IVC thrombosis (0%–30%)
- Recurrent PE (3%–4%)
- IVC perforation by filter struts,[91] or deployment devices
- Filter migration (0%–36%)[a]
- Filter fatigue and fracture
- Filter malfunction: tilt, crossed legs, improper opening
- Technical errors: incorrect size, improper positioning
- Guidewire entrapment during subsequent line placement

[a] Numbers are estimated frequencies of events.

IVC FILTERS CURRENTLY APPROVED FOR USE IN THE UNITED STATES

Please refer to Figure 38–1 in Chapter 38 for identification purposes.

Stainless Steel Greenfield Filter

The Stainless Steel Greenfield over-the-wire filter has been the most widely used filter to date. The 20-year follow-up[48] is the longest for any filter to date. In its original form, the filter was surgically placed through a 24-French system and was first available for use in 1973. The first percutaneous placement was performed by Tadavarthy

---

Table 37–6 • COMPARISON OF FEATURES OF FIVE IVC FILTERS

Filter	PE Recurrence (%)	IVC Patency (%)	Migration (%)	MRI Compatible?
Stainless Steel Greenfield[78,51,72,82-85]	4–7	85–98	0–35	No
Bird's Nest[62,82,85-88]	0.5–3	95.3–98.5	0–9[a]	No
Titanium Greenfield[52,53,82,85,86]	3–3.5	95–99	6–15	Partially
Simon Nitinol[82,85,86,89]	2–4.4	75–93	0–12	Yes
Vena Tech[82,85,86,90]	1–4	70–100	3–36	Yes

Comparison is not reliable as a variety of methods were used in filter studies for establishing outcomes.
[a] Migration rates of 9% are prior to modification.

in 1984.[21] It is the only currently available filter placed over a wire. It is composed of six legs forming the shape of a cone. This design allows progressive vertical filtering as the struts unite at the apex. Because of the cone shape, 80% of the filter may be occluded by clot, but this results in only a 64% decrease in cross-sectional area of the filter.[49] The apex allows a guidewire to pass through it, guiding deployment. The base is the open end, consisting of wires that have hooks curved 180° on their ends for attachment to the caval wall. This is the only part that touches the cava. The filter is 4.9 cm in length, with a diameter of 32 mm at the base. Maximal recommended caval diameter is 28 mm. Its stainless steel fabrication limits MRI examinations of the abdomen by disturbing the magnetic field. A problem unique to the Greenfield design is filter tilt. In animal experiments a filter tilt allowed clots of larger size to pass through, but these were not clinically significant.[50] In general it is recommended that filter tilt greater than 16° be treated with an additional filter because of the increased size of clot allowed through. The placement of two tandem filters in the inferior vena cava is standard in certain circumstances, but the long-term effects of two filters have not been studied. Potentially, the thrombogenic effect would be increased. Based on Greenfield's 20-year follow up study,[48] the rate of recurrent PE was 4% and the caval patency rate was 96%. Filter migration was seen in 8% but was of no clinical significance. In an imaging review study of 46 patients by Lang and coworkers,[51] the struts of the Stainless Steel Greenfield filter were found to penetrate the wall of the cava in 41%, but in no cases was this event of any clinical significance.

Titanium Greenfield Filter

The Titanium Greenfield has been available for use since 1987. It has a similar design to the Stainless Steel Greenfield filter but differs in dimensions, composition, and deployment. The filter is composed of a titanium alloy. There is no central hole for a guidewire during delivery. The diameter at the base is 38 mm and the filter has an overall length of 47 mm. Although originally troubled by migration and caval penetration, the filter was modified and these problems were resolved. Limb asymmetry, seen in 10% of deployments, is not clinically significant.[52] However, we have seen two instances of recurrent PE through asymmetric legs, one of which was fatal and documented on postmortem examination. Also not a self-centering design, the filter may inherently tilt, causing its efficacy to decrease. A more serious problem that may decrease efficacy is leg crossing on deployment, which may be seen in 5.4%.[53] It may be possible to correct this problem at the time of deployment by gentle manipulation with a catheter; otherwise, an additional filter should be placed. Because of its titanium composition, it is less likely to disturb the magnetic field and is therefore less degrading to MRI images than the stainless steel version.

Vena Tech-LGM Filter

The Vena Tech-LGM first became available for use in the United States in 1989. It has a similar design to the Greenfield filters in that the filtering mechanism is a cone; however, it also has side rails that are designed to self-center the filter and prevent tilt. Instead of having hooks on the base, there are small hooks on the side rails that secure it to the caval wall. It is composed of Phynox, an alloy of eight metals, similar to the material used for pacer wires. The alloy has no ferromagnetic properties and therefore is MRI compatible and only results in local magnetic field susceptibility. It is 45 mm in height and has a diameter of 28 mm. An early European study of 100 patients demonstrated a 16% malposition rate, either slight tilting or incomplete opening, and a 13% migration rate.[54] Because of these design problems, it was modified in 1991. Recurrent PE rates of 0% to 3.5% are reported.[55] Caval patency 1 year after placement as followed by venography in 90 patients was 93%.[55]

Bird's Nest Filter

The Bird's Nest became available for use in 1982. Initially plagued by prolapse and migration, it has since been modified. The Bird's Nest filter is the only free-form filter; that is, it has no fixed, predesignated shape. It is composed of two V-shaped struts at each end connected via four 25-cm-long, 0.018-inch-diameter stainless steel wires, which form the so-called nest. The nest itself may be difficult to evaluate fluoroscopically because its wires are so thin, but they are visible on a spot radiograph. Small hooks anchor the nest to the caval wall. The length when deployed is 70 mm. It is the only filter currently available that can be placed into large cavae, up to 40 mm in diameter. The reported rate of recurrent pulmonary embolism is 2.7% and caval patency by clinical follow-up is 97.1%.[56] One patient had severe caval occlusion, leading to phlegmasia cerulea dolens and subsequent demise. Prolapse of wires may be seen in 13% to 45%,[49] but this may not affect acute clot-trapping ability.[57]

Simon Nitinol Filter

The Simon Nitinol was first approved for use in the United States in 1990. Its compact design is 38 mm in length. This is a unique filter in that it is composed of a nickel-titanium alloy that has a characteristic temperature-dependent shape-forming property: it reforms to its original configuration on warming to body temperature. This thermal shape memory allows it to be placed straight and folded in a small flexible delivery system that can even be inserted through an arm vein or via the subclavian approach. It has a dual filtration design, with its six-legged base similar in appearance to that of a Greenfield filter; in addition, it has a second filtration system in the shape of a dome, consisting of seven ovoid loops. There are hooks at the ends of the legs for securing it to the caval wall. The diameter of the dome is 28 mm, and the filter is used in inferior venae cavae up to 28 mm in diameter. Because of its alloy composition, it is MRI compatible and only causes minimal field inhomogeneity in the region of deployment. During deployment, the filter drops 1 to 2 cm. The filter can be repositioned appropriately from the femoral approach before the legs are released, however, anticipation of the caudal drop when placing from the jugular route should be anticipated before any deployment. In individuals in whom the cava is smaller than the dome, the dome cannot reform fully and may end up in a spindle shape.[58] In a multicenter trial of 103 patients, symptomatic recurrent PE rates were 3%, with a caval patency rate of 86%.[59] There have been isolated reports of filter migration to the heart and cases of aortic penetration by the struts.

TrapEase Filter

The TrapEase was approved for use in the United States in 2000. This filter is laser cut from nitinol tubing and is therefore nonferromagnetic and MRI compatible. It has proximal and distal baskets pointing in opposite directions and consists of six diamond-shaped struts, the two baskets being connected by six straight struts containing hooks to anchor the device to the caval wall. It is a self-centering device and is may be used in inferior venae cavae to ranging from 18 to 30 mm in diameter. Of all the FDA-approved IVC filters, the fewest data are available on the results of the TrapEase filter.

PATIENT PREPARATION AND IVC FILTER PLACEMENT

Once filter placement is determined to be indicated, adequate patient preparation is required to ensure safety and minimize potential hazards. Review of filter indications (Table 37–3) and pertinent diagnostic studies are mandatory not only to confirm the need, but also to evaluate possible access sites, evaluate anatomy for significant variants, and determine the extent and location of thrombus. Guidelines for determining the urgency of placement of filters according to our institution are given in Table 37–8. The basis for these guidelines is an early study by Greenfield.[60] Most patients have had lower-extremity ultrasound for evaluation of their DVT, and this is helpful to evaluate the patency of the common femoral veins, the most common access route for IVC filter placement.

In our institution coagulation parameters are measured with the prothrombin time (PT) and the activated partial thromboplastin time (aPTT). In patients on intravenous heparin, the infusion is stopped on call to the angiography suite. Reversal with protamine is not necessary. If necessary, we restart heparin 2 hours after the procedure. For patients on warfarin, the International Normalized Ratio (INR) is manipulated to less than or equal to 2. For patients receiving low-molecular-weight heparin, we usually hold one dose prior to placement. A platelet count is obtained prior to filter placement and should be greater than 50,000/μL. Evaluation of the renal function prior to contrast injection is important, although usually relatively small volumes of contrast medium (20 to 30 mL) are used. With renal dysfunction or severe contrast allergy, an alternative contrast such as carbon dioxide or gadolinium may be used to evaluate the inferior vena cava. Although no clear evidence exists for bacterial seeding of a filter in a septic patient, it is plausible that a filter may become infected in such cases. Although we prefer not to place an IVC filter in the presence of bacteremia, if the patient is receiving adequate antibiotic coverage, we will place the filter. It is obviously essential to explain the entire procedure to the patient and the family and discuss known risks and benefits. Almost all filters are placed with local anesthesia (2% lidocaine) at the puncture site, and intravenous conscious sedation may be used with fentanyl (Sublimaze) and midazolam (Versed) in small divided doses while monitoring vital signs during the procedure. However, IVC filter placement is not painful and is quick to perform, so that intravenous conscious sedation is usually not necessary unless the patient is overly anxious or cannot lie still. The filter can be placed via the common femoral veins or the internal jugular veins, or occasionally via an arm vein.

Unusual circumstances may arise in which a venous anomaly exists and filter placement must be modified to accommodate this see (Table 37–2). In cases of double IVCs, bilateral filters should be placed. In the case of infrarenal IVC thrombus, a suprarenal filter may be placed. Care must be taken not to overlook accessory

Table 37–8 • GUIDELINES FOR DETERMINING THE URGENCY OF IVC FILTER PLACEMENT

Anticoagulation Status	Clinical Circumstance (Indication)				
	Pulmonary Embolism[a]		Deep Venous Thrombus[a]		Prophylactic
	With hemodynamic compromise[b]	Without hemodynamic compromise[b]	Femoro-popliteal	Free-floating iliofemoral (>5 cm long)	
Contraindicated	Emergent	Place within 24 hours	Place within 24 hours	Place within 12 hours	Elective
Failed[c]	Emergent	Place within 24 hours	Place within 24 hours	Place within 24 hours	Elective

Algorithm currently in use at Brigham and Womens Hospital (Boston).
[a] PE or DVT documented by nuclear medicine, CT, MRI, pulmonary angiography, venography, or ultrasonography.
[b] Hemodynamic compromise equals systemic hypotension and/or right ventricular strain on echocardiography.
[c] Failed anticoagulation but currently on anticoagulation.
Modified from Jones TK, Barnes RW, Greenfield LJ. Greenfield vena caval filter: rationale and current indications. Ann Thorac Surg 1986;42: S48–S55, with permission.

renal veins, which may arise below the usual location, and if left unfiltered, provide a bypass conduit for clot. Rarely, large collaterals, particularly the left gonadal vein, may provide a large bypass for clot, in which case a suprarenal filter may be placed. Filters placed into the cava are able to trap clot by obvious means. The filter itself is thrombogenic because of its metallic composition, the reaction in the wall of the cava, and turbulence and hemodynamic changes in caval flow. Flow studies show the Bird's Nest filter to be least disturbing to laminar flow.[38,49] The filters trap emboli of different sizes based upon their configuration. Once an embolus is trapped, the rapid flow of the cava and renal inflow along with the body's own lytic system eventually lyse the clot. Of course, if a large-enough clot or multiple clots are trapped, complete blockage to flow may result, further complicating matters by thrombosing back into the iliac veins. A suprarenal filter location complicated by occlusion may result in renal vein thrombosis.

COMPLICATIONS OF IVC FILTER PLACEMENT

The currently FDA-approved filters are permanent devices and it is difficult to evaluate long-term sequelae. It may be wise to assume that the longer time they are within the body, the greater the potential for complications. Major associated complications are listed in Tables 37–6 and 37–7. As with any angiographic procedure, certain complications are universal. Overall contrast reactions occur in 4%.[61] Lethal contrast reactions are rare and occur in 0.006% of patients who receive intravenous contrast media.[61] Puncture site complications include thrombosis, which is reduced with the lower-profile designs and produces symptoms in only 3%[62] but have been seen in up to 41% of asymptomatic patients after percutaneous placement of the early 24-French Greenfield filter.[63] Venous hemorrhage may be seen in less than 5% and is usually self-limited. Arteriovenous fistula from the puncture may be seen in 1% to 3%.[64] Filter malposition varies with the device and with operator skill, but ranges between 1% and 10%.[54,56,65,66] It most commonly involves the right heart, the right renal vein, and the iliac veins. Filter tilt cannot be assessed on plain film alone, without knowing the actual course of the inferior vena cava. Minor degrees of filter migration are not unusual, but are usually medically insignificant. Significant migration is usually due to a large cava. Vena caval perforation by the filter struts is common, but is usually inconsequential. There have been case reports of aortic, vertebral body, or ureteral penetration. Filter fracture has been described[67] but no serious side effects from it are known, although theoretically it may lose some of its efficacy. The most clinically significant complications are recurrent PE and IVC occlusion with secondary phlegmasia cerulea dolens. Every filter must allow clot of some finite size to pass; otherwise it would rapidly be obstructed with clots. The rates of symptomatic IVC occlusion range widely between studies and filter designs to between 0% and 30%.[55] Large filling defects and caval occlusion are found among the wires of the Birds Nest filter. Asymptomatic caval occlusion is more likely as revealed by many imaging-based follow-up studies.[55] This may be of more concern as clot may propagate through and above the filter, rendering it useless. Concomitant use of anticoagulation should be undertaken if possible to treat the underlying DVT. However, there still is a significantly higher incidence of recurrent DVT at 2-year follow-up in patients with IVC filters (20.8%) compared to those without filters (11.6%) despite anticoagulation in both groups.[4] A recent Japanese study of 42 patients found the incidence of recurrent PE, caval occlusion, and filter thrombus to be lower in patients with filters who had been simultaneously anticoagulated as well.[68] The mortality rate due to filter deployment is extremely low. In a review of 2557 filter placements, only three deaths were reported.[69] Mortality is usually due to contrast medium-induced anaphylaxis, the patient's pre-existing disease, or severe operator error.

SPECIAL FILTER CIRCUMSTANCES

Superior Vena Cava

Filters must be placed cautiously in the superior vena cava as space and margin of error is limited. It is very unusual for a superior vena caval (SVC) filter to be necessary for upper-extremity venous thrombosis. There is limited experience and long-term outcomes are unknown. In a study of six patients, four of whom were followed for up to 14 months, no complications were encountered and there was no evidence of recurrent PE.[70] In a series of 72 SVC Greenfield filters placed and a mean follow-up of 7.8 months, no migration or displacement was seen. Although 34 of the patients died of unrelated causes, the remaining 38 patients had no evidence of recurrent PE.[71]

Suprarenal Filter

There was no difference in the rates of recurrent PE between suprarenal and infrarenal IVC filters in a limited study of Stainless Steel Greenfield filters.[72] Suprarenal filters are safe and effective.[73] There is no evidence that suprarenal placement alters renal function or patency.[72,73] This is the ideal location for placement in patients with infrarenal IVC thrombus, in those with large gonadal collaterals or renal source of emboli, with improper functioning of an infrarenal filter, or pregnant patients.[73]

Pediatric Patients

This field remains controversial as long-term data are nonexistent. It would seem risky in terms of future complications to place a filter in a child. A study of eight pediatric patients aged 6 to 16 years over a 19-month follow-up period demonstrated a 100% technical success rate with no immediate complications. Three patients subsequently died during follow-up, two from their underlying tumors and one from IVC and renal vein thrombosis, which was the indication for filter placement. The remaining five were uncomplicated at 19 months.[74]

Terminally Ill Patients

Placement of filter in a patient with terminal illness as a "last rite" has shown no survival advantage,[75] and may expose the patient to unnecessary stress and risk, although advanced neoplastic disease itself should not be a deterrent if a filter is indicated.[76] The overall health and life span of the patient as well as potential survival must be considered.

Prophylactic Placement

Permanent device placement remains controversial. As any contraindication to anticoagulation may be temporary, a permanent filter with its long-term risks, especially in a young patient, gives cause for concern. However, the rate of pulmonary emboli in high-risk bedridden patients is great, and the use of anticoagulation may prove to be even more complicated. In such a circumstance the safer choice may be a filter. A prospective randomized trial is needed to determine the value of IVC filtration. Patients with severe multiple trauma, especially neurosurgical and orthopedic patients, are at high risk for DVT.[77] In patients who have poor cardiopulmonary reserve and who cannot tolerate a PE, a filter may be of benefit. In a mean follow-up of 28.9 months of 105 filters inserted for trauma, of which 64 were placed prophylactically, no recurrent PE was detected, although one IVC was occluded and 44% of patients developed a DVT. Eleven patients were symptomatic with leg swelling.[78]

Septic Thromboemboli

Traditionally this has been treated with surgical caval interruption. In a study by Peyton and coworkers[79] using a dog model, the Greenfield filter plus antibiotics proved better than caval ligation, and had a lower risk of complicating sequelae.

FUTURE OUTLOOK

There are many studies underway to evaluate temporary filters and their safety. The usual indication for filter placement is a patient who cannot for some reason undergo anticoagulation. Often this is an acute problem. In these circumstances, it would be very useful to have a device that could bridge the gap until anticoagulation became safe. Currently two main temporary filter designs exist: the tethered filters and the retrievable filters. The tethered filters, such as the Tempofilter (Braun Medical Inc., Bethlehem, Pennsylvania), have a permanent attachment by way of a tether to the site of entry. The filter may be left in place for up to 6 weeks prior to its permanent incorporation into the caval wall. The tether is buried in the subcutaneous tissue and when needed is used with a sheath to retrieve the filter. The retrievable filters are not connected to the skin, but instead have a hook on one end, usually opposite the entry site for placement, and a foldable design. An example of a retrievable design is the Gunther Tulip filter (William Cook Europe A/S, Bjaeverskov, Denmark). This design allows deployment from a femoral route and retrieval via the hook from jugular access. Usually retrieval through a sheath must be made within 2 to 4 weeks. The hook is grasped and the filter is folded into the sheath for removal. Problems that may be inherent to these filters include the loss of ability to retrieve due to caval incorporation. Other complications are similar[80] to those of permanent filters, the most worrisome being recurrent pulmonary embolism and filter thrombosis. Additionally, because of their inherent temporary nature, these filters may be more likely to migrate, and fatalities are well-described in the literature. In a study on the Tempofilter, migration, although seen in 7.5% of 66 patients prior to removal, did not preclude removal of the device.[81] One problem unique to temporary filters is how to manage the filter that contains trapped emboli. In the prior mentioned study,[81] removal was not hindered although partial thrombosis of the filter was observed in 15% of patients. If necessary, however, possible solutions include lysis of the thrombus prior to removal, mechanical removal of the thrombus, placement of a permanent filter above the temporary one if thrombus is seen, or nonremoval of the "temporary filter" (i.e., concession to permanence). We should see temporary designs available in the United States within the next few years, although many issues regarding their use and safety remain to be elucidated.

■ REFERENCES

Chapter 37 References

1. Lilienfield DE. Decreasing mortality from pulmonary embolism in the United States, 1979–1996. Int J Epidemiol 2000;29:465–469.
2. Ortega M, Gahtan V, Roberts A, et al. Efficacy of anticoagulation post inferior vena cava filter placement. Am Surg 1998;5:419–423.
3. Streiff MB, Vena caval filters: A comprehensive review. Blood 2000;95:3669–3677.
4. Decousus H, Leizorovicz A, Parent F, et al. A clinical trial of vena caval filters in the prevention of pulmonary embolism in patients with proximal deep vein thrombosis. N Engl J Med 1998; 338:409–415.
5. Hunter J. Observations on inflammation of internal coat of veins. Trans Soc Improve Med Chir Knowledge (London) 1793;1:18–42.
6. Homans J. Thrombosis of deep veins of the lower leg, causing pulmonary embolism. N Engl J Med 1934;211:993–997.
7. Ochsner A, DeBakey M. Intravenous clotting and its sequelae. Surgery 1943;14:679–690.
8. Homans J. Deep quiet venous thrombosis in the lower limb: preferred levels for interruption of veins; iliac sector or ligation. Surg Gynecol Obstet 1944;79:70–82.

9. Nasbeth, DC, Moran JM. Reassessment of the role of inferior vena cava ligation in venous thromboembolism. N Engl J Med 1965;23:1250–1253.
10. Adams JT, Feingold BE, Deweese JA. Comparitive evaluation of ligation and partial interruption of the inferior vena cava. Arch Surg 1971;103:272–276.
11. Amador E, Li TK, Crane C. Ligation of inferior vena cava for thromboembolism: clinical and autopsy correlations in 119 cases. JAMA 1968;8:1758–1760.
12. Schroeder TM, Elkins RC, Greenfield LJ. Entrapment of sized emboli by KMA–Greenfield intracaval filter. Surgery 1978;83: 435–439.
13. Moser KM, Harsany PG, Harvey-Smith W et al. Reversible interruption of the inferior vena cava by means of a ballon catheter. J Thorc Cardiovasc Surg 1971;62;205–212.
14. Eichelter P, Shenk WG. Prophylaxis of pulmonary embolism: a new experimental approach with initial results. Arch Surg 1968: 97;348–356.
15. DeWeese MS, Hunter DC. A vena caval filter for the prevention of pulmonary embolism. Arch Surg 1963;86:852–868.
16. Moretz WH Rhode CM, Shepherd MH. Prevention of pulmonary emboli by partial occlusion of the inferior vena cava. Am Surg 1959;25;617–625.
17. Adams JT, Feingold BE, DeWeese JA. Comparative evaluation of ligation and partial interruption of the inferior vena cava. Arch Surg 1971;103;272–276.
18. Jones TK, Barnes RW, Greenfield LJ. Greenfield vena caval filter: rationale and current indications. Ann Thorc Surg 1986:42; S48–S55.
19. Mobin-Uddin K, Smith PE, Martinez LO, et al. A vena caval filter for the prevention of pulmonary embolus. Surg Forum 1967: 18;209–211.
20. Rutherford RB. Vascular Surgery. 2nd edition. Philadelphia, WB Saunders, 1984.
21. Tadavarthy SM, Castenada-Zuniga WR, Salomonowitz E, et al. Kimray–Greenfield vena cava filter: percutaneous introduction. Radiology 1984;151:525–526.
22. Mejia EA, Saroyan RM, Balkin PW, et al. Analysis of inferior venacavography before Greenfield filter placement. Ann Vasc Surg 1989;3:232–235.
23. Kellman GM, Alpern MB, Sandler MA, et al. Computed tomography of vena caval anomalies with embryologic correlation. Radiographics 1988;8;533–556.
24. Ferris EJ. The inferior vena cava. In: Abrams H (Ed): Abrams Angiography. 3rd edition. Boston, Little Brown, p.939.
25. Dharman K. Transcaval ureter. J Urol 1980;123:575–576.
26. Norris CS, Greenfield LJ; Herrmann JB. Free floating iliofemoral thrombus, a risk of pulmonary embolism. Arch Surg 1985;120: 806–808.
27. Combined staff clinics: Thromboembolism. Am J Med 1947;3: 753–768.
28. Barker NW Anticoagulation therapy in post-operative thrombophlebitis and pulmonary embolism. Minn Med 1946:29;778–782.
29. Coon WW, Willis PW III, Symons MJ. Assesment of anticoagulation treatment of venous thromboembolism. Ann Surg 1969:170; 559–568.
30. Barker NW, Nygaard KK, Walters W, et al. A statistical study of post operative venous thrombosis and pulmonary embolism. Time of occurrence during the post operative period. Proc Staff Meet Mayo Clin 1941;16:17–21.
31. Landefeld CS, Beyth RJ. Anticoagulant related bleeding: clinical epidemiology, prediction, and prevention. Am J Med 1993;95: 315–328.
32. Kakkar VV, Howe CT, Flanc C, et al. Natural history of post operative DVT. Lancet 1969;2:230–232.
33. Khansarinia S, Dennis JW, Veldenz HC, et al. Prophylactic Greenfield filter placement in selected high-risk trauma patients. J Vasc Surg 1995;22:231–236.
34. Knudson MM, Howe CT, Flanc C, et al. Prevention of venous thromboembolism in trauma patients. J Trauma 1994;37:480–487.
35. Dennis JW, Menawat S, Vonthron J, et al. Efficacy of DVT prophylaxis in trauma patients and identifying high risk groups. J Trauma 1993;35:132–139.
36. Shackeford SR. Venous thromboembolism in patients with major trauma. Am J Surg 1990;159:365–369.
37. Greenfield LJ, Proctor MC, Michaels AJ, et al. Prophylactic vena caval filters in trauma: the rest of the story. J Vasc Surg 2000; 32:490–495.
38. Katsamouris AA, Waltman AC, Delichatsios MA, et al. Inferior vena cava filters; in vitro comparison of clot trapping and flow dynamics. Radiology 1988;2:361–366.
39. Simon M, Rabkin DJ. Comparative evaluation of clinically available inferior vena cava filters with an in vitro physiologic simulation of the vena cava. Radiology 1993;189:769–774.
40. Korbin CD, Reed RA, Taylor FC, et al. Comparison of filters in an oversized vena caval phantom: intracaval placement of a Bird's Nest filter versus biiliac placement of Greenfield, Vena Tech-LGM, and Simon nitinol filters. J Vasc Interv Radiol 1992;3: 559–564.
41. Mozes M, Adar R. Vein ligation in the treatment of pulmonary embolism. Surgery 1964;5:621–629.
42. Athanasoulis CA, Kaufman JA, Halpern EF, et al. Inferior vena caval filters: review of a 26-year single center clinical experience. Radiology 2000;216:54–66.
43. Moran JM, Khan PC, Callow AD. Partial versus complete caval interruption for venous thromboembolism. Am J Surg 1969;117: 471–479.
44. Dorfman GS, Cronin JJ, Tupper TB, et al. Occult pulmonary embolism: a common occurrence in deep venous thrombosis. Am J Radiol 1987;148:263–266.
45. Huisman MV, Buller HR, ten Cate JW, et al. Unexpected high prevalence of silent pulmonary embolism in patients with deep venous thrombosis. Chest 1989;95:498–502.
46. Murphy TP, Cronon JJ. Evolution of deep venous thrombosis: a prospective evaluation with ultrasound. Radiology 1990;177: 543–548.
47. Murphy TP, Dorfman GS, Yedlicka JW, et al. LGM vena cava filter: objective evaluation of early results. J Vasc Interv Radiol 1991;2:107–115.
48. Greenfield LJ, Proctor MC. Twenty-year clinical experience with the Greenfield filter. Cardiovasc Surg 1995;2:199–205.
49. Ansell G, Bettmann M, Kaufman J. Complications in Diagnostic Imaging and Interventional Radiology, 3rd edition. Oxford, UK, Blackwell Science, 1996.
50. Thompson BH, Cragg AH, Smith TP, et al. Thrombus-trapping efficiency of the Greenfield filter in vivo. Radiology 1988; 172:979–981.
51. Lang W, Schweiger H, Hoffman-Preiss K. Results of long term venocavography study after placement of a Greenfield vena caval filter. J Cardiovasc Surg 1992;33:573–578.
52. Greenfield LJ, Proctor MC, Cho KJ, et al. Extended evaluation of the titanium Greenfield vena cava filter. J Vasc Surg 1994; 20:458–464.
53. Greenfield LJ, Cho KJ, Proctor MC, et al. Results of a multicenter study of the modified hook titanium Greenfield filter. J Vasc Surg 1991;14:253–257.
54. Ricco JB, Crochette D, Sebilotte P. Percutaneous transvenous caval interruption with the "LGM" filter: Early results of a multicenter trial. Ann Vasc Surg 1988;3:242–247.
55. Baum S, Abrams, H. Abrams Angiography 4th edition. Philadelphia; Lippincott Williams & Wilkins, 1996.
56. Roehm JOF, Johnsrude IS, Barth MH, et al. The Bird's Nest inferior vena cava filter: Progress report. Radiology 1988; 168:745–749.
57. Carlson JE, Yedlicka JW, Castenada-Zuniga WR, et al. Acute clot trapping efficiency in dogs with compacted versus elongated wires in Bird's Nest filters. J Vasc Interv Radiol 1993;4:513–516.

58. Simon Nitinol Filter: Instructions for use. Nitinol Medical Technologies, Bard Radiology, 1997
59. Simon M, Athanasoulis CA, Kim D, et al. Simon nitinol inferior vena cava filter: initial clinical experience. Radiology 1989;172:99–103.
60. Greenfield LJ. Current indications for and results of Greenfield filter placement. J Vasc Surg 1984;1:502–504.
61. Shehadi WH. Contrast media adverse reactions. Radiology 1980;137:299–302.
62. Molgaard CP, Yucel EK, Geller SC, et al. Access-site thrombosis after placement of inferior vena cava filters with 12–14 F delivery sheaths. Radiology 1992;185:257–261.
63. Dorffman GS, et al. Iatrogenic changes at the venotomy site after percutaneous placement of the Greenfield filter. Radiology 1989;173:159–162.
64. Grassi CJ, Bettman MA, Finkelstein J, et al. Femoral arterovenous fistula after placement of a Kimray–Greenfield filter. AJR 1988;151:681–682.
65. Grassi CJ, Matsumoto AH, Teitelbaum GP. Vena caval occlusion after Simon Nitinol filter placement: identification with MR imaging in patients with malignancy. J Vasc Intervent Radiol 1992;3:535–539.
66. Grassi CJ. Inferior vena cava filters: analysis of five currently available devices. Am J Radiol 1991;156:813–821.
67. Lang W, Schweiger H, Fietkau R, et al. Spontaneous disruption of two Greenfield vena caval filters. Radiology 1990;174:445–447.
68. Yazu T, Fujioka H, Nakamura M, et al. Long-term reults of inferior vena cava filters: experiences in a Japanese population. Intern Med 2000;39:707–714.
69. Scurr JH, Jarrett PE, Wastell C. The treatment of recurrent pulmonary embolism: experience with the Kimray–Greenfield vena cava filter. Ann R Coll Surg Engl 1983;65:233–234.
70. Ascer E, Gennaro M, Lorenson E, et al. Superior vena caval Greenfield filters: indications, techniques, and results. J Vasc Surg 1996;3:498–503.
71. Ascher E, Hingorani A, Tsemekhin B, et al. Lessons learned from a 6-year clinical experience with superior vena cava Greenfield filters. J Vasc Surg 2000;32:881–887.
72. Greenfield LJ, Cho KJ, Proctor MC, et al. Late results of suprarenal Greenfield vena cava filter placement. Arch Surg 1992;127:969–973.
73. Matchett WJ, Jones MP, McFarland DR, et al. Suprarenal vena caval filter replacement: follow up of four filter types in 22 patients. J Vasc Interv Radiol 1998;4:588–593.
74. Reed RA, Teitelbaum GP, Stanley P, et al. The use of inferior vena cava filters in pediatric patients for pulmonary embolus prophylaxis. Cardiovasc Intervent Radiol 1996;6:401–405.
75. Rosen MP, Porter DH, Kim D. Reassessment of vena caval filter use in patients with cancer. J Vasc Interv Radiol 1994;5:501–506.
76. Lossef SV, Barth KH. Outcome of patients with advanced neoplastic disease receiving vena caval filters. J Vasc Interv Radiol 1995;2:273–277.
77. Gosin JS, Graham AM, Ciocca RG, et al. Efficacy of prophylactic vena cava filters in high risk trauma patients. Ann Vasc Surg 1997;1:100–105.
78. Wojcik R, Cipolle MD, Fearen I, et al. Long-term follow-up of trauma patients with a vena caval filter. J Trauma 2000;49:839–843.
79. Peyton JW, Hylemon MB, Greenfield LJ, et al. Comparison of Greenfield filter and surgical ligation for experimental septic thromboembolism. Surgery 1983;93:533–537.
80. Linsenmaier U, Rieger J, Schenk F, et al. Indications, management, and complications of temporary inferior vena cava filters. Cardiovasc Interv Radiol 1998;6:464–469.
81. Bovyn G, Gory P, Reynaud P, et al. The Tempofilter: a multicenter study of a new temporary caval filter implantable for up to six weeks. Ann Vasc Surg 1997;11:520–528.
82. Ferris EJ, McCowan TC, Carver DK, et al. Percutaneous inferior vena cava filters: follow-up of seven designs in 320 patients. Radiology 1993;188:851–856.
83. Greenfield LJ, Michna BA. 12 year clinical experience with the Greenfield vena cava filter. Surgery 1988;104:706–712.
84. Greenfield LJ, Delucia A. Endovascular therapy of venous thromboembolic disease. Surg Clin North Am 1992;72:969–989.
85. Mohan CR, Hollballah JJ, Sharp WJ, et al. Comparative efficacy and complications of vena cava filters. J Vasc Surg 1995;21:235–246.
86. Becker DM, Philbrick JT, Selby JB. Inferior vena cava filters: indications, safety, effectiveness. Arch Intern Med 1992;152:1985–1994.
87. Starok MS, Comman AA. Follow-up after insertion of Bird's Nest inferior vena cava filter. Can Assoc Radiol J 1996;47:189–194.
88. Nicholson AA, Ettles DF, Paddon AJ, et al. Long term follow-up of the Bird's Nest inferior vena cava filter. Clin Radiol 1999;54:759–764.
89. Poletti PA, Becker CD, Prina L, et al. Long term results of the Simon Nitinol inferior vena cava filter. Eur Radiol 1998;8:289–294.
90. Crochet DP, Brunel P, Troglic S, et al. Long term follow-up of Venatech-LGM filter: predictors and frequency of caval occlusion. J Vasc Interv Radiol 1992;10:137–142.
91. Cho KJ. Efficacy and problems associated with vena cava filters. In: Cope C (ed.): Current Techniques in Interventional Radiology. Philadelphia, Current Medicine, 1994, pp. 8.1–8.17.

CHAPTER 38

Inferior Vena Caval Filters: A Hematologist's Perspective

Michael Streiff, M.D.

Deep venous thrombosis (DVT) and pulmonary embolism (PE) occur in approximately 800,000 patients in the United States each year.[1] While the vast majority of these episodes are amenable to treatment with anticoagulant or thrombolytic therapy, occasionally situations arise when medical therapy is contraindicated. In these rare instances, inferior vena caval (IVC) filters have been proposed as a useful alternative to prevent recurrent PE. In recent years as filter technology has improved and the ease of insertion has increased (for a discussion of anatomical details, history of IVC filters, and description of their insertion, see Chapter 37), a number of investigators have proposed that the indications for filter insertion be broadened.[2–15] Current estimates indicate that approximately 40,000 IVC filters are inserted annually in the United States (150 filters per million population).[16] In comparison, only 20 to 30 IVC filters are inserted annually in Sweden (three filters per million inhabitants), an industrialized nation with health care of comparable quality.[17] Disparity of this magnitude warrants scrutiny. Do IVC filters significantly reduce morbidity and mortality or do we use these devices primarily because of our insatiable appetite for health care technology?

The results of a 1993 survey of a university-affiliated community hospital suggest that the latter conclusion may account for some of our current usage. The investigators found that 20% of IVC filter recipients had no identifiable contraindication to anticoagulation and 14% had filters placed without even prior confirmation of venous thromboembolism (VTE) by objective testing.[18] The purpose of this chapter will be to review the available literature regarding IVC filters and the traditional and proposed indications for their use, and determine whether the available data support our current practice.

THE SAFETY AND EFFICACY OF IVC FILTERS IN VTE

The modern age of venous interruption began in 1973 when Greenfield and colleagues introduced the original model of the Kimray–Greenfield filter.[19] A cone of stainless steel wires with anchoring hooks for fixation, the Stainless Steel Greenfield filter influenced the design of many of the currently available IVC filters on the market (Fig. 38–1A). The currently available Greenfield filters include the modified-hook Titanium Greenfield filter, first introduced in 1991, and the over-the-wire alternating-hook stainless steel Greenfield filter, approved by the U.S. Food and Drug Administration in 1995. The Titanium Greenfield filter was crafted from titanium with the hope that its improved flexibility and smaller introducer would reduce the incidence of insertion site thrombosis (Fig. 38–1B).[20–32] Problems with filter tilting stimulated the development of the over-the-wire alternating-hook Stainless Steel Greenfield filter, which has an apical aperture through which a guidewire passes, easing placement and centering.[33–35]

Borrowing from the cone-shaped design of the Greenfield filters, the Vena Tech filter consists of a cone of six limbs constructed of Phynox, a nonparamagnetic alloy, stabilized by six barbed side rails (Fig. 38–1E).[16,26–28,30,31,36–44] In contrast, the Simon Nitinol filter consists of an umbrella of seven petal-shaped loops affixed to the caval wall by six hooked legs. Its unique nickel-titanium alloy gives it thermal memory properties. The filter consists of a set of soft wires that open like an umbrella when exposed to body temperature. This capability allows it to be loaded in the smallest introducer catheter of any available filter (9F) (Fig. 38–1D).[26,28,31,32,45–51] As its name suggests, the Bird's

569

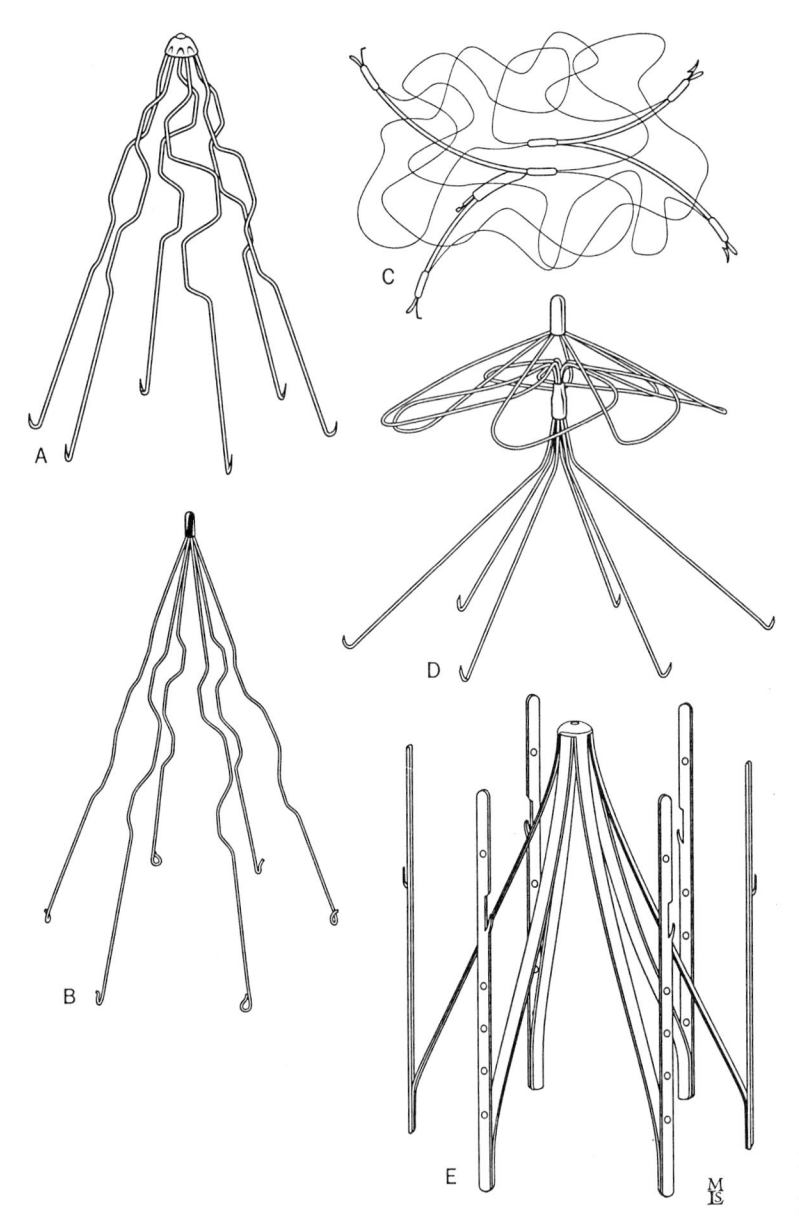

Figure 38–1. Vena caval filter models. **A.** Stainless Steel Greenfield filter. **B.** Titanium Greenfield filter. **C.** Bird's Nest filter. **D.** Simon Nitinol filter. **E.** VenaTech filter.

Nest filter consists of a nest of stainless steel wires attached to V-shaped struts, which anchor it in the inferior vena cava. Its unique design allows it to be placed in cavae as large as 40 mm in diameter (all other filters are limited to cavae of 28 mm or less) (Fig. 38–1C).[16,26,28,30–32,52–63]

Despite considerable design differences, in vivo the filters demonstrate comparable safety and efficacy. Although the original Stainless Steel Greenfield filter is no longer available, data on this device are included because it has been studied in more patients than any other device and serves as a benchmark of comparison for other filters.[2,4,16,28,29,31,32,64–98] When reviewing these data, several study design caveats must be kept in mind. All of the filter studies published to date save one have been prospective or retrospective clinical case series. No randomized trials comparing different filter types exist. Therefore, no filter can claim superiority. Clinical end points of efficacy (PE) and adverse effects (DVT, insertion site thrombosis, inferior vena caval thrombosis, etc.) are often investigated when clinical symptoms suggest their presence. Only a minority of study patients underwent routine radiologic end point assessment. Therefore, it is likely that many of the event rates represent underestimates of their true frequency.

With these limitations in mind, all of the filter types appear to be roughly equivalent in prevention of PE (Table 38–1). Although differences in study design are significant, the rate of PE postfilter insertion compares favorably with that seen with anticoagulation. Therefore, IVC filters appear to be a useful alternative in the prevention of PE when anticoagulation is absolutely contraindicated.

Insertion-site thrombosis (IST) is a DVT that develops at the site of venous access following filter placement. Predictably, studies that used routine screening identified two- to threefold more IST than studies without screening. Nevertheless, while intuitively it makes

Table 38–1 • COMPILATION OF IVC FILTER STUDY DATA

Filter Type	No. Studies	No. Patients	F/U Duration (mos.)	PE	DVT	IVCT	Postphlebitic Syndrome
Stainless Steel Greenfield	40	3184	18 (range, 1–60)	66/2561 (2.6%) (range, 0–9%) 22 fatal (0.9%)	96/1634 (5.9%) (range, 0–18%)	73/2033 (3.6%) (range, 0–18%)	254/1353 (19%) (range, 0–47%)
Over-the-wire alternating-hook Stainless Steel Greenfield	3	646	20.6 (range, 8.5–26)	7/278 (3.1%) 1 fatal (0.4%)	18/240 (7.5%)	6/278 (2.2%)	62/231 (26.8%)
Titanium Greenfield	10	511	5.8 (range, 0–81)	13/422 (3.1%) (range, 0–3.8%) fatal 7 (1.7%)	5/22 (22.7%) (range, 0–36%)	15/230 (6.5%) (range, 1%–31%)	34/236 (14.4%) (range, 9%–20%)
Bird's Nest	16	1487	15.6 (range, 0–72)	32/1186 (2.7%) (range, 0–8.3%) 6 fatal (0.5%)	25/443 (5.6%) (range, 0–20%)	37/1079 (3.4%) (range, 0–15%)	63/485 (13%) (range, 0–41%)
Simon Nitinol	10	417	13.8 (range, 0–62)	12/326 (3.7%) (range, 0–5.3%) 5 fatal (1.5%)	14/186 (7.5%) (range, 8–11%)	22/266 (8.3%) (range, 4%–18%)	16/124 (12.9%) (range, 6%–44%)
Vena Tech	15	1050	12 (range, 0–81)	33/963 (3.4%) (range, 0–8%) 3 fatal (0.3%)	8/25 (32%) (range, 32%)	83/741 (11.2%) (range, 0–28%)	95/232 (41%) (range, 24%–59%)

F/U, follow-up; PE, pulmonary embolism; DVT, deep venous thrombosis; IVCT, inferior vena caval thrombosis.
Note: The denominators of the various complications only include patients who were evaluated. Patients lost to follow-up or dead are not included. Only a portion of the studies evaluated patients for all these events.

sense to identify and treat both symptomatic and asymptomatic thrombi, this strategy remains to be verified in this patient population. More surprising are the comparable rates of IST among the various filter designs. The recognition of this complication was a major force behind the development of smaller introducer systems. Although the idea that smaller insertion systems would result in less venous trauma and fewer IST is theoretically attractive, there is little support for this notion given the IST frequency among various filters. The Simon Nitinol filter, which uses the smallest introducer catheter (9F), has an IST rate comparable to the filter with the largest catheter size (29F), the Stainless Steel Greenfield filter. The currently available data suggest that placement of any available filter is associated with a comparable frequency of subsequent access site thrombus formation (Table 38–2).

DVT is not an infrequent occurrence in patients following IVC filter placement. DVT rates vary widely among the different filter types (Table 38–1). No studies performed routine follow-up radiologic studies so these rates apply only to symptomatic thrombi. In general, higher DVT rates have been noted when small populations have been studied and rates have declined as study populations have increased in size. This trend may reflect more intense observation of smaller populations of patients or alternatively may be due to the disproportionate impact of a few thrombotic events on rates when study populations are small. Since filters are typically placed in patients at high risk for thrombotic events, these data need not necessarily indicate that filters increase the chances of recurrent DVT in patients. However, data from a randomized multicenter trial in France suggest that filters double the risk of recurrent DVT in patients (see below).[99]

Inferior vena caval thrombosis (IVCT) was a common complication of early caval interruption devices, including the Mobin-Uddin umbrella filter. While the incidence of IVCT is less with modern filters, these devices nevertheless are not free of this complication (Table 38–1). As with DVT and IST rates, the rate of IVCT varies greatly between different studies of the same filter and studies of different filters. As with IST rates, surveillance intensity is the most important variable in this equation. Studies using sensitive radiologic methods (inferior vena cavagrams, contrast computed tomography [CT] scans, magnetic resonance angiograms) on a routine basis reveal higher rates of IVCT, while studies using less sensitive methods or using imaging only in symptomatic patients report lower rates. Since the vast majority of studies fall into the latter category, it is likely that the mean rate of IVCT for all the filters is a gross underestimate.

Perhaps the best estimate of this complication comes from the studies of Crochet and coworkers who followed a population of Vena Tech filter patients with routine ultrasonography and/or vena cavography every 2 years. At 9 years of follow-up, only 67% of filters were still patent, with no evidence of a plateau in the incidence curve. Among patients who had PE and failed anticoagulation, the patency rate was only 35%. These data suggest that a progressive decline of filter patency and loss of protection as venous collaterals develop are predictable long-term sequelae of caval interruption. Since these data were obtained in Vena Tech filter patients, it is unclear whether similar results would be obtained with other filtration devices.[42]

Postphlebitic syndrome is a common chronic complication of VTE. It consists of chronic lower-extremity swelling, venous stasis changes, including skin discoloration, and ulceration. In one study of DVT patients treated with standard anticoagulation, only 13% of patients were free of postphlebitic symptoms 10 years after their episode of DVT.[100] Therefore, it is not surprising that many patients develop postphlebitic syndrome after filter placement (Table 38–1). Since follow-up intensity and duration varies, no filter can be reliably asserted to be more or less likely to precipitate this syndrome. Therefore, the high rate of postphlebitic syndrome documented with the Vena Tech filter is more likely secondary to study design characteristics than idiosyncrasies of the device itself (Table 38–1).[37,42]

Although the following events should be mentioned when obtaining the consent of patients prior to filter placement, periprocedural complications (pneumothorax, hemorrhage, wound infection, misplacement) are rare (occurring in less than 1%). Likewise, migration and inferior vena cava perforation/penetration are highly publicized occurrences, which rarely result in clinically significant consequences. Migration is usually defined as movement of the filter more than 10 mm from its original placement location on follow-up abdominal radiographs. Except for the Titanium Greenfield filter (12.8%) and the Vena Tech filter (8.3%), migration is an uncommon event, occurring in 2% to 5% of filter recipients. Design differences or follow-up intensity may be responsible for these disparities. Less than 1% of filter recipients experience complications from filter migration. There is a wide variation among filter types of the frequency of inferior vena cava penetration (0% for Vena Tech filter versus 37% for Bird's Nest and Simon

Table 38–2 • INSERTION SITE THROMBOSIS RATES FOR IVC FILTERS

Filter Type (size)	IST—No Surveillance	IST—Routine Surveillance
Stainless Steel Greenfield (29F)	87/898 (9.6%) (range, 1%–47%)	50/217 (23%) (range, 14%–41%)
Over-the-wire alternating-hook Stainless Steel Greenfield (12F)	10/231 (4.3%)	NA
Titanium Greenfield (14F)	35/267 (13.1%) (range, 2%–50%)	23/82 (28%) (range, 25%–50%)
Bird's Nest (14F)	31/417 (7.4%) (range, 0–33%)	23/101 (23%) (range, 0–33%)
Simon Nitinol (9F)	22/252 (8.7%) (range, 0–64%)	11/36 (31%) (range, 16%–64%)
Vena Tech (12F)	36/215 (16.7%) (range, 8%–44%)	16/44 (36%) (range, 34%–44%)

IST, insertion site thrombosis.

Nitinol filters), which varies considerably depending upon what imaging modalities are used to demonstrate it. CT scans are the most sensitive technique. Although case reports have documented occasions when filters have perforated the inferior vena cava and invaded adjacent structures (duodenum, aorta, ureter, etc.), the vast majority of inferior vena cava perforations are asymptomatic.[101-104] Although filter tilting (5% to 12%) and leg fracture (1% to 14%) could conceivably contribute to decreased performance, proof that these complications are linked to any clinical events is lacking.

A RANDOMIZED TRIAL OF IVC FILTERS IN THE PREVENTION OF PULMONARY EMBOLI

The first and only randomized study of IVC filters in the prevention of PE was conducted by by Decousus et al.[99] They randomized 400 patients with a proximal DVT in a two-by-two factorial design to receive a IVC filter or no filter and unfractionated heparin or enoxaparin. Four different types of IVC filters were used and all were placed within 48 hours of randomization. Ventilation/perfusion scans were performed at baseline and after 8 to 12 days of anticoagulation. IVC filters were associated with a significant decrease in the incidence of PE compared with anticoagulation alone (1.1% versus 4.8%). At 2 years of follow-up this difference was no longer significant although the trend still favored IVC filters (3% versus 6%) (Fig. 38-2). Fatal emboli were also more common in patients treated solely with anticoagulation (0.5% versus 2.5%).[99] However, IVC filters were associated with significantly more recurrent DVT than anticoagulation alone (20.8% versus 11.6%) (Fig. 38-3). No difference in bleeding or mortality was documented. Sixteen of the 37 patients (43.2%) with IVC filters who had recurrent DVT also had IVCT.[99]

These data suggest that IVC filters are effective in the immediate prevention of pulmonary emboli and, when combined with anticoagulation, may be superior to anticoagulation alone in the short term. Unfortunately, these benefits do not persist over the long term and filters are associated with an increase in recurrent DVT. However, these data provide no guidance as to the safety and efficacy of filters in the typical patient who should not be anticoagulated. In addition, the question as to whether IVC filters are superior to anticoagulation still remains unanswered.

ANTICOAGULATION AFTER IVC FILTER PLACEMENT: IS IT NECESSARY?

If possible, many investigators recommend routine anticoagulation following placement of an IVC filter for 3 months until endothelialization has occurred.[105,106] Understandably, many patients who get IVC filters cannot be placed on anticoagulants because of the very contraindications that led to their insertion. In the published series to date that recorded anticoagulation status, only 44.7% of patients were on anticoagulant therapy during follow-up. Several authors have attempted to determine whether anticoagulants are in fact necessary after Greenfield filter placement. Ortega and coworkers conducted a retrospective chart review of 240 consecutive patients who had Greenfield filters placed. Half of the patients were discharged on warfarin. The mean period of warfarin treatment was 2 weeks, with a range of 1 to 8 weeks. Duplex ultrasound follow-up documented recurrent DVT in four anticoagulated patients and five on no anticoagulant.[94] Jones and coworkers also conducted a retrospective comparison of their group of Greenfield filter patients, some of whom received warfarin or heparin for 4 to 6 months. No difference in the

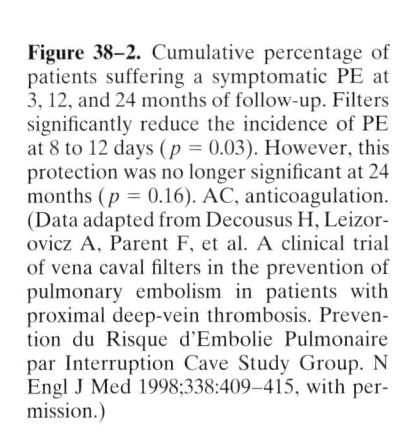

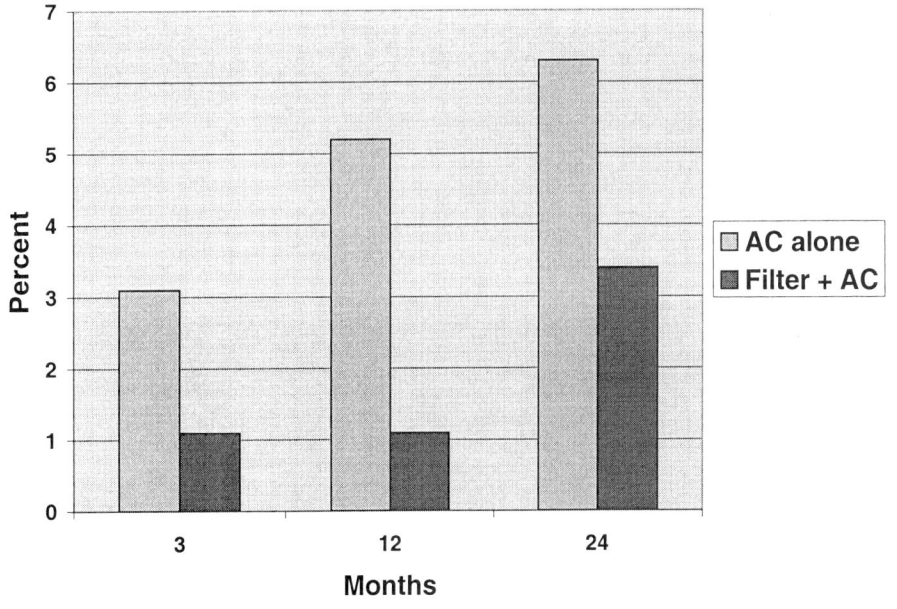

Figure 38-2. Cumulative percentage of patients suffering a symptomatic PE at 3, 12, and 24 months of follow-up. Filters significantly reduce the incidence of PE at 8 to 12 days ($p = 0.03$). However, this protection was no longer significant at 24 months ($p = 0.16$). AC, anticoagulation. (Data adapted from Decousus H, Leizorovicz A, Parent F, et al. A clinical trial of vena caval filters in the prevention of pulmonary embolism in patients with proximal deep-vein thrombosis. Prevention du Risque d'Embolie Pulmonaire par Interruption Cave Study Group. N Engl J Med 1998;338:409–415, with permission.)

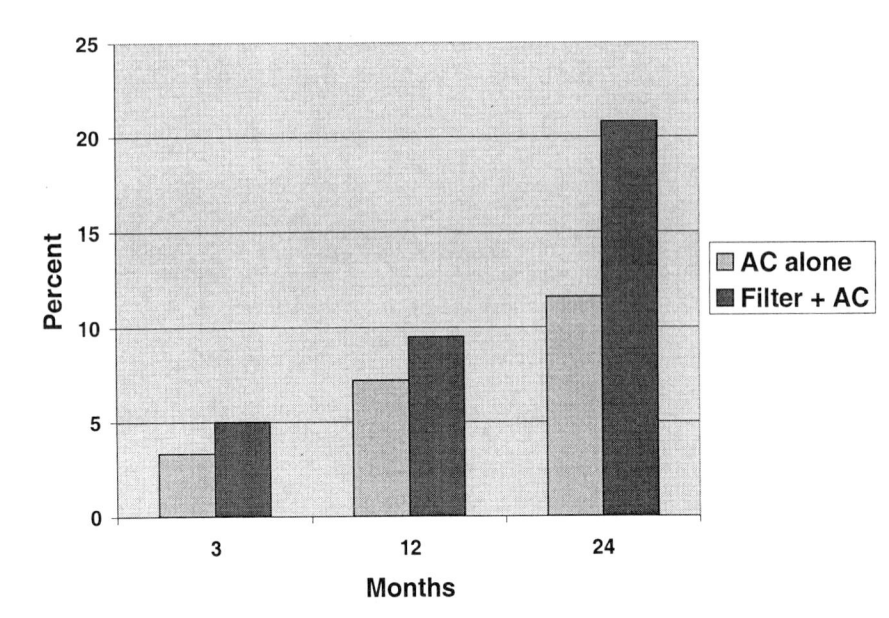

Figure 38–3. Cumulative percentage of patients with and without a filter suffering a DVT during follow-up. A significantly higher percentage of patients with vena caval filters developed a DVT during 24 months of follow-up ($p = 0.02$). (Data adapted from Decousus H, Leizorovicz A, Parent F, et al. A clinical trial of vena caval filters in the prevention of pulmonary embolism in patients with proximal deep-vein thrombosis. Prevention du Risque d'Embolie Pulmonaire par Interruption Cave Study Group. N Engl J Med 1998;338:409–415, with permission.)

rate of recurrent DVT between the anticoagulated and nonanticoagulated patients as documented by physical examination or telephone interviews was noted at 18 months of follow-up.[80] Both papers suggested that there is no evidence that anticoagulation reduces the risk of thrombotic complications. Greenfield and Michna as well as Lang and coworkers reached similar conclusions after reviewing patient outcomes in their retrospective case series.[76,90] Unfortunately, none of these studies are randomized and several used ineffective schedules of anticoagulation. Therefore, the utility of postplacement anticoagulation in filter patients still remains to be determined.

ANTICOAGULATION VERSUS IVC FILTERS FOR VTE

The only published literature examining this issue comes from Jones and Fink, who performed physical examinations, impedance plethysmography (IPG), and venous duplex scanning of patients who were treated for VTE during an 18-month period in 1990–1991 with either anticoagulation or Greenfield filters. No randomization scheme was utilized and patient selection criteria were not specified. Nineteen patients with Greenfield filters and 44 patients treated with anticoagulation were enrolled. No significant differences were noted between the groups at 6 months on IPG or ultrasonographic testing or on prevalence of lower-extremity symptoms. Although the investigators suggest that both treatments appear equivalent, serious design flaws (unrandomized, small study population, short follow-up) hamper any attempt to draw a definitive conclusion from these data.[64] Given the obvious ethical issues associated with any randomized study of these alternative approaches to VTE, it is likely that this question will remain unanswered.

SUPRARENAL IVC FILTERS

Vena caval filters are generally placed below the renal veins to avoid the possibility of renal insufficiency that might result if IVCT occurs. Occasionally, however, anomalous venous anatomy, pre-existing IVCT or anticipated pregnancy make it necessary to place filters in the suprarenal inferior vena cava. Greenfield and colleagues have the largest experience, consisting of 148 patients of their total registry population of 1932 (7.6%).[70,89,107] Several other groups have published experiences with smaller numbers of patients.[72,88,108,109]

The primary purpose for filter insertion is the prevention of PE. In this respect, suprarenal devices do not appear to perform as well as infrarenal devices (Table 38–3). Although this difference may reflect physiologic differences between the infrarenal and suprarenal IVC, several alternative explanations exist. The mean follow-up duration in the largest series was 81.6 months, substantially longer than that of comparable infrarenal filter studies. In addition, five of the six patients in the study of Greenfield and coworkers who did develop a PE had their suprarenal filters placed for this diagnosis. Undoubtedly, these patients a represent a group at especially high risk for PE. Furthermore, when compared to the infrarenal filter population, the suprarenal filter population had a higher percentage of patients with malignant disease, a group of patients known to be at high risk for recurrent thromboembolic events.[107]

The longer period of follow-up probably also contributed to the higher frequency of venous insufficiency experienced by this subgroup of patients. Migration of filters was also noted to be higher in these studies, although no symptoms were attributable to any of these episodes. While longer follow-up may be responsible for this finding, the caudal pressure generated by upper abdominal organs and the diaphragm also has been suggested as a possible cause.[107] Although many have expressed concern that renal dysfunction may result from

Table 38-3 • SUPRARENAL IVC FILTER STUDIES

Study	No. Patients	Chart/Clinical F/U	Radiology F/U	Mean F/U Duration	PE	IST/DVT	IVCT	Venous Stasis
Stewart et al., 1982[70]	12	91%	58%	17 mos.	1/11 (9%)	NA/ 2/11 (18%)	NA	1/11 (9%)
Orsini and Jarrell, 1984[72]	11	100%	82%	12.3 mos.	0	0	0	0
Brenner et al., 1992[88]	6	100%	100%	12.5 mos.	0	NA/1/6 (16.7%)	1/6 (16.7%)	
Greenfield et al., 1992[89]	71	85%	34%	53 mos.	3/60 (5%)	NA	0/22	16/39 (41%) present prior to filter
Greenfield and Proctor, 1998[107]	148	49%	49%	81.6 mos.	6/73 (8%)	NA	2/73 (2.7%)	55/73 (75%)
Matchett et al., 1998[108]	22	100%	82%	36 mos.	1/22 (4.5%)	NA	1/22 (4.5%)	NA
Athanasoulis et al., 2000[109]	33	100%	44%	16 mos.	6.5%	NA	NA	NA

F/U: follow-up; PE, recurrent pulmonary embolism; DVT, deep venous thrombosis; IST, insertion site thrombosis; IVCT, inferior vena caval thrombosis; NA, not assessed.
Note: Greenfield and Proctor's 1998 publication is an update of a series of patients first reported by Stewart and coworkers in 1982 and previously updated by Greenfield and coworkers in 1992.

suprarenal IVC filter placement, only one study found any evidence of this complication. Brenner and coworkers inserted suprarenal IVC filters into six patients prior to or during unilateral nephrectomies for renal cell carcinoma. Four of their patients had elevated serum creatinine levels (1.7 to 2.1 mg/dL) postoperatively; no baseline serum creatinine values were given. Since these data have yet to be replicated, it is likely they are unique to this patient group and do not represent the typical outcome of patients with suprarenal IVC filters.[88]

SUPERIOR VENA CAVAL FILTERS

The published experience of filters placed in the superior vena cava is extremely limited and consists of a few case reports and two case series.[110–116] Although some have suggested that filters in this location are safe and effective, longer and more intense follow-up are needed before definitive statements on filters in this location can be made.

EXPANDED INDICATIONS: IVC FILTERS IN HIP AND KNEE ARTHROPLASTY

With the increasing ease of insertion and a growing number of vena caval filters to choose from, a number of investigators have endorsed expanding the indications for IVC filter insertion.[2,3] Among these expanded indications is prophylaxis against PE in hip and knee arthroplasty. In the absence of prophylaxis, 50% to 80% of patients develop DVT and 5% to 10% sustain PE. Medical prophylaxis with warfarin or low-molecular-weight heparin (LMWH) can reduce the incidence of VTE by 20% to 60% and 50% to 70%, respectively.[117] Use of IVC filters for the prevention of PE in this population has only been investigated in a few studies encompassing 143 patients.[15,118–120] All are unrandomized case series in which filters were used as primary or secondary prophylaxis. Follow-up for an average of 32 months was obtained by chart review or telephone. No routine radiology studies were obtained. While PE and adverse side effects of IVC filter implantation were rare, the absence of randomization precludes any meaningful comparisons with standard medical management. Furthermore, recent LMWH trials in the prophylaxis of VTE in hip and knee surgery patients have demonstrated venographic DVT rates as low as 6% and PE rates of 0 to 2.8%. Many trials have had no episodes of nonfatal or fatal PE.[117] In light of these data, placement of a large number of Greenfield filters cannot be considered cost effective or worth the potential and largely undocumented long-term complications of these devices. In the absence of a randomized trial demonstrating greater efficacy and safety of IVC filters for PE prophylaxis in hip and knee arthroplasty patients, these devices should be reserved for rare treatment situations where anticoagulant therapy is clearly contraindicated.

IVC FILTERS FOR PREVENTION OF VTE IN TRAUMA PATIENTS

An area where the use of prophylactic IVC filters has been extensively studied is the prevention of PE in trauma patients (Table 38–4).[6,8–11,121–137] VTE is extremely common among trauma patients. The incidence of DVT is as high as 60% with 2% to 10% developing symptomatic PE, which are fatal in 1% to 2% of patients. Many episodes of DVT are clinically silent; therefore effective prophylaxis is crucial. Approaches to prophylaxis have included anticoagulation (subcutaneous unfractionated heparin or LMWH), mechanical devices (antiembolism stockings, pneumatic compression devices [PCD], IVC filters), and intensive radiologic screening (Doppler ultrasonography, magnetic resonance venography [MRV]).[134]

While there is some evidence that noninvasive forms of prophylaxis are effective, no strategy is universally effective and applicable to all trauma patients. The incomplete protection afforded by pharmacologic and noninvasive mechanical methods has led many trauma surgeons to advocate the routine placement of IVC filters for PE prophylaxis in the trauma population. Sixteen studies examining the use of IVC filters in the prophylaxis of PE in major trauma patients have been published (Table 38–4).[6,8–11,121–131] IVC filters were only placed in patients considered at high risk for VTE, which constituted 1.5% ($n = 995$) of a total trauma study population of 59,969 patients. The criteria used to define high-risk status varied somewhat from study to study and were often based upon retrospective reviews of the trauma population. Commonly cited high-risk identifiers include spinal cord injuries, age above 55, long bone fractures, head injuries, complex pelvic fractures, an injury severity scale (ISS) score above 16, and fractures of pelvis or long bones in conjunction with prolonged bed rest.

Concomitant use of alternative forms of prophylaxis varied between studies from no prophylaxis to use of venous compression boots, compression stockings, aspirin, warfarin, low-dose subcutaneous heparin (5000 U q12h or q8h), enoxaparin (30 mg SC bid), pneumatic compression devices, and combinations of these modalities. Screening for thromboembolic events varied from no screening to use of impedance plethysmography or ultrasonography. The frequency of screening varied from once during the hospital stay to once or twice a week.

To assess the effectiveness of IVC filters in the prevention of PE, nine studies included historical comparison groups.[6,8–11,122,123,125,128] By these criteria, IVC filters do appear to reduce the incidence of PE in the trauma population. Among controls the frequency of PE varied from 3.3% to 17.5% compared with 0% to 2.9% among patients receiving IVC filters. However, the use of historical controls instead of a randomized concurrent control group significantly limits the strength of this conclusion. Illustrative of this limitation is the considerable variation in the PE frequency between the historical and contemporary low-risk groups (0.5% versus 0.1%) in

Table 38-4 • PROPHYLACTIC IVC FILTER STUDIES IN TRAUMA PATIENTS

Study	No. Patients	Prophylaxis	Screening	Follow-up	PE	DVT	IVCT
Webb et al., 1992[121]	24 VCF 27 No VCF	UFH, ASA, CS	None	Clinical 100% 18 mos.	VCF 0 No VCF 2/27 (7.4%) 1 fatal	VCF 1/24 (4.2%) No VCF 1/27 (3.7%)	NA
Rogers et al., 1993[6]	Hist. controls 2525 Hist. high risk 428 Prospective 792 High risk 35	VCB	IPG q7d	U/S at 30 d and 1 yr. 50%	Hist. high risk 3.3% Hist. low risk 0.1% Prospective VCF 0/34 Prospective low risk 2/757 (0.3%)	VCF 6/34 (17.6%)	2/17 (11%)
Leach et al., 1994[10]	10,948 VCF 201	None	None	Chart review 201/201 100%	VCF 0 Others 4/10747 (0.04%) Hist. control 11/1257 (0.9%)	None reported	0
Rosenthal et al., 1994[122]	Hist. controls 94 Prospective 67 VCF 29	UFH, PCD None in VCF group	None	Chart review 100% U/S 21/29 (72%) 32 mos.	Hist. controls 22/94 (23%) Prospective 1/67 (1.5%) VCF 0	Hist. controls 19/94 (20%) Prospective 9/67 (13%) VCF 0	0/21
Wilson et al., 1994[123]	Hist. controls 111 Prospective 15	UFH, VCB	IPG q7d	U/S at 30 d. and 1 yr. 9/15 (60%) Chart review 100% 15 mos.	Hist. controls 7/111 (6.3%) 3 fatal Prospective 0	None	2/9 (22%)
Winchell et al., 1994[124]	65/9721 trauma patients with PE or VCF studied retrospectively	None, PCD, PCD+UFH and VCF	NA	Retrospective chart review	36/9721 (0.4%) fatal 8 (.08%) None 7/36 (19.4%) PCD 21/36 (58%) PCD+UFH 8/36 (22%) VCF 0/29	IST 1/29 (3.4%)	NA
Khansarinia et al., 1995[9]	Hist. controls 216 VCF 108	UFH or PCD	U/S 1-2 ×/wk.	NA	VCF 0 Hist. controls 13/216 (6%) Fatal 9 (4.2%)	VCF 1/108 (0.9%)	NA
Rogers et al., 1995[125]	Hist. controls 2525 High risk 428 Prospective 3151 High risk 71 VCF 63	VCB	IPG q7d	U/S at 30 d and then q yr. 1 yr. 36/63 (57%) 2 yr. 16/63 (25%) 3 yr. 8/63 (12.7%)	VCF 1/63 (1.6%) fatal Hist. controls High risk 14/428 (3.3%) 2 fatal low risk 11/2097 (0.5%)	VCF 19/63 (30.2%)	2/36 (5.5%)

Table continued on following page

Table 38-4 • PROPHYLACTIC IVC FILTER STUDIES IN TRAUMA PATIENTS (*Continued*)

Study	No. Patients	Prophylaxis	Screening	Follow-up	PE	DVT	IVCT
Zolfaghari et al., 1995[126]	29	UFH or PCD	None	None	0	NA	NA
Patton et al., 1996[127]	110	UFH or PCD	None	Telephone 45/110 (41%) Exam/U/S 30/110 (27%) 19 mos.	0	14/30 (47%)	1/110 (0.9%)
Rodriguez et al., 1996[11]	Hist. controls 80 VCF 40	UFH, PCD, both	None	U/S 38/40 (95%) 11 mos.	VCF 1/40 (2.5%) Controls 14/80 (17.5%) 8 fatal	VCF 6/40 (15%) Controls 15/80 (19%)	VCF 4/40 (10%) Controls 0/80
Gosin et al., 1997[8]	Prospective 1630 High risk 250/1630 VCF 99/250 Hist. controls 249	UFH, PCD or both	None	Chart review 100%	VCF 0 High risk No VCF 4/151 (2.6%) Hist. controls 12/250 (4.8%)	NA	NA
Rogers et al., 1997[28]	Prospective 940 High risk 41 VCF 35 Retrospective 1150 High risk 83	PCD if possible	IPG q wk.	U/S at 1 mo., 6 mos. and q yr. in VCF group	Prospective VCF 1/35 (2.9%) No VCF 1/905 (0.1%) Retrospective HR 6/83 (7.2%) Others 5/1067 (0.5%)	IST 2/35 (5.7%)	6.4% at 2 yrs.
Rogers et al., 1998[29]	132 VCF pts. of 5280 total	PCD	IPG q wk. first 2 years of study	U/S at 1 mo., and q yr. in VCF group 47/132 (35.6%) Mean F/U 20 mos.	3/132 (2.3%) 1 fatal (0.8%)	IST 4/132 (3%) DVT 6/132 (4.5%)	1/47 (2.1%)
Greenfield et al., 2000[130]	249	UFH, PCD, or CS in 24%	NA	Clinical 59% CT/cavagram 19% Autopsy 2% Mean F/U 28 mos.	3/197 (1.5%)	IST 3/197 (1.5%) DVT 39/197 (15.2%)	5/197 (2.5%)
Wojcik et al., 2000[131]	191 VCF 64 prophylactic	PCD, LMWH, warfarin	U/S if symptomatic	U/S, abdominal X-ray exam 105/191 (55%)	0	IST 28/64 (44%) DVT 2/4 (50%)	1/105 (0.95%)

VCF, vena caval filter; UFH, unfractionated heparin; ASA, aspirin; CS, compression stockings; VCB, venous compression boots; IPG, impedance plethysmography; U/S, ultrasonography; PCD, pneumatic compression device; PE, recurrent pulmonary embolism; DVT, deep venous thrombosis; IST, insertion site thrombosis; IVCT, inferior vena cava thrombosis; NA, not assessed.

the absence of any intervention and the extraordinarily high incidence of PE in some of the historical high-risk control groups (17.5% reported by Rodriguez and coworkers).[11,128]

Follow-up screening for complications of vena caval filters was also suboptimal in these studies.[6,11,121,123,125,127,129] Most studies did not conduct routine follow-up procedures for patients after discharge; thus only 36% of the IVC filter population was available for follow-up for a mean duration of 25 months. Ultrasonography was performed in 50% of the follow-up population, although it is unclear in some of the studies if both the lower extremities and inferior vena cava were imaged. Few patients had definitive imaging for IVCT performed (CT scans, inferior vena cavagrams). The remainder had either clinical or telephone follow-up. IST occurred in 9.1%, while 14.1% developed a subsequent DVT unrelated to the insertion procedure. IVCT developed in 3.6% of patients.[121,124] Postphlebitic syndrome occurred in equal numbers of patients in the filter (26.6%) and control groups (29.8%), although few studies provided data on this outcome.[11,121,127] Misplacement of filters occurred in fewer than 1% of insertions.[10,127,130] Migration occurred in four patients (0.75%), two of whom required an operative procedure to remove the wayward device and place a second filter.[10,127,130] Since routine follow-up studies for the presence of these complications was variable, it is likely that these frequencies represent an underestimate.

Instead of prophylactic IVC filters, several investigators have attempted to use radiologic surveillance with serial duplex ultrasonography or MRV to restrict filters to patients with documented DVT (Table 38–5).[135–137] Although one study demonstrated a reduction in PE compared to a historical control group, others' experience with this strategy has been less satisfactory. Furthermore, some have questioned the broad applicability of ultrasound surveillance in trauma patients given its poor sensitivity in asymptomatic patients and the frequency of lower-extremity injuries, which makes comprehensive examinations impossible.[130,134,137] MRV looks promising but requires further study in a larger population of patients.

Despite the fact that a considerable number of studies of IVC filters in PE prophylaxis in the trauma population have been performed, nagging questions remain about the efficacy and long-term safety of these devices. Furthermore, the appropriate target population remains to be clearly identified. Using current criteria and estimates of the incidence of PE in the trauma population, placement of 1000 filters would be required to prevent 40 pulmonary emboli and 7 fatal pulmonary emboli (assuming 100% protection).[134] A recent analysis of a statewide hospital database found only 0.3% of all trauma patients suffered a pulmonary embolus. The highest rate, in patients with extremity injuries, was only 0.53%.[138] While these discharge data may represent an underestimate of the incidence of PE in the trauma population, the fact remains that the current approach requires the placement of a large number of filters to prevent a few fatal events. Given that the long-term complications of these devices remains unclear, a more selective approach to the placement of filters is needed until well-designed studies of IVC filters in the trauma population are performed. Further investigation of MRV DVT surveillance with selective use of IVC filters is warranted. Future research efforts should also be directed at developing an effective temporary IVC filter, which could provide the benefits of acute PE protection without the long-term risks of a permanent device.

Until these data are available, it would seem prudent to carefully assess each patient's risk of hemorrhage and thrombosis, to use as many forms of prophylaxis (LMWH or UFH with or without PCD, or PCD alone) as deemed reasonable for the particular clinical situation. If feasible, DVT surveillance (MRV or ultrasonography) in high-risk patients is probably worthwhile in the early days of hospitalization when anticoagulant therapy is most often contraindicated. At the present, IVC filters probably should be reserved for those patients who develop DVT despite prophylaxis and have absolute contraindications to anticoagulation.

Table 38–5 • STUDIES USING DVT SURVEILLANCE TO SELECT TRAUMA PATIENTS FOR VENA CAVAL FILTERS

Study	Patient #	Prophylaxis	Screening	PE	DVT	IVCT
Piotrowski et al.,[135] 1996	343 HR of 3154 total	UFH, TED stockings, and/or PCD	Duplex U/S at 48 hrs., q wk. ×3, then q2wk. ×3 then q mo.	3/343 (0.9%) 1 despite filter	20/343 (5.8%) 1 after filter	NA
Headrick et al., 1997[136]	228 HR of 1566 total Hist. controls 234 HR	PCD and/or UFH	Duplex U/S at 72 hrs. Then q wk.	1/228 (0.4%) Study VCF 0.29 Study AC 1/10 Controls 6/234 (2.6%)	Study group 39/228 (17%) Controls 15/234 (6.4%)	0?
Montgomery et al., 1997[137]	101 hip fracture	UFH, warfarin	MRV within 48 hrs., at 7 d U/S or venogram postop	1/101 (1%)	37/101 (37%) 26 VCF 8 AC	NA

HR, high risk; UFH, unfractionated heparin (5000 U sc q12h); PCD, pneumatic compression devices; U/S, ultrasound; NA, not assessed; VCF, vena caval filter; AC, anticoagulation; MRV magnetic resonance venogram.

IVC FILTERS FOR VTE IN CANCER PATIENTS

Treatment of VTE in patients with malignancies is another area where some investigators have suggested that routine use of IVC filters should be considered. Seventeen studies have been performed to examine the effectiveness of IVC filters in this population involving 810 patients (Tables 38–6 and 38–7).[12–14,60,139–152] All are retrospective chart reviews of case histories, four of which include telephone follow-up data.[140,143–145] Six studies compare the outcome of patients treated with anticoagulation or IVC filters as primary therapy.[14,139,143,144,146,148] No randomization was used in any study. Mean follow-up duration was 11.5 months. The frequency of recurrent PE was 3.2% among patients receiving anticoagulation and 6.1% among patients with IVC filters. However, the frequency of recurrent PE (2.2%) among filter patients is much lower in the case series that examine IVC filters exclusively. When all the studies are combined, the frequency of recurrent PE among patients who received IVC filters is 3%, not significantly different from the rate among patients receiving anticoagulation. Fatal PE was rare, with one episode occurring in each of the treatment groups. Bleeding was more common in patients treated with anticoagulants (16.3% versus 1.2%). Three patients treated with anticoagulation had fatal episodes of bleeding. None occurred in the IVC filter group.

In contrast, recurrent DVT occurred more commonly in patients receiving IVC filters (13.7%) than in anticoagulated patients (5.6%). Almost 7% of patients receiving filters developed an IVCT. None occurred in the anticoagulated patients. Other complications of IVC filter placement such as migration (1.2%), misplacement (1.4%), IVC perforation (2.8%), and wound infection (0.6%) were documented in a few studies and occurred infrequently.[13,141,147,149,150] Only a single episode of cardiac arrhythmia, arteriovenous fistula, and periprocedural death were noted.[141,149]

In light of the available data, it is difficult to build a strong case for routine placement of IVC filters for thromboembolic disease in cancer patients. Although they appear to be effective in preventing PE and are not associated with bleeding complications, IVC filters do so at a cost of more recurrent DVT and IVCT. Many proponents of routine IVC filter use in this population have cited studies such as that of Moore and coworkers, which noted a 25% incidence of major hemorrhage in this population, to justify an aggressive approach to IVC filter use.[152] However, this study, which included only 32 patients, and many of the IVC filter studies reviewed above were conducted in the era before the international normalized ratio (INR) was used for routine mon-

Table 38–6 • IVC FILTERS IN THE MANAGEMENT OF VENOUS THROMBOEMBOLIC DISEASE IN CANCER PATIENTS

Study	Patient #	F/U Population	F/U Duration	PE	IST/DVT	IVCT	Venous Stasis
Cantelmo et al., 1982[13]	70	Chart review 93%	16 mos.	0	NA	1/70 (1.4%) M-U Filter	10/70 (14%) filter type?
Walsh et al., 1987[150]	41	Chart review 100%	20.6 mos.	0	NA/1/41 (2.4%)	NA	NA
Whitney and Kerstein, 1987[151]	10	Chart review 100% autopsy in 3	11 mos.	0	0	NA	0
Muchmore et al., 1989[12]	5	Chart review	5 mos.	1/5 (20%)	1/5 (20%) Phlegmasia cerulea dolens	NA	NA
Martin et al., 1990[60]	5	Chart review	1–4 mos.	0	0	0	NA
Cohen et al., 1991[14]	41	Chart review/ telephone	6.4 mos.	1/41 (2.4%) fatal	NA/1/18 (5.5%)	NA	2/18 (11%)
Hubbard et al., 1994[142]	31	Chart review 100%	12.3 mos.	0	NA/4/31 (13%)	2/31 (6.5%)	8/31 (26%)
Rosen et al., 1994[147]	61	Chart review	up to 3 weeks after D/C	5/61 (8.2%) 4 fatal	1/61 (1.6%)/0	NA	NA
Lossef and Barth, 1995[145]	34	Chart review/ telephone	5.2 mos.	0	NA	1/34 (2.9%)	NA
Schwarz et al., 1996[149]	182	Chart review	NA	4/182 (2.2%)	NA/1/182 (6%)	NA	NA
Greenfield et al., 1997[141]	166	Chart review	10 mos.	3/166 (1.8%)	1/166 (0.6%)/ 51/166 (31%)	NA	NA

F/U, follow up; PE, recurrent pulmonary embolism; DVT, deep venous thrombosis; IST, insertion site thrombosis; IVCT, inferior vena cava thrombosis; NA, not assessed.

Table 38-7 • STUDIES OF ANTICOAGULATION AND IVC FILTERS IN THE TREATMENT OF VENOUS THROMBOEMBOLIC DISEASE IN CANCER PATIENTS

Study	Patient #	F/U Population	F/U Duration	PE	DVT	IVCT	Bleeding	Venous Stasis
Olin et al., 1987[146]	50 pts. with brain tumors	Chart review 49/50 (98%)	NA	AC group 0 VCF group 1/24 (5%)	NA	NA	AC group 4/25 (16%) VCF group 0	NA
Cohen et al., 1992[140]	29 cancer pts.	Chart review 100%	7 mos.	AC 1/11 (9.1%) VCF 0	NA	NA	AC 3/11 (27.3%) VCF 0	AC 0 VCF 2/18 (11%)
Levin et al., 1993[144]	49 pts. with brain tumors	Chart review/ telephone AC 93% VCF 83%	AC >6 mos. VCF?	AC 1/15 (7%) VCF 5/42 (12%)	AC 1/15 (7%) VCF 9/42 (12%)	AC 0 VCF 11/42 (26%)	AC 0 VCF 0	AC 0 VCF 4/42 (10%)
Schiff and DeAngelis, 1994[148]	51 brain tumor pts.	Chart review	NA	AC 2/42 (5%) VCF 2/10 (20%)	AC 4/42 (10%) VCF 2/10 (20%)	NA	AC 9/42 (21%) VCF 0	NA
Ihnat et al., 1998[143]	60 cancer pts.	Chart review/ telephone 100%	AC 10.6 mos. VCF 13.1 mos.	AC 2/138 (1%) VCF 2/60 (3%)	AC 5/138 (4%) VCF 6/60 (10%)	AC 0 VCF 1/60 (2%)	AC 18/138 (13%) VCF 2/60 (3%)	AC 0 VCF 2/60 (3%)

F/U, follow-up; PE, recurrent pulmonary embolism; DVT, deep venous thrombosis; IST, insertion site thrombosis; IVCT, inferior vena cava thrombosis; AC, anticoagulation group; VCF, vena caval filter group; NA, not assessed.

itoring of warfarin anticoagulation. Therefore, it is likely that most of the participants were overanticoagulated, contributing to the high incidence of bleeding complications. Several recent prospective studies of anticoagulation in cancer patients have found no difference in major bleeding rates between cancer patients and patients without cancer.[153,154] Therefore, anticoagulation should still be considered the primary therapy for VTE in cancer patients. The oncology population that generates the most anxiety among physicians regarding anticoagulation is patients with central nervous system (CNS) malignancies. Despite the understandable concern that use of anticoagulation in these patients evokes, the published literature, though limited, is reassuring. Most patients with CNS malignancies can be safely treated with anticoagulation.[144,146,148,157] Exceptions to this rule would be patients with metastatic melanoma and choriocarcinoma and any patients with evidence of hemorrhage on CT imaging.[146,148,158–160] Most cases of CNS hemorrhagic complications in patients with brain tumors were associated with excessive anticoagulation.[148,157–159] Therefore, as with all patients on anticoagulant therapy, close monitoring is essential to minimize bleeding complications. Clearly, further studies are needed to guide management in these difficult situations. Until these data are available, anticoagulation should be considered primary therapy for cancer patients with VTE. Until their utility outside of standard indications for their use is demonstrated in well-controlled randomized trials, IVC filters should be considered as a therapeutic option only when anticoagulation is strictly contraindicated.

FREE-FLOATING THROMBUS: AN INDICATION FOR IVC FILTER PLACEMENT?

The presence of a free-floating thrombus also has been held as an indication for IVC filter placement.[3] In 1985, Norris and coworkers retrospectively reviewed 78 patients with venographically documented iliofemoral thrombi and found that patients with free-floating thrombus were much more likely to suffer a PE (3 of 5; 60%) than those with adherent thrombi (5.5%) despite adequate anticoagulation.[160] Subsequently, a number of studies have re-examined this issue, with varying conclusions. No study has rigorously examined the utility of IVC filters in this situation although several have endorsed their use (Table 38–8).[161–165] Recently, Pacouret and coworkers performed a prospective study of PE in patients with adherent and free-floating thrombi. All patients had baseline and follow-up lung scans and pulmonary angiograms (when the lung scan was abnormal) after 10 days of anticoagulation. No increase in PE was

Table 38–8 • STUDIES OF PE IN PATIENTS WITH FREE-FLOATING THROMBUS

Study	Patient #	Screening	PE
Norris et al., 1985[160]	78 FFT 5/78 (6.4%) AT 73/78 (93.6%)	None Dx confirmed with biplanar venography and V/Q scan	FFT 3/5 (60%) AT 4/73 (5.5%)
Radomski et al., 1987[163]	467 total 44 IVC thrombus 26 FFT	None DVT dx by monoplanar venogram PE dx by angiogram or V/Q scan	Admit PE FFT 13/26 (50%) Attached 2/13 (15%) F/U PE FFT 7/26 (27%) Attached 1/8 (16%) None after VCF
Monreal et al., 1989[165]	121 34 FFT 87 AT	Biplanar venography for DVT dx Routine lung scan on admit and day 8	FFT 7/34 (21%) AT 5/87 (5.7%)
Berry et al., 1990[161]	399 DVT 74 FFT	Duplex U/S for DVT dx Lung scan, autopsy clinical suspicion for PE dx	FFT 17/65 (26%) Bilateral FFT 6/14 (43%) 1 after VCF
Baldridge et al., 1990[162]	732 DVT 73 FFT	DVT dx by duplex U/S PE dx by lung scan or angiogram F/U U/S 33/73 (45%) at 1–2 weeks	9/73 (12%) 7/9 (78%) PE before DVT dx 2/9 (22%) after
Voet and Afschrift, 1991[164]	76 DVT 39 FFT	Duplex U/S at DVT dx and 2 weeks and 3 mos. PE dx by lung scan, angiogram, and autopsy	FFT 13/39 (33%) 4/39 (10%) PE after DVT dx
Pacouret et al., 1997[166]	276 DVT FFT 62 AT 28	Venogram, duplex U/S lung scan on admit and after days 9–11 of treatment (angiogram if lung scan abnormal)	Admit PE F/U PE FFT 64% 3.3% AT 50% 3.7%

FFT, free-floating thrombus; AT, adherent thrombus; DVT, deep venous thrombosis; PE, pulmonary embolism; U/S, ultrasonography; VCF, vena caval filter; F/U, follow-up.

identified among patients with free-floating thrombi (3.3% versus 3.7% for adherent thrombi).[166]

Several differences between this study and previous ones deserve mention. Pacouret and coworkers used monoplanar instead of biplanar venography, which may have influenced the number of thrombi designated as free floating. The high percentage of patients diagnosed with free-floating thrombi in this study (69% versus 6.4% in the study by Norris and coworkers) tends to support this contention although one previous study that supported their findings had nearly as high a proportion of free-floating thrombi (59%).[163] Unlike previous investigators, Pacouret and coworkers used rigorous criteria to diagnose PE and used LMWH in the vast majority of their patients. Whether study design or patient population differences are responsible for the dissimilar conclusions, it is clear that a randomized study of the utility of anticoagulation and IVC filters would do much to settle this controversy. In the interim, the superiority of IVC filters or anticoagulation in this situation still remains undecided.

IVC FILTERS FOR VTE IN OTHER PATIENT POPULATIONS

Several investigators have also suggested that IVC filters be used for VTE patients with limited cardiopulmonary reserve, chronic obstructive pulmonary disease or post-pulmonary embolectomy, or in pregnant patients.[3,17,167] However, only a small number of reports exist to support these recommendations.[2,4,73,86,168] Further data demonstrating the superiority of IVC filters to anticoagulation in these situations are needed before these endorsements can be considered acceptable practice.

TEMPORARY/RETRIEVABLE IVC FILTERS

Since the long-term safety of permanent IVC filters remains unknown and many patients have only temporary contraindications to anticoagulation, there has been considerable interest in developing effective temporary filtration devices. Several are currently being investigated, including the Tempo filter (B. Brown Medical, Evanston, Illinois), and the Gunther Tulip filter (Cook Inc., Bloomington, Indiana). The cone-shaped Tempo filter is attached to a catheter, which is anchored in the subcutaneous tissue at the insertion site. It can be left in place for up to 6 weeks prior to removal.[169] Preliminary studies in Europe have demonstrated it to be safe and effective.[171] The Gunther Tulip filter is a permanent IVC filter that can be retrieved if desired during the first 10 days after implantation. A small European study demonstrated an 80% success rate when retrieval was performed within 12 days.[169,171] If shown to be safe and effective, these devices could prove to be valuable tools in the treatment and prevention of VTE, especially in patients with transient risks such as trauma patients.

INDICATIONS FOR IVC FILTER PLACEMENT

In light of the published data on IVC filters, what are appropriate indications for their use? Traditional indications for placement of an IVC filter include an absolute contraindication to anticoagulation, a life-threatening complication from anticoagulation, or a failure of adequate anticoagulation in the setting of active VTE (Table 38–9). While filters are an appropriate consideration in each of these situations, each patient must be evaluated on an individual basis. Conclusive documentation of thrombus is a *must*. In patients with acute submassive PE and no evidence of residual lower-extremity clot, withholding anticoagulation is a viable option that deserves further study.[172] As noted above, many patients with CNS malignancies (excluding metastatic melanoma, choriocarcinoma, hemorrhagic metastases) may be safely anticoagulated. Therefore, the actual number of patients with an absolute contraindication to anticoagulation is fewer than previously believed.

Likewise, failure of adequate anticoagulation is actually an infrequent event and undertreatment or noncompliance must be excluded. In addition, any patient with warfarin resistance must be evaluated for the presence of Trousseau syndrome, the hypercoaguable state associated with malignant tumors. These patients are characterized by migratory thrombophlebitis in the venous and arterial systems, nonbacterial thrombotic endocarditis, and laboratory evidence of disseminated intravascular coagulation. Since thromboses in this syndrome are not limited to one vascular bed, local prophylactic measures such as an IVC filter are useless. Heparin anticoagulation and/or eradication of the underlying neoplasm are the only effective therapies.[173]

With the increased ease of IVC filter placement, the number of proposed indications has expanded dramatically (Table 38–10). As detailed in the previous sections, the data supporting these indications are inconclusive. Thus, in this author's opinion, routine placement of filters for these indications awaits definitive demonstration of their superior efficacy, safety, and cost effectiveness.

Table 38–9 • TRADITIONAL INDICATIONS FOR IVC FILTER PLACEMENT

- Absolute contraindication to anticoagulation
  - CNS hemorrhage
  - Overt gastrointestinal bleeding
  - Retroperitoneal hemorrhage
  - Massive hemoptysis
  - Cerebral metastases[a]
  - Massive cerebrovascular accident
  - CNS trauma or surgery
  - Significant thrombocytopenia (< 50,000/μL)
- Life-threatening hemorrhage with anticoagulation
- Failure of adequate anticoagulation

[a] Particularly true for melanoma, choriocarcinoma, and hemorrhagic metastases.

Table 38–10 • INVESTIGATIONAL INDICATIONS FOR IVC FILTER PLACEMENT

- Prophylaxis for PE in trauma patients
- Treatment of venous thromboembolism in cancer patients
- Prophylaxis for PE in high-risk orthopedic patients
- Pre- or postpulmonary embolectomy
- Prevention of PE in patients with extensive free-floating iliofemoral thrombi
- Prevention of PE in patients with COPD and DVT
- Prevention of PE in patients with minimal cardiopulmonary reserve and DVT
- Treatment of venous thromboembolism in pregnancy
- Treatment of venous thromboembolism in organ transplant patients

CONCLUSION

Since Trousseau first proposed that venous interruption might serve as a useful maneuver in the prevention of PE, techniques of venous interruption have evolved tremendously.[174] Despite these advances, most questions about this technology still remain unanswered. Only one randomized trial of IVC filters has been performed. No statistically sound data exist to compare the efficacy of these devices to one another or with standard anticoagulation. Furthermore, the long-term safety of these permanent implants remains to be clarified. Therefore, until better data are available, the use of IVC filters should be restricted to these rare situations in which standard anticoagulation is contraindicated. More liberal application of IVC filters should be considered experimental and should only occur as part of well-designed prospective clinical trials. Temporary filters, which may provide any advantages of permanent filters without the potential long-term side effects, are currently being tested. Multicenter randomized studies have done much to refine the use of anticoagulants in clinical medicine. Clearly, the time is long overdue for scrutiny of similar rigor to be applied to permanent and temporary IVC filters. Until these studies are performed, the potential misapplication of this technology will undoubtedly continue to the detriment of patients, physicians, and society.

■ REFERENCES

Chapter 38 References

1. Bick RL. Hereditary and acquired thrombophilia: preface. Semin Thromb Hemost 1999;25:251–253.
2. Golueke PJ, Garrett WV, Thompson JE, et al. Interruption of the vena cava by means of the Greenfield filter: expanding the indications. Surgery 1988;103:111–117.
3. Jones TK, Barnes RW, Greenfield LJ. Greenfield vena caval filter: rationale and current indications. Ann Thorac Surg 1986;42:S48–S55.
4. Rohrer MJ, Scheidler MG, Wheeler HB, et al. Extended indications for placement of an inferior vena cava filter [see comments]. J Vasc Surg 1989;10:44–49.
5. Sarasin FP, Eckman MH. Management and prevention of thromboembolic events in patients with cancer-related hypercoagulable states: a risky business. J Gen Intern Med 1993;8:476–486.
6. Rogers FB, Shackford SR, Wilson J, et al. Prophylactic vena cava filter insertion in severely injured trauma patients: indications and preliminary results. J Trauma 1993;35:637–641.
7. Britt LD, Zolfaghari D, Kennedy E, et al. Incidence and prophylaxis of deep vein thrombosis in a high-risk trauma population. Am J Surg 1996;172:13–14.
8. Gosin JS, Graham AM, Ciocca RG, et al. Efficacy of prophylactic vena cava filters in high-risk trauma patients. Ann Vasc Surg 1997;11:100–105.
9. Khansarinia S, Dennis JW, Veldenz HC, et al. Prophylactic Greenfield filter placement in selected high-risk trauma patients. J Vasc Surg 1995;22:231–235.
10. Leach TA, Pastena JA, Swan KG, et al. Surgical prophylaxis for pulmonary embolism. Am Surg 1994;60:292–295.
11. Rodriguez JL, Lopez JM, Proctor MC, et al. Early placement of prophylactic vena caval filters in injured patients at high risk for pulmonary embolism. J Trauma 1996;40:797–802.
12. Muchmore JH, Dunlap JN, Culicchia F, et al. Deep vein thrombophlebitis and pulmonary embolism in patients with malignant gliomas. South Med J 1989;82:1352–1356.
13. Cantelmo NL, Menzoian JO, Logerfo FW, et al. Clinical experience with vena caval filters in high-risk cancer patients. Cancer 1982;50:341–344.
14. Cohen JR, Tenenbaum N, Citron M. Greenfield filter as primary therapy for deep venous thrombosis and/or pulmonary embolism in patients with cancer. Surgery 1991;109:12–15.
15. Emerson RHJ, Cross R, Head WC. Prophylactic and early therapeutic use of the Greenfield filter in hip and knee joint arthroplasty. J Arthroplasty 1991;6:129–135.
16. Magnant JG, Walsh DB, Juravsky LI, et al. Current use of inferior vena cava filters. J Vasc Surg 1992;16:701–706.
17. Bergqvist D. The role of vena caval interruption in patients with venous thromboembolism. Prog Cardiovasc Dis 1994;37:25–37.
18. Arnold TE, Karabinis VD, Mehta V, et al. Potential of overuse of the inferior vena cava filter. Surg Gynecol Obstet 1993;177:463–467.
19. Greenfield LJ, McCurdy JR, Brown PP, et al. A new intracaval filter permitting continued flow and resolution of emboli. Surgery 1973;73:599–606.
20. Greenfield LJ, Cho KJ, Pais SO, et al. Preliminary clinical experience with the Titanium Greenfield vena caval filter. Arch Surg 1989;124:657–659.
21. Harris EJJ, Kinney EV, Harris EJS, et al. Phlegmasia complicating prophylactic percutaneous inferior vena caval interruption: a word of caution. J Vasc Surg 1995;22:606–611.
22. Greenfield LJ, Cho KJ, Proctor MC, et al. Results of a multicenter study of the modified-hook titanium Greenfield filter. J Vasc Surg 1991;14:253–257.
23. Lim MC, Tan HC, Choo MH. The new titanium Greenfield vena cava filter: initial experience and review. Singapore Med J 1994;35:622–625.
24. Greenfield LJ, Proctor MC, Cho KJ, et al. Extended evaluation of the titanium Greenfield vena caval filter [published erratum appears in J Vasc Surg 1995 Jan;21:162]. J Vasc Surg 1994;20:458–464.
25. Thomas LA, Summers RR, Cardwell MS. Use of Greenfield filters in pregnant women at risk for pulmonary embolism. South Med J 1997;90:215–217.
26. Ferris EJ, McCowan TC, Carver DK, et al. Percutaneous inferior vena caval filters: Follow-up of seven designs in 320 patients. Radiology 1993;188:851–856.
27. Wittenberg G, Kueppers V, Tschammler A, et al. Long-term results of vena cava filters: Experiences with the LGM and the Titanium Greenfield devices. Cardiovasc Intervent Radiol 1998;21:225–229.
28. Mohan CR, Hoballah JJ, Sharp WJ, et al. Comparative efficacy and complications of vena caval filters. J Vasc Surg 1995;21:235–245.

29. Lagattolla NR, Burnand KG, Irvine A, et al. Twelve years experience of vena cava filtration [published erratum appears in Ann R Coll Surg Engl 1997 Jan; 79:27]. Ann R Coll Surg Engl 1994;76:336–339.
30. Molgaard CP, Yucel EK, Geller SC, et al. Access-site thrombosis after placement of inferior vena cava filters with 12–14F delivery sheaths. Radiology 1992;185:257–261.
31. Blebea J, Wilson R, Waybill P, et al. Deep venous thrombosis after percutaneous insertion of vena caval filters. J Vasc Surg 1999;30:821–829.
32. Aswad MA, Sandager GP, Pais SO, et al. Early duplex scan evaluation of four vena caval interruption devices. J Vasc Surg 1996;24:809–818.
33. Cho KJ, Greenfield LJ, Proctor MC, et al. Evaluation of a new percutaneous stainless steel Greenfield filter. J Vasc Interv Radiol 1997;8:181–187.
34. Johnson SP, Raiken DP, Grebe PJ, et al. Single institution prospective evaluation of the over-the-wire Greenfield vena caval filter. J Vasc Interv Radiol 1998;9:766–773.
35. Greenfield LJ, Proctor MC. The percutaneous Greenfield filter: Outcomes and practice patterns. J Vasc Surg 2000;32:888–893.
36. Taylor FC, Awh MH, Kahn CEJ, et al. Vena Tech vena cava filter: experience and early follow-up [see comments]. J Vasc Interv Radiol 1991;2:435–440.
37. Crochet DP, Stora O, Ferry D, et al. Vena Tech-LGM filter: long-term results of a prospective study. Radiology 1993; 188:857–860.
38. Murphy TP, Dorfman GS, Yedlicka JW, et al. LGM vena cava filter: objective evaluation of early results. J Vasc Interv Radiol 1991;2:107–115.
39. Cull DL, Wheeler JR, Gregory RT, et al. The Vena Tech filter: evaluation of a new inferior vena cava interruption device. J Cardiovasc Surg (Torino) 1991;32:691–696.
40. Ricco JB, Crochet D, Sebilotte P, et al. Percutaneous transvenous caval interruption with the LGM filter: Early results of a multicenter trial. Ann Vasc Surg 1988;3:242–247.
41. Ricco JB, Dubreuil F, Reynaud P, et al. The LGM Vena-Tech caval filter: results of a multicenter study. Ann Vasc Surg 1995;9 (Suppl):S89–100.
42. Crochet DP, Brunel P, Trogrlic S, et al. Long-term follow-up of Vena Tech-LGM filter: predictors and frequency of caval occlusion. J Vasc Interv Radiol 1999;10:137–142.
43. Millward SF, Peterson RA, Moher D, et al. LGM (Vena Tech) vena caval filter: experience at a single institution. J Vasc Interv Radiol 1994;5:351–356.
44. Millward SF, Marsh JI, Peterson RA, et al. LGM (Vena Tech) vena cava filter: clinical experience in 64 patients [see comments]. J Vasc Interv Radiol 1991;2:429–433.
45. Simon M, Athanasoulis CA, Kim D, et al. Simon nitinol inferior vena cava filter: initial clinical experience. Work in progress. Radiology 1989;172:99–103.
46. Poletti PA, Becker CD, Prina L, et al. Long-term results of the Simon nitinol inferior vena cava filter. Eur Radiol 1998;8: 289–294.
47. McCowan TC, Ferris EJ, Carver DK, et al. Complications of the nitinol vena caval filter. J Vasc Interv Radiol 1992;3:401–408.
48. Hawkins SP, al-Kutoubi A. The Simon nitinol inferior vena cava filter: preliminary experience in the UK. Clin Radiol 1992; 46:378–380.
49. Engmann E, Asch M. Clinical experience with the antecubital Simon Nitinol IVC filter. J Vasc Interv Radiol 1998;9:774–778.
50. Grassi CJ, Matsumoto AH, Teitelbaum GP. Vena caval occlusion after Simon nitinol filter placement: identification with MR imaging in patients with malignancy. J Vasc Interv Radiol 1992; 3:535–539.
51. Kim D, Edelman RR, Margolin CJ, et al. The Simon nitinol filter: evaluation by MR and ultrasound. Angiology 1992;43:541–548.
52. Roehm JOJ. The bird's nest filter: a new percutaneous transcatheter inferior vena cava filter. J Vasc Surg 1984;1:498–501.
53. Firkin A, Walters N, Thomson K, et al. Inferior vena cava "birds nest" filters—2 year follow-up. Australas Radiol 1992;36: 286–288.
54. Nicholson AA, Ettles DF, Paddon AJ, et al. Long-term follow up of the Bird's Nest IVC filter. Clin Radiol 1999;54:759–764.
55. Thomas JH, Cornell KM, Siegel EL, et al. Vena caval occlusion after bird's nest filter placement. Am J Surg 1998;176:598–600.
56. Smith JA, Atkinson NR, Walters NA, et al. Early experience with the bird's nest inferior vena-caval filter [letter]. Med J Aust 1989;150:164–165.
57. Hicks ME, Middleton WD, Picus D, et al. Prevalence of local venous thrombosis after transfemoral placement of a Bird's Nest vena caval filter. J Vasc Interv Radiol 1990;1:63–68.
58. Lord RS, Benn I. Early and late results after Bird's Nest filter placement in the inferior vena cava: clinical and duplex ultrasound follow up. Aust N Z J Surg 1994;64:106–114.
59. Starok MS, Common AA. Follow-up after insertion of Bird's Nest inferior vena caval filters. Can Assoc Radiol J 1996; 47:189–194.
60. Martin B, Martyak TE, Stoughton TL, et al. Experience with the Gianturco–Roehm Bird's Nest vena cava filter. Am J Cardiol 1990;66:1275–1277.
61. Reed RA, Teitelbaum GP, Taylor FC, et al. Use of the Bird's Nest filter in oversized inferior venae cavae. J Vasc Interv Radiol 1991;2:447–450.
62. Wojtowycz MM, Stoehr T, Crummy AB, et al. The Bird's Nest inferior vena cava filter: review of a single-center experience. J Vasc Interv Radiol 1997;8:171–179.
63. Young N: Clinical follow-up of patients with percutaneously inserted inferior vena caval filters. Australas Radiol 1995; 39:233–236.
64. Jones BT, Fink JA. A prospective comparison of the status of the deep venous system after treatment with intracaval interruption versus anticoagulation. J Am Coll Surg 1994;178:220–222.
65. Scurr JH, Jarrett PEM Wastell C. The treatment of recurrent pulmonary embolism: experience with the Kimray–Greenfield vena cava filter. Ann R Coll Surg Engl 1983;65:233–234.
66. Wingerd M, Bernhard VM, Maddison F, Towne JB. Comparison of caval filters in the management of venous thromboembolism. Arch Surg 1978;113:1264–1271.
67. Berland LL, Maddison FE, Bernhard VM. Radiologic follow-up of vena cava filter devices. AJR 1980;134:1047–1052.
68. Cimochowski GE, Evans RH, Zarins CK, et al. Greenfield filter versus Mobin-Uddin umbrella: the continuing quest for the ideal method of vena caval interruption. J Thorac Cardiovasc Surg 1980;879:358–365.
69. Greenfield LJ, Peyton R, Crute S, et al. Greenfield Vena Caval Filter Experience: Late results in 156 patients. Arch Surg 1981;116:1451–1456.
70. Stewart JR, Peyton JWR, Crute S, et al. Clinical results of suprarenal placement of the Greenfield vena cava filter. Surgery 1982;92:1–4.
71. Gomez GA, Culter BS, Wheeler HB. Transvenous interruption of the inferior vena cava. Surgery 1983;93:612–619.
72. Orsini RA, Jarrell BE. Suprarenal placement of vena caval filters: indications, techniques and results. J Vasc Surg 1984;1:124–135.
73. Hux CH, Wapner RJ, Chayen B, et al. Use of the Greenfield filter for thromboembolic disease in pregnancy. Am J Obstet Gynecol 1986;155:734–737.
74. Carabasi RA, Moritz MJ, Jarrell BE. Complications encountered with the use of the Greenfield filter. Am J Surg 1987;154:163–168.
75. Rose BS, Simon DC, Hess ML, et al. Percutaneous transformal placement of the Kimray–Greenfield vena cava filter. Radiology 1987;165:373–376.
76. Greenfield LJ, Michna BA. Twelve-year clinical experience with the Greenfield vena caval filter. Surgery 1988;104:706–712.

77. Pais SO, Tobin KD, Austin CB, et al. Percutaneous insertion of the Greenfield inferior vena cava filter: Experience with ninety-six patients. J Vasc Surg 1988;8:460–464.

78. Todd GJ, Sanderson J, Nowygrod R, et al. Recent clinical experience with the vena cava filter. Am J Surg 1988; 156:353–358.

79. Welch TJ, Stanson AW, Sheedy II PF, et al. Percutaneous placement of the Greenfield vena caval filter. Mayo Clin Proc 1988;63:343–347.

80. Jones B, Fink JA, Donovan DL, Sharp WV. Analysis of benefit of anticoagulation after placement of Kimray–Greenfield filter. Surg Gynecol Obstet 1989;169:400–402.

81. Richenbacher WE, Atnip RG, Campbell DB, et al. Recurrent pulmonary embolism after inferior vena caval interruption with a Greenfield filter. World J Surg 1989;13:623–628.

82. Hye RJ, Mitchell AT, Dory CE, et al. Analysis of the transition to percutaneous placement of Greenfield filters. Arch Surg 1990;125:1550–1553.

83. Kolachalam RB, Julian TB. Clinical presentation of thrombosed Greenfield filters. Vasc Surg 1990;24:666–670.

84. Fink JA, Jones BT. The Greenfield filter as the primary means of therapy in venous thromboembolic disease. Surg Gynecol Obstet 1991;172:253–256.

85. Hlavaty TS, McCowan TC, Ferris EJ, et al. Experience with the Kimray–Greenfield inferior vena caval filter. J Ark Med Soc 1991;88:215–217.

86. Pomper SR, Lutchman G. The role of intracaval filters in patients with COPD and DVT. Angiology 1991;42:85–89.

87. Braverman SJ, Battey PM, Smith RB. Vena caval interruption. Am Surg 1992;58:188–192.

88. Brenner DW, Brenner CJ, Scott J, et al. Suprarenal Greenfield filter placement to prevent pulmonary embolus in patients with vena caval tumor thrombi. J Urol 1992;147:19–23.

89. Greenfield LJ, Cho KJ, Proctor MC, et al. Late results of suprarenal Greenfield vena caval filter placement. Arch Surg 1992; 127:969–973.

90. Lang W, Schweiger H, Hofmann-Preiss K. Results of long-term venacavography study after placement of a Greenfield vena caval filter. J Cardiovasc Surg 1992;33:573–578.

91. Alexander JJ, Yuhas JP, Piotrowski JJ. Is the increasing use of prophylactic percutaneous IVC filters justified? Am J Surg 1994;168:102–106.

92. Sullivan TM, Martinez BD, Lemmon G, et al. Clinical experience with the Greenfield filter in 193 patients and description of a new technique for operative insertion [see comments]. J Am Coll Surg 1994;178:117–122.

93. Greenfield LJ, Proctor MC. Twenty-year clinical experience with the Greenfield filter. Cardiovasc Surg 1995;3:199–205.

94. Ortega M, Gahtan V, Roberts A, et al. Efficacy of anticoagulation post-inferior vena caval filter placement. Am Surg 1998;64: 419–423.

95. Kantor A, Glanz S, Gordon DH, et al. Percutaneous insertion of the Kimray–Greenfield filter: incidence of femoral vein thrombosis. AJR 1987;149:1065–1066.

96. Dorfman GS, Cronan JJ, Paolella LP, et al. Iatrogenic changes at the venotomy site after percutaneous placement of the Greenfield filter. Radiology 1989;173:159–162.

97. Mewissen MW, Erickson SJ, Foley WD, et al. Thrombosis at venous insertion sites after inferior vena caval filter placement. Radiology 1989;173:155–157.

98. Tobin KD, Paris SO, Austin CB. Femoral vein thrombosis following percutaneous placement of the Greenfield filter. Invest Radiol 1989;24:442–445.

99. Decousus H, Leizorovicz A, Parent F, et al. A clinical trial of vena caval filters in the prevention of pulmonary embolism in patients with proximal deep-vein thrombosis. Prevention du Risque d'Embolie Pulmonaire par Interruption Cave Study Group [see comments]. N Engl J Med 1998;338:409–415.

100. Saarinen J, Sisto T, Laurikka J, et al. Late sequelae of acute deep venous thrombosis: Evaluation five and ten years after. Phlebology 1995;10:106–109.

101. Goldman HB, Hanna K, Dmochowski RR. Ureteral injury secondary to an inferior vena caval filter. J Urol 1996;156:1763.

102. Dabbagh A, Chakfe N, Kretz JG, et al. Late complication of a Greenfield filter associating caudal migration and perforation of the abdominal aorta by a rutured strut. J Vasc Surg 1995;22: 182–187.

103. Bianchini AU, Mehta SN, Mulder DS, et al. Duodenal perforation by a Greenfield filter: endoscopic diagnosis. Am J Gastroenterol 1997;92:686–687.

104. Miller CL, Wechsler RJ. CT evaluation of Kimray–Greenfield filter complications. AJR 1986;147:45–50.

105. Ballew KA, Philbrick JT, Becker DM. Vena cava filter devices. Clin Chest Med 1995;16:295–305.

106. Kanter B, Moser KM. The Greenfield vena cava filter. Chest 1988;93:170–175.

107. Greenfield LJ, Proctor MC. Suprarenal filter placement. J Vasc Surg 1998;28:432–438.

108. Matchett WJ, Jones MP. McFarland DR, Ferris EJ. Suprarenal vena caval filter placement: follow-up of four filter types in 22 patients. J Vasc Interv Radiol 1998;9:588–593.

109. Athanasoulis CA, Kaufman JA, Halpern EF, et al. Inferior vena caval filters: Review of a 26 year single center clinical experience. Radiology 2000;216:54–66.

110. Ascher E, Hingorani A, Tsemekhin B, et al. Lessons learned from a 6-year clinical experience with superior vena cava Greenfield filters. J Vasc Surg 2000;32:881–887.

111. Paris SO, Orchis DF, Mirvis SE. Superior vena caval placement of Kimray–Greenfield filter. Radiology 1987;165:385–386.

112. Ascer E, Gennaro M, Lorensen E, Pollina RM. Superior vena caval Greenfield filters: indications, techniques, and results. J Vasc Surg 1996;23:498–503.

113. Lidagoster MI, Widman WD, Chevinski AH. Superior vena caval occlusion after filter insertion. J Vasc Surg 1994;20:158–159.

114. Owen EWJ, Schoettle GPJ, Harrington OB. Placement of a Greenfield filter in the superior vena cava. Ann Thorac Surg 1992;53:896–897.

115. Black MD, French GJ, Rasuli P, et al. Upper extremity deep venous thrombosis: underdiagnosed and potentially lethal. Chest 1993;103:1887–1890.

116. Hoffman MJ, Greenfield LJ. Central venous septic thrombosis managed by superior vena cava Greenfield filter and venous thrombectomy: a case report. J Vasc Surg 1986;4:606–611.

117. Geerts WH, Heit JA, Clagett GP, et al. Prevention of venous thromboembolism. Chest 2001;119:132S–175S.

118. Vaughn BK, Knezevich S, Lombardi A VJ, et al. Use of the Greenfield filter to prevent fatal pulmonary embolism associated with total hip and knee arthroplasty. J Bone Joint Surg [Am] 1989;71:1542–1548.

119. Bicalho PS, Hozack WJ, Rothman RH, et al. Treatment of early symptomatic pulmonary embolism after total joint arthroplasty. J Arthroplasty 1996;11:522–524.

120. Woolson ST, Harris WH. Greenfield vena caval filter for management of selected cases of venous thromboembolic disease following hip surgery. Clin Orthop Rel Res 1986;204:201–206.

121. Webb LX, Rush PT, Fuller SB, et al. Greenfield filter prophylaxis of pulmonary embolism in patients undergoing surgery for acetabular fracture. J Orthop Trauma 1992;6:139–145.

122. Rosenthal D, McKinsey JF, Levy AM, et al. Use of the Greenfield filter in patients with major trauma. Cardiovasc Surg 1994;2: 52–55.

123. Wilson JT, Rogers FB, Wald SL, et al. Prophylactic vena cava filter insertion in patients with traumatic spinal cord injury: preliminary results. Neurosurgery 1994;35:234–239.

124. Winchell RJ, Hoyt DB, Walsh JC, et al. Risk factors associated with pulmonary embolism despite routine prophylaxis: implications for improved protection. J Trauma 1994;37:600–606.

125. Rogers FB, Shackford SR, Ricci MA, et al. Routine prophylactic vena cava filter insertion in severely injured trauma patients decreases the incidence of pulmonary embolism. J Am Coll Surg 1995;180:641–647.

126. Zolfaghari D, Johnson B, Weireter LJ, et al. Expanded use of inferior vena cava filters in the trauma population. Surg Annu 1995;27:99–105.

127. Patton JHJ, Fabian TC, Croce MA, et al. Prophylactic Greenfield filters: acute complications and long-term follow-up [see comments]. J Trauma 1996;41:231–236.

128. Rogers FB, Shackford SR, Ricci MA, et al. Prophylactic vena cava filter insertion in selected high-risk orthopaedic trauma patients. J Orthop Trauma 1997;11:267–272.

129. Rogers FB, Strindberg G, Shackford SR, et al. Five-year follow-up of prophylactic vena cava filters in high-risk trauma patients. Arch Surg 1998;133:406–411.

130. Greenfield LJ, Proctor MC, Michaels AJ, et al. Prophylactic vena caval filters in trauma: the rest of the story. J Vasc Surg 2000;32:490–497.

131. Wojcik R, Cippolle MD, Fearen I, et al. Long-term follow up of trauma patients with a vena caval filter. J Trauma 2000;49:839–843.

132. Velmahos GC, Kern J, Chan LS, et al. Prevention of venous thromboembolism after injury: An evidence-based report—Part I: Analysis of risk factors and evaluation of the role of vena caval filters. J Trauma 2000;49:132–139.

133. Velmahos GC, Kern J, Chan LS, et al. Prevention of venous thromboembolism after injury: An evidence-based report–Part II: Analysis of risk factors and evaluation of the role of vena caval filters. J Trauma 2000;49:140–144.

134. Montgomery KD, Geerts WH, Potter HG, et al. Thromboembolic complications in patients with pelvic trauma. Clin Orthop 1996;329:68–87.

135. Piotrowski JJ, Alexander JJ, Brandt CP, et al. Is deep vein thrombosis surveillance warranted in high-risk trauma patients? Am J Surg 1996;172:210–213.

136. Headrick JR, Barker DE, Pate LM, et al. The role of ultrasonography and inferior vena caval filter placement in high-risk trauma patients. Am Surg 1987;63:1–8.

137. Montgomery KD, Potter HG, Helfet DL. The detection and management of proximal deep venous thrombosis in patients with acute acetabular fractures: a follow-up report. J Orthop Trauma 1997;11:330–336.

138. Tuttle-Newhall JE, Rutledge R, Hultman CS, et al. Statewide, population-based, time-series analysis of the frequency and outcome of pulmonary embolus in 318,554 trauma patients [see comments]. J Trauma 1997;42:90–99.

139. Calligaro KD, Bergen WS, Haut MJ, et al. Thromboembolic complications in patients with advanced cancer: anticoagulation versus Greenfield filter placement. Ann Vasc Surg 1991;5:186–189.

140. Cohen JR, Grella L, Citron M. Greenfield filter instead of heparin as primary treatment for deep venous thrombosis or pulmonary embolism in patients with cancer. Cancer 1992;70:1993–1996.

141. Greenfield LJ, Proctor MC, Saluja A. Clinical results of Greenfield filter use in patients with cancer. Cardiovasc Surg 1997;5:145–149.

142. Hubbard KP, Roehm JOJ, Abbruzzese JL. The Bird's Nest filter. An alternative to long-term oral anticoagulation in patients with advanced malignancies. Am J Clin Oncol 1994;17:115–117.

143. Ihnat DM, Mills JL, Hughes JD, et al. Treatment of patients with venous thromboembolism and malignant disease: should vena cava filter placement be routine? J Vasc Surg 1998;28:800–807.

144. Levin JM, Schiff D, Loeffler JS, et al. Complications of therapy for venous thromboembolic disease in patients with brain tumors. Neurology 1993;43:1111–1114.

145. Lossef SV, Barth KH. Outcome of patients with advanced neoplastic disease receiving vena caval filters. J Vasc Interv Radiol 1995;6:273–277.

146. Olin JW, Young JR, Graor RA, et al. Treatment of deep vein thrombosis and pulmonary emboli in patients with primary and metastatic brain tumors. Arch Intern Med 1987;147:2177–2179.

147. Rosen MP, Porter DH, Kim D. Reassessment of vena caval filter use in patients with cancer. J Vasc Interv Radiol 1994;5:501–506.

148. Schiff D, DeAngelis LM. Therapy of venous thromboembolism in patients with brain metastases. Cancer 1994;73:493–498.

149. Schwarz RE, Marrero AM, Conlon KC, et al. Inferior vena cava filters in cancer patients: indications and outcome. J Clin Oncol 1996;14:652–657.

150. Walsh DB, Downing S, Nauta R, Gomes MN, Metastatic cancer: A relative contraindication to vena caval filter placement. Cancer 1987;59:161–163.

151. Whitney BA, Kerstein MD. Thrombocytopenia and cancer: use of the Kim-Ray Greenfield filter to prevent thromboembolism. South Med J 1987;80:1246–1248.

152. Moore FD Jr., Osteen RT, Karp DD, et al. Anticoagulants, venous thromboembolism and the cancer patient. Arch Surg 1981;116:405–407.

153. Bona RD, Sivjee KY, Hickey AD, et al. The efficacy and safety of oral anticoagulation in patients with cancer. Thromb Haemost 1995;74:1055–1058.

154. Landefeld CS, Goldman L. Major bleeding in outpatients treated with warfarin: incidence and prediction by factors known at the start of outpatient therapy. Am J Med 1989;87:144–152.

155. Prandoni P, Lensing AWA, Cogo A, et al. The long-term clinical course of acute deep venous thrombosis. Ann Intern Med 1996;125:1–7.

156. Altschuler E, Moosa H, Selker RG, et al. The risk and efficacy of anticoagulant therapy in the treatment of thromboembolic complications in patients with primary malignant brain tumors. Neurosurgery 1990;27:74–77.

157. Norris LK, Grossman SA. Treatment of thromboembolic complications in patients with brain tumors. J Neurooncol 1994;22:127–137.

158. Wolfe MW. Intracranial hemorrhage during systemic anticoagulation in patients with cerebral metastases. Arch Intern Med 1988;148:1878–1879.

159. So W, Hugenholtz H, Richard MT. Complications of anticoagulant therapy in patients with known central nervous system lesions. Can J Surg 1983;26:181–183.

160. Norris CS, Greenfield LJ, Herrmann JB. Free-floating iliofemoral thrombus: A risk of pulmonary embolism. Arch Surg 1985;120:806–808.

161. Berry RE, George JE, Shaver WA. Free-floating thrombus: A retrospective analysis. Ann Surg 1990;211:719–723.

162. Baldridge ED, Martin MA, Welling RE. Clinical significance of free-floating venous thrombi. J Vasc Surg 1990;11:62–69.

163. Radomski JS, Jarrell BE, Carabasi RA, et al. Risk of pulmonary embolus with inferior vena cava thrombosis. Am Surg 1987;53:97–101.

164. Voet D, Afschrift M. Floating thrombi: diagnosis and follow-up by duplex ultrasound. Br J Radiol 1991;64:1010–1014.

165. Monreal M, Ruiz J, Salvador R, et al. Recurrent pulmonary embolism: A prospective study. Chest 1989;95:976–979.

166. Pacouret G, Alison D, Pottier J-M, et al. Free-floating thrombus and embolic risk in patients with angiographically confirmed proximal deep venous thrombosis: A prospective study. Arch Intern Med 1997;157:305–308.

167. Greenfield LJ, Peyton MD, Brown PP, Elkins RC. Transvenous management of pulmonary embolic disease. Ann Surg 1974;180:461–468.

168. Greenfield LJ, Scher LA, Elkins RC. KMA-Greenfield filter placement for chronic pulmonary hypertension. Ann Surg 1979;189:560–565.
169. Millward SF. Temporary and retrievable inferior vena cava filters: Current status. J Vasc Interv Radiol 1998;9:381–387.
170. Bovyn G, Gory P, Reynaud P, et al. The Tempo filter: a multicenter study of a new temporary caval filter implantable for up to six weeks. Ann Vasc Surg 1997;11:520–528.
171. Ponchon M, Gofette P, Hainaut P. Temporary vena caval filtration: Preliminary clinical experience with removable vena caval filters. Acta Clin Belg 1999;54:223–228.
172. Stein PD, Hull RD, Raskob GE. Withholding treatment in patients with acute pulmonary embolism who have a high risk of bleeding and negative serial noninvasive leg tests. Am J Med 2000;109:301–306.
173. Sack GH, Levin J, Bell WR. Trousseau's syndrome and other manifestations of chronic disseminated coagulopathy in patients with neoplasms: clinical, pathophysiological and therapeutic features. Medicine 1977;56:1–37.
174. Trousseau A. Phlegmasia alba dolens. In Cormack SJR (Ed): Lectures on Clinical Medicine, Delivered at the Hotel-Dieu, Paris—Volume V. Philadelphia, Lindsay and Blakiston, 1872, p. 281.

CHAPTER 39

Neuraxial Anesthesia and the Anticoagulated Patient: Balancing the Risks and Benefits

Terese T. Horlocker, M.D.
John A. Heit, M.D.

Regional anesthesia and analgesia consist of central neuraxial (epidural or spinal) and peripheral nerve block. Neuraxial anesthesia may be given as a single injection or as a continuous infusion through an indwelling neuraxial catheter. Epidural anesthesia has the potential advantage of continued postoperative analgesia. The infusion may contain opioids and/or local anesthetics. For selected procedures, neuraxial anesthesia and/or analgesia provide several advantages over general anesthesia and systemic narcotic analgesia. One of the most serious risks of neuraxial block is spinal hematoma and associated paraplegia. Fortunately, this risk is very low, with an estimated incidence of about 1 in 190,000 epidural anesthetics, and 1 in 220,000 spinal anesthetics.[1,2] However, the flurry of reports of spinal hematoma after the 1993 release of low-molecular-weight heparin in the United States has focused attention on the complex medical decisions associated with concurrent neuraxial anesthesia and antithrombotic therapy. In this chapter, we review the pathophysiologic effects of surgery and general anesthesia and their role on adverse outcomes after surgery, the potential benefits of neuraxial anesthesia and analgesia in blocking these pathophysiologic effects, and the risk factors for spinal hematoma, including the estimated incremental risk for specific classes of antithrombotics. Finally, we provide recommendations for minimizing this risk among patients receiving concurrent neuraxial anesthesia and/or analgesia and antithrombotic therapy. With this information as well as knowledge regarding the pharmacokinetics of antithrombotic medications, the hematologist can tailor an individualized anticoagulant-based prophylaxis strategy or an antithrombotic therapy that both minimizes the risk of thrombosis and bleeding, and provides the most appropriate anesthesia and analgesia. In general, recommendations reported in this chapter

follow the consensus statements on Neuraxial Anesthesia and Anticoagulation published by the American Society of Regional Anesthesia.[3–7]

HISTORICAL OVERVIEW

The first spinal anesthetic was administered in 1898. The first spinal hematoma after neuraxial anesthesia was reported 10 years later, and involved a patient with spina bifida occulta and a spinal vascular malformation.[8] Sixty-one cases of spinal hematoma associated with epidural or spinal anesthesia were subsequently reported from 1906 to 1994.[9] Of these, 42 (68%) occurred in patients with impaired hemostasis: 30 patients had received intravenous or subcutaneous (standard or low molecular weight) heparin, and 12 had evidence of coagulopathy or thrombocytopenia, or were treated with antiplatelet medications (aspirin, indomethacin, ticlopidine), oral anticoagulants, thrombolytic agents (urokinase), or dextran 70. Needle and catheter placement was reported as difficult or bloody in 15 (25%) patients each. Overall, 53 of the 61 cases (87%) had either impaired hemostasis or difficult needle placement. A spinal anesthetic was performed in 15 patients. The remaining 46 patients received an epidural anesthetic, including 32 patients with an indwelling catheter. In 15 of these 32 patients, the spinal hematoma occurred immediately after removal of the catheter; nine catheters were removed during therapeutic levels of heparinization. A 1997 U.S. Food and Drug Administration (FDA) Public Health Advisory called attention to 43 additional patients from the United States who developed spinal hematoma after receiving low-molecular-weight heparin (enoxaparin sodium).[10] These spinal hematoma cases were reported to the FDA in the 5-year period after the release of enoxaparin sodium in 1993. Nearly 90% of cases occurred in patients receiving low-molecular-weight heparin as prophylaxis after surgery, primarily total knee or hip replacement surgery or spinal surgery.

PHYSIOLOGIC RESPONSES TO SURGERY

Surgical stress activates the sympathetic nervous system and causes release of neuroendocrine hormones (e.g., epinephrine, norepinephrine, cortisol, renin), and may indirectly cause adverse vascular, cardiac, pulmonary, and gastrointestinal outcomes.[11] For example, arterial vasoconstriction and venodilation induced by surgery may predispose to deep venous thrombosis because of venous overdilatation and endothelial injury, tissue factor exposure or expression and activation of coagulation, and reduced blood flow (see Chapter 30). Plasma procoagulant clotting factors also increase after surgery as an acute phase response, and may predispose to thrombosis. Vasoconstriction and reduced arterial blood flow may predispose to bypass graft thrombosis after vascular surgery. Sympathetic activation causes an increase in heart rate, cardiac inotropy, and blood pressure as well as coronary artery vasoconstriction, all of which predispose to myocardial ischemia, infarction, and dysrhythmias. Pain and abnormal diaphragmatic function from upper-abdominal and thoracic incisions cause impaired pulmonary function (atelectasis and ventilation–perfusion abnormalities), which may persist for up to 2 weeks after surgery. Abdominal pain after general surgery activates a spinal reflex arc that inhibits intestinal mobility and predisposes to postoperative ileus. Finally, general anesthesia may cause a prolonged impairment in cognitive function, which predisposes to such postoperative complications as depression, decubitus ulcers, stroke, urologic complications, and longer hospitalizations.

BENEFITS OF NEURAXIAL ANESTHESIA AND ANALGESIA

Neuraxial anesthesia and analgesia reduces many of the adverse physiologic responses to the stress of surgery and general anesthesia. However, there are few studies demonstrating that blocking these adverse responses translates into improved outcomes after surgery. In the following sections, we discuss the available outcome data for the procedures in which neuraxial block has been frequently used.

Total Hip or Knee Replacement Surgery, or Surgery for Hip Fracture

Blood loss and transfusion requirements during total hip replacement are reduced with spinal or epidural anesthesia compared to general anesthesia.[12] These differences are even more apparent if epidural analgesia is continued postoperatively.[13] Pain management also is a significant issue for patients undergoing major orthopedic surgery. Severe or moderate postoperative pain affects up to 90% of total knee arthroplasty patients and retards mobility. Two to three days of epidural analgesia facilitates physical rehabilitation and results in improved joint range of motion and reduced hospital stay.[14] Neuraxial anesthesia also may reduce the incidence of deep venous thrombosis after total hip replacement surgery (either elective or after hip fracture); however, the relative risk reduction is modest and primary prophylaxis is still indicated.[15]

Major Abdominal Aorta and Lower-Extremity Vascular Bypass Surgery

In one of the few available randomized clinical trials, Tuman and coworkers evaluated the effect of anesthetic technique on outcomes in patients undergoing major abdominal aorta surgery or lower-extremity vascular bypass surgery.[16] Patients were randomly allocated to receive general anesthesia combined with epidural anesthesia and analgesia versus general anesthesia combined with on-demand opioid analgesia. Patients receiving epidural anesthesia and analgesia had a lower incidence of myocardial infarction, prolonged intubation, and acute vascular graft occlusion. These differences were most apparent for patients with significant pre-existing cardiac or pulmonary disease who underwent major abdominal aorta procedures.

Cardiac Surgery

Selective blockade of cardiac sympathetic innervation via thoracic epidural anesthesia mitigates the adverse cardiac physiologic responses to surgery. Although the profound analgesia, attenuation of the stress response, and thoracic cardiac sympathectomy theoretically may be beneficial, there are few randomized clinical trials that evaluated neuraxial block in patients undergoing cardiac surgery and none used clinical outcomes as primary endpoint measures.[17] Additional studies are needed to determine the impact of neuraxial block on mortality and the incidence of complications after cardiac surgery.

General Surgery

Neuraxial analgesia improves gut motility after surgery by blocking both the pain afferent pathways as well as the sympathetic efferent pathways. The epidural solution should contain a local anesthetic (with or without an opioid) and should be continued until postoperative bowel function has returned.[18]

Parturition

Neuraxial techniques such as single-dose spinal, continuous epidural, and combined spinal–epidural anesthesia provide more effective intrapartum pain relief than nonpharmacologic methods, intramuscular/intravenous opioids, and inhalational agents (nitrous oxide).[19] Superior analgesia results in additional benefits, which include improved uteroplacental perfusion and increased oxygen delivery to the fetus.[20]

RISK FACTORS FOR SPINAL HEMATOMA

Impaired hemostasis from either congenital or acquired causes increases the risk of spinal hematoma associated with neuraxial anesthesia. For the purposes of this review, we will concentrate on the risk associated with drugs that impair hemostasis. The magnitude of this risk cannot be quantified currently. We provide qualitative estimates of the risk based on reported clinical case series as well as expert opinion.

Standard (Unfractionated) Heparin

Both the reported experience as well as a vast clinical experience suggests that neuraxial anesthesia is relatively safe following preoperative thromboprophylaxis doses (e.g., up to 5000 units) of subcutaneous heparin. In two case series, there were no spinal hematomas in 204 epidural and 119 spinal anesthetics performed on patients who had received 5000 units of unfractionated subcutaneous heparin started 2 hours prior to needle placement.[21,22] In an extensive literature review, Schwander and coworkers found no reported spinal hematomas in over 5000 patients who received varying doses of subcutaneous heparin in combination with spinal or epidural anesthesia.[23] Spinal hematoma also is extremely rare in patients who undergo major conduction blocks while receiving low-dose heparin. Only three such cases have been reported, and two occurred with a continuous epidural anesthetic technique.[24–26] The risk of neuraxial bleeding may be increased in debilitated patients or after prolonged subcutaneous heparin prophylaxis.

Elective neuraxial procedures should be avoided in patients who are therapeutically anticoagulated with heparin (or with oral anticoagulants) because of the substantially increased risk of spinal hematoma. Moreover, commencing therapeutic anticoagulation immediately after needle placement and without adequate time for hemostasis also should be avoided. Ruff and coworkers reported documented spinal hematomas in 7 of 342 patients (2%) who underwent a diagnostic lumbar puncture either during therapeutic heparin anticoagulation or when anticoagulation was started within 1 hour after lumbar puncture; 5 patients developed paraparesis.[27] Eighteen additional patients had severe radicular back pain lasting more than 48 hours after the lumbar puncture. Two of these patients died of unrelated causes and underwent autopsy; one patient had a chronic epidural hematoma, while the other had an organized subdural hematoma. The investigators identified traumatic needle placement, initiation of therapeutic anticoagulation within 1 hour of lumbar puncture, and concomitant aspirin therapy as risk factors for spinal hematoma in anticoagulated patients.

In contrast to the substantial risk of spinal bleeding during neuraxial block in the anticoagulated patient, a brief period of intraoperative heparin anticoagulation beginning *after* needle placement has been performed and *after* allowing sufficient time for neuraxial hemostasis appears to be relatively safe. Rao and coworkers evaluated 3164 patients who had continuous epidural anesthesia and 847 patients who had continuous spinal anesthesia for lower extremity vascular procedures.[28] Patients with a history of pre-existing coagulation abnormalities, thrombocytopenia, or preoperative anticoagulation therapy were excluded. In four patients, blood was freely aspirated following insertion of the needle into the epidural space. For these patients, surgery was postponed until the following day and the patients were given general anesthesia. For the remaining patients, heparin was administrated as an intravenous bolus beginning 50 to 60 minutes after catheter placement and the dose was adjusted to therapeutic levels by maintaining the activated clotting time (ACT) twice the baseline value. The bolus heparin dose was repeated every 6 hours following measurement of the ACT throughout the period of anticoagulation therapy. The catheters were removed the following day and 1 hour prior to administration of the next maintenance dose of heparin. No patient developed signs or symptoms of epidural or subarachnoid hematoma, including four patients who had traumatic needle placement and subsequently received general anesthesia. Similarly, Baron and coworkers reported no neurologic sequelae in 912 vascular surgical patients who received continuous epidural anesthesia and underwent transient intraoperative anticoagulation with heparin (ACT above 100 seconds).[29] The catheters were removed immediately after surgery. Finally, Mathews and coworkers reported no neurologic complications in 40 cardiac surgical patients who received intrathecal morphine through 20- to 25-gauge needles beginning 50 minutes prior to cardiopulmonary bypass and systemic anticoagulation with heparin.[30] There currently are no data to suggest that perioperative outcomes are improved with either single-dose or continuous neuraxial techniques compared to systemic opioids in patients undergoing cardiac revascularization.[17] However, surgery may be canceled or delayed because of a bloody return during needle or catheter placement.

The rarity of spinal bleeding makes it difficult to assess the incremental risk and risk factors for spinal hematoma among patients receiving continuous catheter neuraxial anesthesia and a brief course of intraoperative intravenous heparin therapy. Risk factors for spinal hematoma in this setting likely include a pre-existing coagulopathy, thrombocytopenia, concomitant aspirin or other antiplatelet therapy, traumatic or difficult needle placement, therapeutic heparinization within 1 hour of spinal or epidural puncture, and no or inappropriate monitoring of the heparin effect.[9,27,28,30]

Low-Molecular-Weight Heparin

Low-molecular-weight heparin (LMWH) (e.g., enoxaparin sodium) was first introduced in the United States in 1993 for venous thromboembolism prophylaxis after total hip replacement surgery. In the next 5 years, 43 cases of spinal hematoma associated with neuraxial anesthesia and concurrent LMWH thromboprophylaxis were reported to the manufacturer (Table 39–1).[31] From these data, the incidence of spinal hematoma in patients receiving enoxaparin while undergoing spinal or epidural anesthesia has been estimated as 1 in 3100 continuous epidural anesthetics and 1 in 41,000 spinal anesthetics.[32] Many of these events occurred when LMWH was administered intraoperatively or early postoperatively to patients undergoing continuous epidural anesthesia and analgesia (Table 39–2). The median age of these 43 patients was 78 years (range, 28 to 90) and 78% were women. Some patients had pre-existing spinal abnormalities and a third received concurrent medications including nonsteroidal anti-inflammatory agents (NSAIDs) that impair hemostasis. Nearly 90% of cases received enoxaparin as prophylaxis after surgery, primarily total knee or hip replacement surgery or spinal surgery. Factors suspected of predisposing patients to perispinal hematoma are listed in Table 39–3.

In contrast, LMWH has been used extensively in Europe since the early 1980s, most often as thromboprophylaxis for elective surgery. Despite the frequent use of concurrent neuraxial anesthesia (e.g., up to 1.5 million neuraxial blocks per year in Germany alone), the reported incidence of spinal hematoma is extremely low.[1,9,33,34] The difference in the spinal hematoma incidence between Europe and the United States cannot be accounted for by differences in neuraxial block technique. At least 75% of neuraxial blocks in Europe, and 70% of blocks in the United States, are single-dose spinal blocks. However, there are important differences in the LMWH dose schedule between North America and Europe.[34] In Europe, the first LMWH thromboprophylaxis dose is given the night (e.g., at least 10 to 12 hours) before surgery. Thus, the neuraxial block is administered at the nadir of LMWH plasma concentration. The subsequent LMWH dose is administered at least 4 hours after the neuraxial block. Thus, the peak concentration of LMWH occurs at least 6 to 8 hours after the spinal puncture and after sufficient time for normal neuraxial hemostasis. Finally, practice guidelines for the concurrent use of neuraxial anesthesia and LMWH thromboprophylaxis have been used extensively in Europe. We believe these differences in dose schedule, the use of practice guidelines, and proper patient selection may account for the apparent difference in the incidence of spinal hematoma in Europe compared to the United States.

LMWH also has been approved in the United States as inpatient therapy for acute deep venous thrombosis with or without pulmonary embolism (enoxaparin or tinzaparin), outpatient treatment of acute deep venous

Table 39–1 • SPINAL HEMATOMA CASES WITH LOW-MOLECULAR-WEIGHT HEPARIN REPORTED THROUGH THE MEDWATCH SYSTEM BETWEEN 1993 AND 1998

Etiology	Number of Patients
Spontaneous	1
Major spine surgery	2
Neuraxial block	39
Attempted spinal/epidural	3
Epidural steroid injection	2
Spinal	6 (including one continuous spinal)
Epidural (continuous)	23
Unspecified continuous	2
Unknown technique	3

Adapted from Horlocker TT, Wedel DJ. Neuraxial block and low molecular weight heparin: balancing perioperative analgesia and thromboprophylaxis. Reg Anesth Pain Med 1998;23:164–177, with permission.

Table 39–2 • FACTORS AMONG 26 PATIENTS DEVELOPING SPINAL HEMATOMA WITH CONCURRENT NEURAXIAL ANESTHESIA/ ANALGESIA AND LOW-MOLECULAR-WEIGHT HEPARIN PROPHYLAXIS

Variable	Number of Patients
Initiation of LMWH dosing	
Preoperative	4
≤12 h postoperatively	11
24 h postoperatively	5
Unknown	6
LMWH administered with catheter indwelling[a]	17
Concomitant antiplatelet/anticoagulant medications	
Antiplatelet therapy	7
Warfarin	2
Multiple medications	3
Onset of symptoms[b]	
Catheter indwelling	4
Within hours of catheter removal	7
>12 hours after catheter removal	10
Undetermined	5

[a] A minimum of 17 patients received LMWH with an indwelling neuraxial catheter. Only two patients had documented catheter removal occur prior to initiation of LMWH, including one patient who received warfarin in the postanesthesia care unit.
[b] Four patients reported minor deficits prior to catheter removal, including two patients who became acutely paraplegic upon catheter removal. While paralysis occurred shortly after catheter removal in at least seven patients, 24 hours or more often elapsed between catheter removal and the onset of neurologic dysfunction.
Adapted from Horlocker TT, Wedel DJ. Neuraxial block and low molecular weight heparin: balancing perioperative analgesia and thromboprophylaxis. Reg Anesth Pain Med 1998;23:164–177, with permission.

Table 39–3 • RISK FACTORS FOR SPINAL HEMATOMA ASSOCIATED WITH NEURAXIAL ANESTHESIA AND LOW-MOLECULAR-WEIGHT HEPARIN THROMBOPROPHYLAXIS

- Underlying hemostatic disorder
- Traumatic needle or catheter insertion, or blood return
- Improper anticoagulant dosage or dose schedule
- Use of continuous epidural catheter
- Concurrent medications that impair hemostasis
- Vertebral column abnormalities
- Older patient age
- Female gender

thrombosis without pulmonary embolism (enoxaparin sodium), and therapy for acute coronary syndromes (e.g., unstable angina and non-Q-wave myocardial infarction) in combination with aspirin (dalteparin sodium; enoxaparin sodium). Moreover, LMWH increasingly is used as "bridging" therapy for the chronically anticoagulated patient who requires anticoagulation reversal for an operative procedure and yet is at high risk for an intercurrent thrombosis. Compared to venous thromboembolism prophylaxis, the intensity of anticoagulation during LMWH therapy is much higher (e.g., peak LMWH concentration of 0.1 to 0.2 anti-X_a U/mL for prophylaxis versus therapeutic levels of 0.5 to 1.0 anti-X_a U/mL). For these patients, neuraxial anesthesia should be delayed at least 24 hours after the last subcutaneous LMWH dose. For patients with impaired renal function (e.g., serum creatinine 2.0 or above), LMWH clearance is delayed. Thus, neuraxial anesthesia should be delayed even longer for these patients, and it is probably wise to either ensure that the plasma anti-X_a level is no higher than 0.1 IU/mL prior to needle placement or use an alternative anesthesia.

Oral Anticoagulants

Full therapeutic oral anticoagulation (e.g., warfarin) therapy is a relative contraindication to neuraxial anesthesia.[35,36] However, chronically anticoagulated patients frequently require brief anticoagulation reversal in order to undergo a procedure. Usually, an elapsed time of about 4 days is required for the International Normalized Ratio (INR) to return toward normal after stopping oral anticoagulation.[37] The INR is most sensitive to factor VII and X activity, and is relatively insensitive to factor II (prothrombin) activity.[38] In addition, factor VII activity recovers quickly while prothrombin activity recovers slowly after discontinuing oral anticoagulants (e.g., plasma factor VII and II half lives are 4 to 6 hours and 60 to 72 hours, respectively). Thus, the INR may be near normal when factor VII and X activity exceed about 50% to 55% yet the prothrombin activity is still low and inadequate for normal hemostasis. Consequently, we recommend that neuraxial anesthesia be delayed until the INR is normal and for at least 4 days after stopping warfarin, regardless of whether the INR becomes normal sooner than 4 days.

The other circumstance where neuraxial anesthesia may be used concurrently with oral anticoagulation is in the setting of warfarin thromboprophylaxis, which may be started either the night before, or the night of, surgery. Unfortunately, there are few published data regarding the risk of spinal hematoma in such patients. There were no reported spinal hematomas in 192 patients receiving postoperative epidural analgesia in conjunction with low-dose warfarin thromboprophylaxis after total knee arthroplasty.[39] Patients received warfarin to prolong the prothrombin time (PT) to 15.0 to 17.3 seconds, corresponding to an INR of 2.0 to 3.0. Epidural catheters were left indwelling 37±15 hours after surgery (range, 13 to 96 hours). The mean PT at the time of epidural catheter removal was 13.4±2 seconds (range, 10.6 to 25.8 seconds). In another case series, there were no neurologic complications among 459 orthopedic patients who underwent spinal or epidural anesthesia and received warfarin thromboprophylaxis, including 412 patients who received postoperative epidural analgesia.[40] All patients were anticoagulated with warfarin postoperatively; 181 patients also received warfarin preoperatively. The mean duration of epidural analgesia was 43.6±12.5 hours. Patients who had warfarin prophylaxis administered preoperatively had significantly higher prothrombin times at the time of catheter removal. These case series contain too few patients to accurately estimate the risk of spinal bleeding among these patients or to conclude that such a practice is safe. In general, we recommend that oral anticoagulant prophylaxis be started after surgery in patients who will receive a neuraxial block. When a catheter is used, the catheter should be removed before the INR becomes significantly prolonged.

Antiplatelet Therapy

Medications which impair platelet function, including aspirin, NSAIDs, and thienopyridines (ticlopidine and clopidogrel), likely do increase the risk for spinal hematoma associated with neuraxial anesthesia.[9] However, based on a few small studies and a vast clinical experience, the risk increment appears to be relatively small. For example, the Collaborative Low-dose Aspirin Study in Pregnancy (CLASP) Group studied 1422 high-risk obstetric patients who received daily aspirin (60 mg).[41] All patients received epidural anesthesia during delivery and none suffered a spinal hematoma. Horlocker and coworkers reported a retrospective review of the outcomes from 1013 spinal and epidural anesthetics in which antiplatelet drugs were taken by 39% of patients, including 11% of patients who were on multiple antiplatelet medications.[42] While no patient developed a clinically detectable spinal hematoma, patients administered antiplatelet medications experienced a higher incidence of a bloody needle or catheter return (a risk factor for spinal hematoma). There were no spinal hematomas in a subsequent prospective study of 390 neuraxial anesthetics on patients receiving antiplatelet therapy.[43] In this study, however, antiplatelet therapy was not a risk factor for needle or catheter bloody return. Instead, a bloody return was correlated with other patient and anesthetic variables, including female gender, increased age, a history of excessive bruising or bleeding, continuous catheter technique, large needle gauge, multiple needle passes, and difficult needle placement. These data suggest (but do not prove) that preoperative antiplatelet therapy is not a major risk factor for spinal hematoma during spinal or epidural anesthesia.

Newer drugs that inhibit the fibrinogen-binding conformation of the platelet integrin receptor glycoprotein $\alpha_{IIb}\beta_3$ (GP IIb/IIIa; e.g., abciximab [ReoPro], eptifibatide [Integrilin], tirofiban [Aggrastat]) cause profound and sustained impairment of platelet function and usually are given in combination with therapeutic standard heparin or LMWH anticoagulation. We believe the risk of spinal hematoma is likely to be substantial in patients treated with these agents and that neuraxial anesthesia and/or analgesia should be avoided.

Thrombolytic Therapy

As with patients receiving systemic heparin, LMWH, or oral anticoagulation therapy, lumbar puncture is contraindicated in patients receiving thrombolytic therapy. However, thrombolytic therapy is occasionally (and often unexpectedly) necessary after a neuraxial blockade has been given, particularly during vascular surgery. While there are several reported cases of spinal hematoma in patients with indwelling epidural catheters who received thrombolytic therapy, the true incidence of this complication among such patients is unknown. Dickman and coworkers reported a case in which a patient with femoral artery occlusion received an epidural anesthetic for surgical placement of an intra-arterial catheter for infusion of urokinase.[44] Three hours postoperatively, the patient complained of back pain, which progressed to paraplegia despite discontinuation of the urokinase infusion. An emergency decompressive laminectomy was performed, and a large solidified hematoma compressing the thecal sac was evacuated. The patient recovered full neurologic function within 3 days. Onishchuk and Carlsson reported a patient with superficial femoral artery occlusion who underwent epidural catheter placement for femoral–popliteal artery bypass.[45] Blood was noted in the epidural catheter during placement. The patient received a bolus of 6300 units of heparin 90 minutes later, and a single bolus of urokinase was also injected intra-arterially during the surgical procedure. A heparin infusion of 1000 units/h was initiated and continued postoperatively for 24 hours. The patient was taken to the recovery room and the epidural catheter removed. On the fourth postoperative day, the patient became paraplegic. A magnetic resonance imaging scan revealed an epidural hematoma extending from T10 to L2. The patient remained paraplegic despite an emergency decompressive laminectomy. Based on these reports, we believe epidural anesthesia should be avoided in patients who will receive thrombolytic therapy.

New Antithrombotic Agents

The limitations of aspirin and heparin have led to the development of new antithrombotic drugs that target various steps in the hemostatic system, such as inhibiting platelet aggregation, blocking coagulation factors, or enhancing fibrinolysis[46] (see Chapter 24). Many of these antithrombotic agents have prolonged plasma half-lives and are difficult to reverse even with administration of blood components. The administration of these medications in combination with neuraxial anesthesia must be considered very carefully.[47–49] We must learn from our experience with LMWH to review anticoagulant pharmacology, including onset time, plasma-half life, and drug interactions, in order to minimize the risk of spinal hematoma.

CONSULTATION CONSIDERATIONS

Neuraxial anesthesia and/or analgesia should be avoided in patients with impaired hemostasis, thrombocytopenia, spina bifida occulta or other spinal defects, and known vascular malformations. Where possible, medications that impair hemostasis should be stopped in sufficient time before surgery for the antithrombotic effect to resolve. This may be difficult or even contraindicated in patients with significant thrombophilia or those with deep venous thrombosis or pulmonary embolism within 3 to 4 months. In general, neuraxial anesthesia also should be avoided in patients receiving more than one medication that impairs hemostasis (e.g., an antiplatelet drug plus heparin or LMWH regardless of the heparin dose). The guiding principle of concurrent neuraxial block and antithrombotic therapy is that any potential trauma to the spinal canal contents (such as may occur with lumbar puncture, or with spinal catheter placement, re-positioning, or removal) should be minimized and ideally should be timed to occur when there is no anticoagulant effect, or at the nadir of the anticoagulant effect (Tables 39–4 and 39–5). Moreover, subsequent anticoagulant therapy should be withheld until there is adequate time for normal hemostatic repair. A bloody or difficult needle placement may increase the spinal hematoma risk. In this circumstance, the hematologist working with the attending anesthesiologist and surgeon must assess the risks, benefits, and alternatives to neuraxial anesthesia and concurrent anticoagulation, including possibly delaying surgery and monitoring for the development of neurologic deficits. Risks and benefits of continuing and discontinuing anticoagulants must be individualized for any given patient. If the decision is to proceed, especially careful postoperative monitoring is warranted. Other factors suspected of predisposing patients to perispinal hematoma include spinal needle or catheter insertion or removal in the presence of significant levels of anticoagulant agents, use of continuous epidural catheters, older age, and female gender.

Regional Anesthetic Management of the Patient Receiving Standard Heparin

1. While European guidelines recommend that lumbar puncture should be delayed at least 4 hours after a low-dose (e.g., 5000 units or less) subcutaneous heparin injection; this has not been the general practice in the United States.
2. Lumbar puncture for neuraxial regional anesthesia should be avoided in patients receiving systemic heparin therapy.
3. For patients who have received neuraxial anesthesia, subsequent intravenous heparin administration should be delayed for at least 1 hour after needle placement. Indwelling catheters should be removed at least 1 hour before subsequent heparin administration and 2 to 4 hours after the last heparin dose. Evaluation of the activated partial throm-

Table 39-4 • PHARMACOLOGIC VENOUS THROMBOEMBOLISM PROPHYLAXIS REGIMENS FREQUENTLY USED WITH NEURAXIAL ANESTHESIA

Indication and Modality	Regimen
Total Hip or Knee Replacement	
Adjusted-dose unfractionated heparin	3500 units SC q8 h, started 2 hours before surgery; after surgery, the dose is adjusted to maintain the aPTT within the upper normal range
Low-molecular-weight heparin	
Ardeparin sodium (Normiflo)	50 U/kg SC bid, started, 12–24 hours after surgery
Dalteparin sodium (Fragmin)	5000 U SC qd, started 12 hours before surgery, or 2500 U SC given 7 hours after surgery, then 5000 U SC daily.
Danaparoid sodium (Orgaran)	750 U SC bid, started 2 hours before surgery
Enoxaparin sodium (Lovenox)	30 mg SC bid, started 12–24 hours after surgery, or 40 mg SC qd, started 10–12 hours before surgery
Tinzaparin (Innohep)	75 U/kg SC qd, started 10–12 hours before surgery
rHirudin (desirudin, Revasc)	15 mg SC bid, started within 30 minutes of surgery (and after regional anesthesia, if used)
Warfarin sodium	5 mg PO, started the night before or immediately after surgery and adjusted to prolong the INR to 2.0–3.0
General Surgery	
Unfractionated heparin	5000 units SC q8–12 h, started 2 hours before surgery
Low-molecular-weight heparin	
Dalteparin sodium	2500 U SC qd, started 1–2 hours before surgery
Enoxaparin sodium	40 mg SC qd, started 2 hours before surgery

boplastin time (aPTT) may be appropriate prior to catheter removal for patients with excessive heparin anticoagulation or patients receiving high doses of heparin.

4. Prolonged therapeutic anticoagulation appears to increase the risk of spinal hematoma, especially if combined with other agents which interfere with hemostasis. Therefore, neuraxial blocks should be avoided in this clinical setting. If systematic anticoagulation therapy is begun with an epidural catheter in place, catheter removal ideally should be delayed for 2 to 4 hours after stopping the heparin and when the aPTT is near normal or normal.

Regional Anesthetic Management of the Patient Receiving LMWH

The Sixth American College of Chest Physicians (ACCP) Consensus Conference on Antithrombotic Therapy made the following recommendations for venous thromboembolism prophylaxis after major orthopedic surgery of the leg.[50] For routine patients undergoing elective total hip replacement surgery, either subcutaneous LMWH (started either 12 hours before or 12 to 24 hours after surgery), or adjusted-dose warfarin (INR postoperative target = 2.5; range, 2.0 to 3.0; started preoperatively or immediately after surgery), are recommended. Adjusted-dose unfractionated heparin (started preoperatively) is an acceptable alternative. Adjuvant prophylaxis with elastic compression stockings or intermittent pneumatic compression may provide additional efficacy. Although other agents such as low-dose unfractionated heparin, aspirin, dextran, and intermittent pneumatic compression alone reduce the overall incidence of venous thromboembolism, they are less effective and are not recommended to be used alone for total hip replacement surgery.

For patients undergoing elective total knee replacement surgery, either LMWH or adjusted-dose warfarin

Table 39-5 • ANTITHROMBOTIC PEAK EFFECT AND TIME TO NORMAL HEMOSTASIS AFTER DISCONTINUATION

Antithrombotic	Peak Effect	Time to Normal Hemostasis
Standard heparin		
Intravenous	Immediate	2–3 hours
Subcutaneous	40–50 minutes	4–6 hours
Low-molecular-weight heparin	2–4 hours	12+ hours
Heparinoid (danaparoid sodium, Orgaran)	2–5 hours	3–5 days
Warfarin sodium	4–6 days	4–6 days
Antiplatelet agents		
Aspirin	Hours	5–8 days
Thienopyridines (ticlopidine, clopidogrel)	Hours	10 days
NSAIDs	Hours	1–3 days
Thrombolytic agents (rtPA, streptokinase)	Minutes	1–2 days

are recommended. Optimal use of intermittent pneumatic compression is an alternative option but this is a less certain recommendation because of the small sample sizes and few trials using this prophylaxis modality. Low-dose unfractionated heparin is not recommended.

For patients undergoing hip fracture surgery, either LMWH or adjusted-dose warfarin prophylaxis is recommended.

The optimal duration of anticoagulant prophylaxis after total hip or knee replacement surgery is uncertain although at least 7 days of prophylaxis is recommended. Extended out-of-hospital LMWH prophylaxis may reduce the incidence of clinically important thromboembolic events and is recommended at least for high-risk patients.

LMWH prophylaxis for elective hip or knee replacement surgery may be started either the night before surgery or 12 to 24 hours after surgery (Table 39–5). The timing of the first LMWH dose is important when planning neuraxial anesthesia.

1. When LMWH prophylaxis is started before surgery, the first dose should be given 10 to 12 hours (e.g., the night) before the neuraxial block. Neuraxial anesthesia should be avoided if the first LMWH dose is given later (e.g., 2 hours before surgery, as in general surgery patients), since the lumbar puncture would occur at the time of peak anticoagulant concentration. The next dose of LMWH should be given at least 4 hours after the lumbar puncture.
2. When LMWH prophylaxis is started after surgery, the first dose should be given 24 hours after the surgery.
3. A single-dose spinal anesthetic probably is the safest neuraxial technique. If a continuous technique is selected, the epidural catheter should be removed at least 12 hours after the last LMWH dose. An opioid or dilute local anesthetic solution is recommended in order to allow frequent monitoring of neurologic function. If epidural analgesia is anticipated to continue for more than 24 hours, LMWH administration may be delayed, or an alternate method of thromboprophylaxis may be selected (e.g., external pneumatic compression) based on the risk profile for the individual patient. The catheter may be left indwelling overnight and removed the following day. The first dose of LMWH after catheter removal should be given at least 12 to 24 hours later.
4. Monitoring of the anti-X_a level is not generally recommended. At thromboprophylaxis doses, the plasma anti-X_a level is not predictive of the risk of bleeding. Monitoring should be considered in patients with significant renal insufficiency.
5. The decision to implement LMWH thromboprophylaxis in the presence of an indwelling catheter must be made with care. Extreme vigilance of the patient's neurologic status is warranted. These decisions should be made preoperatively to allow optimal management of both postoperative analgesia and thromboprophylaxis.
6. Patients receiving higher (treatment) doses of LMWH require at least 24 hours between dosing of LMWH and needle or catheter placement, or catheter removal.

Regional Anesthetic Management of the Patient on Oral Anticoagulants

1. For the chronically anticoagulated patient undergoing a procedure that will require an elective neuraxial anesthetic, the oral anticoagulant should be stopped at least 4 days prior to the neuraxial block, and even earlier if the baseline INR is excessively prolonged (e.g., 3.0 or higher). The INR should be normal prior to needle placement. In patients at extreme risk of thromboembolism, the need for continued anticoagulation may well require a different mode of anesthesia.
2. When oral anticoagulant thromboprophylaxis is started the night before surgery, the INR should be checked and proved to be normal prior to neuraxial block if the oral anticoagulant was given more than 24 hours earlier or a second dose was given. Extreme care also is necessary for patients who may be particularly sensitive to the effect of an oral anticoagulant, such as the elderly (e.g., 65 years or older), women, underweight patients (e.g., 45 kg or less), patients with poor nutrition, and patients with significantly impaired cardiac, hepatic or renal function.
3. An indwelling catheter should be removed prior to significant prolongation of the INR.
4. The INR should be obtained daily to monitor anticoagulant activity.

Regional Anesthetic Management of the Patient Receiving Antiplatelet Medications

1. If possible, drugs that impair platelet function should be stopped in sufficient time before neuraxial anesthesia to allow return of normal platelet function. Aspirin and thienopyridines (e.g., ticlopidine, clopidogrel) should be stopped for at least 7 to 10 days, and NSAIDs for at least 72 hours, before the neuraxial block to allow return of normal platelet function.
2. When antiplatelet therapy either cannot be stopped or there is insufficient time to stop the therapy, it is probably safe to proceed with neuraxial anesthesia and concurrent antiplatelet therapy as long as there are no other risk factors for spinal bleeding.
3. Assessment of platelet function prior to performance of neuraxial block is not recommended. However, careful preoperative assessment of the patient to identify alterations of health that might contribute to bleeding is crucial.

Regional Anesthetic Management of the Patient on Thrombolytic Therapy

1. Neuraxial anesthesia and analgesia should be avoided in patients receiving thrombolytic therapy.
2. Thrombolytic therapy is relatively contraindicated for at least 10 days after lumbar puncture.
3. There is no definitive recommendation for removal of neuraxial catheters in patients who receive thrombolytic therapy during a neuraxial catheter infusion. Caution must be exercised in making decisions about removing or maintaining these catheters. Determination of the PT, aPTT, and fibrinogen level may be helpful in guiding a decision about the timing of catheter removal. Fibrinogen levels of 50 mg/dL or higher are sufficient to support hemostasis.

Table 39-6 • NEUROLOGIC OUTCOME IN PATIENTS WITH SPINAL HEMATOMA FOLLOWING NEUROSURGERY[a]

Interval Between Onset of Paraplegia and Neurosurgery	Good N = 15	Partial N = 11	Poor N = 29
< 8 hours (N = 13)	6	4	3
Between 8 and 24 hours (N = 8)	1	2	4
> 24 hours (N = 11)	2	0	10
No surgical intervention (N = 13)	4	1	8
Unknown (N = 10)	2	4	4

[a] Neurologic outcome was reported for 55 of 61 cases of spinal hematoma following neuraxial blockade
Adapted from Vandermeulen EP, Van Aken H, Vermylen J. Anticoagulants and spinal-epidural anesthesia. Anesth Analg 1994;79:1165-1177, with permission.

SIGNS AND SYMPTOMS OF SPINAL HEMATOMA AFTER NEURAXIAL ANESTHESIA

Hemorrhage into the spinal canal most commonly occurs in the epidural space because of the prominent epidural venous plexus. Spinal cord compression from spinal hematoma may result in neurologic ischemia and paraplegia. Among patients who develop spinal hematoma after neuraxial anesthesia, neurologic compromise usually presents as progression of the sensory or motor block (e.g., progression of lower-extremity numbness or weakness) or bowel/bladder dysfunction, rather than severe radicular back pain. All patients should be monitored carefully and frequently for the new onset of back pain and symptoms or signs of cord compression. For patients in whom spinal hematoma is suspected, diagnostic imaging (e.g., MRI) and definitive surgical therapy must be performed as rapidly as possible in order to avoid permanent paresis. Decompressive laminectomy was undertaken in 65% of the patients reported in the FDA Public Health Advisory, but permanent paraplegia still occurred in 37%. Paraplegia was more likely to be reversible in patients who underwent laminectomy within 8 hours of onset of neurologic dysfunction (Table 39-6). The decision to perform neuraxial anesthesia should include the degree and duration of anticoagulation, availability of MRI, and availability of prompt neurosurgical consultation.

In summary, the decision to perform spinal or epidural anesthesia/analgesia and the timing of catheter removal in a patient receiving thromboprophylaxis should be made on an individual basis, weighing the small but definite risk of spinal hematoma with the benefits of regional anesthesia for the individual patient. Alternative anesthetic and analgesic techniques exist for patients considered to be at an unacceptable risk such as patients who require a high degree of thromboprophylaxis because of their thromboembolic history. The patient's coagulation status should be optimized at the time of spinal or epidural needle/catheter placement, and the level of anticoagulation must be carefully monitored during the period of epidural catheterization. Indwelling catheters should not be removed in the presence of therapeutic anticoagulation. In addition, communication between clinicians involved in the perioperative management of patients receiving anticoagulants for thromboprophylaxis is essential. Patients should be monitored closely in the perioperative period for early signs of cord compression. If spinal hematoma is suspected, the treatment of choice is immediate decompressive laminectomy. Recovery of neurologic compromise is unlikely if surgery is postponed for more than 8 to 12 hours.

REFERENCES

Chapter 39 References

1. Tryba M. Epidural regional anesthesia and low molecular weight heparin: Pro. Anästh Intensivmed Notfallmed Schmerzther 1993;28:179-81.
2. Wulf H. Epidural anesthesia and spinal hematoma. Can J Anaesth 1996; 43:1260-1271.
3. Liu SS, Mulroy MF. Neuraxial anesthesia and analgesia in the presence of standard heparin. Reg Anesth Pain Med 1998;23:157-163.
4. Horlocker TT, Wedel DJ. Neuraxial block and low molecular weight heparin: balancing perioperative analgesia and thromboprophylaxis. Reg Anesth Pain Med 1998;23:164-177.
5. Enneking KF, Benzon HT. Oral anticoagulants and regional anesthesia: a perspective. Reg Anesth Pain Med 1998;23:140-145.
6. Rosenquist RW, Brown DL. Neuraxial bleeding: fibrinolytics/thrombolytics. Reg Anesth Pain Med 1998;23:152-156.
7. Urmey WF, Rowlingson JC. Do antiplatelet agents contribute to the development of perioperative spinal hematoma? Reg Anesth Pain Med 1998;23:146-151.
8. Usubiaga JE. Neurologic complaints following epidural anesthesia. Int Anesthesiol Clin 1975;13:1-553.
9. Vandermeulen EP, Van Aken H, Vermylen J. Anticoagulants and spinal-epidural anesthesia. Anesth Analg 1994;79:1165-1177.
10. Wysowski DK, Talarico L, Bacsanyi J, et al. Spinal and epidural hematoma and low-molecular-weight heparin. N Engl J Med 1998;338:1774.

11. Liu S, Carpenter RL, Neal JM. Epidural anesthesia and analgesia. Their role in postoperative outcome. Anesthesiology 1995;82:1474–1506.
12. Modig J, Borg T, Karlstrom G, et al. Thromboembolism after total hip replacement: role of epidural and general anesthesia. Anesth Analg 1983;62:174–180.
13. Keith I. Anaesthesia and blood loss in total hip replacement. Anaesthesia 1997;32:444–450.
14. Capdevila X, Barthelet Y, Biboulet P, et al. Effects of perioperative analgesic technique on the surgical outcome and duration of rehabilitation after major knee surgery. Anesthesiology 1999;91:8–15.
15. Prins MN, Hirsh J. A comparison of general anesthesia and regional anesthesia as a risk factor for deep vein thrombosis following hip surgery: a critical review. Thromb Haemost 1990;64:497–500.
16. Tuman KJ, McCarthy RJ, March RJ, et al. Effects of epidural anesthesia and analgesia on coagulation and outcome after major vascular surgery. Anesth Analg 1991;73:696–704.
17. Chaney MA. Intrathecal and epidural anesthesia and analgesia for cardiac surgery. Anesth Analg 1997;84:1211–1221.
18. Bradshaw BG, Liu SS, Thirlby RC. Standardized perioperative care protocols and reduced length of stay after colon surgery. J Am Coll Surg 1998;186:501–506.
19. Abboud TK, Afrasiabi A, Sarkis F, et al. Continuous infusion epidural analgesia in parturients receiving bupivacaine, chloroprocaine, or lidocaine: maternal, fetal, and neonatal effects. Anesth Analg 1984;63:421–428.
20. Hollmen AI, Jouppila R, Jouppila P, et al. Effect of extradural analgesia using bupivacaine and 2-chloroprocaine on intervillous blood flow during normal labour. Br J Anesth 1982;54:837–842.
21. Lowson SM, Goodchild CS. Low-dose heparin therapy and spinal anesthesia. Anaesthesia 1989;44:67–68.
22. Allemann BH, Gerber H, Gruber UF. Rückenmarksnahe anaesthesie und subkutan verabreichtes low-dose heparin-dihydergot zur thromboembolieprophylaxe. Anaesthetist 1983;32:80–83.
23. Schwander D, Bachmann F. Heparine et anesthesies medullaires: analyse de decision. Ann Fr Anesth Reanim 1991;10:284–296.
24. Darnat S, Guggiari M, Grob R, et al. Un cas d'hematome extradural rachidien au cours de la mise en place d'un catheter peridural. Ann Fr Anesth Reanim 1986;5:550–552.
25. Dupeyrat A, Dequire PM, Merouani A, et al. Hematome sousarachnoidien et rachianesthesie. Ann Fr Anesth Reanim 1990;9:560–562.
26. Metzger G, Singbartl G. Spinal epidural hematoma following epidural anesthesia versus spontaneous spinal subdural hematoma. Two case reports. Acta Anaesthesiol Scand 1991;35:105–107.
27. Ruff RL, Dougherty JH. Complications of lumbar puncture followed by anticoagulation. Stroke 1981;12:879–881.
28. Rao TLK, El-Etr AA. Anticoagulation following placement of epidural and subarachnoid catheters: an evaluation of neurologic sequelae. Anesthesiology 1981;55:618–620.
29. Baron HC, LaRaja RD, Rossi G, et al. Continuous epidural analgesia in the heparinized vascular surgical patient: a retrospective review of 912 patients. J Vasc Surg 1987;6:144–146.
30. Mathews ET, Abrams LD. Intrathecal morphine in open heart surgery (letter). Lancet 1980;2:543.
31. Horlocker TT. Heit JA. Low molecular weight heparin: biochemistry, pharmacology, perioperative prophylaxis regimens, and guidelines for regional anesthetic management. Anesth Analg 1997;85:874–885.
32. Schroeder DR. Statistics: Detecting a rare adverse drug reaction using spontaneous reports. Reg Anesth Pain Med 1998;23 Suppl 2:183–189.
33. Bergqvist D, Lindblad B, Mätzsch T. Low molecular weight heparin for thromboprophylaxis and epidural/spinal anaesthesia: is there a risk? Acta Anaesthesiol Scand 1992;36:605–609.
34. Tryba M. European practice guidelines: thromboembolism prophylaxis and regional anesthesia. Reg Anesth Pain Med 1998;23 Suppl 2:178–182.
35. Wille-Jorgensen P, Jorgensen LN, Rasmussen LS. Lumbar regional anaesthesia and prophylactic anticoagulant therapy: is the combination safe? Anesthesia 1991;46:623–627.
36. Gogarten W, Van Aken H, Wulf H, et al. Regional anesthesia and thromboembolism prophylaxis/anticoagulation. Anaesthesiol Intensivmed 1997;12:623–628.
37. White RH, McKittrick T, Hutchinson R, et al. Temporary discontinuation of warfarin therapy: changes in the international normalized ratio. Ann Intern Med 1995;122:40–42.
38. Heit JA, Plumhoff EA, Thompson CK, et al. Monitoring oral anticoagulant therapy: prothrombin time/INR versus factor II activity/native prothrombin antigen. Thromb Haemost 1993;69:2080A.
39. Horlocker TT, Wedel DJ, Schlichting JL. Postoperative epidural analgesia and oral anticoagulant therapy. Anesth Analg 1994;79:89–93.
40. Wu C, Perkins FM. Oral anticoagulant prophylaxis and epidural catheter removal. Reg Anesth 1996;21:503–507.
41. CLASP (Collaborative Low-Dose Aspirin Study in Pregnancy) Collaborative Group. CLASP: a randomized trial of low-dose aspirin for the prevention and treatment of pre-eclampsia among 9364 pregnant women. Lancet 1994;343:619–629.
42. Horlocker TT, Wedel DJ, Offord KP. Does preoperative antiplatelet therapy increase the risk of hemorrhagic complications associated with regional anesthesia? Anesth Analg 1990;70:631–634.
43. Horlocker TT, Wedel DJ, Offord KP, et al. Preoperative antiplatelet therapy does not increase the risk of spinal hematoma associated with regional anesthesia. Anesth Analg 1995;80:303–309.
44. Dickman CA, Shedd SA, Spetzler RF, et al. Spinal epidural hematoma associated with epidural anesthesia: complications of systemic heparinization in patients receiving peripheral vascular thrombolytic therapy. Anesthesiology 1990;72:947–950.
45. Onishchuk JL, Carlsson C. Epidural hematoma associated with epidural anesthesia: complications of anticoagulant therapy. Anesthesiology 1992;77:1221–1223.
46. Weitz JI, Hirsh J. New antithrombotic agents. Chest 1998;114:715S–727S.
47. Eriksson BI, Ekman S, Kälebo P, et al. Prevention of deep-vein thrombosis after total hip replacement: direct thrombin inhibition with recombinant hirudin, CGP 39393. Lancet 1996;347:635–639.
48. Eriksson BI, Ekman S, Lindbratt S, et al. Prevention of thromboembolism with use of recombinant hirudin. J. Bone Joint Surg [Am] 1997;79:326–333.
49. Eriksson BI, Wille-Jørgensen P, Kälebo P, et al. A comparison of recombinant hirudin with a low-molecular-weight heparin to prevent thromboembolic complications after total hip replacement. N Engl J Med 1997;337:1329–1335.
50. Geerts WH, Heit JA, Clagett GP, et al. Prevention of venous thromboembolism. Chest 2001;119:132S–175S.

Index

Note: Page numbers followed by f refer to figures; page numbers followed by t refer to tables.

A

Abciximab
  in cardiovascular disease, 295–296, 296f, 298f, 298t, 300t, 304t, 305f
  thrombocytopenia with, 503
Abscess, drainage of, 174
Accumetrics, 537t
Acquired immunodeficiency syndrome (AIDS), 515–519
  antiphospholipid antibodies in, 517
  hemolytic-uremic syndrome in, 518–519
  Kaposi sarcoma in, 160
  protease inhibitors in, 516–517
  protein S deficiency in, 517
  thrombocytopenia in, 515–516
    vs. immune thrombocytopenic purpura, 120t, 122
  thrombocytopenic purpura in, 518–519
  thrombosis in, 517–518, 518t
ACT II Automated Coagulation Timer, 541t, 543–544
Activated partial thromboplastin time (aPTT), 17–18, 17f, 17t, 32t, 33–34
  during pregnancy, 437–438
  for lupus anticoagulants, 274, 274t
  in clinical decision-making, 18–19, 18t
  in coagulation factor inhibition, 75–76
  in critically ill patient, 493–494, 495t, 496, 496t
  in hemophilia, 47–48
  in liver disease, 485, 485t, 486, 498
  in transfused patient, 500
  preoperative, 469
Activated protein C resistance, 184–185. *See also* Factor V Leiden.
Activation assays, in heparin-induced thrombocytopenia, 363–364
Adenosine diphosphate (ADP), platelet response to, 21, 22f, 23, 23t
Adenosine diphosphate (ADP) receptor antagonists, platelet effects of, 144
Adenosine triphosphate (ATP), platelet response to, 21, 22f, 23, 23t
Adult respiratory distress syndrome (ARDS), disseminated intravascular coagulation and, 174
Afibrinogenemia, 57–59, 59t
  clinical manifestations of, 58
  diagnosis of, 32t, 58–59
  differential diagnosis of, 59
  genetics of, 57–58

Afibrinogenemia (*Continued*)
  pathogenesis of, 57–58
  treatment of, 59, 139
Aggregation assays, in heparin-induced thrombocytopenia, 364
Agnogenic myeloid metaplasia, 139, 140
Air plethysmography, in postphlebitic syndrome, 248, 248t
Airplane travel, venous thromboembolism with, 203
Allergy, in platelet transfusion therapy, 109
Alloimmunization, in platelet transfusion therapy, 108–109
Alphanate SD, 49t
Alphanine, 49t
Ambulatory venous pressure, in postphlebitic syndrome, 248–249
ε-Aminocaproic acid (EACA), 403–406, 404t
  dosage of, 404
  in congenital platelet disorders, 139
  in disseminated intravascular coagulation, 175–176
  in factor XI deficiency, 67
  in von Willebrand disease, 98t, 99
  indications for, 404–406
  thrombosis with, 404
  toxicity of, 404
Aminoglycosides, factor V inhibition in, 84–85
Amniocentesis, in maternal von Willebrand disease, 440
Ampicillin, platelet effects of, 144
Amyloidosis, 157
  factor X deficiency with, 30, 65, 84
Anagrelide
  in essential thrombocythemia, 141, 261–263, 262t
  side effects of, 262–263, 262t
Anemia, aplastic, interleukin-6 effects on, 111
Anesthesia. *See also* Neuraxial anesthesia/analgesia.
  hemostatic effects of, 465
  in maternal von Willebrand disease, 440
Aneurysm, aortic, disseminated intravascular coagulation and, 169–170
Angiography, in pulmonary embolism, 209
Angioma, cherry, 150t, 161
Anisoylated plasminogen streptokinase activator complex, 285, 389
Antibiotics
  factor V inhibitors and, 63
  factor VIII inhibitors and, 79
  platelet effects of, 144

599

Antibody(ies)
    anticardiolipin, 269, 270t, 271, 272–273
    anti-factor V, 52–53, 63, 84–85, 499–500
    anti-factor VIII, 75, 79. *See also* Factor VIII, inhibitors of.
    anti-factor XIII, 68, 85
    antifibrinogen, 61
    anti-idiotypic, 75
    antiphospholipid, 17f, 19, 269, 270t, 271–273, 274t, 275–276, 517
    antiplatelet, 117–118, 118f, 118t, 143
    antiprothrombin, 62, 83–84, 272
Anticardiolipin antibody (ACA), 269, 270t
    disease associations of, 272–273
    thrombocytopenia and, 271
Anticoagulant proteins, assays of, 20
Anticoagulation, 523–531. *See also specific drugs.*
    after atrial fibrillation, 299
    after inferior vena caval filter placement, 573–574
    bleeding during
        evaluation of, 527–528, 528t
        prevention of, 528–531, 529t, 530t
    during invasive procedures, 527, 527t
    in antiphospholipid syndrome, 275
    in axillary vein thrombosis, 235
    in cancer, 331–336, 333t
    in cardiac valve disease, 302, 302t, 303t
    in cardiovascular disease, 285t, 288–290, 289t, 290t
    in cerebral venous thrombosis, 232, 232t
    in deep venous thrombosis, 212, 214
    in hip replacement surgery, 473–474
    in mesenteric vein thrombosis, 228
    in neurosurgical patient, 553–554
    in ovarian vein thrombosis, 237
    in portal vein thrombosis, 229
    in pulmonary embolism, 210–211
    in renal vein thrombosis, 230–231
    in retinal vein thrombosis, 235
    in secondary thromboprophylaxis, 216–218, 216f–219f
    in splenic vein thrombosis, 229
    in subclavian vein thrombosis, 235
    initiation of, 525–526
    International Normalized Ratio for, 524–525, 525t, 526–527, 526t
    invasive diagnostic procedures and, 473–474
    long-term, 192–193
    maintenance dose for, 525–526
    mechanism of action of, 523, 524f
    monitoring of, 524–525, 525t
    neuraxial anesthesia/analgesia and, 591–593, 592t, 595–596
    nontherapeutic International Normalized Ratio with, 526–527, 526t
    patient self-testing for, 529–531, 530t
    pharmacokinetics of, 523
    therapeutic ranges of, 524–525, 525t
    vs. inferior vena caval filter, 574
Antifibrinogen antibodies, 61
Antifibrinolytic therapy, 98t, 99
    in disseminated intravascular coagulation, 175–176
    in factor XI deficiency, 67
    in hemophilia, 51
    in α_2-plasmin inhibitor deficiency, 70
Antigen assays, in heparin-induced thrombocytopenia, 364–365, 365f
Anti-idiotypic antibodies, 75
Antiphospholipid antibodies (APA), 269, 270t, 274t
    assays for, 17f, 19, 273–274, 275–276
    cardiac valve dysfunction and, 271–272
    disease associations of, 272–273
    immunology of, 273
    in acquired immunodeficiency syndrome, 517

Antiphospholipid syndrome, 269–276
    cardiac valve dysfunction and, 271–272
    cardiolipin assay in, 273
    catastrophic, 504
    clinical manifestations of, 269–270, 270t
    fetal loss and, 271
    historical perspective on, 269
    immunology of, 273
    in pregnancy, 454–455, 455t
    infarctive placental dysfunction in, 237–238
    lupus anticoagulant testing in, 273–274, 274t
    medicolegal aspects of, 275–276
    neurologic manifestations of, 270–271, 270t
    pathophysiology of, 273
    primary, 270
    prothrombin deficiency and, 272
    secondary, 270
    stroke in, 270–271, 270t
    terminology for, 269, 270t
    thrombocytopenia in, 271
    treatment of, 274–275
    venous thromboembolism in, 275
Antiplatelet antibodies, 143
    in immune thrombocytopenic purpura, 117–118, 118f, 118t
Antiplatelet therapy. *See also* Aspirin.
    in cardiovascular disease, 285t, 290–299, 291f, 291t, 292f, 293t, 298f, 298t, 299f, 300t
Antiprothrombin antibodies, 83–84
Antithrombin (Antithrombin III)
    assays of, 20
    deficiency of, 181–182, 182t
        acquired, 182, 182t
        evaluation of, 190–192, 191f
        factor V Leiden and, 189, 189t
        heparin resistance in, 192
        in pregnancy, 238, 450
        thrombosis risk in, 187–188, 188t
    in disseminated intravascular coagulation, 175
    normal levels of, 182
Antithrombin III Pittsburgh, 70
Antithrombotic therapy, in cardiovascular disease, 303–306, 304t, 305t
α_1-Antitrypsin Pittsburgh, 58t, 70
Aorta
    abdominal, aneurysm of, 169–170
    ascending, atheroma of, 303
Apolipoprotein E, in cardiovascular disease, 314
Apoptosis, in thrombotic thrombocytopenic purpura, 347
Aprotinin, 406
    in hip replacement, 468
    in liver transplantation, 488, 488t
    in orthopedic surgery, 468
aPTT. *See* Activated partial thromboplastin time (aPTT).
Arachidonic acid, impaired liberation of, in platelet stimulation, 137
AR-C69931MX, in thrombotic thrombocytopenic purpura, 351
Argatroban, 383t, 384
    in cardiovascular disease, 289, 304t
    in heparin-induced thrombocytopenia, 367, 367t, 368t, 501
Arterial thrombosis
    coronary, 282–285, 283f, 284f. *See also* Cardiovascular disease.
    in essential thrombocythemia, 256, 258
    in heparin-induced thrombocytopenia, 360
    in pregnancy, 456
    in protein C deficiency, 190
    in protein S deficiency, 190
    in prothrombin G20210A mutation, 190

Arteriolar-venous malformation, in Osler-Weber-Rendu syndrome, 157, 158
Arterioles, 151
Arthropathy, hemophilic, 45–46
Aspirin
  after coronary artery bypass surgery, 292
  after stroke, 292
  in cardiovascular disease, 280, 280f, 290–293, 291f, 291t, 292f, 304t
  in essential thrombocythemia, 264
  in heparin-induced thrombocytopenia, 368
  in myeloproliferative diseases, 141
  in percutaneous coronary interventions, 292–293
  in pregnancy, 457
  in stroke, 550
  in thrombotic thrombocytopenic purpura, 350
  neuraxial anesthesia/analgesia and, 593, 596
  platelet effects of, 143–144
Atherosclerosis, 281–282. See also Cardiovascular disease.
  subclinical, 313
  von Willebrand factor in, 93
Atrial fibrillation, 299, 301f
Atrophia blanche, 161
Autoantibody. See Antibody(ies).
Axillary vein thrombosis, 235–236
Azathioprine
  in refractory immune thrombocytopenic purpura, 127
  in thrombotic thrombocytopenic purpura, 350, 350t

B

Bacteremia, platelet transfusion therapy and, 107–108, 107t
Bartonella bacilliformis, in thrombotic thrombocytopenic purpura, 347
Bayer Diagnostics, 537t
Bebulin VH, 49t
Bed rest, in deep venous thrombosis, 215
Benefix, 49t
Bernard-Soulier syndrome, 120t, 134–135
  diagnosis of, 138
  laboratory profile in, 32t
  platelet disorders in, 134
Bethesda assay, 20, 36, 76, 77f
  in hemophilia, 48
Biopsy
  bone marrow, 34
  liver, 471, 486
Bird's Nest filter, 561t, 562, 569–570, 570f, 571t
Bivalirudin, 383t, 384–385
  administration of, 385
  adverse effects of, 385
  indications for, 385
Bleeding, 27–38. See also Hemorrhage.
  clinical evaluation of, 27–31, 28t, 29t
    history for, 27–30, 28t, 29t
    physical examination for, 30–31, 31t
  laboratory evaluation of, 31–36, 31t, 32t
    in coagulopathies, 32–34, 32t, 35–36
    in platelet disorders, 32–35, 32t
    screening, 31, 31t
Bleeding time, 32t, 33
  in afibrinogenemia, 58
  in von Willebrand disease, 94–95
  template, 21
β-Blockers, platelet effects of, 144
Blood group, von Willebrand factor level and, 93, 95
Blue toe syndrome, 150t, 160
Bone marrow
  aspiration of, in immune thrombocytopenic purpura, 120

Bone marrow (*Continued*)
  biopsy of, in platelet disorders, 34
  metastases to, pancytopenia in, 105
Bovine collagen–based topical hemostatic agents, 419–420, 420t
Bovine gelatin–based topical hemostatic agents, 420–421, 420t
Branch retinal vein occlusion, 234–235
Breast cancer, treatment of
  interleukin-11 in, 111
  thrombosis with, 332
Brodificoum, 62
Bronchoscopy, 471–472
Bruising, 150t, 153. See also Purpura.
  excessive, 29
  physical examination in, 31
  tendency toward, 30
Budd-Chiari syndrome (hepatic venous thrombosis), 232–234, 233f, 233t, 234f
Busulfan, in essential thrombocythemia, 263, 264

C

Cachectic purpura, 150
Calcium, mobilization of, in platelet disorders, 136
Calf vein thrombosis. See also Venous thromboembolism.
  diagnosis of, 207
  postphlebitic syndrome with, 249
  recurrence of, 212
  treatment of, 211–212, 212t
Cancer
  anticoagulation in, 331–336, 333t
    mortality and, 335–336
  catheter thrombosis in, 332, 335
  disseminated intravascular coagulation in, 328–329
  factor VIII inhibitors in, 78–79
  hemorrhage in, 335
  inferior vena caval filter in, 335, 580–582, 580t, 581t
  interleukin-6 in, 111
  interleukin-11 in, 111–112
  mortality in, 335–336
  procoagulants of, 327–328, 327f
  surgery in, anticoagulant prophylaxis for, 331–332, 336–337
  thrombocytopathy in, 328
  thrombocytopenia in, 105, 328
  thrombocytosis in, 328
  thrombophilia in, 329
  thrombotic disease and, 325–337, 326t, 327t
    catheter-related, 332, 335
    coagulation and, 325–326
    historical perspective on, 325–326, 326t
    pathogenesis of, 326–328, 327f
    prophylaxis for, 331–332
    treatment of, 331–336, 333t
    tumor procoagulants in, 327–328
    Virchow's triad in, 326, 327f
  venous thromboembolism in, 329–331, 331t
    case studies of, 336–337
    inferior vena caval filter in, 335
    prophylaxis against, 331–332, 333t
    secondary prophylaxis against, 333–334
    treatment of, 332–334, 333t
Cancer procoagulant, 327–328, 327f
Capillaries, 151, 151f
  in disseminated intravascular coagulation, 167f
  in thrombocytopenia, 153, 153f
Carbenicillin
  bleeding with, 505
  platelet effects of, 144

Cardiac valves
　dysfunction of
　　antiphospholipid antibodies and, 271–272
　　　embolism with, 301–302, 302t, 303t
　　　platelet destruction in, 105
　　prosthetic, embolism with, 301, 302, 302t, 303t
Cardioembolism, 299, 301, 301f, 301t
Cardiolipin assay, 273
Cardiopulmonary arrest, in heparin-induced thrombocytopenia, 361
Cardiovascular disease, 279–306
　C-reactive protein in, 315–317, 316f
　D-dimer in, 317
　fibrinogen in, 314–315
　fibrinolytic function in, 317
　glycoprotein IIb-IIIa receptor antagonists in, hemorrhagic complications of, 303–306, 304t, 305f, 306t
　hemorrhage in, 303–307, 304t, 305f, 306f
　historical perspective in, 279–281, 280f–282f, 280t
　hormone replacement therapy and, 431
　lipoprotein(a) in, 313–314, 314f
　pathogenesis of, 281–284, 283f, 284f
　plasma homocysteine in, 317–319, 318f
　risk factors for, 311–319, 312t, 314f, 316f, 318f
　subclinical atherosclerosis in, 313
　treatment of, 284–299, 286f, 287f
　　abciximab in, 295–296, 296f
　　anisoylated plasminogen streptokinase activator complex in, 285
　　anticoagulation therapy in, 285t, 288–290, 289t, 290t
　　antiplatelet therapy in, 285t, 290–299, 291f, 291t, 292f, 293t, 298f, 298t, 299f, 300t
　　antithrombotic therapy in, 303–306, 304t, 305t
　　argatroban in, 289
　　aspirin in, 290–293, 291f, 291t, 292f
　　clopidogrel in, 294–295, 294f, 295f
　　emergency coronary bypass surgery in, 306t, 307
　　eptifibatide in, 297–299, 298t, 299f
　　fibrinolytic therapy in, 284–287, 287t, 288t
　　　clinical indications for, 286–287
　　　complications of, 287
　　　mechanisms of, 284
　　hemorrhagic complications of, 303–306, 304t, 305f, 306t
　　heparin in, 288
　　heparinoids in, 288
　　hirudin in, 288–289, 289t
　　historical perspective on, 280–281, 280f–282f
　　lanoteplase in, 286
　　platelet glycoprotein IIb-IIIa receptor antagonists in, 295–299, 296f, 298f, 298t, 300t
　　reteplase in, 286
　　single-chain urokinase-like plasminogen activator in, 285
　　staphylokinase and, 286
　　streptokinase in, 285
　　tenecteplase in, 286, 287t, 288t
　　ticlopidine in, 293–294, 293t
　　tirofiban in, 296–297
　　tissue-type plasminogen activator in, 285–286, 287t
　　urokinase in, 285
　　warfarin in, 289–290, 290t
　von Willebrand factor in, 93
Carotid artery disease, hyperhomocysteinemia and, 188
Catheters, 472–473
　thrombosis with, 52, 235, 332, 335, 507
CD40 ligand, for refractory immune thrombocytopenic purpura, 127
Cefotetan, hemolysis with, 498
Ceftriaxone, hemolysis with, 498
Cellulose-based topical hemostatic agents, 420, 420t

Central nervous system, in disseminated intravascular coagulation, 174
Central retinal vein occlusion, 234–235
Central venous access device, 472–473
　thrombosis with, 52, 235, 332, 335, 507
Cephalosporins, hemolysis with, 498
Cerebral venous thrombosis, 231–232, 231t, 232f
　clinical features of, 231–232, 232lt
　risk factors for, 231
Chemotherapy. See also Cancer.
　interleukin-3 and, 110
　interleukin-11 and, 111–112
　thrombocytopenia with, 105
　thrombosis with, 332
Cherry angioma, 150t, 161
Child-Pugh score, in liver disease, 486
Chlorambucil, in essential thrombocythemia, 263
2-Chlorodeoxyadenosine, in refractory immune thrombocytopenic purpura, 127
Cholesterol emboli syndrome, 160
Chorionic villus sampling, in maternal von Willebrand disease, 440
Chromogenic assay, in hemophilia, 47–48
Chrono-log Corporation, 537t
CirAid legging, 251
Clopidogrel
　in cardiovascular disease, 294–295, 294f, 295f, 304t
　neuraxial anesthesia/analgesia and, 593, 596
　platelet effects of, 144
Cloxacillin, platelet effects of, 144
c-mpl, 103, 112
CoaguChek, 540, 540t
CoaguChek Pro-DM, 541t, 544–545
CoaguChek S, 540, 540t
Coagulation, 15, 16f, 166
　extrinsic, 279–280
　intrinsic, 279
Coagulation factor(s). See at Factor.
Colchicine, in refractory immune thrombocytopenic purpura, 127
Collagen, platelet response to, 21, 22f
Collagen-based topical hemostatic agents, 419–420, 420t
Colonoscopy, 471
Compression stockings, 250
Computed tomography
　in adrenal gland hemorrhage, 236, 237f
　in cerebral venous thrombosis, 231–232
　in hepatic venous thrombosis, 232, 233f, 234f
　in mesenteric vein thrombosis, 226, 227f
　in portal vein thrombosis, 229, 230f
　in pulmonary embolism, 209, 209t, 506
Connective tissue disorders, 157–158
Consultant(s)
　disagreement with, 11–12
　duties of, 8
　lack of diagnosis by, 12
　mismanagement management by, 11
　point of view of, 7–8
　primary care by, 11
　recommendations of, 9–10
　redirection of workup by, 11
　request for additional consultation by, 13
Consultation, 3–13
　brief, 4
　comprehensive, 4
　confirmatory, 4
　curbside, 5
　duration of, 12
　ethical issues in, 10
　extent of, 4–5, 4t

Consultation (*Continued*)
    focus of, 7–8
    for assistance to another physician, 5–6
    for disgruntled patient/family, 6
    for independent medical evaluation, 6, 9
    for second opinion, 6
    for third-party payor, 6
    in catastrophically ill patient, 5
    inappropriate, 7
    outcomes of, 10–12
    process of, 3–4, 4t, 9
    secondary, 13
    supporting, 10–11
    timing of, 8–9
    undiagnosing, 5
    urgent, 5
Consumptive coagulopathy, 165
Contact factors, congenital deficiency of, 67–69
Coronary artery bypass surgery
    aspirin after, 292
    emergency, 306t, 307
    hemostatic effects of, 466–467, 466t, 504
Coronary artery disease. *See* Cardiovascular disease.
Corticosteroids
    in acquired hemophilia, 83
    in hemophilic arthropathy, 45
C-reactive protein, in cardiovascular disease, 315–317, 316f
Creutzfeldt-Jakob disease, 50, 53–54
Critically ill patient, 493–507
    antiphospholipid antibody syndrome in, 504
    bleeding problems in, 493
    cardiac bypass in, 504
    catheter thrombosis in, 507
    disseminated intravascular coagulation in, 497, 497t
    drug-induced hemolytic–disseminated intravascular coagulation syndromes in, 498
    drug-induced platelet disorders in, 503, 503t, 505
    evaluation of, 493–495, 494t, 495t
    factor V inhibitors in, 499–500
    hemolytic-uremic syndrome in, 502
    heparin-induced thrombocytopenia in, 501
    laboratory testing for, 493–495, 495t, 496t
    liver disease in, 498–499. *See also* Liver disease.
    post-transfusion purpura in, 504
    pregnancy and, 500–501, 500t, 503–503
    preprocedure considerations in, 496
    purpura fulminans in, 497–498
    sepsis in, 503–504
    thrombotic thrombocytopenic purpura in, 501–503
    transfusion therapy for, 495–496, 496t, 500
    uremia in, 504–505, 505t, 506t
    venous thromboembolism in, 505–507
        prevention of, 507
        treatment of, 506–507
    vitamin K deficiency in, 499
    warfarin-treated, 494t, 499
Cryoprecipitate, 398
    in acute hemorrhage, 37
    in afibrinogenemia, 58
    in factor XIII deficiency, 69
    in liver disease–related coagulopathy, 489
    in uremia, 142
Cryoprecipitate-based topical hemostatic agents, 421–422, 421t, 422f
Cryosupernatant, in thrombotic thrombocytopenic purpura, 350, 350t
Cyclo-oxygenase, inhibition of, by nonsteroidal anti-inflammatory agents, 144

Cyclophosphamide
    in acquired hemophilia, 83
    in refractory immune thrombocytopenic purpura, 126
Cystathionine β-synthase deficiency, 185–186. *See also* Hyperhomocysteinemia.
Cytokines, in disseminated intravascular coagulation, 169t
Cytomegalovirus infection, with platelet transfusion therapy, 108
Cytoreduction, in myeloproliferative diseases, 140, 141

D

Dade Behring, 537t
Danaparoid sodium, 382–383, 383t
    administration of, 383
    adverse effects of, 383
    in cardiovascular disease, 288, 304t
    in heparin-induced thrombocytopenia, 365–366, 366t, 368t, 501
    in stroke, 550
    indications for, 382–383
    mechanism of, 382
    reversal of, 383
Danazol, in refractory immune thrombocytopenic purpura, 127
D-dimer, in cardiovascular disease, 317
Deep venous thrombosis. *See also* Calf vein thrombosis; Pulmonary embolism; Venous thromboembolism.
    after inferior vena caval filter placement, 571t, 572
    factor V Leiden and, 186
    hyperhomocysteinemia and, 189
    in spinal cord injury, 550–553, 551t, 552t
    in stroke, 549–550, 550t
    postphlebitic syndrome with, 243–252. *See also* Postphlebitic syndrome.
    prevention of, 199–204. *See also* Thromboprophylaxis.
    recurrent
        diagnosis of, 204–207, 205t
        plethysmography for, 206, 207
        risk for, 190
        ultrasound surveillance for, 205–207
        venography for, 206
    risk factors for, 200–201, 201f, 201t
    treatment of, 212–215, 213f, 213t, 214f
        low-molecular-weight heparin in, 281, 282f
        recanalization with, 244
        ultrasound surveillance in, 205–207
        warfarin failure with, 205, 205t
    venous reflux after, 244–245. *See also* Postphlebitic syndrome.
Defibrination syndrome, 165
Dental care
    anticoagulation during, 527, 527t
    in hemophilia, 52, 464, 464t
Dermatan sulfate, in cardiovascular disease, 288
1-Desamino-8-D-arginine vasopressin (DDAVP), 400–403, 401t, 402t
    administration of, 401–402
    dosage of, 401–402, 402t
    during pregnancy, 439–440, 439t
    hemostatic activity of, 400–401
    in acquired hemophilia, 82
    in acute hemorrhage, 37–38
    in afibrinogenemia, 58
    in congenital platelet disorders, 139
    in hemophilia, 51
    in liver disease–related coagulopathy, 489
    in pregnancy, 403, 441, 441t
    in uremia, 142, 505, 505t
    in von Willebrand disease, 98, 98t
    indications for, 402–403
    mechanisms of action of, 401
    preoperative, 402–403

1-Desamino-8-D-arginine vasopressin (DDAVP) (*Continued*)
  tachyphylaxis with, 401
  thrombosis with, 403
  toxicity of, 403
Des-γ-carboxyl prothrombin, in liver disease, 483, 486
Desmopressin
  in acquired hemophilia, 82
  in afibrinogenemia, 58
Diagnostic process, 3
Dialysis, in uremia, 142
Disseminated intravascular coagulation (DIC), 165–177
  abdominal aortic aneurysm and, 169–170
  associated conditions in, 30
  axes of, 168–169, 169t
  causes of, 167, 167t, 169–170
  central nervous system in, 174
  clinical features of, 170, 170t
  closed head injury and, 169
  coagulation physiology and, 166
  consequences of, 173–174, 173t
  consultation considerations in, 176
  cost-containment issues in, 176
  cytokines in, 169t
  diagnosis of, 32t, 170–171, 170t
  differential diagnosis of, 171–173, 172t
  fibrinolytic system activation in, 173
  heart in, 174
  historical overview of, 165–166
  in cancer, 328–329
  in critically ill patient, 497, 497t
  in liver disease, 484, 487, 489, 498
  inhibitor loss in, 166, 166t
  initiation of, 167–169, 168f, 169t
  kidney in, 174
  laboratory findings in, 170–171, 170t
  lethality of, 174
  liver in, 167, 173–174
  mediators in, 169t
  medical-legal considerations in, 176–177
  multiorgan dysfunction syndrome in, 173–174, 173t
  pathophysiology of, 166–167, 166t, 167f, 168, 168f
  purpura in, 158–159
  quinine-induced, 498
  terminology for, 165
  treatment of, 174–176, 175t
  vs. immune thrombocytopenic purpura, 120t, 122
  vs. liver disease, 487
  vs. Trousseau syndrome, 171, 173, 173t
Down syndrome, 134
Drugs. *See specific drugs and types of drug therapy.*
dRVVT (dilute Russell's viper venom time), 19
Duke bleeding time, 33
Dysfibrinogen, in liver disease, 483, 486
Dysfibrinogenemia, 59–61, 187
  clinical manifestations of, 60, 60t
  diagnosis of, 32t, 36, 60
  differential diagnosis of, 60–61
  genetics of, 59–60
  pathogenesis of, 59–60
  treatment of, 61
  variants of, 60t
Dysproteinemia
  in cancer, 328
  platelet defects in, 141
Dysprothrombinemia, 61–63
  clinical manifestations of, 61
  diagnosis of, 61
  differential diagnosis of, 61–62

Dysprothrombinemia (*Continued*)
  genetics of, 61, 62t
  pathogenesis of, 61
  treatment of, 62–63

E

Eastern diamondback rattlesnake envenomation, 171
Ecchymosis, 150t. *See also* Purpura.
  in thrombocytopenia, 153
Economy class syndrome, 203
Ehlers-Danlos syndrome, 32t
Ehrlichiosis, 503
Empty delta sign, in cerebral venous thrombosis, 231
Endoglin gene, in Osler-Weber-Rendu syndrome, 158
Endoplasmic reticulum–Golgi intermediate compartment
    (ERGIC)-53 gene, 69
Endothelial cells, 151, 151f
  microorganism attack on, 155
Enzyme-linked immunosorbent assay (ELISA), of coagulation
    factor inhibitors, 77
Epinephrine, platelet response to, 21, 22f, 23, 23t
Episiotomy, excessive bleeding after, 28
Epistaxis
  in Osler-Weber-Rendu syndrome, 158
  in thrombocytopenia, 153
Eptifibatide
  in cardiovascular disease, 297–299, 298f, 298t, 299f, 300t, 304t,
    305f
  platelet effects of, 144
Erythema, 150t, 161
Erythromelalgia, in essential thrombocythemia, 140, 256
Erythropoietin, 396–397
  in uremia, 142
Esophagastroduodenoscopy, 471
Estrogen, 411
  in liver disease, 489
  in Osler-Weber-Rendu syndrome, 158
  in uremia, 142, 505, 505t
  in von Willebrand disease, 99
Ethanol, platelet effects of, 145
Ethical issues, in consultation, 10
Euglobulin clot lysis assay, 24, 32t, 36
Extracorporeal shock-wave lithotripsy, in factor deficiencies, 464

F

Factor II, VII, IX, X, protein C and S combined deficiency, 69
Factor V
  activation of, 166t
  deficiency of, 58t
    congenital, 63–64, 69
    vs. dysprothrombinemia, 61
    factor VIII deficiency with, 69
    in liver disease, 483, 486
  inhibitors of, 63, 84–85
    in critically ill patient, 499–500
    in hemophilia, 52–53
  origin of, 63
Factor V Leiden, 184
  evaluation of, 190–192, 191f
  idiopathic deep venous thrombosis and, 186
  in pregnancy, 238, 450–451, 457
  thrombosis risk in, 188, 188t, 189, 189t
Factor V–factor VIII combined deficiency, 69
Factor VII
  deficiency of, 58t
    congenital, 64–65
    in pregnancy, 442
  during pregnancy, 437

Factor VIIa, recombinant
  in factor VII deficiency, 65
  in factor XI deficiency, 67
Factor VIII
  activation of, 166t
  assay of, 94, 94t
  deficiency of. See also Hemophilia.
    factor V deficiency with, 69
    in liver disease, 483
    in pregnancy, 440–441, 441t
  during pregnancy, 437
  excess of, 187
  gene for, in hemophilia, 43
  human vs. porcine inhibitor titers of, 81, 81f
  inhibitors of, 75, 77–82. See also Hemophilia, acquired.
    age and gender distribution of, 77, 78f–79f
    bypass agents for, 53, 53t, 81–82
    concomitant conditions with, 77–79, 79f
    drug reactions and, 79
    factor IX complex concentrates for, 82
    immunochemistry of, 79–80
    immunosuppression of, 83
    intravenous immune globulin for, 83
    laboratory diagnosis of, 20, 75–77, 76t, 77f
    natural history of, 77, 78f–79f
    patterns of, 80
    presentation of, 77
    quantitative assays for, 76–77, 77f
    recombinant factor VIIa for, 82–83
    transient titer reduction in, 83
    treatment of, 80–83, 80f
    vs. lupus anticoagulants, 76, 76t
  levels of, in hemophilia, 44
  porcine, replacement therapy with, 80–82, 81f
  postpartum inhibitor to, 77–78
  recombinant, 399
  von Willebrand factor binding to, 93
Factor VIII concentrates
  administration of, 50
  in hemophilia, 48, 49t, 50–51
  plasma levels of, 50
  viral inactivation of, 50
Factor VIII:C chromogenic assay, in hemophilia, 47–48
Factor IX
  deficiency of. See also Hemophilia.
    in pregnancy, 440–441, 441t
  excess of, 187
  inhibitors of, 84
    in hemophilia, 52–53
  levels of, in hemophilia, 44
  recombinant, 399
Factor IX concentrates
  administration of, 50
  in acquired hemophilia, 81
  in hemophilia, 49t, 50–51
  plasma levels of, 50
  viral inactivation for, 50
Factor VIII-related antigen, 91
Factor X
  deficiency of, 58t
    amyloidosis and, 30
    congenital, 65–66
      vs. dysprothrombinemia, 61
  during pregnancy, 437
  inhibitors of, 84
Factor XI
  deficiency of, 58t
    congenital, 66–67

Factor XI (Continued)
    in pregnancy, 441–442
      preconception counseling in, 442
  excess of, 187
  inhibitors of, 67, 84
Factor XII
  congenital deficiency of, 58t, 67–68, 187
  inhibitors of, 67
Factor XIII
  assay of, 20, 34
  deficiency of, 58t
    congenital, 68–69
    in pregnancy, 442
  inhibitors of, 68, 85
Familial combined coagulation deficiencies, 69–70, 69t
  factor II, VII, IX, X, protein C and S, 69–70
  factor V–factor VIII, 69
Fanconi anemia, platelet production defects in, 105
Fat embolism syndrome, 159
Fatty liver, in pregnancy, 500–501, 500t
Febrile nonhemolytic transfusion reaction, 399
Fever, in platelet transfusion therapy, 109
Fibrin clot retraction assay, 37
Fibrin degradation products, 24
  in disseminated intravascular coagulation, 165–166
Fibrin glue, cryoprecipitate-based, 51, 421–422, 422t
Fibrin sealant, 51, 421t, 422–423, 422t
Fibrin(ogen) degradation products, 24, 165–166
Fibrinogen
  concentration of, 19, 32t, 35
  congenital disorders of, 57–61. See also Afibrinogenemia; Dysfibrinogenemia.
  genetics of, 57
  in cardiovascular disease, 314–315
  in liver disease, 483
  inhibitors of, 85
Fibrinolysis, 24, 280
  in cardiovascular disease, 317
  in disseminated intravascular coagulation, 173, 175–176
  in liver disease, 484, 486–487, 489, 498–499
  laboratory evaluation of, 24
Fibrinolytic therapy, 385–392
  administration of, 385–386, 386t
  complications of, 386, 386t, 387t
  contraindications to, 385, 385t
  in cardiovascular disease, 284–287, 287t, 288t
  in deep venous thrombosis, 212–215, 213f, 213t, 214f
  in pulmonary embolism, 210–211
Fibroblasts, in postphlebitic syndrome, 245
Fitzgerald factor, congenital deficiency of, 68
Fletcher factor, congenital deficiency of, 68
Flow cytometry, for platelet evaluation, 23–24
Folate, in pregnancy, 458
Fracture, fat embolism syndrome in, 159
Fresh frozen plasma, 397–398
  in acute hemorrhage, 37
  in congenital dysprothrombinemia, 62
  in critically ill patient, 496, 496t
  in disseminated intravascular coagulation, 175
  in factor V deficiency, 64
  in factor XI deficiency, 67
  in factor XIII deficiency, 69
  in liver disease–related coagulopathy, 488–489, 488t
  in pregnancy, 442
  in thrombotic thrombocytopenic purpura, 349–350, 349t, 502

G

G protein, platelet, activation defects in, 136
Gangrene, venous, 215–216
Gastrointestinal bleeding
  aspirin and, 143–144
  in hemophilia, 47
Gelatin-based topical hemostatic agents, 420–421, 420t
GEM Portable Coagulation Laboratory, 541t, 542
Gene therapy, in hemophilia, 54–55
Genetic counseling, 9
  for hemophilia carriers, 44
Glanzmann thrombasthenia, 32t, 135
  diagnosis of, 138
  treatment of, 139
Glucocorticosteroids
  in refractory immune thrombocytopenic purpura, 126, 126t
  in thrombotic thrombocytopenic purpura, 502
Glycocalicin, plasma, 24, 34
Glycoprotein Ib, von Willebrand factor binding to, 92
Glycoprotein Ib-IXV complex
  disorders of, 134–135
  in platelet response, 133
Glycoprotein IIb-IIIa complex
  activation of, signal transduction defects in, 137
  defect in, 135
  von Willebrand factor binding to, 92
Glycoprotein IIb-IIIa receptor agonists, platelet effects of, 144
Glycoprotein IIb-IIIa receptor antagonists
  hemorrhage with, 303–306, 304t, 305f, 306t
  in cardiovascular disease, 281, 282f, 295–299, 296f, 298f, 298t, 300t
  thrombocytopenia with, 305f, 306, 503
Graft-versus-host disease, transfusion-associated, 109, 399, 400
Gray platelet syndrome, 32t
Gunther Tulip filter, 565, 583

H

Haemoscope, Inc, 537t
Ham test, 34
Hantavirus pulmonary syndrome, 504
Harmony INR Monitoring System, 540–541
Head injury, disseminated intravascular coagulation and, 169
Heart, in disseminated intravascular coagulation, 174
Heckathorn disease, 44
HELLP (*h*emolysis, *e*levated *l*iver enzymes, *l*ow *p*latelets) syndrome, 172t
  in pregnancy, 446–447, 446t, 500, 500t
  platelet destruction in, 105
  vs. disseminated intravascular coagulation, 171, 172t
Hemangioma, 161
Hemarthrosis
  in factor V deficiency, 63
  in factor VII deficiency, 64
  in factor X deficiency, 65
  in hemophilia, 44–46
  without major trauma, 29
Hematoma
  definition of, 150t
  in factor XIII deficiency, 68
  in hemophilia, 44–45
  spinal, 589–590, 591–594, 592t, 597, 597t. See also Neuraxial anesthesia/analgesia.
  without major trauma, 29
Hematopoietic stem cell transplantation, thrombocytopenia in, 113
Hematuria, 46
Hemochron Jr. Signature, 541t, 542–543
Hemochron Response analyzer, 541t, 543
Hemofil, 49t
Hemolysis, drug-induced, 498
Hemolytic-uremic syndrome
  in acquired immunodeficiency syndrome, 518–519
  in critically ill patient, 502
  in pregnancy, 500t, 501
  platelet destruction in, 105
  vs. thrombotic thrombocytopenic purpura, 344, 345, 348, 348t
Hemophilia, 43–55
  acquired, 75. See also Factor VIII, inhibitors of.
    age and gender distribution in, 77, 78f–79f
    bleeding management in, 80, 80f
    corticosteroids for, 83
    cyclophosphamide for, 83
    1-deamino-8-D-arginine for, 82
    exchange plasmapheresis for, 83
    factor IX complex concentrates for, 81
    factor VIII inhibitors in, 80
    factor VIII replacement therapy for, 80–82, 81f
    incidence of, 77
    intravenous immune globulin for, 83
    recombinant factor VIIa for, 82–83
  acquired immunodeficiency syndrome with, 53–54
    protease inhibitors in, 516–517
  carrier testing for, 44
  clinical features of, 45–47
  dental care in, 52
  epidemiology of, 43
  gastrointestinal bleeding in, 47
  genetic basis of, 43–45
  hematuria in, 46
  in pregnancy, 440–441, 441t
  intra-articular bleeding in, 45–46
  intracranial hemorrhage in, 46–47
  intramuscular hemorrhage in, 46
  laboratory studies in, 47–48
  oropharyngeal bleeding in, 47
  postnatal diagnosis of, 44
  postpartum, 28
  prenatal diagnosis of, 44
  prophylaxis in, 51–52
  pseudotumor formation in, 47
  treatment of, 48–51, 49t
    alloantibodies with, 48, 52–53, 53t
    antifibrinolytic agents in, 51
    coagulation factor concentrates in, 48–51, 49t
    complications of, 52–54, 53t
    DDAVP in, 51
    fibrin glue/sealants in, 51
    gene therapy in, 54–55
    treatment centers for, 48
    venous access device in, 52
    viral infection with, 53–54
Hemophilic arthropathy, 45–46
Hemorrhage. See also Bleeding.
  activated partial thromboplastin time and, 18
  acute, management of, 37–38
  circulating platelet count and, 105–107, 106t, 107t
  fibrinolytic therapy and, 287
  glycoprotein IIb-IIIa receptor antagonist–induced, 303–306, 304t, 305f, 306t
  in acquired hemophilia, 80, 80f
  in afibrinogenemia, 58
  in α_1-antitrypsin Pittsburgh, 70
  in dysfibrinogenemia, 61
  in dysprothrombinemia, 61
  in essential thrombocythemia, 256
  in factor V deficiency, 63

Hemorrhage (*Continued*)
   in factor V inhibition, 85
   in factor VII deficiency, 64
   in factor X deficiency, 65
   in factor XIII deficiency, 68
   in immune thrombocytopenic purpura, 124
   in myeloproliferative diseases, 140
   in Osler-Weber-Rendu syndrome, 158
   in α_2-plasmin inhibitor deficiency, 70
   in von Willebrand disease, 93–94
   intracranial
      in hemophilia, 46–47
      in neonatal hemophilia, 44
      in neonatal immune thrombocytopenic purpura, 128
   intramuscular, in hemophilia, 46
   postoperative, 474–476, 475t. *See also* Surgery.
      etiology of, 475–476, 475t
      history of, 27–28, 28t
   warfarin and, 61–62
Hemorrhagic fever, viral, purpura in, 156
Hemostasis, 15, 16f
   laboratory evaluation of, 16–20, 17f, 17t–18t. *See also at* Factor; Platelet(s).
HemoSTATUS assay, 537t, 538–539
Henoch-Schönlein purpura, 149, 150, 155
Heparan sulfate, in cardiovascular disease, 288
Heparin, 378–380, 383t (*See also* Low-molecular-weight heparin)
   administration of, 378–379, 378t, 379t
   adverse effects of, 379–380. *See also* Heparin-induced thrombocytopenia.
   and activated partial thromboplastin time, 18
   in acute thrombosis, 192
   in cancer, 331–336, 333t
   in cardiovascular disease, 288, 304t, 305f
   in cerebral venous thrombosis, 232, 232t
   in deep venous thrombosis, 212, 214, 215
   in disseminated intravascular coagulation, 175
   in pregnancy, 451–454, 452t, 453t, 454t, 457–458
   in recurrent deep venous thrombosis, 204
   in stroke, 550
   in thromboprophylaxis, 201–203
   in Trousseau syndrome, 173, 175, 175t
   indications for, 379
   mechanism of, 378
   monitoring of, 378–379, 379t
   neuraxial anesthesia/analgesia and, 591, 595–596
   pharmacology of, 378
   platelet effects of, 144
   reversal of, 380, 380t
   vs. low-molecular-weight heparin, 382
Heparin cofactor II, deficiency of, 186
Heparin-induced platelet activation assay, in heparin-induced thrombocytopenia, 364
Heparin-induced thrombocytopenia, 355–370
   activation assays in, 363–364
   aggregation assays in, 364
   antigen assays in, 364–365, 365f
   arterial thrombosis with, 360
   cardiac syndromes in, 361
   clinical features of, 357–362, 358t
   differential diagnosis of, 362, 363f, 363t
   enzyme immunoassay in, 364–365, 365f
   frequency of, 356–357, 358f
   heparin re-exposure and, 369
   heparin-related complications in, 361
   historical perspective on, 355
   in critically ill patient, 501
   laboratory findings in, 362–365, 365t

Heparin-induced thrombocytopenia (*Continued*)
   limb ischemia in, 360
   neurologic syndromes in, 361
   nonimmune, 355, 356t
   outpatient presentation of, 362, 362f
   pathogenesis of, 356, 357f
   severity of, 358, 360f
   temporal profile of, 358–358, 359f
   terminology for, 355, 356t
   venous thrombosis in, 358, 360
      subclinical, 369, 370t
      treatment of, 365–368, 370t
         adjunctive therapies in, 368
         argatroban in, 367, 367t, 368t
         caveats in, 368–369
         danaparoid sodium in, 365–366, 366t, 368t
         lepirudin in, 366–367, 367t, 368t
         parenteral anticoagulation in, 367–368, 368t
         prothrombotic complications of, 360–361, 361f, 361t
   warfarin in, 367–368
      complications of, 360–361, 361f, 361t
   washed platelet activation assays in, 364
   with thrombosis, 160
Heparinoids, in cardiovascular disease, 288
Hepatic venous thrombosis (Budd-Chiari syndrome), 232–234, 233f, 233t, 234f
Hepatitis virus
   in hemophiliac patient, 53–54
   inactivation of, in coagulation factor products, 50
   with platelet transfusion therapy, 108
Hepcon HMS Hemostasis Management System, 541t, 544
Hereditary hemorrhagic telangiectasia, 149, 157–158, 158f
Hexilate, 49t
High-molecular-weight kininogen, congenital deficiency of, 68
Hip replacement
   anticoagulation with, 473–474
   aprotinin in, 468
   inferior vena caval filter in, 576
Hippocrates, 3
Hirudin. *See* Lepirudin.
HIV virus. *See* Human immunodeficiency virus (HIV).
Homocysteine, 185, 185f. *See also* Hyperhomocysteinemia.
   in cardiovascular disease, 317–318, 318f
   normal levels of, 186
Hormone replacement therapy, 430–432
   cardiovascular disease and, 431
   venous thromboembolism and, 431–432
Human immunodeficiency virus (HIV), inactivation of, in coagulation factor products, 50
Human immunodeficiency virus (HIV) infection. *See also* Acquired immunodeficiency syndrome (AIDS).
   in hemophilia patient, 53–54
   in platelet transfusion therapy, 108
   Kaposi sarcoma herpes virus with, 160
Humate P, 49t, 399
Hydroxyurea
   in essential thrombocythemia, 141, 260–261
   side effects of, 261
Hypercortisolism, purpura in, 156–157
Hyperfibrinolysis, 172t, 173
Hyperhomocysteinemia, 185–186, 185f, 186t
   acquired, 186
   evaluation of, 190–192, 191f
   in cardiovascular disease, 317–318, 318f
   in pregnancy, 451, 457
   thrombosis risk in, 188–189, 188t
Hypersensitivity reaction, delayed-type, in afibrinogenemia, 58

Hypersplenism, liver disease and, vs. immune thrombocytopenic purpura, 120t, 122
Hypertension, pulmonary, in pulmonary embolism, 210–211
Hypoprothrombinemia, 61–63. *See also* Dysprothrombinemia.

I

Idiopathic thrombocytopenic purpura, 32t, 105, 149, 150, 328
Immune globulin, intravenous
  in factor VIII inhibitor suppression, 83
  in heparin-induced thrombocytopenia, 368
  in HIV-associated thrombocytopenia, 516
  in immune thrombocytopenic purpura, 123, 124
Immune response. *See* Antibody(ies).
Immune thrombocytopenic purpura, 117–128
  asymptomatic thrombocytopenia in, 123–124
  autoantibody-mediated platelet destruction in, 117–118, 118f, 118t
  azathioprine for, 127
  cyclophosphamide for, 126
  danazol for, 127
  definition of, 117
  differential diagnosis of, 120t, 121–123, 121t
  evaluation of, 119–120, 119f, 119t
  glucocorticoids for, 126
  historical aspects of, 117–118, 118f, 118t
  incidence of, 117
  neonatal, 128
  pediatric, 123
  peripheral blood smear in, 119, 119f, 119t
  platelet count in, 123
  pregnancy-associated, 127–128, 443–445
  refractory, 125–127, 126t
  severe thrombocytopenia with, 124, 127
  splenectomy for, 124–125, 127
  symptomatic purpura with, 124
  treatment of, 123–128
    platelet count in, 123–124
  vinca alkaloids for, 126–127
Immune tolerance, induction of, for reduction of alloantibody inhibitors, 53
Immunoadsorption
  in factor VIII inhibition titer control, 83
  in refractory immune thrombocytopenic purpura, 127
Immunodiffusion assay, for coagulation factor inhibitors, 77
Immunoglobulin, factor XIII inhibition by, 85
Immunoglobulin G, in acquired hemophilia, 79
Independent medical evaluation, 6, 9
India rubber man syndrome, 157
Infection
  lupus anticoagulants and, 273
  transfusion-related, 53–54, 399
Inferior vena cava
  anatomy of, 558–559, 558t, 559t
  anomalies of, 558–559, 558t, 559t
  filter-associated occlusion of, 564
Inferior vena caval filter, 557–565, 569–584
  anticoagulation with, 573–574
  Bird's Nest, 561t, 562, 569–570, 570f, 571t
  caval occlusion with, 564
  complications of, 561t, 564, 570–573, 571t
  contraindications to, 559–560, 559t
  deep venous thrombosis after, 571t, 572
  efficacy of, 570, 571t, 573, 573f, 574f
  fracture of, 564
  historical perspective on, 558
  in cancer patients, 335, 580–582, 580t, 581t
  in children, 564–565

Inferior vena caval filter (*Continued*)
  in deep venous thrombosis, 214–215
  in free-floating thrombus, 582–583, 582t
  in hip arthroplasty, 576
  in knee arthroplasty, 576
  in pregnancy, 453–454
  in septic thromboembolism, 565
  in spinal cord injury patient, 552, 552t
  in terminally ill patients, 565
  in thromboprophylaxis, 203–204
  in trauma patients, 576–579, 577t–578t, 579t
  indications for, 559–560, 559t, 583, 583t, 584t
  inferior vena caval thrombosis with, 571t, 572
  insertion-site thrombosis with, 570, 572, 572t
  malposition of, 564
  placement of, 563–564, 563t
  postphlebitic syndrome with, 571t, 572
  prophylactic placement of, 565
  selection of, 560–561, 560t, 561t
  Simon Nitinol, 561t, 562–563, 569, 570f, 571t
  Stainless Steel Greenfield, 561–562, 561t, 569, 570f, 571t
  suprarenal, 574–576, 575t
  temporary, 565, 583
  Titanium Greenfield, 561t, 562, 569, 570f, 571t
  TrapEase, 563
  VenaTech, 561t, 562, 569, 570f, 571t
  vs. anticoagulation, 574
Inflammation, in venous thromboembolism, 198, 198t
INR (International Normalized Ratio), 16–17, 33, 524–525, 525t, 526–527, 526t
Instrumentation Laboratory, 537t
Integrilin, in thrombotic thrombocytopenic purpura, 351
Intensive care unit. *See* Critically ill patient.
Interferon-alpha
  in essential thrombocythemia, 263
  in myeloproliferative diseases, 141
  side effects of, 263
Interleukin-3, 109–110, 110t
Interleukin-3/granulocyte-macrocyte colony-stimulating factor fusion protein, 110
Interleukin-6, 110–111, 110t
Interleukin-11, 110t, 111–112
Interleukin-1, in cancer, 327, 327f
Interleukin-8, in cancer, 327, 327f
Intermittent pneumatic compression, in thromboprophylaxis, 201–202
International Normalized Ratio (INR), 16–17, 33, 524–525, 525t, 526–527, 526t
International Technidyne Corporation, 537t
Intracranial hemorrhage
  in hemophilia, 44, 46–47
  in immune thrombocytopenic purpura, 128
Intramuscular hemorrhage, in hemophilia, 46
Intron 22, in hemophilia, 43
Invasive diagnostic procedures, 470–473
  anticoagulation and, 473–474

K

Kaolin clotting time, for lupus anticoagulants, 274, 274t
Kaposi sarcoma, 160–161
Kasabach-Merritt syndrome, 105
Ketorolac, bleeding with, 505
Kidneys, in disseminated intravascular coagulation, 174
Knee arthroplasty, inferior vena caval filter in, 576
Koate DVI, 49t
Kogenate, 49t
Konyne, 49t

L

Labor. *See also* Pregnancy.
　disseminated intravascular coagulation and, 174
　episiotomy at, 28
Laboratory testing, 15–24. *See also specific factors and proteins.*
　of fibrinolytic system, 24
　of natural anticoagulants, 20
　of platelet function, 20–21, 22f, 23t
　of procoagulant system, 16–20, 17f, 17t, 18t
β-Lactam antibiotics, platelet effects of, 144
Lactate dehydrogenase, in critically ill patient, 494
Lamifiban, in cardiovascular disease, 305f
Lanoteplase, in cardiovascular disease, 286
Left-sided portal hypertension, 228
Lepirudin, 383–384, 383t
　administration of, 383
　adverse effects of, 384
　in cardiovascular disease, 288–289, 289t, 304t
　in disseminated intravascular coagulation, 175
　in heparin-induced thrombocytopenia, 366–367, 367t, 368t, 501
　indications for, 383
　pharmacology of, 383
　reversal of, 384
Leptospirosis, purpura in, 156
Leukemia
　acute promyelocytic, 175, 176
　chronic myelogenous, 139, 140
　platelet defects in, 141
　platelet transfusion in, 106
　thrombocytopenia in, 105
Leukostasis syndromes, 159
LifeScan, Inc., 537t
Lipodermatosclerosis, in postphlebitic syndrome, 246, 246f
Lipoprotein(a), in cardiovascular disease, 313–314, 314f
Livedo reticularis, 150t, 161
　vs. purple (blue) toe syndrome, 160
Livedo vasculitis, 161
Liver
　biopsy of, 471, 486
　disease of, 481–490. *See also* Liver disease.
　in disseminated intravascular coagulation, 167, 173–174
　transplantation of, 487–488, 487t
　　hemostatic effects of, 467–468, 468t, 487t, 488–488, 488t
Liver disease, 481–490
　biopsy in, 471, 486
　bleeding in, 484–485, 485t
　Child-Pugh score in, 486
　coagulopathy with, 482–487, 498–499
　　diagnosis of, 485–486, 485t
　　pathophysiology of, 482–484, 483t
　　treatment of, 488–489, 488t
　des-γ-carboxyl prothrombin in, 483, 486
　diagnosis of, 484–485, 485t
　disseminated intravascular coagulation in, 484, 487, 498
　drug toxicity in, 489
　dysfibrinogen in, 483, 486
　factor deficiencies in, 64, 65, 482–483, 483t, 486
　fibrinolysis in, 484, 486–487, 498–499
　historical perspective on, 481–482, 482f
　hypersplenism in, vs. immune thrombocytopenic purpura, 120t, 122
　in dysfibrinogenemia, 60–61
　platelet defects in, 483–484, 486
　vitamin K deficiency in, 483, 486
Low-molecular-weight heparin, 380–382, 383t (*See also* Heparin)
　adverse effects of, 382
　clinical use of, 381–382, 381t

Low-molecular-weight heparin (*Continued*)
　in cancer, 331–336, 333t
　in cardiovascular disease, 288, 304t
　in deep venous thrombosis, 212, 214, 215, 281, 282f
　in pregnancy, 451–454, 452t, 453t, 454t, 457–458
　in stroke, 550
　in thromboprophylaxis, 201–203, 203t
　in venous thromboembolism, 506–507
　mechanisms of, 380–381, 380t
　neuraxial anesthesia/analgesia and, 591–593, 592t, 595–596
　pharmacokinetics of, 382
　pharmacology of, 380–381, 380t
　vs. heparin, 382
Lumbar puncture, 472
Lung, transfusion-related injury to, 399–400
Lupus anticoagulants, 269, 270t
　assays for, 17f, 19, 273–274, 274t, 275–276
　disease associations of, 272–273
　prothrombin deficiency and, 272
　vs. coagulation inhibitors, 76, 76t
Lymphedema, vs. postphlebitic syndrome, 246
Lysine analog antifibrinolytic agents, 403–406, 404t
　dosage of, 404
　indications for, 404–406
　thrombosis with, 406
　toxicity of, 406

M

Magnetic resonance angiography, in renal vein thrombosis, 230, 231f
Magnetic resonance imaging
　in calf vein thrombosis, 207
　in cerebral venous thrombosis, 232, 232f
Malignancy. *See* Cancer.
May-Hegglin anomaly, 134
Medtronic Perfusion Systems, 537t
Megakaryocyte(s). *See also* Platelet(s).
　acquired pure aplasia of, 120t, 123
　burst-forming units of, 103–104
　colony-forming units of, 103
　differentiation of, 103
　historical perspective on, 103
　interleukin-6 effects on, 110–111
Megakaryocyte high-proliferative-potential colony-forming cells, 103
Megakaryocytopoiesis, 103–104, 111
Melphalan, in essential thrombocythemia, 263
Menorrhagia, history of, 29
Menstrual cycle, von Willebrand factor levels in, 93
Mesenteric vein thrombosis, 226–228, 226t, 227f
　diagnosis of, 227f, 228
　symptoms of, 228
　treatment of, 228
Metalloproteinases
　in postphlebitic syndrome, 246
　in thrombotic thrombocytopenic purpura, 346, 350–351
Methylenetetrahydrofolate reductase (MTHFR) deficiency, 186. *See also* Hyperhomocysteinemia.
Mezlocillin, platelet effects of, 144
Microcirculation, 150–151, 151f
Microthrombus, purpura with, 158–160
Mixing studies, 17–18, 32t, 35–36
Monarc M, 49t
Monoclate, 49t
Monoclonal antibodies, in thrombotic thrombocytopenic purpura, 351
Monocytes, in postphlebitic syndrome, 245–246
Mononine, 49t

Mopidamol, in cancer patient, 335
Morbus maculosus Werlhofii, 150
c-*Mpl* protein, in essential thrombocythemia, 256
Multiorgan dysfunction syndrome, in disseminated intravascular coagulation, 173–174, 173t
Mural thrombosis, 303
Myeloblastemia, 159
Myelodysplastic syndromes, 111, 120t, 122, 141
Myeloproliferative diseases, 139–141
　clinical features of, 140
　morphologic abnormalities in, 140
　thrombosis risk in, 140
　treatment of, 140–141
Myelosuppressive drugs, thrombocytopenia with, 105
Myocardial infarction. *See also* Cardiovascular disease.
　antiphospholipid-protein antibodies and, 272
　hyperhomocysteinemia and, 188
　mural thrombosis after, 303
　oral contraceptives and, 428–429, 433t
　reperfusion after, 280–281, 281f

N

Nadroparin, in stroke, 550
Nafcillin, platelet effects of, 144
Near-site testing, 535–545, 537t. *See also specific instruments*.
　clot-detection analyzers for, 539–545, 540t, 541t, 542t
　costs of, 535
　evaluation of, 536
　indications for, 535
　platelet function analyzers for, 536–539, 537t
Nephrotic syndrome, renal vein thrombosis in, 229–230
Neuraxial anesthesia/analgesia, 589–597
　benefits of, 590–591
　consultation considerations in, 594–597, 595t
　historical perspective on, 589–590
　in abdominal aorta surgery, 590
　in antiplatelet-treated patient, 596
　in arthroplasty, 590
　in cardiac surgery, 590
　in general surgery, 590
　in heparin-treated patient, 594–596, 595t
　in parturition, 590–591
　in thrombolytic therapy–treated patient, 597
　in vascular bypass surgery, 590
　in warfarin-treated patient, 596
　spinal hematoma with, 591–594, 592t
　　signs and symptoms of, 597, 597t
Neurologic disorders
　in antiphospholipid syndrome, 270–271, 270t
　in essential thrombocythemia, 256, 257t
　in heparin-induced thrombocytopenia, 361
Neurosurgery. *See also* Surgery.
　consultant's role in, 554–55
　thromboprophylaxis for, 553
　venous thromboembolism with, 553–554
Neutrophils, in postphlebitic syndrome, 245–246
Nonsteroidal anti-inflammatory agents
　neuraxial anesthesia/analgesia and, 593, 596
　platelet effects of, 143–144
Normal perfusion pressure breakthrough syndrome, 476

O

Obliterative hepatocavopathy, 232–234, 233t
Oral contraceptives, 427–430, 428t, 433t
　myocardial infarction and, 428–429, 433t
　stroke and, 429, 433t
　thrombophilia and, 429–430
　venous thromboembolism and, 429–430, 433t
Oropharyngeal bleeding, in hemophilia, 47
Orthopedic surgery. *See also* Surgery.
　aprotinin in, 468
Osler-Weber-Rendu syndrome, 149, 157–158, 158f
Osteoporosis, low-molecular-weight heparin and, 453
Ovarian vein thrombosis, 237, 455, 456t
Oxacillin, platelet effects of, 144
Oxford assay, 36

P

PAI-1 gene, obstetric complications and, 457
Paracentesis, 471
Paroxysmal nocturnal hemoglobinuria, 34
Parvovirus B19
　inactivation of, in coagulation factor products, 50
　purpura with, 156
　transmission of, in hemophiliac patient, 53–54
PEG-rHuMGDF, 112–113
Pemphigus vulgaris, coagulation factor inhibition in, 78
Penicillin, platelet effects of, 144
Pentoxifylline, in postphlebitic syndrome prevention, 252
Percutaneous coronary interventions, aspirin for, 292–293
Peripheral blood smear
　in essential thrombocythemia, 259
　in immune thrombocytopenic purpura, 119, 119f, 119t
Petechiae, 150t, 151f. *See also* Purpura.
　appearance of, 31
　in fat embolism syndrome, 159
　in thrombocytopenia, 153
PFA-100 Platelet Function Analyzer, 537t, 538
Pharmanetics, 537t
Phlegmasia cerulea dolens, 215–216
Phosphatidylcholine, platelet, 137
Phosphatidylethanolamine, platelet, 137
Phosphatidylserine, platelet, 137
Phospholipase C, defects in, in platelet disorders, 136
Piperacillin, platelet effects of, 144
Pipobroman, in essential thrombocythemia, 264
Pituitary gland, thrombosis of, 236
Placenta, infarctive dysfunction of, 237–238
Plaque, 282, 283f. *See also* Cardiovascular disease.
Plasma clot solubility assay, 32t, 34
Plasma glycocalicin, 24, 34
Plasmapheresis
　hemostatic effects of, 400
　in factor VIII inhibitor titer reduction, 83
　in factor XI deficiency, 67
　in heparin-induced thrombocytopenia, 368
　in thrombotic thrombocytopenic purpura, 349–350, 349t, 502
Plasmin
　in coagulation, 168, 168f
　in disseminated intravascular coagulation, 166, 166t
α_2-Plasmin inhibitor deficiency, 70
Plasminogen activator, tissue-type, 317, 388–389, 388t
Plasminogen activator inhibitor type 1
　in cardiovascular disease, 317
　in disseminated intravascular coagulation, 167–168
Plasminogen deficiency, 186–187
Platelet(s). *See also* Thrombocythemia; Thrombocytopenia.
　acquired disorders of, 139–145, 139t
　adhesion of, disorders of, 134–135, 134f
　aggregation of, 133
　　disorders of, 134f, 135, 136–137
　　evaluation of, 21, 22f, 23, 23t, 32t, 35
　in essential thrombocythemia, 259
　in myeloproliferative diseases, 140

Platelet(s) (*Continued*)
   antibodies against, 143
      in immune thrombocytopenic purpura, 117–118, 118f, 118t
   antimicrobial agent effects on, 144
   antiphospholipid-protein antibody binding to, 273
   apheresis effects on, 400
   aspirin effects on, 143–144
   clopidogrel effects on, 144
   collection of, for transfusion therapy, 107
   concentration of, evaluation of, 20–21, 23–24
   congenital disorders of, 134–139, 134f, 135t
      classification of, 134, 135t
      consultation considerations in, 138–139, 138f
      diagnosis of, 138–139, 138f
      frequency of, 137–138
      treatment of, 139
   count of, 32–33, 32t
      hemorrhage and, 105–106, 106t
      in essential thrombocythemia, 259
      in immune thrombocytopenic purpura, 123
      in secondary thrombocythemia, 259
      thrombopoietin and, 112
   decreased production of, 104t, 105
   dense granules of, deficiency of, 135, 138, 142
   disorders of, 133–145, 134f, 135t, 138f, 139t, 143t
      acquired, 139–145, 139t
      congenital, 134–139, 134f, 135t
      consultation considerations in, 145
      drug-induced, 143–145, 143t, 505
         neuraxial anesthesia/analgesia and, 593–594, 596
      in acute leukemia, 141
      in cancer, 328
      in dysproteinemia, 141
      in liver disease, 484, 486
      in myelodysplastic syndromes, 141
      in myeloproliferative diseases, 139–141
      in uremia, 141–142
      laboratory tests in, 32–35
      purpura with, 154
   factor V origin and, 63
   fetal, in maternal immune thrombocytopenic purpura, 444–445
   flow cytometric evaluation of, 23–24
   G protein activation defects on, 136
   glycoprotein IIb-IIIa receptor agonist effects on, 144
   historical perspective on, 103, 280
   in blood vessel injury, 133, 134f
   in myeloproliferative diseases, 139–141
   interleukin-3 effects on, 110
   β-lactam antibiotic effects on, 144
   nonsteroidal anti-inflammatory drug effects on, 143–144
   normal responses of, 133, 134f
   physiology of, 133, 134f
   procoagulant activities of, disorders of, 137
   secretions of, disorders of, 134, 135–137
   sequestration of, 104–105, 104t
   signal transduction in, disorders of, 136
   thrombolytic agent effects on, 144
   ticlopidine effects on, 144
   transfusion of. *See* Platelet transfusion.
   von Willebrand factor binding to, 92
Platelet serotonin release assay, in heparin-induced thrombocytopenia, 364
Platelet transfusion, 397
   allergic reactions to, 109
   alloimmunization with, 108–109
   bacteremia with, 107–108
   cost of, 109
   cytomegalovirus infection with, 108

Platelet transfusion (*Continued*)
   fever in, 109
   graft-versus-host disease with, 109
   hepatitis with, 108
   human immunodeficiency virus infection with, 108
   in acute hemorrhage, 37
   in congenital platelet disorders, 139
   in critically ill patient, 495–496, 496t
   in disseminated intravascular coagulation, 175
   in factor V deficiency, 64
   in heparin-induced thrombocytopenia, 369
   in immune thrombocytopenic purpura, 124
   in liver disease–related coagulopathy, 489
   in uremia, 142
   platelet collection for, 107
   prophylactic, 105–107, 107t
   risks of, 107–109, 107t
   thrombocytopenia and, 105–107, 106t, 107t
   trigger point for, 105–106, 106t, 107t
   viral infection with, 108
Plateletpheresis, in essential thrombocythemia, 264
Pleckstrin phosphorylation, defects of, 136
Plethysmography
   in postphlebitic syndrome, 248, 248t
   in recurrent deep venous thrombosis, 206, 207
Point-of-care testing. *See* Near-site testing.
Polycythemia vera, 139
Portal vein thrombosis, 226t, 229, 230f
Postphlebitic syndrome, 243–252
   air plethysmography in, 248, 248t
   ambulatory venous pressure in, 248–249
   blood flow regulation in, 245
   CEAP classification of, 246, 247t
   clinical manifestations of, 243, 246, 246f, 247t
   consultation considerations in, 252
   diagnosis of, 247–249, 248t, 249f
   differential diagnosis of, 246
   duplex scanning in, 247–248
   epidemiology of, 243
   medical treatment of, 250–251
   outflow obstruction and, 245
   pathophysiology of, 244–246
   pharmacologic treatment of, 252
   prevention of, 249–250
   risk factors for, 247
   site-specific factors in, 245
   surgical treatment of, 251–252
   treatment of, 250–252
   vena caval filters and, 245
   venography in, 248, 249f
   venous reflux and, 244–245
   with inferior vena caval filter, 571t, 572
Potassium, serum, in essential thrombocythemia, 259
Pravastatin, in cardiovascular disease, 316–317
Preconception counseling, 442–443
Prednisone
   in acquired hemophilia, 83
   in congenital platelet disorders, 139
   in immune thrombocytopenic purpura, 124
Pregnancy, 437–447, 500–501, 500t
   activated protein C resistance in, 450–451
   acute fatty liver in, 500–501, 500t
   alloimmune thrombocytopenia in, 445–446
   antiphospholipid syndrome in, 271, 454–455, 455t
   antithrombin III deficiency in, 450
   antithrombotic therapy in, 457–458
   arterial thrombosis in, 456
   coagulation factors during, 437–438

Pregnancy (*Continued*)
  counseling before, 442–443
  DDAVP in, 439–440, 439t
  essential thrombocythemia and, 265
  factor V Leiden in, 450–451, 457
  factor VII deficiency in, 442
  factor XI deficiency in, 441–442
  factor XIII deficiency in, 442
  folate in, 458
  HELLP syndrome in, 446–447, 446t, 500, 500t
  hemolytic uremia in, 500t, 501
  hemophilia in, 440–441, 441t
  hyperhomocysteinemia in, 451, 457
  immune thrombocytopenic purpura in, 127–128, 443–445
  ovarian vein thrombosis after, 455, 456t
  protein C deficiency in, 450
  protein S deficiency in, 450
  prothrombin G20210A mutation in, 451, 457
  recurrent loss of, 456–457
  thrombocytopenia in, 443, 445–446
    vs. immune thrombocytopenic purpura, 120t, 121–122
  thrombophilia in, 450–451, 456–457
    fetal loss and, 456–457
    management of, 451–454, 452t, 453t, 454t
  thrombotic thrombocytopenic purpura in, 500t, 502–503
  vena caval filter in, 453–454
  venous thromboembolism in, 449–451, 450f, 450t
    prevention of, 451–454, 452t, 453t, 454t
    treatment of, 452–454, 453t
  von Willebrand disease in, 438–440
    prenatal testing and, 440
    regional anesthesia and, 440
    treatment of, 99, 439–440, 439t
  von Willebrand factor levels in, 93, 438–439
Prekallikrein, congenital deficiency of, 68
Preoperative testing, 468–470, 469t, 470t
Priapism, 236–237
Prion diseases, transmission of, 54
Procoagulants, 15
  laboratory evaluation of, 16–20, 17f, 17t–18t
Profilnine, 49t
Proplex T, 49t
Propranolol, platelet effects of, 144
Protamine, 411–412
Protease inhibitors
  bleeding with, 516–517
  thrombosis with, 517
Protein A, staphylococcal, in factor VIII inhibition titer control, 83
Protein C
  assays of, 20
  in disseminated intravascular coagulation, 175
  normal levels of, 183
  warfarin effects on, 159
Protein C deficiency, 182–183, 182t, 183t
  acquired, 182t, 183
  evaluation of, 190–192, 191f
  factor V Leiden and, 189, 189t
  fetal loss and, 238
  in pregnancy, 450
  skin necrosis in, 236
  thrombosis risk in, 187–188, 188t
  type I, 183, 183t
  type II, 183, 183t
  warfarin-induced skin necrosis in, 192
Protein S
  assays of, 20
  normal levels of, 184
Protein S deficiency, 182t, 183–184
  acquired, 182t, 184
  evaluation of, 190–192, 191f
  factor V Leiden and, 189, 189t
  fetal loss and, 238
  in acquired immunodeficiency syndrome, 517
  in pregnancy, 450
  in warfarin skin necrosis, 159
  skin necrosis in, 236
  thrombosis risk in, 187–188, 188t
Protein Z deficiency, 57, 58t, 70
Protein Z-dependent protease inhibitor, 58t, 70
Prothrombin
  deficiency of, 61–63. *See also* Dysprothrombinemia.
    lupus anticoagulants and, 272
  in liver disease, 483, 486
  inhibitors of, 62, 83–84, 272
  variants of, 62t
Prothrombin complex concentrates, 398–399
  in congenital dysprothrombinemia, 62–63
  in factor XI deficiency, 67
Prothrombin G20210A mutation, 185
  evaluation of, 190–192, 191f
  fetal loss and, 238
  in pregnancy, 451, 457
  thrombosis risk in, 188, 188t
Prothrombin gene, mutations in, 61, 62t
Prothrombin time (PT), 16–17, 17f, 17t, 32t, 33
  drug-related increases in, 494t
  during pregnancy, 437–438
  in clinical decision-making, 18–19, 18t
  in coagulation factor deficiency, 75–76
  in coagulation factor inhibition, 75–76
  in critically ill patient, 493–494, 495t, 496, 496t
  in factor VII deficiency, 64
  in liver disease, 485, 485t, 486, 498
  in transfused patient, 500
  patient self-testing of, 529–531, 530t, 539–541, 540t
  point-of-care testing of, 529–531, 530t
ProTime microcoagulation analyzer, 539–540, 540t
Proton nuclear magnetic resonance spectroscopy, in cardiovascular disease, 314
P-selectin, in essential thrombocythemia, 256
Pseudo–heparin-induced thrombocytopenia, 362, 363f, 363t
Pseudothrombocytopenia, 20–21
  vs. immune thrombocytopenic purpura, 120t, 121
Pseudothrombocytosis, 259
Pseudotumor, in hemophilia, 47
Pseudotumor cerebri, 231
Psoralen-treated pooled plasma, for acute hemorrhage, 37
Psoriasis, coagulation factor inhibition in, 78
PT. *See* Prothrombin time (PT).
PTT. (*See* Activated partial thromboplastin time)
Pulmonary angiography, in pulmonary embolism, 209
Pulmonary embolism. *See also* Deep venous thrombosis; Venous thromboembolism.
  angiography in, 209
  computed tomography in, 209, 209t
  diagnosis of, 207–210, 208f, 209t, 505–506
  differential diagnosis of, 209–210
  in heparin-induced thrombocytopenia, 361
  in spinal cord injury, 550–553, 551t, 552t
  prevention of, 199–204. *See also* Inferior vena caval filter; Thromboprophylaxis.
  pulmonary hypertension and, 210–211
  renal vein thrombosis and, 230
  risk factors for, 200–201, 201f, 201t, 208–209, 208f
  shock with, 211
  treatment of, 210–211, 507

Purple toe syndrome, 150t, 160
Purpura, 149–162
  actinic, 157
  atrophic, 157
  cachectic, 150
  classification of, 152t
  consultation considerations in, 161–162
  costs of, 162
  definition of, 149, 150t
  factitious, 152
  historical perspective on, 149–150
  in amyloidosis, 157
  in cholesterol emboli syndrome, 160
  in disseminated intravascular coagulation, 158–159
  in fat embolism syndrome, 159
  in heparin-induced thrombocytopenia, 160. *See also* Heparin-induced thrombocytopenia.
  in heritable connective tissue disorders, 157–158
  in hypercortisolism, 156–157
  in leptospirosis, 156
  in parvovirus B19, 156
  in rickettsial diseases, 155–156
  in Rocky Mountain spotted fever, 155–156
  in scurvy, 156
  in viral hemorrhagic fever, 156
  laboratory evaluation of, 162
  mechanical, 152
  medical-legal considerations in, 162
  microvascular structure and, 150–151, 151f
  palpable, 154–155, 154f, 154t
  pathophysiologic categories of, 152–161, 152t
  post-transfusion, 399, 400, 504
  progressive pigmented, 153
  psychogenic, 152
  red blood cell extravasation in, 151, 151f
  senile, 157
  thrombocytopenic, 153–154, 153f
    idiopathic, 32t, 105, 149, 150, 328
    immune, 117–128. *See also* Immune thrombocytopenic purpura.
    thrombotic, 159–160, 172t. *See also* Thrombotic thrombocytopenic purpura.
  treatment of, 162
  vs. Kaposi sarcoma, 160–161
  with abnormal platelet function, 154
  with microbial endothelial damage, 155–156
  with microthrombi, 158–160
  with microvascular mechanical strength compromise, 156–158, 158f
  with no known microvascular pathology, 152–153
  with vascular malignancy, 160–161
Purpura fulminans, 158, 236
  in critically ill patient, 497–498
Purpura haemorrhagica, 150
Purpura rheumatica, 150, 154
Purpura simplex, 31, 152–153

Q

Quebec platelet disorder, 135
Questionnaire, for work-up of bleeding disorders, 27–30
Quinine, disseminated intravascular coagulation with, 498

R

Radiation therapy, thrombosis with, 332
Radionuclide synovectomy, in hemophilic arthropathy, 45–46
Radiophosphorus, in essential thrombocythemia, 263–264
Raloxifene, 433, 433t
Rapidpoint Coag Analyzer, 541–542, 541t

Rattlesnake envenomation
  hyperfibrinolysis with, 173
  vs. disseminated intravascular coagulation, 171
Re Facto, 49t
Recombinate, 49t
Red blood cells
  extravasation of, 151, 151f
  for transfusion, 396–397
  in uremia, 142
Referring physician, duties of, 8
Renal vein thrombosis, 226t, 229–231
Reo-Pro, in thrombotic thrombocytopenic purpura, 351
Reptilase time, 36
Reteplase, 389
  in cardiovascular disease, 286
Retinal vein thrombosis, 234–235
all-trans-Retinoic acid, in acute promyelocytic leukemia, 176
Retroperitoneal hematoma, without major trauma, 29
Rheumatoid arthritis, with factor VIII inhibitor development, 78
Rickettsial diseases, purpura with, 155–156
Ristocetin cofactor assay, 20, 94
Ristocetin-induced platelet aggregation, 92t, 95
Rituxan, in refractory immune thrombocytopenic purpura, 127
Roche Diagnostics Corporation, 537t
Rocky Mountain spotted fever, purpura with, 155–156
Rodenticides, hemorrhage with, 62
Russell viper venom time (RVVT), 19
  for lupus anticoagulants, 274, 274t
  in coagulation inhibitor specificity, 76

S

Scott syndrome, 134, 137
Scurvy
  purpura in, 156
  vs. idiopathic thrombocytopenic purpura, 149, 150
Second opinion, consultation for, 6
Selective estrogen receptor modulators, 432–433
Sepsis
  disseminated intravascular coagulation with, 174
  inferior vena caval filter in, 565
  thrombocytopenia with, 503
Serum thrombopoietin, 23
Sienco Inc., 537t
Signal transduction, in platelet disorders, 137
Simon Nitinol filter, 561t, 562–563, 569, 570f, 571t
Single-chain urokinase-like plasminogen activator, in cardiovascular disease, 285
Skin
  heparin-induced lesions of, 361
  microvascular thrombosis of, 236
  necrosis of, 236
  warfarin-induced necrosis of, 150t, 159, 377
    in heparin-induced thrombocytopenia, 360–361, 361f
    in protein C deficiency, 192
SonoClot Coagulation Analyzer, 545
Spiders, 150t, 161
Spinal cord injury
  inferior vena caval filter in, 552, 552t
  venous thromboembolism with, 550–553
    prophylaxis against, 550–552, 551t
Splenectomy
  in immune thrombocytopenic purpura, 124–125, 127
  in thrombotic thrombocytopenic purpura, 350, 350t
Splenic vein thrombosis, 228–229
Splenomegaly
  in immune thrombocytopenic purpura, 119–120
  platelet sequestration in, 105

Stainless Steel Greenfield filter, 561–562, 561t, 569, 570f, 571t
Staphylokinase, 286
Stasis, in venous thromboembolism, 197–198, 198t
Storage pool deficiency, 135
    acquired, 142
    diagnosis of, 138
    treatment of, 138
Streptokinase, 285, 386–387, 388t
Stroke, 299, 301, 301f, 301t
    aspirin after, 292
    deep venous thrombosis with, 549–550, 550t
    hyperhomocysteinemia and, 188
    in antiphospholipid syndrome, 270–271, 270t
    in heparin-induced thrombocytopenia, 361
    oral contraceptives and, 429
Subclavian vein thrombosis, 235–236
Subfascial endoscopic perforator surgery, in postphlebitic syndrome prevention, 251
Sucrose hemolysis test, 34
Superficial vein thrombosis. See also Deep venous thrombosis.
    treatment of, 211–212, 212t
Superior vena caval filter, 564, 576
Superwarfarins, hemorrhage with, 62
Suprarenal filter, 564
Surgery, 463–476
    anticoagulation during, 527, 527t
        in cancer patient, 331–332, 336–337
    consultation considerations for, 474–476, 475t
    hemostatic defect screening before, 468–470, 469t, 470t
    hemostatic effects of, 368t, 465–468, 465t, 466t
    in congenital hemostatic defects, 463–465, 464t
    neuraxial anesthesia/analgesia for, 589–597. See also Neuraxial anesthesia/analgesia.
    thrombotic disorder screening before, 470
Synovectomy, radionuclide, in hemophilic arthropathy, 45–46
Systemic inflammatory response syndrome, disseminated intravascular coagulation and, 174
Systemic lupus erythematosus
    cardiac valve dysfunction in, 271–272
    lupus anticoagulants in, 272
    with factor VIII inhibitor development, 78

T

Tamoxifen, 332, 336, 432–433, 433t
Tangier disease, 314
Telangiectasia, 31, 149, 150t, 157–158, 158f
Template bleeding time, 21
Tempofilter, 565
Tenecteplase, 389
    in cardiovascular disease, 286, 287t, 288t
Terminally ill patient. See also Critically ill patient.
    inferior vena caval filter in, 565
Third-party payor, consultation request by, 6
Thoracentesis, 471
Thoracic outlet syndrome, 236
Thrombectomy, in deep venous thrombosis, 250
Thrombin
    discovery of, 279, 280t
    factor VIII activation by, 79
    in coagulation, 166, 168, 168f
    in disseminated intravascular coagulation, 166, 166t
    inhibitors of, 83–84
    topical bovine, factor V inhibitors with, 63, 84–85
Thrombin clotting time, 19, 32t, 36
Thrombin-activatable fibrinolysis inhibitor, 187
Thrombin:thrombomodulin complex, 168, 168f

Thrombocythemia
    essential, 139
        clinical features of, 140, 257, 258t
        diagnosis of, 258–259, 259t
        laboratory findings in, 259
        life expectancy in, 256
        neurologic disorders in, 256, 257t
        pathogenesis of, 255–257
        platelet abnormalities in, 256
        pregnancy and, 265
        prognostic factors in, 257–258
        risk stratification for, 257–258, 261f
        thrombosis in, 140, 256, 258
        treatment of, 140–141, 259–265, 260t
            alkylating agents in, 263
            anagrelide in, 261–263, 262t
            aspirin in, 264
            hydroxyurea in, 260–261
            plateletpheresis in, 264
            radiophosphorus in, 263–264
            recombinant interferon-alpha in, 263
            strategies for, 265
    hereditary (familial), 256
Thrombocytopenia
    after GP11b/IIIa receptor antagonists administration, 305f, 306
    amegakaryoctyic, congenital, 105
    anticardiolipin antibody and, 271
    asymptomatic, in immune thrombocytopenic purpura, 123–124
    classification of, 104–105
    congenital, 104t, 105, 120t, 122
    definition of, 104
    differential diagnosis of, 104, 104t, 119–122, 120t
    drug-induced, 105, 503, 503t
        interleukin-6 effects on, 111
        interleukin-11 for, 112
        vs. immune thrombocytopenic purpura, 120t, 121
    hemorrhage risk and, 105–106, 106t
    heparin-induced, 355–370. See also Heparin-induced thrombocytopenia.
    history of, 29t
    HIV-associated, 120t, 122, 515–516
    immune-mediated, 104t, 105, 117–128. See also Immune thrombocytopenic purpura.
    in acquired pure megakaryocytic aplasia, 120t, 123
    in afibrinogenemia, 58
    in antiphospholipid syndrome, 271
    in cancer, 328
    in critically ill patient, 493, 494, 495t
    in disseminated intravascular coagulation, 122
    in hematopoietic stem cell transplantation, 113
    in liver disease, 483–484, 486
    in myelodysplastic syndromes, 120t, 122, 141
    in pregnancy, 120t, 121–122, 443, 445–446
    in sepsis, 503
    infection-related, 120t, 122, 515–516
    neonatal, 128
    nonimmune-mediated, 104t, 105
    pathophysiology of, 104–105
    platelet destruction in, 104t, 105
    platelet production defects in, 104t, 105
    platelet sequestration in, 104–105, 104t
    post-transfusion, 504
Thrombocytopenia with absent radii (TAR), 105, 120t, 122
Thrombocytopenic purpura, 153–154, 153f
    idiopathic, 32t, 105, 149, 150
        in cancer, 328

Thrombocytopenic purpura (Continued)
  immune, 117–128. See also Immune thrombocytopenic purpura.
  thrombotic, 159–160, 343–352. See also Thrombotic thrombocytopenic purpura.
Thrombocytosis, 255–265. See also Thrombocythemia.
  differential diagnosis of, 259, 260t
  in cancer, 328
  primary, 255, 256t
  secondary, 255, 256t, 259, 260t
Thromboelastogram, 545
  in liver disease, 486–487
Thromboembolectomy, in heparin-induced thrombocytopenia, 368
β-Thromboglobulin, in essential thrombocythemia, 256
Thrombolytic Assessment System, 544
Thrombolytic therapy
  adjunctive therapy with, 389–390
  bleeding with, 390–392, 390t, 391f
  catheter-directed, 389
  in heparin-induced thrombocytopenia, 368
  in postphlebitic syndrome, 249–250
  in pulmonary embolism, 507
  neuraxial anesthesia/analgesia and, 587, 594
  α_2-plasmin inhibitor deficiency in, 70
  platelet effects of, 144
  regional, 389
Thrombophilia. See also Deep venous thrombosis; Thrombosis; Venous thromboembolism.
  hereditary, 181–193. See also specific disorders.
    evaluation of, 190–192, 191f
    thrombosis risk in, 187–189, 188t, 189t, 191, 191f
    treatment of, 192–193
  in cancer, 329
  in pregnancy, 450–451, 456–457
  oral contraceptives and, 429–430
Thromboplastin inhibition assay, for lupus anticoagulants, 274, 274t
Thrombopoiesis
  decreased, 105. See also Thrombocytopenia.
  increased, 255. See also Thrombocythemia.
  physiologic, 103–104
Thrombopoietic growth factors, 109–113, 110t
  recombinant, 112
Thrombopoietin, 111–112
  historical perspective on, 103
  in essential thrombocythemia, 256
  recombinant, for pediatric tumors, 113
  serum, 23
Thromboprophylaxis, 199–204
  heparin in, 201–203
  in airline traveler, 203
  in general medical patients, 200–201, 201f, 202–203, 203t
  in neurosurgical patient, 553
  in spinal cord injury patient, 550–552, 551t, 552t
  in surgical patients, 200–201, 201t
  inferior vena caval filter in, 203–204. See also Inferior vena caval filter.
  low-molecular-weight heparin in, 201–203, 203t
  medical-legal aspects of, 554
  methods of, 201–202
  secondary, 216–218, 216f–219f
Thrombosis. See also Arterial thrombosis; Deep venous thrombosis; Venous thromboembolism.
  coronary, 282–285, 283f, 284f. See also Cardiovascular disease.
  diagnosis of, 189–192, 189t
    laboratory evaluation in, 190
    patient history in, 189–190
    physical examination in, 190
  mural, 303
  treatment of, 192–193

Thrombotic microangiopathy, vs. thrombotic thrombocytopenic purpura, 345
Thrombotic storm, 172t
Thrombotic thrombocytopenic purpura, 159–160, 343–352
  apoptosis and, 347
  Bartonella bacilliformis and, 347
  case studies of, 347–348
  clinical manifestations of, 344
  consultation considerations in, 352
  cost containment issues in, 351
  diagnosis of, 351
  differential diagnosis of, 348, 348t
  etiology of, 347–348
  features of, 172t
  historical perspective on, 343–344
  immunology of, 347–348, 350–351
  in acquired immunodeficiency syndrome, 518–519
  in critically ill patient, 501–502
  in pregnancy, 500t, 502–503
  laboratory findings in, 344, 344t, 345f
  medical-legal issues in, 351–352
  pathogenesis of, 350–351
  pathophysiology of, 345–347
  peripheral blood smear in, 344, 345f
  ticlopidine-induced, 294
  treatment of, 349–351, 349t
  types of, 344–345, 344t, 345t
  von Willebrand factor in, 345–347
  vs. disseminated intravascular coagulation, 171
Thrombotic thrombocytopenic purpura/hemolytic-uremic syndrome
  in critically ill patient, 502
  vs. immune thrombocytopenic purpura, 120t, 122
Thromboxane β-2, in essential thrombocythemia, 256
Thromboxane A_2
  disorders of, 137
  in platelet disorders, 136–137
Thyroid hormone, in von Willebrand factor regulation, 93
Ticarcillin, platelet effects of, 144
Ticlopidine
  in cardiovascular disease, 293–294, 293t, 304t
  neuraxial anesthesia/analgesia and, 593, 596
  platelet effects of, 144
Tirofiban
  in cardiovascular disease, 296–297, 298f, 298t, 300t, 304t, 305f
  platelet effects of, 144
Tissue factor
  in hemostasis, 15, 166
  in recombinant factor VIIa, 82
  of tumors, 327–328, 327f
Tissue factor pathway inhibitor, 82
Tissue thromboplastin inhibition test, 19
Tissue-type plasminogen activator, 166t
  in cardiovascular disease, 285–286, 287t
  platelet effects of, 144
Titanium Greenfield filter, 561t, 562, 569, 570f, 571t
Toes, purple (blue), 150t, 160
Topical hemostatic agents, 419–424
  cellulose-based, 420, 420t
  collagen-based, 419–420, 420t
  commercial fibrin for, 422–423, 422t
  cryoprecipitate-based, 421–422, 421t, 422f
  factor V inhibitors with, 63, 84–85
  gelatin-based, 420–421, 420t
Tranexamic acid, 403–406, 404t
  dosage of, 404
  in acute hemorrhage, 38
  in congenital platelet disorders, 139
  in factor XI deficiency, 67

Tranexamic acid (*Continued*)
  in hemophilia, 51
  indications for, 404–406
  thrombosis with, 406
  toxicity of, 406
Transforming growth factor-β, in postphlebitic syndrome, 245
Transfusion, 395–412, 412t
  adverse effects of, 399–400, 500
  commercial plasma fractions for, 398–399
  cryoprecipitate for, 398. *See also* Cryoprecipitate.
  fresh frozen plasma for, 397–398. *See also* Fresh frozen plasma.
  hemostatic effects of, 400
  historical perspective on, 395–396
  in critically ill patient, 495–496, 496t
  in liver transplantation, 488, 488t
  infection with, 53–54, 399
  massive, in critically ill patient, 500
  platelets for, 397. *See also* Platelet transfusion.
  purpura with, 399, 400, 504
  red cells for, 396–397
Transfusion reaction, 399–400
  in porcine factor VIII replacement therapy, 81–82
Transplantation, liver, 467–468, 468t, 487–488, 487t, 488t
TrapEase filter, 563
Trauma
  in venous thromboembolism, 198, 198t
  inferior vena caval filter and, 576–579, 577t–578t, 579t
  minor, excessive bleeding after, 29
Travel, venous thromboembolism with, 203
Trousseau syndrome
  features of, 172t, 173, 173t
  heparin for, 175
  vs. disseminated intravascular coagulation, 171, 173
Tumor. *See* Cancer.
Tumor necrosis factor, in cancer, 327, 327f

U

Ultegra Rapid Platelet Function Assay, 536, 537t
Ultrasonography
  in postphlebitic syndrome, 247–248
  in recurrent deep venous thrombosis, 204, 205–207
Unna boot, in postphlebitic syndrome prevention, 250–251
Uremia, 504–505, 505t
  bleeding in, 141
  platelet disorders in, 141–142
Urokinase, 387–388, 388t
  in cardiovascular disease, 285
Uterus, evacuation of, in disseminated intravascular coagulation, 174

V

Vaginal bleeding, history of, 28
Variceal hemorrhage
  in portal vein thrombosis, 229
  in splenic vein thrombosis, 228
Vascular endothelial growth factor
  in cancer, 327, 327f
  in Kaposi sarcoma, 160
Vasculitis
  cutaneous, 154–155
    by age groups, 154–155, 154t
    disorders associated with, 154, 154t
    laboratory evaluation for, 155, 155t
    primary, 154–155
    secondary, 155
  definition of, 150t
  leukocytoclastic, 154, 154f
  necrotizing, 150t, 154

Vena caval filter. *See* Inferior vena caval filter; Superior vena caval filter.
VenaTech filter, 561t, 562, 569, 570f, 571t
Venography
  in calf vein thrombosis, 207
  in postphlebitic syndrome, 248, 249f
  in recurrent deep venous thrombosis, 206
Venostat, in postphlebitic syndrome prevention, 252
Venous insufficiency, chronic, 243
  primary, 244
  secondary. *See* Postphlebitic syndrome.
Venous limb gangrene
  in heparin-induced thrombocytopenia, 360–361, 361t
  treatment of, 215–216
Venous pressure, ambulatory, in postphlebitic syndrome, 248–249
Venous thromboembolism, 197–219. *See also* Deep venous thrombosis; Pulmonary embolism.
  antiphospholipid syndrome and, in pregnancy, 454–455, 455t
  coagulability in, 198, 198t
  consultation considerations in, 238
  cost considerations in, 238
  diagnosis of, 204–210, 505–506
  historical perspective on, 225–226
  hormone replacement therapy and, 431–432
  idiopathic, 198–199
    in cancer, 329–331
    recurrence of, 18f, 217–218, 219f
  in acquired immunodeficiency syndrome, 517–518, 518t
  in antiphospholipid syndrome, 275
  in critically ill patient, 505–507
  in essential thrombocythemia, 256, 258
  in neurologic patient, 549–555, 550t, 551t, 552t
  in pregnancy, 449–451, 450f, 450t
  inflammation in, 198, 198t
  of adrenal veins, 226t, 236, 237f
  of axillary vein, 226t, 235–236
  of cerebral veins, 226t, 231–232, 231t, 232f
  of hepatic vein, 226t, 232–234, 233f, 233t, 234f
  of mesenteric vein, 226–228, 226t, 227f
  of ovarian veins, 237
  of portal vein, 226t, 229, 230f
  of renal vein, 226t, 229–231
  of retinal vein, 226t, 234–235
  of splenic vein, 226t, 228–229
  of subclavian vein, 226t, 235–236
  oral contraceptives and, 429–430, 433t
  pathogenesis of, 197–199, 198t
  postoperative, 470
  prevention of, 199–204
    in airline traveler, 203
    in general medical patients, 200–201, 201f, 202–203, 203t
    in surgical patients, 200–201, 201t
    inferior vena cava filters in, 203–204
    methods of, 201–202
    secondary, 216–218, 216f–219f
  raloxifene and, 432–433, 433t
  recurrence of, 198–199
    prevention of, 216–218, 216f–219f
  risk factors for, 200–201, 201f, 201t
  stasis in, 197–198, 198t
  tamoxifen and, 432–433, 433t
  trauma in, 198, 198t
  treatment of, 123f, 210–218, 212t, 213t, 214f, 506–507
Vinblastine, in refractory immune thrombocytopenic purpura, 126–127
Vincristine
  in refractory immune thrombocytopenic purpura, 126–127
  in thrombotic thrombocytopenic purpura, 350, 350t

Viral infection
  factor VIII inhibition in, 79
  in hemophilia patient, 53–54
  in platelet transfusion therapy, 108
  thrombopoiesis effects of, 105
Virchow's triad, 197–199, 198t, 326, 327f
Vitamin B_{12}
  deficiency of, 105
  hyperhomocysteinemia with, 186
Vitamin B_6, hyperhomocysteinemia with, 186
Vitamin C, in refractory immune thrombocytopenic purpura, 127
Vitamin K, 406–411
  administration of, 408
  anaphylactic reaction to, 410–411
  deficiency of
    factor VII deficiency and, 64
    factor X deficiency and, 65
    in critically ill patient, 499
    in liver disease, 483, 486, 489
    vs. dysprothrombinemia, 62
  dosage of, 408
  indications for, 408–409, 409t
  mechanism of action of, 407–408
  replacement of, 499
  toxicity of, 410–411
Von Willebrand disease, 85–86, 91–100
  acquired, 97, 98t, 99, 142
  bleeding in, 93–94
  classification of, 95–97, 96t
  clinical presentation of, 93–94
  diagnosis of, 44, 48, 94–95, 94t, 95f, 138
  historical overview of, 91
  laboratory studies in, 32t, 35
  physiology of, 91–93, 92t, 93f
  platelet disorders in, 134
  pregnancy-associated, 28, 99, 438–440
  surgery in, 464–465
  treatment of, 97–100, 98t, 139
    antifibrinolytic therapy in, 98t, 99
    desmopressin in, 98, 98t
    estrogen in, 98t, 99
    practical considerations in, 99–100
    topical agents in, 98t, 99
    von Willebrand factor concentrates in, 98–99, 98t
  type 1, 96, 96t
  type 2A, 96, 96t
  type 2B, 96, 96t
  type 2M, 96–97, 96t
  type 2N, 96t, 97
  type 3, 96t, 97
  vs. hemophilia, 44, 48
Von Willebrand factor, 92t
  assay of, 20, 94–95, 94t, 95f
  during pregnancy, 437, 438–439
  factor VIII interactions with, 79, 93

Von Willebrand factor (*Continued*)
  function of, 91–92, 92t, 93f
  genetics of, 92, 93f
  in atherosclerosis, 93
  in platelet response, 133
  in thrombotic thrombocytopenic purpura, 345–347
  in uremia, 141
  inhibitors of, 85–86
  levels of, 93
  nomenclature for, 91, 92t
  platelet-related functions of, 92–93
  synthesis of, 91–92, 93f
Von Willebrand factor antigen, 92t, 94, 94t
Von Willebrand factor concentrates, 98–99, 98t
Von Willebrand factor multimers, 92t, 95, 95f

W

Warfarin, 375–378, 376t
  administration of, 375–376
  adverse effects of, 377
  after atrial fibrillation, 299
  bleeding with, 61–62, 192
  drug interactions with, 494t, 524
  factor VII deficiency from, 64
  in cancer patient, 334, 335
  in cardiovascular disease, 289–290, 290t
  in critically ill patient, 499
  in heparin-induced thrombocytopenia, 360–361, 361f, 361t, 367–368
  in hip replacement surgery, 473–474
  in pregnancy, 453
  in recurrent deep venous thrombosis, 205, 205t
  in secondary thromboprophylaxis, 216–218, 216f–219f
  indications for, 376–377, 376t
  mechanism of, 375
  monitoring of, 375–376, 376t, 525–527, 525t, 526t
  neuraxial anesthesia/analgesia and, 593, 596
  pharmacology of, 375
  reversal of, 377–378, 377t, 408–409, 409t, 410f, 499
    for emergency surgery, 474
  skin necrosis with, 159, 360–361, 361f, 361t, 377
    definition of, 150t
    in protein C deficiency, 192
Washed platelet activation assays, in heparin-induced thrombocytopenia, 364
Werlhof disease, 150. *See also* Idiopathic thrombocytopenic purpura.
Western diamondback rattlesnake envenomation, 173
White clot syndrome, 360
Whole Blood Aggregometer, 536, 537t, 538
Williams factor, congenital deficiency of, 68
Wiskott-Aldrich syndrome, 137
  laboratory profile in, 32t
  platelet production defects in, 105

Z

Zymogen, 58t

ISBN 0-7216-8264-2